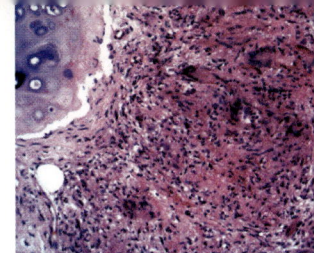

PRINCIPLES OF RESPIRATORY MEDICINE

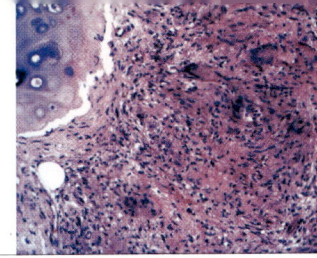

PRINCIPLES OF RESPIRATORY MEDICINE

Farokh Erach Udwadia

MD, FRCP (London & Edinburgh), Master FCCP, FAMS, FCPS, D.sc
Emeritus Professor of Medicine, Grant Medical College & JJ Group
of Hospitals, Mumbai;
Consultant Physician and Director in Charge of the ICU, Breach
Candy Hospital, Mumbai;
Consultant Physician, Parsee General Hospital, Mumbai

Zarir F. Udwadia

MD, DNB, FRCP (London), FCCP (USA)
Consultant Chest Physician, Hinduja Hospital, Mumbai;
Consultant Physician, Breach Candy Hospital and Parsee General
Hospital, Mumbai

Anirudh F. Kohli

MD, DNB, DMRD
Head of Imaging, Breach Candy Hospital, Mumbai;
Consultant Radiologist, Jaslok Hospital, Mumbai

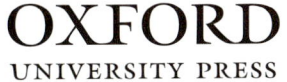

OXFORD

UNIVERSITY PRESS

OXFORD

UNIVERSITY PRESS

YMCA Library Building, Jai Singh Road, New Delhi 110001

Oxford University Press is a department of the University of Oxford. It furthers the
University's objective of excellence in research, scholarship, and education
by publishing worldwide in

Oxford   New York
Auckland   Cape Town   Dar es Salaam   Hong Kong   Karachi
Kuala Lumpur   Madrid   Melbourne   Mexico City   Nairobi
New Delhi   Shanghai   Taipei   Toronto

With offices in
Argentina   Austria   Brazil   Chile   Czech Republic   France   Greece
Guatemala   Hungary   Italy   Japan   Poland   Portugal   Singapore
South Korea   Switzerland   Thailand   Turkey   Ukraine   Vietnam

Oxford is a registered trade mark of Oxford University Press
in the UK and in certain other countries

Published in India
by Oxford University Press, New Delhi

ISBN-13: 978-0-19-807155-6
ISBN-10: 0-19-807155-8

Typeset in Berling LT Std 9.5/11.4
by Eleven Arts, Keshav Puram, New Delhi 110 035
Printed in India at Thomson Press, New Delhi 110 020
Published by Oxford University Press
YMCA Library Building, Jai Singh Road, New Delhi 110 001

To
Vera, Gool, Malavika and our children
for their love and support

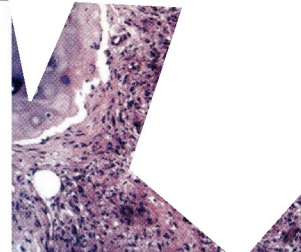

Contents

Contents

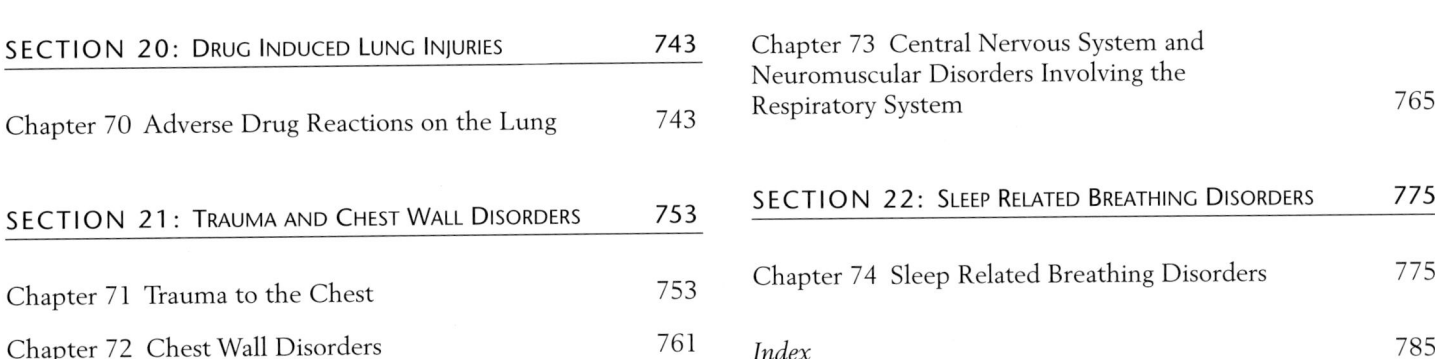

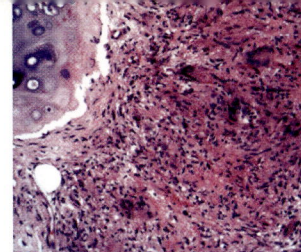

Preface

The prime reason for writing a book on pulmonary medicine is our firm conviction that a description of respiratory diseases occurring in India is best written by experienced physicians working for decades in the same country. The contents of such a text we felt would also by and large be applicable to other developing and poor countries of the world. Considering the fact that far more people live in the underprivileged regions of the world compared to the affluent West, the raison d'être for such a text seemed unquestionable.

We knew that our task was indeed daunting and we made it doubly so by deciding not to invite contributions from colleagues working in various regions of the country. We were determined to accomplish the work by ourselves, so as to finish the task quickly, and to ensure a uniformity of style, language, content and a focussed dedication, all so essential to achieve what we set out to do. The work started in the spring of 2009 and was submitted for publication by August 2010. We however allowed for two exceptions when we invited Dr Thirumalai Rajgopal to contribute two chapters on 'Common Occupational Lung Diseases' and 'Environmental Pollution' and Dr Camilla Rodrigues to write on 'Antibiotic Resistance and its Management'.

In India we encounter almost all the respiratory diseases found in the West. In addition, we live among respiratory diseases which are peculiar only to India and other developing tropical countries, that are uncommon in the West. It is therefore important that physicians practising in these countries are trained in the understanding, diagnosis, and management of both these groups of diseases. The authors sincerely hope that this book achieves this objective. We have not compromised on the generally accepted description of respiratory diseases common to both the affluent West and to poor tropical countries. However, the epidemiology of these diseases, their often subtle variations in clinical presentation, and natural history as observed in the Indian and South-east Asian context have been clearly emphasized.

Respiratory disorders peculiar to India and other tropical countries have, for obvious reasons, been dealt with in considerable detail. For example, pulmonary infections in the tropics, together with pulmonary complications of tropical diseases is a subject that deserves far more attention than what has been accorded by western authors. Parasitic infections of the lungs, the lung in fulminant malaria, in amoebic infection, in salmonellosis, leptospirosis, dengue, in other fulminant, and not so fulminant infections in the tropics, have been discussed in special detail because they are both frequent and important.

The increasing menace of lung cancer in India has been given special emphasis; with a comparison of recent epidemiological data on lung cancer in various parts of India vis-à-vis South-east Asia, China, and several other countries of the world.

Both chronic obstructive pulmonary disease as well as asthma have a significant morbidity and mortality rate in India, South-east Asia, and also in the West. These topics have been discussed at length with special reference to India and South-east Asia.

A highlight of the book is a discussion on the threat of pulmonary tuberculosis and its unsolved challenges. Pulmonary tuberculosis dominates medicine in India and other developing countries. It exists on an epic scale with India accounting for a third of the world's TB burden. Every aspect of this disease has been dealt with, including a detailed epidemiological description, MDR and XDR tuberculosis, tuberculosis in relation to the HIV epidemic, the new diagnostic aids involving the use of genetics and molecular biology, and also the future needs to counter the unsolved challenges of this disease.

We have also included, among others, sections on basic 'Lung Physiology', 'Clinical Approach to Respiratory Disease-Symptoms and Signs', 'Occupational and Environmental Lung Diseases', 'Infectious Diseases' and a section on 'HIV and the Lung'.

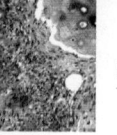
The volume begins with the section 'Imaging Techniques and Imaging of the Chest'. Of all the recent discoveries in respiratory medicine, the most iconic is the discovery of spiral computed tomography in the 1990s. Continuing technological advances have further enhanced the imaging of the microarchitecture of the lung and have enabled a reconstruction of images that allow a three-dimensional view of a lung pathology and of pathologies involving the mediastinum. The advent of virtual bronchoscopy permits a view of the whole bronchial tree and its surrounding structures. These, together with the use of ultrasonography, ventilation-perfusion lung scans, magnetic resonance imaging (MRI), and positron emission tomography (PET scans) in respiratory medicine have been briefly described with suitable illustrations in this section. What is more, every single chapter of every section is illustrated wherever necessary with high quality images that contribute to the further understanding of different respiratory diseases. We feel that the visual image is as important as the written word and often is longer lasting in the mind's eye.

Principles of Respiratory Medicine is a book written by clinicians for clinicians, and though not encyclopaedic in content, is comprehensive in its scope. The varying emphasis given to different respiratory diseases is related to respiratory medicine as observed and practiced in India and to an extent in South-east Asia and other tropical countries. In this respect, the book differs significantly from many others written by western authors.

This is a landmark book not only in India but probably also in South-east Asia. It will prove to be of considerable benefit to medical registrars, registrars in pulmonary medicine, post graduate students, medical practitioners, consultants in general medicine, and to pulmonologists practising in these countries as well as to some extent in Africa and South America. It will also be of interest to our colleagues in the West, for surely they would be keen to know the pattern of respiratory diseases in the other half of the world—in the teaming populations of poor tropical countries. Also, ours is a shrinking world and the frequency and the ease of travel from one continent to another has increasingly resulted in the need for a global awareness—an awareness of different diseases in different parts of the world.

We have based this book on current knowledge, evidence, experience, and recent advances, all perhaps in equal measure. Yet it behoves the reader to bear in mind that what is true today may not be true tomorrow, for the history of medicine, including respiratory medicine, is a chronicle of change. We leave the reader with the words of Sir Francis Bacon... 'Read not to contradict and confute, nor to believe and take for granted, nor to find talk and discourse, but to weigh and consider'.

We owe a great deal of gratitude to a number of individuals, some of whom deserve special mention. We owe an immense debt of gratitude to Mr Shreyas Doshi of Shrenuj & Company who has been kind enough to give an extraordinarily generous subsidy towards the publication of this work. The price of the book has thereby been substantially reduced to bring it within the reach of all students and colleagues in the profession.

Our sincerest thanks above all to Dr Khyati Mehta, our research assistant, without whose devotion, diligence, cheerful disposition, and invaluable help this book would never have been possible. She has been largely responsible for the organization of the numerous sections and chapters, the insertion of so many images and illustrations at appropriate places throughout the volume and meticulous attention to detail in the production of this work. Her help with the page-proofs, with the huge number of references, and her cordial liaison with our publishers have been of immense help. She indeed is as much a part of the book as the authors inscribed on the cover.

Our sincerest thanks to Dr Thirumalai Rajgopal for his chapters on 'Common Occupational Lung Diseases' and 'Environmental Pollution'. We also thank Dr Camilla Rodrigues for her chapter on 'Antibiotic Resistance and its Management'.

We are grateful to AV Graphic Designers Pvt. Ltd. (Mumbai) for creating excellent illustrations and tables that have been used throughout the book. Their cooperation and punctuality during the production of this work was outstanding. Our thanks to Dr Maansi Parekh for her help with the images and to Ms Kinni Makwana who has provided us with four special illustrations.

We thank Mrs Vera F. Udwadia for her help in the correction of the page-proofs. We also thank Mr Neeraj Chavan for his help in typing the manuscript. We thank the many authors whose work we have consulted during the preparation of this book, in particular the text on *Clinical Respiratory Medicine* edited by Albert R.K., Spiro S.C. and Jett R. We would also like to extend our thanks to those publishers and authors who have granted permission for some figures, images, and tables from their books/journals.

Finally, our sincerest thanks to the team at Oxford University Press in Delhi and Mumbai for their unstinted help and cooperation in publishing this work.

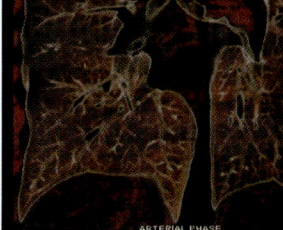
CHAPTER **1**

Imaging Techniques and Imaging of the Chest

INTRODUCTION

The chest radiograph remains the primary imaging investigation in the evaluation of diseases of the respiratory system. It is a low-radiation, cheap and easily available imaging technique, providing invaluable information regarding the lung parenchyma, pleura, mediastinum and chest wall. It has its share of limitations being a projectional two-dimensional imaging modality. Computed tomography (CT), a cross-sectional imaging modality provides excellent detail of the lung, pleura, mediastinum as well as chest wall to compensate for the limitations of chest X-ray. The chest X-ray as well as the CT scan suffice for all imaging needs in the chest. Ultrasonography (USG)/magnetic resonance imaging (MRI)/positron emission tomography (PET) have complementary roles in the evaluation of chest diseases.

CHEST RADIOGRAPHS

Even after 100 years of technological developments, the chest X-ray remains the primary imaging modality for diseases of the chest. It is obtained with the patient erect, facing the cassette, with the X-ray beam directed from behind the patient, from a distance of six feet to avoid magnification of mediastinal structures. The X-ray is obtained at deep inspiration. A film obtained in expiration will result in alteration of the mediastinal contour as well as a misleading appearance of diffuse lung disease. It is important to position the patient well such that he

or she is not rotated. A well-centred X-ray will demonstrate the medial ends of the clavicles to be equidistant from the transverse processes of the vertebrae. Rotation to the right results in the manubrium sternum, superior vena cava (SVC) and great vessels appearing prominent—this may simulate a mediastinal mass. Rotation may also result in one lung appearing more or less translucent. To minimize the shadow of the scapula on the lungs, the arms are placed on the sides and shoulders rotated forward so as to rotate the scapula laterally.

A large part of the lungs on a frontal radiograph are obscured by the bony rib cage. To be able to visualize larger areas of lung parenchyma free from significant obscuration by the ribs, high Kvp (peak kilo voltage) techniques are used. As the co-efficient of X-ray absorption of soft tissue and bone approach each other at high Kvp, the bony rib cage no longer obscures the lungs to the same extent as on lower Kvp films. The mediastinum is also penetrated better in high-Kvp films, thereby allowing more details to be viewed of the mediastinum and large airways. Scattered radiation is higher at high Kvp, causing significant degradation of image quality. To minimize this effect a grid or an air gap of 15 cm between the patient

Fig 1.1: PA view of the chest: Positioning for a PA view of the chest with patient facing the cassette and arms rotated forward to take the scapulae off the film.

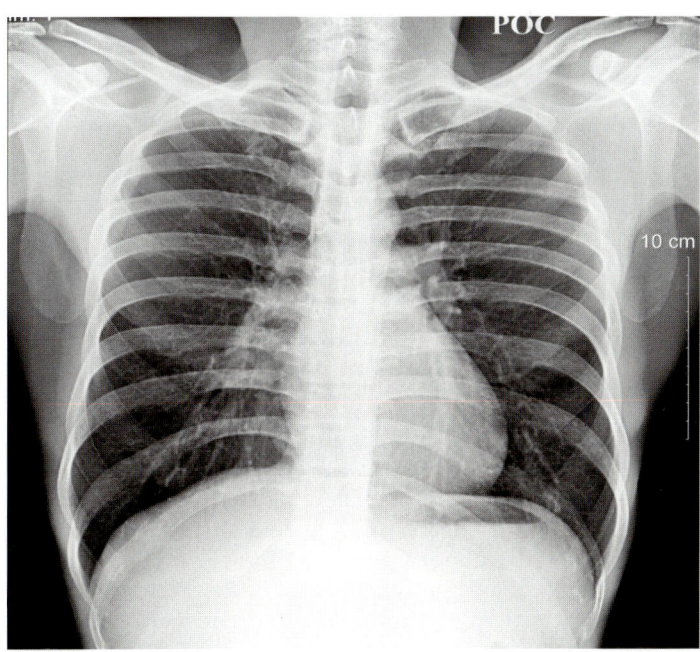

Fig 1.2: PA view of the chest: Normal chest X-ray, note scapulae have been rotated off the chest so as to avoid obscuration of lung parenchyma.

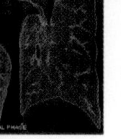

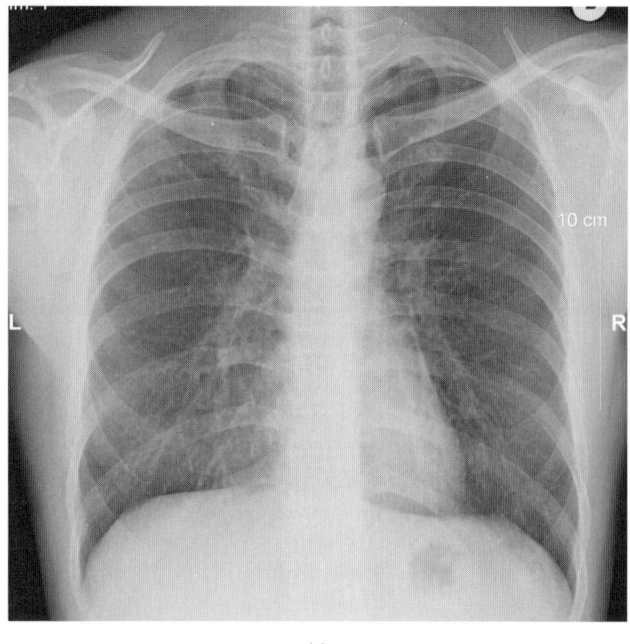

(a)

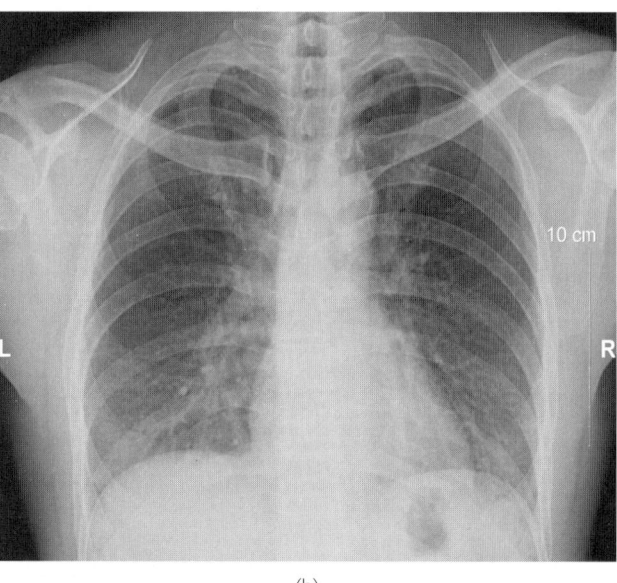

(b)

Fig 1.3: Inspiratory and expiratory views: PA view of the chest in inspiration (a) and in expiration (b) of same patient. Note change in mediastinal contour as well as diffuse haziness in both lung bases on expiratory view simulating interstitial lung disease.

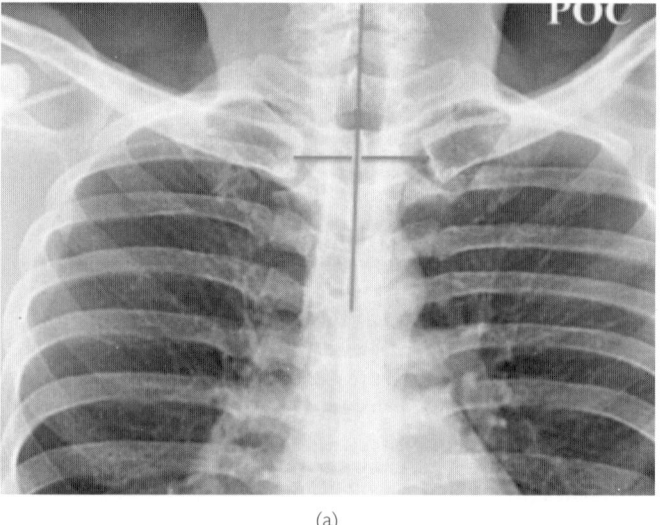

(a)

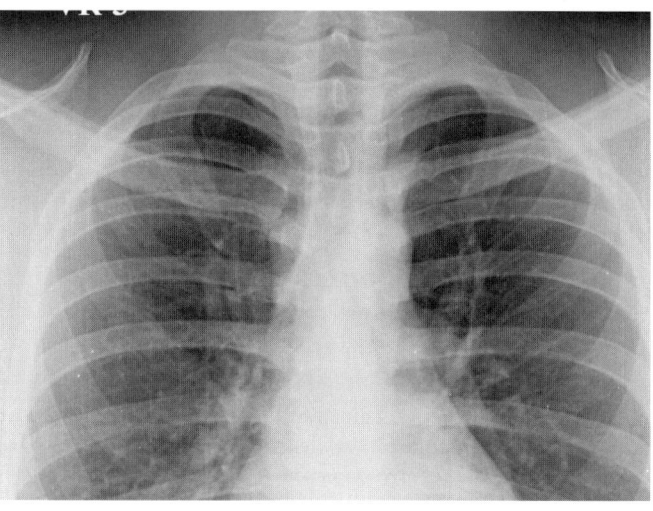

(b)

Fig 1.4: Rotation: (a) To check for rotation on a PA view, a vertical line is drawn along the spinous processes of the vertebrae (blue). Horizontal line is drawn between the medial ends of the clavicles so as to cut the vertical line. The medial ends of the clavicles should be equidistant when there is no rotation (b) Note rotation to left as medial end of right clavicles further away, resulting in right paratracheal opacity representing SVC shadow. This opacity may simulate a mass or adenopathy.

and cassette is used, thereby improving image quality. If an air gap is used, the distance between patient and X-ray beam is increased to 12 feet to avoid magnification of the mediastinum. A drawback of high Kvp is a lack of demonstration of calcified lesions and small pulmonary nodules. Low-Kvp films have the advantage of providing excellent detail in the unobscured lung, as there is excellent contrast resolution between vessels and aerated lung.

Digital chest radiography has now nearly totally replaced analog radiography modalities. There have been compelling reasons for this shift. The availability of data in an electronic form makes it possible to post-process the image data so as to present optimal image quality, view the images on large high-resolution workstations, archive as well as distribute images across a hospital network or to any remote location. Computed radiography or CR, the first commercially available digital X-ray imaging technique is still the most popular digital imaging technique available today. In this technique, conventional X-ray film is replaced by a phosphor plate. This phosphor plate when exposed to X-rays, stores the X-ray radiation as energy. This phosphor plate is read by a laser beam which releases the energy stored on the phosphor plate as light, producing an image. Recently, flat panel detectors have been introduced.

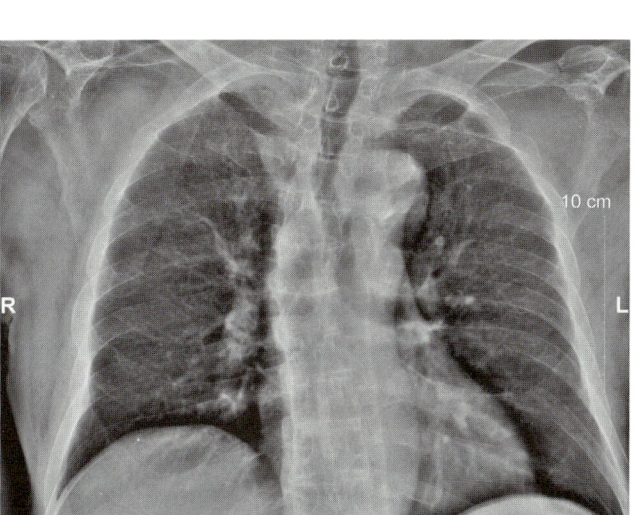

Fig 1.5: High-Kvp X-ray demonstrates the lung fields well, the opacity of overlying ribs is reduced considerably; note the detail of the mediastinum and trachea. A disadvantage of this technique is a lower detection rate of pulmonary nodules and calcified granulomas as compared to low-Kvp X-ray.

These do away with the need to have a cassette containing the phosphor plate. The images are instantly available as soon as the X-ray is exposed. The image quality is superior and as no cassette is involved, the work flow is much faster.

ADDITIONAL VIEWS

Lateral

The utility of this view is to check whether an equivocal frontal chest X-ray shadow is actually present, to position an abnormality seen on a frontal X-ray, and define as to which lobe it is located in. The patient stands perpendicular to the cassette with arms held high and well away from the thorax. The lateral

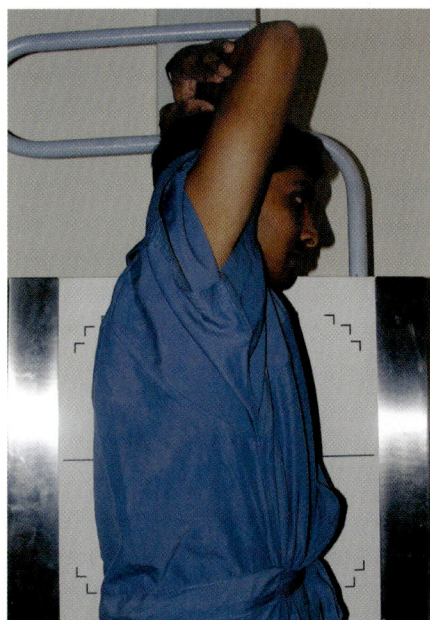

Fig 1.6: Lateral view of chest and positioning for a lateral view: Left side of chest is in contact with the cassette, as this reduces cardiac magnification as compared to right side; arms are held up.

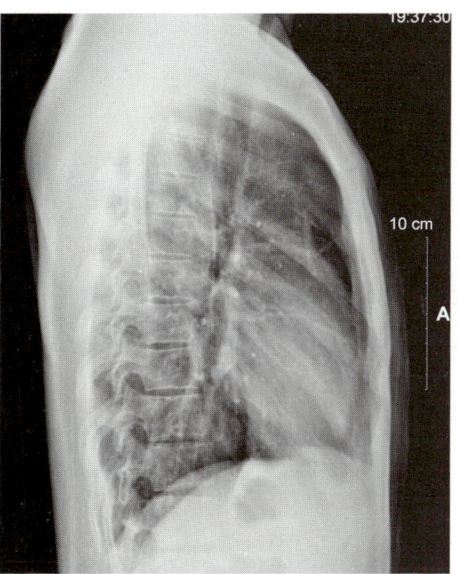

Fig 1.7: Lateral X-ray of chest—A normal lateral X-ray of the chest. Important points to note are the increasing lucency of the descending dorsal vertebrae. Loss of this progressive lucency is indicative of a pathological process in this location. Note the homogenous cardiac opacity as well as aerated retrosternal region. Loss of homogeneity in this region would indicate the presence of a pathological process.

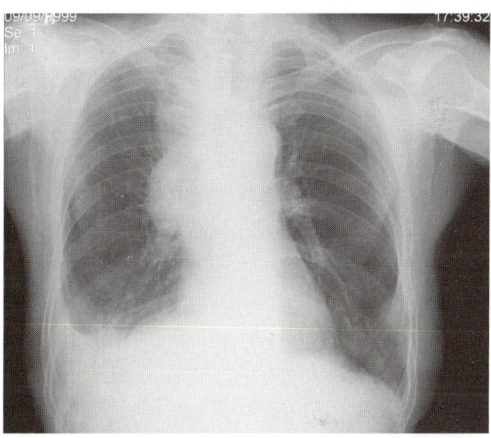

(a)

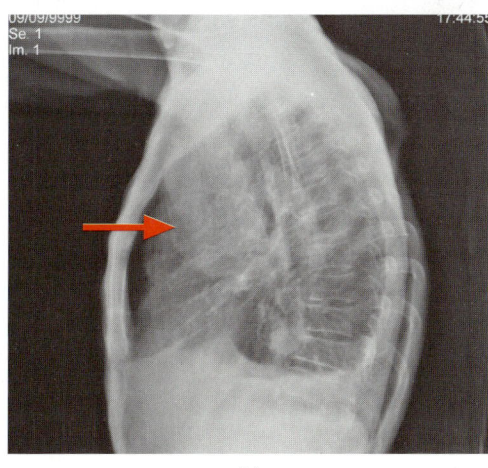

(b)

Fig 1.8: (a) PA view of the chest demonstrates a large mass lesion in the right upper and middle zone, silhouetting the right mediastinal border, with a small right pleural effusion (b) Lateral X-ray demonstrates the large opacity overlying the upper cardiac silhouette as well as partly obliterating the retrosternal air space. The translucency over the lower dorsal vertebrae is lost due to presence of pleural fluid. Note well-defined lower zone pulmonary nodule overlying anterior end of lower dorsal vertebra. This lesion was not appreciated on the PA view.

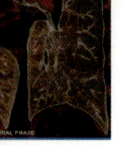

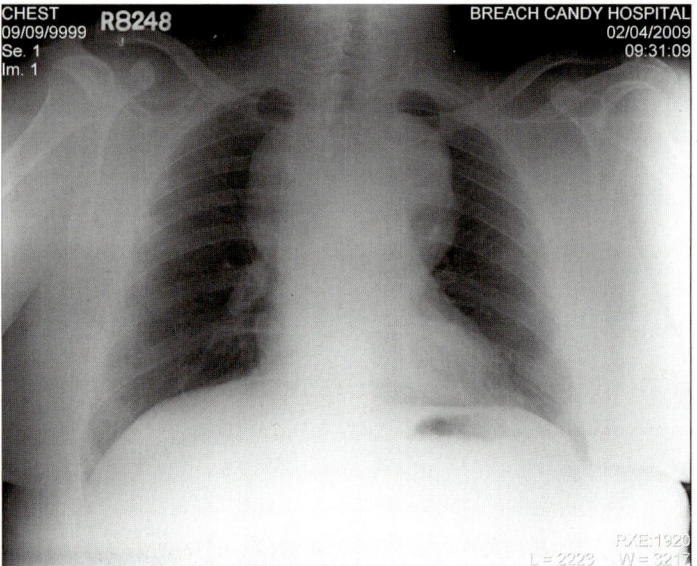

(a)

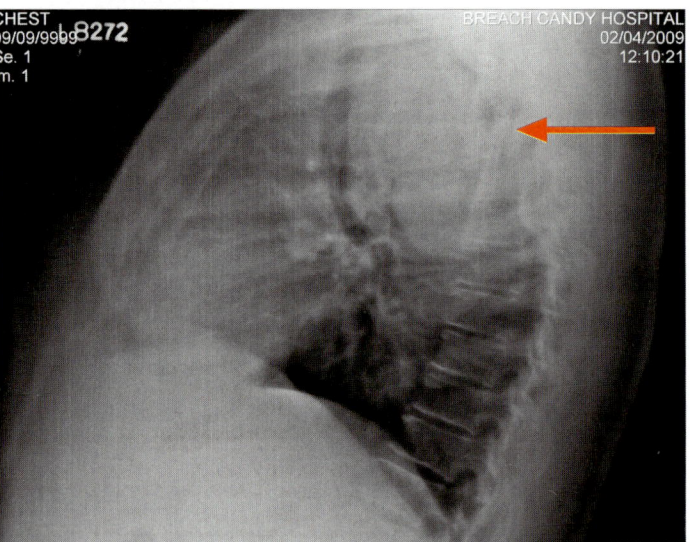

(b)

Fig 1.9: Posterior mediastinal mass: (a) PA view of the chest reveals a large mass lesion occupying and extending beyond the confines of the mediastinum (b) Lateral view localizes the mass to the posterior mediastinum. The mass lesion is seen as a homogenous opacity posterior to the trachea as well as displacing the trachea anteriorly.

chest X-ray is not of much use in evaluating the apices, as the shoulders overlap this region.

Lateral Decubitus

Lateral decubitus is a useful view to demonstrate a small pleural effusion which is not visible on the PA view, or differentiate a free pleural effusion from loculated pleural fluid or pleural thickening. A frontal radiograph is obtained with the patient lying in a decubitus position with the side suspected to have pleural effusion down. Free fluid gravitates along the dependent chest wall between the lungs and chest wall.

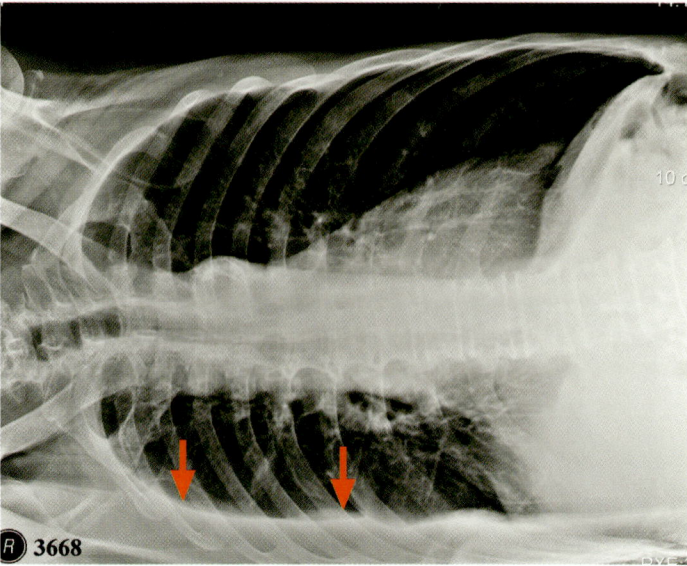

Fig 1.10: Lateral decubitus: PA view of the chest had demonstrated a right basal opacity, ? collapse consolidation, ? pleural fluid. X-ray taken with patient lying on his right side; there is fluid layering along the chest wall indicating a free pleural effusion.

Lateral Shoot Through

This view is useful to demonstrate a small anterior pneumothorax in a supine patient. The X-ray beam is directed horizontally from one lateral chest wall and the cassette is placed along the other lateral chest wall.

Lateral Oblique

This view is used to demonstrate rib fractures and rib lesions. The axillary course of a rib is obscured on a frontal radiograph; on oblique view these are well visualized. The patient is rotated by 45 degrees and a frontal radiograph is obtained.

Lordotic View

On a frontal radiograph the apices are often obscured by the clavicle and first rib thereby obscuring a lesion in this location. Subtle tubercular lesions hidden beneath the first rib/clavicle can be well demonstrated on this view. Additionally, on a PA view it may be difficult to discern between a fibrotic tubercular lesion and costochondral cartilage; a lordotic view would be able to differentiate the two. The patient is positioned upright and the X-ray beam is angled 15 degrees upwards or alternatively the X-ray beam is kept horizontal and the patient arched backwards resembling the posture of a 'lord'.

PORTABLE RADIOGRAPHS

These are extremely useful as they are performed at the patient's bedside. They do have their share of limitations. Due to the shorter tube focus distance, there is mediastinal magnification. High-Kvp techniques are not possible as the output of these machines is limited, the exposure time is longer, so that patients may be unable to hold their breath, resulting in motion artifacts. The positioning of these patients is also a challenge as they are often half upright or rotated. Patients also find it difficult to take a deep breath in a semi-erect position. Digital X-rays have fortunately helped considerably to improve image quality of portable X-rays. Similar to X-rays taken in the imaging department using CR, the same CR cassettes can be used in the intensive care unit (ICU), and processed in the same readers available in the imaging department. DR or digital radiography units which do not require a cassette and which are available for an imaging department are also available for portable radiography. These have a great advantage; they provide an instant image, thereby saving precious time—time taken to transport a cassette to the imaging department, process it, archive the image and transport it back. These however at present are extremely expensive. As a bridge, portable CR readers are being developed, so that at the bedside itself the CR cassette can be read, producing a quick image.

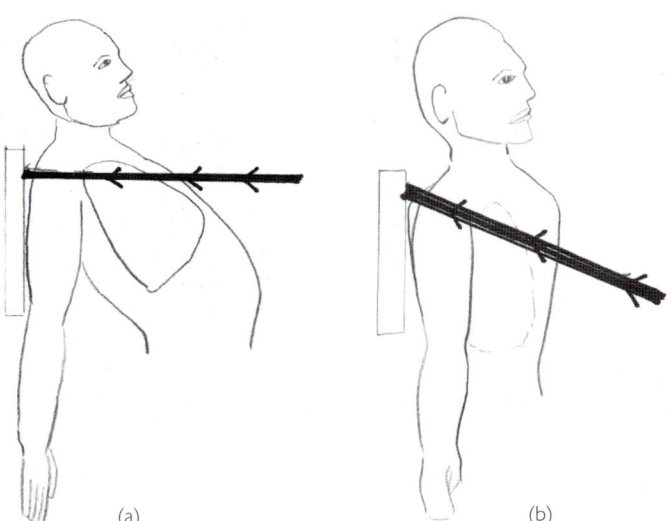

(a) (b)

Fig 1.11: Lordotic X-rays demonstrate two methods of demonstration of the apices without overlap of first rib, in (a) the X-ray beam is horizontal, the patient is arched back simulating a 'lord'. In the other method (b) the X-ray beam is angled upwards by 15 degrees to the apex, the patient stands straight with back to the cassette.

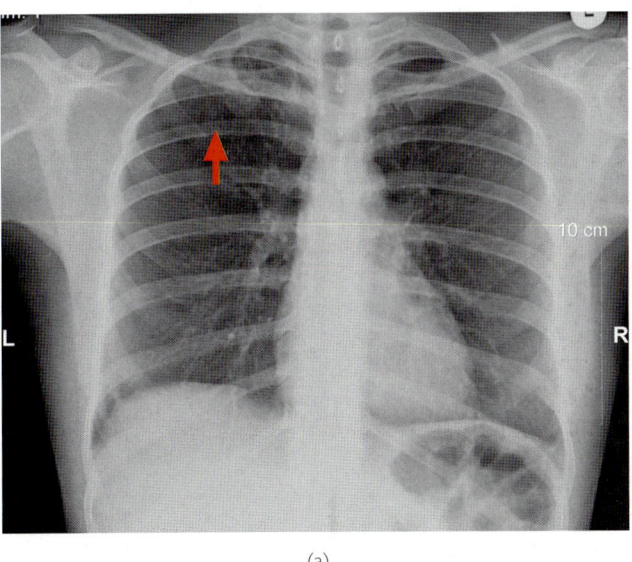

(a)

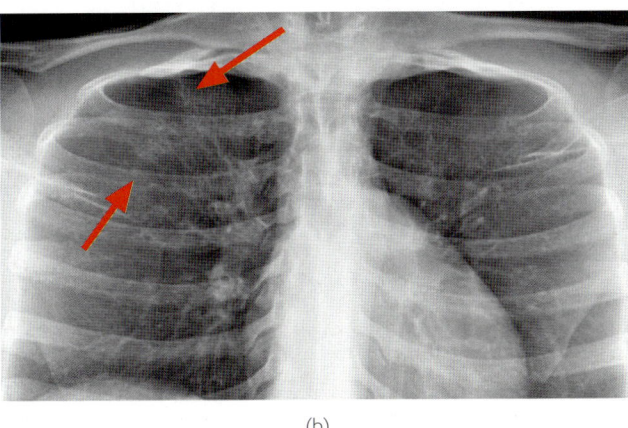

(b)

Fig 1.12: Lordotic view: (a) PA view of the chest reveals a questionable opacity underlying the first rib on the right side (b) Lordotic view uncovers the first rib demonstrating ill-defined soft opacities in the right apex due to active tuberculous infection.

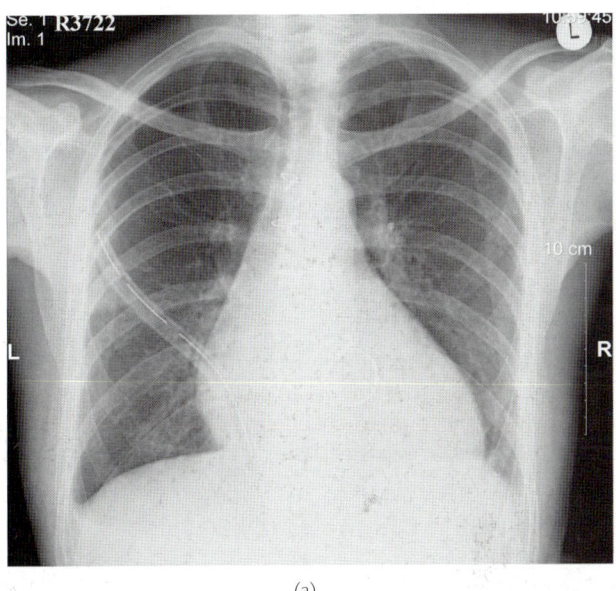

(a)

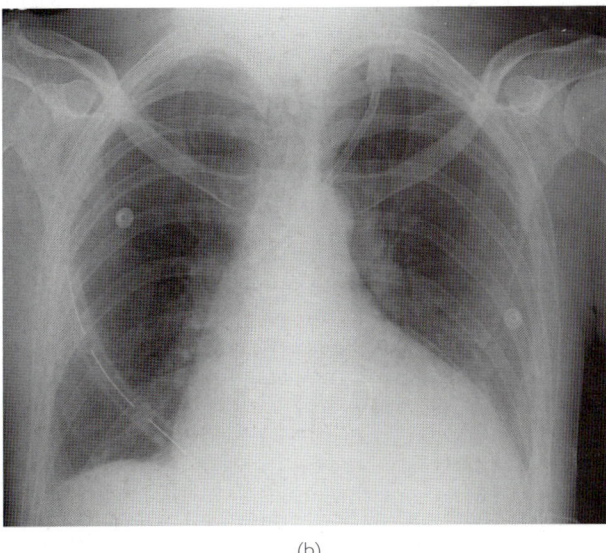

(b)

Fig 1.13: Portable chest radiograph: (a) PA view and (b) portable AP view of the chest. Note the change in cardiac outline between a PA view and an AP view. Commenting on cardiomegaly on an AP view may be hazardous.

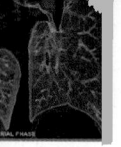

There are newer novel applications developing in digital radiography—Dual Energy, Tomosynthesis and Temporal Subtraction.

Dual-Energy Subtraction Imaging

The absorption of X-ray by tissues depends upon the Kilo voltage used, as well as on the consistency of the tissues. When Kv is varied the response of tissues changes; as a result tissues can be separated from each other at different Kv. In the chest, bone and soft tissue both appear bright on low Kv, so that a pulmonary nodule underlying a rib will be obscured due to their similar densities. At higher Kv the attenuation of calcium and soft tissue to X-rays differs. This principle is used to generate images using different Kvs. The images are subtracted to provide images with only soft tissue. This helps to improve detection of a solitary pulmonary nodule as only soft tissue is seen and no bone.

Digital Tomosynthesis

Digital tomosynthesis is a technique where images of a certain depth in the chest are obtained. The tissues above and below this level are blurred, only tissue at that depth is visualized. This is similar to tomography of the olden days, now using digital techniques to enhance the evaluation.

Temporal Subtraction

This technique utilizes subtraction of a previous image from the present image. If there is any interval change it will be demonstrated. Inaccuracies do occur in terms of positioning as well as differences in breath-hold.

Computer-Aided Diagnosis (CAD)

This is a technique which relies on a pattern recognition approach using artificial intelligence to help detect lesions which may be missed by radiologists. The main applications being evaluated at present are detection of pulmonary nodules, as well as pulmonary emboli. These techniques are yet to become popular, as there is a high rate of false-positive detection; also the detection rate is similar to that observed by radiologists.

LIMITATIONS OF CHEST X-RAY

The limitations of a chest X-ray relate essentially to the fact that the chest X-ray is a two-dimensional (2D) modality, imaging a three-dimensional structure. Nearly 75% of the lungs are covered by ribs, mediastinum and diaphragm; as a result a number of anatomical structures are superimposed reducing the detectability of lesions. From a technical aspect since the chest is a large region to be imaged, approximately 40 cm, as the whole of this area has to be radiated, there is significant scatter radiation resulting in degradation of image quality.

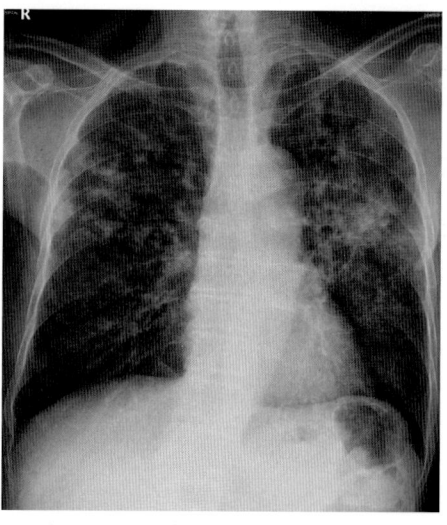

(a)

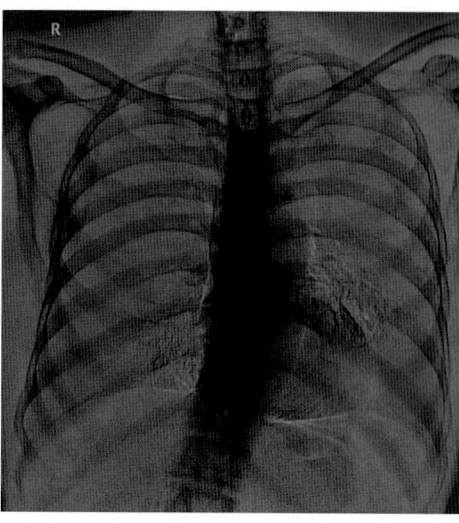

(b)

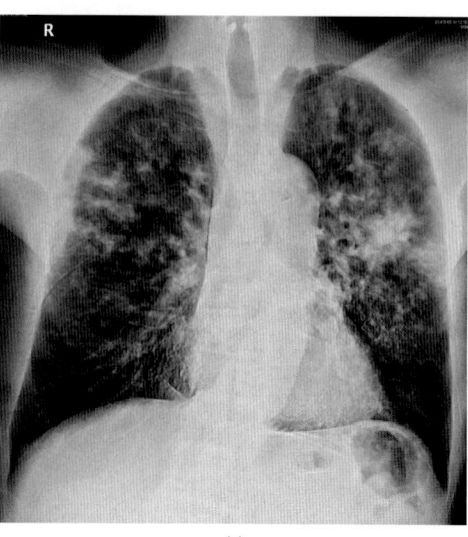

(c)

Fig 1.14: Dual-energy subtraction: (a) PA view of the chest (b) following dual-energy subtraction all tissues other than bone subtracted (c) following dual energy, bone is subtracted leaving behind only soft tissue, no bone obscures visualization of the lungs.

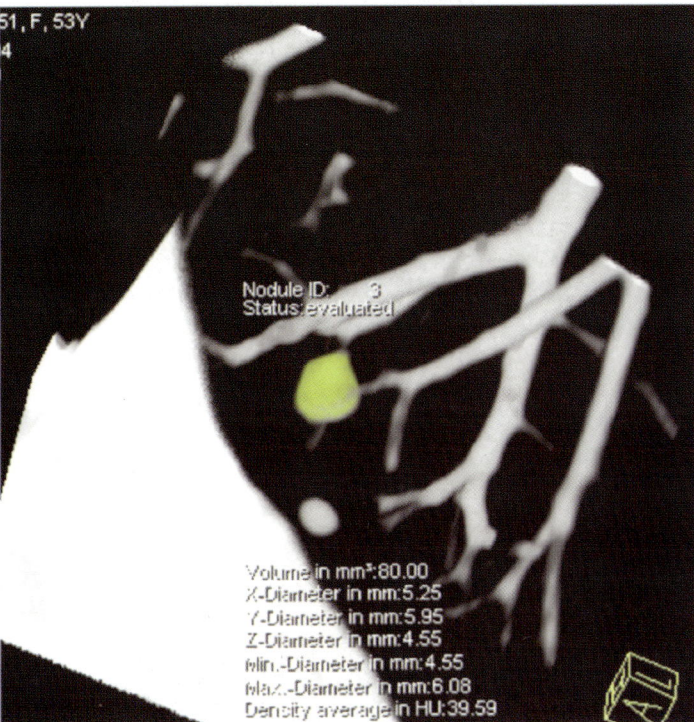

51, F, 53Y

Nodule ID: 3
Status: evaluated

Volume in mm³: 80.00
X-Diameter in mm: 5.25
Y-Diameter in mm: 5.95
Z-Diameter in mm: 4.55
Min.-Diameter in mm: 4.55
Max.-Diameter in mm: 6.08
Density average in HU: 39.59

Fig 1.15: Computer-aided diagnosis: CAD demonstrates a pulmonary nodule coloured in yellow, separate from adjacent vessels. The volume of this nodule can be easily determined. The nodule can be followed up on subsequent examinations to determine rate of growth. CAD helps in detecting lesions which may have been missed by radiologists; at present CAD has a high false-positive detection rate; however, it is extremely useful for volume measurements.

COMPUTED TOMOGRAPHY

CT has been heralded as the greatest discovery in medicine following the discovery of X-rays. The history of the development of the CT scanner is extremely unique. Electrical and musical industries (EMI) became famous in the 1960s as they were the record label for the Beatles. At their Abbey Road studios they recorded enough Vinyl for the Beatles to go around the earth's circumference. They became a cash-rich company. Godfrey Hounsfield an eminent scientist with EMI who had already developed the first all-transistor computer was keen to develop a product which would more effectively evaluate the attenuation of X-rays through soft tissues. This research was funded directly by profits from the Beatles. In 1972 Godfrey Hounsfield unveiled the first CT scanner to the world named as EMI. That scanner took four minutes to acquire a single slice and a further seven minutes to reconstruct the image. CT has come a long way since those days with the entire thorax being scanned with a dual-source CT in under a second in 2010. Not only did the Beatles spawn an entire shift in musical tastes, outlook, physical appearance and hairstyles for nearly the entire globe, they contributed to one of the greatest advances in medicine since the discovery of X-rays.

CT scanners are based on the same principles as X-ray. Tissues attenuate X-rays differently depending on their composition i.e. atomic number; thereby a CT scanner is able to detect minute differences in attenuation by tissues,

providing extremely high anatomical detail. A CT scanner consists of an X-ray tube which emits X-rays, and a detector opposite to the X-ray tube. This combined assembly rotates 360 degrees around the patient acquiring data. Data from one 360-degree rotation produces a single image. Present-day scanners are helical scanners; data is acquired simultaneously with the table moving and X-ray tube rotating during a single breath-hold. This technique has significant advantages over the previous non-helical scanners. As scans are acquired in a single breath-hold, the possibility of missing a pulmonary nodule due to respiratory misregistration does not arise. Data is acquired as a volume and therefore can be reconstructed at any slice thickness as well as in any plane which is desired. Additionally, as the scan time is shorter, less intravenous contrast medium is required. Helical scanners have advanced technologically from being single-detector to multidetector scanners (MDCT). These MDCT scanners may have from 2 to 64 rows of detectors. Increasing the number of rows of detectors enables faster scans, reducing respiratory and motion artifacts. Angiographic images may be obtained as well as larger volumes may be covered, with thinner sections obtained. A CT image is a 2D image, but there is a third dimension, depth or slice thickness. A thick slice contains different tissues within the section, which will be averaged to produce the final image. To obtain a high degree of anatomical detail as with high-resolution CT (HRCT) very thin sections are required, 1mm or less, so that there is no averaging of tissues. These scanners have further revolutionized the diagnostic potential of CT, especially the 16,64 slice scanners, as these produce thin slices (0.6–0.75 mm) which are isotropic, i.e. reconstruction of these slices in any plane results in no loss of resolution. These scanners have essentially converted CT from an axial cross-sectional technique to a true three-dimensional technique allowing arbitrary selection of scan planes, and volumetric display of data. Newer scanners with 128,256,360 rows and dual-source CT have been introduced essentially to facilitate CT coronary angiography. The dual-source CT houses two CT scanners in one CT gantry. The advantage of this is in the performance of CT coronary angiograms without the need to use beta-blockers. As dual-source CT scanners have two X-ray tubes,

Problems of Conventional CT...

Misregistration due to different levels of respiration

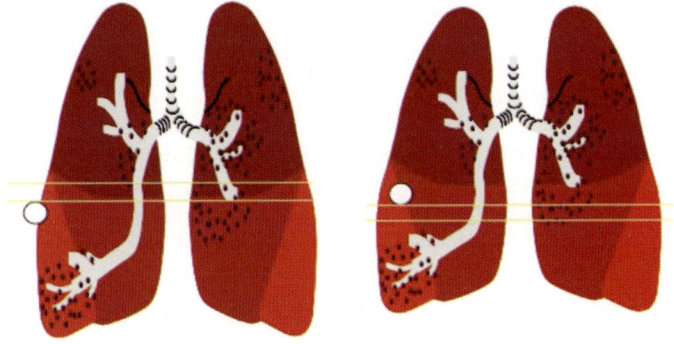

Deep inspiration   Moderate inspiration

Fig 1.16: Problems of conventional CT scan.

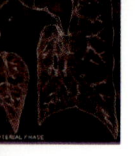

they can fire at different energies resulting in dual-energy scans. This is useful in obtaining lung perfusion scans. These help in the detection of pulmonary embolism. Segmental and sub-segmental emboli may only be detected by demonstrating a perfusion defect on dual-energy scans.

Respiratory Misregistration

Conventional CT scanned the chest slice by slice. With every slice, the patient was asked to hold his or her breath, the table then moved to the next table position and another slice was obtained. The illustration demonstrates respiratory mis-registration. In the first section, due to an increased inspiratory effort the nodule goes below the slice; in the next slice where the nodule should be visualized, it is not, as the patient has taken only a moderate inspiratory effort. This resulted in a lower accuracy for CT in detecting pulmonary nodules.

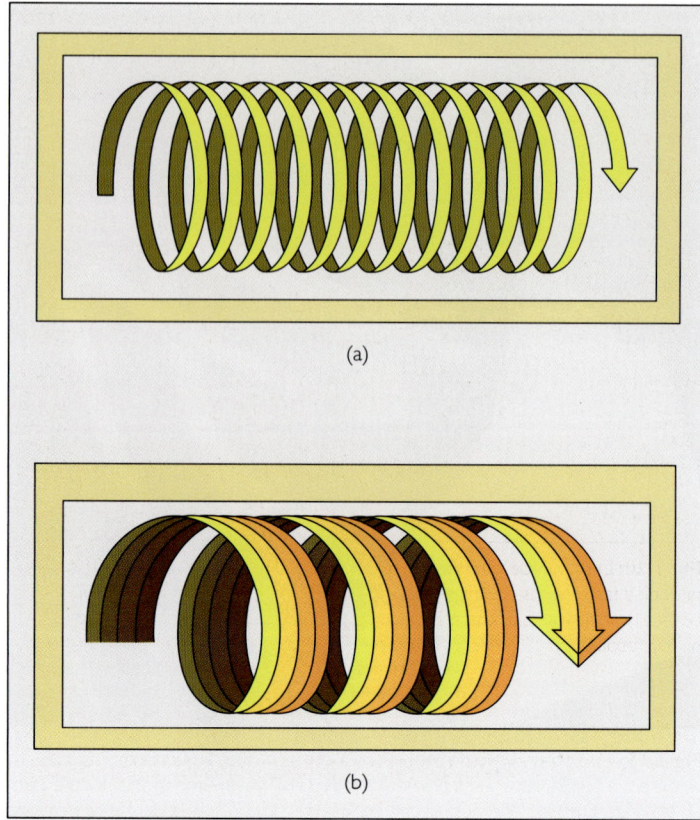

Fig 1.18: Multidetector CT: (a) demonstrates a single-slice helical CT rotation, (b) demonstrates a multidetector helical CT rotation.

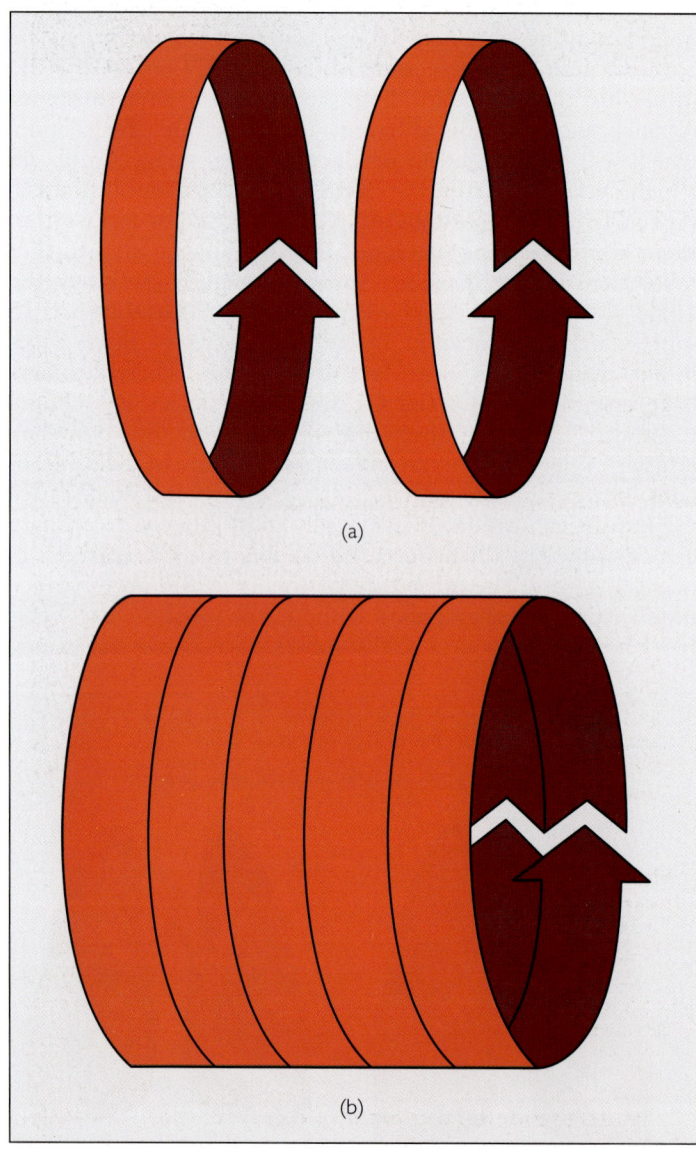

Fig 1.17: Helical CT: (a) demonstrates a conventional CT which obtained slices one by one (b) demonstrates a helical CT, all slices are obtained simultaneously in one breath-hold.

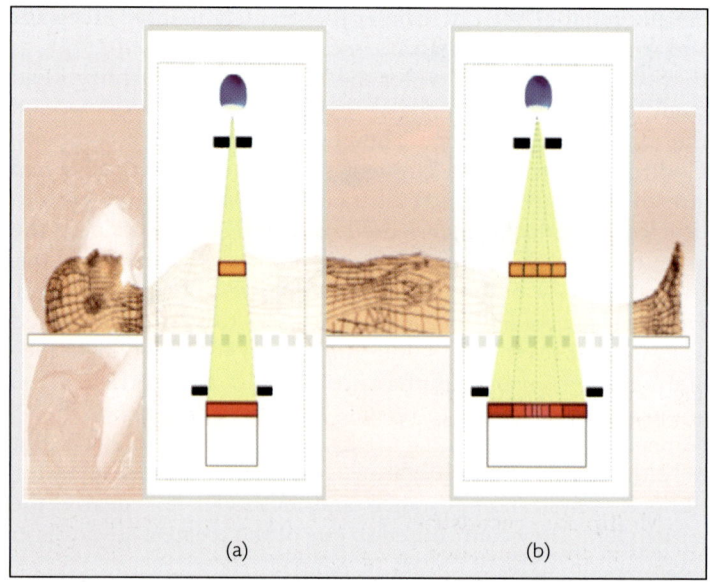

Fig 1.19: Multidetector CT: Comparison between a single-detector CT and a multidetector CT. (a) single-detector (b) Multidetector CT. Note the increased coverage in a single rotation with a multidetector CT allowing for large volume coverage in shorter time with thinner slices.

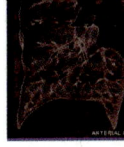

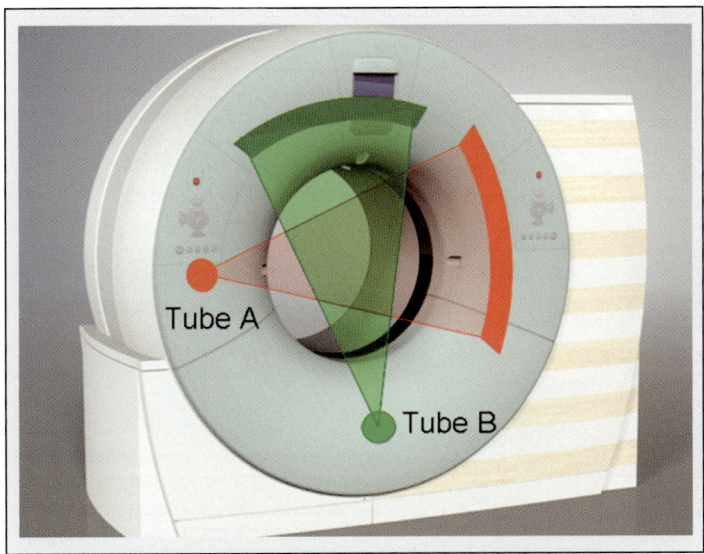

Fig 1.20: Dual-source CT: New generation of CT scanners with two CT tubes, providing faster scans and higher temporal resolution, of particular value in coronary angiograms as there is no need of beta-blockers, and images are of higher resolution.

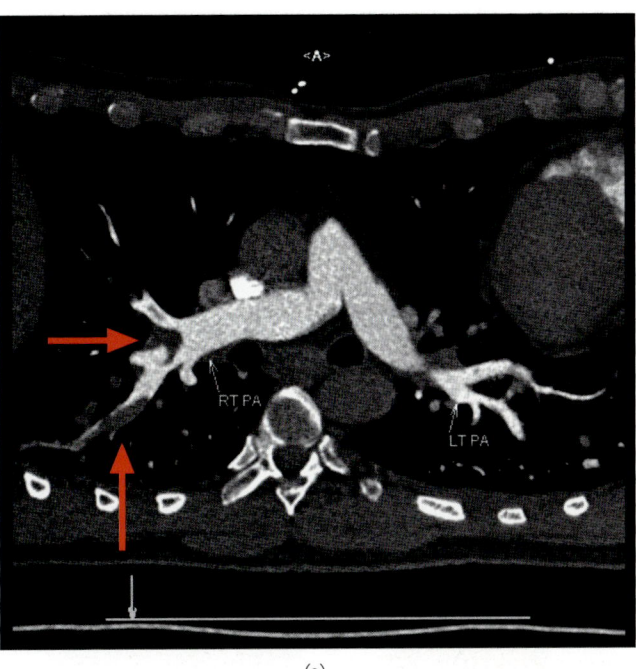

(a)

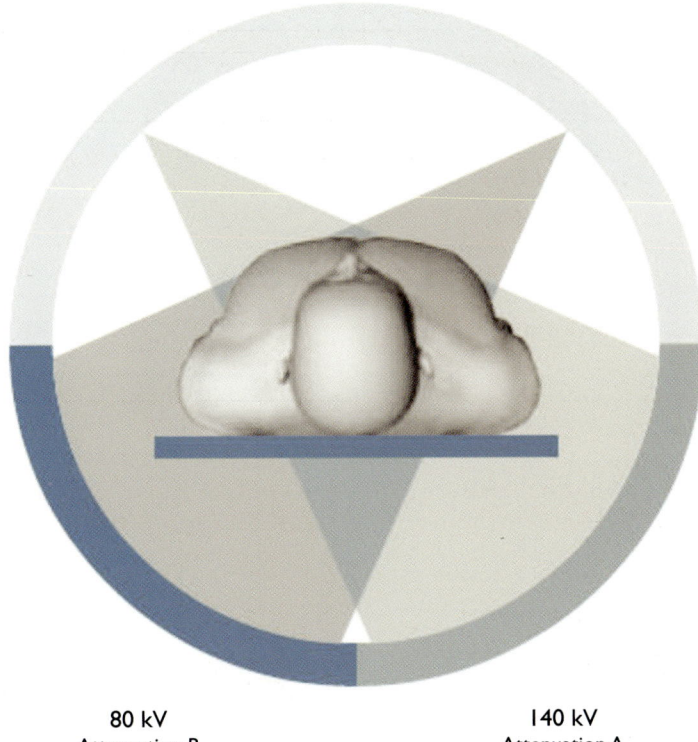

80 kV
Attenuation B

140 kV
Attenuation A

Fig 1.21: Dual-energy CT: Schematic diagram of a dual-energy CT scan, two tubes firing at different KVs, one at 80 and other at 140 KV simultaneously.

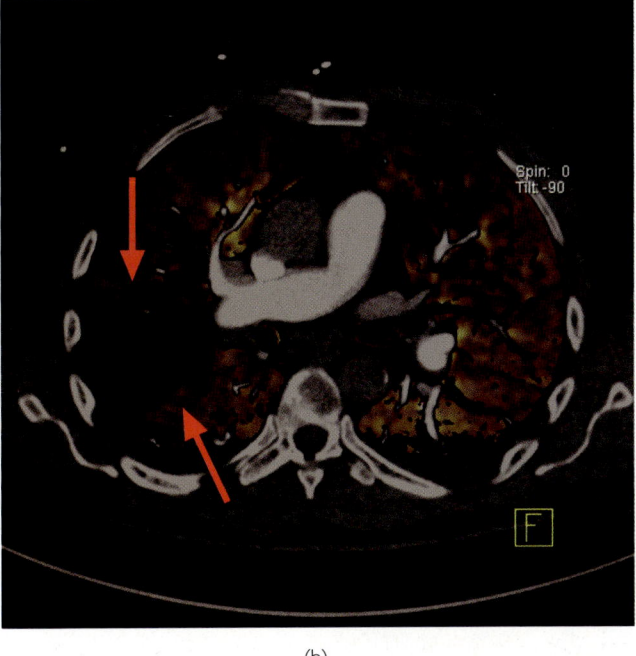

(b)

Fig 1.22: Dual-energy CT: CT pulmonary angiogram (a) demonstrates bilateral pulmonary emboli, particularly on the right side. Dual-energy CT (b) demonstrates perfusion defects, particularly wedge-shaped defect in right mid-zone. Dual-energy CT provides a CT angiography with a perfusion scan, thereby increasing accuracy in detection of pulmonary embolism, especially sub-segmental emboli. CT data in MDCT scanners is acquired as a data volume; this data can be post-processed to provide a variety of different images.

Multiplanar reconstructions (MPR) allow reconstruction of images in any plane such as the coronal, sagittal or any oblique plane. Curved multiplanar reconstructions are also possible where a curved structure such as a vessel or airway may be straightened out; its diameter as well as extent of stenosis may be quantified.

Volume-rendered techniques (VRTs) are three-dimensional (3D) techniques which provide a rendering of the surface of the organ. These are useful for demonstrating the tracheobronchial tree, as well as vasculature, especially the aorta and

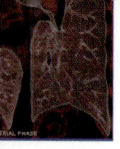

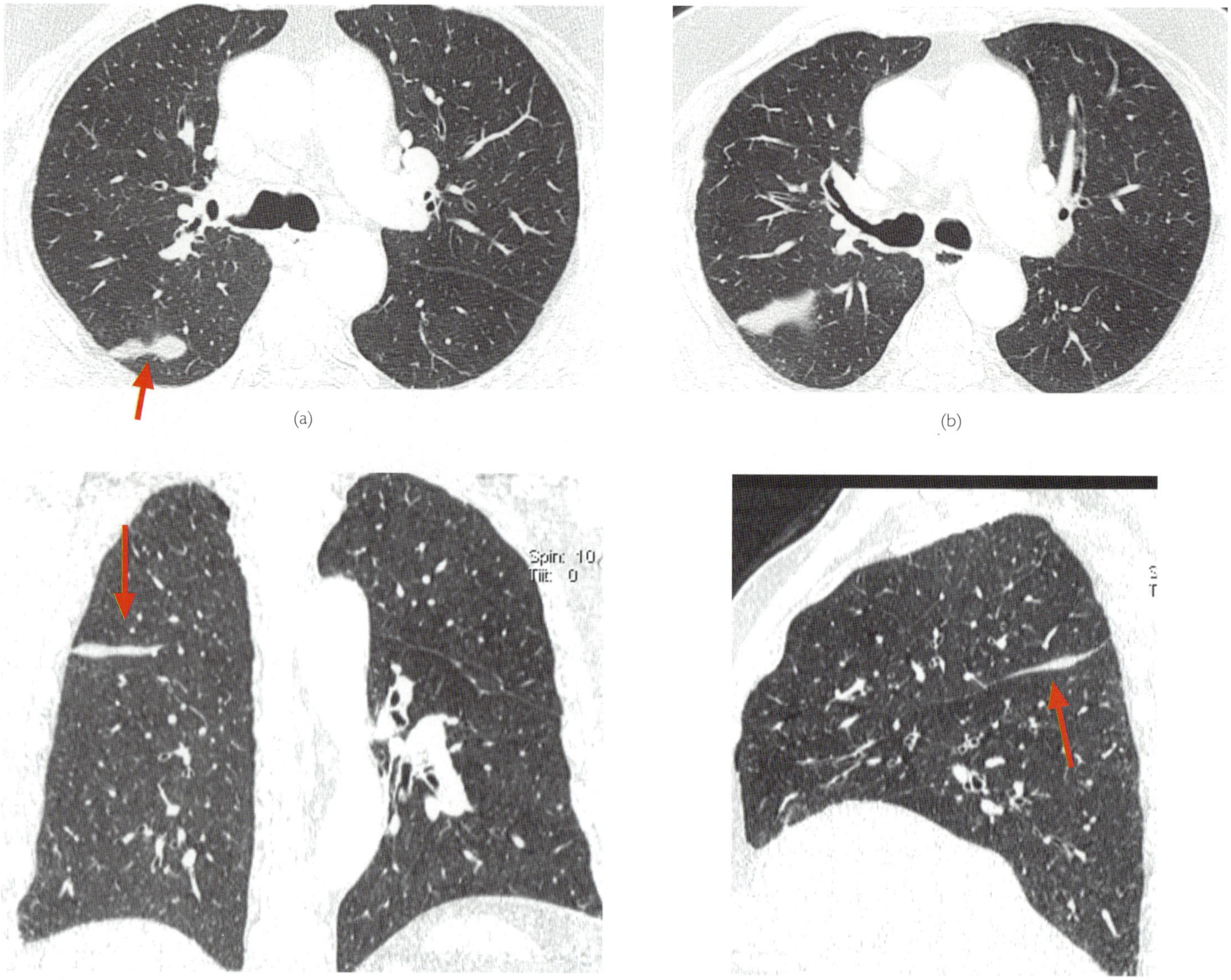

(a)

(b)

(c)

(d)

Fig 1.23: (a and b) Axial CT scans reveal an opacity in the right upper lobe. On the axial scans it is difficult to determine the aetiology of the lesion (c and d) Coronal and sagittal reconstructions demonstrate that the opacity represents fluid in the interlobar fissure. An example of how visualization of an abnormality in multiple planes may help establish the location, extent and aetiology of the lesion.

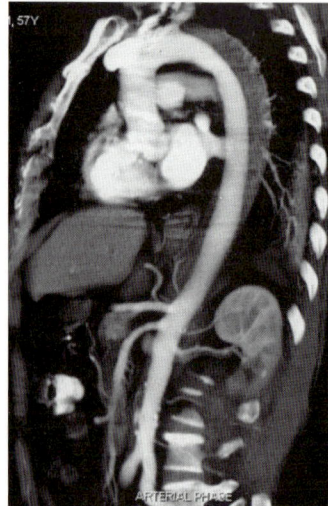

Fig 1.24: Curved MPR: Curved MPR of aorta demonstrates an aortic dissection with thrombosis of the false lumen. The advantage of a curved MPR is that a curvilinear structure can be straightened out.

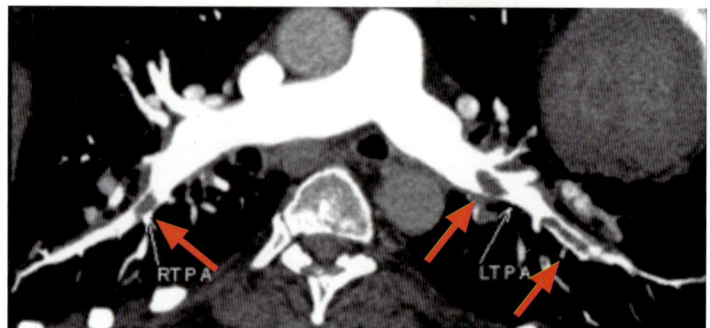

Fig 1.25: Curved MPR of pulmonary arteries: Curved MPR demonstrates main pulmonary artery and both right and left pulmonary arteries in one image. Note multiple pulmonary emboli in right and left pulmonary arteries. The advantage of a curved MPR is that the main, right and left pulmonary arteries can be demonstrated in a single image.

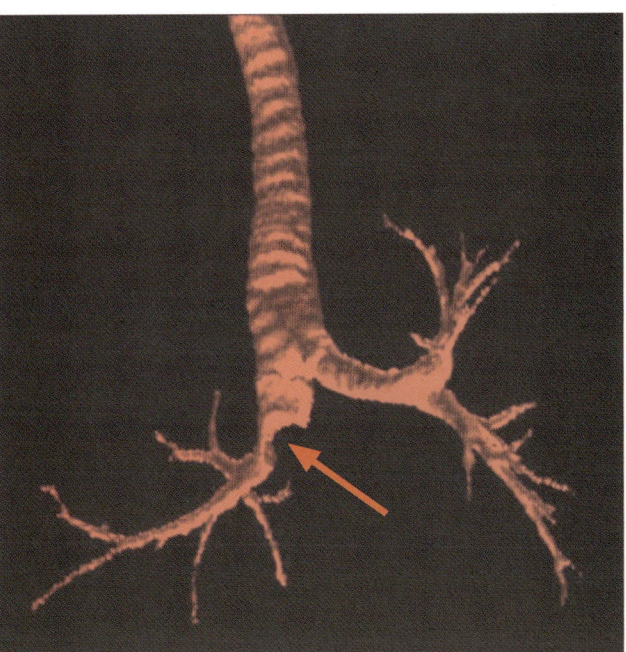

Fig 1.26: VRT of trachea: Volume-rendered image of the trachea demonstrates an extrinsic mass lesion indenting the right main bronchus, causing significant narrowing of its lumen.

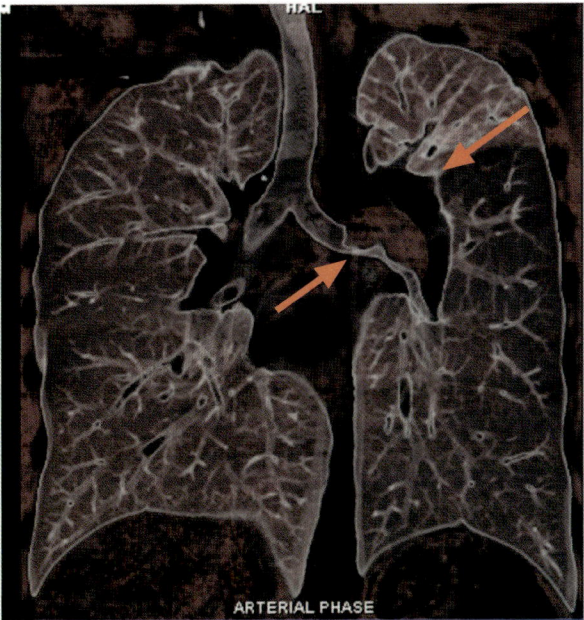

Fig 1.28: VRT tracheobronchial tree: Volume-rendered image of tracheobronchial tree and lung parenchyma. Mass lesion seen in left upper lobe infiltrates the left upper lobe bronchus causing significant narrowing of its lumen.

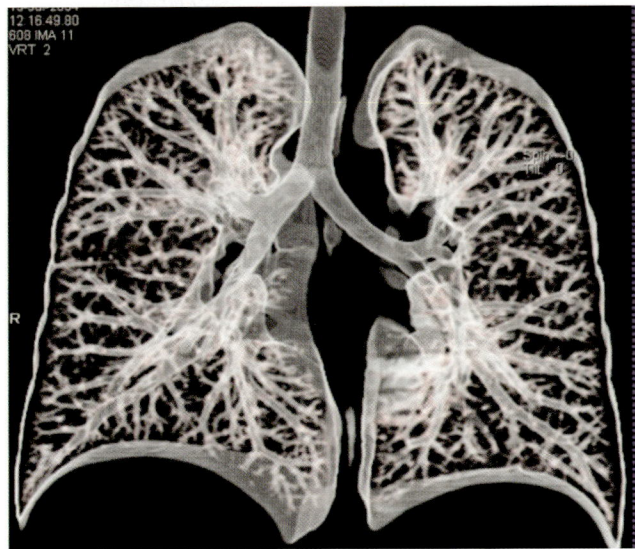

Fig 1.27: VRT tracheobronchial tree. Volume-rendered 3D image of the tracheobronchial tree, no abnormality was detected. Note the visualization of not only the tracheobronchial tree, but also segmental and sub-segmental bronchi.

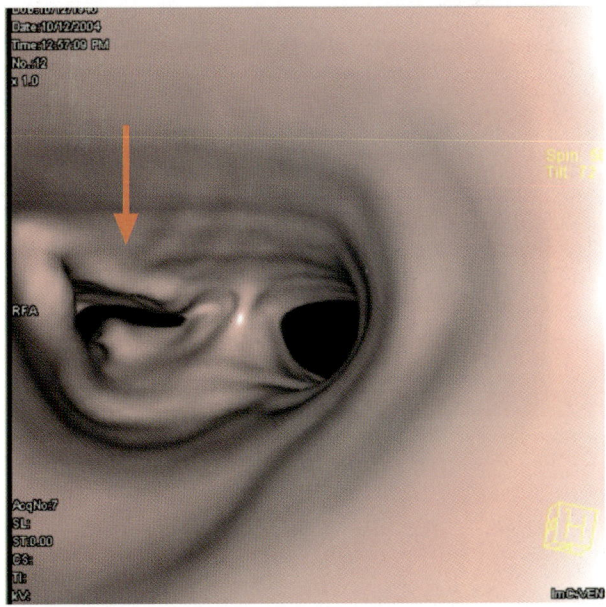

Fig 1.29: Virtual bronchoscopy. Virtual bronchoscopy at the level of the carina reveals marked irregularity and narrowing of the right main bronchus due to a bronchogenic carcinoma.

coronary arteries. An adaptation of this technique is virtual bronchoscopy. A 3D volume of the tracheobronchial tree is obtained, utilizing a fly-through software. The internal contents of the tracheobronchial tree can be visualized similar to an optical bronchoscopy, the advantages of a virtual bronchscopy being the ability to demonstrate tracheobronchial stenosis, extrinsic compression, intraluminal masses, foreign bodies or intraluminal extension of extrinsic lesions. Internal measurements of the tracheobronchial tree are also possible. This helps to determine the length and size of stents required in planning surgery. The main disadvantage is the inability to obtain biopsies and lavages.

Maximum Intensity Projections

The disadvantage of thin-section CT is the inability to differentiate small nodules from vessels. On thicker sections it is possible to differentiate these as the branching appearance

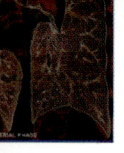

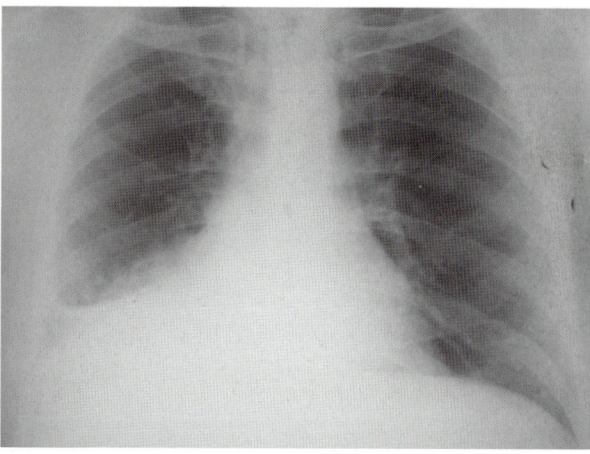

(a)

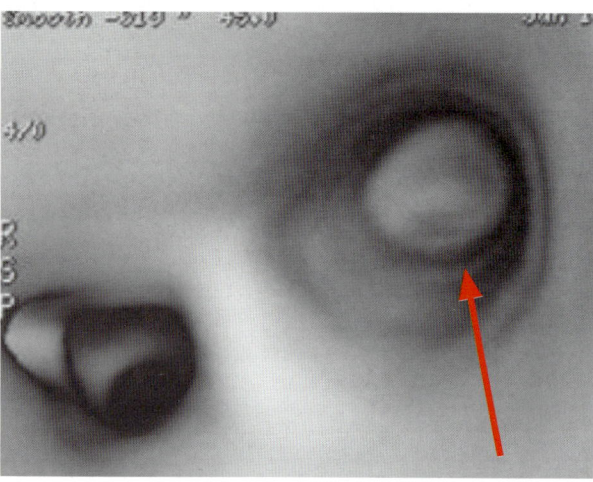

(b)

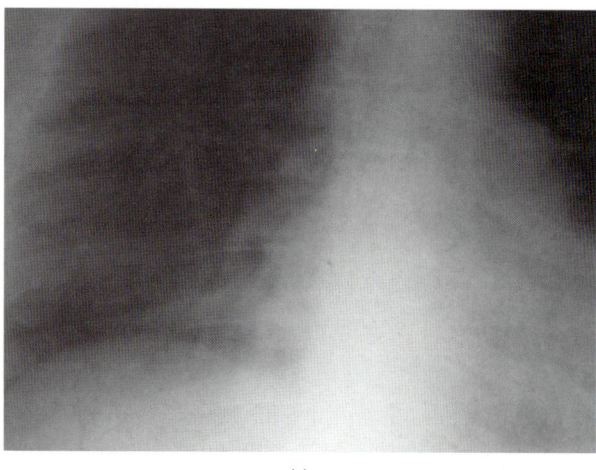

(c)

Fig 1.30: Virtual bronchoscopy: (a) Chest X-ray reveals an area of collapse consolidation in the right lower zone (b) Virtual bronchoscopy reveals a well-defined foreign body in the right bronchus (image orientation is flipped horizontally). On optical bronchoscopy the lesion seen was a betel nut; this was removed. (c) Post procedure, chest X-ray reveals clearing of collapse consolidation.

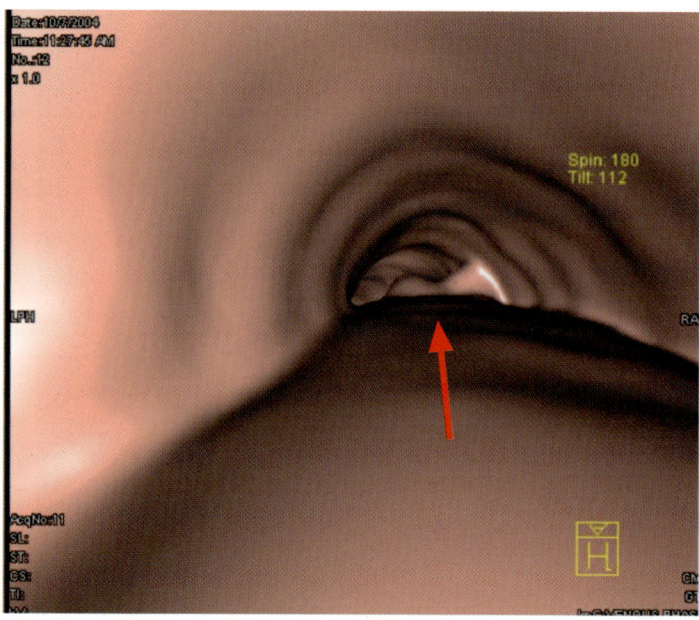

Fig 1.31: Virtual bronchoscopy: Virtual bronchoscopy in an individual with carcinoma oesophagus. The oesophageal mass indents the posterior surface of the trachea as well as infiltrates into the lower trachea. Seen as small nodular lesions projecting into the distal aspect of the trachea. This is an excellent non-invasive technique to determine local extension into the tracheobronchial tree.

of vessels is easily appreciated. Maximum intensity projections (MIPs) create a thicker slab of tissue and highlight structures with high intensity such as vessels and nodules. As the slab is thicker, the branching nature of the vessels is well appreciated, the detection of nodules is much easier. The ideal thickness is 3 mm; an additional benefit beyond precise detection is an accurate characterization of the location of the nodules in relation to the vessels—whether centrilobular or perivascular. For detection of miliary nodules or pulmonary metastatic deposits this technique is ideal.

Minimum Intensity Projections

In emphysema, bronchiolitis obliterans, the contrast between normal and low-attenuation lung parenchyma may be subtle on inspiratory HRCT. Such subtle regional density differences can be highlighted by minimum intensity projections (MinIPs). MinIPs correlate excellently with pulmonary function tests. Another useful application of MinIP is demonstration of tracheobronchial tree stenosis /occlusions. A window width of 350–500 HU and a window level of -750 to -900 HU is ideal.

Window Settings

To visualize body structures the CT images are 'windowed'. Two variables are used to select the densities to be viewed. Window width and window level. CT density is measured in HU values. Arbitrarily, water is considered as zero and air as -1000. Window width determines the number of Hounsfield units to be demonstrated. Any densities greater than the upper limit of the window width are displayed as white and any below are displayed as black. Between these two levels all densities are demonstrated in shades of grey.

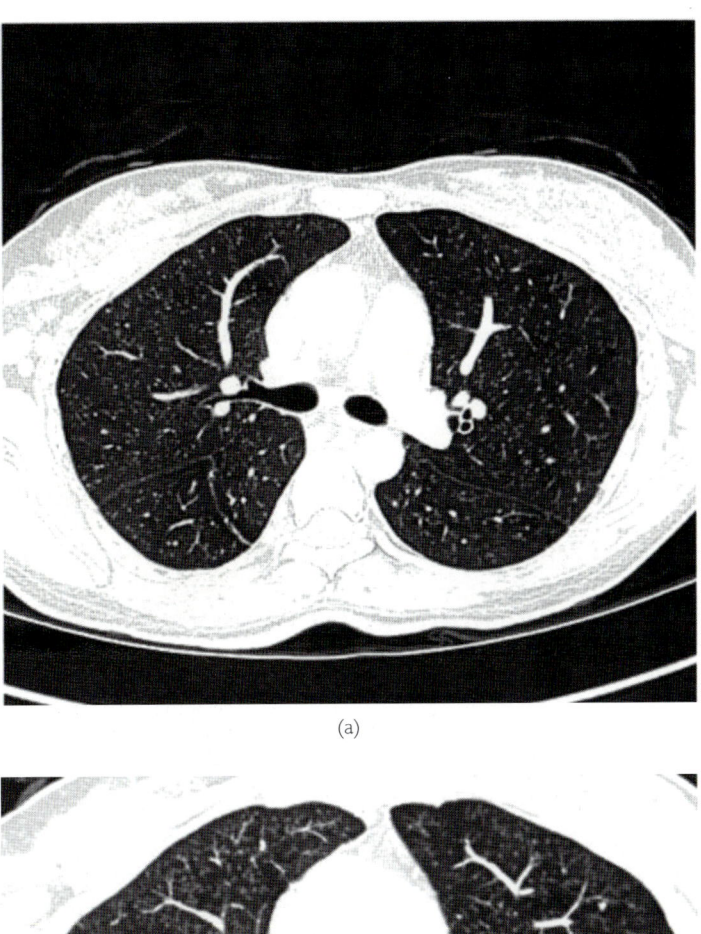

(a)

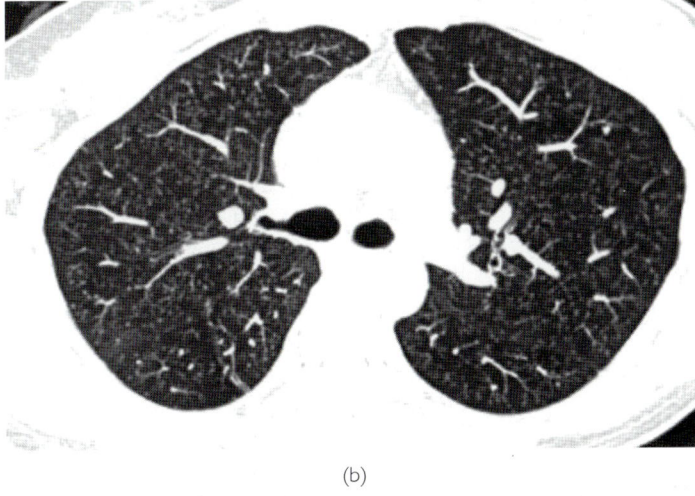

(b)

Fig 1.32: MIP (a) Routine HRCT reveals suspicious small nodules in the lung parenchyma. As the slice thickness is very thin, it is difficult to be certain whether these represent nodules or vessels (b) MIP demonstrates vessels very well as branching structures. The fine nodules are seen well separate from the vessels. This technique is very useful in detecting subtle military nodules.

CONTRAST MEDIA

Intravenous contrast enhancement is required to enhance mediastinal vasculature and separate vessels from mediastinal masses as well as demonstrate enhancement within mass lesions. Ionic contrast mediums which had a significant incidence of mild, moderate as well as severe reactions have now been nearly universally replaced by non-ionic contrast media which are far safer. Other than anaphylactic reactions, contrast-induced nephropathy (CIN) is an important adverse event.

CIN is an exacerbation of previously demonstrated impairment in renal function occurring within three days following

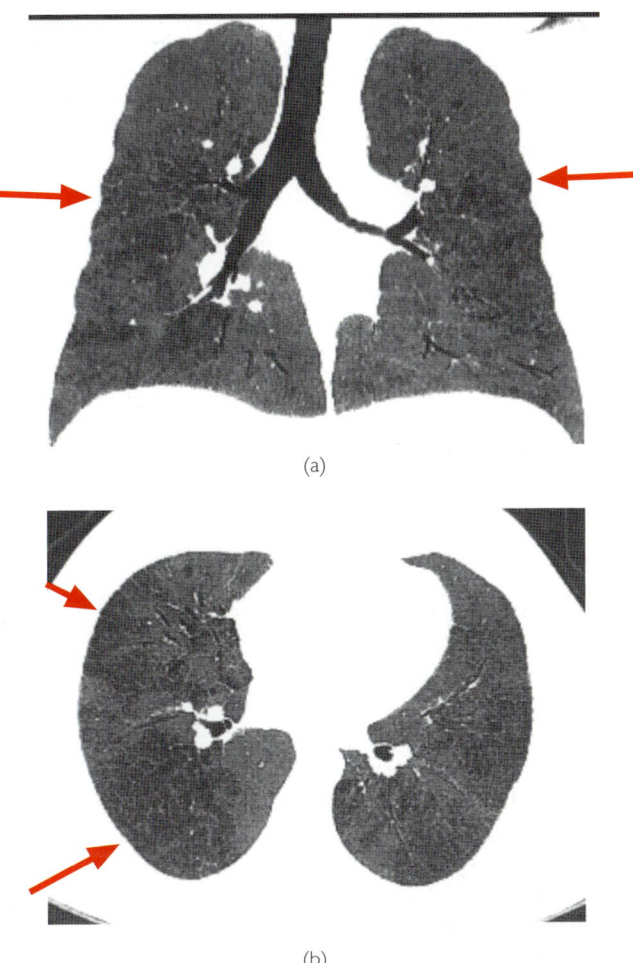

(a)

(b)

Fig 1.33: Minimum intensity projection: (a) coronal and (b) axial minimum intensity projections demonstrate ill-defined areas of decreased attenuation in the lung fields representing areas of emphysema.

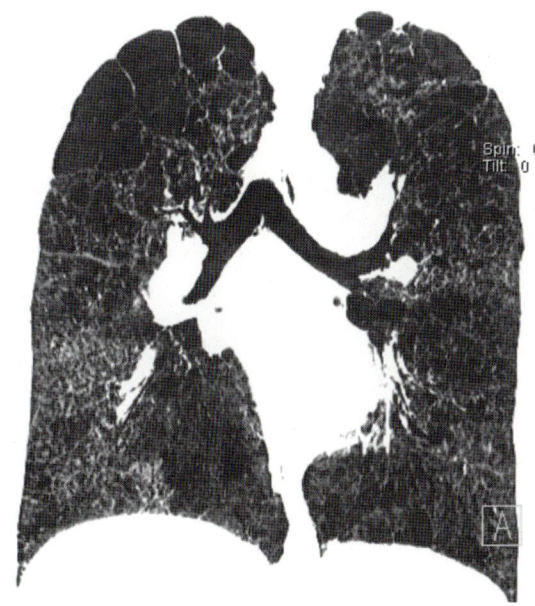

Fig 1.34: Minimum intensity projections: HRCT demonstrates extensive emphysema; narrow window settings demonstrate emphysematous changes very well. Minimum intensity projections demonstrate the involvement extremely well, providing a global view.

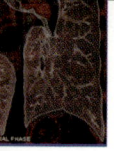

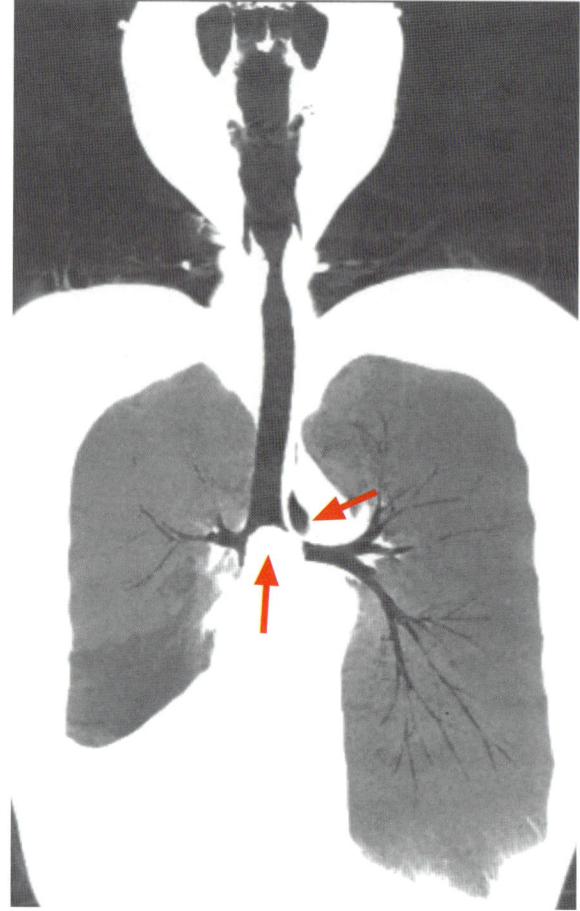

Fig 1.35: Minimum intensity projection of tracheobronchial tree. The entire tracheobronchial tree is demonstrated from the level of the pharynx. There is a mass lesion at the carina indenting the carina, extending to engulf the right lower lobe bronchus with resultant right lower lobe collapse; there is extension to the left to encase the left main bronchus narrowing and obliterating the left main bronchus. Note right lower lobe collapse with elevation of diaphragm.

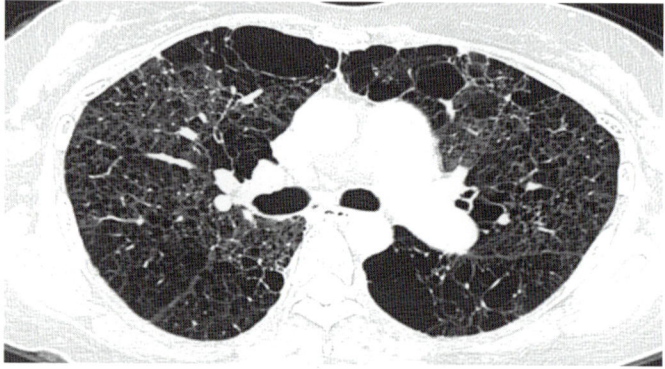

Fig 1.36: Ideal window settings displaying emphysema.

intravascular administration of contrast medium. This is in the absence of an alternative aetiology for the deteriorating renal function. An increase in serum creatinine of more than 0.5 mg/dl or 25% above the baseline serum creatinine is considered the criterion to determine the presence of contrast-induced nephropathy. CIN is by no means uncommon. It is the third

most common cause of acute renal failure in patients admitted to hospital. The incidence is estimated to be 1% with intravenous contrast medium, and 2–7% with intra-arterial contrast medium. In diabetics with normal renal function it rises to 16%. In patients with pre-existing renal insufficiency prior to receiving contrast media, the incidence of developing CIN is 33%. Diabetics with associated renal insufficiency are at the greatest risk for developing CIN. Other risk factors for developing CIN are dehydration, hypotension, nephrotic syndrome, multiple myeloma, use of higher dose of contrast media, repeated doses of contrast media within 48 h, use of higher osmolar contrast media and concurrent use of nephrotoxic drugs.

To minimize the risk of CIN, universal use of non-ionic contrast media, a volume expansion and the use of N-acetyl cystine are recommended. If the serum creatinine is > 1.4 mg/dl the possibility of another imaging modality should be considered. If a CT with contrast is considered imperative, the risk-benefit ratio should decide the issue.

SUPPORTIVE IMAGING TECHNIQUES

Sonography

This is a very useful imaging modality to demonstrate pleural fluid, especially at the bedside. Fluid manifests as an anechoic area separating the echogenic margin of lung and diaphragm. The contents of pleural fluid can also be estimated depending upon its echogenicity. Pleural fluid is usually anechoic; exudates are also anechoic but usually have internal septae. Empyemas have echoes within and a haemothorax has echogenic fluid. Sonography is very useful to determine whether a basal opacity on an X-ray is due to pleural fluid or collapse consolidation.

Sonography is also an excellent guide for paracentesis, reducing the incidence of post-aspiration pnuemothorax.

RADIONUCLIDE IMAGING

The main utility of radionuclide imaging in the respiratory system is in the detection of pulmonary embolism. Ventilation/

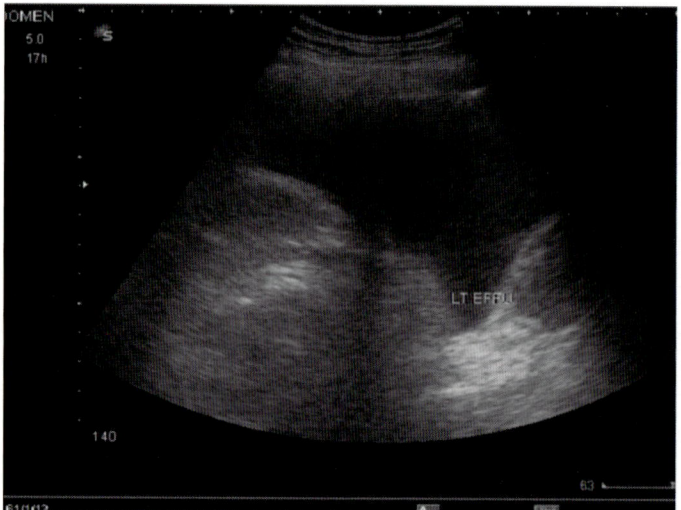

Fig 1.37: USG of the chest demonstrates a hypoechoic area representing a pleural effusion.

Perfusion scans also known as V/Q scans simultaneously image the pulmonary blood flow as well as alveolar ventilation.

Perfusion imaging is performed by intravenous injection of microparticles or human protein-labelled technetium (Tc – 99). These are trapped in the pulmonary capillaries on their first pass. In patients with a right to left shunt there is a small possibility of the particles occluding systemic vessels with resultant tissue ischemia/necrosis. Similarly, in patients with pulmonary hypertension there is a risk of further occlusion of an already depleted vascular bed. In both these situations the quantum of radiotracer particles injected should be reduced, though there is usually a wide safety margin. The radiotracer has a half-life of 6–8 hours; by 24 hours, most of the activity is only visible in the kidneys and gut. The radiotracer is injected with the patient in the supine position; this limits the effect of gravity on regional blood flow. The particles mix in the heart and consequently are trapped by pulmonary pre-capillary arterioles. The distribution of the particles is proportional to the regional blood flow. At least six views are obtained—anterior, posterior, right lateral, left lateral, right posterior oblique, left posterior oblique. Additionally, right anterior oblique and left anterior oblique views may be obtained, if required. Even though multiple projections are obtained, perfusion scans underestimate perfusion abnormalities. For example, the medial basal segment of the right lower lobe is completely surrounded by normal lung; consequently, a perfusion defect is not detected on planar perfusion imaging.

All parenchymal diseases cause a reduction in pulmonary blood flow in the affected lung zone. In pulmonary embolism, perfusion is reduced whereas ventilation is preserved. Parenchymal lung diseases cause both a ventilation and a perfusion defect. Tc-99m radio-labelled aerosols are used for ventilation scans. Approximately 30 mCi of radiotracer in 3 ml of saline is placed within a nebulizer. Oxygen is forced through the nebulizer at high pressure to form aerosolized droplets which are inhaled by the patient via a mouthpiece. The distribution of the radiotracer is proportional to regional ventilation. Images are obtained in multiple planes similar to perfusion imaging.

In pulmonary embolism there are perfusion defects which may be sub-segmental, segmental or even involve an entire lobe or lung. The ventilation scan in these patients is normal; thereby there are mismatched defects. In patients who have pulmonary embolism with infarcts there would also be a ventilation defect;

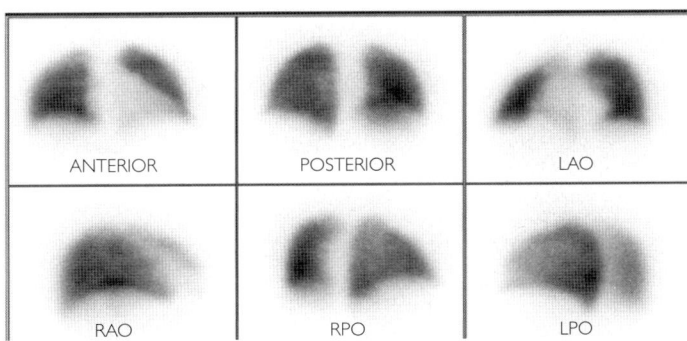

Fig 1.39: Perfusion scan: Perfusion scan demonstrates no evidence of perfusion defect. A normal perfusion scan virtually rules out the possibility of a pulmonary embolism.

however, the ventilation defect is smaller in size than the perfusion defect. Matched defects occur in chronic obstructive pulmonary disease (COPD) as there is a ventilation defect as well as reflex hypoperfusion.

CT angiography has virtually replaced ventilation-perfusion scans as the modality of choice in the detection of pulmonary embolism.

	V/Q scan	**CT angio**
Non-diagnostic	26.5%	6%
Sensitivity	77%	83%
Specificity	98%	96%
Definitive Diagnosis	74%	94%

Table 1.1: Differences between V/Q scan and CT angiography

Source: Acute pulmonary embolism: Sensitivity and specificity of ventilation-perfusion scintigraphy in PIOPED II study; Dirk Sostman: *Radiology* Volume 246 number 3 941–946, March 2008.

CT angiography has additional advantages. It is available at most institutions round the clock; many institutions may not have nuclear medicine facilities. Clinical mimics of pulmonary embolism such as aortic dissection and pneumonia can be detected by CT. Concurrent venous imaging to detect lower limb/pelvic venous thrombosis is possible with CT angiography, increasing the sensitivity of CT angiography, though at the cost of a higher radiation dose. The requirement to use contrast in CT angiography is a potential disadvantage, especially in individuals with renal impairment or in patients with a history of anaphylaxis to non-ionic contrast media. Another debatable issue is the quantum of radiation dose in these two modalities. CT angiography has a higher radiation dose ranging from 2.7 mSev to 10.2 mSev depending on the type of scanner and technique used, as compared to radiation dose in V/Q, ranging from 1.2 to 6.8 mSev. The newer dual-source CT scanners utilize a much lower radiation dose, 1.9 to 2.7 mSev, similar to the radiation dose of V/Q scan. In pregnancy the radiation dose to the foetus in V/Q scans is 0.1 to 0.8 milligrey as compared to CT angiography, 0.01 to 0.6 milligrey. CT

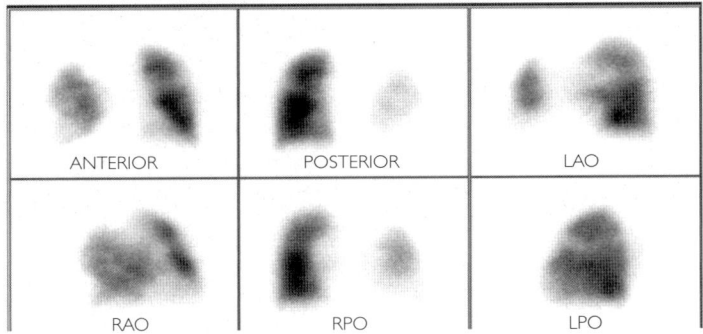

Fig 1.38: Perfusion scan: Perfusions scans demonstrate multiple perfusion defects bilaterally, ventilation scan revealed no abnormality, indicative of ventilation-perfusion mismatch due to pulmonary embolism.

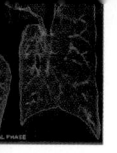

angiography is thus preferred over V/Q scan in pregnancy. The dose to maternal breasts is much higher using CT angiography than V/Q scan; however, this can easily be minimized by using bismuth breast shields. In view of these significant advantages with a positive benefit over risk ratio, CT angiography is the preferred modality.

MAGNETIC RESONANCE IMAGING

Magnetic resonance imaging (MRI) is making rapid strides in the evaluation of the abdominal pathologies. Its utility in imaging the brain, spine, musculoskeletal system and pelvis is well established. Evaluation for pulmonary pathologies is limited by

a number of factors–the lower proton density of lung, and by cardiac and respiratory motion. These limitations are magnified with increasing field strength; the recent shift to 3T by institutions has not helped. Outside the lung parenchyma, MRI can be a useful alternative to CT, especially when intravenous (IV) contrast is contraindicated such as in patients with renal failure or history of anaphylaxis to contrast media. MRI is useful in the evaluation of the chest wall and mediastinum, to detect mass lesions, as well as demonstrate their local extension. It is also useful to evaluate the pulmonary arteries, aorta and heart. IV contrast may be used if serum creatinine is not elevated. Advances are occurring rapidly using newer sequences as well as experimenting with gases for ventilation scans.

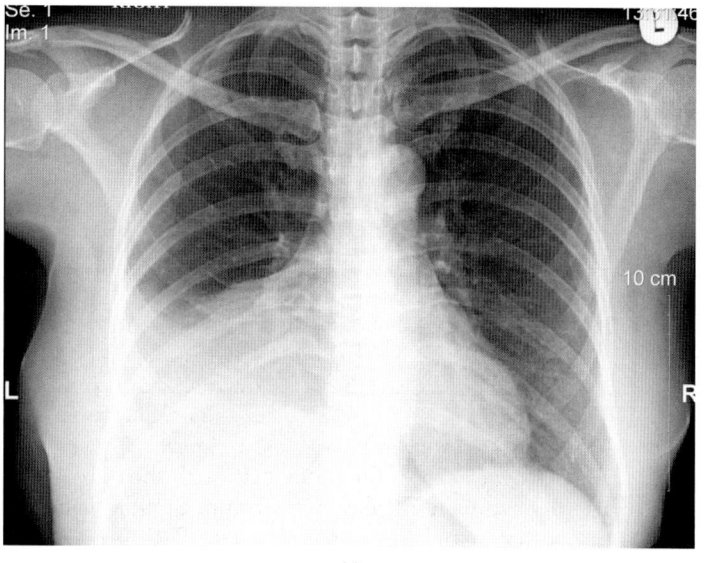

(a)

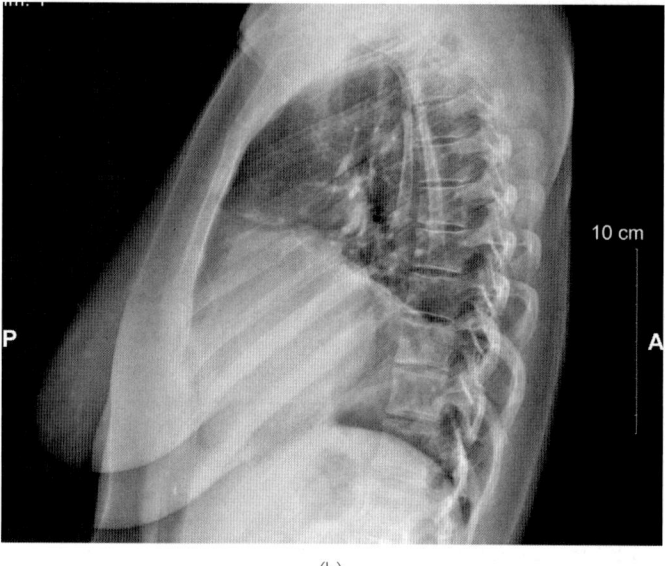

(b)

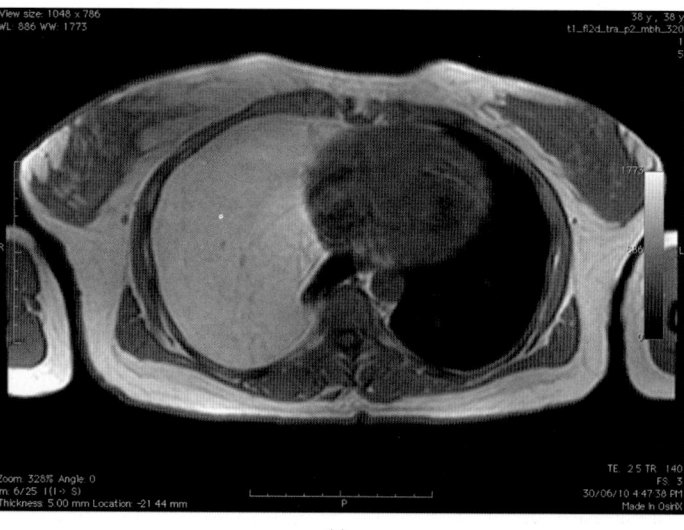

(c)

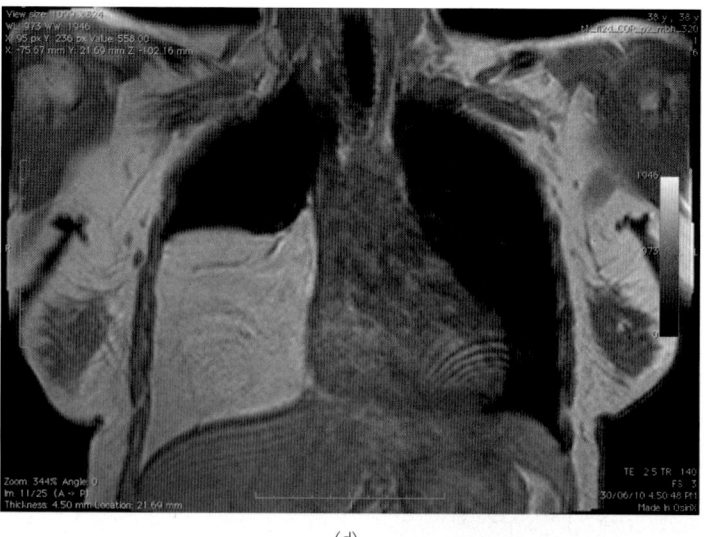

(d)

Fig 1.40: Lipoma: (a) Chest X-ray demonstrates a large homogenous mass in the right lower zone with no shift of the mediastinum (b)Lateral X-ray demonstrates opacity in an anterior location (c and d) MRI characterizes the lesion as a lipoma, as the mass is of fat density.

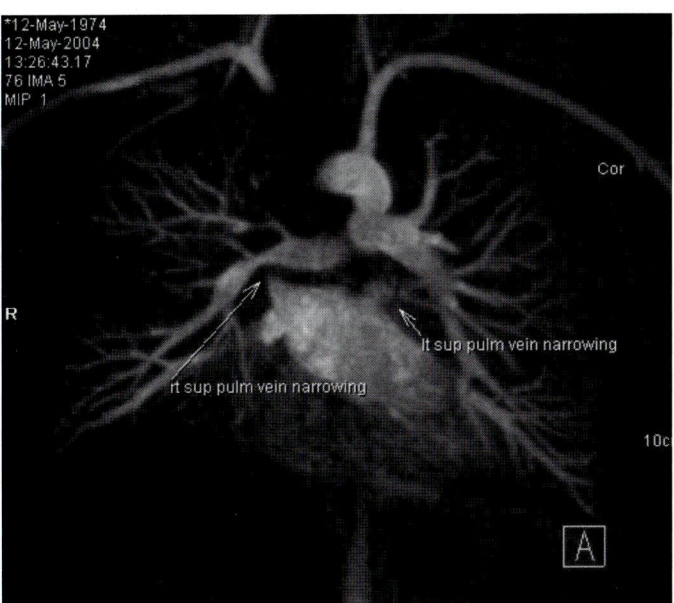

Fig 1.41: Mediastinal fibrosis: Contrast-enhanced MRI reveals bilateral superior pulmonary vein narrowing due to mediastinal fibrosis.

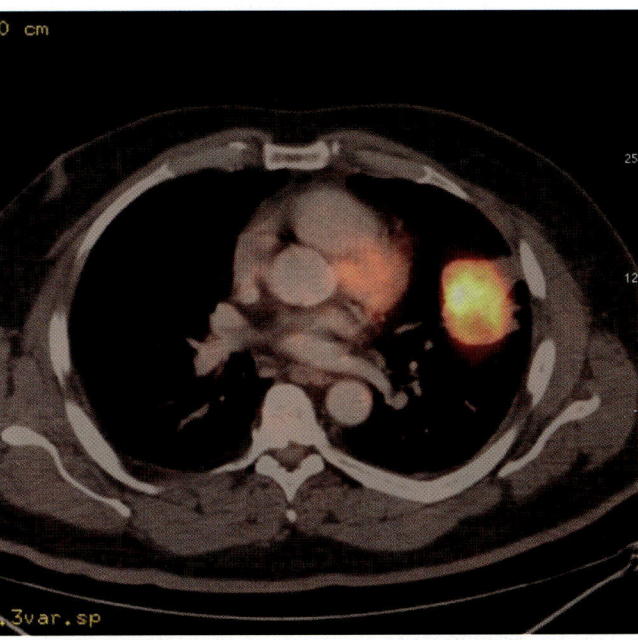

Fig 1.43: PET-CT demonstrates marked uptake in the left lung mass lesion representing a primary lung neoplasm.

POSITRON EMISSION TOMOGRAPHY— COMPUTED TOMOGRAPHY

Positron Emission Tomography–Computed Tomography (PET-CT) combines a PET scanner and a CT scanner in one gantry. Images acquired from both devices can be obtained sequentially in the same session and images superimposed in a single image.

PET imaging is based on the fact that metabolically active cells take up glucose. PET-CT fuses anatomical and functional data to provide an excellent correlation of anatomic and metabolic information. A radionuclide-labelled glucose analogue Fluorine 18–deoxyglucose (FDG) is taken up by malignant tumours, inflammation/infection and active tissue repair. Sixty minutes after IV FDG, a CT is acquired over approximately 30 seconds, followed by a slow transit of the patient through the bore of the PET. This data acquisition takes 30–40 min. Standard uptake values can be calculated from the PET data. This is useful as a value above 2.5 SUV is considered significant. The main utilities of PET-CT in respiratory medicine are in the staging of neoplastic processes, including lymphoma and mesothelioma. It is also useful in the detection of inflammatory processes which are not detected by other imaging modalities.

PULMONARY ANGIOGRAPHY

Pulmonary angiography is considered to be the gold standard in the evaluation of pulmonary thromboembolism. This is an invasive procedure with an incidence of 1.5% serious complications. Acute pulmonary emboli are demonstrated as intraluminal filling defects, peripheral occlusion of pulmonary vessels and/or wedge-shaped perfusion defects. To improve the detection of small pulmonary emboli, dedicated techniques are now available, such as cine angiography, balloon occlusion angiography and superselective angiography.

Many studies using spiral CT angiography have demonstrated a sensitivity and specificity for spiral CT angiogram to match that of pulmonary angiogram. The limitations of both spiral CT angiography and pulmonary angiography are also comparable. It is reported that 10% of spiral CT examinations will be inconclusive compared to 12% for pulmonary angiograms. Three per cent of spiral CT angiograms will be technically inadequate compared to 4% for pulmonary angiograms. In view of the less invasiveness and similar sensitivity and specificity of spiral CT

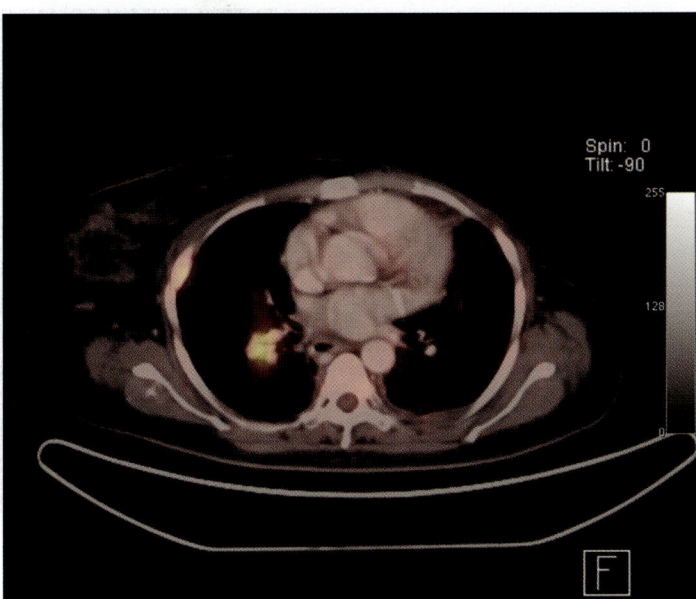

Fig 1.42: PET-CT: A patient with nasopharyngeal cancer for staging. PET-CT demonstrates uptake in the right hilum and right rib indicating metastatic deposits.

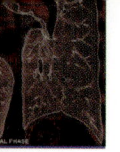

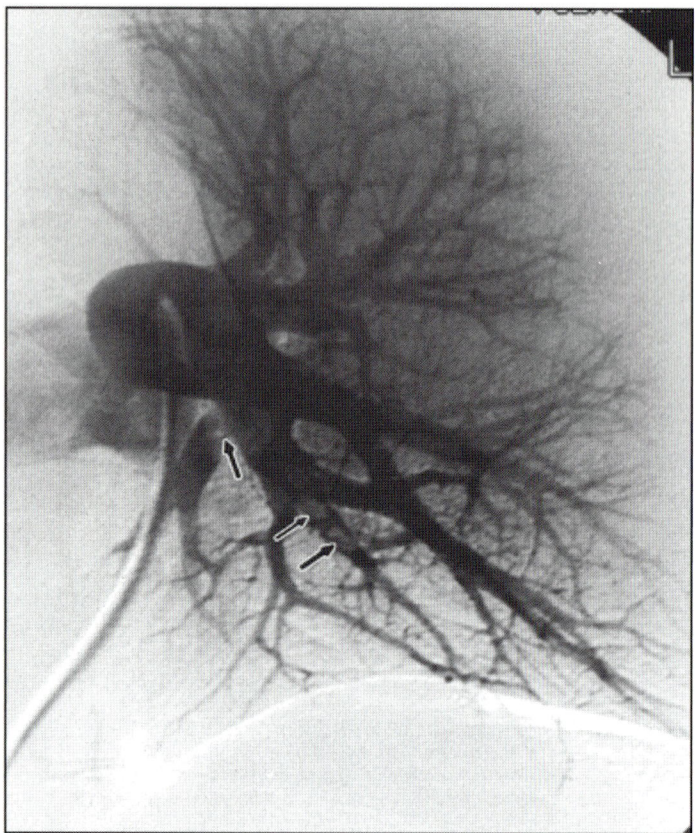

Fig 1.44: Pulmonary angiogram: Selective injection of left pulmonary angiogram demonstrates multiple filling defects in lower branch pulmonary arteries.

angiogram as compared to pulmonary angiograms, spiral CT angiograms have by and large replaced pulmonary angiograms in the detection of pulmonary emboli.

BRONCHIAL ARTERY EMBOLIZATION

Bronchial artery embolization is performed to stop massive haemoptysis. The bronchial arteries arise from the intercosto-bronchial trunk which arises from the aorta at T5. There is a single bronchial artery on the right side and two on the left side. As with most anatomical structures there are variations in the anatomy of the bronchial arteries. These vessels are selectively cannulated and if on angiography, there is extravasation of the dye from an artery or its branch, that vessel is selectively embolized using polyvinyl alcohol or gel foam. Serious complications following bronchial artery embolization are rare. Patients mainly complain of occasional haemoptysis, transient fever and chest pain.

APPEARANCES OF A NORMAL CHEST RADIOGRAPH

Lung Parenchyma

The lung markings seen on a chest X-ray represent vascular shadows. Occasionally, an accompanying bronchus may be visualized along with the vessels as an air-filled thin tube. Bronchi are best demonstrated end on with the accompanying vessel. In the erect

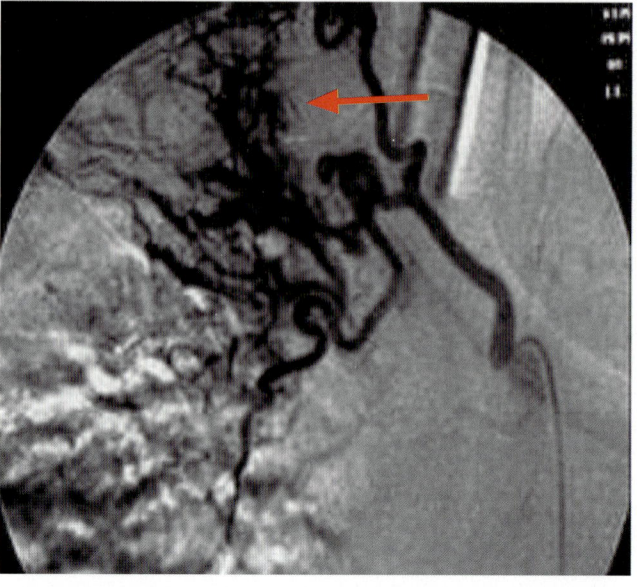

(a)

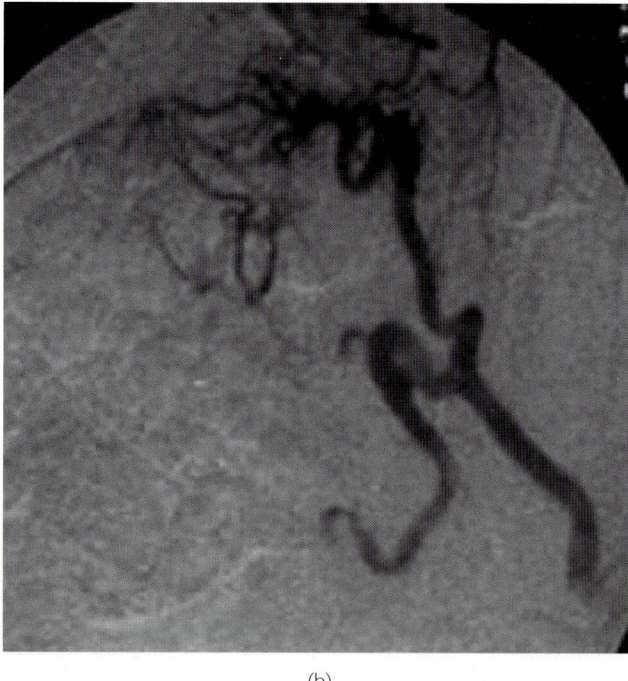

(b)

Fig 1.45: Bronchial artery angiogram: A patient with active tuberculosis presented with massive haemoptysis. Bronchial arteriogram (a) demonstrates large feeding vessels with extravasation of contrast, indicative of bleeding vessel (b) The large feeder vessel was occluded with coils to stop the bleeding.

position the vascular markings are more prominent in the lower zones as the diameters of vessels are larger in the lower zones. In the supine position there is an equalization of the diameters of the vessels in the apices and bases. The vascular markings are a combination of pulmonary arteries and veins. In the upper zones it is not possible to differentiate these as they course similarly in a curvilinear fashion; in the lower zones they may be separated as veins course horizontally and arteries more vertically.

Trachea

The trachea enters the thorax 1–3 cm above the level of the suprasternal notch, the intrathoracic portion is 6–9 cm in length. The trachea contains 16–20 incomplete or horseshoe-shaped cartilage rings giving the trachea a corrugated outline—calcification of the cartilage rings occurs after the age of 40 years. The trachea deviates mildly to the right to accommodate the left-sided aortic arch. With unfolding and ectasia of the aorta the trachea deviates more to the right.

The trachea divides into the two mainstem bronchi at the carina, approximately at the level of the T5. The left main bronchus extends up to twice as far as the right main bronchus before giving off its upper lobe division. The right main bronchus is approximately 25-mm long; the left main bronchus is approximately 50-mm long. In children the angles between the bronchi are symmetric, but in adults the right mainstem bronchus has a steeper angle than the left. The segmental bronchi are not well demonstrated on the X-ray unless seen end on; they are well-demonstrated on CT.

Hilum

The hilar opacity is mainly due to pulmonary arteries and to a lesser extent due to the pulmonary veins. There is a small contribution by adenopathy, fat and bronchial walls. The left hilum is higher in position than the right hilum; this is because the left pulmonary artery arches over the left bronchus and descends posterior to the left bronchus while the right pulmonary artery extends directly inferiorly, anterior to the right bronchus. In 5% of individuals they may be at the same level. If the left hilum is found to be lower than the right hilum, it is useful to evaluate for left lower lobe collapse or a right upper lobe collapse. There is usually a wide variation in size of the hilum in normal individuals. If there is prominence of a hilar shadow, the possibility that this is due to a technical factor such as rotation or scoliosis should be first excluded. The margins of the hilum are usually smooth; if there is a lobulated contour a mass should be suspected.

The pulmonary arteries descend vertically downwards; the size of the descending vessels is relatively equal to a little finger. If the descending pulmonary artery is not visualized on the right side always check for right lower lobe collapse. A mass lesion at the hilum in contact with the hilar vessels will result in a loss of the hilar silhouette. If the hilum is well-visualized through a mass lesion then the mass has not silhouetted the hilum, indicating that the mass is anterior or posterior to the hilum.

Diaphragm

The right dome is normally at the level of the sixth rib anteriorly. The left dome is usually about 1.5–2.5 cm below the right dome. There may be variations in the position of the diaphragm; they may be one interspace higher or lower, they may be at the same level or occasionally, the left is higher than the right but not more than 1 cm. During a respiratory cycle the diaphragm may move between 2.5 and 8.0 cm.

Nipples

These may be visualized as bilaterally symmetric dense well-defined spherical shadows with a sharp and a non-sharp margin. If they are asymmetric they may be mistaken for a pulmonary nodule. To clarify whether a shadow is a nipple or a pulmonary nodule, a marker may be placed on the nipple, or in a female the breasts are manually elevated. If a nipple casts a shadow, the

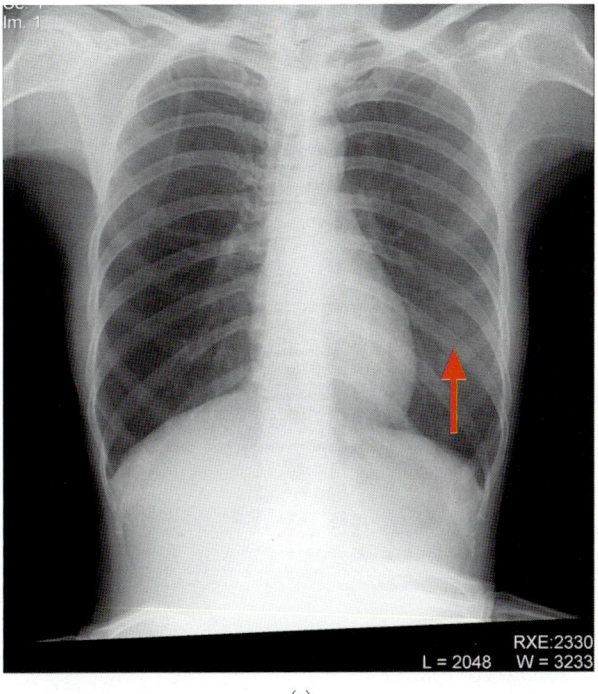

(a)

Fig 1.46: Nipple shadow: PA view of the chest demonstrates a well-defined nodular lesion in the left lower zone, this may represent a nipple shadow or a nodular lesion.

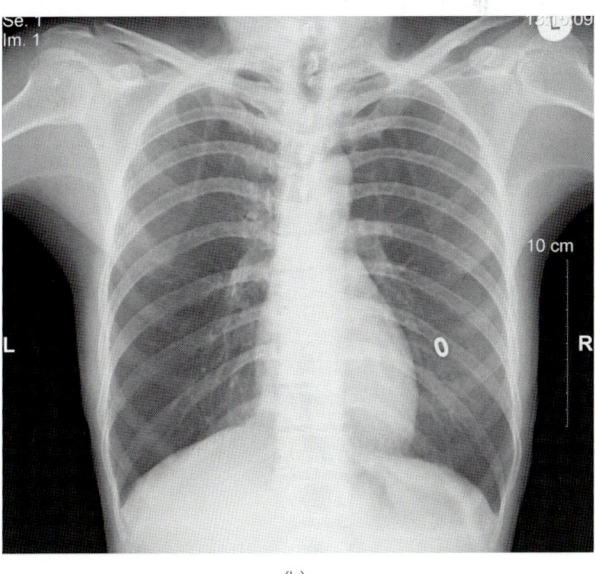

(b)

Fig 1.47: Nipple shadow: PA view of the chest shows a nipple marker placed at the nipple. The nipple marker coincided with the nodular lesion indicating that the shadow was a nipple.

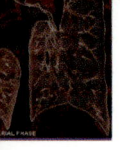

marker will be on the opacity; if the breasts have been elevated, the nipple will move up, the pulmonary nodule will remain in the same location.

Fissures

Major fissures are present bilaterally and separate the upper from the lower lobes. The fissures run obliquely forward and downward crossing the hilum. They arise from the fifth thoracic vertebrae and end at the diaphragm approximately 3 cm behind the sternum. On a lateral radiograph, often parts or the whole of a fissure may be visualized. On a frontal radiograph the major fissures are rarely visualized.

A minor fissure is present on the right side dividing the upper and middle lobes. The fissure extends from the hilum anteriorly and laterally. On a frontal radiograph it is seen in nearly 50% of individuals, contacting the lateral chest wall at or near the axillary portion of the sixth rib. It is also seen on the lateral chest radiograph in approximately 50% of individuals extending anteriorly from the hilum.

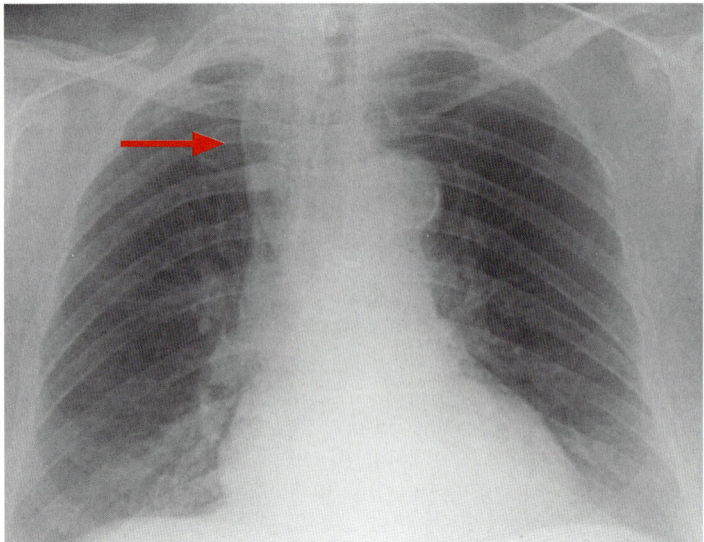

Fig 1.49: Azygous lobe: PA view demonstrates an azygous fissure in the right upper zone.

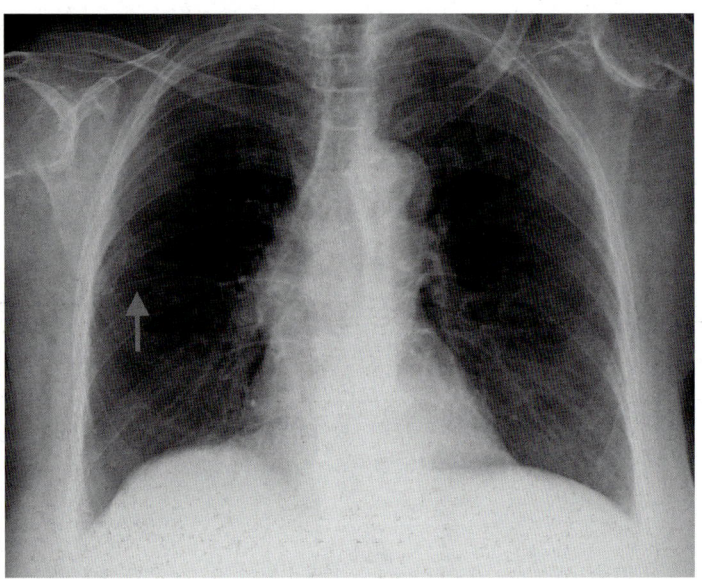

Fig 1.48: Minor fissure: PA view of the chest demonstrates the minor fissure on the right side.

Azygous Lobe Fissure

This fissure develops due to failure of the azygous vein to migrate from the chest wall through the lung into its location at the tracheobronchial angle. The invaginated visceral and parietal pleura persist to form a fissure, at the bottom of which lies the azygous vein. This may be occasionally seen on the left side with the left superior intercostal vein occupying the bottom of the fissure.

Mediastinum

The left mediastinal border above the level of the aortic arch is constituted by the left subclavian and carotid arteries. The left wall of the trachea is not visualized as it is in contact with the vessels. From the level of the aortic arch inferiorly the border is constituted by the aorta, main pulmonary artery, and heart. A small nodular well-defined opacity may be seen just below the aortic knuckle; this represents the left superior intercostal vein as it arches around the aorta before entering the left brachiocephalic vein. This should not be misinterpreted for a lymph node. The left border of the descending aorta is visualized through the main pulmonary artery and heart down to the aortic hiatus in the diaphragm.

The right mediastinal border is formed by the right brachiocephalic vein, SVC and right atrium. The right paratracheal stripe consisting of the tracheal wall and adjacent fat is seen through the brachiocephalic vein and SVC as the lung is in contact with the posterior wall of the trachea. The presence of this stripe excludes the possibility of a paratracheal mass lesion. This stripe is visible in two-thirds of individuals. At the lower end of this stripe is the azygous vein in the tracheobronchial angle.

Lateral View

On the lateral view there are three zones to observe. The vertebrae, each thoracic vertebra appears more translucent than the one above. The cardiac shadow is visualized as a homogenous opacity. The retrosternal space is well-aerated, any alteration in this pattern indicates an abnormality.

The two domes of the diaphragm overlap each other. It is fairly easy to separate the two. The right is visualized all the way from front to back. The left is only seen from the costophrenic recess posteriorly to the point where it meets the cardiac silhouette. Anterior to this point, it is not visualized as the lung/diaphragm interface is obliterated by the cardiac silhouette. Occasionally, it may be difficult to separate the two domes as they totally overlap. If the diaphragm silhouette is lost, an abnormality in the lower lobes should be suspected.

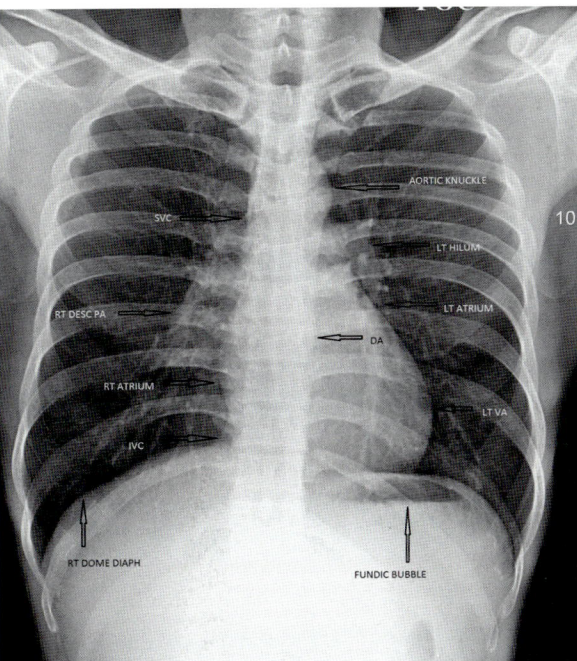

(a)

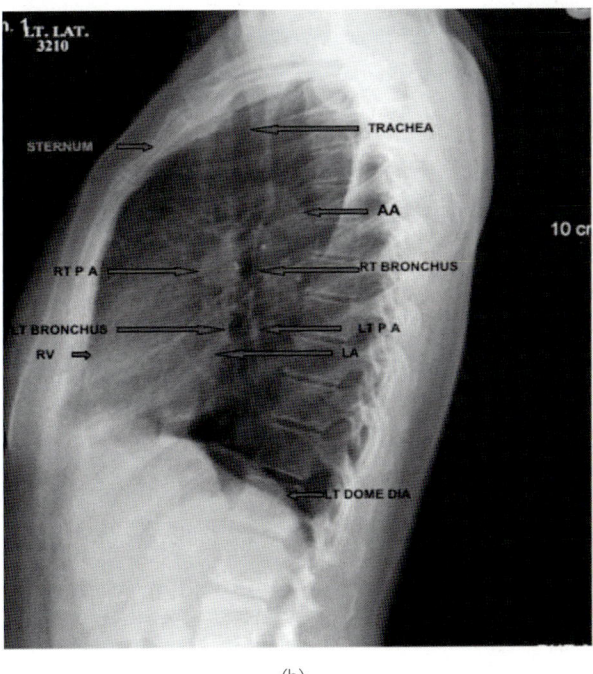

(b)

Fig 1.50: (a) PA and (b) lateral views of chest demonstrating anatomy.

It is difficult to differentiate the right from the left hilum as they totally overlap each other. The right pulmonary artery traverses anterior to the right bronchus and the left pulmonary artery hooks over and is posterior to the left bronchus. The bronchi are seen end on, the higher ring is the right and the lower the left bronchus. If the hilum is considerably prominent, large in size and lobulated in contour, a hilar mass should be suspected.

The mediastinal opacity is occupied by the heart. The portion behind the hila is the left atrium; the posterior border below the hilum is constituted by the left ventricle, the anterior surface

of the shadow constitutes the right ventricle. If the cardiac silhouette does not appear to be homogenous, the possibility of a superimposed pulmonary pathology may be considered.

The aortic arch is well-visualized with the brachiocephalic artery often being visualized arising and extending anterior to the trachea. The left and right brachiocephalic veins are often visualized as an extra-pleural bulge beneath the manubrium sternum and should not be mistaken for a sternal/chest wall mass. Similarly, in the inferior part of the chest, the anterior paracardiac fat may simulate a mass lesion posterior to the chest wall. This is because the two lungs do not meet in the midline, the heart and paracardiac fat being interposed.

The horizontal fissure is seen on most lateral chest X-rays. Oblique fissures appear like the blades of a propeller. The right oblique fissure at its most posterior position lies 4–5 cm behind the sternum, the left oblique is positioned slightly more superior.

The IVC may be visible as a well-defined vertical line which meets the posterior and inferior aspect of the heart.

Interpreting Chest Radiographs

A systematic approach to the interpretation of a chest radiograph is very important. This is particularly so when an obvious abnormality is present. The PA view of the chest is printed as if the patient is facing the interpreter, with the right side facing the interpreter's left side. It is important first to evaluate the radiograph from a technical quality perspective. Important factors to evaluate are:

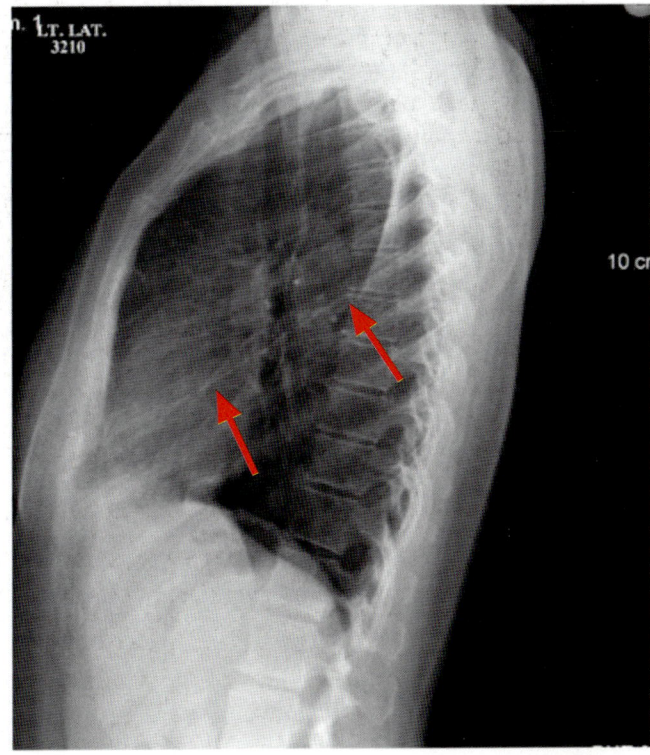

Fig 1.51: Lateral view of chest demonstrates the normal oblique fissures extending from the fifth dorsal vertebra posteriorly to the cardiophrenic angle crossing the hilum.

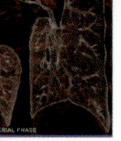

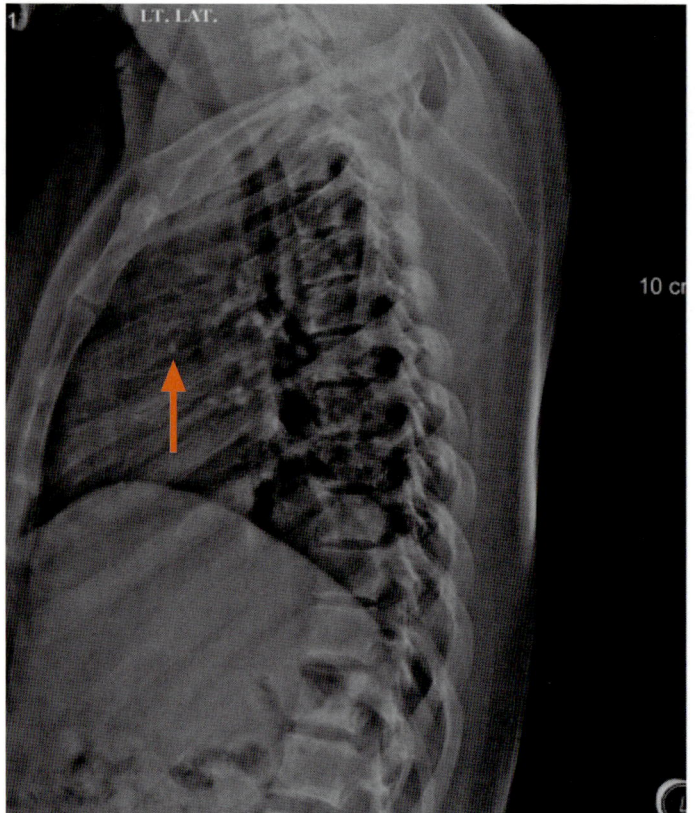

Fig 1.52: Minor fissure: Lateral view of chest reveals minor fissure as a horizontal line extending from the hilum anteriorly.

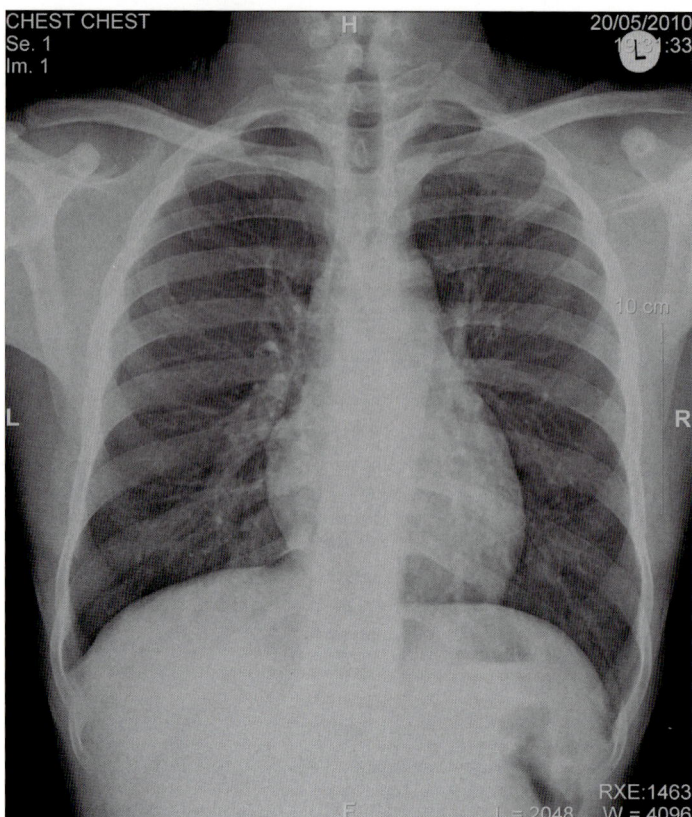

Fig 1.53: Normal chest X-ray: A perfectly exposed X-ray as the dorsal interspaces are just visualized. There is no rotation as the clavicles are equidistant from the cervical spinous processes; the inspiratory effort is adequate, as the anterior ends of the sixth ribs are at the mid-diaphragmatic level.

Exposure   In a well-exposed radiograph the dorsal intervertebral discs should just be visible through the cardiac shadow. In an overexposed X-ray the vertebral bodies are well-outlined, the lung fields are darkened. The risk of overexposure is that parenchymal lung lesions may not be visible, though the retro-cardiac regions are well-visualized. In an underexposed X-ray the mediastinum appears brighter than usual; also, there is no visualization of the dorsal intervertebral discs.

Inspiratory Effort   Chest X-rays are obtained in deep inspiration; the midpoint of the right hemidiaphragm should be at the anterior end of the sixth rib.

Rotation   The medial ends of the clavicle should be equidistant from the spinous processes of the cervical vertebrae.

Evaluation of Different Structures on a Chest X-ray

Start with the trachea, note its position, mass effect, deviation and calibre. Then evaluate the mediastinal silhouette, the right border, then the left border from above downwards. Note any loss of silhouette, cardiomegaly. Next evaluate the hilum, again one at a time, position of hilum, right in relation to left, equality in size and density. If a hilum appears larger or denser, a lateral view is very useful to confirm or exclude a mass lesion. For example, if the right hilum is prominent, presence

of a mass will be seen on the lateral view as being posterior to the trachea, since the right pulmonary artery is anterior to the trachea. For the left, it is converse as the left pulmonary artery is posterior to the trachea. The lower lobe pulmonary vessels are well-visualized on a radiograph. Absence of this leash of vessels on a well-centred X-ray is a useful clue to lobar collapse. Evaluate the diaphragms for position, contour any loss of silhouette. Now evaluate the lungs. A useful method is to examine them in a zigzag fashion from below upwards. Evaluate each zone from a size, transradiancy perspective. The position of the horizontal fissure if visible should be noted, as this may also be a clue towards lobar collapse. Finally, evaluate the ribs and chest wall. Before concluding, pitfall areas where abnormalities may lurk should be evaluated. These include the central mediastinum, lungs behind the diaphragm and heart, lung apices, lung and pleura along the inner surface of the chest wall.

CT Anatomy of Normal Mediastinum and the Lung

The normal mediastinal structures, heart, blood vessels, tracheobronchial tree, oesophagus are always identified on cross-sectional imaging.

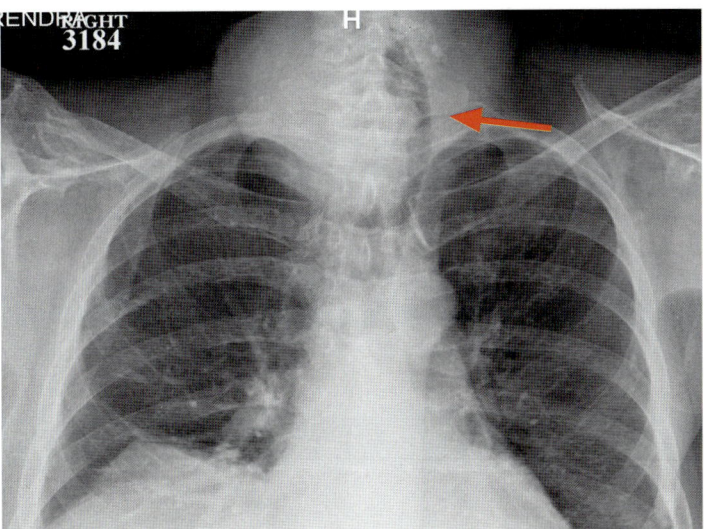

Fig 1.54: Tracheal deviation: PA View of the chest demonstrates tracheal deviation as a result of a mass lesion in the neck arising from the thyroid causing significant displacement and compression to the left.

MEDIASTINAL VASCULATURE

The vertical portions of the ascending and descending aorta are well-visualized as spherical tubes, the diameter of the ascending aorta is 3.5 cm and of the descending aorta 2.5 cm. The descending aorta descends to the left of the vertebrae and then takes a more midline course to enter the abdomen anterior to the vertebrae. The arch of the aorta is seen in cross-section traversing from the ascending aorta to the descending aorta right to left, anterior to the trachea. Above the level of the aortic arch the great vessels are well-visualized in an arc anterior and to the left of the trachea. The left common carotid artery lies to the left of the trachea, left subclavian artery to the left or posterior to the trachea. The brachiocephalic artery is larger than the left common carotid and left subclavian artery. In 0.5% of the population the right subclavian artery has an anomalous origin arising distal to the left subclavian artery. It courses from left to right, posterior to the oesophagus at the level of the aortic arch; it then ascends in the right paravertebral space to the root of the neck. The brachiocephalic in this situation becomes the right common carotid artery, with a size similar to that of the left common carotid artery. A barium swallow will demonstrate the posterior indentation of the oesophagus caused by the anomalous right subclavian artery. Pressure on the oesophagus by this artery may cause dysphagia.

The right subclavian and jugular vein unite to form the right brachiocephalic vein, which descends vertically in the mediastinum to continue as the superior vena cava (SVC) following its union with the left brachiocephalic vein. The SVC is usually half to two-thirds the diameter of the ascending aorta. The left brachiocephalic vein courses through the mediastinum from the left to the right, anterior to the great vessels. In 0.3–0.5% of the population a left SVC is present. This is more commonly seen in individuals with congenital heart disease. The left SVC is formed by the union of the left jugular and subclavian veins, and descends vertically in the left mediastinum to open into the coronary sinus. Due to the increased blood flow, the coronary sinus is increased in size in this situation.

The azygous vein ascends from the diaphragm in the prevertebral space to the right or posterior to the oesophagus; it arches over the right main bronchus to open into the posterior wall of the SVC. In 1% of individuals the azygous penetrates the lung as it arches over the bronchus resulting in an azygous lobe. Occasionally, the IVC does not develop, the azygous becomes the conduit to drain blood back to the heart, and is then termed as the azygous continuation of the IVC. The hepatic veins then open directly into the right atrium and the azygous vein dilates. Variants in vascular anatomy such as left-sided SVC, azygous continuation of IVC, left superior intercostal vein, may be mistaken for a mass lesion or adenopathy on an unenhanced scan or chest X-ray. The hemiazygous and accessory hemiazygous veins ascend posterior to the descending aorta. The accessory hemiazygous may cross to the right to open into the azygous or open into the left superior intercostal vein. The left superior intercostal vein is a small vein, which arches around the aorta at the level of the arch and descending aorta to open into the left brachiocephalic vein. It is only occasionally identified on X-ray/CT.

Pulmonary Artery

The main pulmonary artery runs backward and upward obliquely to the left of the ascending aorta. The right branch travels horizontally to the right between the ascending aorta and tracheobronchial tree; it then descends anterior to the right bronchus. The left branch curves upwards and posteriorly over the left main bronchus and descends posterior to the left main bronchus. The main pulmonary artery diameter is approximately 2.8 cm. A main pulmonary artery/aortic ratio greater than 1 indicates pulmonary hypertension. The pulmonary artery branches are two-thirds the diameter of the main pulmonary artery.

Thymus

The thymus is best visualized in a section at the level of the aortic arch, anterior to the aorta and pulmonary artery, inferior to the left brachiocephalic vein, and superior to the right pulmonary artery. Till puberty the thymus occupies most of the anterior mediastinum with a density of soft tissue. After puberty the gland starts to get replaced by fatty tissue; by 40 the gland is not visualized as it is replaced by fatty tissue. In individuals on chemotherapy the thymus may be visualized in adults, termed as thymic rebound.

Mediastinal lymph nodes

Ninety-five per cent of normal mediastinal lymph nodes measure less than 10 mm in short axis diameter. Mediastinal lymph nodes are chiefly located in the paratracheal, prevascular, pretracheal, subcarinal and aortopulmonary regions.

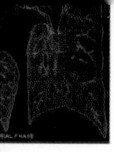

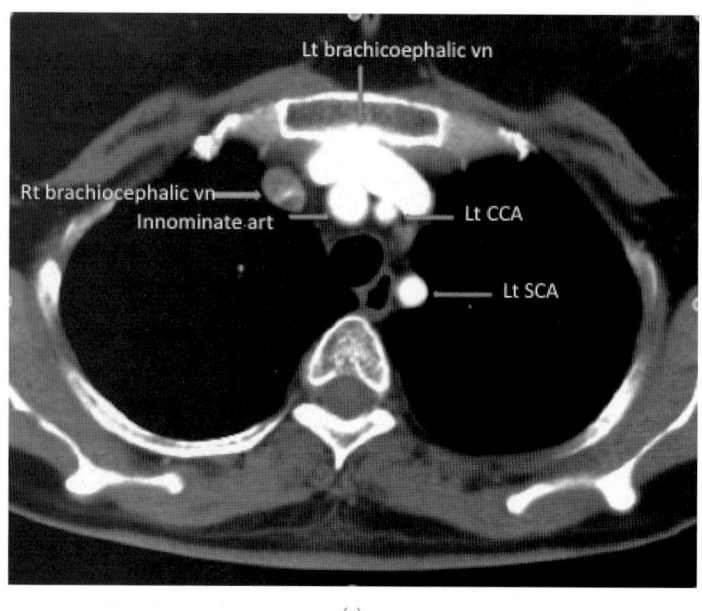

(a)

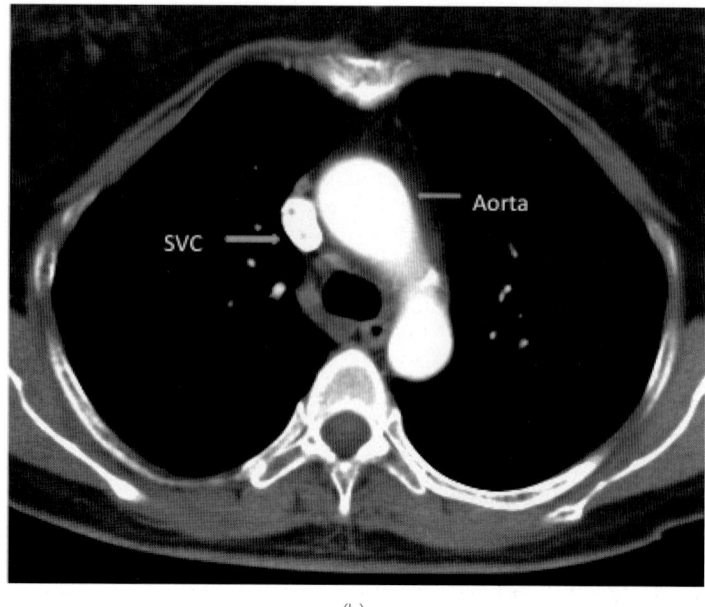

(b)

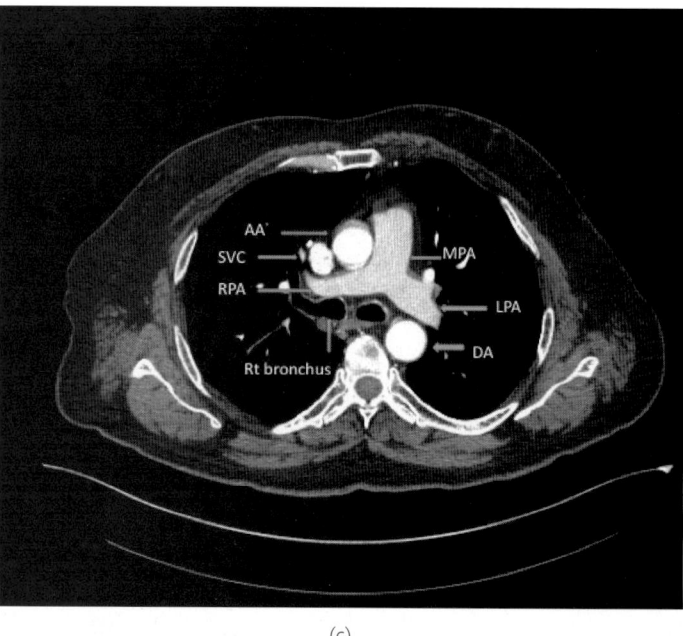

(c)

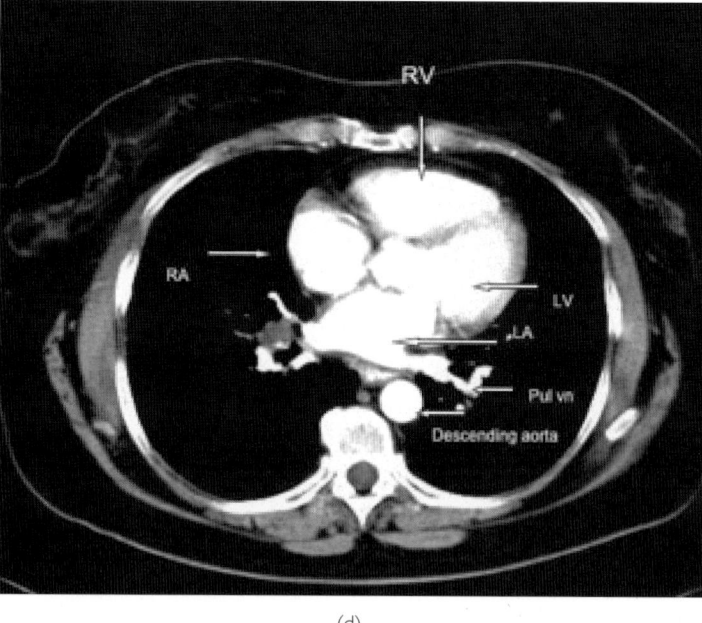

(d)

Fig 1.55: (a–d) CT anatomy of normal mediastinal structures.
RV—right ventricle; RA—right atrium; LV—left ventricle; LA—left atrium; SVC—superior vena cava.

Trachea

In cross-section, the trachea is round or oval with a flattened posterior margin formed by the fibromuscular membrane. On expiration there is a significant change in the diameter of the trachea. This is due to forward motion of the posterior wall of the trachea; there is consequent reduction in the AP diameter of the trachea.

The trachea divides into the two mainstem bronchi at the carina, approximately at the level of T5. The left main bronchus extends up to twice as far as the right main bronchus before giving off its upper lobe division. The right main bronchus

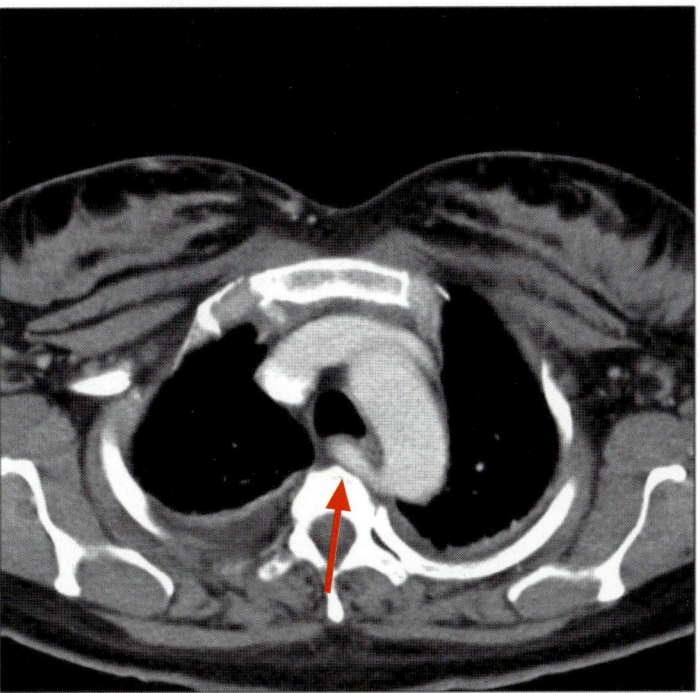

(a)

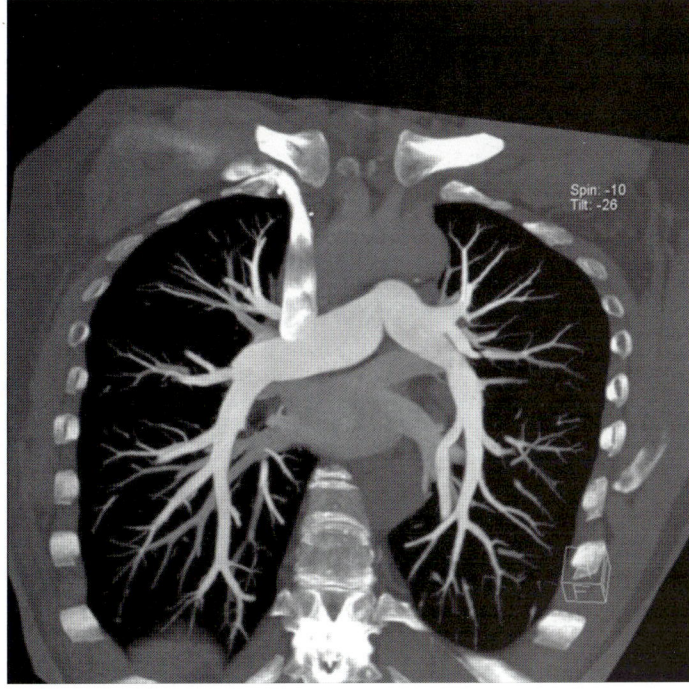

Fig 1.57: CT pulmonary angiogram demonstrates a normal pulmonary angiography.

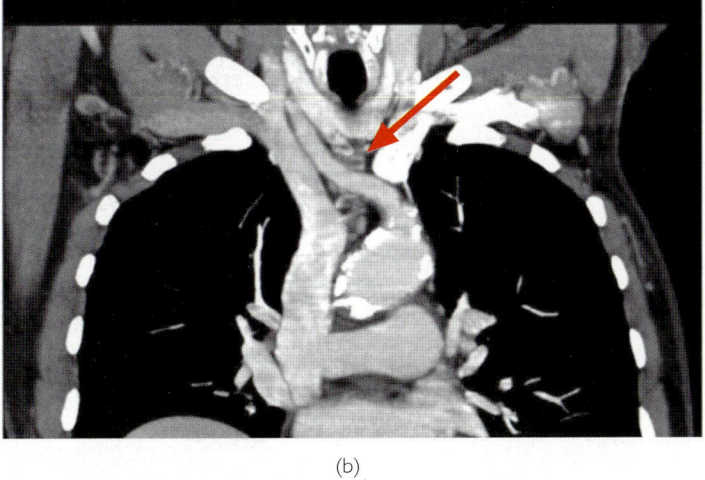

(b)

Fig 1.56: Aberrant right subclavian artery: (a) Axial and (b) Coronal CT chest with contrast; right subclavian artery arises distal to the left subclavian and courses from left to right, posterior to the trachea and oesophagus.

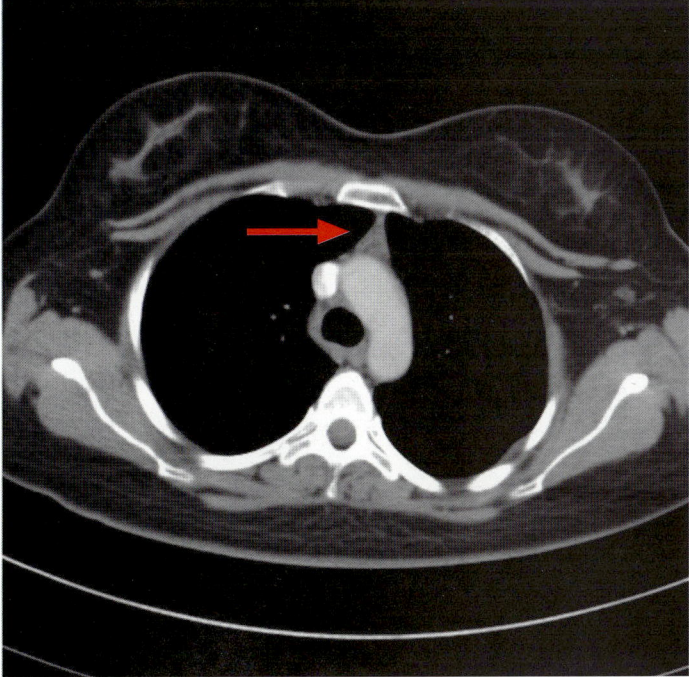

Fig 1.58: Thymus: CT scan chest demonstrates a normal thymus. Seen as a triangular well-defined soft-tissue density with internal fat densities.

is approximately 25 mm long, the left main bronchus is approximately 50 mm long. In children the angles between the bronchi are symmetric, but in adults the right mainstem bronchus has a steeper angle than the left. The segmental bronchi are well-demonstrated on CT.

The right upper lobe bronchus divides into the right apical, posterior and anterior segmental upper lobe bronchi.

The right lower lobe bronchus divides into right lower lobe superior segment bronchus, (middle lobe medial and lateral) segmental bronchi and anterior, lateral, posterior and medial lower lobe segmental bronchi.

On the left side the upper lobe bronchus divides into apico-posterior and anterior upper lobe segmental bronchi as well as the lingular superior and inferior segmental bronchi. The left lower lobe bronchus divides into superior segmental and anterior medial basal, posterior and lateral basal segmental bronchi.

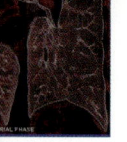

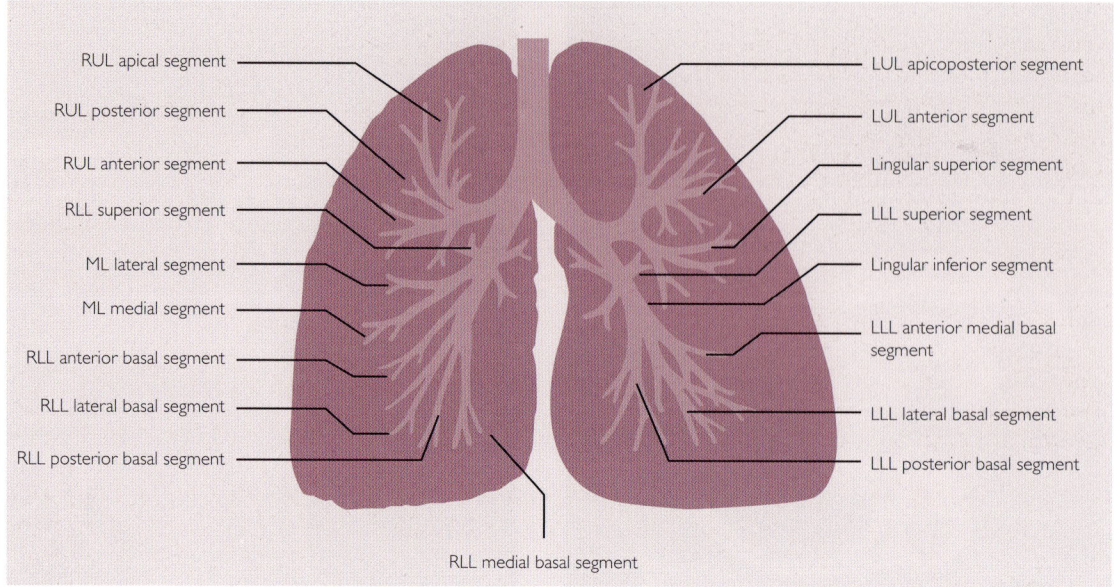

Fig 1.59: Anatomy of tracheobroncial tree: AP view of branches of airways beyond the segmental bronchi.

VARIATIONS

1. Common origin of right upper/middle bronchus
2. Tracheal bronchus—either a segmental or the entire right upper lobe bronchus arises from the trachea; there may be a displaced or supernumerary bronchus
3. Accessory cardiac bronchus arising from the medial aspect of the right main bronchus, usually blind-ended but may supply a small lobule
4. Lateral inversion of right and left-sided airways in *Situs Invertus*
5. *Situs Ambigus*—airway has either bilateral right-sided or left-sided configuration
6. Bridging bronchus—right lower lobe bronchus arises from the left main bronchus, crosses the mediastinum to reach the right lung.

The segmental bronchi divide progressively into smaller airways till after 6–20 divisions become bronchioles which further divide till terminal bronchioles. These are the last of the conducting airways. Beyond the terminal bronchioles lie the gas exchange units, the acini. The anatomy of the secondary lobule is discussed under the HRCT section of this chapter.

Diaphragm

The diaphragm consists of a large dome-shaped central tendon with radiating striated muscle attached to the xiphisternum

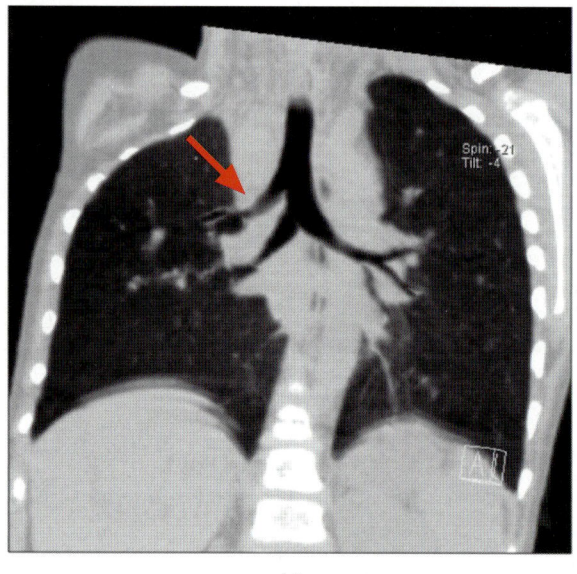

(a)

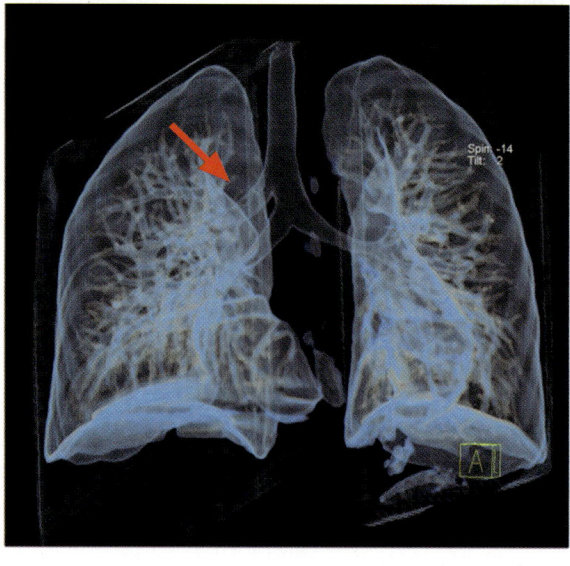

(b)

Fig 1.60: Tracheal Bronchus: (a) Minimum intensity projection and (b) Volume-rendered images of the tracheobronchial tree demonstrate a tracheal bronchus. The right upper lobe bronchus is seen to arise directly from the trachea.

and to the 7th to12th ribs. The two crura arise from the first three lumbar vertebrae forming the lateral walls of the aortic hiatus. The aorta, azygous, hemiazygous veins and thoracic duct pass through this hiatus. There are two more hiatuses anterior to the aortic hiatus in the diaphragm--the oesophageal hiatus through which pass the oesophagus, oesophageal arteries and vagus nerve, and the hiatus for the IVC.

Fissures

The major fissures are well visualized as thin white lines traversing from posterior to anterior and from cephalad to caudal. The minor fissure lies in the plane of the scanning, therefore the fissure per se is not visualized. Its position can be inferred as there is an avascular zone in the subpleural regions.

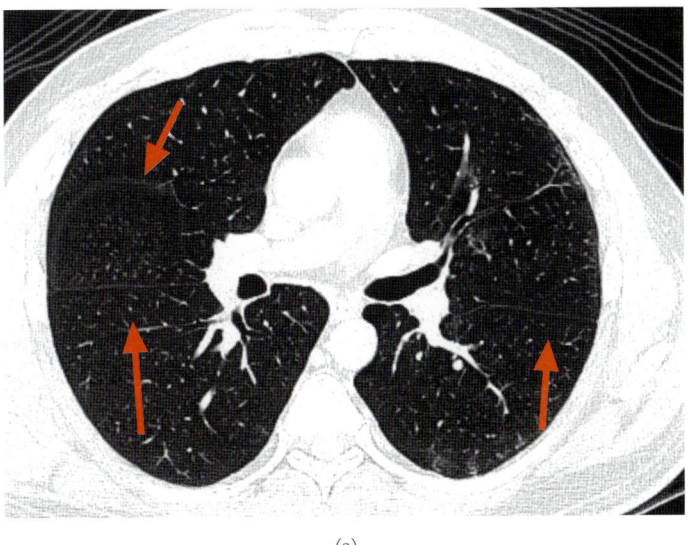

(a)

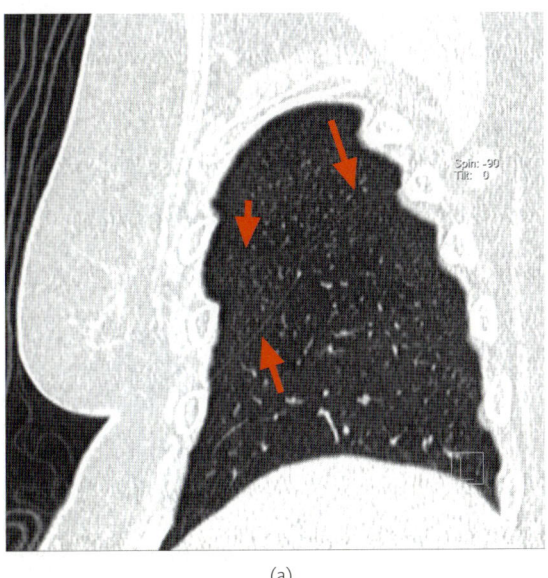

(a)

Fig 1.61: Fissures: (a) Axial and (b) sagittal reconstructions demonstrate major interlobar fissures. The minor fissure is not seen on the axial scan as it is in the same plane as the slices. The position of this fissure is inferred on the axial images as a zone of avascularity.

An avascular zone in the right middle lobe points to the site of the minor fissure.

Interstitium—Normal HRCT Anatomy

The lung is supported by a network of connective tissue fibres known as the interstitium of the lung. The interstitium is divided into three components, the axial interstitium, the peripheral interstitium and the intralobular interstitium which communicates between the axial and peripheral interstitium. The peripheral interstitium is located beneath the visceral pleura; it envelops the lung like a fibrous sac from which connective tissue septae penetrate into the lung parenchyma. Between each interlobular septa lies a secondary lobule. The axial interstium consists of the peribronchovascular interstitium which is strong connective tissue encasing the central bronchi and arteries. This interstitium extends from the level of the pulmonary hila to the periphery of the lung, encasing the centrilobular arteries and bronchioles in the secondary lobules. The secondary lobule is the smallest unit of lung structure varying in size from 1–2.5 cm containing 10–12 acini. It is polygonal in shape, with its apex pointing to the hilum and base towards the pleural surface. Each is supplied by a small bronchiole and pulmonary arterial branch—centrilobular artery. This is visualized on HRCT sections as a small dot; however, the bronchus is not visualized as it is below the resolution of present-day HRCT scans. The interlobular septae which marginate the secondary lobules contain pulmonary veins and lymphatics. At the level of the secondary lobule all three connective tissue systems are present.

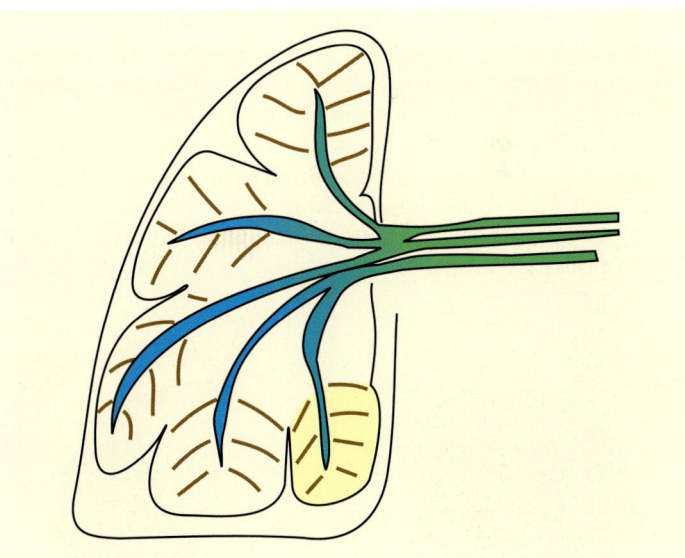

Fig 1.62: Normal anatomy of interstitium: Schematic diagram demonstrates peribronchovascular interstitium in green extending to the secondary lobules. In secondary lobules it forms centrilobular interstitium (blue). The periphery of the secondary lobule is bounded by the interlobular interstitium (yellow). Within the secondary lobule the fine bands in brown represent the intralobular interstitium.

Anatomy of Bronchi and Pulmonary Vessels

The bronchi and pulmonary arteries run parallel to each other. Their appearances depend upon the scan plane they are

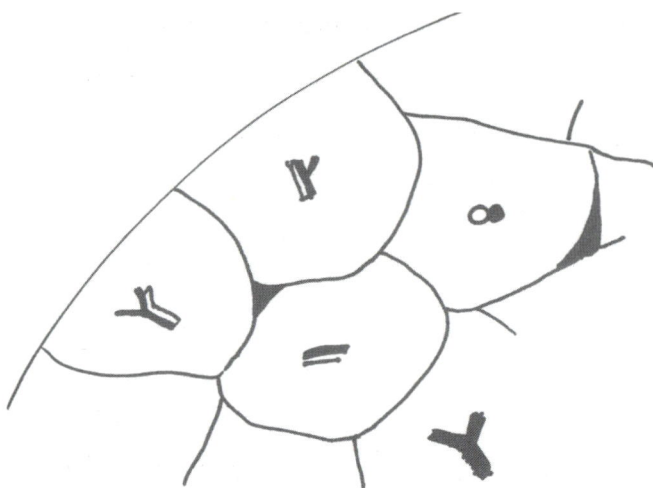

Fig 1.63: Anatomy of secondary lobule—Schematic diagram demonstrates polygonal secondary lobules. The secondary lobules share common walls with lymphatics and pulmonary veins in their walls. The centre of the secondary lobule contains the centrilobular artery and bronchus.

sectioned in. If the scan plane is perpendicular to their course they will appear as well-defined round structures adjacent to each other. If sectioned in the same plane, they will appear as tubular structures running parallel to each other. The artery is seen as a well-defined round homogenous white structure. The accompanying bronchus has a thin well-defined wall with a lucent centre containing air resembling a pipe with air in its lumen. The outer surface of these structures is smooth. The inner diameter of the bronchus to accompanying arterial diameter is usually 0.65/0.7:1. A bronchoarterial ratio of 1:1 is considered normal; greater than this is considered as bronchiectasis. An increased bronchoarterial ratio greater than 1 may be seen in patients who reside at a high altitude; the mild hypoxemia induces mild bronchial dilatation as well as vasoconstriction, resulting in an altered bronchoarterial ratio. Bronchi are visualized till the peripheral 2 cm of the lung. It is rare to see normal bronchi in the peripheral 2 cm of the lung. Normal bronchi may extend till 1 cm of the mediastinal surface.

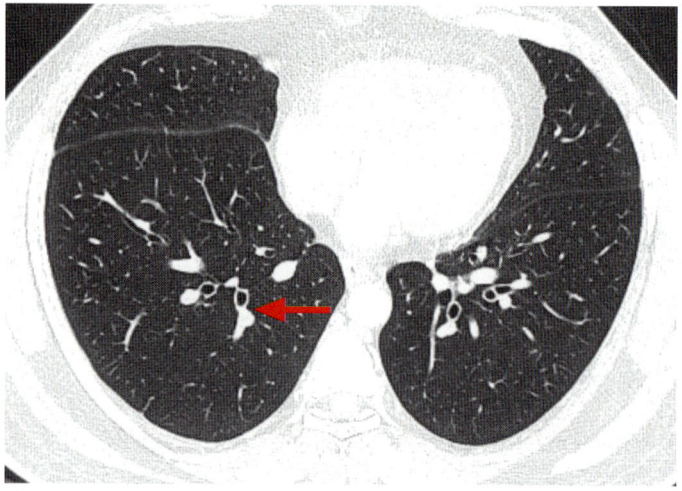

RADIOGRAPHIC PATTERNS OF DISEASE PROCESSES

The most important aspects of imaging are to determine the anatomic location of a lesion, whether in the lungs, mediastinum, pleura or chest wall as well as the nature of the lesion. The most common abnormality visualized on a radiograph is a pulmonary opacity. An opacity is often ill-defined and is more opaque than the surrounding lung. It is useful to categorize the patterns of pulmonary opacities as it helps to narrow the differential diagnostic possibilities.

Table 1.2: Patterns of pulmonary opacities
1. Consolidation or air-space opacities
2. Atelectasis
3. Linear /band-like opacities
4. Nodular/reticulo-nodular opacities
5. Nodules/masses
6. Cavitations
7. Cysts/bullae/Honeycombing
8. Calcifications

Consolidation/Air-Space Opacities

Air-space opacities represent one or more ill-defined areas of increased density in the lung parenchyma. When they abut the pleura they have a sharp margin. Vascular shadows are obscured by the air-space opacity, as the air-filled dark lung does not contrast with the soft tissue density of vessels. Similarly, intrapulmonary airways are rarely visible on chest X-rays. With air-space opacification the air in the airways contrasts with the air-space opacity, so that the airways become visible. This appearance is known as an air bronchogram sign. It also confirms the opacity is intrapulmonary. Another useful sign is the silhouette sign. The borders of the heart and domes of the diaphragm are well-visualized as they are contrasted by the interface with the dark lung. If a pulmonary opacity is in contact with the margins of the heart/diaphragm there is an interruption of the margins resulting in a loss of silhouette. This helps in detecting and localizing the abnormality. Conversely, presence of an opacity with preservations of the silhouette, would indicate that the pulmonary abnormality is not in contact with the heart border or diaphragmatic surface. Cavitation may occur within air-space opacities. The cavity results following expulsion or drainage of necrotic contents via the bronchial tree. A gas-filled space with or without an air-fluid level is seen in the air-space opacity. CT is more sensitive in detection of air-space opacities; it may detect opacities even when the chest X-ray is normal. The causes of air-space opacities are numerous; any pathological process which results in filling of alveoli will result in an air-space opacity. The differential diagnosis of air-space opacities includes pneumonia, atelectasis, infarction, haemorrhage, neoplasm, oedema.

Important points which may help in the differential diagnosis of air-space opacities:

1. Opacities over half a lobe with no loss of lung volume are virtually diagnostic of pneumonia.
2. Widespread pneumonia is invariably accompanied by cough and fever.
3. Lobar consolidation with lobar expansion causing bulging of the fissure is most often seen in infection due to *Klebsiella pneumoniae*. It is also occasionally seen following infection with *Streptococcus pneumoniae*, staphylococcus, and other Gram-negative bacteria.
4. Neoplastic obstruction of a lobar bronchus usually causes some degree of atelectasis. However, bronchoalveolar carcinoma and lymphoma may appear as lobar pneumonia with no evidence of atelectasis, as the neoplastic process spreads in the alveolar spaces without involvement of the bronchi.
5. Aspiration should be suspected with a history of alcoholism, seizures, unconscious state. Air-space opacities with evidence of associated loss of volume is seen in patients with aspiration pneumonia. Air-space opacities with well-marked haemoptysis may occur in intrapulmonary haemorrhage.
6. Cavitation within a consolidated lobe could represent tuberculosis or a necrotizing pneumonia. The latter is commonly caused by *Kl. pneumoniae*, *Ps. aeruginosa*, *Staphylococcus aureus* and anaerobic bacteria. Cavitation could also arise in relation to non-infectious aetiologies such as Wegener's granulomatosis, other forms of vasculitis and in neoplasms.
7. Lucencies seen within an air-space opacity could be due to overlying uninvolved lung, areas of centrilobular emphysema within the abnormal lung, necrosis of tissue with cavitation, pneumatoceles.
8. Rib or vertebral body destruction in the absence of a mass points to a metastatic lesion, though tuberculosis or fungal infections can also present similarly, as destructive bone lesions.

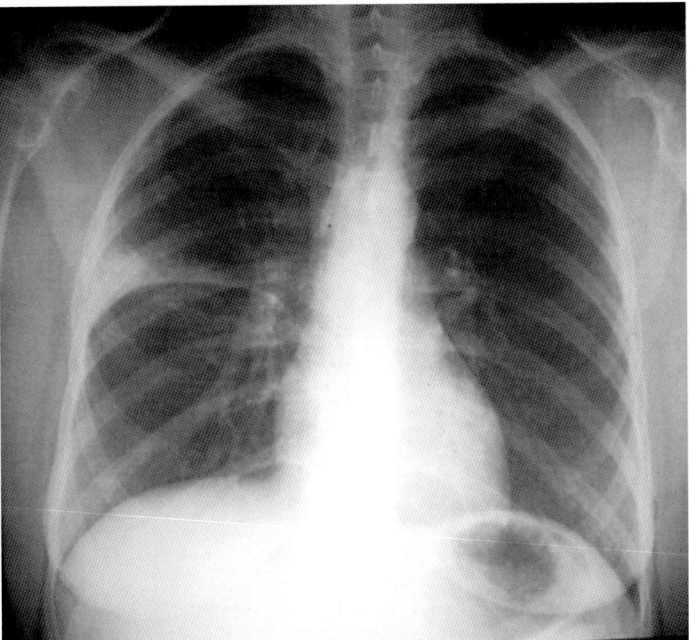

Fig 1.66: Upper lobe consolidation. PA view of the chest reveals an ill-defined air-space opacity in the right upper zone which has an ill-defined superior margin but sharp inferior margin. Air-space opacities are ill-defined; however, when they abut the pleura, as in this case on the minor fissure, they have a sharp margin.

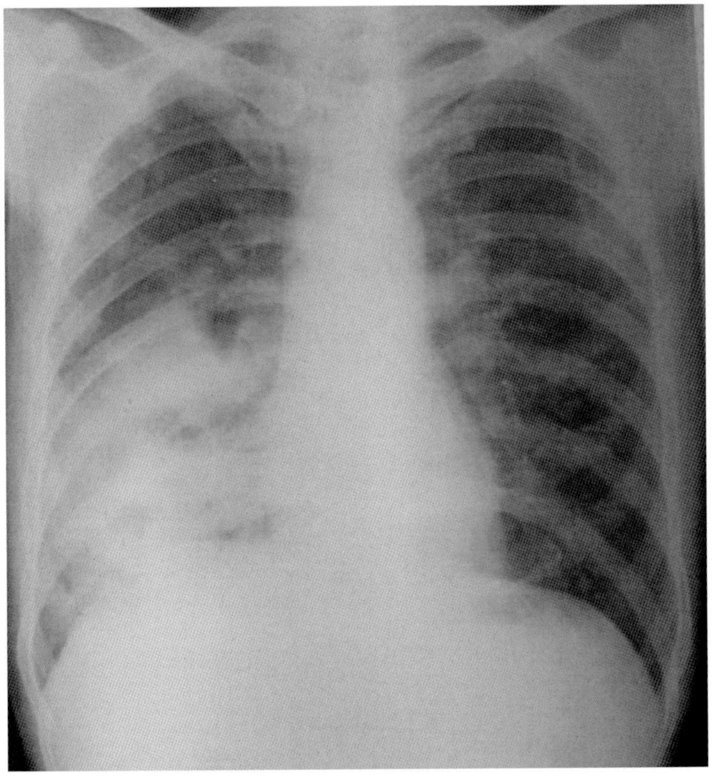

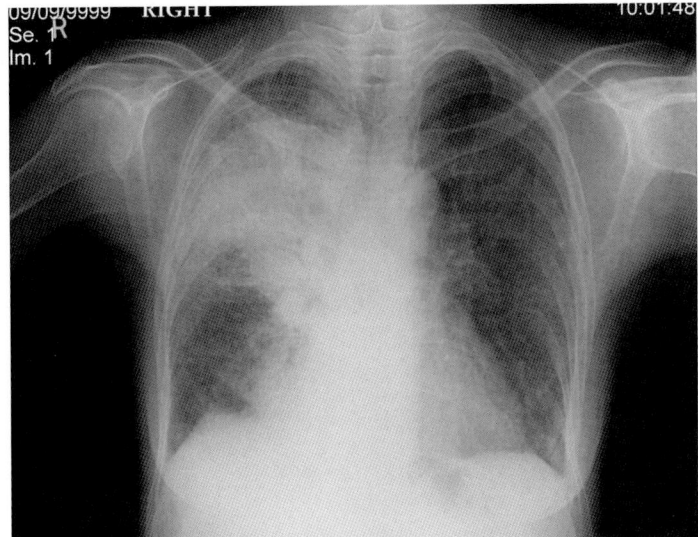

Fig 1.67: Right upper lobe pneumonia. Large area of consolidation in the right upper lobe demonstrates loss of silhouette with right border of heart with subtle air bronchogram; note no evidence of loss of volume or mediastinal shift.

Fig 1.65: Right lower lobe pneumonia: PA view chest X-ray demonstrates a large ill-defined area of consolidation in the right mid and lower zone. Note loss of silhouette with right dome of diaphragm. This consolidation occupies nearly 50% of the lung but there is no loss of volume or shift of mediastinal structures. This is a feature of pneumonia.

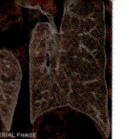

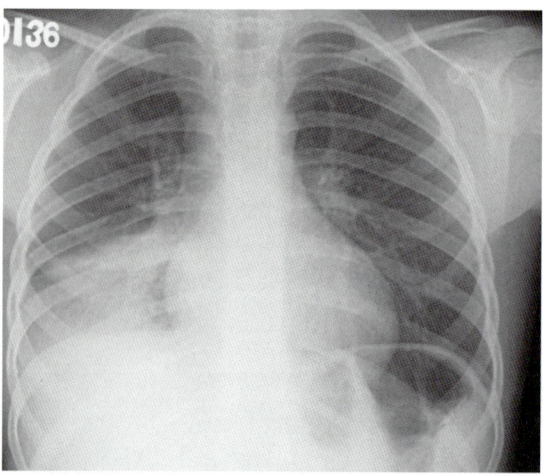

Fig 1.68: Right lower lobe pneumonia. PA view of the chest demonstrates an ill-defined consolidation in the right lower zone preserving silhouette with cardiac margin but loss of silhouette with diaphragm.

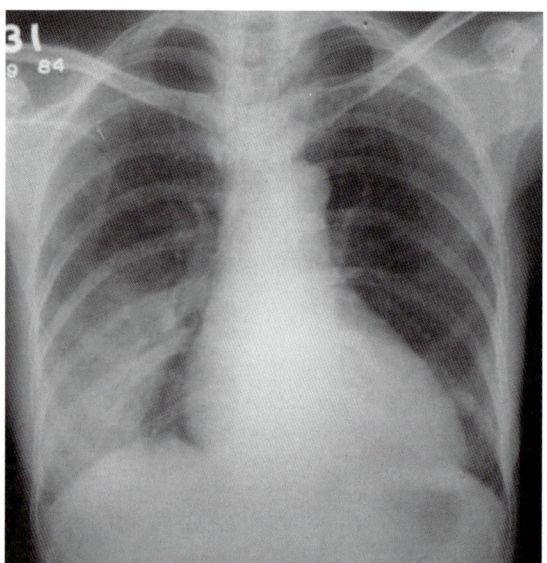

Fig 1.69: Right lower lobe pneumonia. PA view of the chest demonstrates an ill-defined area of consolidation in the right lower zone; there is no loss of the silhouette of the cardiac as well as diaphragmatic surface indicating this consolidation is not in contact with either the diaphragm or cardiac surface.

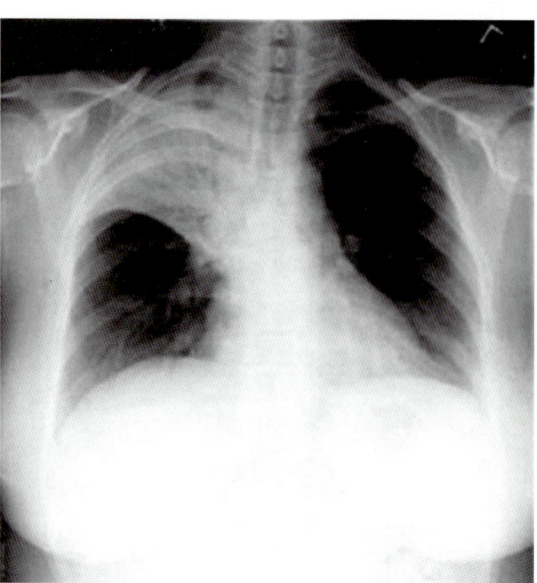

Fig 1.70: Right upper lobe pneumonia. PA view of the chest reveals an ill-defined air space opacity in the right upper lobe with an air bronchogram. There is loss of volume as evidenced by elevation of the minor fissure.

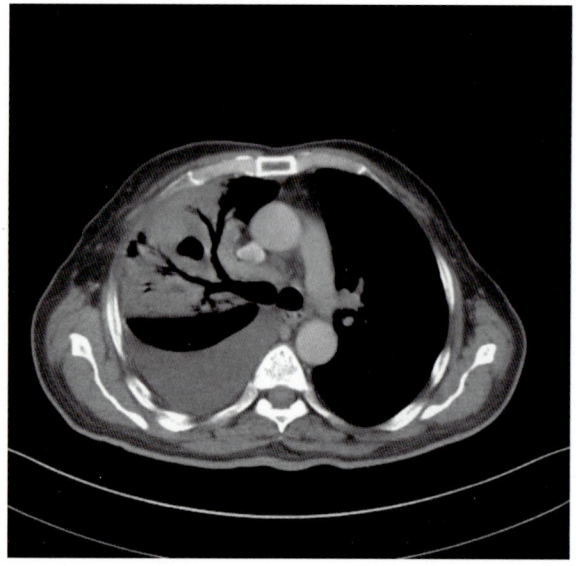

Fig 1.71: Consolidation. CT chest demonstrates a large consolidation in the right middle lobe with an air bronchogram pattern. There is an associated pleural effusion.

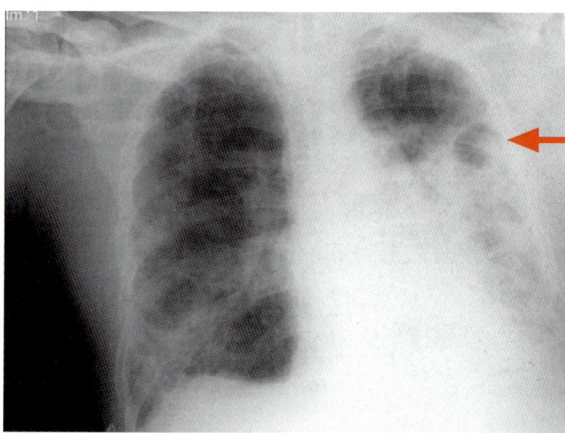

Fig 1.72: Consolidation with cavitation. Portable AP view of chest reveals an ill-defined area of consolidation with cavitation in the left lung. Patchy consolidations in right lower lobe. Causative organism—*Staphylococcus aureus*.

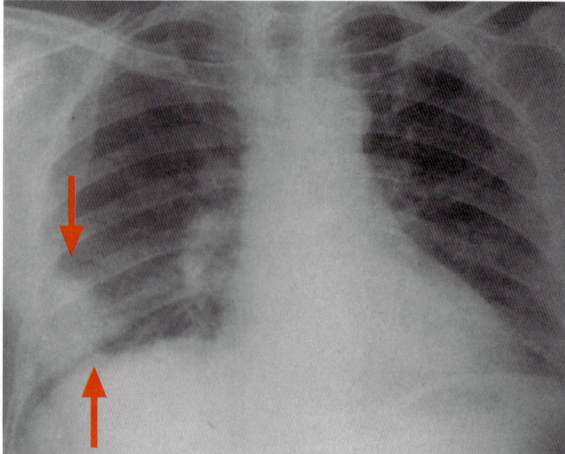

Fig 1.73: Pulmonary infarct. PA view of the chest reveals a wedge-shaped area of consolidation in the right lower zone abutting the pleura. The appearance of a wedge-shaped consolidation should raise the possibility of a pulmonary infarct.

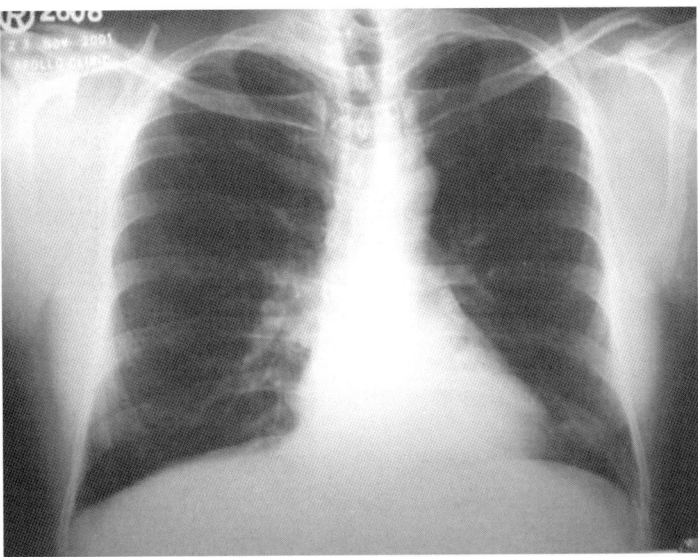

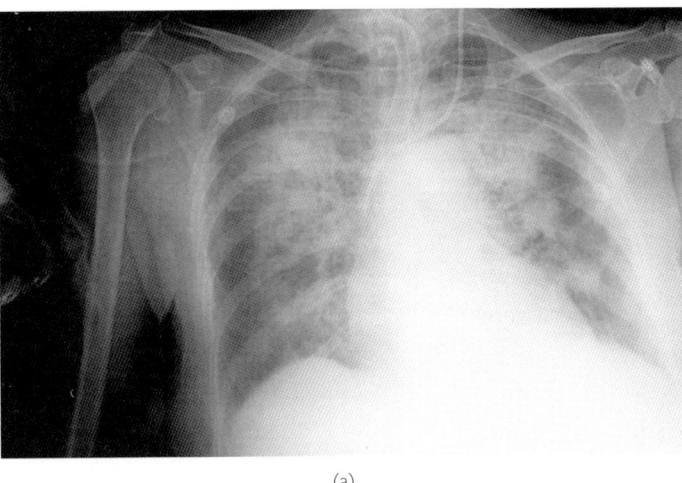

(a)

(a)

(b)

(b)

Fig 1.75: Pulmonary oedema. AP view portable X-ray. (a) demonstrates ill-defined fluffy opacities in both lung fields; within a few hours, on a follow-up X-ray (b) the opacities regressed.

Fig 1.74: (a) X-ray chest in a febrile patient demonstrates no abnormality (b) CT chest reveals multiple bilateral cavitating and subpleural nodular lesions. CT is more sensitive than chest X-rays in detection of focal lesions, as well as demonstrating internal morphology of focal lesions, such as cavitation, necrosis, calcification, air bronchograms.

BAT WING PATTERN OF PULMONARY OPACITY

This is a term used to describe diffuse parahilar opacities which have ill-defined margins. These may be symmetric or asymmetric, being larger on one side. The most common cause for this opacity is pulmonary oedema, especially if associated with cardiomegaly/pleural effusion/Kerly A/B lines. Another feature of pulmonary oedema is the rapid appearance and disappearance of opacities. Other conditions which may present with this type of opacities are aspiration pneumonias, and inhalation exposure to noxious gases. Immunocompromised patients, especially *Pneumocystis carinii* pneumonia can have a similar appearance. Bat wing opacities unchanged over a long period of time with non-specific symptoms, suggest the

possibility of alveolar proteinosis or a neoplastic process such as lymphangitic carcinomatosis.

Peripheral Air-Space Consolidations are considered as a photographic negative of pulmonary oedema as the opacities are in the lung periphery. Especially when present in the upper zones the most common possibility is chronic eosinophilic pneumonia. If the opacities are not predominantly in the upper zones, the possibilities include cryptogenic organizing pneumonia, viral pneumonia or a mycoplasmal pneumonia. Fleeting shadows, shadows which come and go, or appear in different regions of the lungs, raise the possibilities of pulmonary oedema, eosinophilic pneumonia, asthma, ABPA and vasculitis.

White-out lungs are typical for ARDS, especially with associated air bronchograms. Sarcoid may present with patchy opacities in the lungs which may be spherical and have associated mediastinal adenopathy.

COLLAPSE/ATELECTASIS

Often the words collapse and consolidation are used interchangeably. Consolidation is essentially due to replacement of

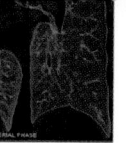

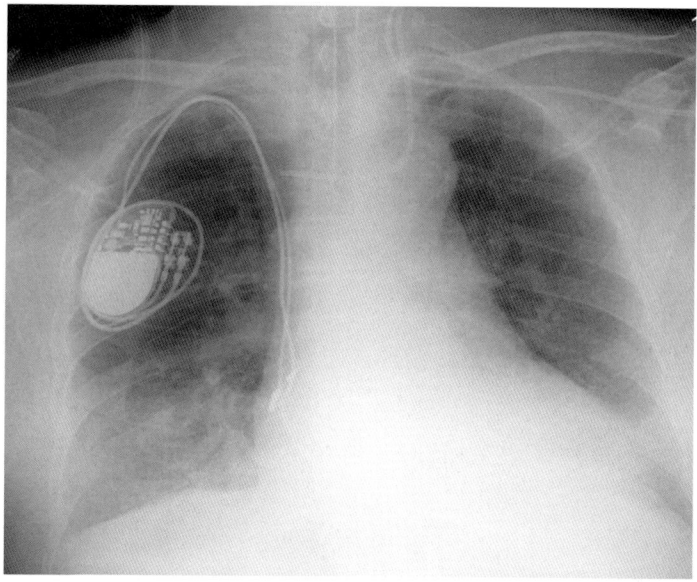

(a)

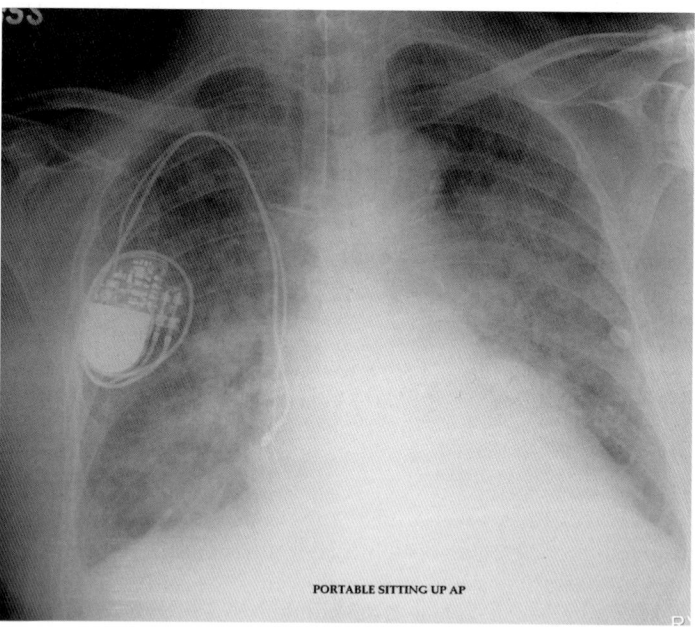

PORTABLE SITTING UP AP

(b)

Fig 1.76: Pulmonary oedema. Portable chest X-rays in a patient with a pacemaker *in situ*. X-ray (a) reveals an ill-defined opacity in the right lower zone (b) subsequent X-ray a few hours later reveals increasing opacities in the left lung. This feature of rapidly appearing and disappearing shadows is highly suggestive of pulmonary oedema.

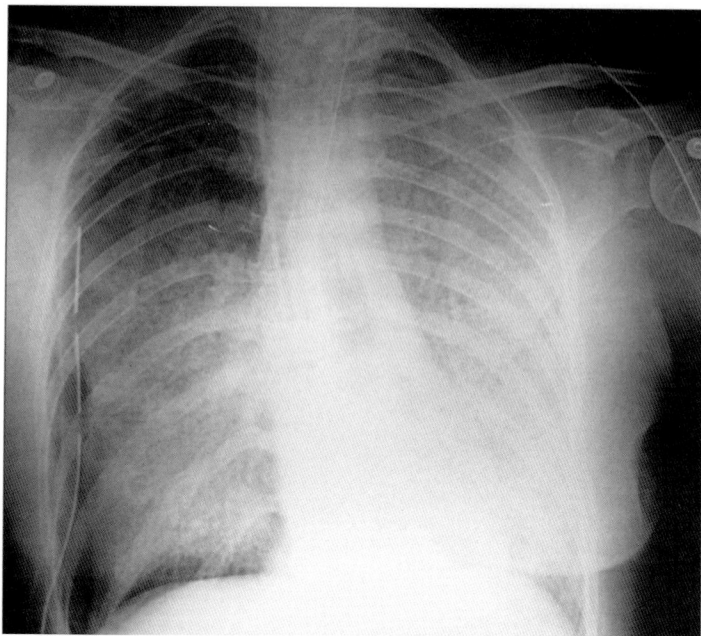

Fig 1.77: Alveolar proteinosis. PA view of the chest demonstrates ill-defined airspace opacities in both lung fields sparing the right upper lobe. ICD seen *in situ* following thoracoscopic biopsy which revealed pulmonary alveolar proteinosis. Patient presented with cough, fever and mild dyspnoea over three months. This is an example of bilateral white-out lungs with subacute to chronic symptoms.

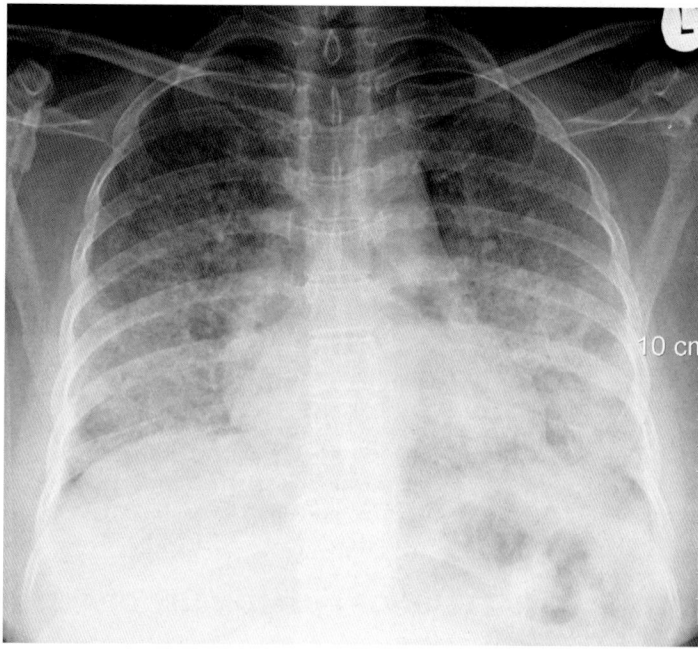

Fig 1.78: PCP: Immunocompromised patient with diffuse ill-defined air-space opacities. In the setting of immunocompromise the most likely aetiology would be *Pneumocystis carinii* pneumonia.

alveolar air by an exudate, transudate or cellular debris resulting in a homogenous opacity with no loss of volume. Atelectasis or its synonym 'collapse' indicates volume loss. The atelectatic/collapsed segment or lobe of the lung will therefore demonstrate a homogenous opacity with accompanying volume loss. Atelectasis is caused by bronchial obstruction which is either due to an intrabronchial pathology, foreign body or extrinsic compression of the bronchus. Compression atelectasis can be due to compression of adjacent lung by tumour, bulla, pneumothorax or pleural effusion.

Cicatrisation Atelectasis

Following resolution of an inflammatory/infective process there may be localized atelectasis. This is due to either direct destruction of lung parenchyma or fibrotic contraction, termed as cicatrisation fibrosis. This is commonly seen in tuberculosis, radiation fibrosis, interstitial pulmonary fibrosis, bronchostenosis.

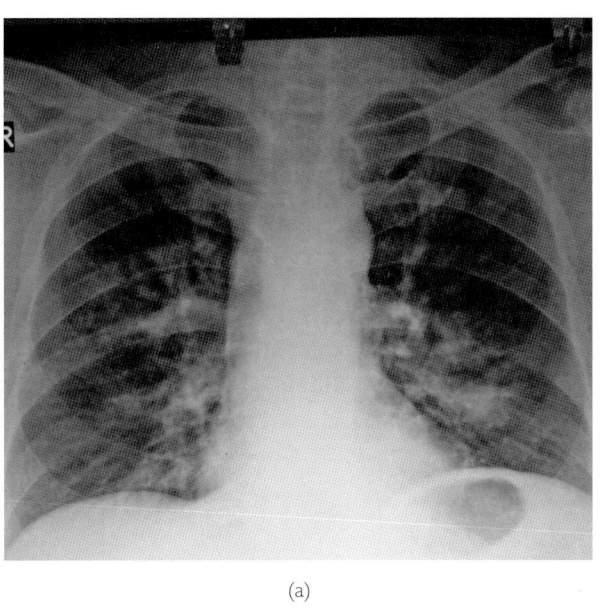

(a)

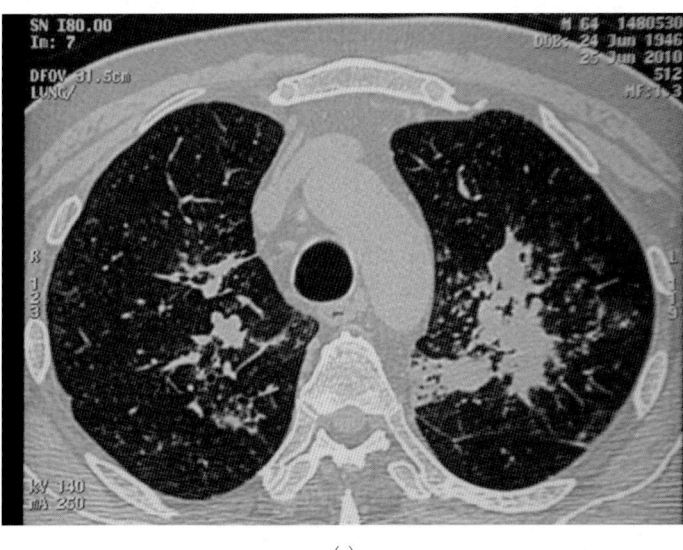

(c)

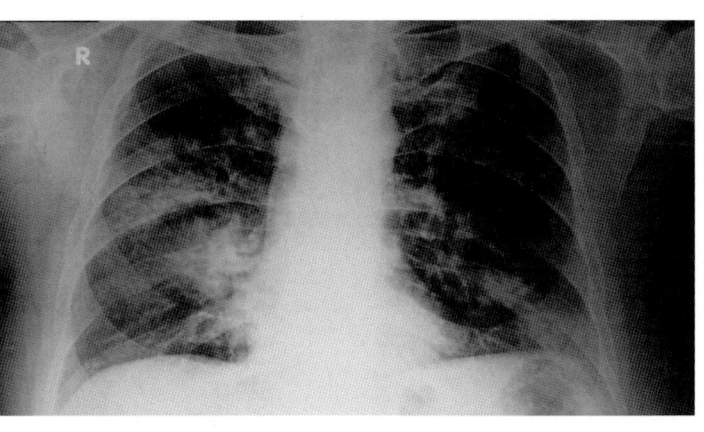

(b)

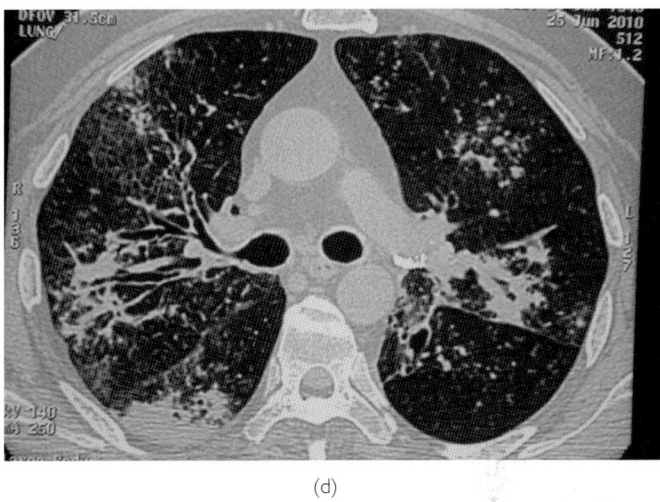

(d)

Fig 1.79: Fleeting opacities. PA view of chest (a) reveals ill-defined consolidation in left lower lobe with patchy consolidations in right lower lobe (b) Follow-up X-ray after three weeks reveals regression of left lower lobe consolidation with fresh right lower lobe consolidation (c and d) CT chest revealed extensive subpleural and parenchymal consolidation. Blood eosinophilia was present, CT biopsy revealed Churg-Strauss syndrome with vasculitis.

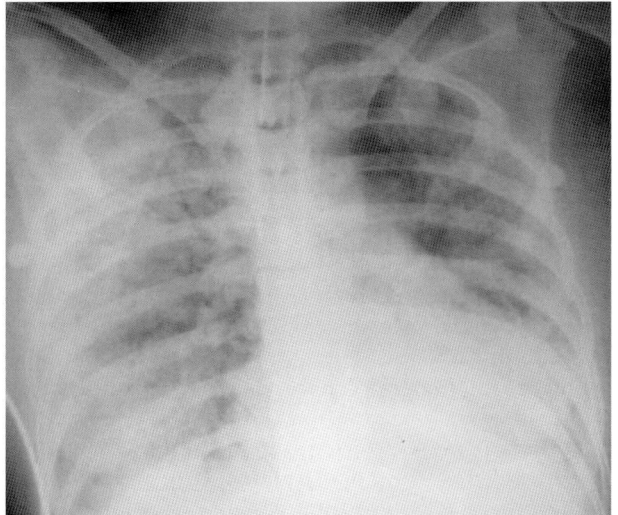

Fig 1.80: Acute lung injury: Typical white-out lung appearance seen in acute lung injury.

Pulmonary fibrosis can cause significant loss of volume due to fibrotic contraction of lung parenchyma.

Plate or Discoid Atelectasis

This is a form of atelectasis, which is due to hypoventilation, leading to alveolar collapse. The alveoli in the lung bases as well as posterior aspects of the lung fields are the most prone to collapse. These appear as linear plate or disc-like opacities in the lower zones, occasionally extending across the whole breadth of the lower lobe. As these are due to hypoventilation they are seen mainly in hospitalized patients, post general anaesthesia and in patients with an acute abdomen where the diaphragm is splinted, resulting in reduced respiratory excursion.

Lobar Collapse/Atelectasis

The imaging features of lobar collapse are a pulmonary opacity with evidence of volume loss. The pulmonary opacity

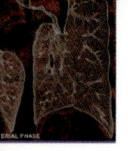

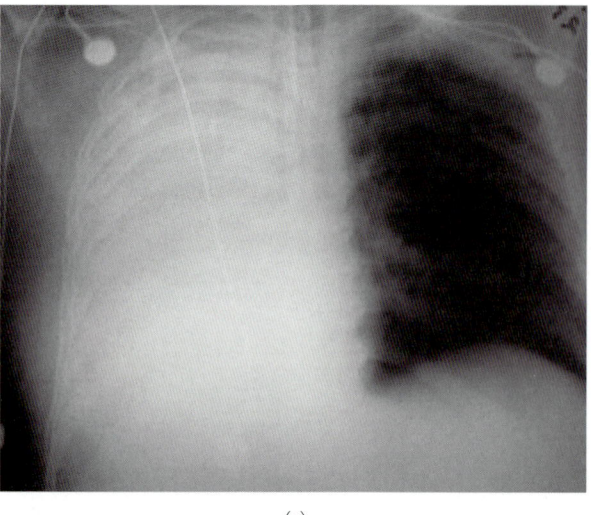
(a)

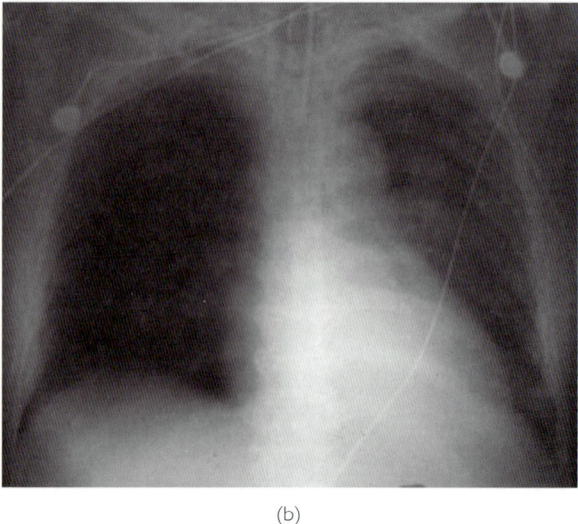
(b)

Fig 1.81: Obstructive atelectasis. Chest X-ray (a) demonstrates an opaque right hemithorax with a shift of the mediastinum to the right indicative of collapse of the right lung. The most likely cause would be an obstruction to the right main bronchus. Bronchoscopy revealed a mucus plug obstructing the right main bronchus (b) After aspirating the mucus plug the right lung expanded fully.

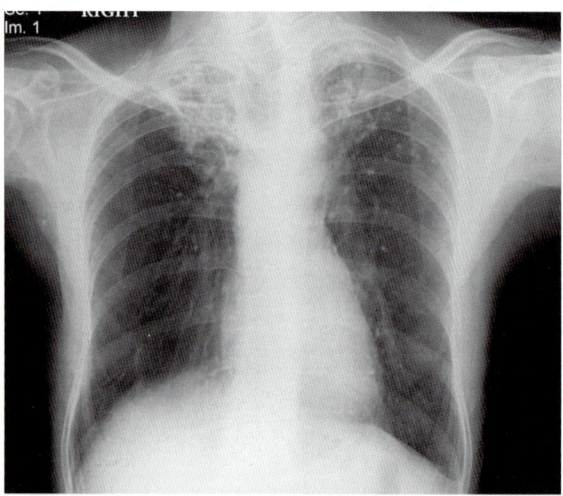

Fig 1.82: Fibrocalcareous TB. PA view of the chest reveals bilateral apical fibrotic lesions with calcified nodular lesions in both apices. These features of reticular opacities with calcified nodules and loss of volume are typical of old healed tuberculosis.

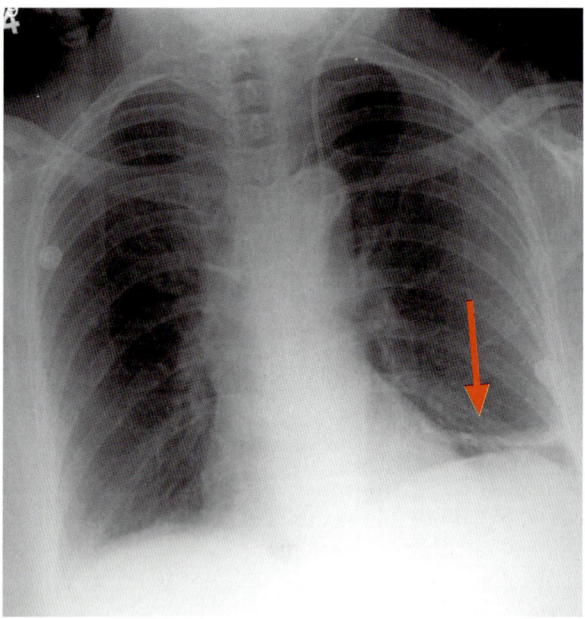

Fig 1.84: Plate atelectasis. PA view of the chest in a postoperative patient reveals a central line *in situ*. Plate atelectasis is seen in the left lower zone with evidence of loss of volume as evidenced by elevation of left dome of diaphragm.

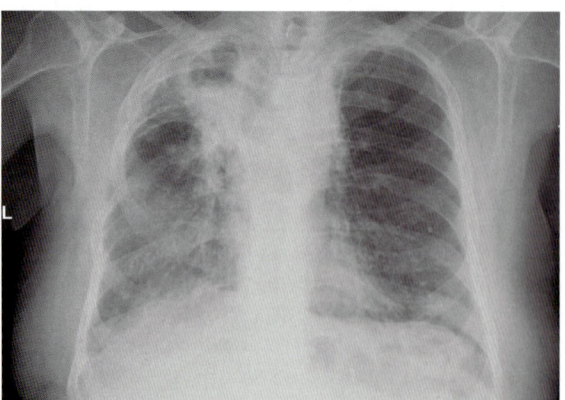

Fig 1.83: Radiation fibrosis. PA view of the chest reveals an ill-defined opacity in the right apical region with associated loss of volume, shift of trachea to the right, with the right hilum pulled up. Patient had received radiation for cancer of the oesophagus with resultant radiation fibrosis.

is due to loss of air in the alveoli of the collapsed segment/lobe and/or due to retained mucus secretions. The loss of volume is demonstrated by a shift of normal structures such as the hilum, interlobar fissures, mediastinum, with crowding of ribs, and of bronchovascular structures and elevation of the dome of the diaphragm. There is hypertranslucency of the normal ipsilateral lung due to compensatory overexpansion, with pulmonary vessels within it being more widely separated when compared to the opposite lung. It is important to note that when there is severe/total collapse of a lobe it may not always be possible to demonstrate the shadow of the lobar collapse on an X-ray, as the signs are too subtle. A shift of the hilum, fissure or the mediastinum should always suggest an underlying atelectasis.

GOLDEN S SIGN

When there is obstructive collapse by a central neoplasm with consequent peripheral collapse—the shape of the fissure assumes an 'S' shape, as the fissure is concave peripherally and convex centrally.

Lower Lobe Atelectasis

The appearances of right and left lower lobe atelectasis are similar. The lobes collapse posteromedially in the lower part of the chest. Left lower lobe atelectasis is often difficult to detect as the collapsed lobe is hidden by the cardiac silhouette. A penetrated X-ray would reveal the opacity of the collapsed lower lobe. As the lobe collapses posterio-medially, the oblique fissure rotates backwards and medially, the upper portion of the oblique fissure swinging downwards. The collapsed lobe is seen as a triangular opacity lying against the mediastinum. On the right side the medial aspect of the diaphragm is obscured, the lateral margin of the adjacent vertebrae is effaced, the ipsilateral hilum is depressed and the ipsilateral lower lobe pulmonary artery is not visualized. Lower lobe atelectasis is better demonstrated on a lateral view. The lung collapses posteriorly, therefore is seen as an opacity overlying the vertebrae. Normally, the vertebrae on a lateral view demonstrate increasing transradiancy of the lower dorsal vertebrae. On CT the collapsed lobe is seen plastered along the vertebral column in a posteriomedial location. The major fissure rotates to lie obliquely.

Right Middle Lobe Atelectasis

The atelectatic right middle lobe on a chest X-ray is seen as an opacity along the right heart border resulting in a loss of the silhouette of the right cardiac border. There is no significant change in the vasculature; the right hilum does not change in position. Right middle lobe atelectasis is best demonstrated on a lateral view as the horizontal fissure descends with increasing atelectasis. The atelectatic lobe is seen as an opaque wedge extending from the hilum anteriorly. Occasionally, when the atelectasis is very severe the appearances may resemble a thickened fissure. On CT, right middle lobe atelectasis is seen as a triangular wedge atelectatic lung, bound by the major fissure posteriorly and minor fissure anteriorly.

Right Upper Lobe Collapse

The right upper lobe collapses against the mediastinum and lung apex. As the lobe collapses the silhouette of the superior vena cava is lost. When there is total collapse a wedge of tissue is seen in the right upper zone along the mediastinum. The right middle and lower lobes demonstrate compensatory expansion and there is elevation of the right hilum. The major and minor fissures move upward and towards each other. This is well seen on the lateral view. The collapsed lobe on the lateral view silhouettes the ascending aorta. On CT, the collapsed right upper lobe appears as a triangular soft tissue density lying against the mediastinum and anterior chest wall.

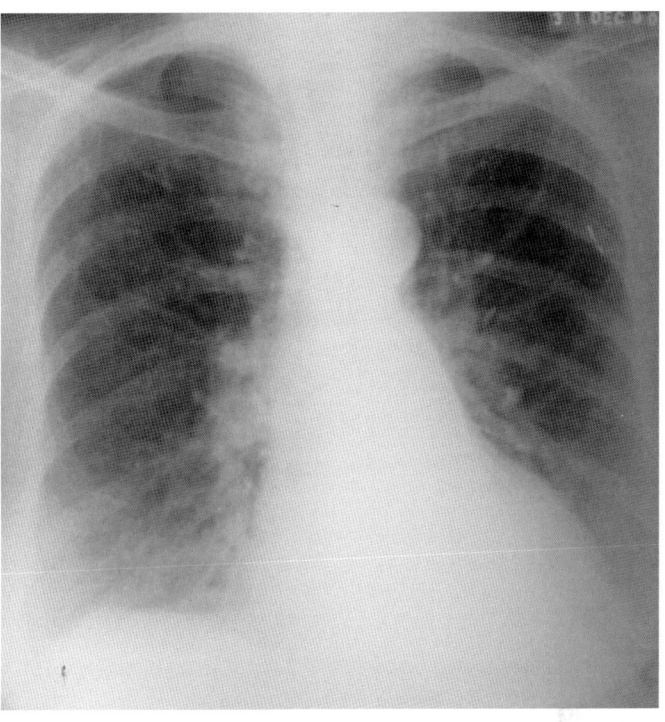

(a)

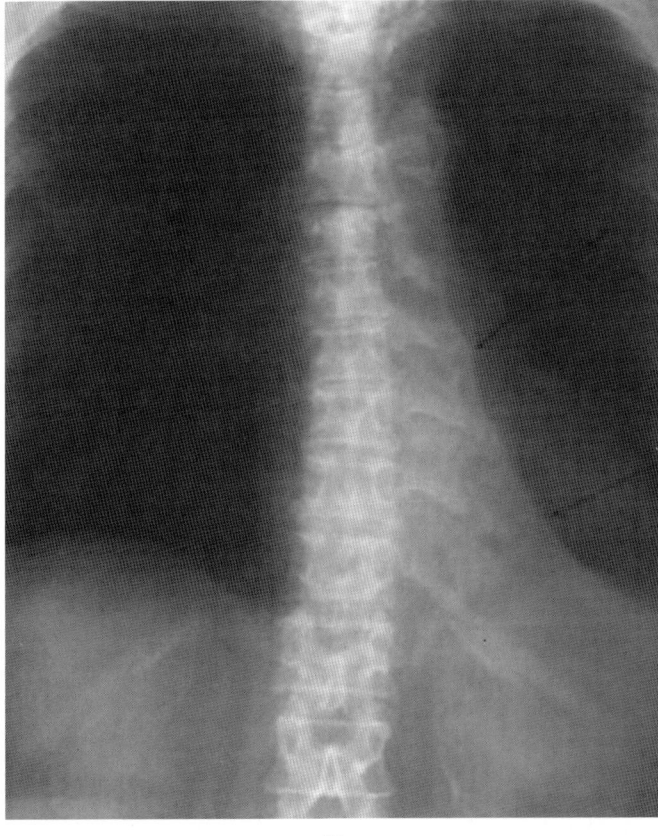

(b)

Fig 1.85: Left lower lobe collapse. (a) PA view of the chest does not reveal any significant abnormality except for the subtle appearance of straightening of the left heart border below the aortic knuckle. A penetrated view (b) demonstrates the collapsed left lower lobe as an opacity along the vertebral column.

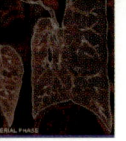
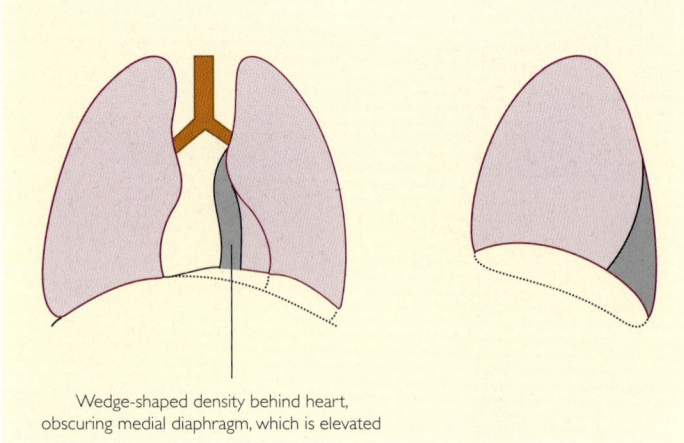

Wedge-shaped density behind heart,
obscuring medial diaphragm, which is elevated

Fig 1.86: Lower lobe collapse—Schematic diagram of left lower lobe collapse.
The lower lobe collapses behind the cardiac silhouette on the PA view.
The diaphragm is mildly elevated and the left lung volume is reduced.
The diagram of the lateral view demonstrates the posterior collapse of the lower
lobe, and a shift of the oblique fissure posteriorly.

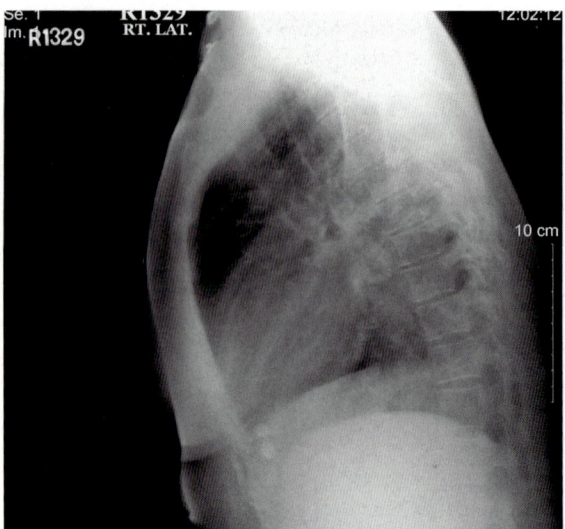

Fig 1.88: Right lower lobe collapse. Lateral view demonstrates
an ill-defined haze overlying the lower dorsal vertebrae. There is
loss of normal increasing translucency of lower dorsal vertebrae
due to the collapsed right lower lobe opacity overlapping the
vertebrae. Note the elevated right dome of the diaphragm.

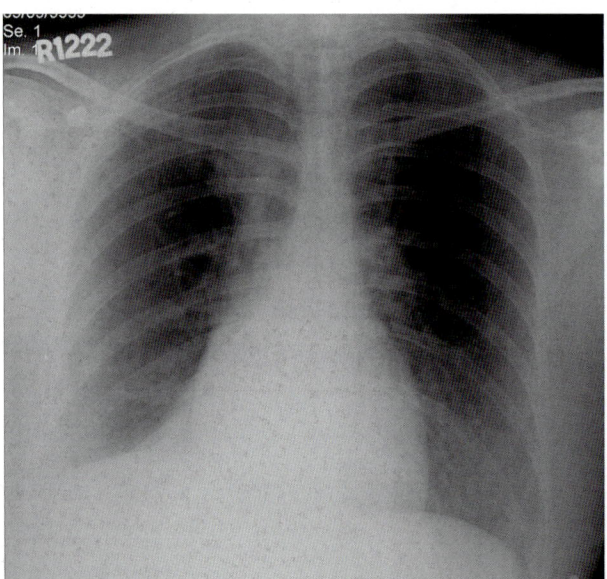

Fig 1.87: Right lower lobe collapse. PA view of the chest demonstrates
a homogenous opacity in the right paracardiac region with loss of
the cardiac and diaphragmatic silhouette. There is evidence of loss of
volume, as the right dome of the diaphragm is elevated and the right
lung is smaller in size as compared to the left.

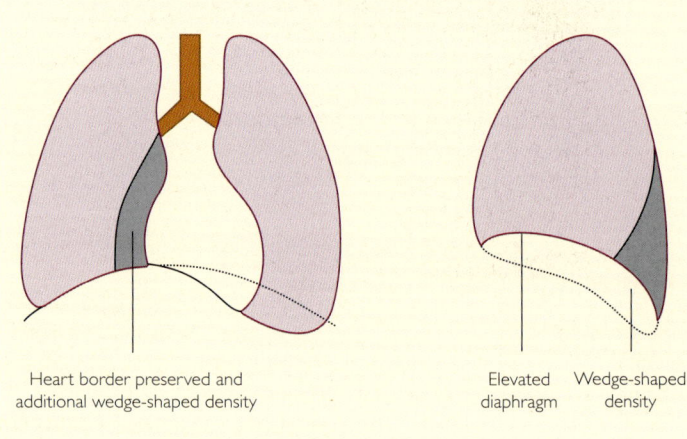

Heart border preserved and   Elevated   Wedge-shaped
additional wedge-shaped density   diaphragm   density

Fig 1.89: Right lower lobe atelectasis: Schematic diagram—PA view demonstrates
collapsed segment along the right heart border abutting the diaphragm. There
is elevation of the right dome of the diaphragm, loss of volume in right lung
and a shift of mediastinum to the right. Lateral view reveals the collapsed lung
posteriorly with a shift of the oblique fissure posteriorly.

Left Upper Lobe Atelectasis

The pattern of collapse is complex, as there is no horizontal
fissure. As the lobe collapses it pulls the major fissure forward
and the lower lobe expands posterior to the major fissure. As the
left lower lobe expands posterior to the collapsing left upper
lobe, on PA radiographs the atelectatic left upper lobe appears
as a diffuse haze overlying the left hilum often extending to the
lung apex, but fading inferiorly and laterally. The left cardiac
and mediastinal silhouette is lost. As the lower lobe expands
the aortic knuckle may be visible and consequently the left
apex and upper mediastinum may be visible as the expanded
lung occupies these regions.

On the lateral view the collapsed lung is seen anteriorly
with the major fissure moving anteriorly to be relatively parallel to the chest wall. As the lower lobe overexpands air may be
seen between the sternum and the atelectatic lung. The appearances on CT are very similar to those seen with right upper lobe
atelectasis.

Right Middle and Lower Lobe Atelectasis

This type of atelectasis is rare considering the distance between
the two bronchi. It may however occur due to separate occlusions
of the right middle and lower lobe bronchi. The appearances
resemble a right lower lobe atelectasis; the extent of involvement
is more extensive, extending to the lateral costophrenic angle on
the PA view and to anterior chest wall on the lateral view.

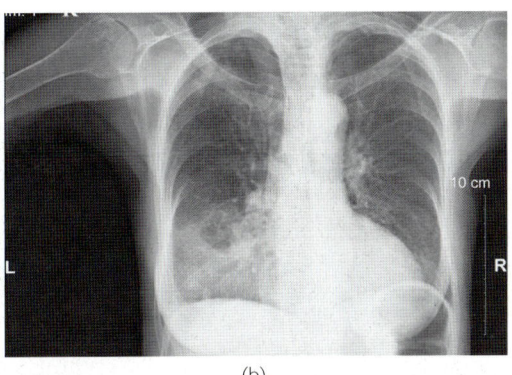

(b)

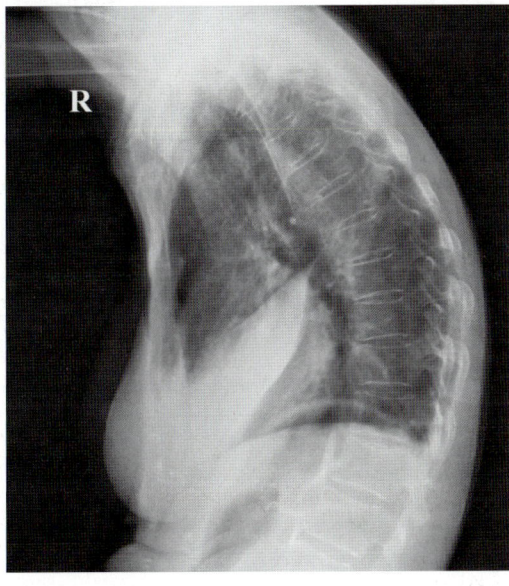

(b)

Fig 1.90: Right middle lobe collapse. (a) PA view demonstrates an ill-defined opacity in the right lower zone (b) lateral view of the chest reveals a homogenous opacity overlying the cardiac silhouette bounded by the interlobar fissures representing right middle lobe collapse. Note the marked downward shift of the lesser fissure.

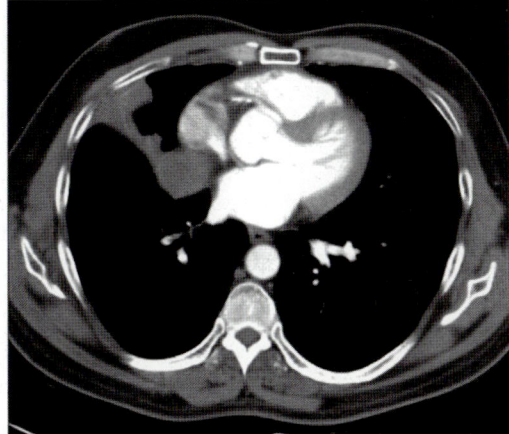

Fig 1.91: Collapse of the lateral segment of the right middle lobe. CT chest reveals a mass lesion in the right hilum causing collapse of the lateral segment of the right middle lobe, seen as a band-like shadow in the right middle lobe.

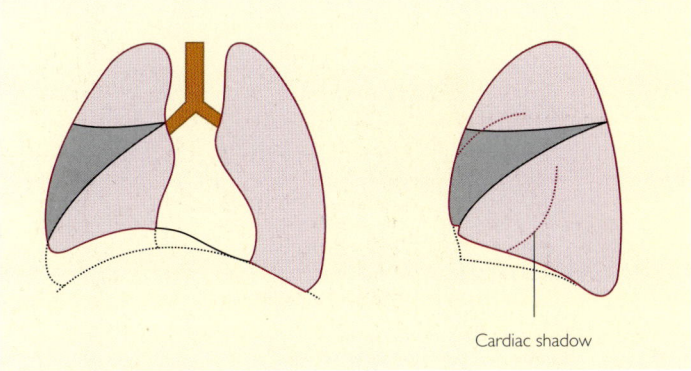

Fig 1.92: Right middle lobe collapse. Schematic diagram demonstrates right lower zone opacity abutting the cardiac silhouette with elevation of the diaphragm, and reduction in right lung volume. Lateral view demonstrates minor and major fissure approximate with each other, with a triangular opacity representing the collapsed middle lobe within.

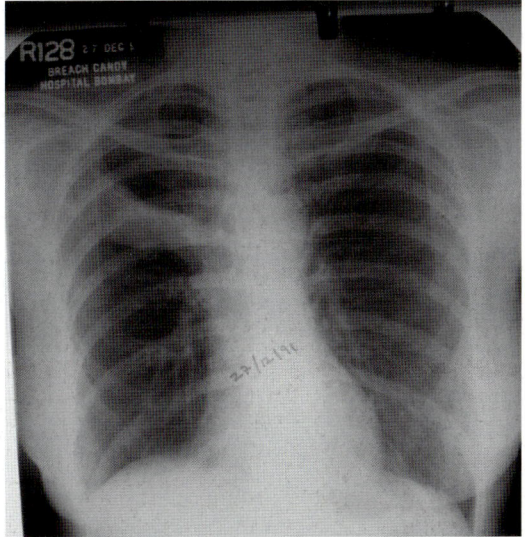

Fig 1.93: Right upper lobe collapse consolidation. PA view of the chest reveals a band-like opacity in the right upper zone with elevation of the minor fissure representing a right upper lobe partial collapse.

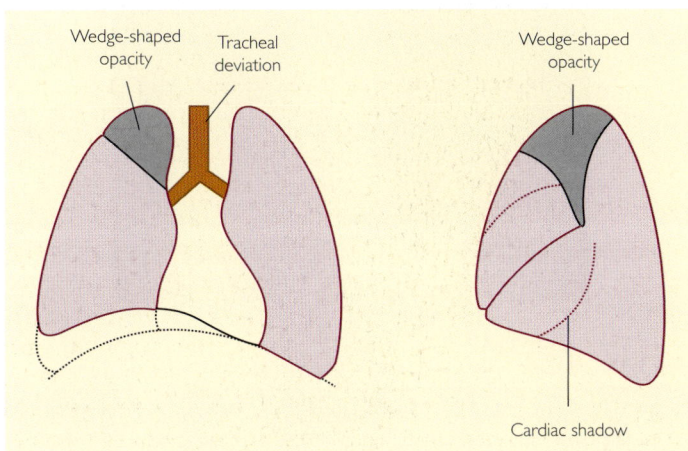

Fig 1.94: Right upper lobe atelectasis. Schematic diagram demonstrates on PA view right upper lobe opacity, elevation of minor fissure, right hilum and right dome of diaphragm. Lateral view demonstrates elevation and backward rotation of minor fissure with collapsed right upper lobe opacity within the two fissures.

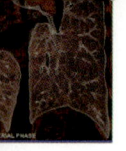

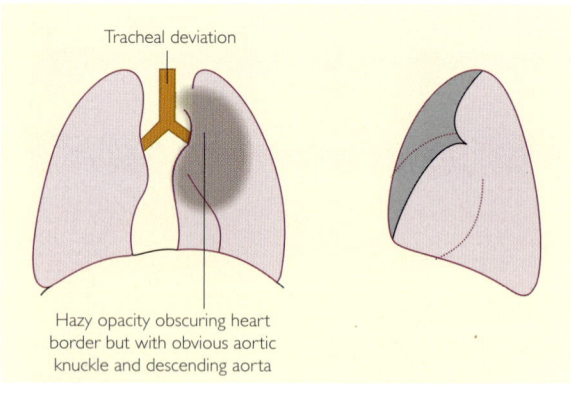

(a)

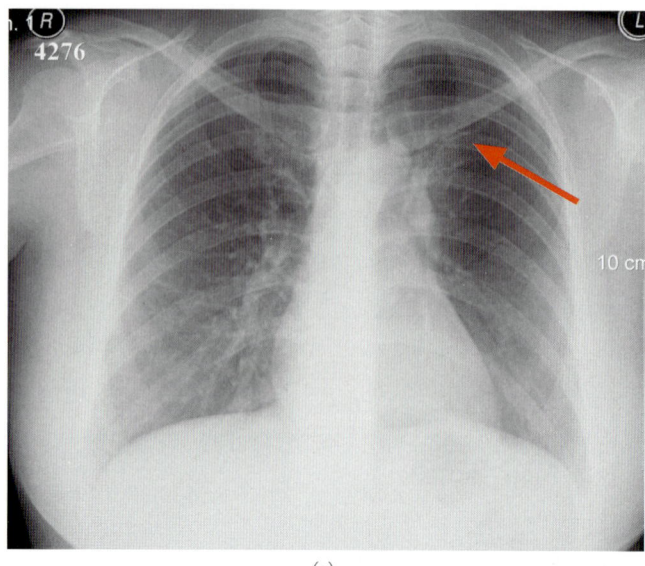

(a)

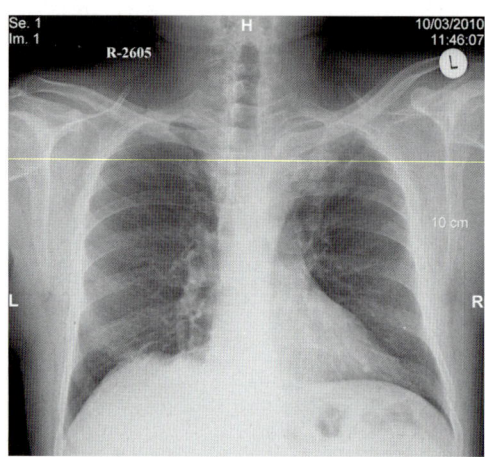

(b)

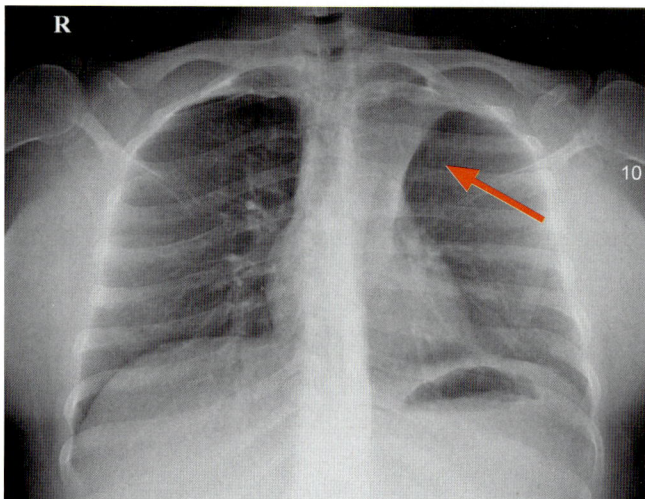

(b)

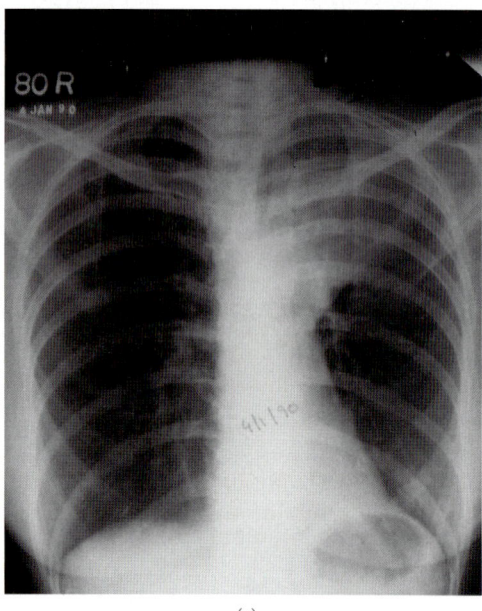

(c)

Fig 1.95: Left upper lobe collapse (a) Schematic diagram (b and c) PA views demonstrate an ill-defined haze overlying the left upper lobe. A homogenous opacity is not seen as in other lobar collapses as the compensatory expansion of the left lower lobe occurs posterior to the collapsed left upper lobe. These opacities are summated on a PA view resulting in only a hazy opacity. On a lateral view the opacity of the collapsed left upper lobe is better visualized, though with marked expansion of the lower lobe, the expanded lower lobe may intersperse between the sternum and collapsed left upper lobe. Note the major fissure moves anteriorly parallel to the anterior chest wall (schematic diagram).

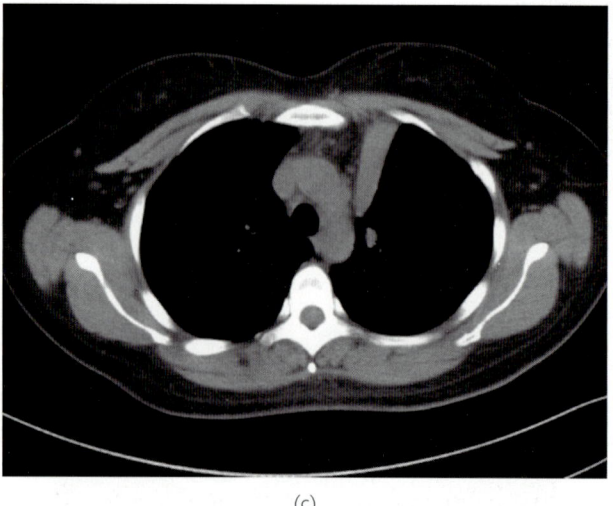

(c)

Fig 1.96: Left upper lobe collapse. PA view of the chest (a) demonstrates an ill-defined opacity in the left suprahilar region. Lordotic view (b) demonstrates a well-defined opacity plastered against the mediastinum. CT chest (c) demonstrates collapsed lobe abutting mediastinum.

Linear and Band-like Opacities

Linear opacities are linear densities less than 5 mm and bands are considered to be linear densities more than 5 mm in thickness. The causes are tabled below.

Table 1.3: Causes of linear opacities
1. Clothing, tubes, etc.
2. Wall of a bleb or pneumatocele
3. Bronchocele (mucoid impaction)
4. Parenchymal or pleuroparenchymal scar
5. Discoid atelectasis
6. Organizing pneumonia (presenting with a band-like pattern)
7. Anomalous blood vessels or feeding and draining vessels to arteriovenous malformations
8. Thickening of pleural fissures
9. Pleural tail associated with pulmonary nodule
10. Septal lines (Kerley lines) as in pulmonary oedema, neoplastic infiltration, lymphangitis carcinomatosis

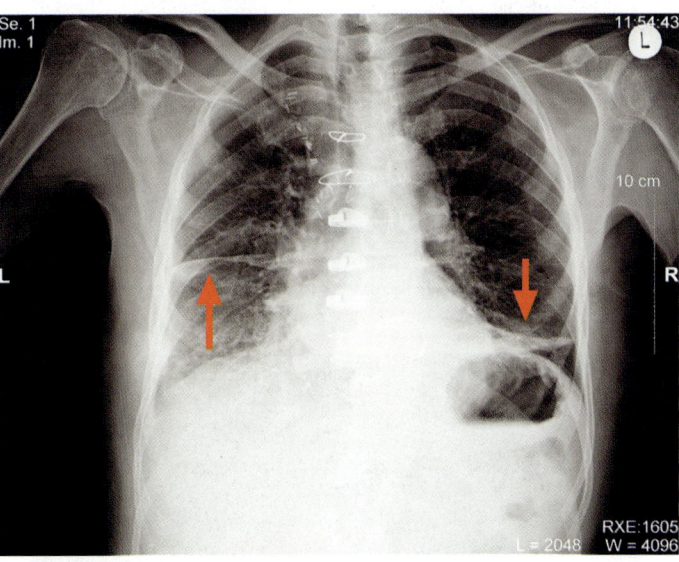

Fig 1.97: Discoid atelectasis. PA view of the chest reveals linear bands in the right mid and left lower zone due to plate atelectasis, following general anaesthesia.

Mucoid Impaction appears as one or more band-like opacities pointing towards the hilum, usually 1.0 cm or more in diameter. The margins are usually sharply demarcated and smooth with a finger-in-glove appearance. This appearance is mainly seen in ABPA but may also be seen as a result of bronchial obstruction in bronchial carcinoid, lung Ca, bronchostenosis, broncholithiasis, and bronchial atresia. If the lung distal to the obstructed segment is consolidated or collapses, the linear bands of mucoid impaction will not be visualized as they are now silhouetted by the collapse/consolidation.

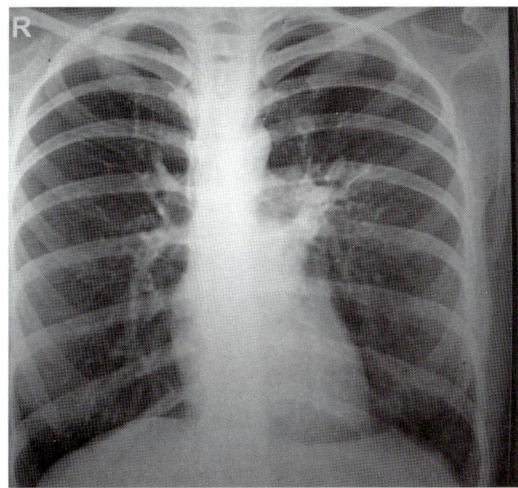

Fig 1.98: Mucoid impaction. Chest X-ray reveals well-defined tubular homogenous opacities in a left parahilar location as a result of allergic bronchopulmonary aspergilliosis.

Septal Lines

Interlobular septa of normal lungs are not visible on chest radiographs or even HRCT. When septa become thickened

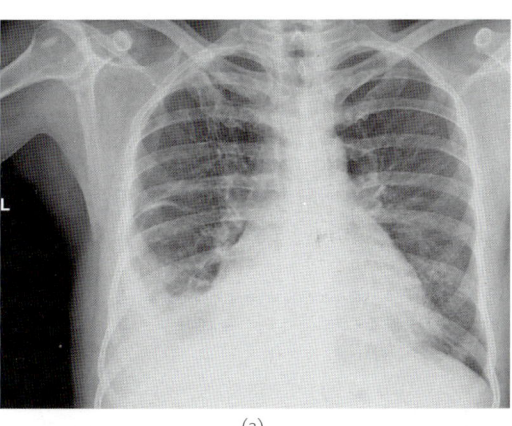

(a)

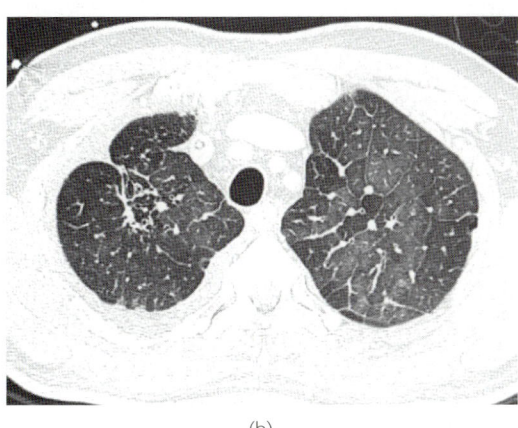

(b)

Fig 1.99: Septal lines: (a) Chest X-ray demonstrates cardiomegaly, right pleural effusion and prominent lung markings (b) CT Chest demonstrates smooth septal thickening with ground-glass densities due to pulmonary oedema secondary to congestive cardiac failure.

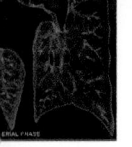

they become visible. Kerley first described septal lines especially in pulmonary oedema. They were named ABC, 'A' referred to septal lines which ranged up to 4.0 cm radiating from the hila into the central portions of the lung, more visible in the upper/mid zones of lung. These are now referred to as deep septa. The 'B' lines are short, less than 1.0 cm in length, are parallel to each other and at right angles to the pleura. They are referred to as peripheral interlobular septa, and are seen most frequently in the lung bases. Kerley 'C' lines have been dropped, as they actually represent many B lines superimposed on each other. It is important to differentiate septal lines from vascular shadows. Kerley B lines are essentially visualized in the last 1 cm of lung parenchyma; lung vessels are not seen in the last 1 cm of the lung. Kerley A lines are differentiated from lung vessels as they are much thinner and do not branch.

Reticular and Reticulonodular opacities

Table 1.4: Reticular and reticulonodular opacities
1. Interstitial lung disease
2. Pulmonary oedema or pneumonia
3. Fever with reticular opacities—mycoplasmic or viral pneumonia
4. Lymphangitis carcinomatosis—unilateral reticular opacities
5. Tuberculosis, rarer causes include fungal disease (histoplasmosis), chronic hypersensitivity pneumonitis, ankylosing spondylitis
6. Sarcoidosis
7. Pneumoconiosis
8. Calcified opacities in both lung fields—miliary metastases due to thyroid carcinoma, osteogenic sarcoma, tuberculosis
9. High-density miliary nodules are observed in silicosis, baritosis, microlithiasis
10. Cloud-like punctate calcification is typically seen in alveolar microlithiasis
11. Conglomerate opacities with fibrosis and military nodules—progressive massive fibrosis with pneumoconiosis

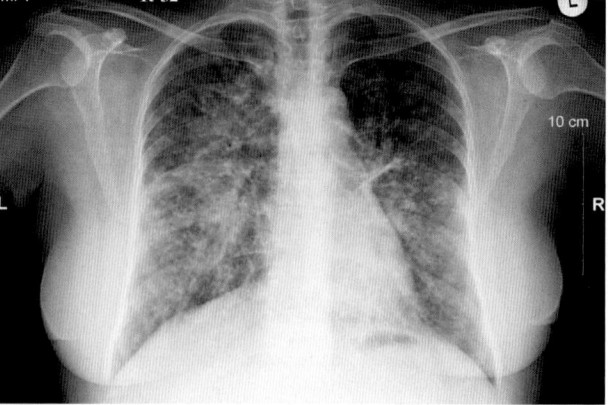

Fig 1.101: Sarcoidosis. PA view of chest reveals multiple small nodular lesions with reticular opacities in both lung fields, especially the perihilar regions. These features are strongly suggestive of sarcoidosis even in the absence of hilar adenopathy.

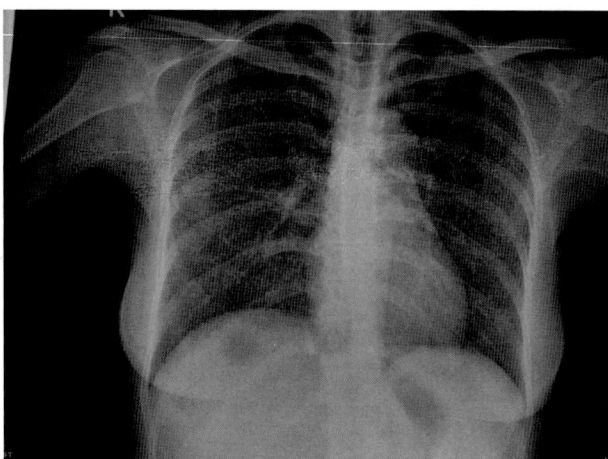

Fig 1.102: Miliary tuberculosis. PA view of the chest reveals multiple small nodules in both lung fields as a result of miliary tuberculosis.

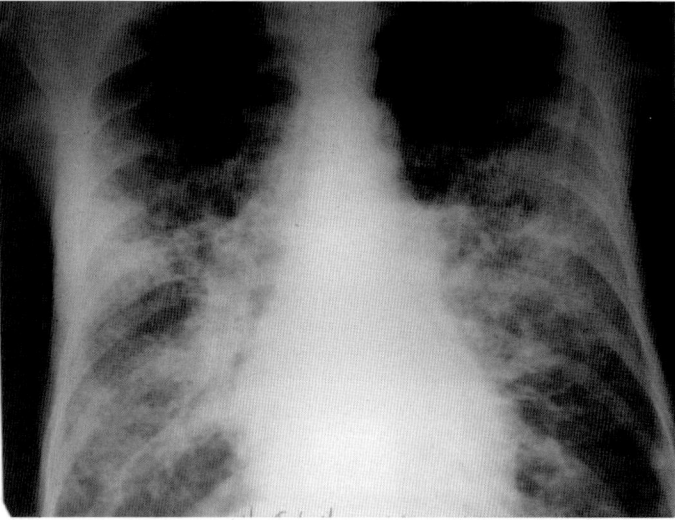

Fig 1.100: Interstitial pneumonia: PA view of chest reveals extensive reticular opacities and ill-defined areas of consolidation as a result of an interstitial pneumonia.

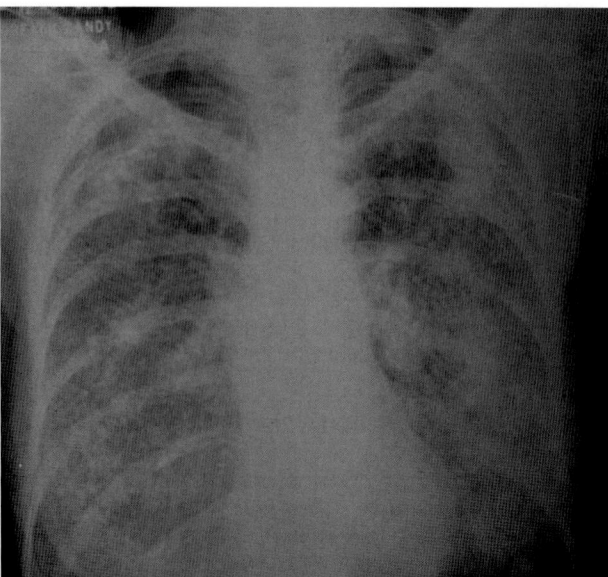

Fig 1.103: Alveolar microlithiasis. PA view of chest reveals extensive small nodular high densities in both lung fields. The very high density is typical of microlithiasis.

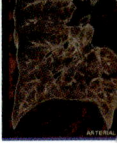

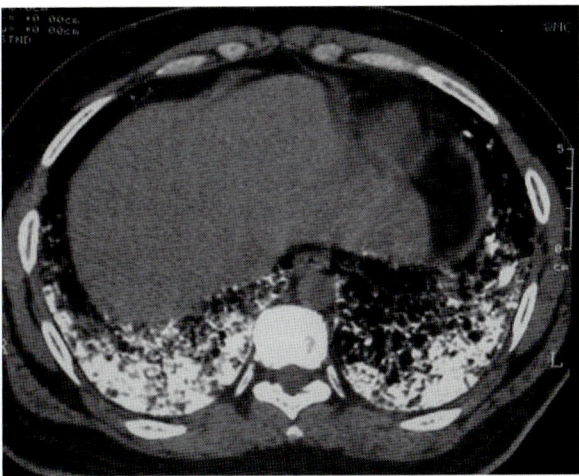

Fig 1.104: Alveolar microlithiasis: Relatively asymptomatic patient reveals on CT chest extensive small nodular high-density calcified lesions in both lung fields as a result of alveolar microlithiasis.

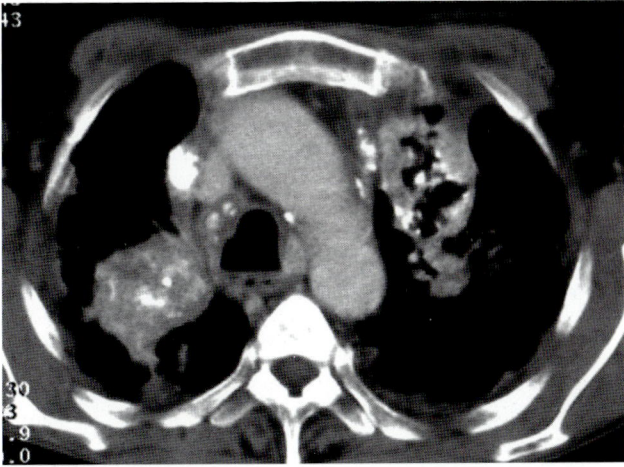

Fig 1.107: Progressive massive fibrosis: CT chest reveals ill-defined soft tissue mass lesions with internal calcification and cavitation in a patient with progressive massive fibrosis secondary to silicosis.

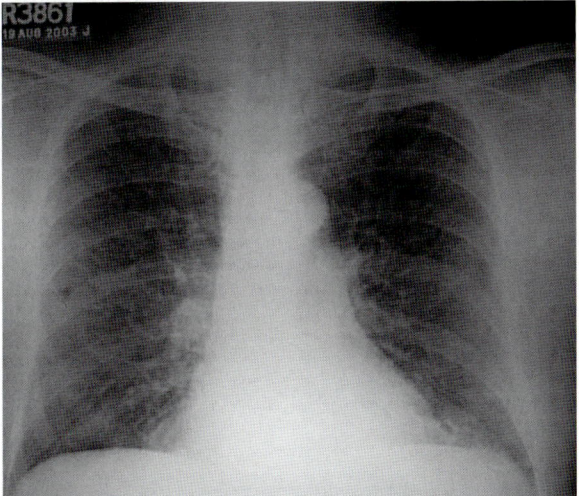

Fig 1.105: Reticular opacities: PA View of chest reveals reticular opacities in both lung fields particularly lung bases. HRCT revealed interstitial pulmonary fibrosis.

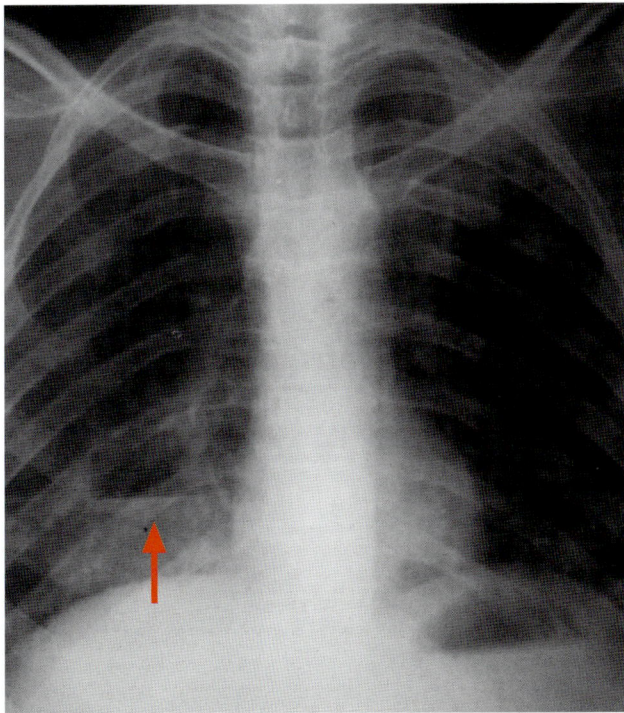

Fig 1.108: Lung abscess: PA view of chest in a patient with fever and expectoration reveals a well-defined rounded opacity with a fluid level in the right lower zone representing a lung abscess.

Unilateral Transradiancy of the Lung

The causes for unilateral transradiancy of the lung are:

1. Radiographic artifact   The radiographic output is usually adjusted to increase the output in the region of the bases as compared to the apices. This is known as a heel-toe effect. If this heel-toe effect is horizontally oriented rather than vertically, it will result in one hemithorax being overpenetrated. A similar effect occurs when the patient is

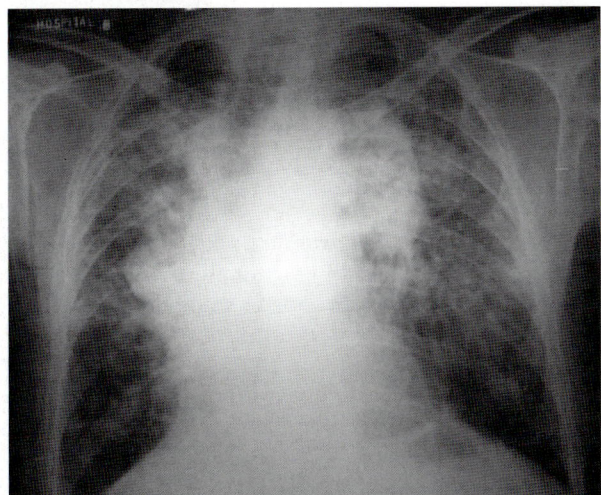

Fig 1.106: Progressive massive fibrosis: PA view of the chest reveals bilateral ill-defined parahilar mass lesions with multiple small ill-defined nodular lesions along the periphery of the lesion.

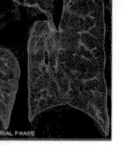

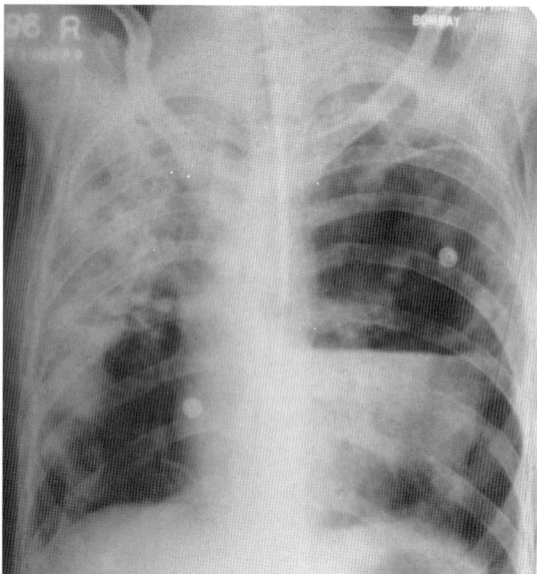

Fig 1.109: Wegener's granulomatosis: Chest X-ray reveals ill-defined areas of consolidation with nodular lesions in the right lung involving the upper and mid-zones. An air-fluid level is seen in the nodular lesion in the right mid-zone. There is evidence of large cavitation with an air-fluid level seen in the left mid-zone. c-ANCA was strongly positive confirming Wegener's granulomatosis.

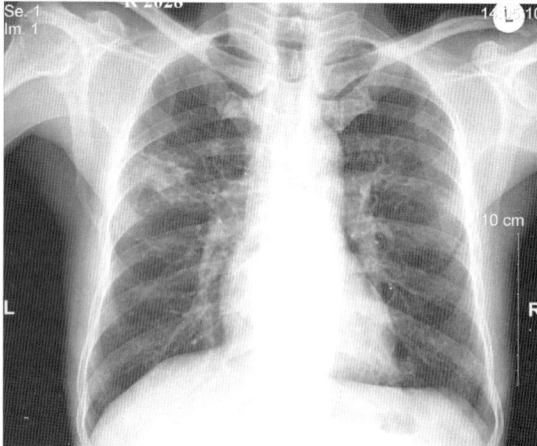

Fig 1.110: Pulmonary tuberculosis. PA view of the chest reveals ill-defined area of consolidation and cavitation in right upper lobe. The presence of cavitation and consolidation in the upper lobe in the Indian subcontinent favours the diagnosis of tuberculosis.

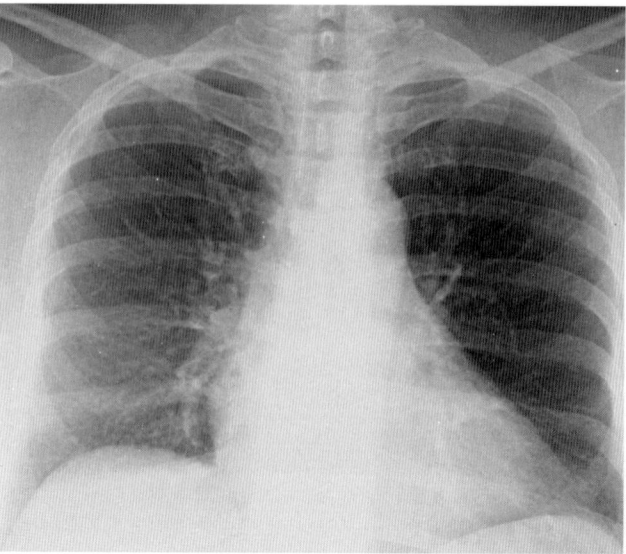

Fig 1.111: Unilateral mastectomy: PA view of chest, note left lung appears more translucent than right lung. This is because there is a mastectomy on the left side.

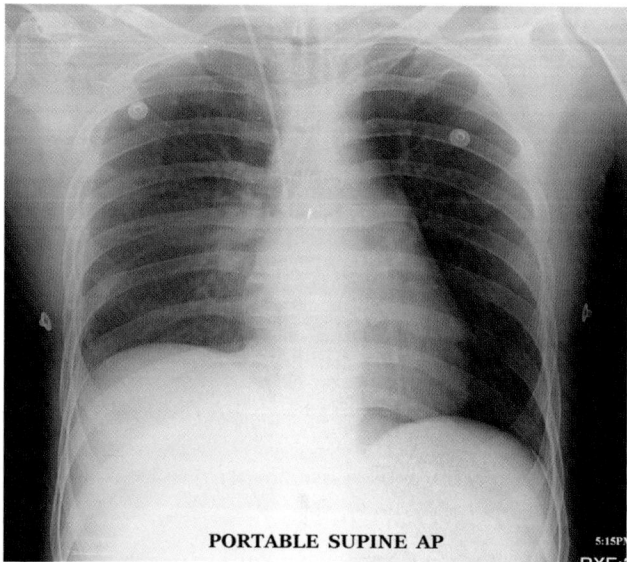

PORTABLE SUPINE AP

Fig 1.112: Unilateral Translucency—Frontal chest X-ray in supine position reveals uniform haziness of right hemithorax with transradiancy of left hemithorax. This is due to a right pleural effusion layering along the chest wall contributing to the right hemithorax opacity and consequent transradiancy of left hemithorax.

rotated. This can be detected by observing the soft tissue in relation to the shoulders; the penetration will be different.

2. Thoracic wall and soft tissue abnormalities
   Unilateral mastectomy or congenital absence of pectoralis muscle (Poland syndrome).

3. Overexpansion or increased translucency of one lung
   - Obstructive emphysema due to a foreign body, or intra-bronchial mass lesion
   - Compensatory emphysema due to severe lobar collapse or lobectomy
   - Pulmonary embolism involving one major pulmonary artery

   - Pleural effusion in a supine patient, causing an ipsilateral increase in density of the hemithorax, consequently the opposite hemithorax appears to be hypertranslucent.
   - Macleod's or Swyer James Syndrome.

4. Increased translucency of both lungs
   - Widespread transradiancy of both lungs may be seen in airway disease such as constrictive bronchiolitis, asthma and emphysema.
   - Obstruction of flow from right side of heart with a right to left cardiac shunt such as Fallot's tetralogy, Eisenmenger's syndrome, severe widespread pulmonary arterial stenosis and massive pulmonary embolism.

Solitary Pulmonary Nodule (SPN)

A pulmonary nodule is referred to as a spherical opacity with relatively well-defined margins with a diameter of up to 3 cm. Lesions more than 3 cm in size are considered as mass lesions. A well-defined spherical opacity below 1 cm in diameter is referred to as a small SPN.

With increasing use of MDCT and its high spatial resolution, small nodules are being detected with an increasing frequency. Though most are benign in aetiology, it is important to remember that 20–30% of lung cancers present as a solitary pulmonary nodule. One of the primary roles of imaging, beyond detection is to accurately differentiate malignant from benign lesions. It is important to obtain 3/5-mm sections as well as thin 1-mm sections through the lung on CT. The thinner sections help to reduce partial volume averaging so as to provide an accurate assessment of the internal contents and margins of the nodule. The thicker 3/5-mm sections are important as it is difficult to differentiate small SPN from vessels in thin 1-mm sections.

The first step in the radiological evaluation is to determine whether the nodule is pulmonary or extra-pulmonary, as the chest X-ray gives a 2D image. Skin, pleural or rib lesions can appear as an intrathoracic lesion. Lateral, oblique X-rays or a CT scan would help to localize the lesion. Once the lesion is confirmed to be intrapulmonary, the possibilities would essentially be an infective lesion, benign lesion or a malignant lesion. There is a significant overlap in the imaging appearances. To help differentiate, it is useful to look at the clinical and morphological features.

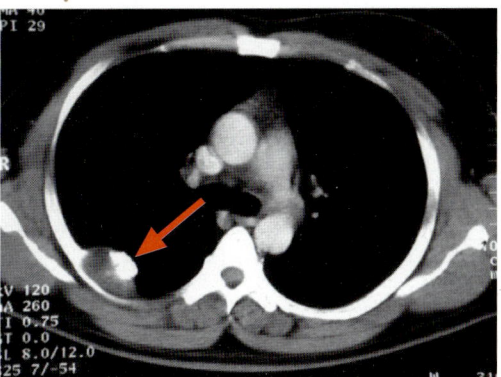

Fig 1.114: Solitary pulmonary nodule: CT demonstrates that the nodule demonstrated on the chest X-ray is not intrapulmonary. It arose from the posterior end of the rib with calcification along its anterior aspect. The histopathology revealed an enchondroma.

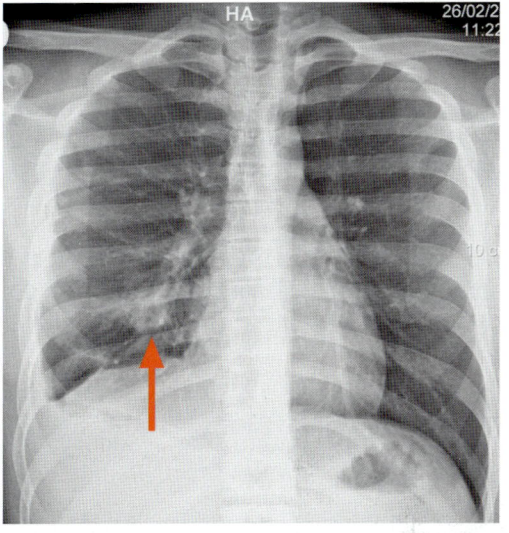

(a)

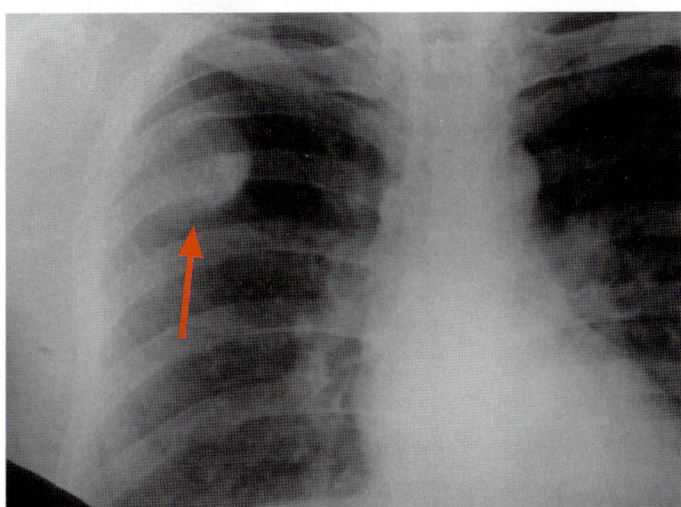

Fig 1.113: Solitary pulmonary nodule: Chest X-ray demonstrates a well-defined nodular lesion with calcification along its medial aspect in the right upper zone. The margins of the lesion appear to have obtuse angels with the chest wall, a sign suggesting that the lesion is extra-pulmonary.

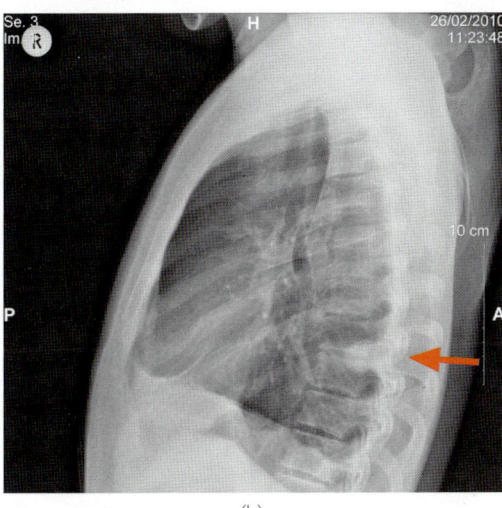

(b)

Fig 1.115: Solitary pulmonary nodule: (a) PA view demonstrates a solitary pulmonary nodule in the right lower zone (b) Lateral view demonstrates nodule is posterior, pleural base with a wide pleural attachment and with obtuse angles against the chest wall. These features favour a pleural/extra-pleural mass lesion rather than an intrapulmonary lesion.

Nodule Morphology

Calcification Presence of calcification in a pulmonary nodule is a useful sign to differentiate benign from malignant nodules. However, 13% of all lung carcinomas demonstrate calcification; only 2% less than 3 cm in size demonstrate calcification. The different types of calcification which may be visualized in

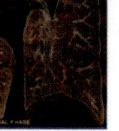

a pulmonary nodule are—concentric, popcorn, punctate/eccentric and uniform.

Concentric The calcification occupies the entire SPN or the entire periphery of the SPN in a laminated manner. This calcification is mainly seen in tuberculous and fungal infections.

Popcorn Calcification Multiple small rings or nodules of calcification which overlap are seen in hamartomas/cartilage tumours.

Punctate/Eccentric Calcification Punctate/Eccentric calcification is suspicious as it may be seen in infections and malignancies. A malignancy may engulf a calcified focus representing an old healed granuloma, with calcification appearing on the periphery of the lesion.

Uniform Calcification The entire SPN is calcified; this is typical of calcified granulomas.

SIZE
Most malignant nodules are larger than 2 cm in size, however 40% are less than 2 cm, 15% are less than 1 cm, 1% of malignant lesions are less than 7 mm in size. Most lesions above 3 cm are likely to be either bronchogenic carcinoma, lung abscess, Wegener's granulomatosis, lymphoma, round atelectasis, focal pneumonia, or hydatid cysts. It is difficult to detect a lesion less than 5 mm in diameter on a chest X-ray. If a lesion which is 5 mm or less is seen on a chest X-ray, it is invariably calcified.

SHAPE
A spiculated margin is very suggestive of carcinoma; the spicules represent spread into the interstitium of the lung. Lobulation

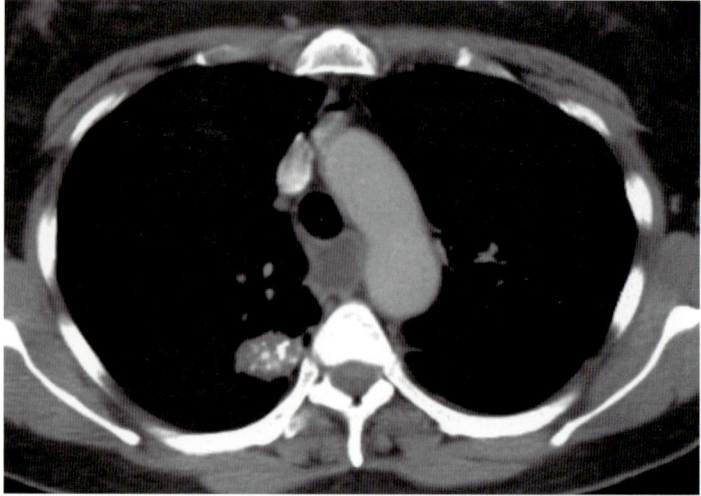

Fig 1.117: Solitary pulmonary nodule: CT chest demonstrates a well-defined nodule in the right upper lobe. There is a popcorn type of distribution of calcification typical of a hamartoma.

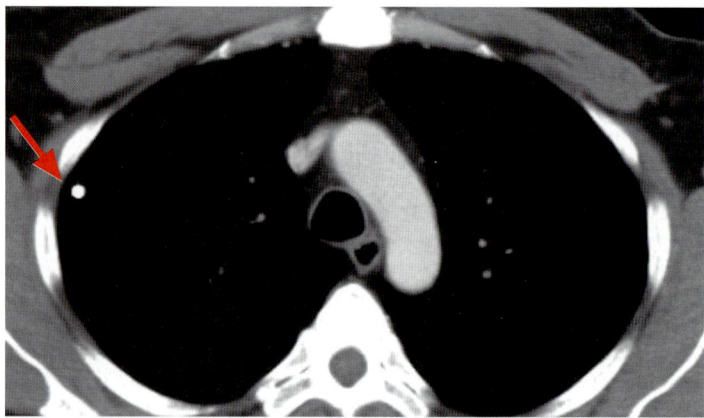

Fig 1.118: Solitary pulmonary nodule: CT chest demonstrates a well-defined pulmonary nodule in the right upper lobe. The nodule is densely calcified, representing a uniform type of calcification, indicating with certainty that the nodule is benign.

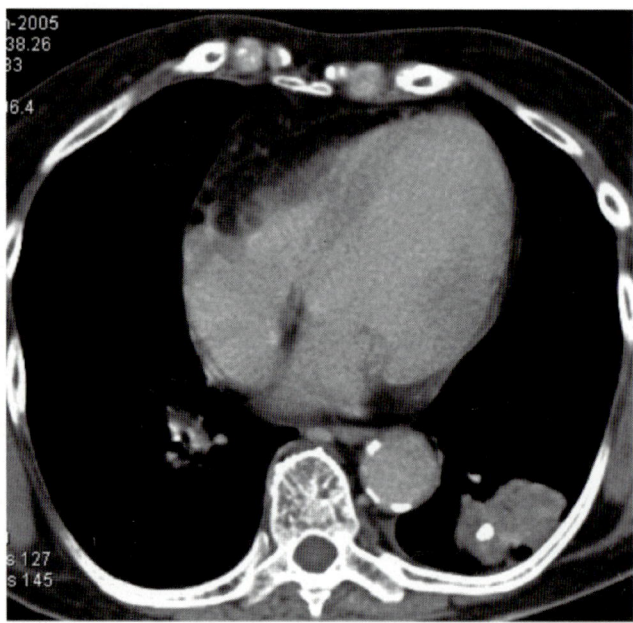

Fig 1.116: Solitary pulmonary nodule: CT chest reveals a nodular mass lesion in the left lower lobe with a calcific speck along its periphery, an example of an eccentric type of calcification. CT-guided biopsy revealed an adenocarcinoma. The calcific density represented an old granuloma which healed with calcification and was engulfed by the neoplasm.

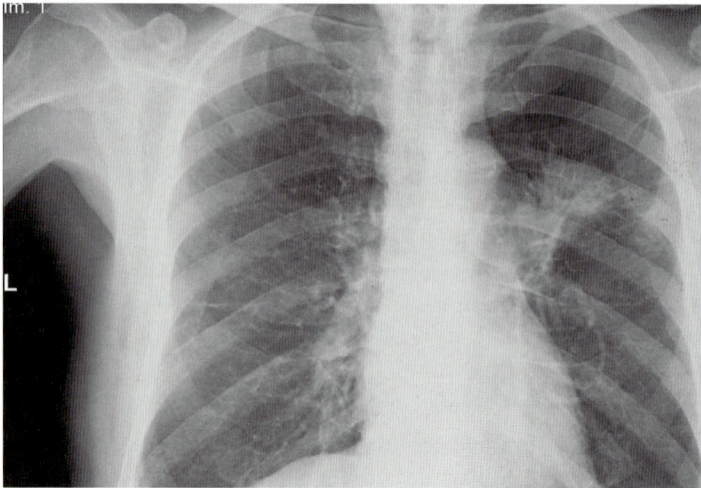

Fig 1.119: Solitary pulmonary nodule: Chest X-ray demonstrates a nodule in the left upper lobe. Note its spiculated margin, a relatively specific sign to indicate malignancy.

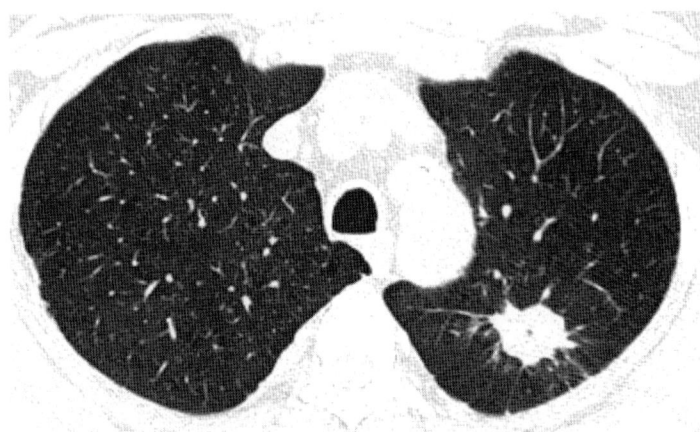

Fig 1.120: Solitary pulmonary nodule: CT chest demonstrates a nodular lesion in the left apex. There are multiple radiating bands arising from the surface of the nodule resulting in a spiculated appearance. This is typical of a malignant lesion. Rarely, an inflammatory lesion may demonstrate spiculation.

and notching which indicate unequal growth are suggestive signs for malignancy but may be seen in inflammatory lesions. There is considerable overlap in the findings between benign and malignant. A spiculated lesion though has a predictive value of 90% to be a malignant lesion. An inflammatory lesion with fibrosis may however have a similar appearance. Benign lesions usually have smooth margins. Conversely 20% of primary lung tumours have smooth margins; most metastatic lesions also have smooth margins.

CAVITATION

Cavitation occurs in inflammatory as well as primary and metastatic tumours. Benign lesions tend to have thinner and smoother walls as compared to malignant lesions, which have thicker and irregular walls.

FAT

Demonstration of fat within a solitary pulmonary nodule is pathognomic of a hamartoma, (50% of hamartomas demonstrate fat in the lesion). Rarely, lipoid pneumonia/metastatic liposarcoma or renal cell carcinoma metastasis may demonstrate fat densities.

SATELLITE NODULES

Multiple small peripheral nodules around an SPN is a very useful sign indicating a benign lesion, especially inflammatory in aetiology. It has a positive predictive value of 90%.

AIR BRONCHOGRAM

Presence of an air bronchogram does not exclude a neoplasm as this may be seen in a bronchoalveolar carcinoma or in lymphoma. Presence of an air crescent is useful to diagnose an aspergillioma.

CT HALO SIGN

Lung cancers can have a halo around them, though such halos may also be seen in inflammatory lesions, especially in invasive aspergillosis.

RATE OF GROWTH

Lung cancers take from 1 to 18 months to double in volume, the average time being 4.2–7.3 months. Volume doubling faster than one month suggests an infection/infarction/aggressive lymphoma. Doubling after 18 months is seen in granuloma/hamartoma/carcinoid/round atelectasis. A lesion which has not grown or has reduced in size in two years is likely to be benign. For a nodule to double in volume, the change in nodule diameter is approximately 26%. A 4-mm nodule which increases to 5 mm would have doubled in volume. Thus accurate measurements are critical in deciding doubling time. There is significant inter- and intra-observer variation in measurements, especially in spiculated lesions. The ideal method to evaluate growth is to evaluate volume, as an irregular-shaped structure is being measured. Automated volume measuring techniques are very useful in this setting. The problems of inter-/intra-observer variations are minimized, as all spiculated and irregular margins are taken into consideration for measurements. Most modern CT workstations have automated software that enables accurate measurements.

NODULE ENHANCEMENT AND METABOLISM

There are numerous reports in Western literature on the utility of contrast enhancement to differentiate between benign and malignant SPN. If the enhancement of a nodule following contrast enhancement exceeds 20 HU then it is most likely malignant, whereas if less than 15 HU it is most likely benign. Enhancement is determined by measuring HU values, post contrast after 1, 2, 3, 4 minutes. The peak HU value is subtracted from the pre-contrast HU value. Sensitivities of 98%, specificity of 73%, positive predictive value of 77%, and negative predictive value of 98% have been reported. However, these findings do not apply to patients in the Indian subcontinent as the most likely differential diagnosis of a malignant SPN is an inflammatory lesion (in particular a tuberculous lesion). A tuberculoma will enhance to a similar extent as a malignant

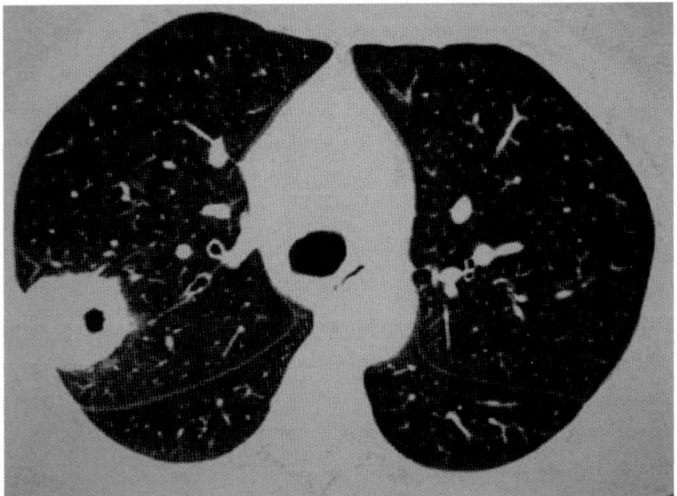

Fig 1.121: Solitary pulmonary nodule: CT chest reveals a well-defined nodular lesion in the right upper lobe abutting the pleura with internal cavitation, the margins of which are smooth. CT-guided biopsy revealed this lesion to be due to *Mycobacterium tuberculosis*.

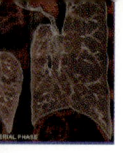

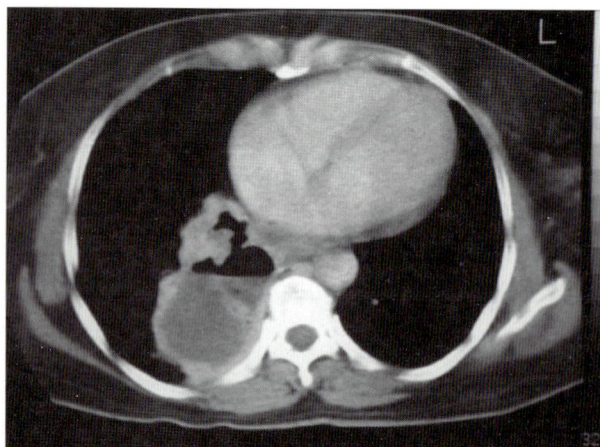

Fig 1.122: Solitary pulmonary nodule: CT chest reveals a large nodular lesion with internal necrosis and cavitation in the right lower lobe. The inner margins of the cavitation are irregular. CT-guided biopsy revealed a squamous carcinoma.

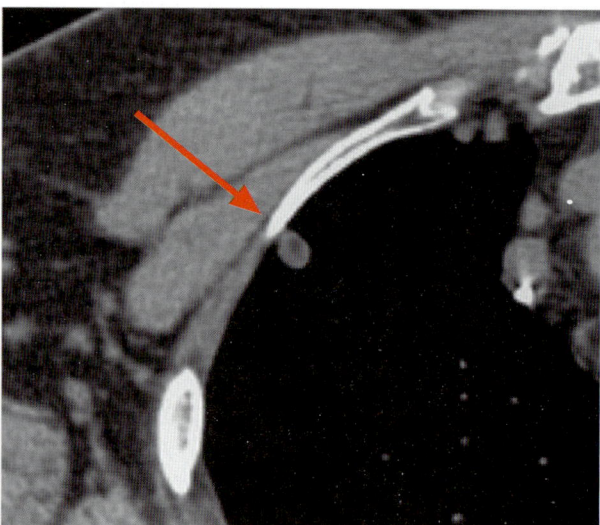

Fig 1.123: Solitary pulmonary nodule: CT chest reveals a small pulmonary nodule in the right chest anteriorly. There is a fat density within the lesion; this is typical of a hamartoma.

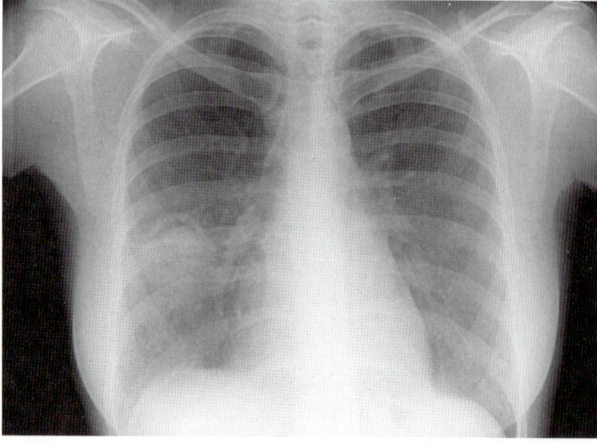

Fig 1.124: Solitary pulmonary nodule: Well-defined solitary pulmonary nodule in right mid-zone with an air crescent along superior surface of nodule. The air crescent indicates that the nodule represents a fungal ball in a cavity—aspergillioma.

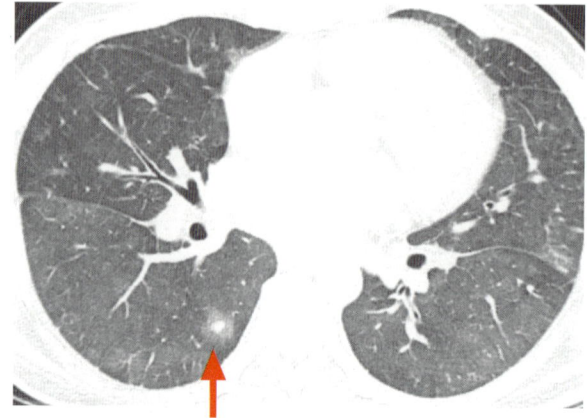

Fig 1.125: Solitary pulmonary nodule: HRCT demonstrates a well-defined nodule in the apical segment of the right lower lobe with an ill-defined halo of ground-glass around the nodule. This appearance is seen in invasive aspergilliosis.

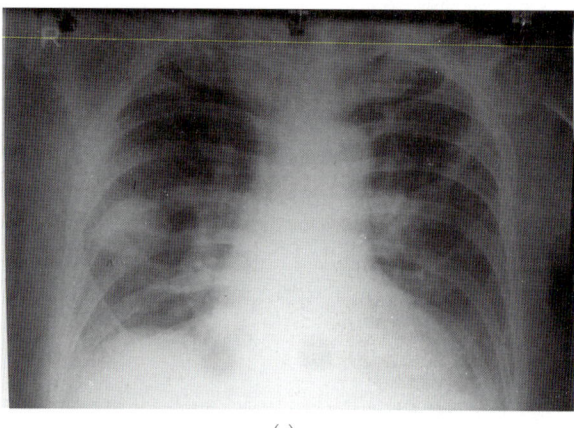

(a)

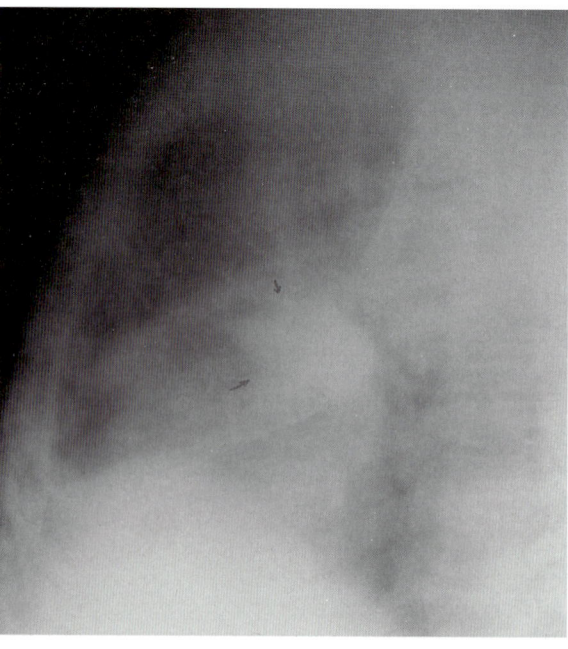

(b)

Fig 1.126: Solitary pulmonary nodule: (a) PA view of chest reveals a well-defined homogenous opacity in the right mid-zone (b) Lateral view reveals that opacity is a loculated effusion in the right minor fissure.

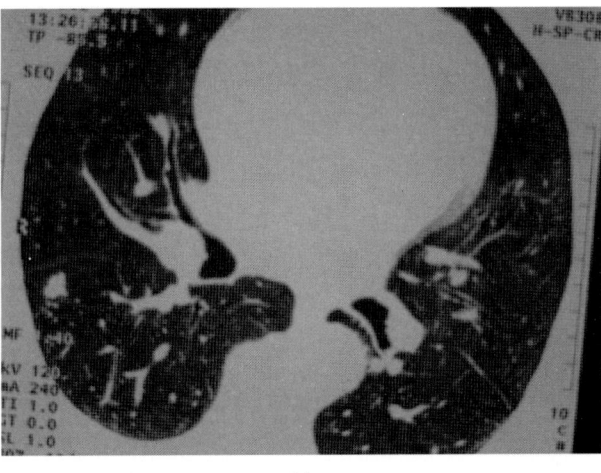

(a)

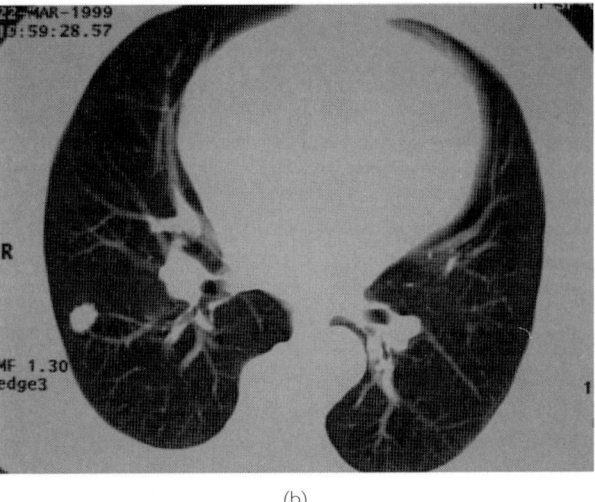

(b)

Fig I.127: Solitary pulmonary nodule: (a and b) CT chest studies done six months apart reveal progression in size of nodule. CT-guided fine needle aspiration cytology (FNAC) of lesion revealed a non-small-cell cancer. This is the most important sign in the evaluation of a pulmonary nodule (its progression in a short period of time). It indicates the need for further intervention, FNAC, biopsy or surgical excision.

nodule. For the same reason the FDG PET is insensitive in differentiating a malignant from a tuberculous or other inflammatory pathology. Further, PET can be quite insensitive in detecting pulmonary nodules, especially metastatic nodules, less than 1 cm in diameter.

HRCT Patterns of Diffuse Lung Disease

The detection and diagnosis of diffuse lung diseases is based on the demonstration and recognition of specific abnormal findings. These findings can be classified into essentially two groups, those with increased lung attenuation and those with decreased lung attenuation. Those with increased lung attenuation can be further subdivided into reticular opacities, nodular opacities and parenchymal opacification. Those with decreased lung attenuation can be subdivided into cystic lesions, emphysema, bronchiectasis, mosaic perfusion/attenuation and air trapping.

RETICULAR OPACITIES

Thickening of the interstitial fibre network of the lung by inflammation, fluid, fibrous tissue or neoplastic infiltration results in linear/reticular opacities. Thickening of the axial interstitium results in thickening of the interstitium along the walls of the bronchovascular structures. Since bronchial walls and vessels have similar densities, it is difficult to differentiate the interstitial thickening from the underlying bronchovascular structures. Consequently, the appearances are of thickening of the bronchial wall and an increase in the vessel diameter.

Thickening of the peripheral interstitium is easy to demonstrate, as septal thickening is seen in the subpleural regions, marginating the secondary pulmonary nodule, and interlobular interstitium. This is manifested as radiating bands extending perpendicular to the pleural surface.

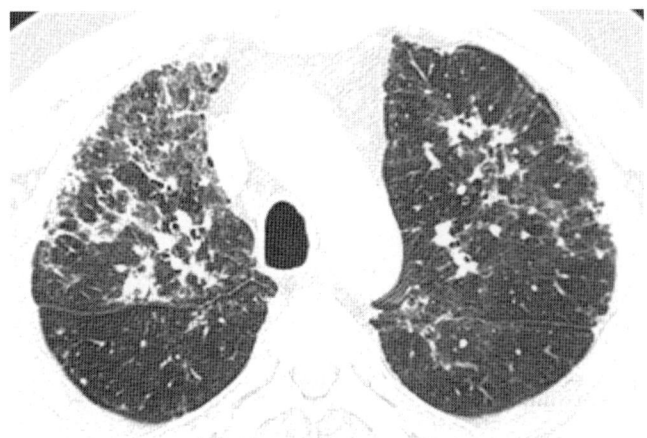

Fig I.128: Peribronchovascular interstitial thickening: The vessels appear to be prominent in size with irregular surfaces. This is due to peribronchovascular interstitial thickening. There is extension of the interstitial thickening extending peripherally into the subpleural regions.

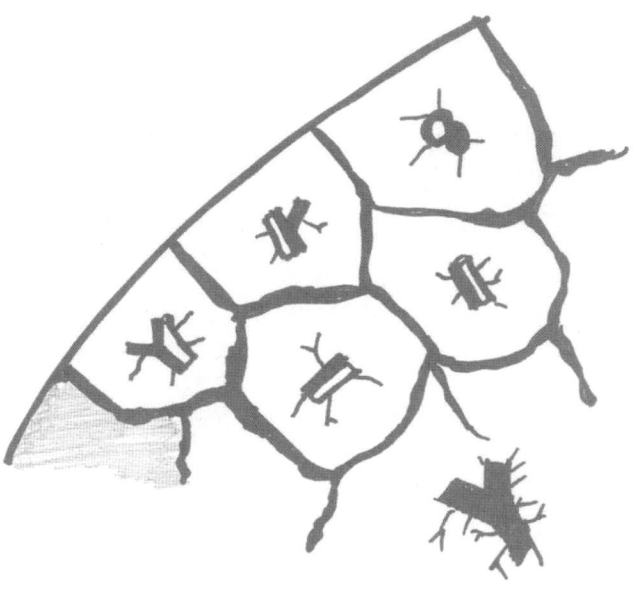

Fig I.129: Interlobular interstitial thickening: Schematic diagram of secondary lobules demonstrates thickening of walls of secondary lobule as well as centrilobular interstitium.

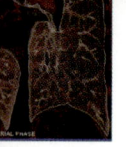

Thickening of the intralobular interstitium, which lies within the secondary lobule, is seen as a fine haze of linear opacities or may appear as ground-glass opacities.

The interstitial thickening may be smooth, nodular or irregular. Smooth thickening is seen in pulmonary oedema, lymphangitis carcinomatosis. Nodular thickening is seen in lymphangitis carcinomatosis, sarcoidosis. Irregular septal thickening is seen mainly in patients with lung fibrosis. Extensive peribronchovascular fibrosis can result in large conglomerate masses of fibrous tissue as seen in sarcoidosis, silicosis, tuberculosis and talcosis. Subtle peribronchovascular interstitial thickening may be difficult to detect.

Involvement of the peribronchovascular interstitium predominantly is seen in non-specific interstitial pneumonias

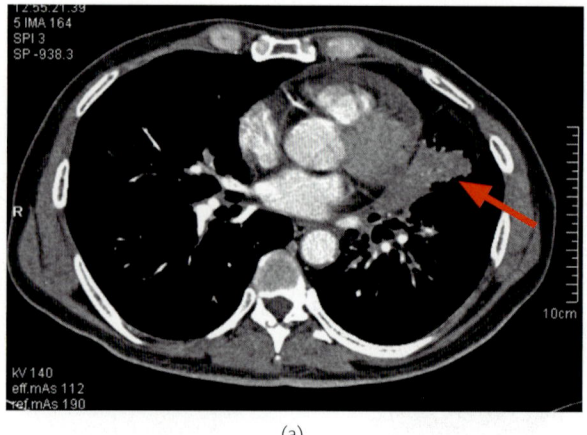

(a)

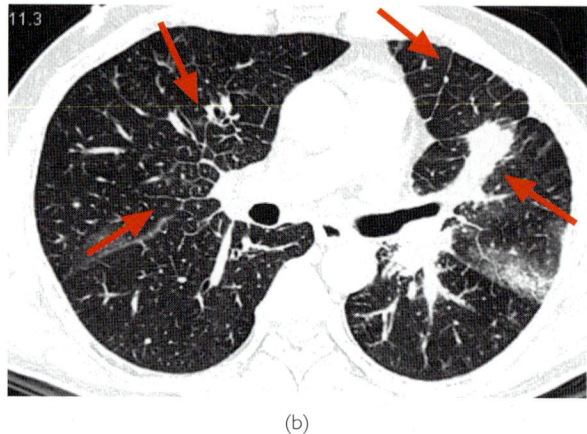

(b)

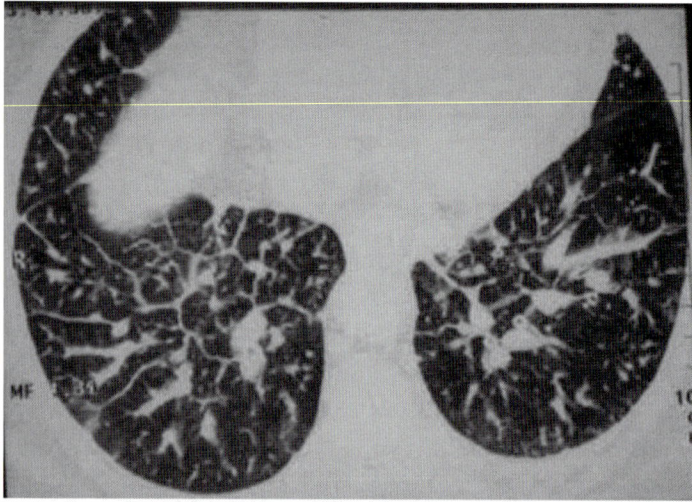

Fig 1.130: Interlobular interstitial thickening: HRCT in a patient with lymphangitis carcinomatosis reveals smooth thickening of the interlobar interstitium. The walls of the secondary lobule are thickened, the internal architecture is preserved, demonstrating the anatomy of the secondary lobule very well.

Fig 1.132: Smooth interstitial thickening: CT chest (a) demonstrates an ill-defined mass lesion in the lingula flush with the pericardium. CT-guided FNAC revealed an adenocarcinoma. HRCT (b) reveals smooth septal thickening from the surface of the mass lesion, this represents lymphatic infiltration by the mass lesion. Smooth septal thickening is also present in the right middle lobe with preservation of the secondary lobule. This is due to lymphangitis carcinomatosis secondary to haematogenous spread.

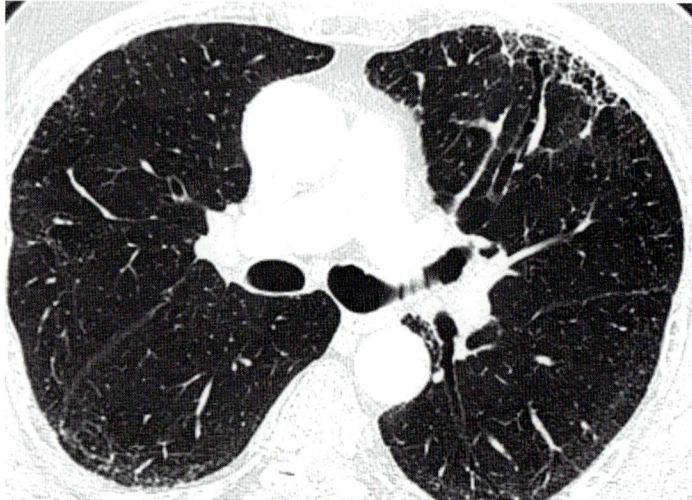

Fig 1.131: Intralobular interstitium: HRCT demonstrates thin lace-like reticular opacities in the left upper lobe anteriorly with thin-walled cysts as well as traction bronchiectasis. The lace-like reticular opacities represent interstitial thickening in the interlobular interstitium; the cystic air spaces represent bronchiolectasis. Similar but less marked changes are seen posteriorly bilaterally. The interstitial fibrosis was due to usual interstitial pneumonia (UIP).

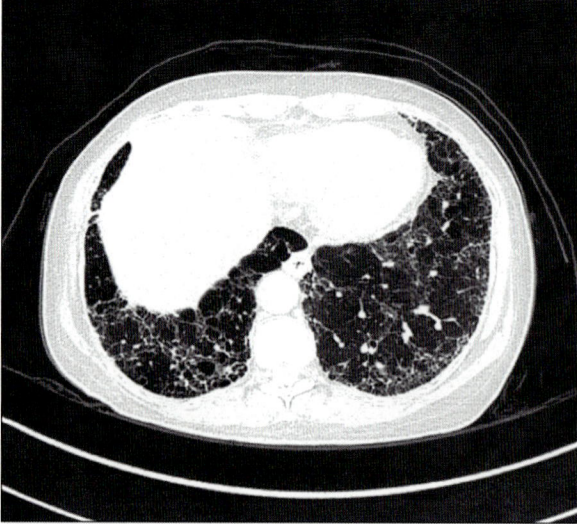

Fig 1.133: Irregular septal thickening: HRCT demonstrates irregular interstitial thickening in both lung bases posteriorly in a subpleural and peribronchovascular location as is seen in usual interstitial pneumonia.

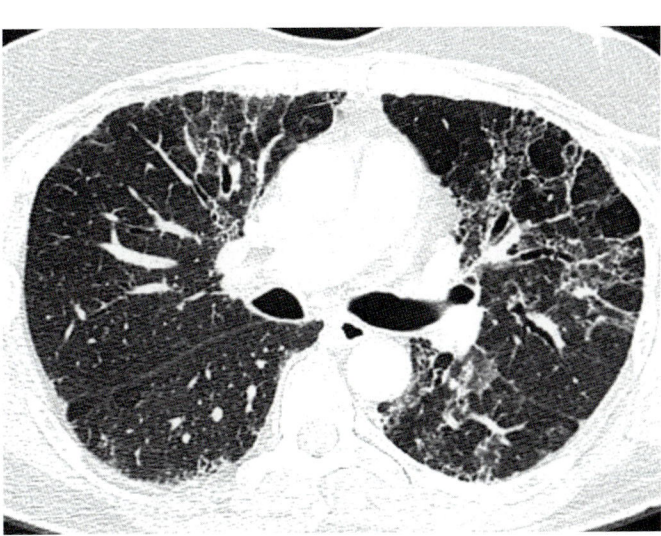

(a)

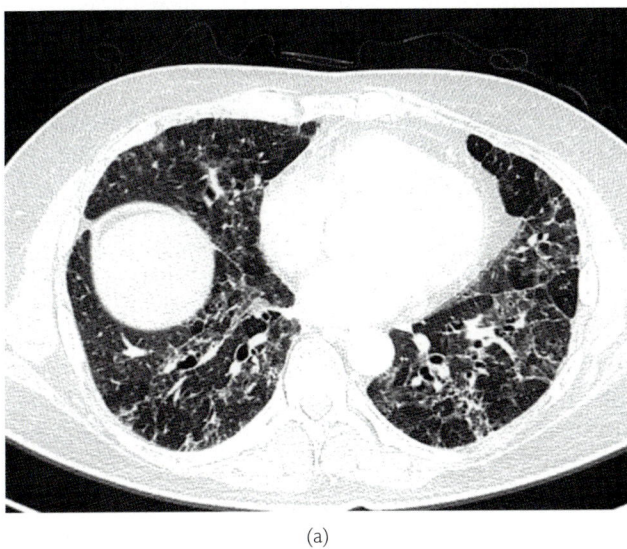

(a)

Fig 1.134: Fibrotic NSIP: (a & b) Extensive interstitial thickening in the lungs anteriorly in the upper lobes and posteriorly in the lung bases. The predominant interstitial thickening is in the peribronchovascular interstitium and not in the subpleural regions.

(NSIPs) as compared to predominantly subpleural interstitial thickening seen in usual interstitial pneumonia. Another differentiating feature is the lack of honeycombing, seen typically in UIP. Also in UIP, there are no significant ground-glass densities and parenchymal opacification which are seen in the cellular variety of NSIP.

Axial Interstitium

In patients with irregular interstitial thickening, fibrotic tissue along the bronchial walls causes traction resulting in **traction bronchiectasis**. A similar involvement of the peripheral bronchioles is termed traction bronchiolectasis. The dilated bronchi have a varicose or a corkscrew appearance.

When there is involvement of the terminal bronchioles, the bronchioles may dilate to occupy the entire secondary lobule,

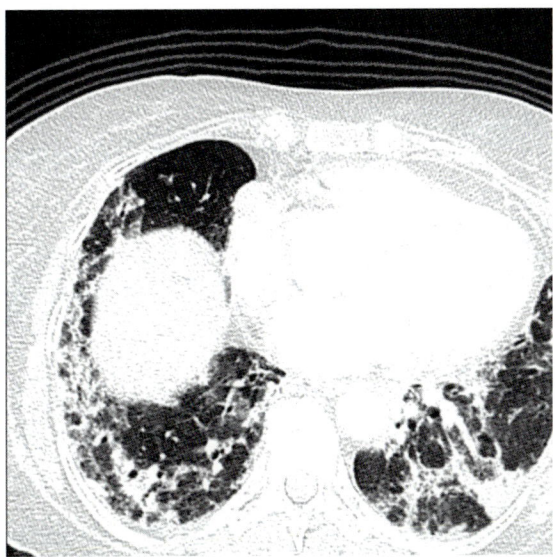

Fig 1.135: Cellular NSIP: HRCT demonstrates ill-defined areas of air-space opacification in the peribronchovascular and subpleural regions of both lung bases. There are no honeycomb changes. In view of the parenchymal opacification, lack of honeycomb changes, and significant fibrotic lesions this would represent the cellular variety of non-specific interstitial pneumonia.

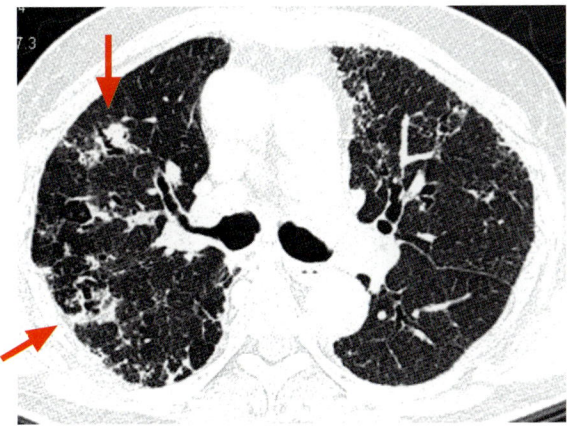

Fig 1.136: Traction bronchiectasis: HRCT demonstrates peribronchovascular interstitial thickening as evidenced by thickening and irregularity of vessels and bronchial walls. There is focal dilatation and irregularity of the bronchi secondary to peribronchial interstitial thickening, representing traction bronchiectasis.

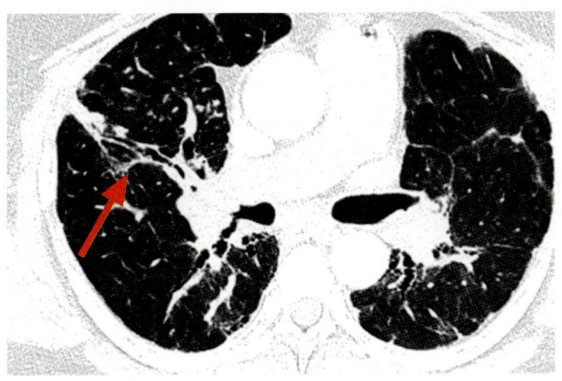

Fig 1.137: Traction bronchiectasis: HRCT demonstrates peribronchovascular interstitial thickening with consequent traction bronchiectasis.

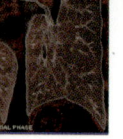

resulting in honeycomb cysts. On HRCT, honeycomb cysts are usually 1.0 cm or more in diameter with thin walls in the subpleural regions. These honeycomb cysts share their walls and occur in several contiguous layers. Honeycombing indicates end-stage lung disease. The location of honeycombing is important in the differential diagnosis of chronic ILD. If the honeycombing

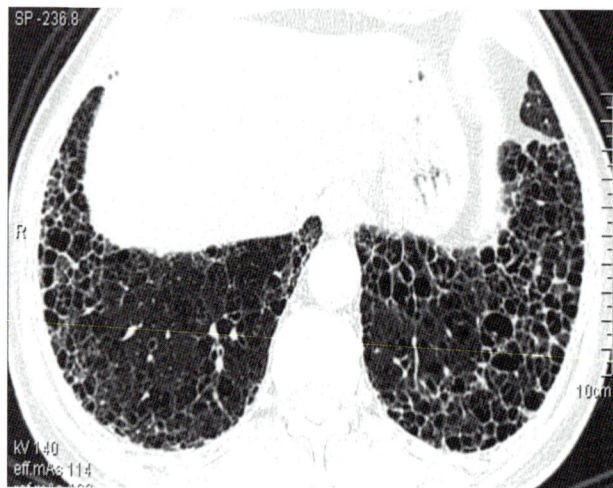

Fig 1.138: Honeycomb cysts: Extensive honeycomb cysts are seen in both lung fields especially the left.

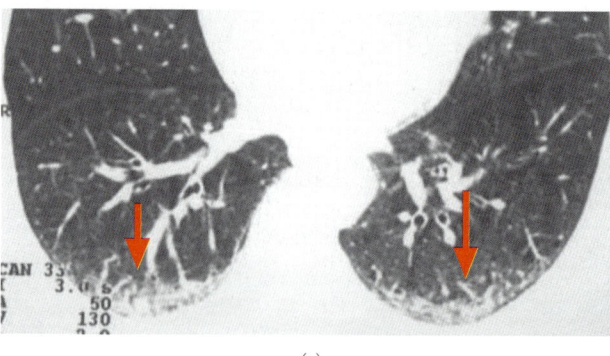

(a)

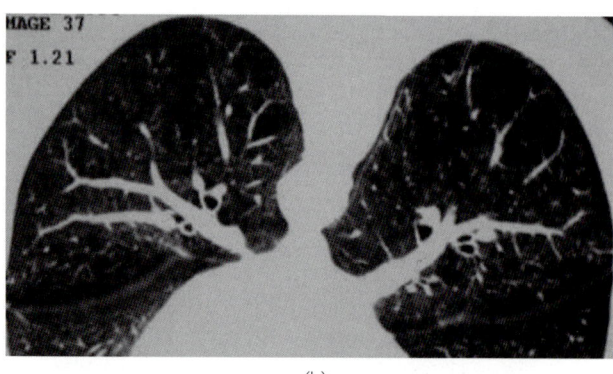

(b)

Fig 1.139: Dependent densities: Supine HRCT reveals ill-defined opacities in the lung bases posteriorly. (a) These appear as reticular opacities due to interstitial fibrosis. Prone scans at the same level (b) demonstrate that the opacities have resolved. These opacities in the lung base on a supine scan represent basal atelectasis. It is important to obtain prone scans in all patients with basal posterior opacities to exclude basal atelectasis.

is basal and posterior with associated significant fibrosis and architectural distortion, the diagnosis is UIP. If honeycomb cysts are seen in the upper zones the possibility of sarcoid should be considered; if in the mid-zone with a patchy distribution, the diagnosis of chronic hypersensitivity pneumonitis should be entertained. Anterior honeycomb cysts with fibrosis are seen in ARDS since the posterior portions of the lungs are protected by collapse/consolidation and are therefore not exposed to the deleterious effects of mechanical ventilation

Nodular Opacities

A nodule is defined as a rounded opacity which can be well- or ill-defined. A small nodule is one which is less than 1.0 cm; a large nodule varies in size between 1.0 and 3.0 cm; nodules above 3.0 cm are termed as masses.

Small nodules are of two types, interstitial and air-space. Interstitial nodules are well-defined and discrete, as seen in sarcoidosis, miliary tuberculosis, silicosis and metastatic lesions. Air-space nodules tend to be ill-defined and conglomerative. Air-space nodules may have a soft tissue density or demonstrate a diffuse ground-glass haze. Examples of air-space nodules are seen in exudative bronchiolitis. Despite these differences in appearance, it is often difficult to differentiate interstitial from air-space nodules on HRCT. The distribution of nodules is extremely useful in establishing the differential diagnosis. Nodules may be perilymphatic, random or centrilobular in distribution. Perilymphatic nodules occur in relation to the lymphatics/interstium i.e. in relation to the perihilar bronchovascular interstitium, interlobular septae, subpleural interstitium. The subpleural distribution of nodules is best demonstrated in relation to fissures. These small nodules in the subpleural regions may coalesce to form pseudo plaques along the pleura. These nodules may also coalesce to form large conglomerative masses. Satellite nodules may be seen in relation to these conglomerative masses giving the appearance of a galaxy. This pattern is seen in sarcoidosis, silicosis/coal workers pnuemoconiosis, lymphangitic carcinomatosis, lymphoproliferative disorders. These diseases demonstrate different patterns of perilymphatic involvement, allowing a distinction.

SARCOIDOSIS

Nodules are seen essentially in relation to the peribronchovascular interstium and subpleural regions. The central bronchovascular structures and fissures have a nodular appearance. An upper lobe preponderance is common, with the lung involved in a patchy asymmetric fashion, groups of nodules occurring in one region, normal lung in other regions.

SILICOSIS/CWP

Nodules are distributed in a subpleural and centrilobular location, rarely in a peribronchovascular location as compared to sarcoidosis. Nodules tend to be more evenly distributed as compared to sarcoidosis.

LYMPHANGITIC CARCINOMATOSIS

There is smooth thickening of the peribronchovascular and interlobular interstitium. Nodules are seen in relation to these thickened septae. The involvement may be unilateral, patchy or bilateral and symmetric.

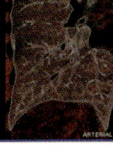

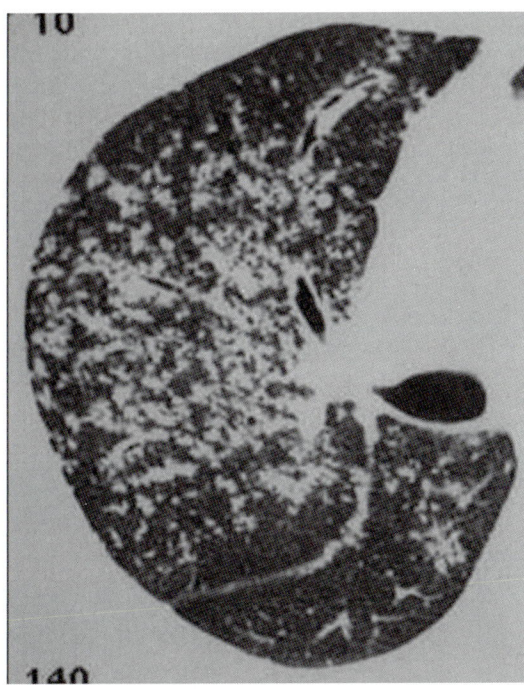

Fig 1.140: Perilymphatic nodules: HRCT demonstrates extensive nodules in a peribronchovascular location along the vascular surfaces as well as the fissures. As the vessels are white and the nodular areas also white, the appearance is of a nodular surface of the vessels.

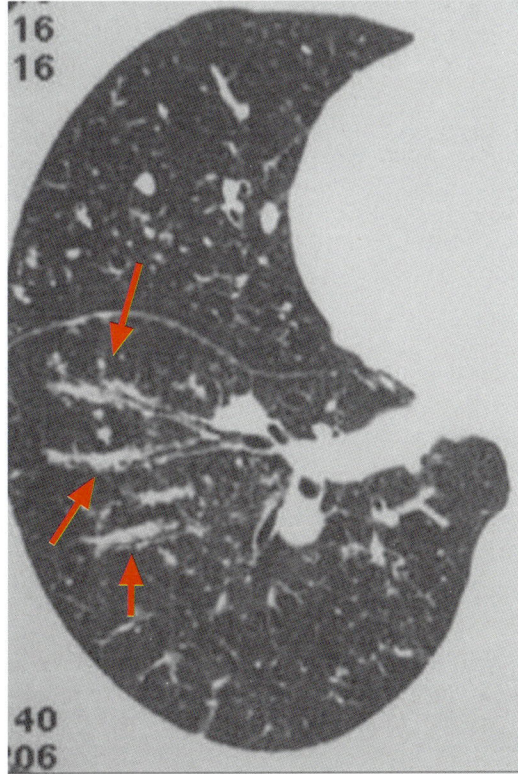

Fig 1.141: Perilymphatic nodules: HRCT demonstrates multiple small well-defined nodules along the surface of the bronchi and vessels. The vessels have a beaded appearance. These represent interstitial nodules along the peribronchovascular interstitium.

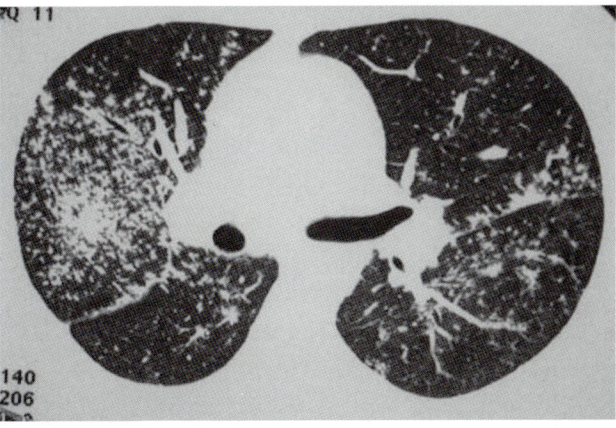

Fig 1.142: Sarcoidosis: HRCT demonstrates multiple small nodules in an interstitial location, along the fissures, vessels and bronchi as well as in the subpleural regions. The distribution is asymmetric and essentially perilymphatic. The nodules are seen to conglomerate in the right middle lobe with a number of satellite nodules resulting in an appearance akin to a galaxy. This distribution pattern is typical of sarcoidosis.

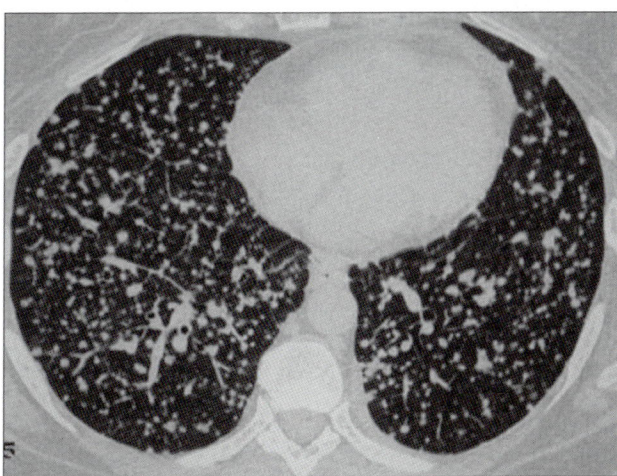

Fig 1.143: Silicosis: HRCT demonstrates multiple small well-defined nodules distributed evenly in both lung fields. These nodules are along the vessels, fissures and in the subpleural regions, i.e. perilymphatic in location. As compared to the asymmetric distribution of nodules in sarcoidosis the distribution is uniform in silicosis.

Patterns of Distribution of Nodules

RANDOM

The distribution is uniform with no predilection for any anatomic structures, bilateral and symmetric as seen in miliary tuberculosis, haematogenous metastasis, fungal infection.

CENTRILOBULAR

Ill-defined small nodules are centred on the centrilobular structures of the secondary pulmonary lobule.

Nodules which are predominantly centrilobular in location are most likely secondary to bronchiolar/peribronchiolar inflammation resulting in infiltration or fibrosis of the surrounding interstitium and alveoli. Angiocentric diseases may also manifest as centrilobular nodules. Bronchiolar diseases manifesting as centrilobular nodules are endobronchial spread of tuberculosis,

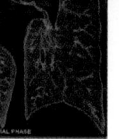

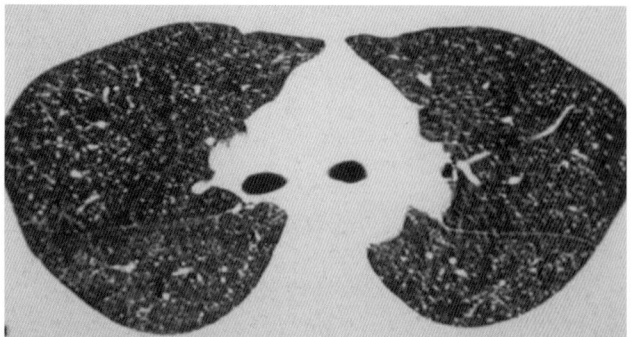

Fig 1.144: Miliary tuberculosis: HRCT demonstrates multiple small nodules in a random distribution. There is no predilection for any anatomic structure; the distribution is uniform. This is typically seen in military tuberculosis.

non-tuberculous mycobacterial infections, granulomatous infections, bronchopneumonia, panbronchiolitis, bronchiectasis, ABPA, hypersensitivity pneumonitis, Langerhans' cell histiocytosis, respiratory bronchiolitis, endobronchial spread of neoplasm. Angiocentric nodules are due to pulmonary oedema and pulmonary haemorrhage.

Centrilobular nodules due to bronchiolar inflammation may have a tree-in-bud appearance; as the bronchioles dilate and are filled with inspissated mucus, a branching pattern is visualized.

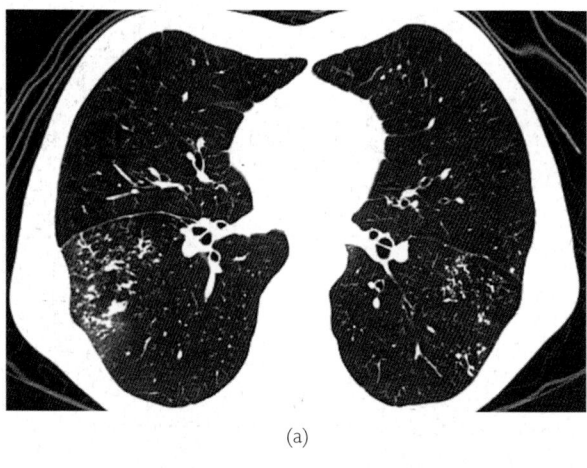

(a)

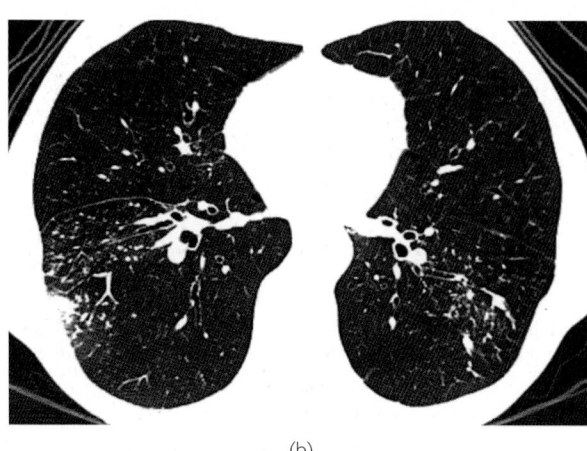

(b)

Fig 1.145: Centrilobular nodules: (a and b) HRCT demonstrates multiple small ill-defined nodular lesions in a centrilobular location.

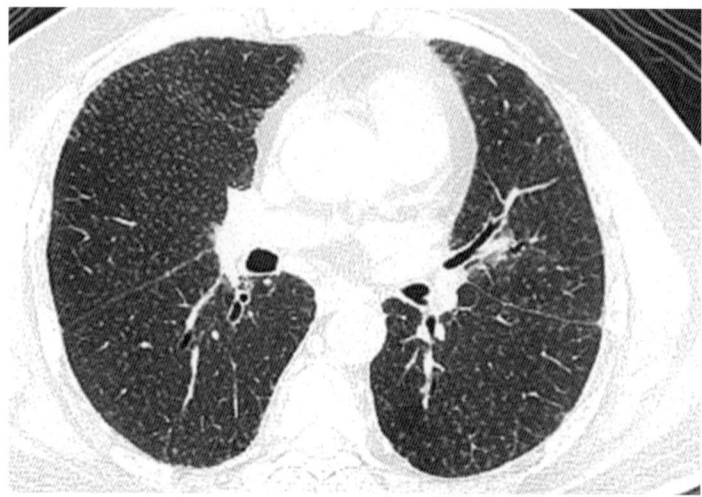

Fig 1.146: Hypersensitivity pneumonitis: HRCT demonstrates multiple small nodules in both lung fields distributed uniformly, evenly spaced, representing centrilobular nodules due to hypersensitivity pneumonitis.

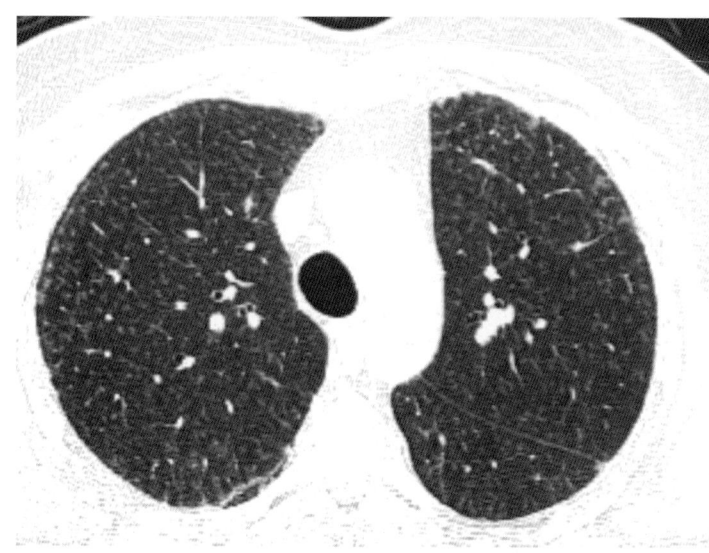

Fig 1.147: Respiratory bronchiolitis: HRCT demonstrates multiple small pulmonary nodules in both lung fields. These nodules are evenly spaced at the centres of the secondary lobule. These represented nodules due to respiratory bronchiolitis.

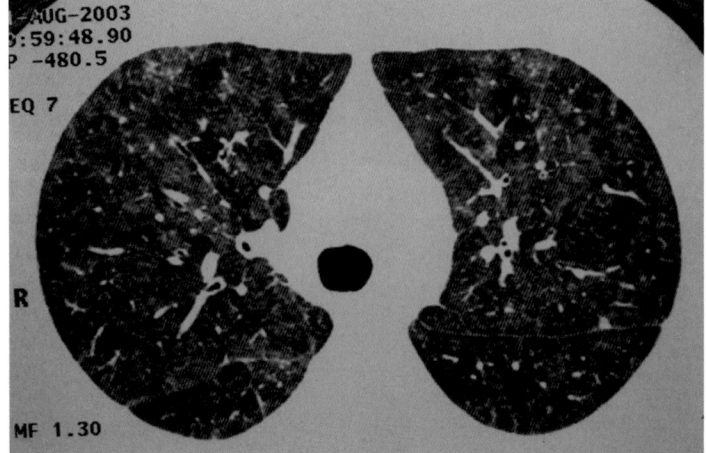

Fig 1.148: Ground-glass pattern of parenchymal opacification. Note vessels are visualised in areas of increased lung attenuation.

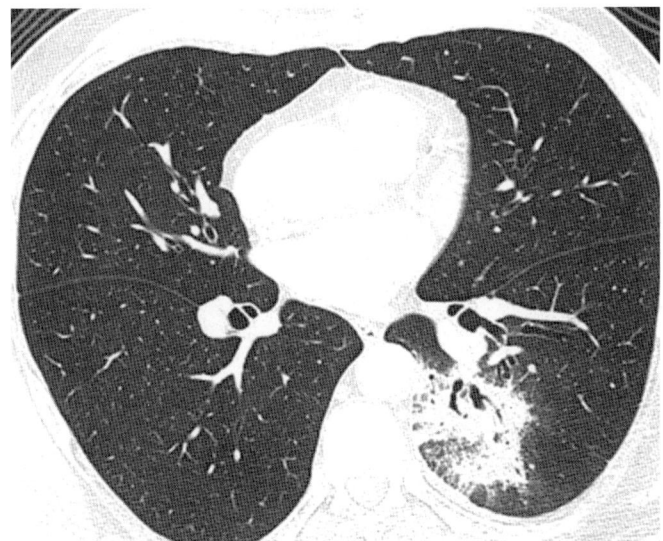

Fig 1.149: CT chest showing consolidation in the left lower lobe with air bronchogram. Note vessels are visualised in areas of increased lung attenuation, indicating consolidation.

Parenchymal Opacification

Diffuse or multifocal increase in lung attenuation is a common finding on HRCT in patients with chronic lung disease. Increased lung opacity may be ground-glass or consolidation. These represent varying degrees of parenchymal opacification, depending upon whether the vessels are obscured or not by the parenchymal opacification. Ground-glass opacity is an area of parenchymal opacification not associated with obscuration of the underlying vessels. Parenchymal consolidation obscures the vessels.

Ground-glass opacity results from either fluid, inflammatory material within the alveoli/interstitium or the presence of fine interstitial fibrosis in the intralobular interstitium of the secondary lobule. The distribution is usually geographic with areas of spared lung interspersed with areas of affected lung. Detection of ground-glass opacity is of significance as this indicates an ongoing active as well as potentially treatable process. Since ground-glass opacity may also be a manifestation of intralobular interstitial thickening, presence of significant areas of fibrosis/lung destruction in other regions would indicate that the ground-glass densities are more likely due to intralobular fibrosis.

Pitfalls in Diagnosis of Ground-Glass Opacity

There is a reduction in the amount of air in the alveoli during expiration; consequently there is an increase in lung attenuation, mimicking the appearance of ground-glass densities. It is useful to check the shape of the trachea to determine whether the scan has an adequate inspiratory effort. If the posterior tracheal surface is seen to bulge into the tracheal lumen, it is an expiratory scan rather than inspiratory. The diagnosis of ground-glass opacity is essentially subjective, based on quantitative assessment of lung attenuation. It is important to maintain consistent window settings. Using too low a window mean with a narrow window width may give an appearance of ground-glass densities. Similar appearances may occur with a wider window width without

changing the window mean. A useful tip is to see the air in the trachea or bronchi. If the air appears grey rather than black, the apparent increase in attenuation of lung parenchyma is usually not genuine. In patients with patchy areas of emphysema or air-trapping, normal lung regions may appear as areas of increased attenuation due to the contrast with darker areas. This can be avoided by using consistent window settings. Additionally in regions of normal lung attenuation, air bronchograms are not visualized as seen in areas of ground-glass density. Expiratory images are also useful in confirming lucent areas to represent areas of emphysema or air-trapping.

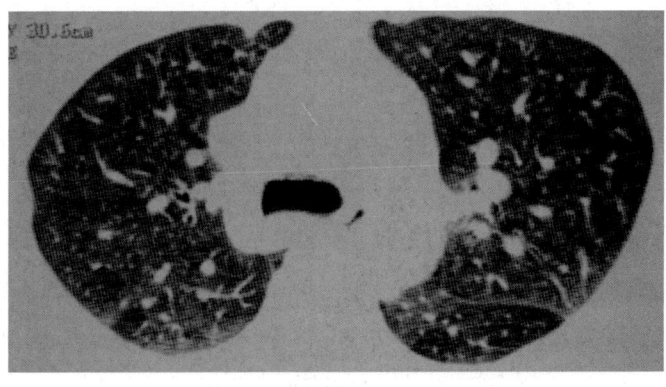

(a)

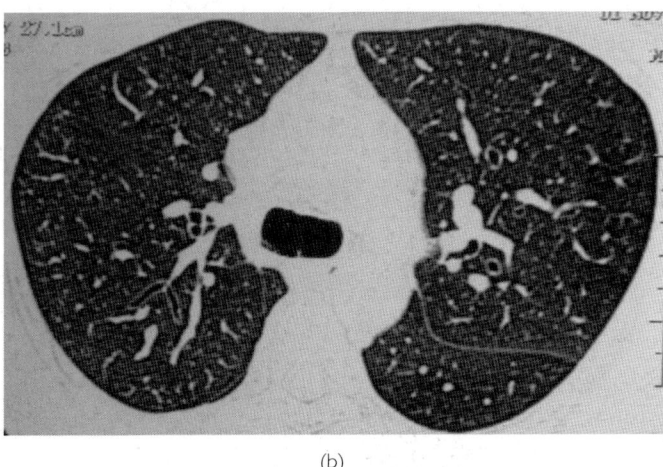

(b)

Fig 1.150: Pitfall in diagnosis: HRCT (a) reveals ill-defined ground-glass densities in both lung fields. Note shape of trachea; the posterior wall is bulging inwards showing that this is an expiratory scan (b) HRCT in deep inspiration in same patient at same level. Note trachea is well-distended and there are no ground-glass densities.

Differential Diagnosis of Ground-Glass Densities

A large number of diseases may be associated with ground-glass opacities on HRCT as the pathological processes in the early stages are similar. These disease processes may be acute, subacute or chronic. Acute disease processes manifesting as ground-glass densities include acute interstitial pneumonia, diffuse alveolar damage, pulmonary oedema, ARDS, pulmonary haemorrhage, pneumonia and early radiation fibrosis. Subacute/chronic disease processes include interstitial pneumonias, especially NSIP, DIP,

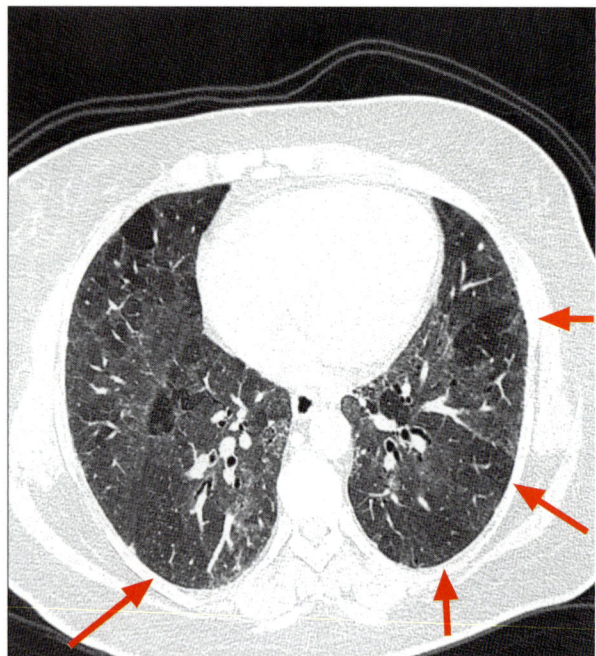

Fig 1.151: Hypersensitivity pneumonitis: Diffuse ground-glass densities with focal areas of air-trapping are seen in both lung fields. This combination of ground-glass densities and focal areas of air-trapping are typical of hypersensitivity pneumonitis. The air-trapping is secondary to endobronchial granulomas.

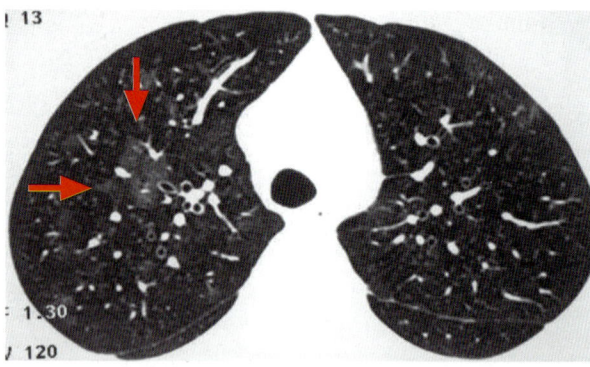

Fig 1.152: Hypersensitivity pneumonitis: HRCT reveals ill-defined areas of ground-glass densities.

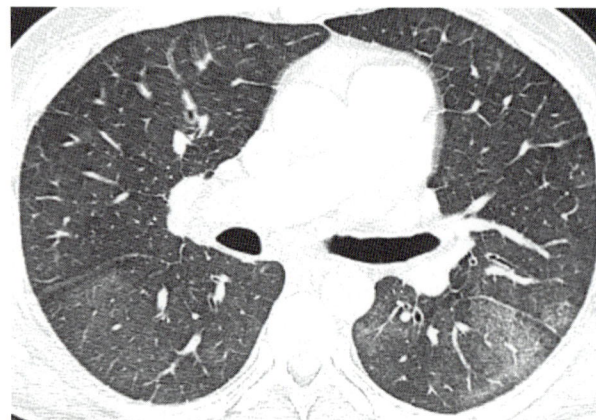

Fig 1.153: *Pneumocytis carinii* pneumonia: Seropositive patient presented with fever and dyspnoea. HRCT revealed diffuse ground-glass densities indicative of PCP. Confirmed on bronchoalveolar lavage.

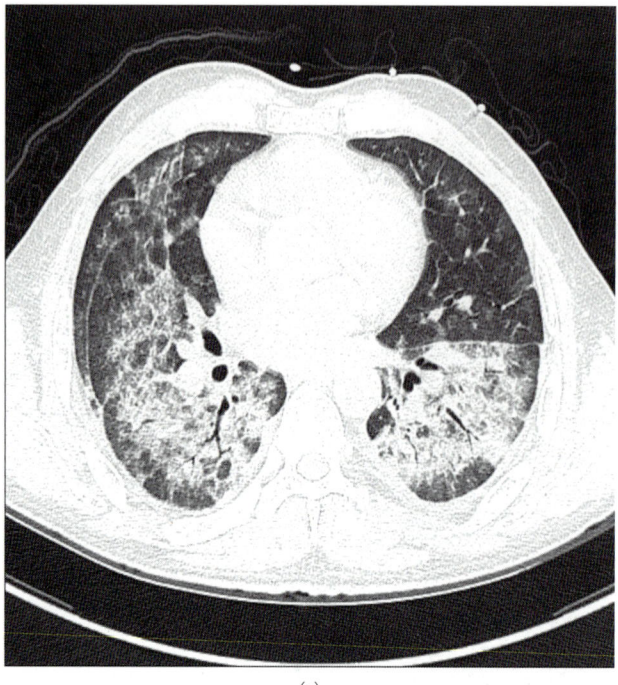

(a)

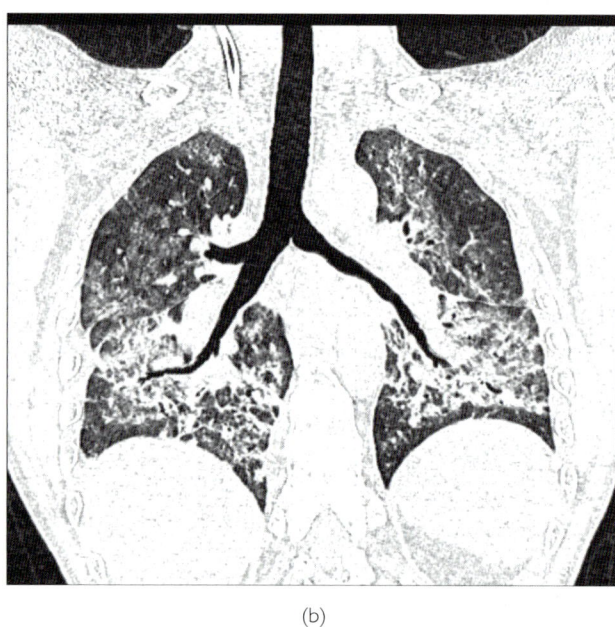

(b)

Fig 1.154: Acute interstitial pneumonia: (a) axial and (b) coronal reconstructions in an acutely breathless patient demonstrates ill-defined areas of increased lung attenuation on HRCT chest.

respiratory bronchiolitis, interstitial lung disease, hypersensitivity pneumonitis, drug reactions, chronic eosinophilic pneumonia, Churg-Strauss syndrome, lipoid pneumonia, sarcoidosis and alveolar proteinosis.

Decreased Lung Attenuation

Pathological processes with decreased lung attenuation may be due to lung cysts, emphysema, bronchiectasis, mosaic attenuation or air-trapping.

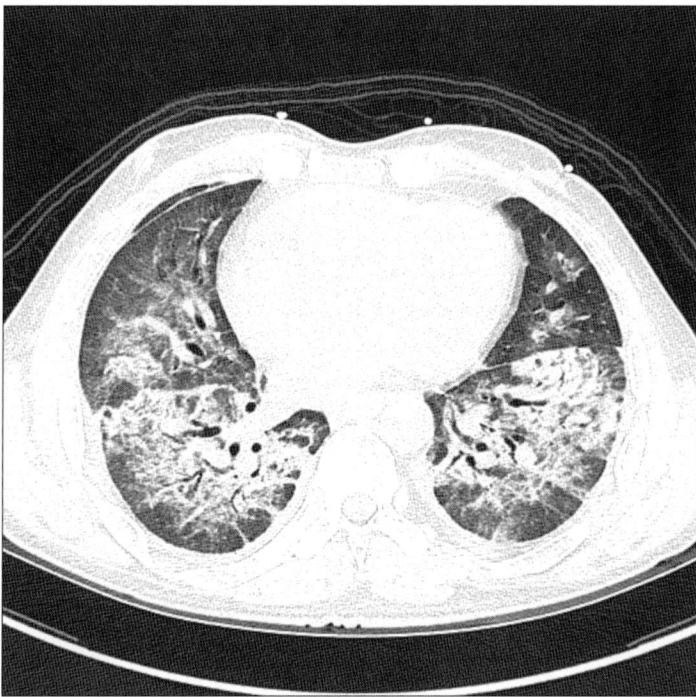

Fig 1.155: Diffuse alveolar damage: Drug-induced diffuse alveolar damage seen on HRCT as diffuse ill-defined areas of increased lung attenuation in both lung fields.

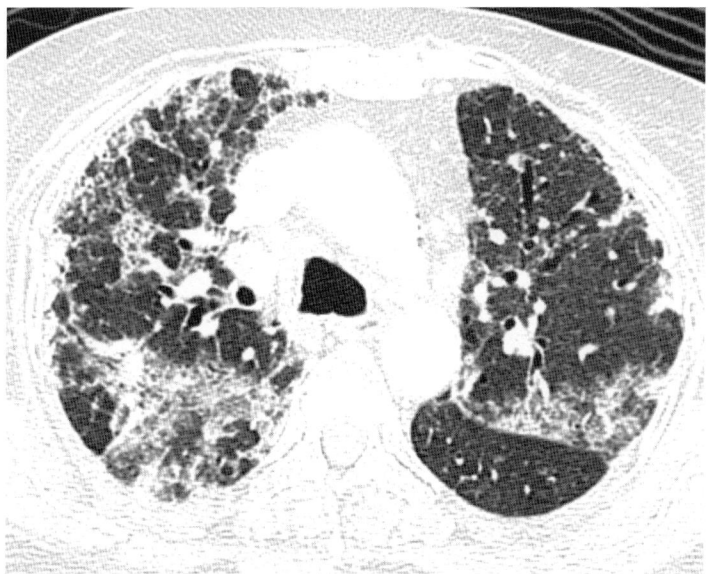

Fig 1.156: Desquamative interstitial pnuemonia: HRCT in a chronic smoker reveals ill-defined areas of parenchymal opacification in the subpleural and peribronchovascular regions. Thoracoscopic biopsy revealed desquamative interstitial pneumonia.

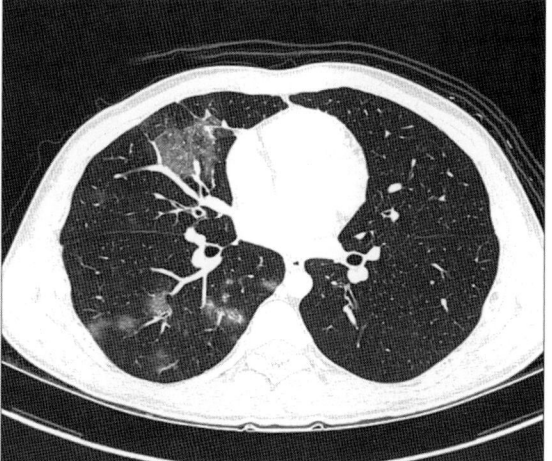

Fig 1.157: Alveolar haemorrhage: HRCT in a patient with haemoptysis demonstrates ill-defined areas of ground-glass density in right middle lobe as well as right lower lobe. The ground-glass densities were due to alveolar haemorrhage.

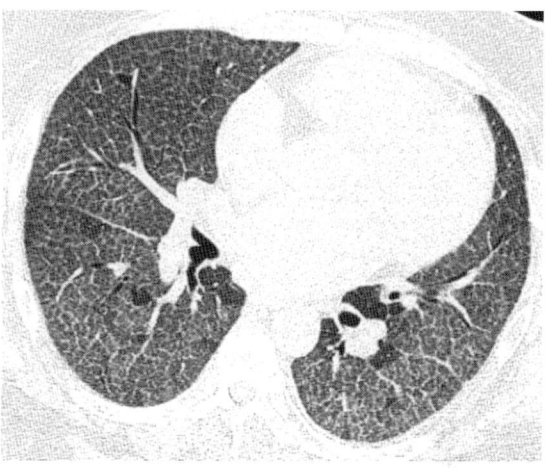

Fig 1.158: Alveolar proteinosis: HRCT reveals ill-defined ground-glass densities in both lung fields with a background of septal thickening. This appearance simulates a crazy pavement appearance, most commonly seen in alveolar proteinosis.

EMPHYSEMA

This is a result of permanent abnormal enlargement of air-spaces with destruction of their walls distal to terminal bronchioles. On HRCT emphysema appears as focal or diffuse areas of decreased attenuation compared to normal lung parenchyma. By modifying the window settings of HRCT (600 to -800 window mean) emphysema can be very well demonstrated. Emphysema is essentially of four types:

1. *Centrilobular*—this occurs predominantly in the upper lobes with lung destruction around the centrilobular arterial branches resulting in lucencies grouped around the centres of the secondary pulmonary lobule. With more severe destruction the appearances resemble panlobular emphysema. Centrilobular emphysema occurs in cigarette smokers due to enzymatic destruction of lung parenchyma as there is an imbalance between lung proteases and antiproteases.

2. Panlobular emphysema—This is characterized by uniform destruction of the pulmonary lobule leading to widespread areas of low attenuation. The pulmonary vessels appear fewer and thinner in appearance, termed as a diffuse simplification of lung architecture. Panlobular emphysema occurs in individuals with alpha-protease inhibitor deficiency and as an extension of centrilobular emphysema in cigarette smokers.

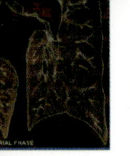
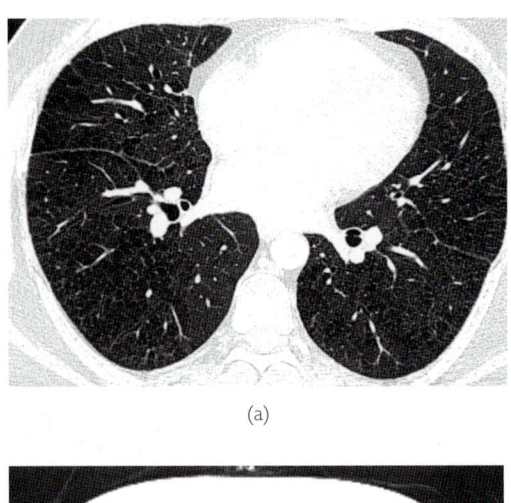

(a)

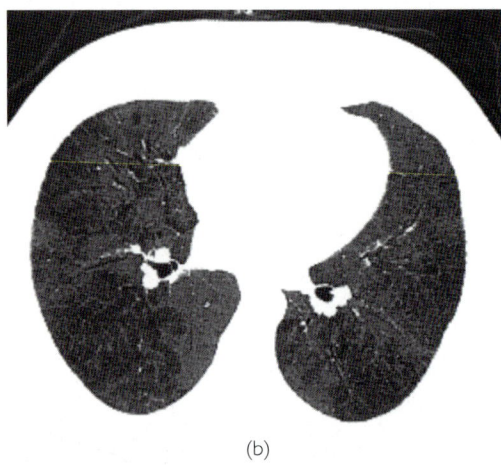

(b)

Fig 1.159: Centrilobular emphysema: (a) multiple thin-walled air spaces in both lung fields due to centrilobular emphysema (b) These are well demonstrated on Minimum Intensity Projection.

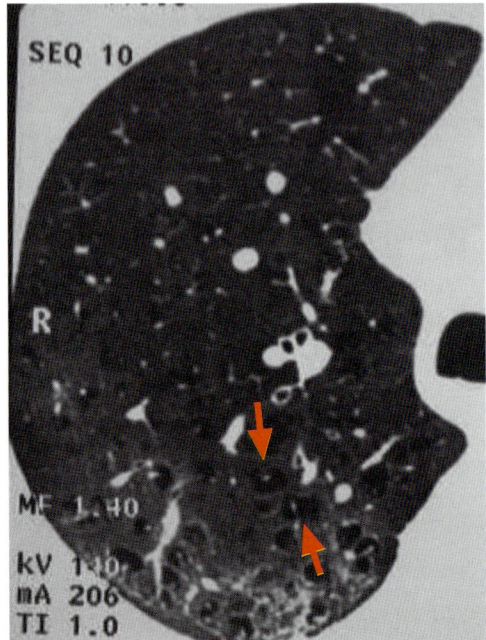

Fig 1.160: Centrilobular temphysema: Multiple well-defined air spaces are seen with a central vessel within. These findings are typical for centrilobular emphysema. Lung destruction is seen to be occurring around the centrilobular vessel.

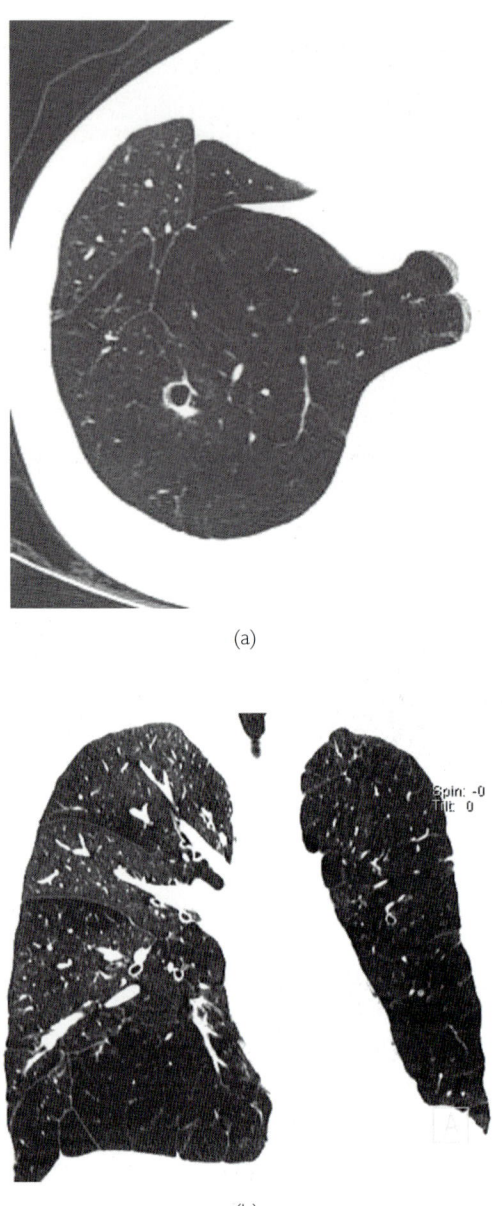

(a)

(b)

Fig 1.161: Panacinar emphysema: (a) Axial and (b) coronal HRCT images demonstrate large area of lung destruction seen in right lower zone. The density of the lung parenchyma is reduced and there is considerable thinning and separation of the vessels.

3. Paraseptal emphysema—The area of destruction involves the alveolar ducts and alveolar sacs marginated by the interlobular septa. On HRCT there are subpleural cysts which share thin walls. These cysts may become fairly large and reach up to a size of 1.0 cm. Paraseptal emphysema may be confused with honeycomb cysts, as both are in a subpleural location. Honeycomb cysts tend to be in several contiguous layers as compared to paraseptal emphysema which tends to occur in a single layer. Additionally, lung fibrosis usually accompanies honeycomb cysts, whereas other forms of emphysema such as centrilobular and panacinar may be present with paraseptal emphysema. Honeycomb cysts tend to be in the lung bases as compared to paraseptal emphysema which tends to be in the upper lobes.

4. *Bullous emphysema* is characterized by large bullae, often associated with centrilobular/paraseptal emphysema.

Bulla represents a sharply demarcated area of emphysema measuring 1.0 cm or more in diameter with a thin wall not more than 1 mm. They may range up to 20 cm in diameter but generally range between 2 and 8 cm in diameter.

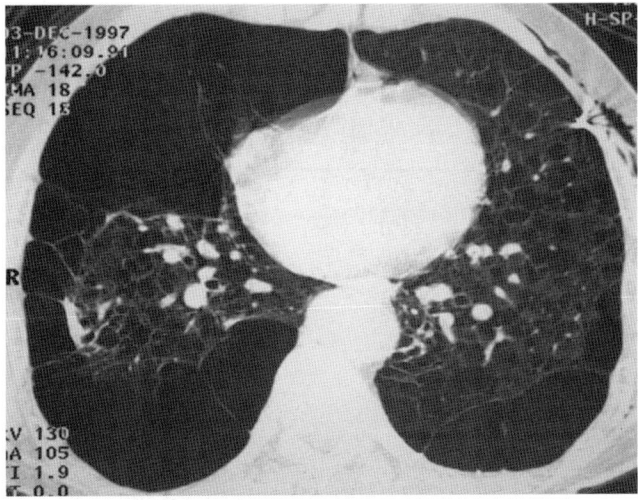

Fig 1.162: Bullous emphysema: HRCT demonstrates extensive bullae in both lung fields, especially right with consequent compression of the lung parenchyma. There is extensive centrilobular emphysema in both lung fields.

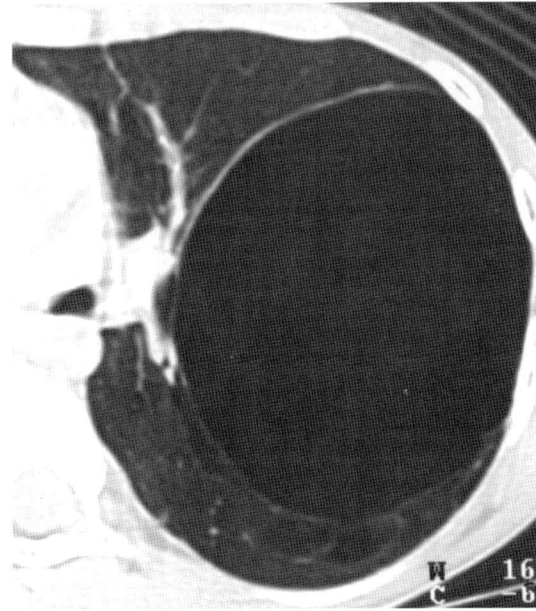

Fig 1.163: Bulla: HRCT demonstrates a huge thin-walled air space representing a bulla.

Bleb—Bleb refers to a gas-containing space within the visceral pleura.

Pneumatocele is a thin-walled gas-filled space within the lung, occurring from lung necrosis and bronchiolar obstruction. It usually occurs in an acute setting following an acute pneumonia and is often transient. Pneumatocele has a similar appearance to lung cyst or bulla.

Differential Diagnosis of Cystic Lesions

The differential diagnosis of diffuse cystic lung diseases includes pulmonary Langerhans' cell histiocytosis, usual interstitial pneumonia, centrilobular emphysema. Langerhans' cell histiocytosis chiefly involve the upper lobes and also show the presence of nodules. UIP chiefly involves the lower lobes with cysts subpleural in location. The cystic spaces in centrilobular emphysema do not have well-defined walls. Lymphangioleiomyomatosis occurs in young females with evenly distributed cysts in both lung fields. Cystic bronchiectasis may also enter into the differential diagnosis and is generally easily identified.

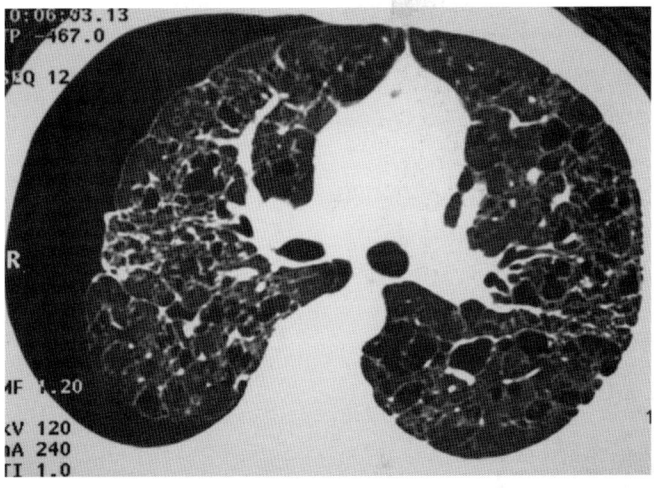

Fig 1.164: Pulmonary Langerhans' cell histiocytosis: HRCT reveals a right-sided pneumothorax with multiple bizarre-shaped cysts in both lung fields. The bizarre shape of the cysts as well as history of exposure to cigarette smoke helps to differentiate from the thin-walled smooth cysts seen predominantly in females in lymphangioleiomyomatosis.

MOSAIC ATTENUATION

The lung may have an inhomogeneous attenuation pattern with ill-defined areas of increased and decreased lung attenuation intermixed. This may be due to infiltrative diseases with areas of ground-glass density, increased lung attenuation with areas of normal lung attenuation intermixed.

Mosaic perfusion is characterized by areas of decreased lung attenuation with areas of normal lung attenuation. Lung density is partially determined by the amount of blood present in lung tissue. Regional perfusion differences may occur due to airway abnormalities or vascular abnormalities. If there is reduced ventilation of a portion of the lung due to narrowing of the airways, there is reflex vasoconstriction resulting in hypoperfusion of the hypoventilated region. This is seen in bronchiolitis obliterans, bronchiolitis, bronchiectasis, cystic fibrosis. If there is vascular obstruction there would be areas of hypoperfusion resulting in areas of low attenuation as seen in acute and chronic pulmonary thromboembolism.

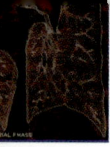

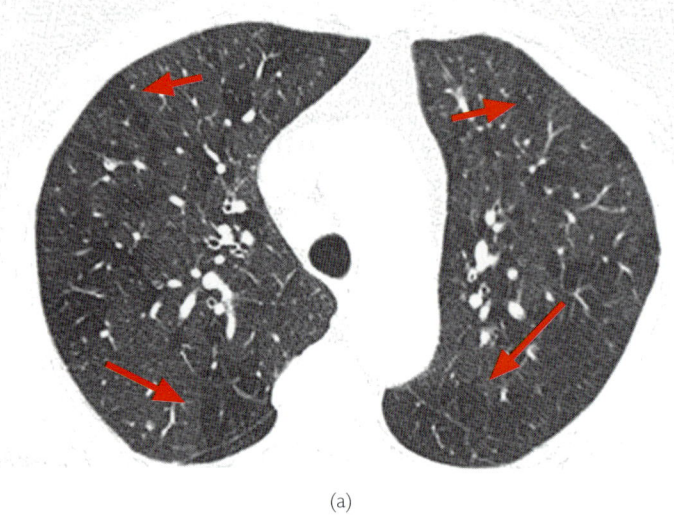

(a)

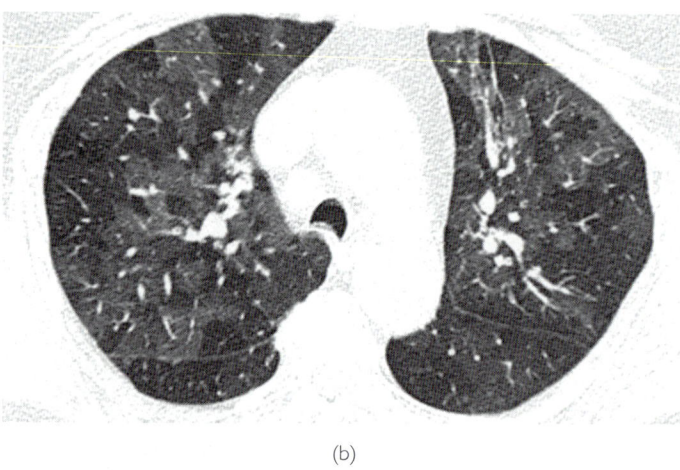

(b)

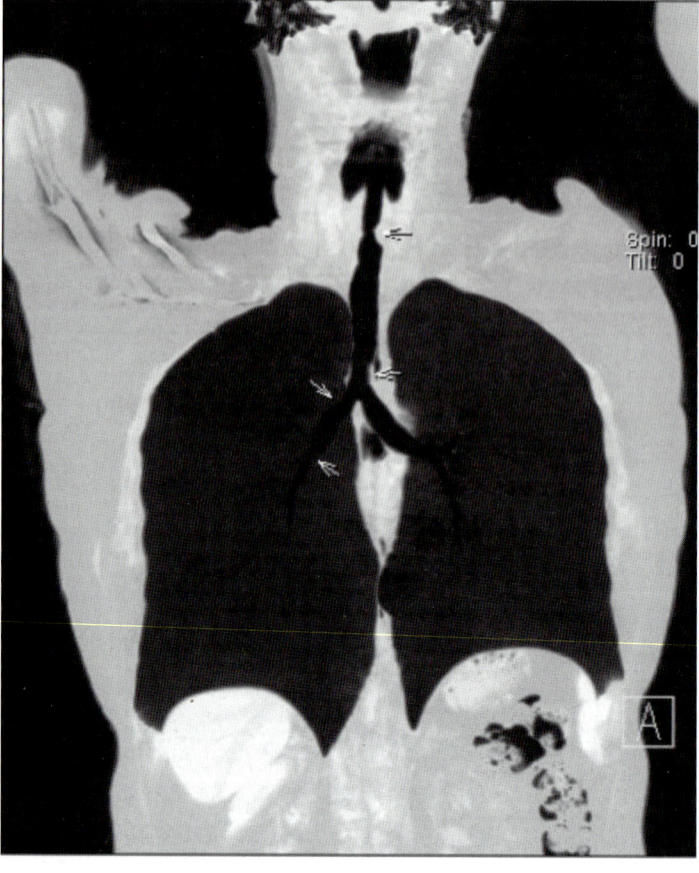

(a)

Fig 1.165: (a) HRCT demonstrates subtle inhomogenous areas of attenuation in both lung fields on inspiratory scan. On expiratory scans (b) there is accentuation of the inhomogenous areas of altered attenuation. Focal areas are seen to be darker and focal areas are brighter. The vessels within the areas which are darker are sparse in distribution and thinner in calibre, representing air-trapping. Mosaic attenuation was due to constrictive bronchiolitis.

Airway Diseases

UPPER AIRWAYS OBSTRUCTION

Tracheal Stenosis   Tracheal stenosis can be related to inflammatory or neoplastic causes and is sometimes due to Wegener's granulomatosis. The lesion may occur anywhere within the trachea and may involve the major bronchi also.

Clinical features include breathlessness, sometimes accompanied by a wheeze. A stridor is often observed when the obstruction is subglottic or if it involves the main trachea. This condition is often mistaken for asthma because of the presence of a wheeze. Even if the wheeze is present, as for example in a patient with obstruction to the right or left bronchus, it is monophonic in nature and not polyphonic as seen in patients with asthma. Flow volume loop confirms the diagnosis. Initially there is flattening of the inspiratory loop but later a flattening of both inspiratory and expiratory loops of the flow volume curve is observed.

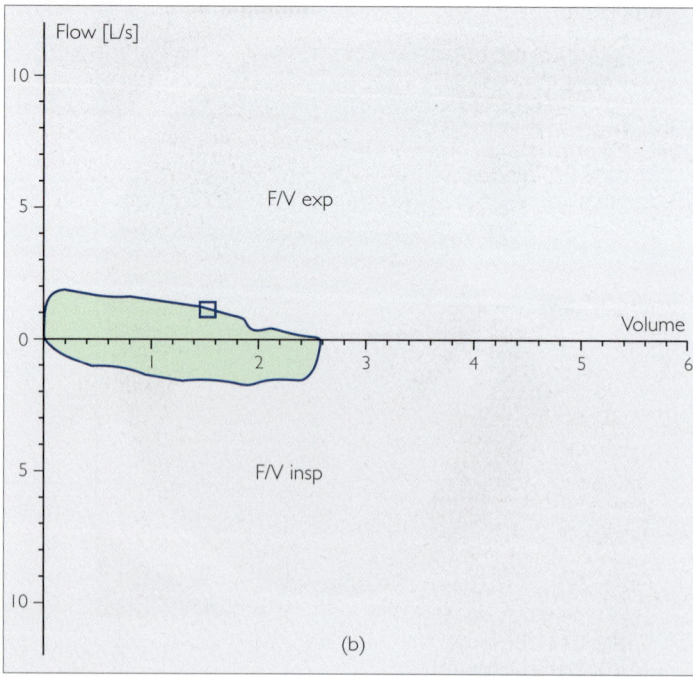

(b)

Fig 1.166: (a) Coronal CT section shows tracheal stenosis at two sites—an upper and a lower one, just above the carina. This patient was a young 23-year-old lady diagnosed as having asthma because of difficulty in breathing and a wheeze on auscultation. Clinical examination revealed noisy breathing, often amounting to a stridor. Auscultation revealed a monophonic wheeze (b) The flow volume loop demonstrated a marked flattening of the inspiratory and expiratory curve. Surgical correction of this disorder was successfully done. The aetiology of this tracheal stenosis was uncertain. It was probably related to Wegener's granulomatosis.

Bronchiectasis Bronchiectasis is defined as localized irreversible dilatation of the bronchial tree. There are a wide variety of causes. It is usually as a result of acute, chronic or recurrent infection. Bronchiectasis is classified on the basis of its severity as cylindrical (the walls of the bronchi are dilated but parallel), varicose (there is dilatation of the bronchi with focal constrictions, thereby giving a varicose appearance), and cystic, where the bronchi are ballooned.

On HRCT the dilated bronchi are visualized depending on the plane they are traversing in. If perpendicular to the plane of CT, i.e. running vertically down, they are visualized in cross-section. This appearance has been likened to a signet ring appearance—the dilated bronchus as the ring and the accompanying pulmonary artery as the jewel on the ring. If the bronchi are running parallel to the scan plane, i.e. horizontal they are visualized as tram tracks or parallel lines. There may be associated atelectasis resulting in the bronchi being bunched up, this gives an appearance of multiple cysts. Bronchial wall thickening may also be seen as well as air-fluid levels, especially in cystic bronchiectasis.

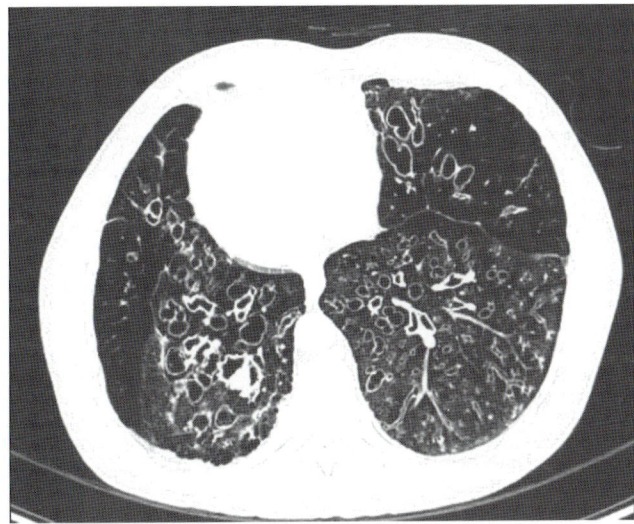

Fig 1.169: Bronchiectasis: HRCT demonstrates dilated bronchi in both lung fields, note dextrocardia in a case of Kartagener's syndrome.

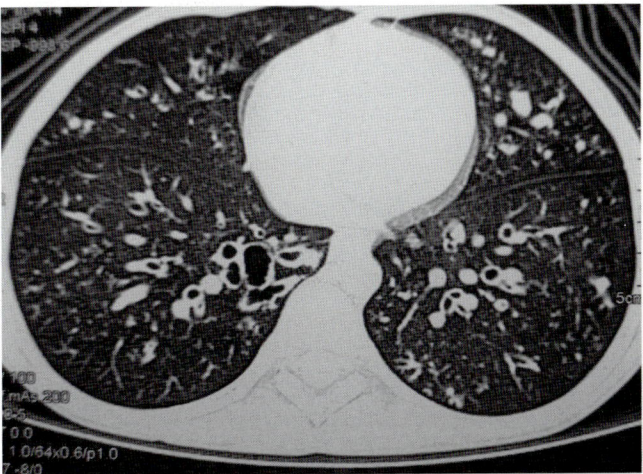

Fig 1.167: Bronchiectasis: HRCT chest demonstrates dilated bronchi representing bronchiectasis.

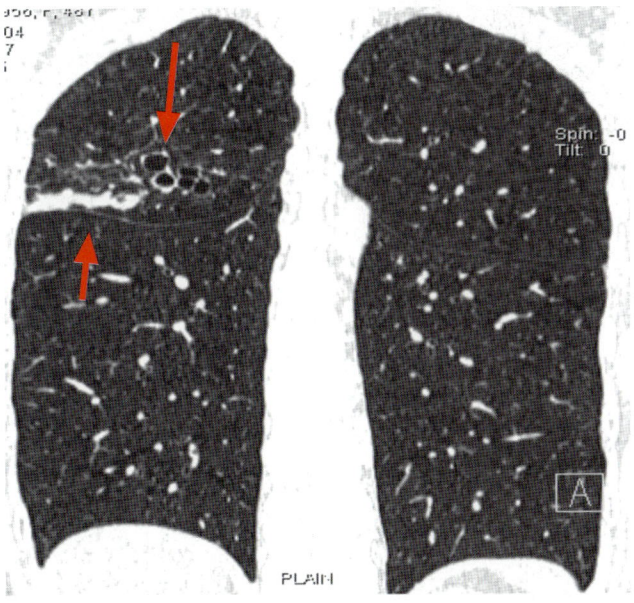

Fig 1.170: Bronchiectasis: Coronal HRCT demonstrates dilated bronchi in the right upper lobe. There is a linear well-defined tubular opacity extending to the subpleural region representing mucoid impaction in dilated bronchus.

Small Airway Diseases—Bronchiolar Diseases

HRCT has revolutionized our ability to diagnose small airway disease. The HRCT findings can be divided into two groups based on the imaging findings:

– Constrictive bronchiolitis
– Exudative bronchiolitis.

Constrictive bronchiolitis Constrictive bronchiolitis is concentric fibrosis involving the submucosal and peribronchial tissues of the terminal bronchioles resulting in bronchial narrowing and obliteration. The HRCT findings reflect the

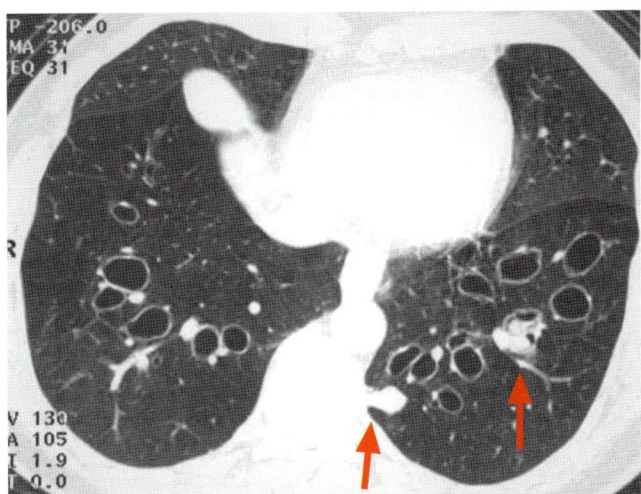

Fig 1.168: Bronchiectasis: HRCT demonstrates dilated bronchi in both lung bases. Note marked difference in the diameter of the bronchus and accompanying artery. A few dilated bronchi in the left lower lobe demonstrate soft tissue within their lumen representing mucoid impaction.

pathophysiology that causes airflow limitation. There is both hypoventilation of the involved segments of the lung as well as air-trapping. This is seen as areas of mosaic attenuation. The affected segments are dark and demonstrate air-trapping on expiratory scans. Hypoventilation of the involved areas of the lung results in reflex hypoperfusion so that vessels in the involved segments appear attenuated and sparse. The airways in these segments may also demonstrate abnormalities in the form of focal bronchial dilatation and wall thickening.

Exudative bronchiolitis There is mucoid impaction in the terminal bronchioles. On chest X-ray these are seen as

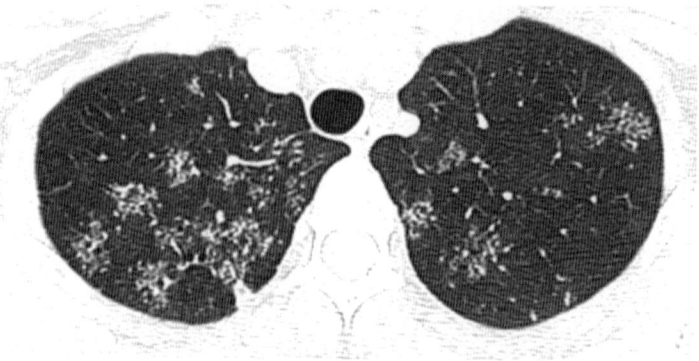

Fig 1.172: Exudative bronchiolitis: HRCT demonstrates multiple small conglomerated nodular lesions representing mucoid impaction in terminal bronchioles as a result of exudative bronchiolitis.

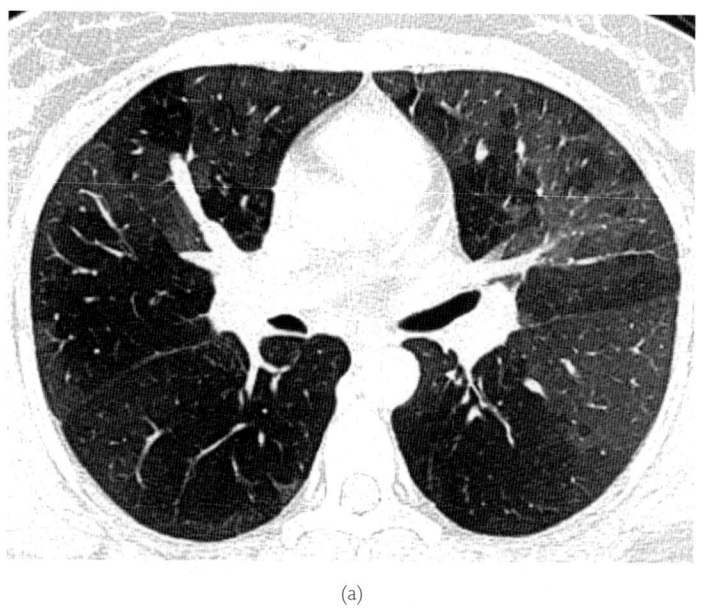

(a)

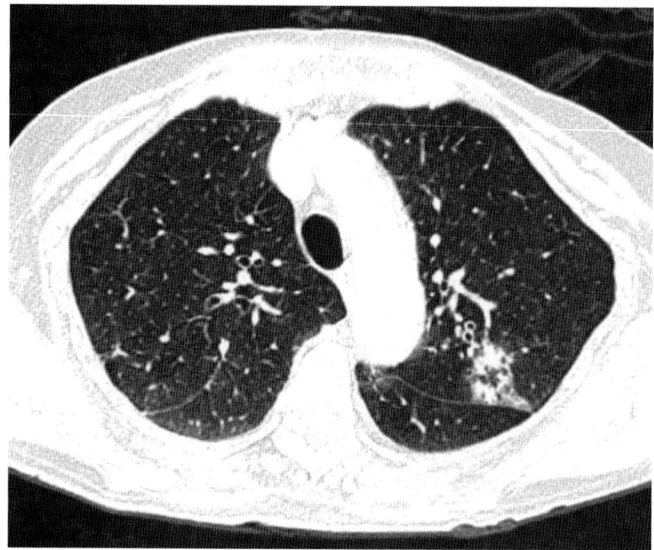

Fig 1.173: Exudative bronchiolitis: HRCT demonstrates multiple small conglomerated nodular lesions representing mucoid impaction in terminal bronchioles with associated ground-glass densities as a result of exudative bronchiolitis with peri-bronchiolar inflammation.

numerous small (5 mm) ill-defined nodules. On HRCT the areas of mucoid impaction are seen as tubular branching structures in the peripheral lung parenchyma resembling toy jacks also termed as tree-in-bud appearance. When seen in cross-section they appear as centrilobular nodules.

Swyer James Syndrome

This condition is usually caused by a viral infection to the immature lung, before it has completed development (below eight years of age). There is obliterative bronchiolitis involving the distal airways. Usually, an entire lung is involved, occasionally segments are spared. There is hypoplasia of the lung together with hypoplasia of the pulmonary artery to the involved lung.

On the chest X-ray there is unilateral transradiancy, the opposite lung appears to be plethoric. The ipsilateral hilum may be small chiefly because of a hypoplastic pulmonary artery supplying the involved lung.

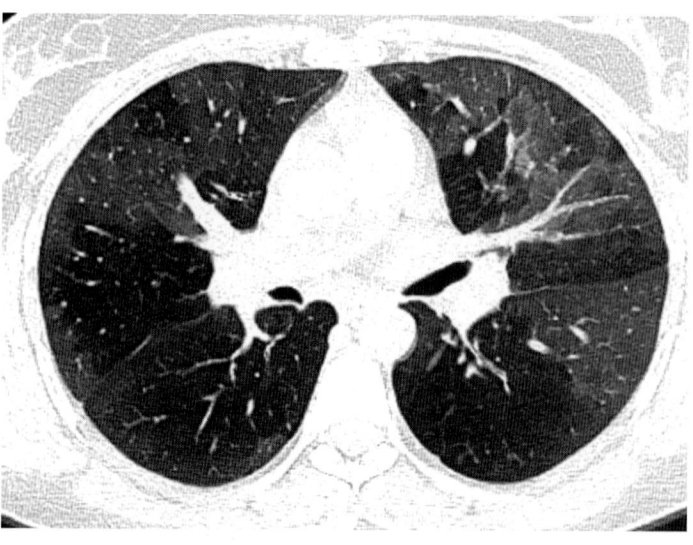

(b)

Fig 1.171: Constrictive bronchiolitis: (a) Inspiratory CT chest: areas of inhomogenous attenuation with areas of increased and decreased attenuation (b) Expiratory scans reveal air-trapping as the areas of decreased attenuation retain their attenuation whereas the areas of increased attenuation become brighter. The air-trapping indicates small-airway disease.

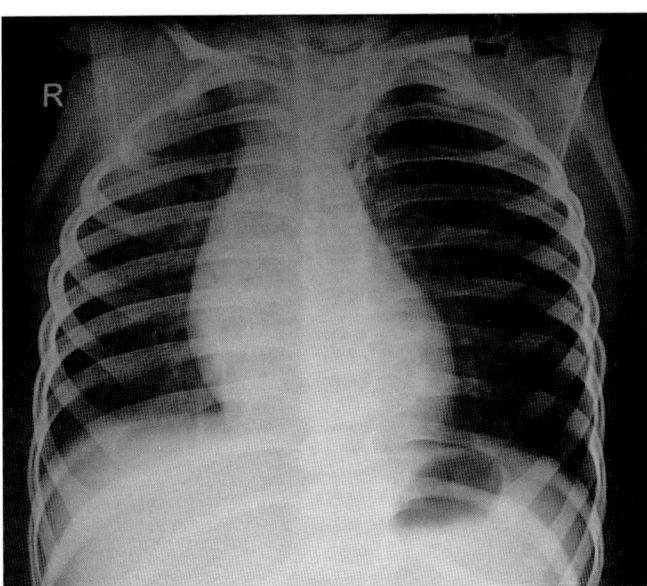

Fig 1.174: Swyer James Syndrome: Chest X-ray demonstrates unilateral transradiancy on the left side due to infantile bronchiolitis resulting in a Swyer James Syndrome.

IMPORTANT CONGENITAL MALFORMATIONS AND ANOMALIES

Pulmonary Arteriovenous Malformations

Nearly 70% of cases with PAVM are associated with hereditary haemorrhagic telengiectasia (HHT or Rendu-Osler-Weber disease). This is an autosomal dominant disorder characterized by the triad of telengiectasia, recurrent epistaxis and a family history of the disease. There is a wide spectrum of presentations. Patients may be asymptomatic, lesions being detected incidentally on a chest X-ray. If the AVM is large enough to cause a marked right to left shunt, the patient may present with cyanosis, dyspnoea, clubbing, haemoptysis, and cardiac failure. Usually, in these cases a distinct bruit is heard over the hemithorax. Patients may also present with cerebral abscesses and cerebral infarction due to paradoxical embolism. An important clinical finding in PAVMs is orthodexia—there is a drop in oxygen saturation from the supine to erect position. This is because PAVMs are mainly in the lower zones; this results in an increased right to left shunting of blood within the lungs in the erect position.

On chest radiographs AVMs are seen as well-defined nodules ranging in size from one cm to more cm. Peripheral AVMs usually demonstrate feeding arteries and draining veins as curvilinear structures. The more central AVMs are more difficult to detect as they may be overlapped by the hilum; the feeding draining vessels may not be visualized as they traverse a short distance.

CT is extremely sensitive and specific in demonstrating pulmonary AVMs. It is able to demonstrate feeding as well as draining vessels. There is intense enhancement of these lesions; CT scans are also able to detect the presence of multiple lesions. Remy Jardin and colleagues in fact found CT more sensitive than pulmonary angiograms, which have been considered the gold standard for the diagnosis of AVMs. CT detected AVMs in 98% of cases compared to pulmonary angiograms, which detected AVMs in 60%. CT additionally assists in deciding further management of these lesions. Using 2D and 3D reconstructions the feeding arteries can be demonstrated. Feeding arteries greater than 3 mm in diameter are embolized interventionally using coils, detachable balloons, to decrease the right to left shunting. Contrast echocardiography can be used to demonstrate complex angioarchitecture as well as provide a road map of the extent of the right to left shunt. MRI is useful in demonstrating larger PAVMs but smaller PAVMs may not be as well detected as in a CT.

Congenital Diaphragmatic Hernia

The classical congenital diaphragmatic hernia results from failure of the pleuro-peritoneal cavity to close with resultant herniation of abdominal contents into the thorax. The incidence is 1:2400 births, and is most commonly left-sided (90%). In the neonatal period these present as respiratory distress, as the herniated abdominal contents cause compressive effects on the lung and mediastinum. The diagnosis is fairly easy on the chest X-ray as there is evidence of soft tissue and air-filled bowel loops in the left hemithorax. When the stomach is included in the hernial sac, the nasogastric tube rather than descending in the abdomen is seen to take a turn upwards into the thorax from the gastro-oesophageal junction.

Hernias on the right side may be difficult to detect as there is usually herniation of liver; the chest radiograph demonstrates a soft tissue opacity in the lower right hemithorax.

Bochdalek Hernia

These result from herniation through a posterior diaphragmatic defect close to the crura. They tend to manifest later in life and may be bilateral and symmetric. The liver prevents herniation on the right side. Occasionally, kidney and /or stomach may herniate on the left side.

Morgagni's Hernia

These are due to herniation between sternal and costal attachments usually developing in the right anterior cardiophrenic sulcus. On the left herniation is impeded by the heart. Visual contents of the hernia are liver and omentum, occasionally transverse colon. On chest X-ray herniation of liver and omentum is visualized as a paracardiac mass with a D/D of pericardial cyst, paracardiac fat pad or a pleural/pulmonary mass. When there is herniation of colon, the presence of a gas-filled viscus makes the diagnosis easy. A lateral view of the chest helps to localize the hernia anteriorly. CT is diagnostic as CT demonstrates the herniation of liver/omentum and bowel.

ABSENCE OF LUNG OR LOBES OF LUNGS

Unilateral agenesis is a rare congenital anomaly presenting with minimal clinical problems. It is frequently associated with other congenital anomalies particularly tracheo-oesophageal fistula and the VACTERL association (non-random association of birth defects). When the bronchus is absent, it is termed as agenesis.

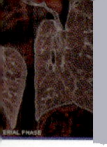

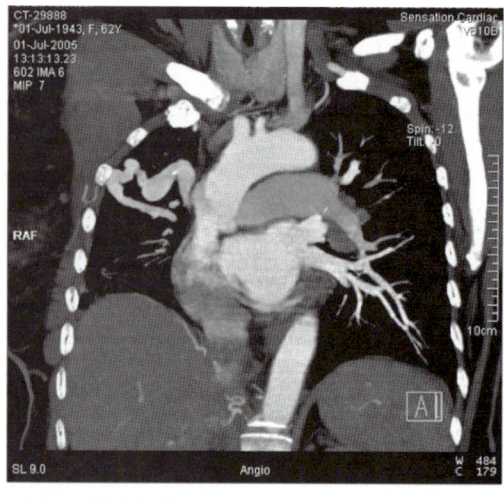

(a)

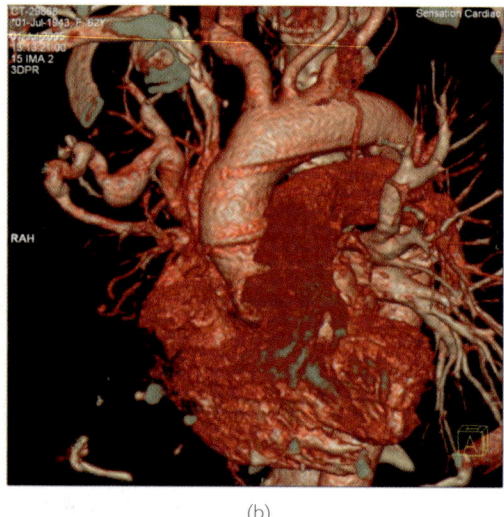

(b)

Fig 1.175: Pulmonary arteriovenous malformation: (a) MIP and (b) VRT images of CT angiography demonstrate an arteriovenous malformation in the right upper zone with feeding arteries and draining veins.

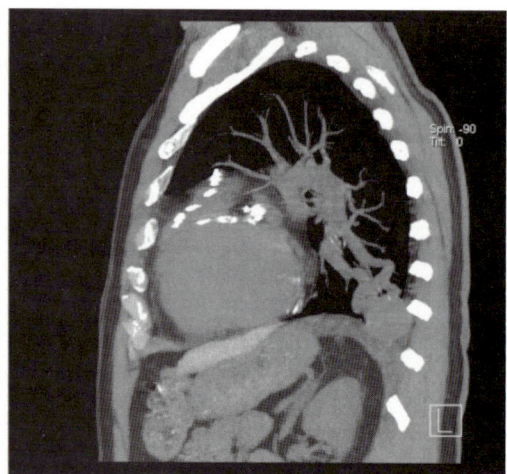

Fig 1.176: Pulmonary arteriovenous malformation: Sagittal MPR demonstrates feeding arteries and draining vein of pulmonary arteriovenous malformation.

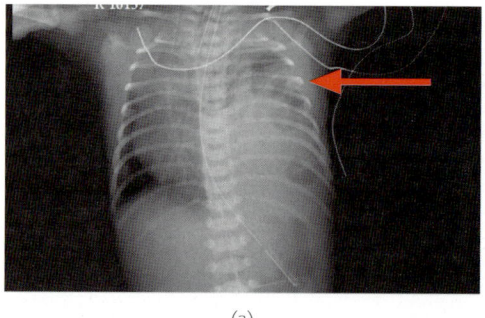

(a)

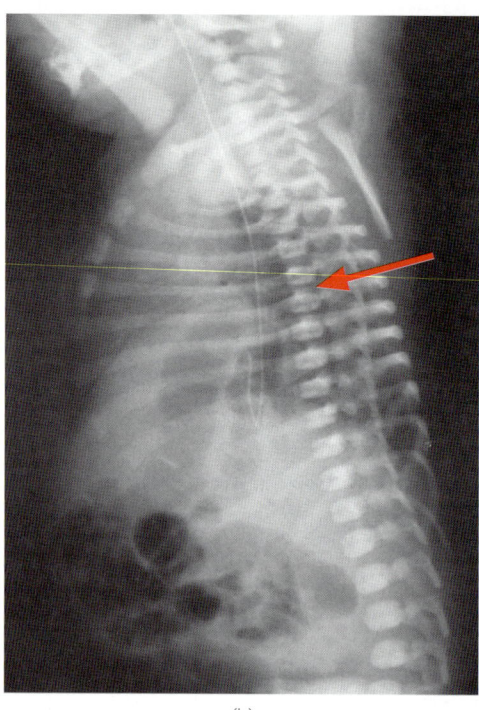

(b)

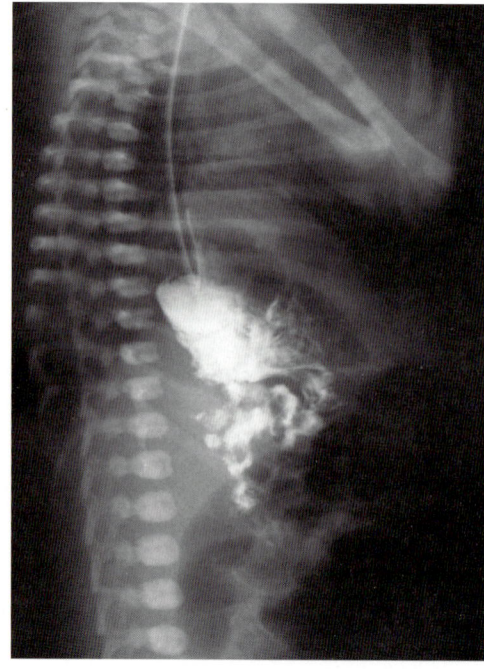

(c)

Fig 1.177: Diaphragmatic hernia: (a) AP and (b) oblique views demonstrate soft tissue opacity and bowel loops in the left hemithorax with shift of the mediastinum to the right (c) Barium study confirms bowel loops in the hemithorax.

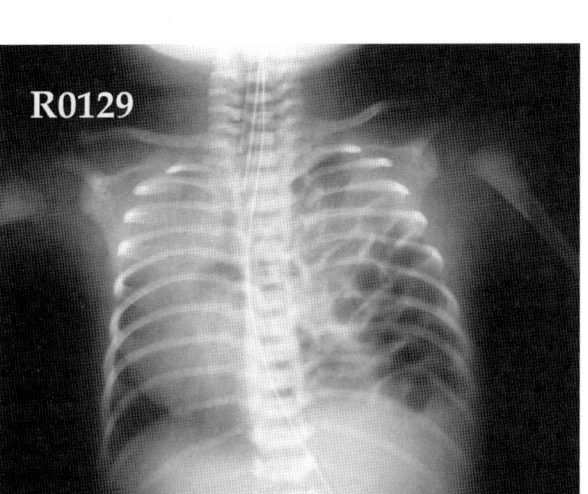

Fig 1.178: Diaphragmatic hernia: Chest X-ray in a neonate reveals ill-defined opacities in the left hemithorax with multiple air-filled loops representing a diaphragmatic hernia. There is consequently a shift of the mediastinum to the right.

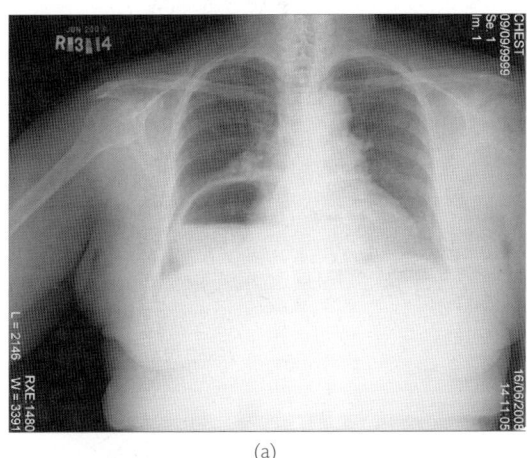

(a)

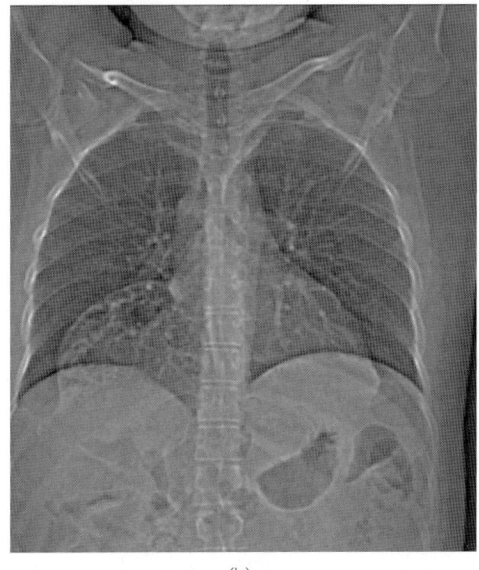

(b)

Fig 1.179: Morgagni's hernia: (a) PA view and (b) topogram of the chest reveals a bowel loop with an air-fluid level in the right hemithorax.

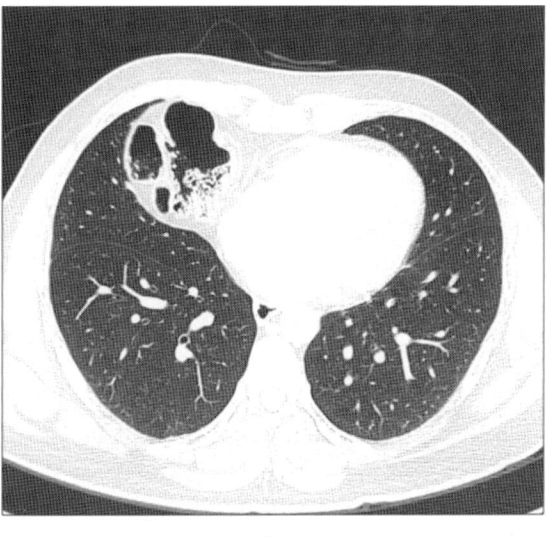

(a)

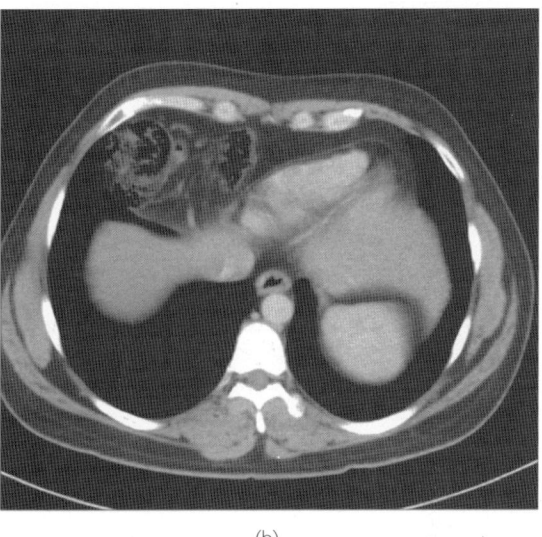

(b)

Fig 1.180: Morgagni's hernia: (a and b) CT scans show herniation of colon through an anterior abdominal wall defect into the anterior hemithorax, representing a Morgagni's hernia.

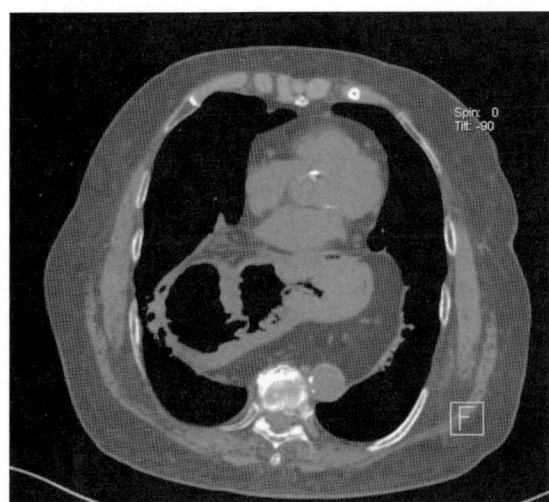

Fig 1.181: Hiatus hernia: CT demonstrates a huge hiatus hernia with the stomach extending into the thoracic cavity.

When the bronchus is present but rudimentary, it is termed aplasia. The ipsilateral pulmonary artery develops but is usually hypoplastic.

Agenesis of the right lung is often accompanied by oesophageal atresia and is twice as common as left lung agenesis. Left lung agenesis is often accompanied by tracheo-oesophageal fistula. On imaging there is loss of aeration and volume on the ipsilateral side as evidenced by elevation of the diaphragm, shift of the mediastinum to the ipsilateral side and increase in extrapleural fat to fill the space due to congenital hypoplasia.

Absence of individual lobes is a form of hypoplastic lung syndrome. When there is absence of a lobe there is compensatory expansion of the rest of the lung, distorting bronchovascular structures. This overexpansion is never adequate to revert the lung to normal size. The size of the ipsilateral lung is always smaller, similar to what is seen in pulmonary hypoplasia. The difference is easily determined on CT as a bronchus is absent, whereas in hypoplasia all segments are present but the tracheobronchial tree is stunted and underdeveloped.

Tracheo-Oesophageal Fistula

Tracheo-oesophageal fistulas are associated with oesophageal atresia and are usually diagnosed in the neonatal period. Rarely, tracheo-oesophageal fistulas are not diagnosed till later in life as the symptoms may be non-specific. These fistulas are of the 'H' type—a short horizontal communication between the trachea and oesophagus—the horizontal communication being represented by the H bar. Symptoms are due to recurrent aspiration, paroxysmal cough, feeding difficulties and recurrent pneumonia. The appearances on chest radiographs are of aspiration, excessive air may also pass from the trachea into the oesophagus as well as into the gut. This may be visualized also on an X-ray as air in the oesophagus and/or gaseous distension of the bowel. An obvious tracheo-oesophageal fistula is fairly easy to demonstrate. A small tracheo-oesophageal fistula, especially the 'H' variety is best demonstrated in the prone position using a feeding tube which is slowly withdrawn while a non-ionic water soluble contrast is injected to demonstrate the fistulous communication. The 'H' type of tracheo-oesophageal fistulas are usually associated with other congenital anomalies—these have been designated by acronyms: VATER—vertebral, anal, tracheo-oesophageal, renal; VACTEL—vertebral, anal, cardiac, tracheo-oesophageal and limb. Pulmonary hypoplasia, tracheal stenosis and pulmonary sequestration may also be associated.

Bronchial Atresia

There is a short segment of atresia involving a segment or subsegmental bronchus. There is consequently dilatation of the bronchus distal to the atresia, resulting in accumulation of mucus in the dilated bronchus. This mucocele is seen on imaging as a mass-like structure; there may be a branching configuration which helps establish the diagnosis. The surrounding lung in the affected segment is hypertranslucent as the lung beyond the atretic segment is aerated by collateral drift and because there is reflex hypoperfusion of the vessels in the affected segment. The vessels appear thinner and less is number in the affected segment. Most patients are asymptomatic. Bronchial atresia has limited clinical significance; the only issue is that it may

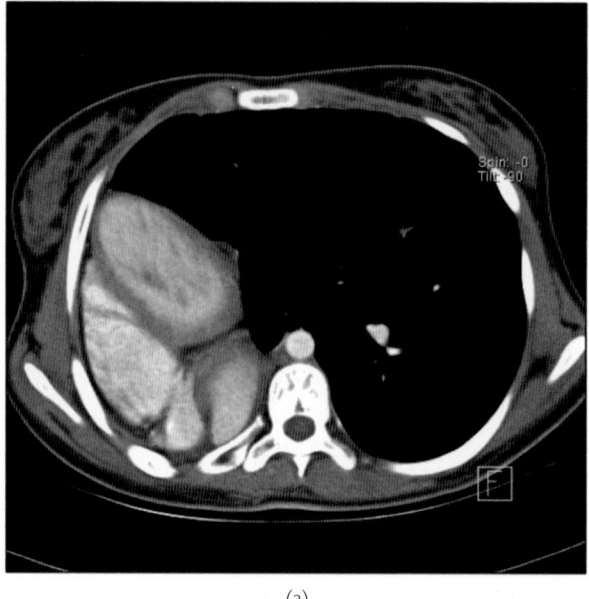

(a)

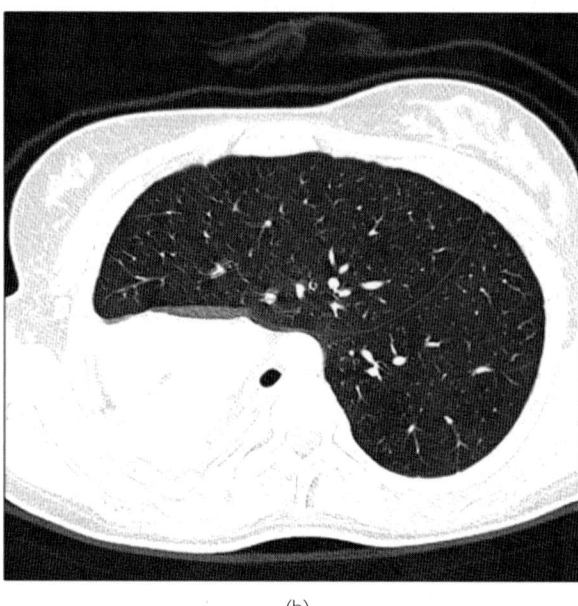

(b)

Fig 1.182: Agenesis of right lung: (a) CT chest reveals a marked shift of mediastinum to the right with no lung tissue seen in right hemithorax (b) There is compensatory expansion of left lung. The right pulmonary artery was absent.

be mistaken for a mass. CT very effectively demonstrates the central mucus-filled mass, atresia of the segmental bronchus, and the hypertranslucent lung segment.

Pulmonary Sequestration

Pulmonary sequestration is characterized by the presence of pulmonary tissue which does not communicate with the central airways through a normal bronchial connection and receives its blood supply via an anomalous systemic artery. Pulmonary sequestration is divided into intralobar and extralobar varieties, based on venous drainage. If the venous drainage is to the pulmonary veins, it is termed intralobar sequestration. If the drainage is to the systemic veins, it is termed extralobar sequestration.

Extralobar sequestrations are congenital abnormalities usually associated with other congenital abnormalities, such as congenital heart disease, diaphragmatic hernia, or cystic adenomatoid malformation. They are asymptomatic and therefore discovered incidentally on antenatal ultrasound, chest X-ray, sonography, CT, angiography or during surgical repair of a congenital diaphragmatic hernia with which they are commonly associated. An extralobar sequestration has a complete serosal covering; it may have a narrow vascular pedicle as it is separate from the normal lung. Extralobar sequestrations in 90% of cases occur on the left side. Torsion is a complication and this may result in a tension hydrothorax.

Extralobar sequestrations are seen on imaging as mass lesions of homogenous density. They have well-defined margins, in particular the lateral margin which is covered by pleura. The medial margin may be difficult to discern as it abuts the mediastinum, often giving the appearance of a mediastinal mass. Sequestration may be seen in relation to the pericardium, diaphragm, and the retroperitoneum, occasionally communicating with the oesophagus or stomach, which can be demonstrated by barium studies.

As compared to extralobar sequestration which is a congenital abnormality, intralobar sequestration is being considered to be more likely an acquired lesion rather than a congenital abnormality. Chronic bronchial obstruction due to foreign body, carcinoid tumour and post-obstructive pneumonia are considered to be causes of intralobar sequestration. The chronic inflammatory process 'parasites' its blood supply from the systemic circulation, often a branch from the descending aorta or branches from the inferior pulmonary ligament. Therefore 98% of all sequestrations occur in the lower lobes. As compared to extralobar sequestrations which are asymptomatic, intralobar sequestrations present as an infective lesion or sequelae of an infective lesion. On imaging they appear as round, oval, lobulated mass lesions simulating an intra-pulmonary mass lesion. Air and air-fluid levels may be seen within these masses due to communication with bronchi

secondary to episodes of infection. CT appearances are similar to those of a chest X-ray; however CT more frequently detects air, air-fluid levels, and the presence of emphysema adjacent to the sequestration. The emphysema occurs due to impaired ventilatation secondary to chronic obstruction with consequent collateral air drift and air-trapping. Occasionally, a pure cystic form of sequestration is detected with air-trapping, focal emphysema and bulla formation. The key in differentiating from other cystic masses is the demonstration of a systemic arterial supply. CT angiography on MDCT scanner has replaced the need for invasive angiography to demonstrate systemic arterial supply, the key to the diagnosis of sequestration. The differential diagnosis of sequestration encompasses infective lesions, pulmonary masses, mediastinal and pleural masses. The clue to the correct diagnosis is location, arterial supply, venous drainage, and a history of repeated infections.

Congenital Lobar Over-inflation (CLO)

Previously known as congenital lobar emphysema, it is now termed as congenital lobar over-inflation. The pathophysiology of this condition is characterized by over-inflation of normal alveoli most likely due to central airway obstruction, presumably due to aplasia, hypoplasia or dysplasia of the bronchial support structures. A clinically similar condition is polyalveolar lobe—the lobe contains four to five times the number of alveoli normally present, resulting in a large lobe having all the compressive effects seen in CLO. CLO manifests in the neonatal period with respiratory distress. On chest X-ray there is hyper-expansion of a lobe of the lung, usually upper or middle lobe. Involvement of more than one lobe or the lower lobe is extremely rare. The hyper-expanded lobe causes mass effect on the adjacent structures, heart, mediastinum and diaphragm. The main differential diagnosis is obstruction to the bronchus by a foreign body, mucus plug, endobronchial mass, extrinsic compression of the airway or a localized pneumothorax. CT is useful to confirm the diagnosis of hyperinflation of a lobe. CT angiography differentiates CLO from other forms of pulmonary hypoplasia.

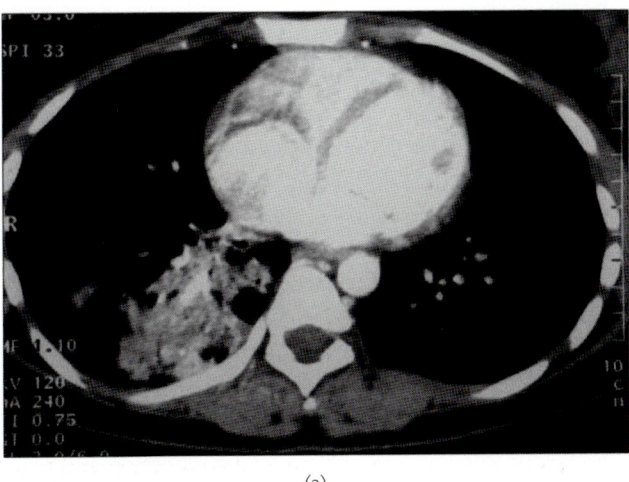

(a)

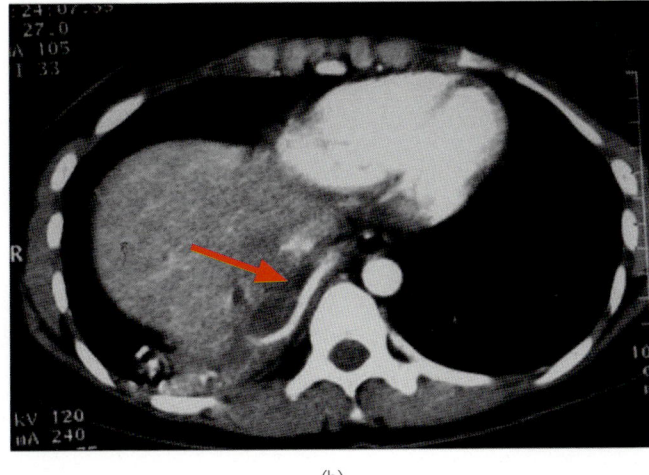

(b)

Fig 1.183: Pulmonary sequestration: (a) CT scan demonstrates an ill-defined consolidation (b) CT angiography demonstrates arterial branch arising from aorta feeding the consolidation representing an intralobar sequestration.

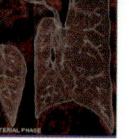
Pulmonary Hypoplasia

Primary unilateral pulmonary hypoplasia is usually associated with the scimitar syndrome or with other vascular malformations. Patients present with repeated episodes of wheezing and pneumonia. The affected lung is small in size, the mediastinum is displaced towards the ipsilateral hemi-thorax and the pulmonary vasculature is reduced in size. On the lateral chest X-ray, a sharply marginated opacity is seen behind and parallel to the sternum. This is due to the displacement of the heart and mediastinum into the ipsilateral thorax. Primary bilateral pulmonary hypoplasia is very rare. Chest X-ray reveals bilateral small lungs with a normal-sized abdominal cavity, presenting a bell-shaped appearance of the chest and abdomen.

Unilateral Absence of Pulmonary Artery

This is a rare anomaly characterized by the absence of a short segment or atresia of the proximal left or right pulmonary artery; the more distal segments are usually present. Chest radiographs demonstrate reduction in lung volume, shift of mediastinum, small-sized or absent pulmonary hilum; peripheral pulmonary perfusion is reduced. There may be reticular opacities in the affected lung due to pulmonary–systemic collaterals. The normal lung may be plethoric as the entire cardiac output is shunted through the lung. CT will demonstrate the absence of the pulmonary artery and the presence of systemic pulmonary collaterals.

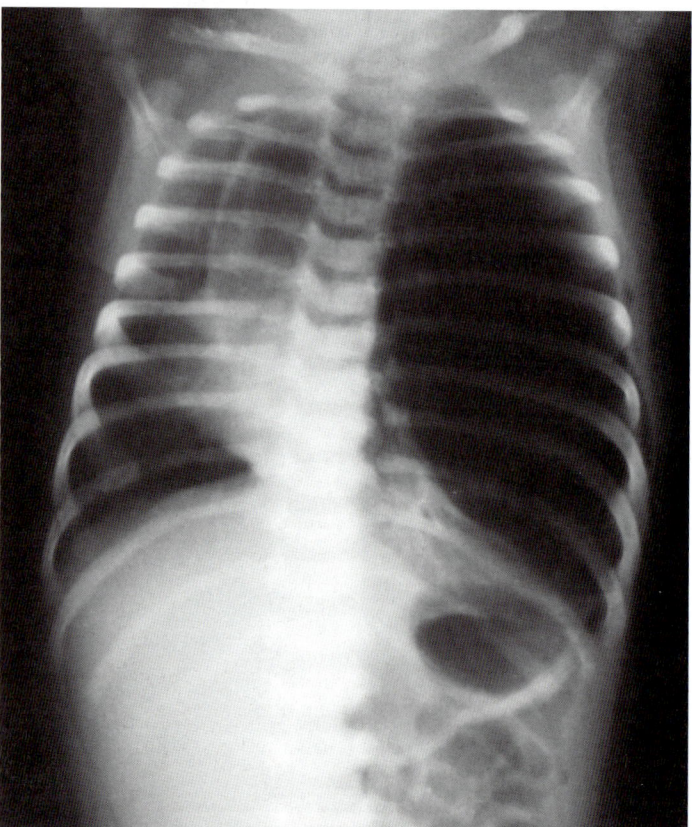

Fig 1.184: CLO. Chest X-ray demonstrates marked over-inflation of the left upper lobe causing a shift of the mediastinum to the right and collapse of the left lower lobe. Collapsed left lower lobe is seen along the left cardiac border.

Scimitar Syndrome

This is a condition involving essentially the right lung which is hypoplastic, with underdevelopment of the airways as well as vasculature. The characteristic finding which in turn contributes to its name is anomalous pulmonary drainage. A large anomalous pulmonary vein descends vertically inferiorly to open into the inferior vena cava above or below the diaphragm. The vein broadens as it curves medially to enter into the vena cava, thereby simulating the appearance of a Turkish sword--scimitar. The anomalous vein may also drain into the coronary sinus, right atrium, or rarely into hepatic veins. The scimitar syndrome may be associated with other congenital anomalies such as septal defects, eventration, Bochdalek hernia, bronchiectasis and tracheal diverticuli. On a chest radiograph, the key feature is the presence of the anomalous draining vein. Additional features are a small-sized right lung, shift of the mediastinum to the right and a small ipsilateral pulmonary artery. CT is useful to confirm the diagnosis, demonstrating the anomalous draining vessel and its termination, tracheobronchial anomalies, small ipsilateral pulmonary artery, as well as associated abnormalities such as tracheal diverticuli and bronchiectasis.

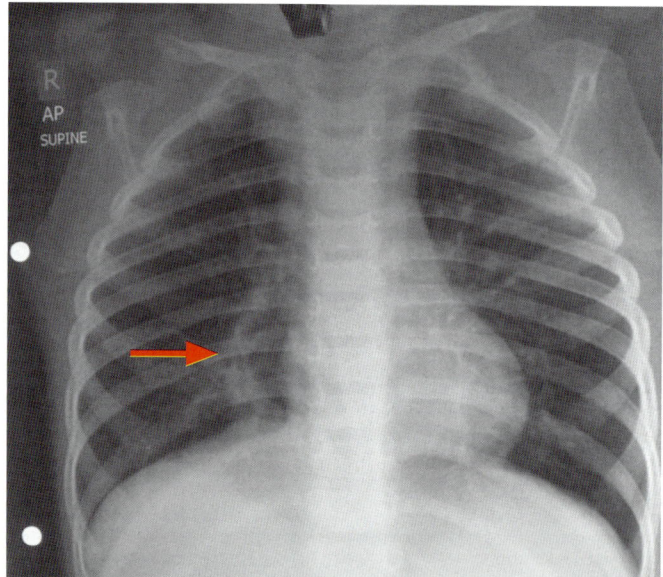

Fig 1.185: Scimitar syndrome: AP view demonstrates typical curvilinear vascular opacity in right paracardiac region.

Imaging of Pleura

PLEURAL EFFUSIONS

Free pleural effusions tend to gravitate to the most dependent portions of the pleural cavity. On erect chest X-rays these are seen as homogenous densities in the lower zone with a typical concave or upward-sloping contour, the lateral margin being higher than the medial margin. Fluid collects in the subpulmonic space then spills into the posterior and finally lateral costophrenic sulcus. The posterior costophrenic (CP) sulcus is the deepest portion of the pleura. This is the site where the fluid tends to first accumulate. Radiologically, this is seen as blunting of the costophrenic angle on the lateral view.

At least 200 ml of fluid is required to cause obliteration of the CP angle on a PA view of the chest, though in some cases there is no blunting of the angle even when 500 ml of fluid is present. The lateral decubitus view is the most sensitive X-ray to demonstrate free fluid. Fluid is seen layering the dependent part of the chest wall as a thin uniform opacity. This view however may be technically difficult to obtain in a patient who is critically ill. In patients who are too critically ill to sit erect, a diagnosis of pleural effusion has to be made on a supine X-ray chest. The findings in moderate-sized or large effusions are a homogenous opacity of the affected hemithorax with absence of the vascular markings. This is because the fluid is layering posteriorly along the chest wall. Fluid also tends to accumulate along the apex, like an apical pleural cap, and in the base, as these are the most dependent areas on a supine film. Small pleural effusions can be easily missed on a supine radiograph. In fact only 67% sensitivity and 70% specificity have been reported for the detection of a pleural effusion on supine chest X-ray as opposed to a lateral decubitus view.

In critically ill patients who cannot be positioned for a lateral decubitus view, or if a supine radiograph shows equivocal or negative findings, sonography is an excellent means for demonstrating pleural fluid. This imaging modality is portable and can be easily performed at the bedside. Pleural fluid is seen as an anechoic area separating the echogenic line of the diaphragm and the echogenic inferior margin of the lung. Sonography is also useful in differentiating a pleural effusion from atelectasis/consolidation which may simulate an effusion on the chest X-ray. Further, it is an excellent guide for thoracocentesis, markedly reducing the incidence of iatrogenic pneumothorax.

Occasionally, free pleural fluid may accumulate in a subpulmonic location between the lung and diaphragm, with the lung floating on the fluid. The upper margin of the fluid may then take the appearance of the diaphragm. There is however a subtle difference from the normal appearance of the diaphragm in a subpulmonic effusion. The peak of the diaphragm is more lateral, the medial aspect has a more gradual slope and the lateral aspect a steeper slope. On a lateral X-ray the posterior costophrenic sulcus is obliterated. Left-sided subpulmonic effusions may be detected by noting the wide distance between the stomach air bubble and diaphragm. On the right side differentiation from an enlarged liver pushing the diaphragm upwards may be difficult. In these cases either a lateral decubitus view or sonography is useful to clinch the diagnosis. A loculated effusion may occur when there are adhesions between the visceral and parietal pleura, as a result of which the fluid does not shift with change of the patient's position. Empyema and haemothorax may appear as loculated effusions. Sonography will demonstrate the fluid is echogenic rather than anechoic in empyemas/haemothorax.

CT is extremely sensitive in detecting even small pleural fluid collections. With the patient supine, free fluid accumulates posteriorly as a hypodense layer conforming to the contour of the chest wall. The presence of septae in the pleural fluid (denoting a likely exudate), is however brought out by a sonographic study rather than by a CT scan. Acute haemorrhage in the pleural space can be well-identified by the hyperdensity of blood. CT is also useful in the assessment of the site, extent and wall thickening of loculated effusions, and for loculated interlobar effusions. These may simulate a mass lesion

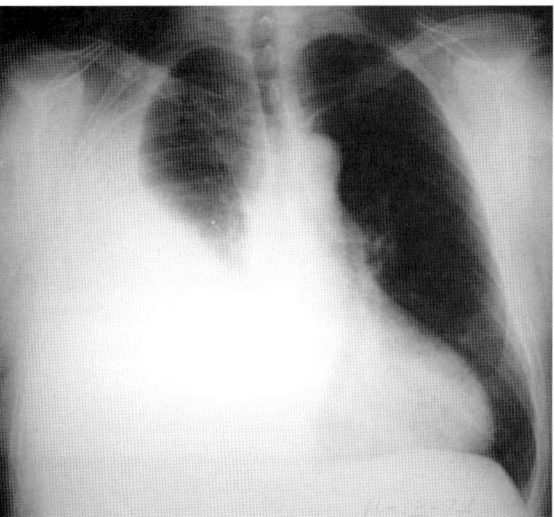

Fig 1.186: Pleural effusion: PA view of the chest reveals a large homogenous opacity in the right hemithorax extending along the right lateral chest wall to the apex. There is a shift of the mediastinum to the left. This is diagnostic of a pleural effusion.

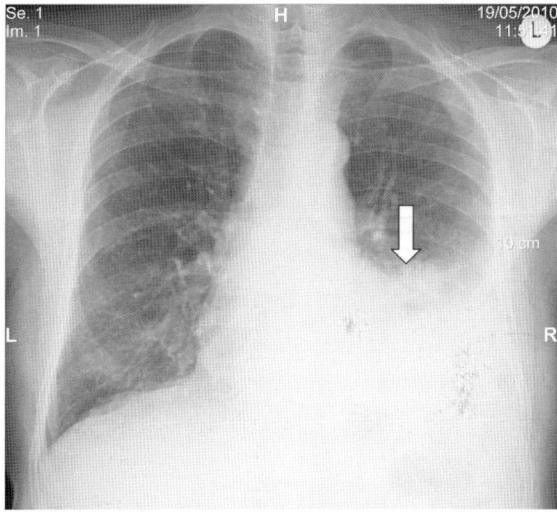

Fig 1.187: Pleural effusion: PA view of chest reveals a left-sided pleural effusion. There is also an underlying spiculated mass which on biopsy was proven to be an adenocarcinoma of lung.

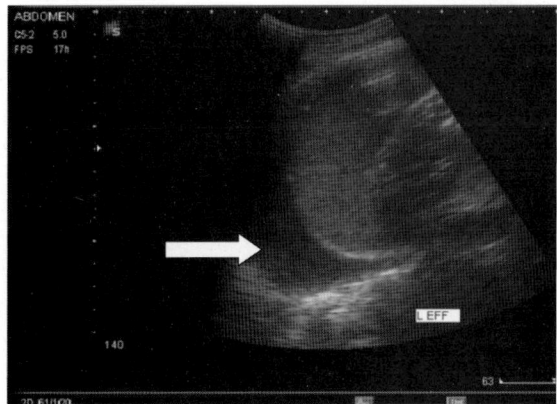

Fig 1.188: Pleural effusion: Sonography demonstrates an hypoechoic appearance of pleural fluid layering above diaphragm.

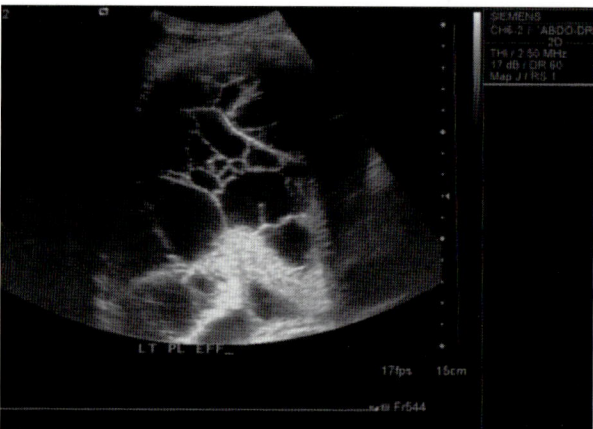

Fig 1.189: Pleural effusion: Sonography demonstrates pleural effusion as an echoic fluid collection. There are multiple linear bands within this fluid collection; these represent septae. Presence of septae is highly suggestive of the effusion being an exudate.

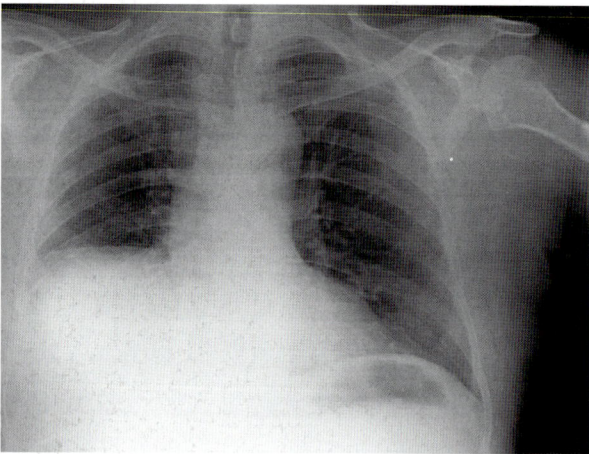

Fig 1.190: Subpulmonic pleural effusion: PA view of the chest demonstrates a homogenous opacity in the right lower zone, appearing as an elevated flattened dome of the diaphragm. This appearance is suggestive of a subpulmonic pleural effusion. Sonography confirmed the presence of a pleural effusion.

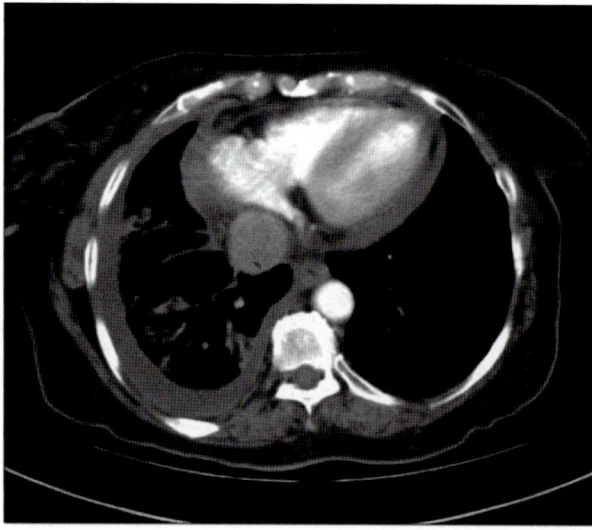

Fig 1.191: Pleural effusion: CT is extremely sensitive in detecting small pleural and pericardial effusion.

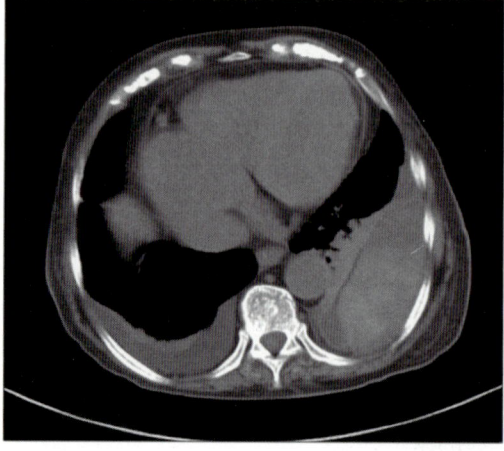

Fig 1.192: Hemorrhagic pleural effusion: CT chest without IV contrast reveals a thin pleural effusion on the right side and a moderate-sized pleural fluid collection on the left. The pleural fluid collection on the left is hyperdense indicating haemorrhage and the right side hypodense indicating fluid. CT is useful in differentiating pleural effusion from a haemothorax.

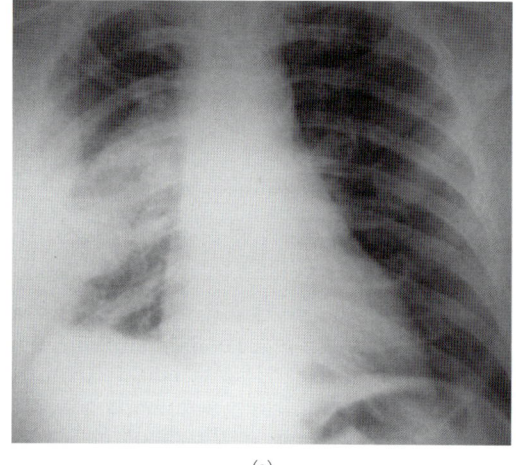

(a)

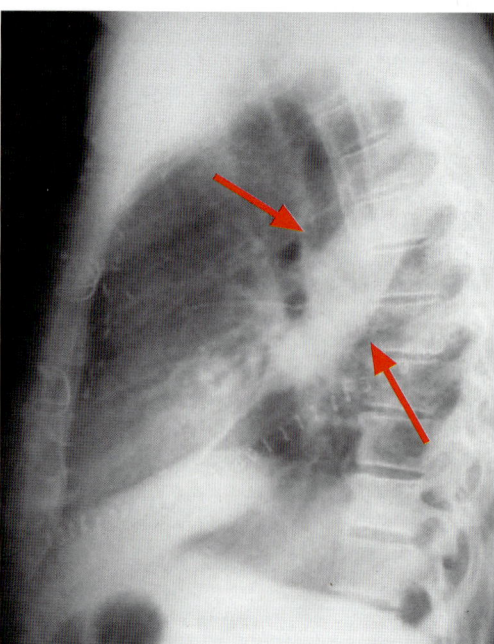

(b)

Fig 1.193:
Interlobar effusion:
(a) PA view
demonstrates a
well-defined opacity
in the right mid-
zone (b) Lateral
view demonstrates
the homogenous
opacity seen on the
PA view, represents
loculated fluid in
the major interlobar
fissure. The inferior
part of the fissure
as well as the
minor fissure are
mildly thickened.
The homogenous
appearance on
the PA view of
an opacity in the
location of the
fissure would
suggest the need
for a lateral view to
localize the lesion.

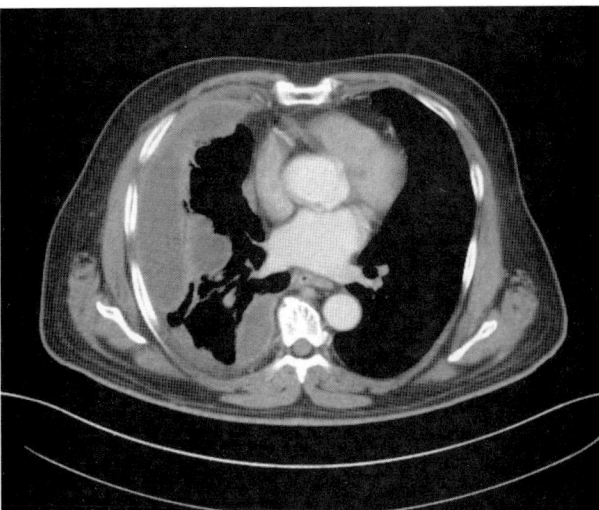

Fig 1.194: Loculated pleural effusion: CT chest demonstrates pleural fluid in the right hemithorax loculated along the right lateral chest wall with multiple loculations.

on plain X-ray but can easily be differentiated on CT. CT with intravenous contrast medium is very useful in differentiating parenchymal from pleural lesions, especially when a plain radiograph has not been helpful.

Empyema

On a chest radiograph an empyema is usually seen as a loculated fluid collection. It tends to be lenticular in shape as compared to a lung abscess which is rounded. Further, an empyema usually forms an obtuse angle with the chest wall while a lung abscess forms an acute angle. CT is very useful in the diagnosis and management of empyema. On CT an empyema appears

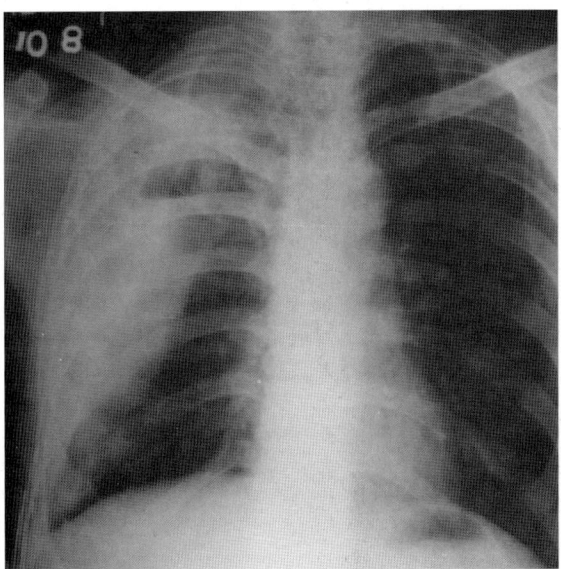

Fig 1.195: Empyema: PA view of the chest demonstrates a homogenous lenticular fluid collection along right lateral chest wall with an air-fluid level. Sonography confirmed the homogenous opacity was fluid with internal echoes. An aspiration revealed an empyema.

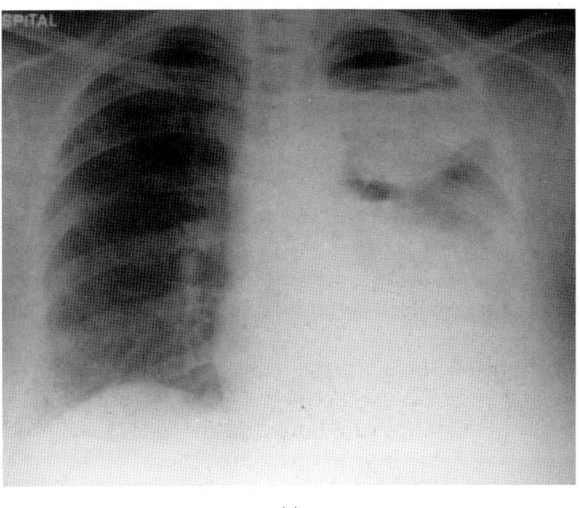

(a)

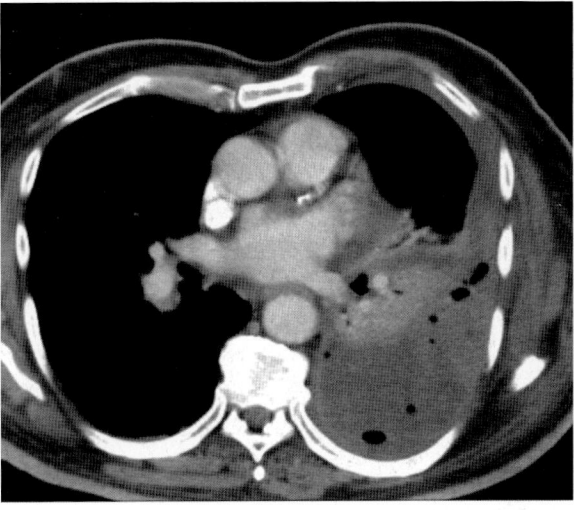

(b)

Fig 1.196: Empyema: (a & b) Chest X-ray and CT chest demonstrates a loculated fluid collection in the left hemithorax. There are multiple specks of air in the fluid collection. The presence of air in a pleural collection is highly suggestive of infection in the pleural fluid. Air may also be present in pleural fluid if it has been inadvertently introduced during aspiration of the fluid.

as a well-defined fluid collection with enhancing parietal and visceral pleura. This sign of separation of the pleura is known as the split pleura sign.

Traditionally, empyemas have been treated with insertion of chest tubes. The success rate with chest tube drainage is 35–71%. However, 35% of all patients treated with conventional chest tubes are found to subsequently require either open chest tube drainage or decortication. Several studies have estimated the success rate of fluoroscopy, sonography and CT in image-guided percutaneous insertion of chest tubes to be between 70–90%. Under imaging guidance, the chest tube can be placed accurately in the fluid collection. In fact image-guided percutaneous drainage of empyemas is advocated as the primary method of treating empyemas. Patients who show inadequate drainage or progressive persistent pleural thickening may finally require decortication.

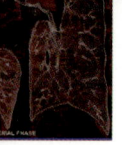

Pneumothorax

Pnuemothorax may be spontaneous, either primary or secondary. A rupture of an apical pleural bleb is the most likely cause for a primary spontaneous pnuemothorax.

The radiographic appearances depend upon the patient's position (air is seen in the most nondependent portion of the pleural cavity) as well as the presence or absence of loculations. In an erect patient, air rises in the pleural space to the apicolateral regions, separating lung from chest wall, allowing the visceral pleural line to become visible. The visceral pleural line separates the vessel-containing lung from the avascular pneumothorax. This line remains parallel with the chest wall; therefore in a shallow pneumothorax it may be difficult to separate the visceral pleural line from the chest wall, especially if covered by ribs. To demonstrate these questionable or

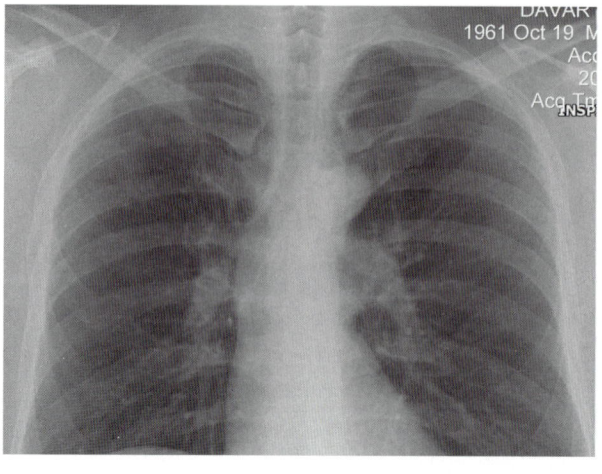

(a)

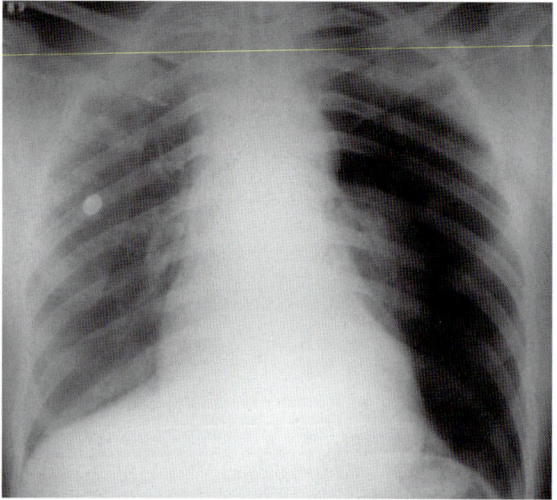

Fig 1.197: Pneumothorax: PA view of the chest demonstrates a large left pneumothorax with total collapse of left lung.

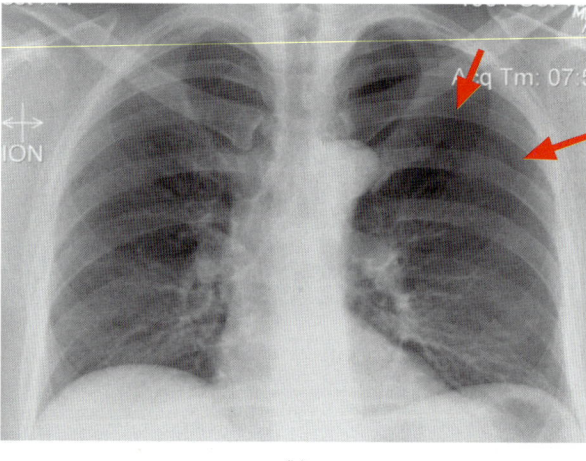

(b)

Fig 1.199: Pneumothorax: (a) Inspiratory PA view demonstrates a suspicious thin visceral pleural line at the right apex (b) Expiratory view demonstrates a large pneumothorax with a well-defined visceral pleural line. Expiratory X-rays are very useful to demonstrate a suspicious pneumothorax as well as the extent of the pneumothorax.

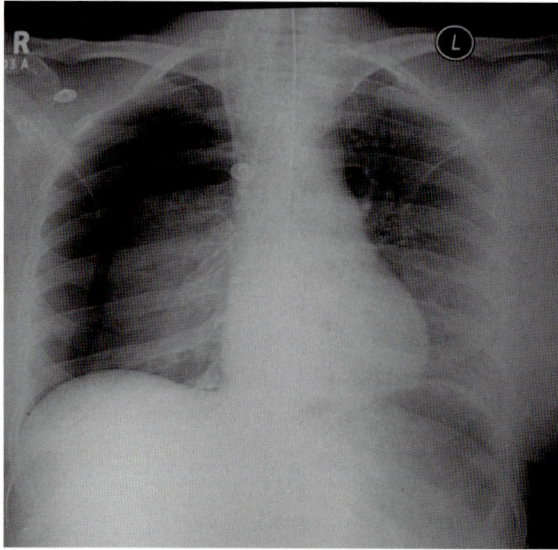

Fig 1.198: Pneumothorax: AP portable erect X-ray reveals a large pneumothorax on the right side with partial collapse of right lung. A central line is seen *in situ* on the right side. The pneumothorax occurred following placement of the central line.

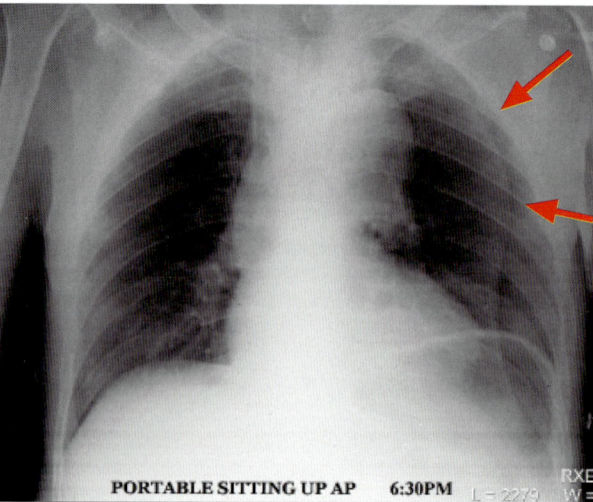

Fig 1.200: PA view of the chest revealed a well-defined line in the left hemithorax simulating a pneumothorax. This however is a skin fold resembling a pneumothorax as the line is seen to extend beyond the confines of the thorax into the abdomen.

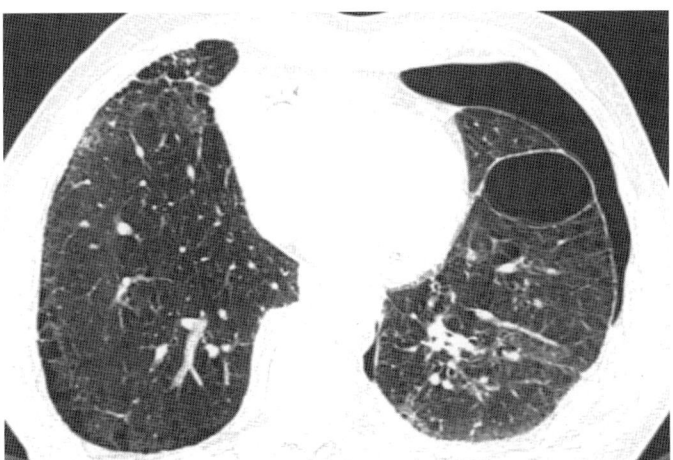

Fig 1.201: Pneumothorax: CT lung window demonstrates a left pneumothorax with a large thin-walled bulla in the left lingula.

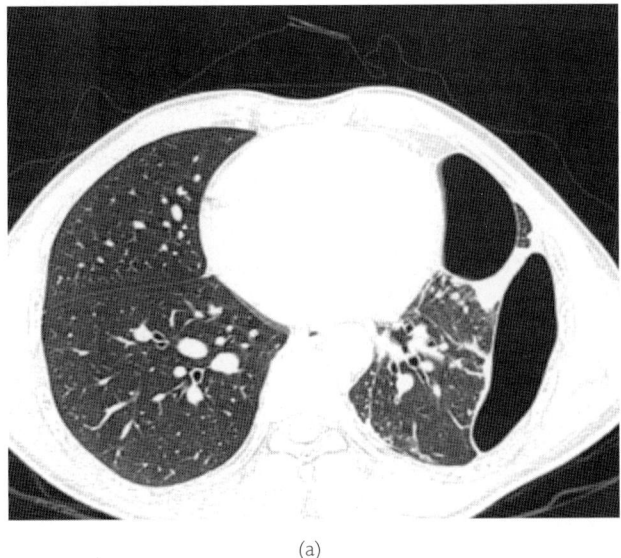

(a)

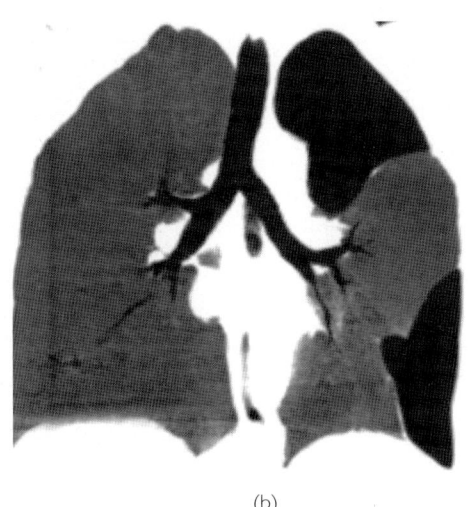

(b)

Fig 1.202: Pneumothorax: (a) CT lung window and (b) minimum intensity projection demonstrate a loculated pneumothorax with adhesions along the left anterior lateral parietal pleura.

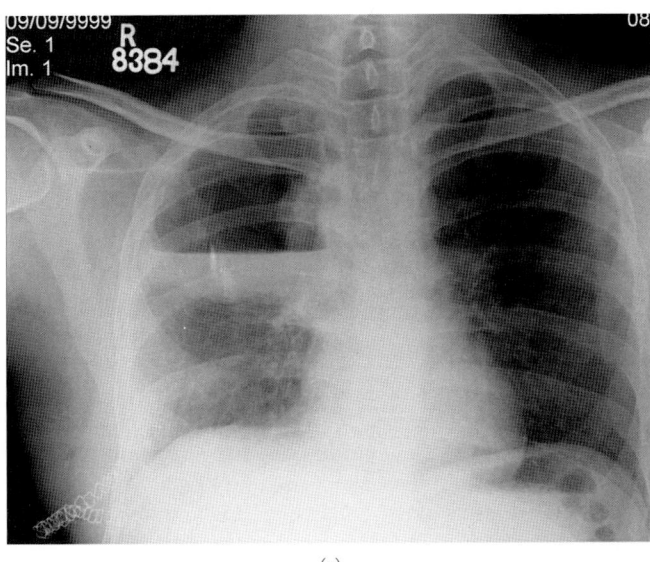

(a)

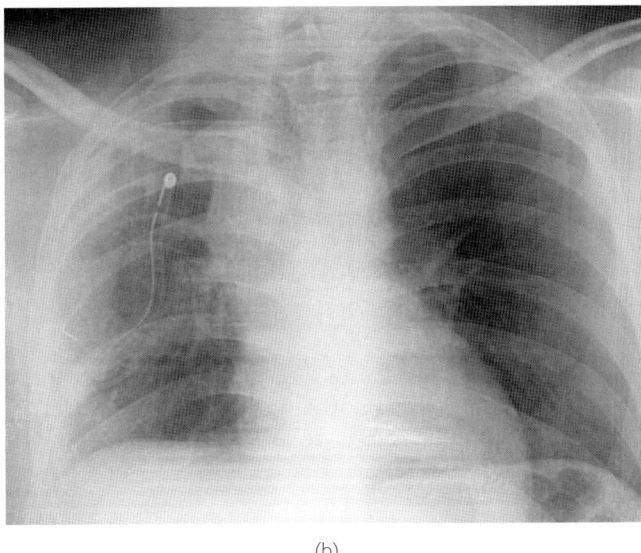

(b)

Fig 1.203: Hydropneumothorax: (a) Chest X-ray demonstrates a right upper zone pneumothorax with an air-fluid level representing a hydropneumothorax. ICD was placed to drain the hydropneumothorax (b) Chest X-ray demonstrates total evacuation of hydropneumothorax.

subtle pneumothoraxes an expiratory film is very useful. This increases the volume of the pneumothorax as well as changes the orientation of the ribs.

There are a number of mimics of a pneumothorax on a chest X-ray. Any curvilinear shadow projected over the lung, especially the apex, may mimic a visceral pleural line. Skin folds, tubes, vascular lines, clothing, scapulae, walls of bulla/cavities all may mimic a visceral pleural line. One of the most helpful differentiators is to follow the so-called visceral pleural line beyond the margins of the chest wall. Other helpful differentiators are when the orientation of the line is not in the orientation of the collapsed lung, or vessels are seen beyond the line. The above circumstances negate the diagnosis of a pneumothorax.

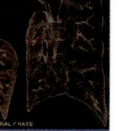

Skin folds appear as thick linear bands with a sharp outer margin and a fading medial margin. The outer margin is transradiant due to air trapped between skin fold and skin. The scapula edge is a common mimic and must be looked out for. Extrapleural dissection of air from a pneumo-mediastinum may also be mistaken for a pneumothorax, the linear abnormality is confined to the lung apex and does not progress in size. The most difficult to differentiate are bullae as they appear translucent/ avascular, and have thin well-defined margins. One differentiating feature is that the inner margin of a bulla is concave as compared to a pneumothorax, which would be convex, in line with the chest wall. CT is very helpful in excluding these mimics of a pneumothorax.

As the pneumothorax increases in size and the lung collapses, the density of the underlying lung increases, till finally in total collapse it appears like a fist-like opacity overlying the hilum. As the density of the collapsing lung increases it becomes easier to detect aetiological causes for the pnuemothorax. For this reason, apical pleural blebs, the most common cause of a primary spontaneous pnuemothorax are visible only on 15% of chest X-rays at the time of the pneumothorax. These blebs are best seen on a CT scan, being detected in 85% of cases. On both X-rays and CT scans other causes such as cysts/bullae/bronchiectasis, etc. should also be looked for. It is also important from a management perspective to estimate the size of a pnuemothorax. A simple method is to measure hemithorax distance, interpleural distance.

$$\% \text{ of pneumothorax} = 100 - \frac{(\text{Hemithorax} - \text{interpleural distance})^3}{\text{Hemithorax distance}^3} \times 100$$

For example, if the hemithorax distance is 10 cm and the interpleural distance is 2 cm, the size of the pneumothorax is 50%, an indication that the pneumothorax is much larger than what might be apparent on an X-ray chest.

PNEUMOTHORAX IN A SUPINE PATIENT

In a number of patients in a critical care setting X-rays can only be done in a supine position. It is important to recognize the signs of a pnuemothorax in a supine patient. Air collects in the highest portion of the pleural cavity which in the supine position is anterior or anteriomedially at the base. The displaced visceral pleural line is difficult to demonstrate on a supine X-ray. In the absence of this specific sign other signs to demonstrate the collection of air are important. As air collects in the anterior costophrenic sulcus there is transradiancy in the hypochondrial region overlying the diaphragm. There is increased sharpness of the adjacent mediastinal margin and diaphragm. The costophrenic sulcus becomes deep with a well-defined margin. The inferior edge of collapsed lung becomes visible. The ipsilateral hemidiaphragm is depressed. Cardiac margins become sharp and pericardial fat pads become well-outlined.

A pneumothorax suspected on a supine film can be confirmed on a cross-table lateral view or lateral decubitus with suspect side uppermost. If there is any doubt a CT will be very useful, as it would be confirmatory.

Tension pneumothorax is an absolute emergency and if untreated results in death. A tension pneumothorax occurs when

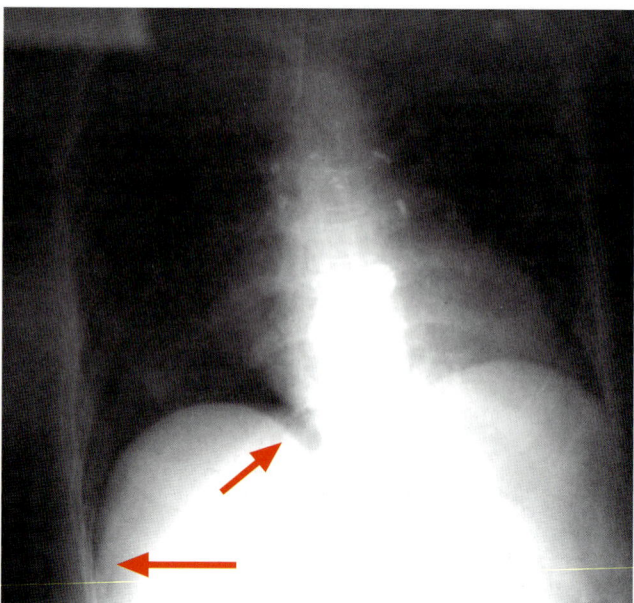

Fig 1.204: Pneumothorax: Supine AP view in a patient who was haemodynamically unstable; an erect view was not possible. The costophrenic and cardiophrenic recess on the right side are deep and well-outlined. The right dome of the diaphragm is well-outlined as compared to the left. These are all features of a pneumothorax in a supine patient.

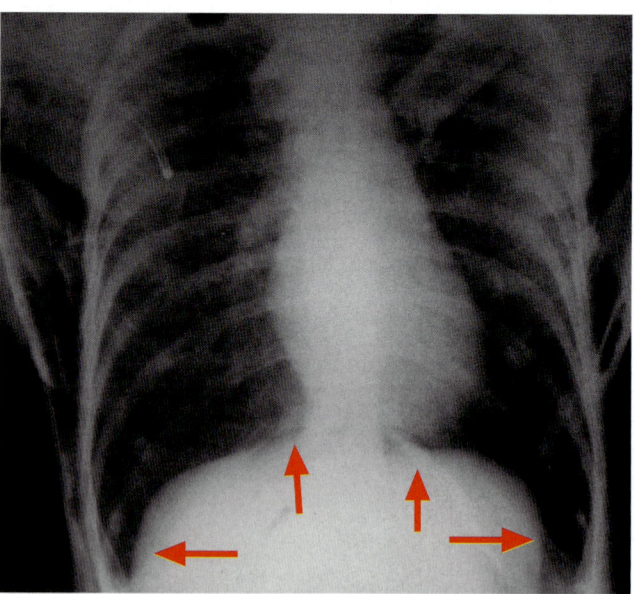

Fig 1.205: Pneumothorax: Supine AP view reveals bilateral pneumothorax as evidenced by a sharp diaphragmatic contour and sharp deep bilateral costophrenic sulci. There is extensive surgical emphysema.

air enters during inspiration but cannot exit during expiration due to a check valve mechanism. On a chest X-ray, the entire hemithorax is hypertranslucent, the mediastinum is shifted to the opposite side and the ipsilateral lung is compressed. In addition the diaphragm on the affected side may be deeply inverted.

MANAGEMENT OF PNEUMOTHORAX

Not every pneumothorax requires drainage. An asymptomatic pneumothorax with interpleural distance less than 2.0 cm may be successfully managed by observation with or without oxygen therapy. Larger symptomatic pneumothoraces may resolve if the air is totally aspirated and the two pleural surfaces appose each other.

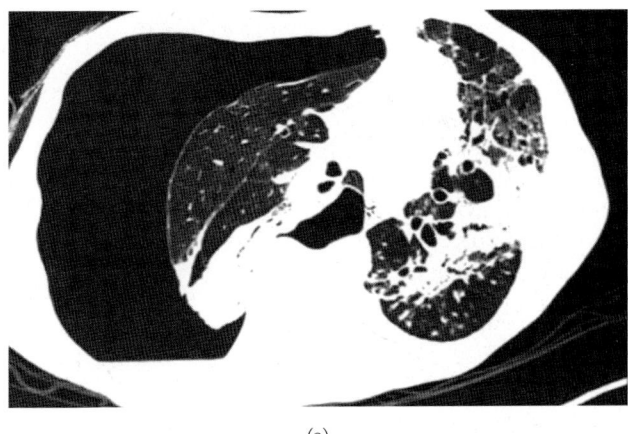

(a)

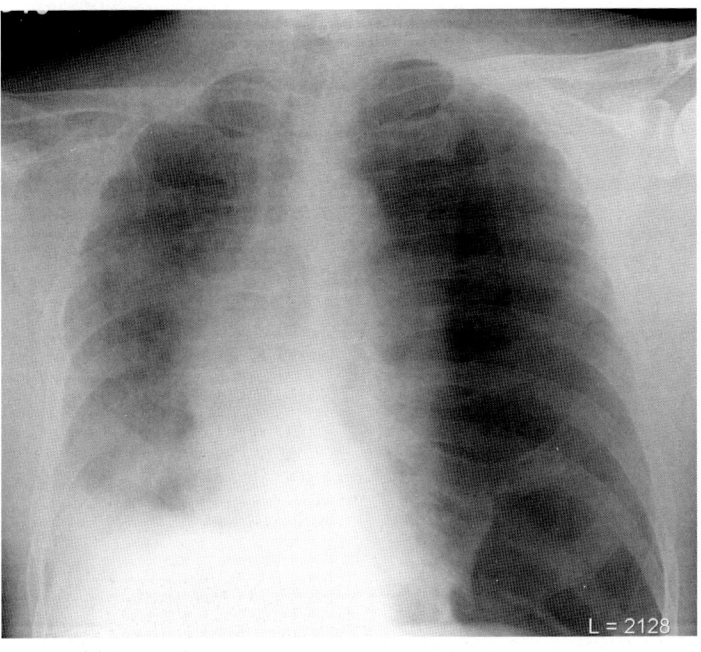

(a)

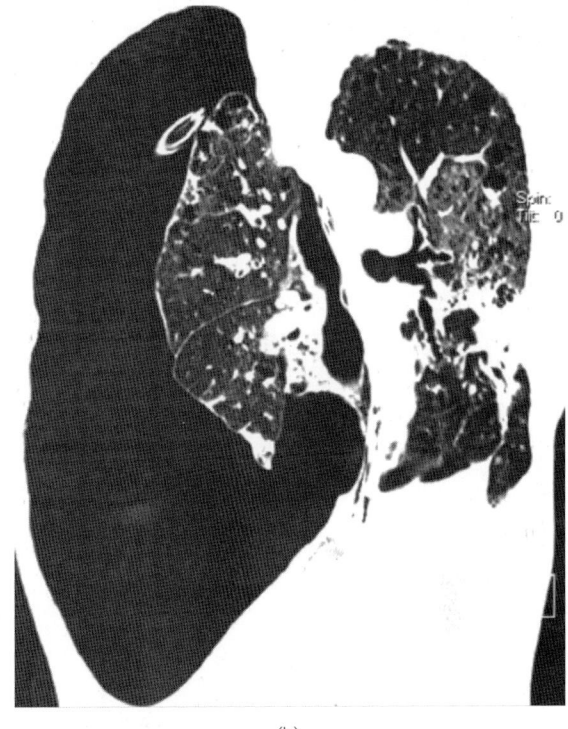

(b)

Fig 1.207: Tension pneumothorax: (a) Axial and (b) coronal CT demonstrate a large pneumothorax on the right side. The pneumothorax is under tension as evidenced by inversion of the right dome of the diaphragm and displacement of the mediastinum. Extensive centrilobular emphysema is seen in both lung fields.

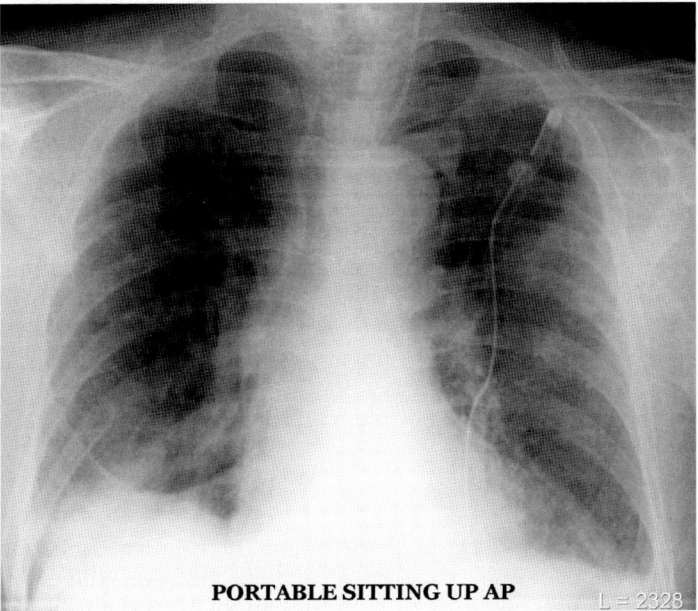

(b)

Fig 1.206: Tension pneumothorax: (a) PA view of the chest reveals a translucency in the left hemithorax due to a large pneumothorax. There is a shift of the mediastinum to the right with herniation of lung to the right side. These are features of a tension pnuemothorax (b) After insertion of ICD tube, there is expansion of lung with a return of mediastinal structures to their normal position.

Bronchopleural Fistula (BPF)

A bronchopleural fistula may be central when the communication is between the bronchus and pleura. A peripheral BPF exists when the communication is between lung parenchyma or a peripheral bronchus and the pleura. The chest radiography signs of a bronchopleural fistula are an increase in air in a pneumonectomy space, with a loss of normal mediastinal shift towards the operated side. Occasionally, the only sign is a persistence of air following pnuemonectomy. CT is useful to demonstrate the bronchopleural fistula, but may do so in only 30–50% of cases.

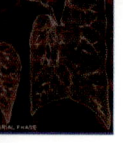

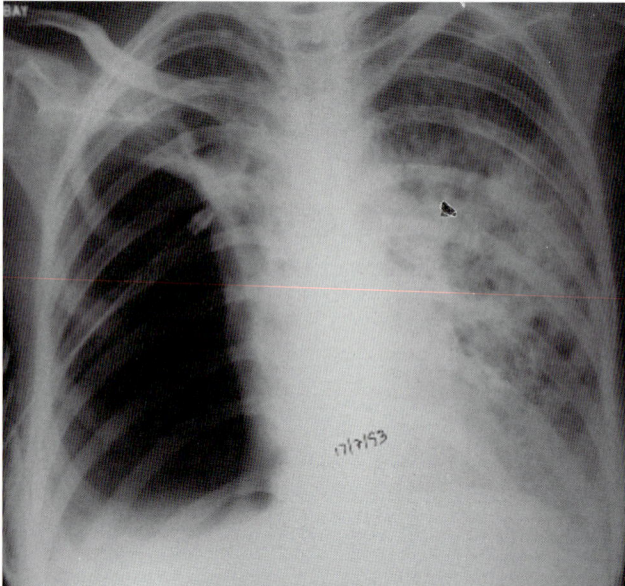

Fig 1.208: Bronchopleural fistula: PA view of the chest demonstrates a large pnuemothorax on the right side with a shift of the mediastinum to the left. There are extensive consolidations in the left lung. An ICD is seen *in situ* in the right pleural space. The pneumothorax is seen to persist even after the ICD has been placed. This is an important sign of a bronchopleural fistula.

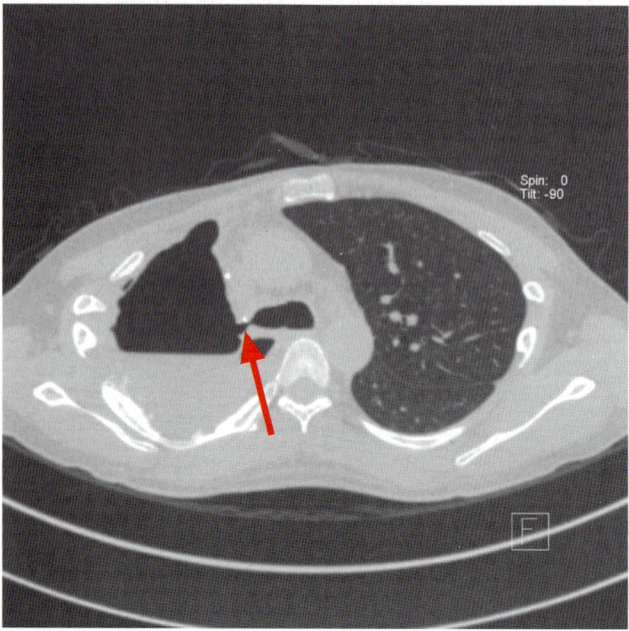

Fig 1.209: Bronchopleural fistula: Persistent hydropneumothorax following a right pneumonectomy. HRCT chest reveals a small persistent communication between the bronchial stump and the pleural space.

Pleural Thickening

Pleural thickening is seen as a veil-like opacity along the inner margins of the chest wall, sharply marginated along its inner aspect and fading into the chest wall along its lateral aspect. Pleural thickening involving the costophrenic angle is seen as an angular opacity differentiating it from pleural fluid which is seen as a smooth curvilinear margin. In cases of difficulty, a

lateral decubitus or ultrasound would help in differentiation. CT is very sensitive in the detection of pleural thickening. Extrapleural fat can mimic pleural thickening; this is also well-differentiated on CT.

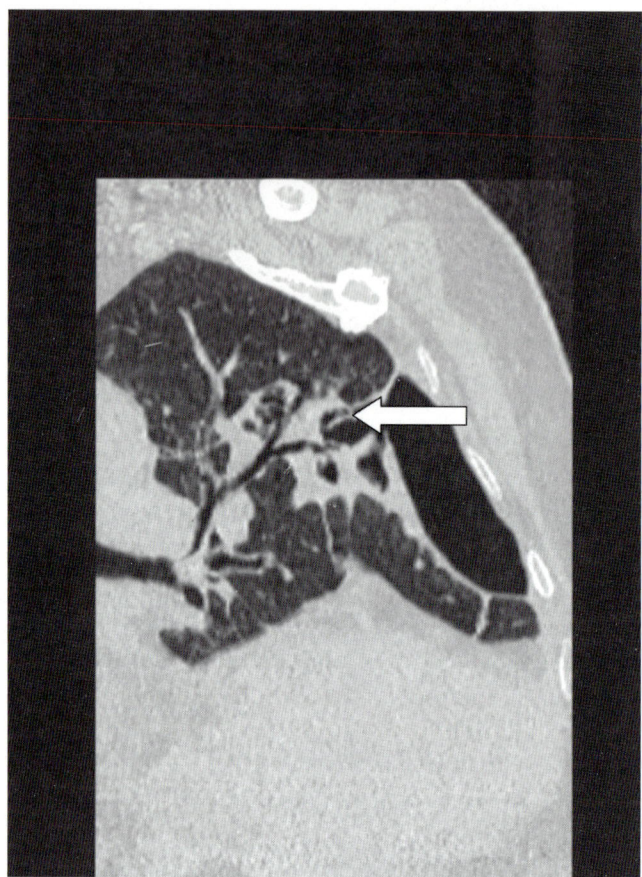

Fig 1.210: Bronchopleural fistula-MPR demonstrates a communication between a left upper lobe bronchus and a loculated pneumothorax.

Pleural Calcification

Pleural calcification is visualized as a sheet of calcification. When visualized en face, it appears as a veil-like opacity; when visualized in profile it is seen as a linear dense band parallel to the inner chest wall. Following resolution of an empyema, calcification may be seen as a double layer due to calcification of visceral and parietal pleura. This is well appreciated on CT.

Mesothelioma

On imaging, there are plaques/nodules on visceral/parietal pleura forming a lobular sheet of tumour up to several cm thick encasing the lung and growing into the interlobar fissure. Invasion of the mediastinum, diaphragm, lung may occur, though late. An important sign is the loss of lung volume on the ipsilateral side, because the mesothelioma grows as a sheet entrapping the lung. These appearances are very well demonstrated on a CT, which is useful for detection, as also for demonstration of chest wall and or mediastinal invasion. Occasionally, the only finding may

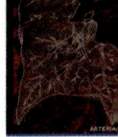

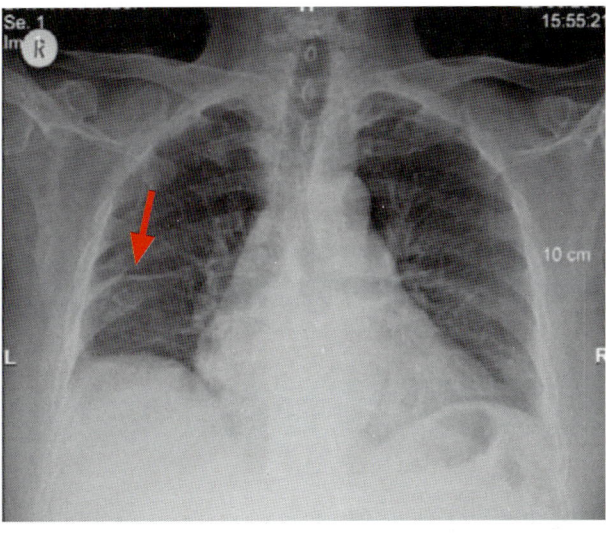

(a)

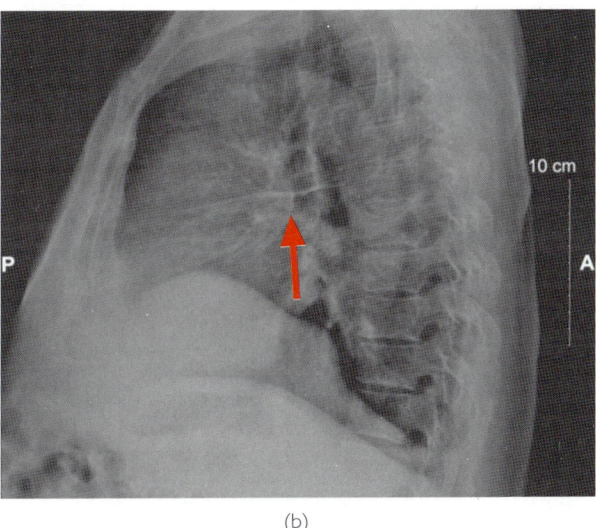

(b)

Fig 1.211: Pleural Thickening: (a) PA and (b) lateral views demonstrate thickening of the minor fissure following resolution of a interlobar effusion.

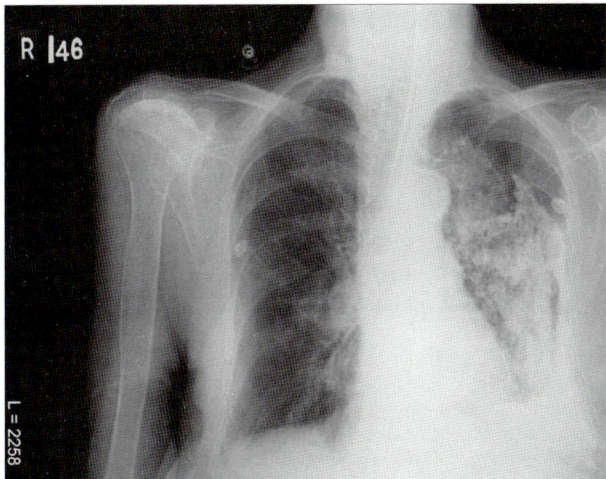

Fig 1.212: Pleural calcification: AP view of chest reveals veil-like calcification in the left hemithorax.

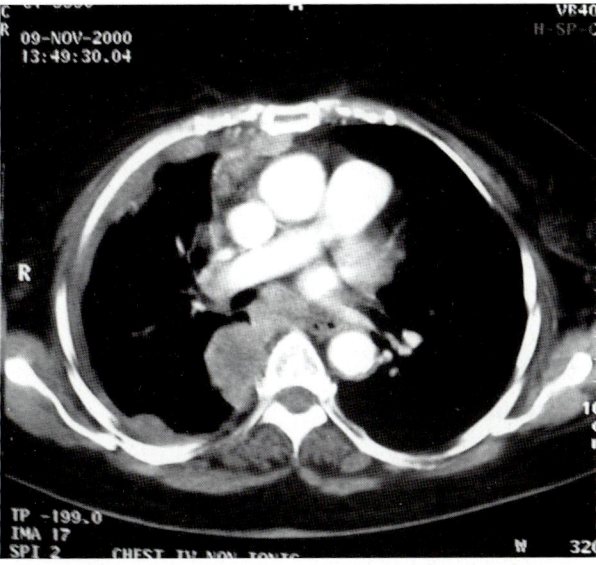

Fig 1.213: Pleural mesothelioma: CT chest shows presence of multiple lobulated enhancing lesions along the entire right pleural surface.

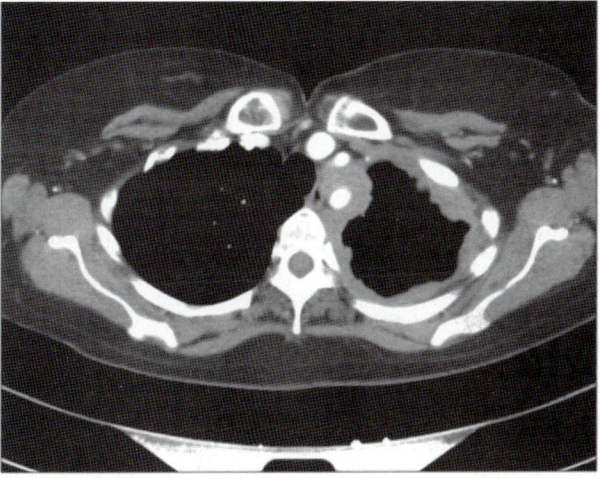

Fig 1.214: Mesothelioma: CT chest reveals plaque-like thickening of pleural surface with nodularity of surface in left apical region. Biopsy revealed a mesothelioma. Note vascular encasement of the great vessels by the mesothelioma.

be pleural thickening with a small-sized ipsilateral hemithorax. The pleural masses are seen to creep along the pleural surfaces. MRI is also useful for demonstrating chest wall and mediastinal involvement.

THE MEDIASTINUM

The chest radiograph is usually the first investigation performed for a suspected mediastinal/hilar mass lesion. Mediastinal masses may also be detected incidentally on X-rays done for other reasons. If a mediastinal pathology is suspected and the chest X-ray reveals no abnormality, a cross-sectional imaging technique, ideally a CT scan is required. Medastinal pathology may be obscured by mediastinal vasculature on an X-ray. A CT scan is very useful to characterize the mass lesion; it also serves as a guide for biopsy of a mediastinal mass. Mediastinal masses appear on chest X-rays as projections

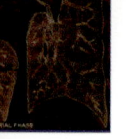

from the mediastinal silhouette. Hilar masses are visualized as prominence and or enlargement of the hilum. The first step in the differential diagnosis is to determine if the lesion arises from the mediastinum or lung. A spiculated mass lesion will nearly always be of pulmonary origin. Homogenous masses which project beyond the confines of the mediastinum, have a broad base and form obtuse angles with the mediastinum, arise from the mediastinum or mediastinal pleura. The differential diagnosis of mediastinal masses is based on their location and internal morphology.

LOCATION

Prevascular Masses

Prevascular masses are located anterior to the ascending aorta and its branches. These are most commonly thymic masses, thyroid masses, germ cell tumours or lymphadenopathy. Thyroid masses are easy to diagnose as they are seen in the superior mediastinum contiguous with the thyroid in the neck. On unenhanced scans they are of a higher attenuation than adjacent skeletal muscle in view of their iodine content. Internally, thyroid masses are heterogeneous with calcific densities and cysts. Thyroid masses are the most common lesions to cause deviation of the trachea. Thymic and germ cell tumours appear similar on imaging; their differentiation is based on clinical and laboratory features. Thymomas may be clinically associated with myasthenia gravis, red cell aplasia, hypogammaglobinemia. An elevated HCG or alpha feto protein levels are indicative of a germ cell tumour. Thymoma, germ cell tumours may demonstrate calcification. Presence of fat, cartilaginous calcification, teeth or a fat fluid level are indicative of a mature teratoma.

Unusual causes of prevascular masses are parathyroid adenoma (usually evidence of hyperparathyroidism). Lymphangioma (cystic with multiple internal septations). Cystic hygroma should be considered when a cystic mass is seen extending from the neck into the mediastinum.

Paracardiac Masses

Chiefly include pericardial cyst, diaphragmatic hernia and lymphadenopathy.

Pericardial cysts are easily diagnosed as they are homogenous, of water attenuation, with thin walls. Diaphragmatic hernia, Morgagni's hernia, are due to a defect in the diaphragm with herniation of a pad of fat and or bowel loops into the thorax. Occasionally, germ cell tumours and thymomas may be visualized in a paracardiac location.

Paratracheal, Subcarinal and Paraesophageal Masses

These are considered together as they are contained in one fascial sheath. The group includes lymphadenopathy, foregut malformations, oesophageal tumours, thyroid mass lesions, hiatus hernia, aneurysms, vascular anomalies and pancreatic pseudocyst. The commonest of these is lymphadenopathy. Oesophageal carcinoma presents early as dysphagia and generally results in a small mass lesion. Vascular anomalies and aneurysms are visualized

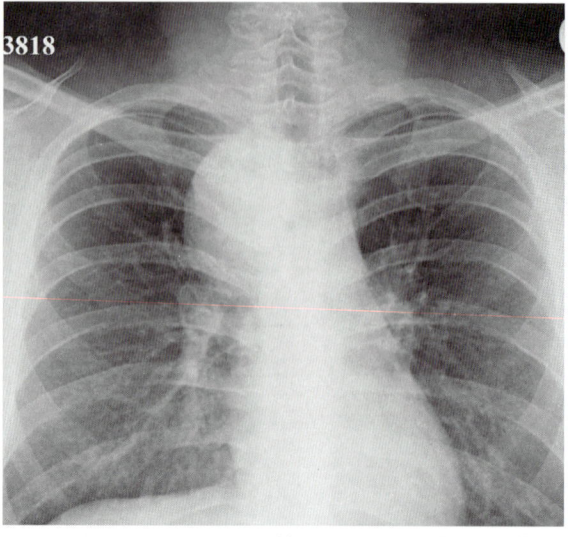

(a)

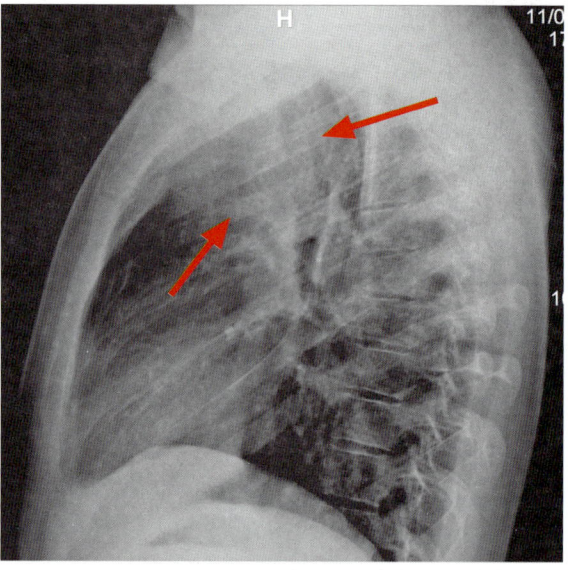

(b)

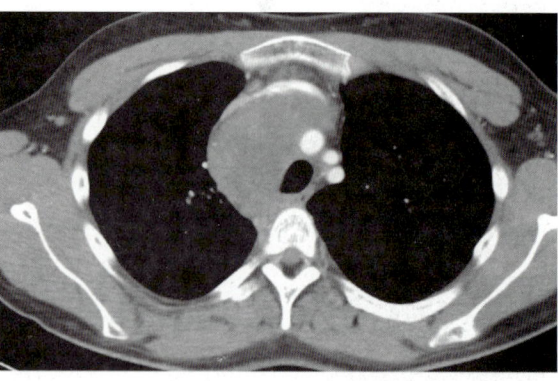

(c)

Fig 1.215: Mediastinal adenopthy: Chest X-ray (a) reveals a large right paratracheal mass lesion. Note it is homogenous with a wide mediastinal base and obtuse angles with the lung indicating a medistinal mass lesion. Lateral view (b) demonstrates the mass lesion to be anterior mediastinum. CT chest (c) confirms that the mass lesion is a large necrotic adenopathy. CT-guided aspiration confirmed the adenopathy to be of tubercular origin.

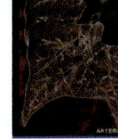

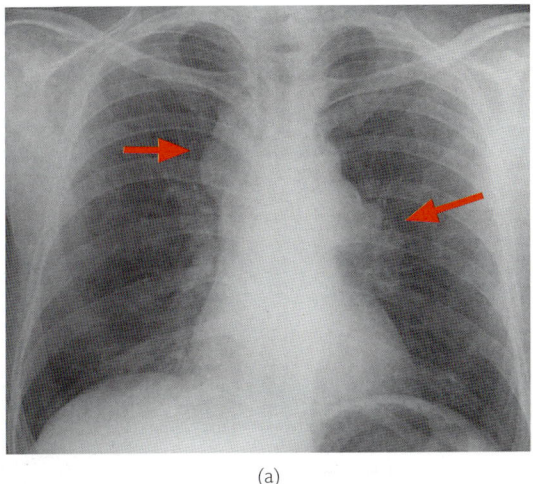

(a)

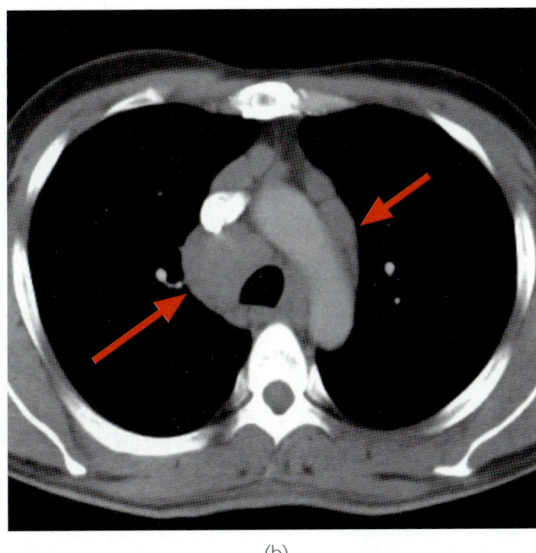

(b)

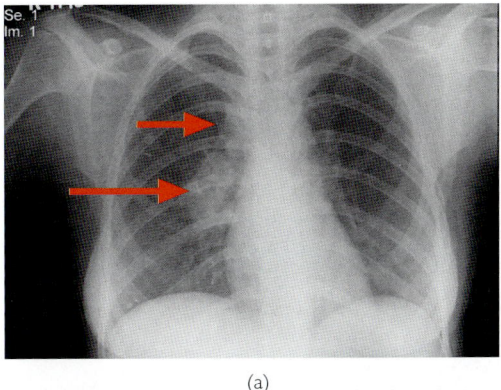

(a)

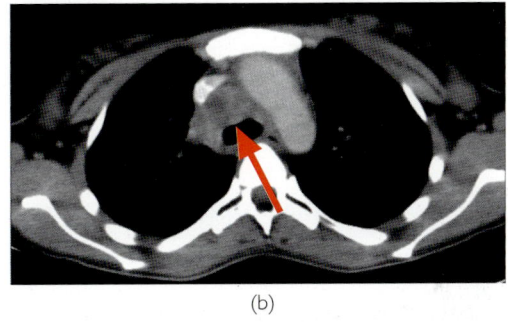

(b)

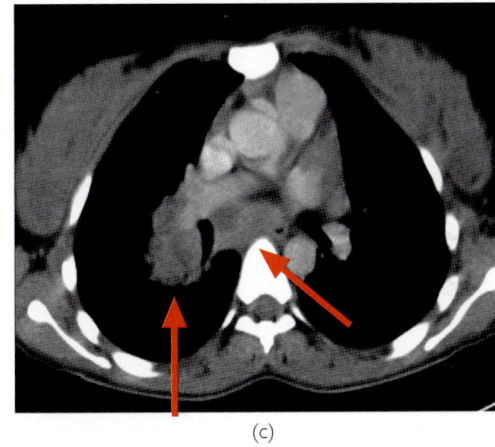

(c)

Fig 1.217: Mediastinal adenopthy: (a) Chest X-ray demonstrates large right paratracheal and hilar adenopathy (b) CT chest (c) confirm adenopathy, which are necrotic, indicating tuberculosis.

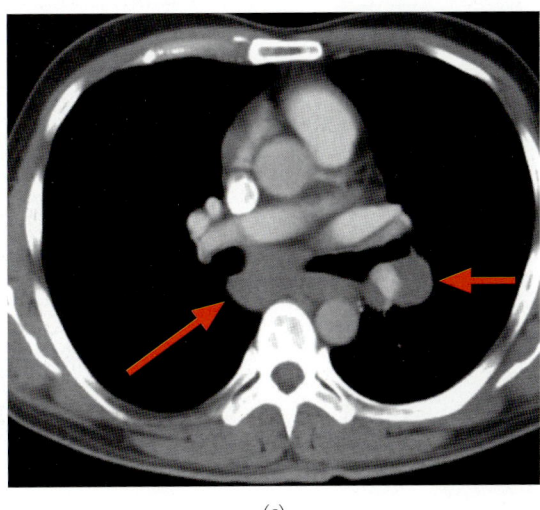

(c)

Fig 1.216: Mediastinal adenopathy: (a) Chest X-ray reveals right paratracheal and left hilar adenopathy (b & c) CT chest confirms adenopathy as well as demonstrates small left prevascular adenopathy and large subcarinal adenopathy, not detected on the X-ray as these were covered by the mediastinum.

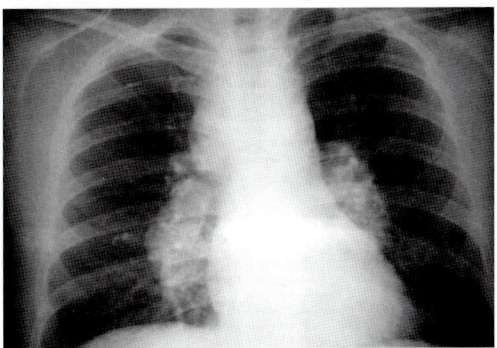

Fig 1.218: Mediastinal adenopathy: Chest X-ray demonstrates large hilar and right paratracheal mass lesions representing adenopathy.

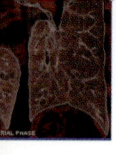

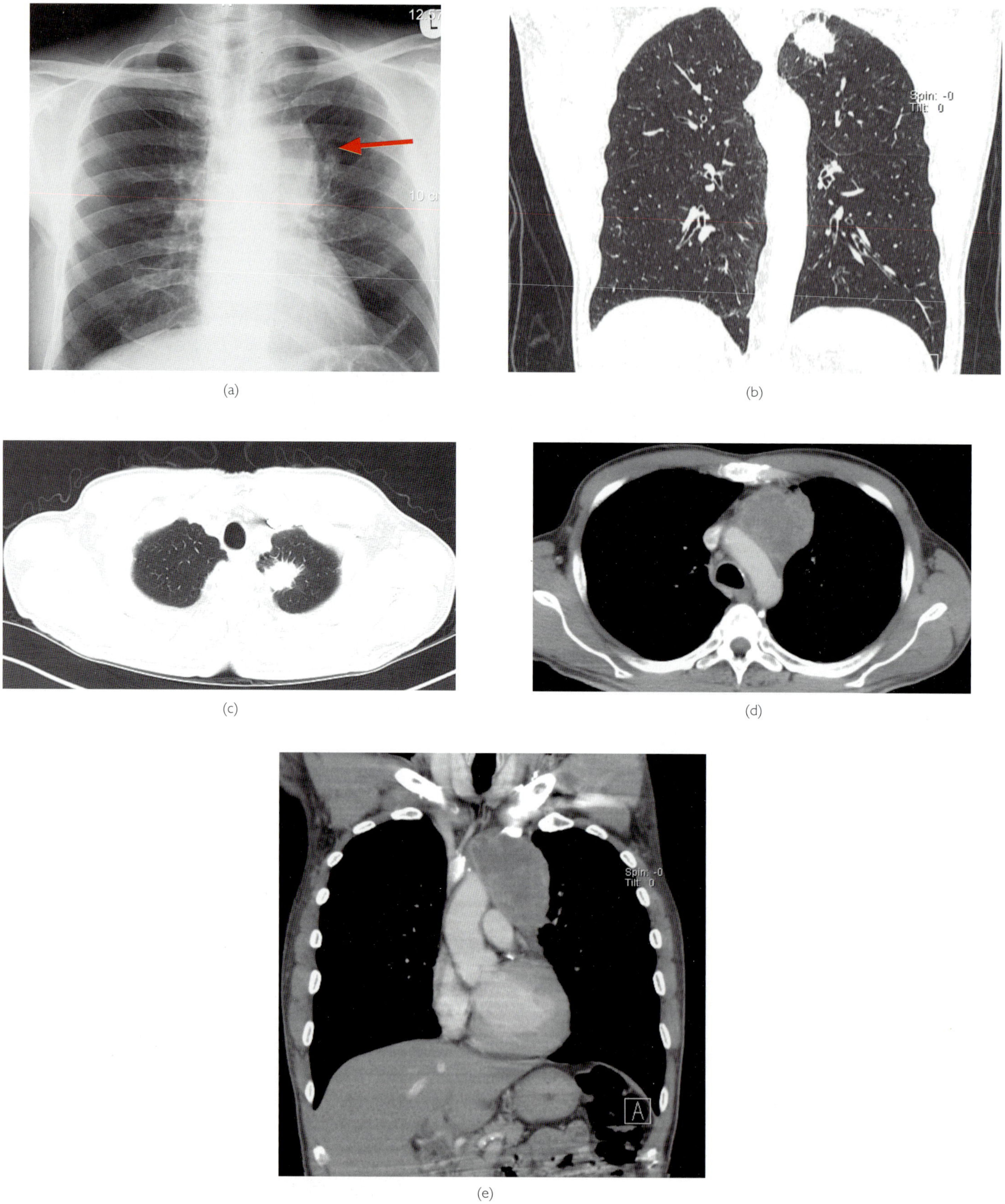

(a)

(b)

(c)

(d)

(e)

Fig 1.219: Metastatic mediastinal adenopathy: (a) Chest X-ray reveals an opacity in the left para-aortic region, however, not silhouetting the aorta (b) Coronal CT demonstrates a spiculated mass lesion in the left apex (c) axial CT demonstrates spiculated apical mass lesion very well. CT-guided FNAC revealed mass to be squamous cell carcinoma (d) axial post-contrast CT reveals large anterior mediastinal mass lesion representing metastases adenopathy (e) coronal reconstruction demonstrates large anterior mediastinal adenopathy.

as homogenous enhancing structures. Foregut malformations are fluid-filled well-defined lesions in relation to the vertebrae, oesophagus or tracheo-bronchial tree.

Prevertebral Masses

These are most commonly neurogenic tumours, or lymph gland masses. Other pathologies include mesenchymal tumours, lesions arising from the pharynx, or vertebra. A paraspinal abscess and an aneurysm of the descending aorta are also observed in the prevertebral location.

Imaging studies of prevascular masses, of paracardiac masses, of paratracheal, subcarinal, paraesophageal masses and of prevertebral masses have been amply illustrated in the chapter on 'Diseases of the Mediastinum' and therefore do not bear repetition.

SUGGESTED READING

Bhalla Sanjiv. Thoracic MDCT Comes of Age. *Radiologic Clinics of North America*. 2010; 48.

Hansell David M, Amstrong Peter, Lynch David, and McAdams Page. *Imaging of the Diseases of the Chest*. 2005, fourth edition: Elsevier Mosby.

Phillippe A Grenier. Imaging of Airway Diseases. *Radiologic Clinics of North America*. 2009; 47.

Richard Webb, Nestor L Muller, and David P. Naidich. *High Resolution CT of the Lung*. 2008, fourth edition, Lippincott Williams & Wilkins.

CHAPTER **2**

Mechanics of Ventilation

This chapter starts by describing lung volumes and then deals with the basic action of respiratory muscles. It goes on to explain the physical properties of the lung and chest wall and the interaction between the two that influences the movement of air in and out of the lungs during the cyclic process of ventilation. Next, the chapter explains the regional differences in ventilation, airway resistance and its measurement and the physiological factors that affect airway resistance. It goes on to explain the dynamic compression of the airways during a forced expiration and finally considers the work required to move the lung and chest wall during ventilation.

LUNG VOLUMES

The total gas-containing capacities can be partitioned into different volumes which when combined give lung capacities.

Total lung capacity (TLC) is the largest amount of air held within the lungs at maximum inspiration. The residual volume (RV) is the amount of air left within the lung after a maximal forced expiration. The greatest volume of air that can be inspired or expired is the vital capacity (VC). The VC is therefore the difference between the TLC and RV.

Tidal volume (TV) is the inspiratory or expiratory volume during normal breathing at rest. It constitutes about 10% of the VC. Tidal volume increases with strenuous exercise, but even so does not exceed 50–60% of VC. The volume of air contained in the lung at end-expiratory position is termed the functional residual capacity (FRC). The FRC is roughly about 50% of the TLC. The FRC consists of the expiratory reserve volume

plus residual volume. The volume of air that can be maximally inspired from the resting end-inspiratory level is the inspiratory reserve volume (IRV). The maximal volume of air inspired

Table 2.1: Glossary for static lung volumes and capacities		
Term	**Abbreviation**	**Definition**
Volumes		
Residual volume	RV	Volume of air remaining in the lungs after maximal expiration
Expiratory reserve volume	ERV	Maximal volume of air expired from the resting end-expiratory level
Tidal volume	TV	Volume of air expired or inspired with each breath during normal breathing
Inspiratory reserve volume	IRV	Maximal volume of air inspired from the resting end-inspiratory level
Capacities		
Inspiratory capacity	IC	Maximal volume of air inspired from the end-expiratory level
Vital capacity	VC	Maximal volume of air expired from the maximal inspiration
Functional residual capacity	FRC	Volume of air remaining in the lung at the end-expiratory level
Total lung capacity	TLC	Volume of air in the lungs after maximal inspiration

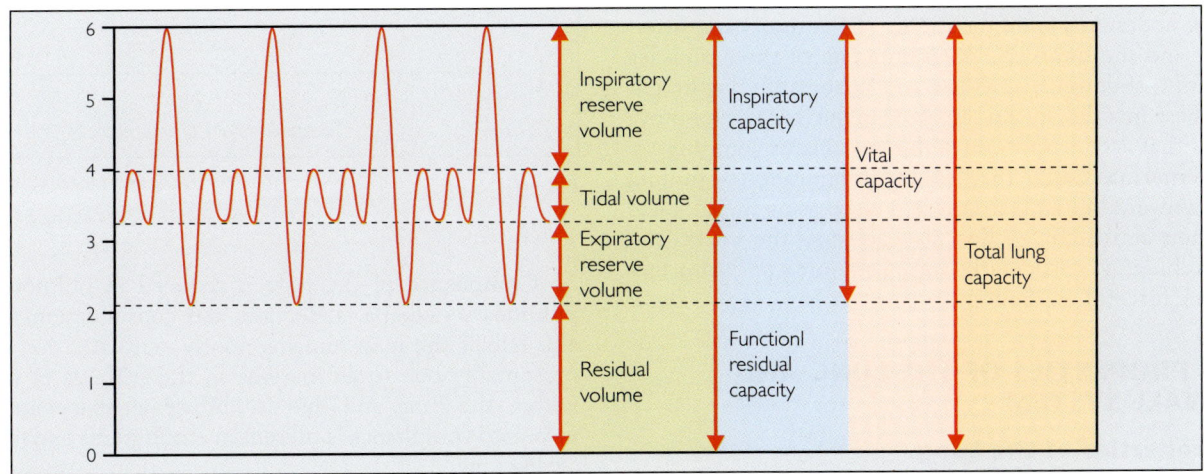

Fig 2.1: Lung volumes and capacities as recorded by a spirometer. The definitions of these subdivisions are found in Table 2.1.

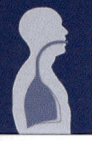

from the end-expiratory level is the–inspiratory capacity (IC). Lung volumes and capacities are defined in Table 2.1 and are depicted schematically in Figure 2.1 and which have been obtained using a spirometer.

RESPIRATORY MUSCLES

Inspiration

The most important muscle of inspiration is the diaphragm, which is a dome-shaped sheet of muscle attached to the lower ribs. The diaphragm contracts on inspiration, pushing the abdominal contents downwards and forwards (the upper abdominal wall in the supine posture is seen to bulge upwards on inspiration) and also increasing the vertical dimension of the chest cavity. In addition the rib margins are lifted upwards and outwards thereby increasing the transverse diameter of the chest wall.

The diaphragm is supplied by the phrenic nerve from cervical segments 3, 4, 5. When the diaphragm is paralysed it is drawn upwards during inspiration because of the increased negativity of the intrapleural pressure. This is termed a *paradoxical movement*. It can be diagnosed at the bedside when the upper abdomen moves inwards rather than outwards on inspiration Diaphragmatic paralysis is best proven by the 'sniff test' (a sharp inspiratory sniff through the nostrils with the mouth closed). Fluroscopic examination during the sniff shows paradoxical upward movement of the diaphragm instead of the usual downward movement. Patients with diaphragmatic paralysis are unable to lie down flat; they become breathless and hypoxic. Substantial relief is observed on sitting or standing.

The external intercostal muscles also help with inspiration. They slope downwards and forward and on contraction pull the ribs upwards and forward increasing both the transverse and the anteroposterior diameter of the chest. The lateral expansion of the chest is due to a 'bucket-handle' movement of the ribs. The intercostal muscles are supplied by the intercostal nerves arising from the spinal cord segments at the same level.

Expiration

Expiration is a passive process during quiet breathing. Expiration becomes active during exercise and during purposeful hyperventilation. The most important muscles of expiration are those of the abdominal wall, the rectus, the external and internal oblique and the transversalis. Contraction of these muscles raises the intra-abdominal pressure and pushes the diaphragm upwards. These muscles are also involved in the forced expiratory movements that accompany coughing, sneezing or vomiting.

The internal intercostal muscles help in expiration by pulling the ribs downwards and inward thereby decreasing the thoracic volume. Their active contraction also prevents the intercostal spaces from bulging, particularly during straining or during any act involving forceful expiration.

ELASTIC PROPERTIES OF THE LUNG AND CHEST WALL SYSTEM

Elastic Properties of the Lung

The lung is a structure with inherent elasticity so that it tends to recoil to a volume equal to (in fact a little less than) residual volume. To increase the volume of the lung from this resting state requires a force that should distend the lung. This force, termed the transpulmonary pressure, is the difference between the alveolar pressure and the pressure surrounding the lung which is the intrapleural pressure. The relation between lung volume and transmural pressure is illustrated in Figure 2.2. The graph illustrates the elastic properties of the lung and its tendency to recoil. This graph is applicable to an excised lung inflated by a pump, to an *in vivo* lung inflated by a ventilator or to a normal lung inflated by a normal physiological inspiration. In each case the graph of volume vs. transpulmonary pressure remains the same.

The slope of the pressure volume curve is a measure of the compliance of the lung. Compliance is defined as the change in volume per unit change in pressure.

$$C = \Delta V/\Delta P$$

In the normal range (intrapleural pressure –5 to –10 cm of H_2O) the lung is markedly compliant or distensible. The compliance of the normal human lung is 200 ml per cm H_2O. The compliance as seen from the graph is more at the beginning of the curve and decreases with greater distending pressure when lung volume approaches TLC. Compliance is obviously dependent on the lung size, so that the small lungs of a child are less compliant than those of an adult. A patient living on one lung following a pneumonectomy will obviously have a lower compliance (half of normal) even though the lung is perfectly healthy. For this reason compliance is often divided by lung volume to give the volume-independent specific compliance.

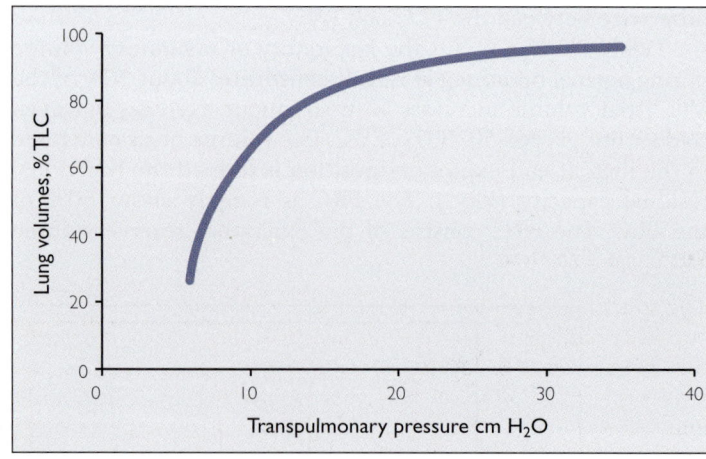

Fig 2.2: Pressure-volume curve of the lung during inspiration.

Compliance of the lung is reduced in pulmonary fibrosis, pulmonary oedema, atelectasis and consolidation. Compliance also falls if the lung remains poorly ventilated for a long time, presumably due to an increase in the stiffness of elastic tissue within the lung and due to diffuse air-space atelectasis. An increased compliance is present in emphysema and in the normal ageing lung.

It should be noted that the pressure surrounding the lung (i.e. the intrapleural pressure) is less than atmospheric pressure because of the elastic recoil of the lung. The tendency of the lung to return or rather recoil to its resting volume is related to the presence of elastic tissue (elastin) visible on histological studies in alveolar walls and around bronchi and vessels. West believes that the elastic behaviour of the lung has less to do with simple elongation of these fibres than it does with their geometric arrangement.

The earlier figure illustrates the pressure volume curve during inspiration. Figure 2.3 shows the pressure volume curves during inspiration and expiration. It will be noted that the curves which the lung follows are different in inspiration and expiration or during inflation and deflation. This phenomenon is termed hysteresis. It is also noted that for any given pressure the lung volume is more in expiration or deflation than in inspiration or inflation. The curve further shows that even without any expanding pressure the lung has some air within it.

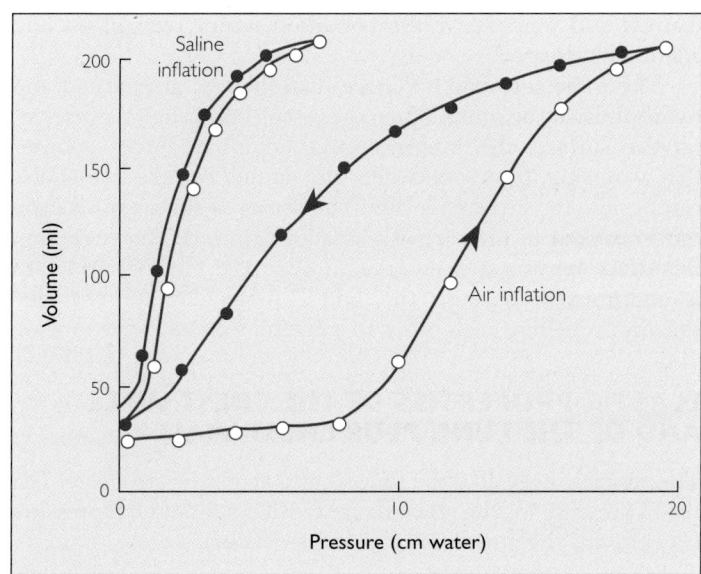

Fig 2.4: Comparison of pressure volume curves of air-filled and saline-filled lung(cat). Open circles, inflation; closed circles deflation. Note that the saline-filled lung has a higher compliance and also much less hysteriesis than the air-filled lung. (With permission from *Respiratory Physiology The Essentials* by John B. West, seventh edition. Lippincott William and Wilkins).

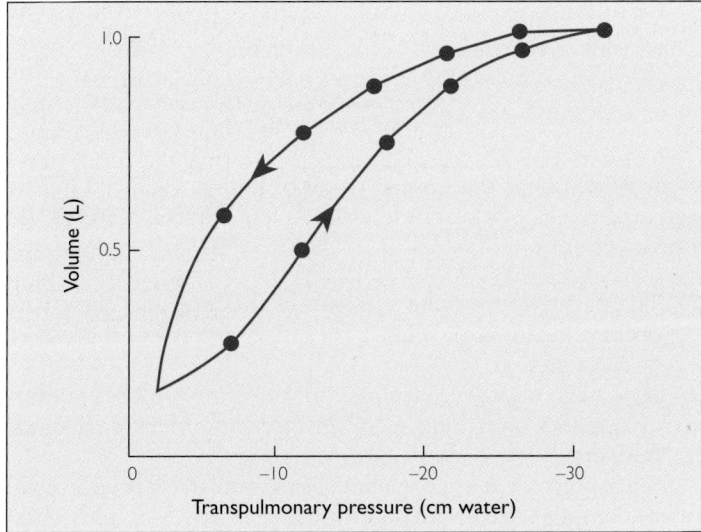

Fig 2.3: Curves which the lung follows during inflation and deflation are different. This behaviour is known as hysteresis.

Surface Tension

The elastic properties of the lung seen in pressure volume curves are influenced by the surface tension of the liquid lining the alveolar walls. Surface tension is produced because the attractive forces between the adjacent molecules of the liquid lining the alveolar walls are much greater than those between liquid and gas. The liquid area as a result shrinks and becomes small. A lung filled with saline so that surface tension forces are thereby abolished will have a different pressure volume curve reflecting only the tissue properties of the lung (Figure 2.4). The saline-filled curve is shifted to the left showing that the lung can be distended with much less pressure. The air-containing lung requires greater pressure for distension and as remarked earlier shows hysteresis—the volume curve during deflation following a different course than that observed during inflation. Also, the deflation curve of the air-filled lung is close to the volume curve of the saline-filled lung at low volumes, indicating that the pressure within alveoli from surface tension is reduced at low volumes. This seems paradoxical for according to Laplace's

law, pressure within a sphere should increase if the radius is reduced, P= 2T/r. This paradox is explained by the presence of a unique fluid lining the alveoli, termed surfactant. Surfactant is responsible for reducing surface tension in a volume-dependent manner so that as the volume of the alveoli decreases, surface tension also decreases, the surface tension being almost absent at residual volume.

The role of surfactant in the alveoli of the lung is important for the following reasons:

1. It prevents collapse and ensures stability of the alveoli. If pressure within alveoli with smaller volume were to increase as per Laplace's Law, they would empty into interconnecting larger alveoli with lower pressure. Surfactant prevents this by paradoxically reducing the pressure within the low-volume alveoli through reduction of surface tension.
2. A low surface tension in the alveoli increases the compliance of the lung and reduces the work of breathing.
3. The force of surface tension at the corners of the alveoli tends to draw fluid inwards into the alveoli from outside capillaries and the interstitium. Surfactant, by lowering surface tension, prevents pulmonary oedema.

Surfactant is secreted by Type II alveolar epithelial cells. These are compact cells which on electron microscopy show lamellar bodies. These bodies are extruded into the alveolar lining fluid as tubular myelin which spreads as a thin layer at the air-liquid interface. The component of the surfactant known to produce a surface tension-lowering effect is dipalmitoyl phosphatidylcholine (DPPC). DPPC is synthesized within the lungs from fatty acids that are either extracted from the blood or synthesized within the lung itself. DPPC has a rapid turnover and is synthesized quickly. Surfactant is produced late in foetal life. Babies born without surfactant develop severe respiratory

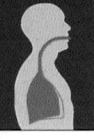

distress and may die if the condition is not recognized and adequately treated.

The molecules of DPPC are hydrophobic at one end and hydrophilic at the other. When these molecules align themselves on the surface, the intermolecular repulsive forces counter the attracting forces between the liquid surface molecules responsible for surface tension. The action of surfactant is even more marked in alveoli with smaller volumes. The reduction in surface tension is even greater when the film of surfactant is compressed, because the DPPC molecules are crowded together repelling each other to a greater extent.

ELASTIC PROPERTIES OF THE CHEST WALL AND OF THE LUNG PLUS CHEST WALL

The thoracic cage, like the lung, is also an elastic structure. The recoil pressure for the relaxed chest wall equals pleural pressure (Ppl) minus the atmospheric pressure (Patm).

$$\text{Elastic recoil of chest wall} = Ppl - Patm$$

Since Patm is taken as zero, elastic recoil of the chest wall equals the pleural pressure (Ppl). When the recoil pressure of the chest wall is zero, the chest wall moves outwards so that its 'unstressed' volume is quite high. This is illustrated in Figure 2.5 when a pneumothorax is produced by introducing air into the pleural space raising the pleural pressure to the atmospheric. The lung is then observed to collapse and moves inwards and the chest wall moves outwards. It follows that under conditions of equilibrium the chest wall is pulled inwards and the lung pulled outwards, the two pulling forces balancing each other.

Figure 2.6 shows the pressure volume curve of the lung alone, the chest wall alone and the lung plus chest wall together. The pressure volume curve of the lung alone is similar to that illustrated in Figure 2.4, only for clarity no hysteresis is shown. The curve shows the airway pressure determined at different volumes. The chest wall pressure volume curve is for the chest wall only and one has to imagine a normal chest wall with no lung within! It is noted that at FRC the recoil pressure is negative (about –5 cm H_2O) so that the chest wall would tend to move outwards. It is only when the volume of the chest wall has increased to 75% of the VC that the recoil pressure is atmospheric.

The pressure volume curve of the combined lung and chest wall is of considerable interest. For this curve, the individual inspires or expires from a spirometer and for each individual volume the airway pressure is measured with respiratory muscles relaxed. Relaxing the respiratory muscles during each airway pressure measurement requires some training and practice. At every volume the relaxation pressure of the lung and chest wall equals the sum of the pressure of the lung and chest wall measured separately. The lung + chest wall curve shows that at FRC the relaxation pressure i.e. the recoil pressure is atmospheric (i.e. zero). Therefore FRC is the 'equilibrium volume' where the elastic recoil pressure of the lung is balanced by the elastic recoil pressure of the chest to move outwards. At FRC the alveolar pressure = atmospheric pressure = zero. The pleural pressure is roughly'– 5 cm H_2O.

Thus lung recoil pressure at FRC = Alveolar pressure – pleural pressure
= 0 – (– 5)
= 5 cm H_2O

Chest wall recoil pressure = Pleural pressure – Atmospheric pressure
= – 5 – 0
= – 5 cm H_2O

It is seen how the inward recoil of lung is balanced by the outward recoil of the chest wall. A few further features are worthy of note.

1. The negative opposing pressure of the lung and chest wall produce a sub-atmospheric (negative) intrapleural pressure (– 5 cm H_2O).
2. It is this negative intrapleural pressure which counters or opposes both lung recoil inwards and chest wall recoil outwards.
3. Since pressure at a particular volume is inversely proportional to compliance, the total compliance of the lung plus chest wall is equal to the sum of the reciprocal of the compliance of the lung and chest wall measured separately

$$1/C_{\text{(lung + chest wall)}} = 1/C_{\text{lung}} + 1/C_{\text{chest wall}}$$

It will be noted from Figure 2.6 that at FRC the lung is distended above its low unstressed volume and the chest wall

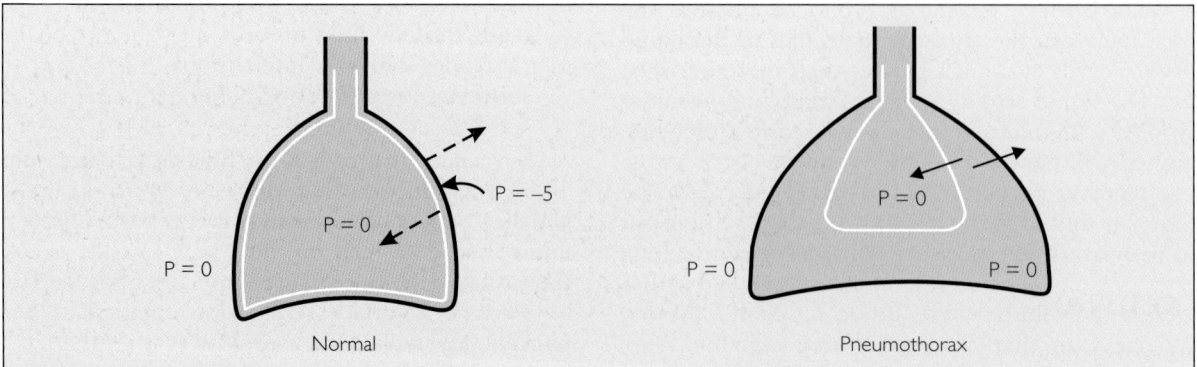

Fig 2.5: The tendency of the lung to recoil to its deflated volume is balanced by the tendency of the rib cage to bow out. As a result, the intrapleural pressure is sub-atmospheric. Pneumothorax allows the lung to collapse and the thorax to spring out.

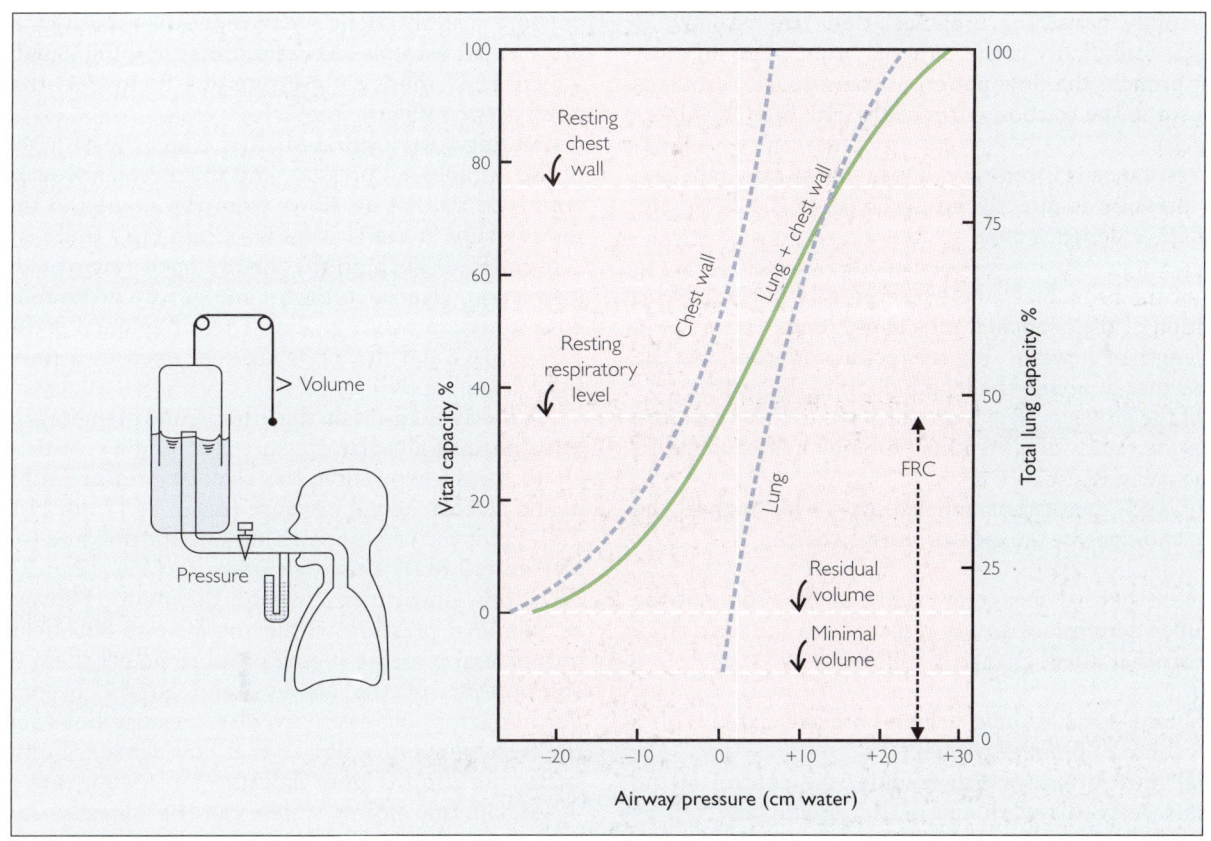

Fig 2.6: The graph in this figure gives the pressure volume curves of the lung, chest wall and the lung + chest wall taken as one unit. The lung + chest wall curve is obtained by the individuals inspiring a certain volume from the spirometer, the pressure at that volume being measured with the respiratory muscles relaxed. The recoil pressure of the lung + chest wall acting as one is equal to the sum of the recoil pressure of the lung and of the chest wall measured separately. (With permission from Respiratory Physiology The Essentials by John B. West, seventh edition. LIppincott Williams and Wilkins).

is held distended below its relatively high unstressed volume. Any change in the unstressed volume or compliance of either lung or chest wall will lead to a new FRC. Thus emphysema leads to both an increase in lung compliance together with increase in unstressed volume of the lung, thereby leading to a higher FRC. Obesity on the other hand reduces the unstressed volume of the chest wall and thereby leads to a reduced FRC.

Recoil pressure of lung, chest wall and lung-chest wall combined. Recoil pressure (transmural pressure) of

Lungs	=	$(P_A) - (Ppl)$
Chest wall	=	$(Ppl) - (Patm)$
	=	(Ppl), since Patm is zero
Lungs + chest wall	=	$(P_A - Ppl) + (Ppl - Patm)$
	=	$P_A - Patm$

where P_A = Alveolar pressure, Ppl = intrapleural pressure; Patm = atmospheric pressure

AIRWAY RESISTANCE

Airflow during expiration from alveoli will depend on the driving pressure (i.e. pressure difference between alveoli and the atmosphere) and the airway resistance.

$$\text{Airflow} = \dot{V} = \frac{\text{Pressure difference between alveoli and atmosphere } (\Delta P)}{\text{Resistance } (R_{aw})}$$

Normal airway resistance (R_{aw}) during quiet breathing is less than 2 cm H_2O/L/second. If air flows through a tube (and the airways approximate to tubes), the pressure difference depends on the rate and the pattern of flow. If the flow rate is slow the stream of air flowing through the tube is parallel to the sides of the wall. This pattern is termed as *laminar* flow (Figure 2.7A). A rather unique feature of laminar flow is that the gas in the centre of the flow moves twice as fast as the average velocity. There is therefore a 'spike' of moving gas along the axis of the tube. This change in velocity across the diameter of the tube is termed the *velocity profile*. If the flow rate increases, eddies tend to form particularly at the branching of the tubes and the pattern is termed *transitional* flow (Figure 2.7C). At high flow rates the stream of flow is disorganized and the pattern of flow is termed *turbulent* flow (Figure 2.7B). Turbulent flow has different properties from laminar flow. Pressure is not proportional to the flow but is approximately equal to its square. Pressure (P) = kV^2, where k is a constant. Also, turbulent flow does not have the high central or axial flow velocity observed in laminar flow.

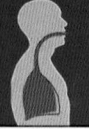

In the rapidly branching bronchial tree, laminar flow is probably to be found only in the terminal bronchioles. In most of the other bronchi the flow pattern is transitional. Turbulent flow may occur in the trachea, particularly with high flow rates as with exercise.

Airway resistance is inversely proportional to flow rate, and the driving pressure is directly proportional to the flow rate. Airway resistance depends on—

1. Calibre of the bronchial tube which is again dependent on the position of the bronchial tube in the lung.
2. On the length of airways R_{aw} is directly proportional to the length, so that doubling the length doubles the resistance.
3. Radius of the airways R_{aw} is proportional to $1/r^4$. Therefore reducing the radius of a breathing tube by half causes a 16 fold increase in R_{aw}.
4. Viscosity and density of inhaled gas The higher the viscosity and density, the greater the resistance.

Of all these factors, change in calibre or the radius of the breathing tubes determines airway resistance to the maximum extent. Factors that affect change in calibre are—

1. Lung volume—smaller lung volumes are associated with a smaller calibre of breathing tubes.
2. Bronchial muscle tone which is under the control of the autonomic nervous system and is also directly affected by histamine and other related substances.
3. Secretions partially blocking the breathing tube.
4. Pressure across the airway wall.

The last point is of importance and needs further explanation. Figure 2.8 schematically shows the forces acting across an airway within the lung. Just before inspiration at FRC the alveolar pressure = atmospheric pressure (at the mouth) = zero. Airway pressure all along is also zero. Because intrapleural pressure is – 5 cm H_2O, there is a pressure of + 5 cm H_2O that keeps the airways open (Figure 2.8A).

During quiet inspiration there is an increase in the negativity of the intrapleural pressure and the alveolar pressure (by say 5 cm H_2O) so that air flows from the mouth to the alveoli. If the pressure in the airways is – 2 cm H_2O there is pressure of + 8 cm H_2O keeping the airway open (Figure 2.8B). At end inspiration, alveolar pressure and airway pressure are equal to atmospheric pressure = zero. The intrapleural pressure is say – 12 cm H_2O and the airway is kept open by a pressure 12 cm H_2O (Figure 2.8C).

In passive expiration the intrapleural pressure is less negative but a positive alveolar pressure is caused by elastic recoil.

In forced expiration, the alveolar pressure is high because of the alveolar recoil pressure (taken at 12 cm H_2O in Figure 2.8D) plus the very positive intrapleural pressure (+25 cm H_2O in Figure 2.8D). This high pressure (25+ 12 = 37 cm H_2O) drives flow downstream towards the mouth. However, once the intraluminal pressure within the airways falls below the high intrapleural pressure (equal pressure point) there is a dynamic compression of the airways, and airflow becomes limited. Further effort increases alveolar pressure but again increases the force of compression so that flow remains limited however strong the effort (Figure 2.8D).

Maximum airflow rates can be directly measured by recording a flow volume loop through a spirometer. Maximum flow rates for any volume except at the highest volume at the very start of exhalation remain the same even with submaximal effort and cannot increase with increased effort (Figure 2.9). The mechanism for flow limitation is dynamic compression of the airways as explained above. This compression as already explained occurs just beyond the point where the pressure

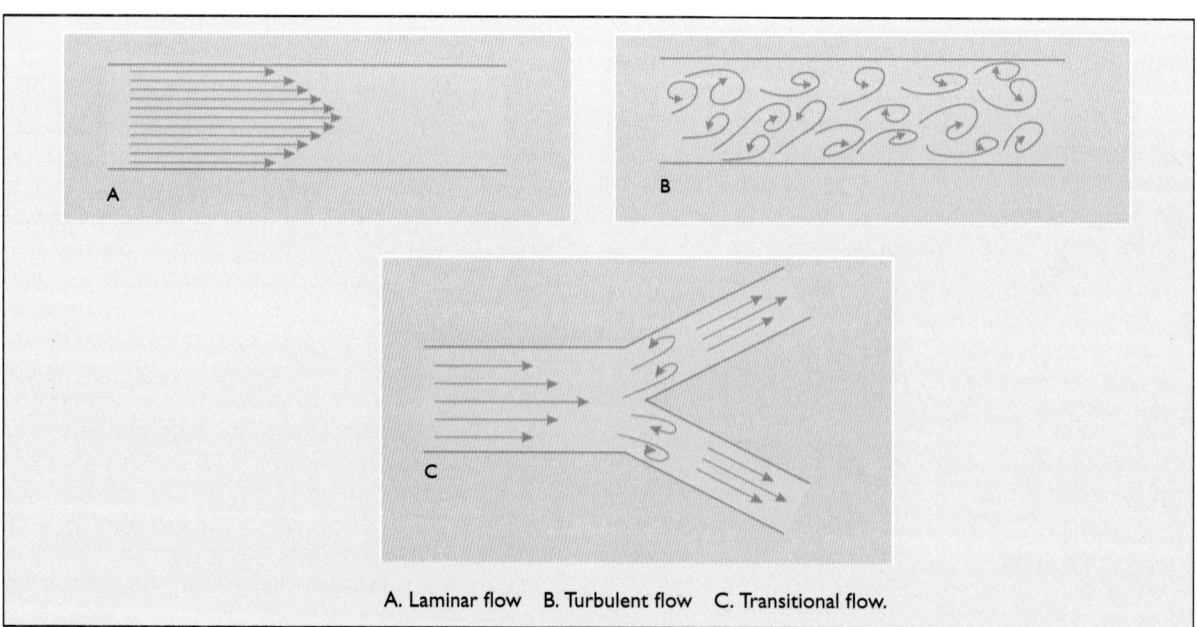

A. Laminar flow B. Turbulent flow C. Transitional flow.

Fig 2.7: Patterns of airflow. A. Laminar flow. B. Turbulent flow. C. Transitional flow.

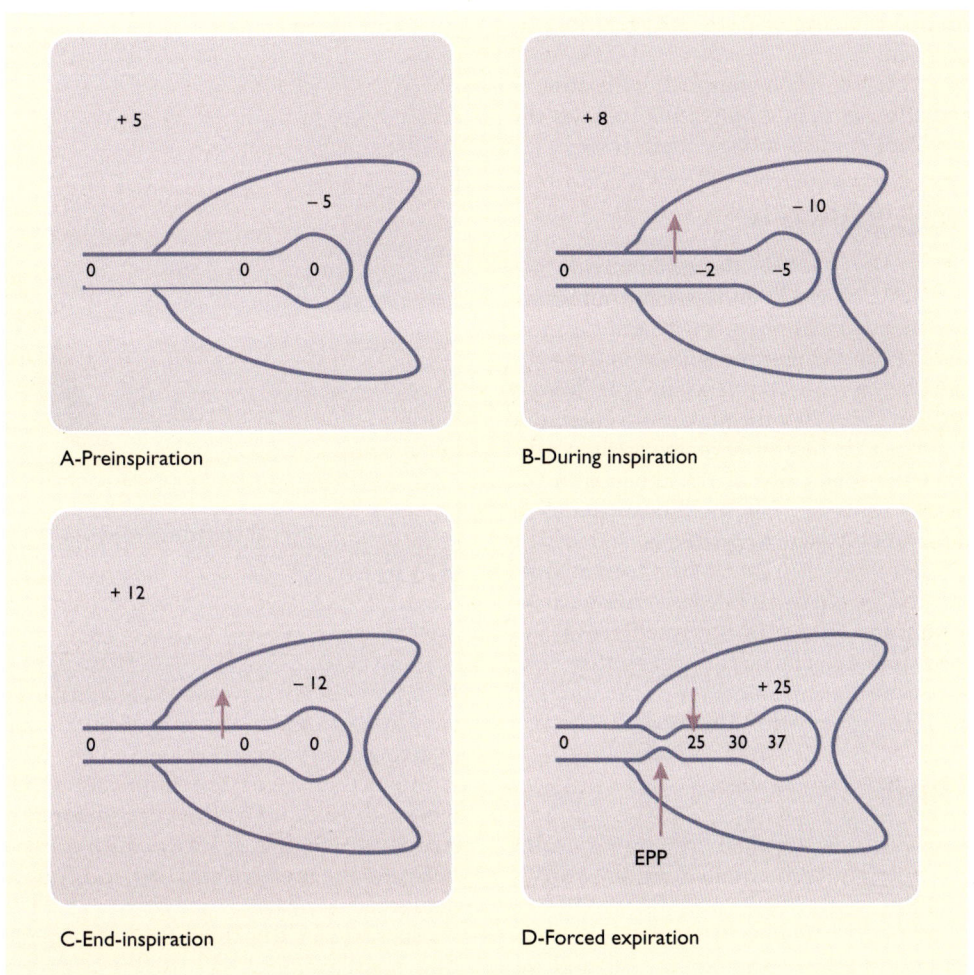

A-Preinspiration

B-During inspiration

C-End-inspiration

D-Forced expiration

EPP

Fig 2.8: Scheme showing airways compression during forced expiration. Note that the pressure difference across the airways is holding it open, except during a forced expiration. (See text)
EPP = Equal pressure point.

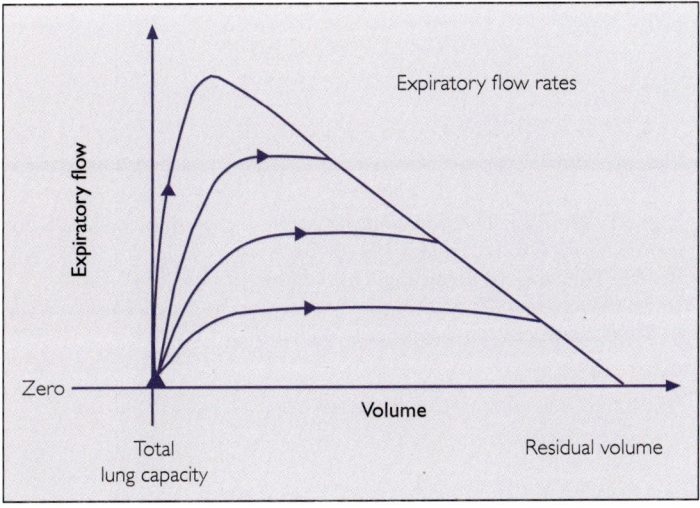

Expiratory flow rates

Zero

Volume

Total
lung capacity

Residual volume

Note that at submaximal efforts the descending portion of the flow volume curve takes the same path.

Fig 2.9: Flow volumes curves at different levels of effort.

within the airways is just below the intrapleural pressure. The driving pressure up to this point is the difference between the intraalveolar pressure and the pleural pressure: P_A– Ppl i.e. 37 cm H_2O–25 cm H_2O (in the above diagram) which equals 12 cm H_2O. This is equal to the elastic recoil pressure of the lung in the illustrative diagram, and the elastic recoil pressure is related to volume of the lung and not to effort. If the individual doubles his expiratory effort so that the intrapleural pressure is 50 cm H_2O at the same lung volume, the driving pressure will be 62 cm H_2O (in the alveoli) – 50 cm H_2O (intrapleural pressure) which still remains at 12 cm H_2O so that the flow rate remains unchanged.

There are certain points worth stressing—

1. Maximal flow rates decrease with lung volume as the pressure difference between alveolar pressure and intrapleural pressure decreases.
2. An increase in resistance of peripheral airways leads to an increase in the magnitude of the pressure drop within the lumen of the airways during forced expiration with a sharper

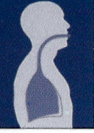

decrease in intraluminal pressure, thereby exaggerating the flow-limiting mechanism.

3. Loss of or impaired elastic recoil coupled with loss of support to the alveolar walls as in emphysema reduces the driving pressure and leads to early airflow limitation.

Major Sites of Airways Resistance

The airways, to start with, are large but divide and subdivide into narrow and narrower tubes ultimately ending into numerous respiratory bronchioles. Resistance as mentioned earlier is most influenced by calibre of the breathing tubes so that halving the radius of the breathing tube increases the resistance 16 fold. It used to be thought till recent times that the maximum resistance was in the very small airways. It has however been shown by actual measurement that the major site of resistance is in the medium-sized bronchi and that the very small bronchioles or airways contribute comparatively little to resistance. In fact, the small airways contribute not more than 20% of the total airways resistance. This is of clinical importance because there can be fairly extensive and significant disease in the small airways of the lung without it being detected clinically or on routine lung function tests. For this reason the small airways of the lung are often referred to as the silent zone within the lung.

WORK OF BREATHING

Work is necessary to move the chest wall and the lungs during inspiration. Work performed is best equated to pressure × volume.

In the pressure volume curve (Figure 2.10), the intrapleural pressure during inspiration follows the curve ABC and the work during inspiration is given by the area OABCDO. Of this area the quadrilateral OAECDO represents the work done to overcome the elastic forces and the coloured area ABCEA represents the work done to overcome airway and tissue resistance. If the airway resistance were to increase, the coloured areas would increase in size due to an associated increase in the negative intrapleural pressure.

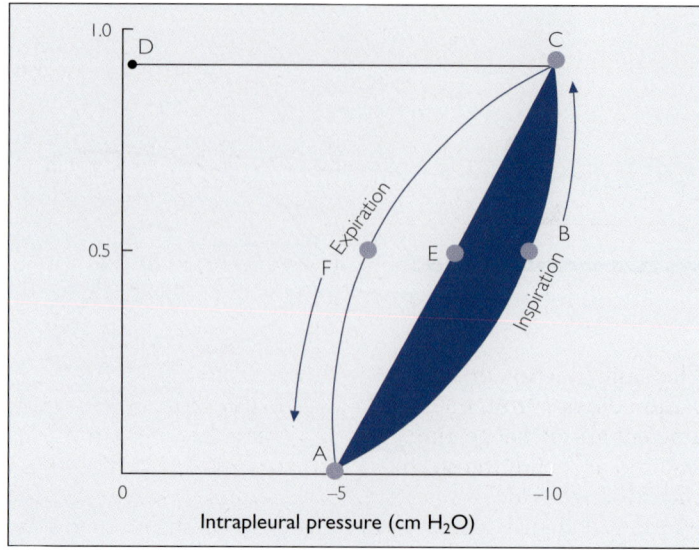

Fig 2.10: Pressure volume curve of the lung showing the inspiratory work done overcoming elastic forces (area OAECDO) and viscous forces (coloured area ABCEA).

On expiration, the area AECFA is the work required to overcome airways resistance. This however is encompassed within the area of the trapezoid OAECDO. Therefore this work can be done by the energy stored in the expanded elastic structure which is released during expiration. The difference between the areas OAECDO and AECFA represents the work dissipated as heat.

Increase in the frequency of respiration leads to increased flow rates leading to increased resistive work with increase in the area ABCEA. Increase in tidal volume would lead to increase in elastic work, with a corresponding increase in the area OACDO.

Patients with interstitial pulmonary fibrosis who have lowered compliance and stiff lungs tend to have an increased respiratory rate, while patients with airways obstruction tend to breathe slowly. These patterns of breathing reduce the workload on the lung.

SUGGESTED READING

Bachofen H, Hildebrandt J, Bachofen M. Pressure-volume curves of air and liquid filled excised lungs. Surface tension in situ. *J Appl Physiol*. 1970; 29:422–31.

De Troyer A. The respiratory muscles. In Crystal RG, West JB, Barnes PJ, Weibel ER (eds). *The Lung Scientific Foundations*. 1997, Second edition, Lippincott-Raveen Press.

Hyatt RE, Black LF. The flow volume curve. A current perspective. *Am Rev Respir Dis*. 1973; 107:191–9.

Otis AB. The work of breathing. *Physiol Rev*. 1954; 34:449–58.

West JB. Mechanics of breathing. In *Respiratory Physiology The Essentials*. 2006, Sixth edition, Lippincott Williams and Wilkins.

CHAPTER **3**

Gas Exchange in the Lung

The basic function of the lung is to provide oxygen and remove carbon dioxide from the blood perfusing the lung. This involves efficient gas exchange, the oxygen reaching the alveoli from the inspired air being transferred to the capillaries perfusing them and carbon dioxide from the capillaries around the alveoli being transferred to the alveoli and then to the outside air during expiration. This gas exchange occurs during each cycle of ventilation—inspiration and expiration and the basic principles of the exchange will be described below.

THE ANATOMY OF THE GAS EXCHANGE AREA OF THE LUNG

The lung can be divided into two zones: a conducting zone which merely serves to conduct or transport inspired and expired gas in and out of the lungs, and a gas exchange zone where oxygen from the outside air reaching the gas exchange zone is transferred to blood perfusing the lungs and carbon dioxide from the blood reaching the gas exchange zone is expired into the outside air.

The conducting zone of the lung consists of the upper respiratory tract, the trachea, the bronchi, the subdivisions of the bronchi, the bronchioles which again divide, right up to the terminal bronchioles. These conducting passages take no part in gas exchange.

The terminal bronchioles divide into two to five generations of respiratory bronchioles, which have increasing number of alveoli on their walls. The respiratory bronchioles divide further into alveolar ducts which also have alveoli on their walls; the alveolar ducts open into large air spaces called alveoli. The gas exchange unit therefore extends only from the respiratory bronchioles to the alveoli. The unit of lung supplied by one terminal bronchiole is termed the acinus. Several acini close to each other form a lung lobule. There is a collateral flow of gas and blood within the lobules and to a lesser extent between lobules. The main gas exchange occurs in the alveoli which are irregular spaces about 250 μm in diameter. There are over 300 million alveoli within the lungs and if they were to be stretched out would cover the size of a tennis court. Eighty-five to ninety per cent of the total alveolar surface is covered by capillaries providing an excellent surface area of 70 m^2 for gas exchange between the alveolar surface and the blood (Figure 3.1).

The alveolar surface is covered by epithelial cells; these are of two types—Type I and Type II. The alveolar cells are attached directly to a thin basement membrane. The alveoli are perfused

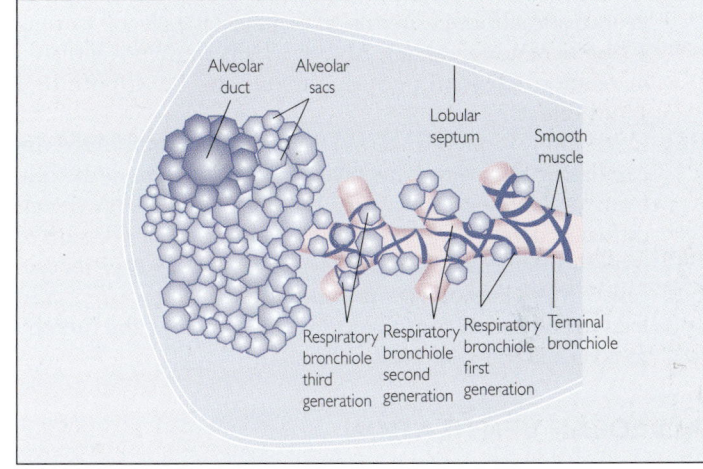

Fig 3.1: Gas exchange zone of the lung.

by capillaries which surround them. The capillaries are lined by endothelial cells and again rest on the basement membrane. Over the greater part of the gas exchange area the basement membrane of the alveolar cells and the basement membrane of capillary endothelial cells are fused with no intervening space between them. For oxygen exchange, oxygen from the alveolus needs to go through the alveolar wall, the basement membranes (of both alveoli and capillary walls), the endothelial lining of the capillaries into their lumen where oxygen is taken up by the haemoglobin of the blood perfusing the capillaries. Carbon dioxide has a reverse process going from the capillaries through the basement membrane, alveolar walls into the alveolus to be expired to the outside.

PHYSIOLOGIC CONCEPT

The volume of air breathed in and out during quiet resting respiration is termed the tidal volume. If, for example, the tidal volume is taken as 500 ml and the individual breathes 14 breaths per minutes, the minute ventilation is 500 × 14 = 7 litres. It is important to realize that not all 500 ml of air inhaled in one breath participates in gas exchange. Only that portion of air reaching perfused alveoli does so. Alveolar ventilation is therefore related to that portion of inspired air or gas reaching perfused alveoli and taking part in gas exchange. This takes us to the concept of dead space which is dealt with just a little later.

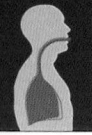

Efficient gas exchange in the lungs requires—

(i) Adequate alveolar ventilation evenly distributed to both lungs

(ii) Even ventilation-perfusion ratios of 0.8 to 1. Uneven ventilation-perfusion ratios or ventilation-perfusion mismatch is an important cause of hypoxia or poor arterial oxygenation. A ventilation-perfusion mismatch is characterized clinically and physiologically by two features: (a) An increase in dead space—ventilation of unperfused or poorly perfused alveoli which are hyperventilated in relation to the blood perfusing them; (b) an increase in venous admixture i.e. perfusion of atelectatic alveoli causing a true right to left shunt. Alveoli which are hypoventilated in relation to blood perfusing them, also contribute to a shunt effect.

(iii) Diffusion of oxygen across the alveolar wall into the capillaries perfusing the alveoli, and of carbon dioxide from the capillaries out into the alveolar space. A severe diffusion defect may contribute to a low partial pressure of oxygen in arterial blood (PaO_2) but is hardly ever its sole cause. Most pathologies producing a diffusion defect also lead to an uneven compliance within the lungs and thereby to a ventilation-perfusion mismatch.

ALVEOLAR VENTILATION

The partial pressure of carbon dioxide in arterial blood ($PaCO_2$) is the best indicator of alveolar ventilation. This basic fact in respiratory physiology is explained below. Consider for purposes of illustration an alveolus of volume $\dot{V}_A$ (Figure 3.2). It contains a volume of CO_2 i.e. $\dot{V}CO_2$. The fractional concentration of CO_2 in this alveolus ($FACO_2$) is given by the volume of CO_2 divided by the volume of the alveolus (V_A).

$$FACO_2 = \frac{\dot{V}CO_2}{\dot{V}_A}$$

The CO_2 released into the alveolus from the blood perfusing it, will be cleared from the alveolus by ventilation; the greater the ventilation the lower the concentration of CO_2 in the alveolus. The alveolar concentration will be a balance between the alveolar ventilation and the rate at which the CO_2 is evolved ($\dot{V}CO_2$). Let us again consider the equation:

$$FACO_2 = \frac{\dot{V}CO_2}{\dot{V}_A}$$

The fractional concentration of CO_2, $FACO_2$ (0.05–0.06), exerts a pressure equal to the same fraction of the barometric pressure (P_B).

$$\frac{P_ACO_2}{P_B} = \frac{\dot{V}CO_2}{\dot{V}_A}$$

$$P_ACO_2 = \frac{\dot{V}CO_2}{\dot{V}_A} \times 0.863$$

0.863 is the correction factor that takes into account the barometric pressure and the different units in which $\dot{V}CO_2$

and $\dot{V}_A$ are expressed. This is the alveolar ventilation equation. It shows that the P_ACO_2 is directly proportional to the CO_2 produced, and inversely proportional to alveolar ventilation ($\dot{V}_A$). If $\dot{V}CO_2$ is constant, then P_ACO_2 is inversely proportional to $\dot{V}_A$.

$$P_ACO_2 \; \alpha \; \frac{1}{\dot{V}_A}$$

There is good evidence to show that $PaCO_2$ (arterial PCO_2) is very close to the average alveolar PCO_2 i.e. P_ACO_2. Thus

$$P_ACO_2 = PaCO_2 = \frac{\dot{V}CO_2}{\dot{V}_A} \times 0.863$$

The $PaCO_2$ is thus inversely related to $\dot{V}_A$. A high $PaCO_2$ (> 48 mm Hg) denotes hypoventilation; a low $PaCO_2$ (< 35 mm Hg) denotes hyperventilation; a normal $PaCO_2$ (35–45 mm Hg) denotes normal alveolar ventilation. It should be evident from the above equation that if the normal $PaCO_2$ of 40 mm Hg is doubled to 80 mm Hg, it means that the alveolar ventilation is just half of what is normally necessary to deal with the CO_2 produced by the body. It is to be also noted that the $PaCO_2$ may rise if the $\dot{V}CO_2$ rises and if the patient for some reason cannot increase his alveolar ventilation to get rid of the extra CO_2.

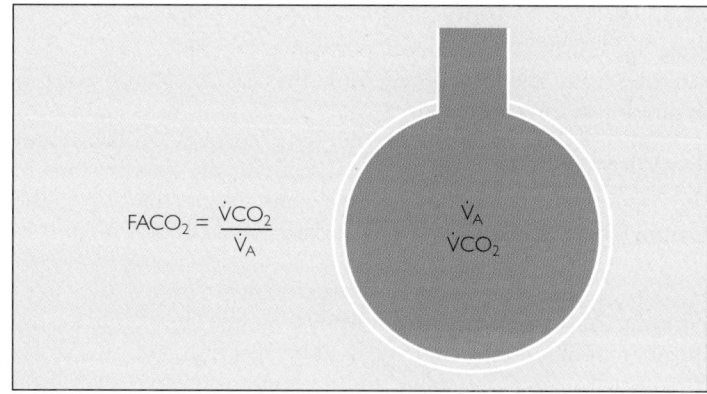

Fig 3.2: Concept of alveolar ventilation.

CONCEPT OF DEAD SPACE

The anatomical dead space is that constituted by the trachea and the bronchi right up to, but not including, the gas exchange unit of the lung. It is the volume of inspired air which fills the airways and is breathed out unchanged. Air entering alveoli which have no blood perfusing them, also does not take part in gas exchange and is breathed out unchanged. This is wasted ventilation and constitutes alveolar dead space. The sum of the anatomical dead space and the alveolar dead space is termed the physiological dead space, though admittedly there is nothing physiological about this dead space. Figure 3.3 illustrates the concept of anatomical and alveolar dead space.

Effective alveolar ventilation is only that ventilation entering perfused alveoli. Hyperventilated alveoli will contribute to the overall concept of alveolar dead space.

Ordinarily, as much as 30% of tidal volume is dead space ventilation. This may increase considerably in patients with diseased lungs. The quantum of dead space can be calculated by the following equation—

$$\frac{\dot{V}_D}{\dot{V}_T} = \frac{PaCO_2 - P_ECO_2}{PaCO_2}$$

where P_ECO_2 is the pressure of CO_2 in expired gas.

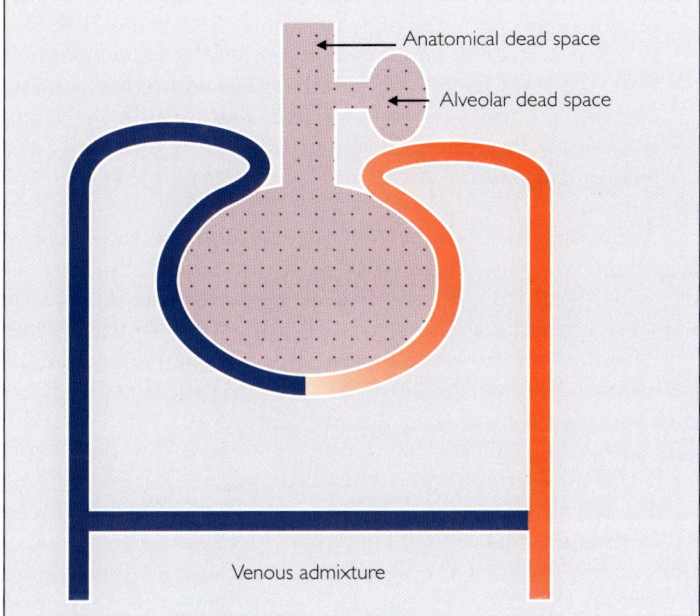

Fig 3.3: Concept of anatomical and alveolar dead space and venous admixture (right to left shunt within the lungs). (From Udwadia FE. (2005). *Principles of Critical Care Medicine*, second edition, Oxford University Press, New Delhi).

ALVEOLAR OXYGEN

Fresh oxygen from inspired gas enters alveoli during ventilation; the oxygen diffuses through the alveolar wall into the blood perfusing the alveoli. For any given concentration of oxygen in inspired gas (FIO_2), the alveolar concentration of oxygen (FAO_2) will be a balance between alveolar ventilation (V_A) and the oxygen taken up (VO_2) by the blood perfusing ventilated alveoli.

$$FIO_2 - F_AO_2 = \frac{\dot{V}O_2}{\dot{V}_A}$$

In terms of partial pressure,

$$PIO_2 - P_AO_2 = \frac{\dot{V}O_2}{\dot{V}_A} \times 0.863$$

We have already defined $\dot{V}_A$ (under Alveolar Ventilation) in terms of $PaCO_2$.

$$P_AO_2 = PIO_2 - P_ACO_2 = \frac{\dot{V}O_2}{\dot{V}CO_2} \times 0.863$$

The ratio $\dot{V}CO_2/\dot{V}O_2$ is in fact the respiratory exchange ratio R, and R in a steady state equals the metabolic respiratory quotient. Thus $P_AO_2 = PIO_2 - PaCO_2 \times 1/R$

If carbohydrates are preponderantly burnt as fuel, R = 1; if fats are burnt as fuel R = 0.7; if carbohydrates and fats are both burnt as fuel, as is usually the case, R = 0.8.

The above equation is a simplified form of the alveolar air equation. It is of great use because:

(a) It allows a quick determination of alveolar oxygen pressure (P_AO_2) if the PIO_2 and the $PaCO_2$ are known.

(b) If the P_AO_2 is known and the PaO_2 is available through an arterial blood gas measurement, the alveolar-arterial oxygen gradient can be calculated as the difference between P_AO_2 and PaO_2. The upper normal of this gradient is 15 to at the most 20 mm Hg. In most normal individuals it averages 10 mm Hg.

(c) The alveolar equation points to a linear relationship between P_AO_2 and $PaCO_2$. The O_2–CO_2 diagram (Figure. 3.4) or line is further elaborated upon in the chapter on 'Acute Respiratory Failure in Adults'. From this diagram one can quickly plot the expected P_AO_2 if the $PaCO_2$ is known for any given inspired oxygen concentration. If the alveolar arterial oxygen gradient is taken as 10–15 mm Hg, then for any given $PaCO_2$ one can read off the PaO_2. This is true provided the alveolar-arterial oxygen gradient is not abnormally increased.

(d) A consideration of the alveolar air equation shows that at a given inspired oxygen concentration and a given respiratory quotient, the alveolar PO_2 is dependent on alveolar ventilation. A lower alveolar ventilation would thus lead to a lowered alveolar PO_2, and hence a lowered arterial PO_2.

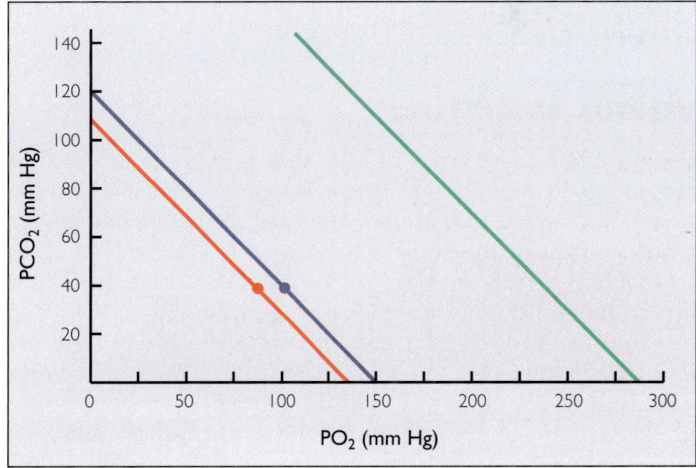

Fig 3.4: O_2–CO_2 diagram.

The blue line represents the relationship between alveolar PO_2 and alveolar PCO_2 with a RQ of 0.8 and when breathing air (PIO_2) = 149 mm HG. The circle marked on this line presents the normal P_AO_2 and P_ACO_2.
The green line illustrates the PO_2–PCO_2 relationship with an RQ of 0.8 when breathing 40% oxygen (PIO_2 = 285 mm Hg).
The red line gives the relationship between arterial PaO_2 and arterial carbon dioxide pressure $PaCO_2$ provided the alveolar arterial gradient is normal (10–15 mm Hg). Therefore from the above diagram if the P_AO_2 is known the expected PaO_2 and the corresponding P_ACO_2 can also be determined.
(From Udwadia FE. (2005). *Principles of Critical Care Medicine*, second edition, Oxford University Press, New Delhi).

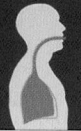

(e) The alveolar air equation helps the physician to check on blood gas measurements. If the value of the measured $PaCO_2$ is taken as correct, the alveolar equation allows one to compute the P_AO_2. If the PaO_2 reported by the laboratory is higher than the P_AO_2, it is obviously incorrect.

THE ALVEOLAR-ARTERIAL OXYGEN GRADIENT

The normal range of the alveolar-arterial oxygen gradient has already been mentioned. An increased alveolar-arterial oxygen gradient denotes an impairment of gas exchange across the alveolar capillary membrane. When, however, a low PaO_2 is due to hypoventilation, or is related to breathing at high altitudes then there is no increase in the alveolar-arterial oxygen gradient since the P_AO_2 is also proportionately low. A lowered PaO_2 from any other cause (V/Q mismatch, increased shunt, impaired diffusion), is always associated with an increased alveolar-arterial oxygen gradient. Also, the greater the alveolar-arterial oxygen gradient, the greater the disturbance in gas exchange within the lungs. This observation should however be viewed in its proper perspective. Thus an alveolar-arterial gradient of 20 mm Hg (upper limit of normal), occurring on the steep part of the oxygen dissociation curve will denote a gross disturbance in pulmonary gas exchange. Let us consider a patient with chronic bronchitis in severe hypercapnic respiratory failure. If the P_AO_2 of this patient is 50 mm Hg and the PaO_2 is 30 mm Hg, the gradient of just 20 mm Hg (upper limit of normal) would suggest that the hypoxia is chiefly due to alveolar hypoventilation. However at a PO_2 of 50 mm Hg the oxygen saturation is 85%; at a PO_2 of 30 mm Hg the oxygen saturation is about 55%. Thus the oxygen saturation has fallen 30% between the alveoli and the arterial blood. Normally, the fall in oxygen saturation does not exceed 2%. It is evident that there is a serious disturbance in gas exchange in this patient, even though the alveolar-arterial oxygen gradient is not unduly increased.

VENOUS ADMIXTURE

Venous admixture (Figure 3.5) is that portion of the cardiac output which does not take part in the gas exchange within the alveoli and which is therefore returned unoxygenated to the left side of the heart. An increase in venous admixture leads to arterial hypoxemia and is one of the chief causes of respiratory failure. A number of unrelated pathological conditions involving the lung can lead to an increase in venous admixture resulting in arterial hypoxemia and respiratory failure. The total venous admixture or shunt may be contributed to by—

1) Anatomical shunt; 2) Intrapulmonary capillary shunt

1. Anatomical shunt. Normally this is constituted by the bronchial veins, pleural veins and thebesian veins; it generally does not cause shunting to a degree exceeding 2%. Only in the presence of large pathological arterio-venous communication, arteriovenous aneurysms or a substantial right to left cardiac shunt will an anatomical shunt give rise to a marked increase in venous admixture so as to cause arterial hypoxemia.
2. Intrapulmonary capillary shunt. The respiratory physician is more concerned with venous admixture due to an intrapulmonary capillary shunt. If unoxygenated blood perfuses atelectatic alveoli, the oxygen content of the blood leaving the atelectatic alveoli will be less than that leaving alveoli which are normally ventilated and perfused. This constitutes the concept of venous admixture. Venous admixture at the bedside has two components—(i) a true right to left shunt due to perfusion of totally atelectatic alveoli, and (ii) a shunt effect observed in alveoli which are hypoventilated in relation to the blood perfusing them i.e. alveoli with low ventilation-perfusion ratios. This is not a true right to left shunt (as with atelectasis), but it is assumed for conceptual reasons that the portion of the blood which remains unoxygenated after perfusing these alveoli behaves in a way similar to an equivalent amount of blood shunted from the right to left. The total venous admixture consists of both (i) and (ii). Some would also include the small anatomical shunt in total venous admixture. Ordinarily, the anatomical shunt as mentioned above is negligible.

A true right to left shunt (also called a true venous admixture) is unchanged by increasing inspired concentration of oxygen. In other words the PaO_2 does not rise to any appreciable extent even with a significant increase in the inspired oxygen concentration. The shunt effect produced by alveoli with lowered ventilation-perfusion ratios will however be abolished, so that the PaO_2 rises sharply on increasing the inspired oxygen concentration. The simple bedside test of noting the degree of rise in PaO_2 with 100% inspired oxygen, thus distinguishes between a true right to left shunt within the lungs, and a shunt effect produced by ventilation-perfusion inequalities. More often than not, a right to left shunt as also ventilation-perfusion inequalities are present in the same patient. This is further elaborated upon in the chapter on 'Acute Respiratory Failure in Adults'. The mathematical calculation of the venous admixture or shunt is given by the following equation:

$$\frac{Q_S}{Q_T} = \frac{C_CO_2 - CaO_2}{C_CO_2 - C_VO_2}$$

where Qs is the shunt fraction, Q_T the cardiac output, CcO_2 the capillary oxygen content, CaO_2 the arterial oxygen content and CvO_2 the mixed venous oxygen content.

In practice, end-capillary oxygen content is calculated from the alveolar PO_2 by assuming that P_AO_2 is equal to end-capillary PO_2. Arterial oxygen content is either derived from the PaO_2, or estimated by an oximeter. Mixed venous oxygen content is obtained by sampling blood from the pulmonary artery through a Swan-Ganz catheter.

The normal Q_S/Q_T is generally not more than 5%. A shunt fraction exceeding 30% is serious, and a shunt fraction approaching 50% indicates a gross degree of venous admixture, and carries a grim prognosis.

REGIONAL GAS EXCHANGE IN THE LUNG

Ventilation-perfusion ratios are not exactly identical in all parts of the lung. In a standing individual, ventilation increases slowly from top to bottom of the lung whereas blood flow increases from top to bottom more rapidly. As a result ventilation blood flow ratios are very high at the top of the lung (blood flow

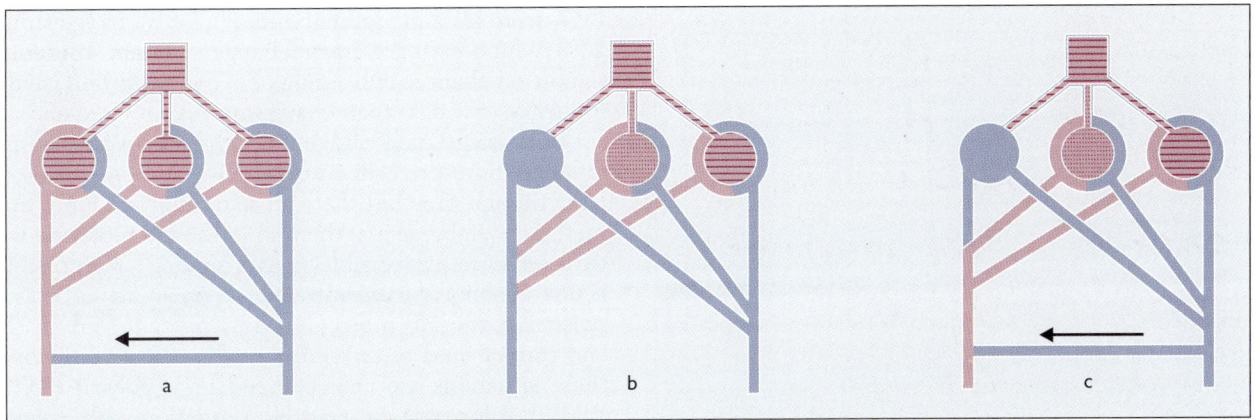

Fig 3.5: (a) Anatomical shunt (portion of cardiac output bypassing pulmonary capillaries). (b) Intrapulmonary capillary shunt produced by perfusion of atelectatic alveoli (as in the alveolus to the left) or when V_A/Q_C ratio is reduced (middle alveolus). (c) Overall physiological shunt which include a true right to left shunt, as also a shunt effect produced by perfusion of poorly ventilated alveoli. (From Udwadia FE. (2005). *Principles of Critical Care Medicine*, second edition, Oxford University Press, New Delhi).

very less) and much lowered at the base of the lung (blood flow more in proportion to the ventilation). The ventilation-perfusion differences can be plotted on an O_2–CO_2 diagram to illustrate the resulting difference in gas exchange.

The lung in a standing individual (Figure 3.6) divided into horizontal sections, each of which is located on the ventilation perfusion line (i.e. the O_2–CO_2 diagram) determined by its own ventilation-perfusion ratio. This ratio is high at the apex so that the V/Q point is to the right of the line. The ratio is comparatively low at the bottom so that the V/Q point is to the left.

Effects on Arterial Blood Gases in Patients with well-marked Ventilation-Perfusion Inequality

When there are a number of alveoli with low V/Q ratios, the blood leaving these alveoli will have a low oxygen concentration and a low PaO_2. Even if there are other remaining alveoli which hyperventilate (as compensation) they cannot compensate for low PaO_2 of alveoli with a low V/Q ratio. This is because even if the hyperventilated alveoli have comparatively high PaO_2 (say 110 mm Hg), the haemoglobin (Hb) in the blood is already fully saturated at a PaO_2 of 100 mm Hg so increasing PaO_2 pressure further cannot increase O_2 saturation. On the other hand the high $PaCO_2$ present in blood leaving alveoli with low V/Q ratios (i.e. hypoventilated alveoli) can be compensated for by other hyperventilating alveoli. Hyperventilation is induced by stimulation of the chemoreceptors by the raised $PaCO_2$. It ceases once the $PaCO_2$ is within normal limits.

DISTRIBUTIONS OF VENTILATION-PERFUSION RATIOS

The distribution of ventilation-perfusion ratios in patients with lung disease can be measured by infusing inert dissolved gases with varying solubilities and measuring the concentration of these gases in arterial blood and expired gas. A distribution of ventilation and blood flow plotted against ventilation-perfusion ratios with 50 compartments equally spaced on a log scale is obtained.

Figure 3.7 illustrates the V/Q ratios with regard to distribution of ventilation and perfusion in a normal adult. The V/Q ratios are close to 1.0 and there is no blood flow to unventilated areas.

Figure 3.8 shows the same distribution curves in a patient with chronic bronchitis and emphysema. It is noted that there is an increased blood flow to poorly ventilated or non-ventilated units leading to decreased V/Q ratios.

CONCEPT OF OXYGEN CONTENT AND OXYGEN TRANSPORT

The heart-lung combine working in unison ensures oxygenation of arterial blood. But this is not enough. Blood should have adequate oxygen content, and what is more the oxygen within the blood should be efficiently delivered or transported to tissue cells all over the body. This principle should never be lost sight of in the management of critically ill patients in the ICU.

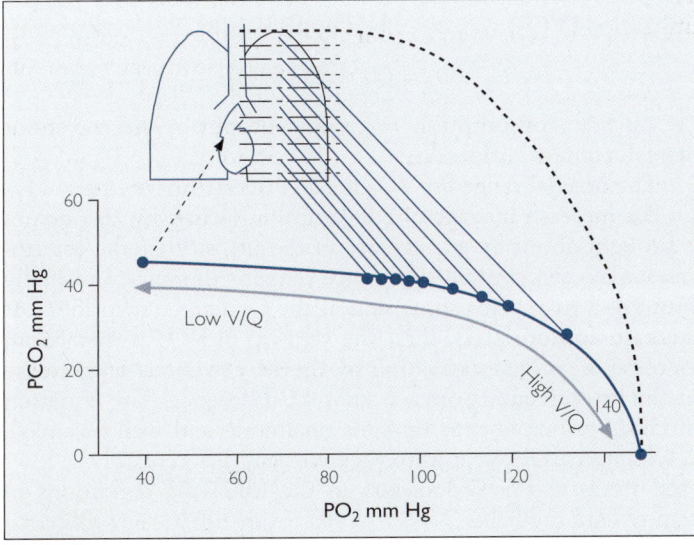

Fig 3.6: High ventilation-perfusion ratio at the apex results in a high PaO_2 and low PaO_2. The low ventilation-perfusion ration at base result in low PaO_2. (With permission from *Respiratory Physiology The Essentials* by John B. West, seventh edition. Lippincott Williams and Wilkins).

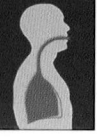
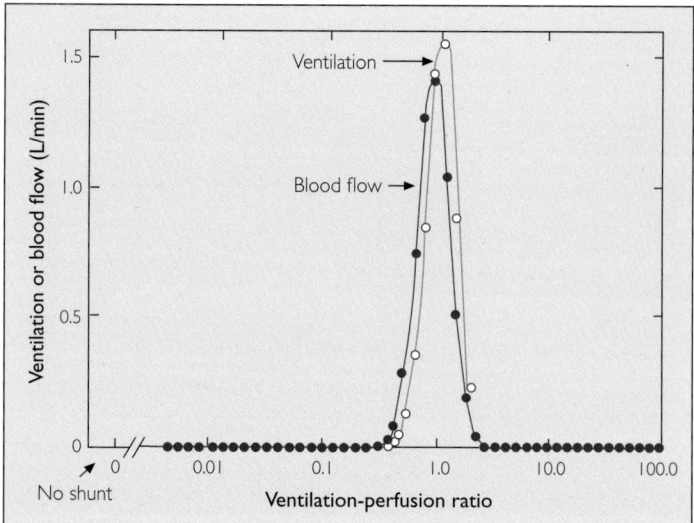

Fig 3.7: Distribution of ventilation-perfusion ratios in a young normal subject. (Adapted from *Respiratory Physiology The Essentials* by John B. West, seventh edition, Lippincott Williams and Wilkins).

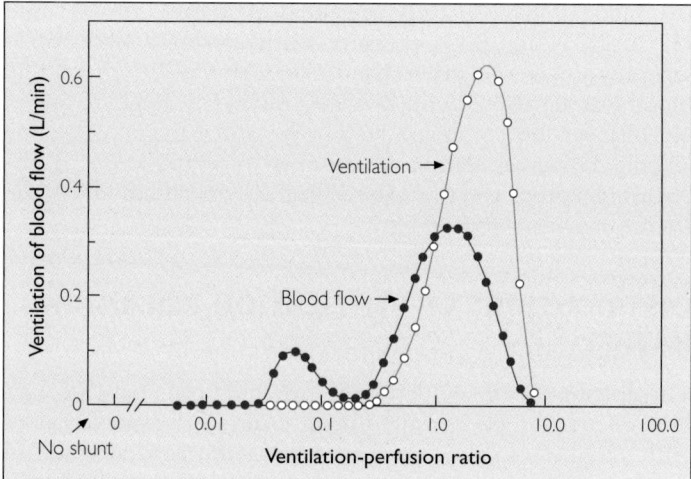

Fig 3.8: Distribution of ventilation-perfusion ratios in a patient with chronic bronchitis and emphysema. (Adapted from *Respiratory Physiology The Essentials* by John B. West, seventh edition, Lippincott Williams and Wilkins).

OXYGEN CONTENT

1 g of Hb combines with 1.39 ml of oxygen at full saturation

$$O_2 \text{ Content} = 1.39 \times Hb \times (\% \text{ saturation}/100) + 0.003 \times PO_2$$

where the solubility coefficient of oxygen at 37°C is 0.003 ml/100 ml blood/mm Hg.

The per cent saturation of Hb in arterial blood is related to the PaO_2. Oxygen content thus depends on Hb concentration and the PaO_2. The amount of oxygen in solution in plasma is very low (0.3 ml) due to its relative insolubility. Anaemia will decrease O_2 content in a linear fashion so that a reduction in Hb from 15 g to 7.5 g/100 ml will reduce arterial oxygen content by one half—i.e. from 21 ml to 10.5 ml. However, a fall in

PaO_2 from 90 mm Hg to 45 mm Hg i.e. by 50% results in just a 20% reduction in the arterial oxygen content. It is evident that significant changes in haemoglobin concentration have a greater influence on CaO_2 than changes in PaO_2

It is mentioned above that the PaO_2 has an important influence on arterial Hb saturation. There are two other situations (rare though they be) that can also influence Hb saturation. In methaemoglobinaemia, the iron in the Hb molecule is oxidized to its ferric state; reversible oxygen binding is not possible and Hb is unavailable for oxygen transport. Again, in carbon monoxide poisoning, the Hb molecule avidly binds to carbon monoxide, and cannot bind to oxygen nor offer effective transport. Both these situations are characterized by a normal Hb, a normal PaO_2, but lowered per cent Hb saturation with oxygen, a poor oxygen content and transport.

OXYGEN TRANSPORT

Transport of oxygen to tissues is a vital function of the cardiorespiratory system. A normal arterial oxygenation or oxygen content does not ensure adequate oxygen transport. The latter is crucially dependent on cardiac output.

$$\text{Oxygen Transport (DO2)} = \text{Cardiac Output (Q)} \times \text{Arterial Oxygen Content (CaO}_2\text{)}$$

$$DO_2 = Q \, CaO_2 = Q \times (1.39 \times Hb \, SaO_2) \times 10$$

It is to be noted that the dissolved oxygen component is removed and that the factor 10 converts the result to ml/minute. If the cardiac index (cardiac output/body surface area) is used instead of the cardiac output, the DO_2 is expressed as ml/minute/m². The normal range for DO_2 is 520-570 ml/minute/m².

It is obvious that both a good cardiac output and satisfactory CaO_2 are necessary for adequate oxygen transport.

THE FICK PRINCIPLE

The interrelationship between oxygen transport and oxygen utilization ($\dot{V}O_2$) was described by Fick in 1872.

$$\dot{V}O_2 = Q_T \times C(a\text{-}v)O_2$$

i.e. oxygen consumption = cardiac output × arteriovenous oxygen content difference.

The normal range for $\dot{V}O_2$ is 110-160 ml/minute/m².

An increase in oxygen consumption ($\dot{V}O_2$) by the tissues is brought about by an increase in the Q_T, so that the arteriovenous oxygen content difference remains the same (normally about 4–5 ml). If for some reason the cardiac output does not increase appropriately, then the step-up in $\dot{V}O_2$ is met by an increase in oxygen extraction by the tissues i.e. by an increase in the arteriovenous oxygen content difference. The equation in Fick's principle thus remains unaltered, and well balanced. A widened arteriovenous oxygen content difference (i.e. a lowered PvO_2 and SvO_2) occurs in the following conditions in critical care medicine.

(i) An inadequate cardiac output for tissue needs.
(ii) Very low arterial oxygen content, as with severe anaemia.

(iii) When tissue demands for oxygen are so great that the normal circulatory system cannot keep pace with excessive tissue demands. This could happen for example in patients with uncontrolled seizures in fulminant tetanus.

As mentioned above, the increased extraction of oxygen by tissues from the blood, leads to a lowered PvO_2 and SvO_2. The normal PvO_2 is 35–40 mm Hg, and the SvO_2 is 75%. There is a reserve which allows for a fall in PvO_2 to 15–20 mm Hg, and the SvO_2 to 25–30%, in conditions characterized by a very low cardiac output, while still enabling diffusion of oxygen at a level that prevents cellular death (Figure 3.9).

In critical care settings, the PvO_2 and the SvO_2 can thus act as indicators for adequacy or inadequacy of cardiac output and tissue perfusion (Table 3.1).

Underlying Fick's principle is the concept that $\dot{V}O_2$ is governed by tissue needs and not by oxygen delivery (DO_2). However, below a critical level of oxygen delivery, $\dot{V}O_2$ *does* depend on oxygen supply. It was earlier believed that in certain pathological states like sepsis, septic shock, acute respiratory distress syndrome, $\dot{V}O_2$ was dependent on DO_2 at all levels of oxygen delivery. The current though not universal consensus is that this is not really so. Nevertheless, the importance of ensuring adequate oxygen transport in the management of critically ill patients cannot be overemphasized.

OXYGEN EXTRACTION RATIO (O_2 ER)

The oxygen extraction ration O_2 ER is the ratio of oxygen uptake to oxygen delivery ($\dot{V}O_2/DO_2$). It signifies the fraction of oxygen taken up by the tissues; the normal O_2 ER is 0.2–0.3 i.e. 20–30%. Oxygen extraction can vary. It increases when the increased demand for oxygen by tissue is not met by an increase in cardiac output. In trained athletes the O_2 ER may be as high as 0.8 at maximal exercise. In diseased states like severe sepsis, multiple organ dysfunction, acute respiratory distress syndrome, oxygen extraction by tissue cells can be poor in spite of adequate oxygen supply.

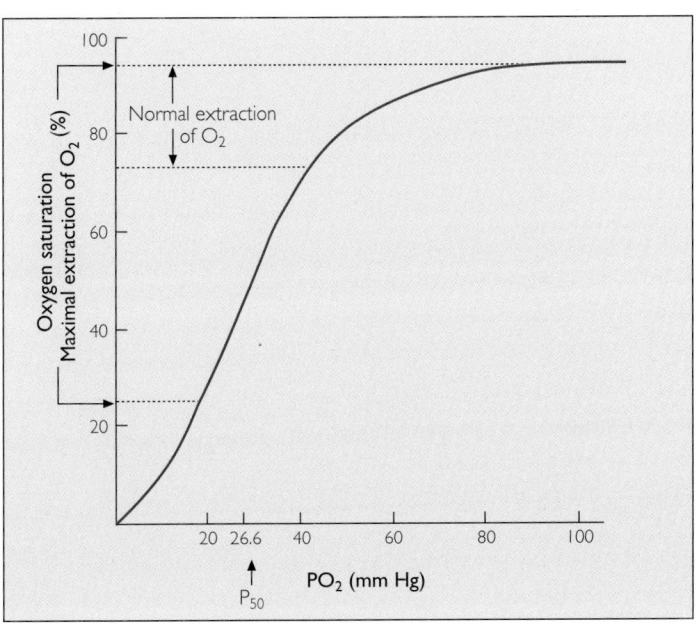

Fig 3.9: The normal oxyhaemoglobin dissociation curve (P_{50} = 26.6 mm Hg). At a normal PaO_2, O_2 saturation is close to 100%. At a PaO_2 of 40 mm Hg (venous blood), O_2 saturation is about 75%. Maximum O_2 extraction allows a reserve down to about 25%, corresponding to a PaO_2 of 15–20 mm Hg. (From Udwadia FE. (2005). *Principles of Critical Care Medicine*, second edition, Oxford University Press, New Delhi).

Table 3.1: PvO2 and SvO2 as indicators of cardiac output and tissue perfusion adequacy		
PvO_2 (mm Hg)	SvO_2 (%)	Clinical State
36–42	71–79	Normal Range
> 45	> 80	Septic Shock
< 30	< 50	Lactic Acidosis
< 17	< 20	Neural Damage

SUGGESTED READING

Udwadia FE. Basic Cardiorespiratory physiology in the intensive care unit. In *Principles of Critical Care*. 2005, second edition, Oxford University Press, New Delhi.

West JB. Ventilation-Perfusion Relationship in *Respiratory Physiology The Essentials*. 2006, sixth edition, Lippincott Williams and Wilkins.

West JB. Gas transport by the blood in *Respiratory Physiology The Essentials*. 2006, sixth edition, Lippincott Williams and Wilkins.

West JB. *Ventilation/Blood Flow and Gas Exchange*. 1990, fifth edition, Oxford, Blackwell, UK.

CHAPTER **4**

Acid-Base Balance and Control of Ventilation

GENERAL CONSIDERATIONS

The maintenance of normal acid-base balance (pH 7.35–7.45) in the blood is of crucial importance and is a vital homeostatic function of the body. Any variation from the normal constitutes an emergency in that a significant change in the H^+ ion concentration of the plasma or the extracellular fluid is incompatible with life; a pH < 7, or a pH > 7.8 spells imminent danger and death.

Acid-base disturbances occur very frequently in patients who are critically ill. It is of vital importance to bear in mind the fact that in patients with respiratory disease, acid-base disturbances and changes in pH may not solely be related to respiratory failure and adverse alterations in lung function. Many of these patients, particularly when critically ill, have associated metabolic problems as also problems associated with other organ systems that can independently influence and alter acid-base equilibrium. These independent alterations in acid-base balance may at times worsen alterations produced by respiratory disease, yet at times may counter them. Hence the great importance for respiratory physicians to have an overall perspective of acid-base disturbances rather than a mere awareness of changes seen in respiratory failure and respiratory disease. This chapter first deals with the basic physiology underlying acid-base balance. It then goes on to briefly describe acid-base disturbances with special reference to those caused by respiratory diseases. It then gives a brief discussion based on illustrative case studies on mixed acid-base disturbances often encountered in patients with respiratory disease and respiratory failure.

The manifestations of an altered acid-base homeostasis in such patients are often subtle, virtually impossible to clinically detect, and are often masked by the clinical features of the illness. There are no barriers to these disturbances; they are encountered in all fields and all specialities of medicine and surgery. Not uncommonly, the realization that sudden clinical deterioration or death in a particular patient may have been related to acid-base disturbances dawns on the physician a trifle too late. An early diagnosis of a change in acid-base equilibrium demands a sharp clinical acumen, a grasp of the physiopathology underlying these changes, and an intelligent interpretation of laboratory data.

No satisfactory assessment of the presence and degree of acid-base disturbances can be made without measuring the pH of the blood by the pH electrode. It is imperative that the importance of pH and acid-base measurements through a blood gas machine using the Astrup technique is universally recognized in all developing countries. Today, though many critical care units in the large metropolitan cities of India provide this very necessary facility, most critical care units in smaller cities lack this basic amenity. It is also unfortunate that many doctors are unable to correctly appreciate the results provided by this technique. Most students and doctors are taught to interpret arterial blood gases and acid-base disturbances by rule of the thumb or by reference to standard charts and graphs which allow a prompt solution for the basic problem. This may be satisfactory—but only to a point. Correct interpretation of blood gases and acid-base disturbances necessitates a familiarity with the basic physiology in this field. Then only can altered physiology be better understood. Intelligent and in-depth interpretation leads to a more rational management of the patient as a whole.

BASIC CONCEPTS

Concept of an Acid

An acid is a potential H^+ ion or proton donor. Conversely a base is a potential proton acceptor.

The strength of an acid (HA) is measured by the extent to which it dissociates in an aqueous solution.

$$HA \rightleftharpoons [H^+] + [A^-]$$

When the above reaction is in equilibrium, for a strong acid $[H^+] + [A^-]$ will be in a greater concentration than HA in the undissociated form. Also, at equilibrium, the product of the concentration on one side of the equation will bear a constant relationship to the product of concentration on the other.

$$Ka = \frac{[H^+] \, [A^-]}{[HA\}}$$

where Ka is the acid dissociation constant. Strong acids have a high Ka. Similar equations would apply to the dissociation of a base.

Concept of pH

The acidity of an aqueous solution is measured by its hydrogen (H^+) ion concentration or activity. The H^+ activity is expressed as pH. This terminology was introduced to simplify the expression of a wide range of H ions found in various fluids within the body. A quantification of H ions in various fluids in moles, would have been cumbersome and difficult. The notation pH is the negative logarithm of H ion concentration. This allows a large range of H^+ concentrations to be simply expressed and measured. Thus

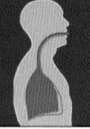

$$pH = \frac{1}{[H^+]}$$

$$= -\log 10 \, [H^+]$$

$$= \text{negative exponent of an expression of } [H^+]$$
$$\text{to the power 10}$$

Thus a pH of 7.4 = $[H^+] \times 10^{-7.4}$

The normal H ion concentration of blood is 40 nanomoles/l or 40×10^{-9} moles/l. This is equivalent to a pH of 7.4. Changes in acid-base balance can be looked upon either as changes in the H ion concentration or changes in pH. Table 4.1 given below shows the H ion concentration in relation to the corresponding pH values.

Table 4.1:
Correlation between H$^+$ ion concentration and pH values

H ion concentration (nmoles/l)	pH
10	8.00
20	7.70
30	7.52
40	7.40
50	7.30
60	7.22
70	7.15
80	7.10
90	7.05
100	7.00

The Henderson-Hasselbalch Equation

In the earlier section on the Concept of an Acid, it has been noted that

$$Ka = \frac{[H^+][A^-]}{[HA]}$$

If we wish to express H ion concentration (H^+) as pH (log 1/H), we may rewrite the above

$$[H^+] = Ka \frac{[HA]}{[A^-]}$$

Taking reciprocals,

$$\frac{1}{[H^+]} = \frac{1}{Ka} \times \frac{[A^-]}{[HA]}$$

Taking logs,

$$\log \frac{1}{[H^+]} = \log \frac{1}{Ka} + \log \frac{[A^-]}{[HA]}$$

i.e.
$$pH = pKa + \log \frac{[A^-]}{[HA]}$$

where pKa is the negative logarithm of the dissociation constant Ka. The above is the Henderson-Hasselbalch Equation.

Buffers

Buffers are substances which react with an acid or base and thereby minimize changes in pH. The metabolic processes within the body add a daily load of H ions to the body. These H ions if not properly dealt with within the body would produce a disastrous rise in H ion concentration, and a catastrophic fall in the pH. The homeostasis of acid-base balance however remains unchanged because of the buffering systems within the body and due to the role of the kidneys.

The main buffer systems of the body are:

(i) Haemoglobin and to a much lesser extent organic phosphates within the red blood cells.
(ii) Bicarbonates and inorganic phosphates within the blood.
(iii) Plasma Proteins.
(iv) Tissue Proteins.
(v) Minerals (phosphates, carbonates) within the bones.

It is only possible in this chapter to deal with the bicarbonate-carbonic acid buffer systems. The reader is referred to a standard textbook on Physiology for a more thorough understanding of the subject.

The bicarbonate-carbonic acid reaction is important in regulating acid-base balance. It constitutes a weak buffer system which can be used as a measure or reflection of all acid-base reactions within the body, because buffer systems are in dynamic equilibrium, and carbon dioxide diffuses freely across all tissues and membranes. Also, these chemical reactions occur very rapidly.

The carbon dioxide (CO_2) produced by tissue metabolism diffuses into plasma and the red blood cells (RBCs). The enzyme carbonic anhydrase within the RBCs catalyses the formation of carbonic acid

$$H_2O + CO_2 = H_2CO_3$$

The carbonic acid within the RBCs is dissociated thus:

$$H_2CO_3 \rightarrow H^+ + HCO_3^-$$

The bicarbonate within the RBCs diffuses out into the plasma, while the H ions are mopped up by the haemoglobin which acts as a buffer base. The loss of one ion from the cell has to be compensated by the entry of an equivalent ion. Thus chloride ions (Cl^-) from the plasma enter the red blood cells in place of the bicarbonate ions which have diffused out into the plasma.

When the blood reaches the lungs, the chloride shift is reversed and bicarbonate enters the red blood cells. The bicarbonate within the RBCs breaks down into H_2O and CO_2. The CO_2 diffuses out through the capillaries into the alveoli, and is washed out into the outside air.

The bicarbonate-carbonic reaction can be looked at from another angle as regards the role it plays in controlling acid-base balance. Thus when H^+ enters tissue fluids

$$H^+ + HCO_3^- \rightarrow H_2CO_3 \rightarrow CO_2 + H_2O$$

The CO_2 is rapidly washed out via the lungs leading to a rapid control of H ion production, but of course at the expense of a fall in $[HCO_3^-]$.

The Henderson-Hasselbalch equation for the bicarbonate-carbonic acid reaction aptly illustrates the role played by this reaction in regulating acid-base balance.

$$pH = pK + \log \frac{HCO_3}{H_2CO_3}$$

$$= 6.1 + \log \frac{HCO_3}{H_2CO_3}$$

$$= 6.1 + \log \frac{HCO_3}{0.03 \times PCO_2}$$

where 0.03 is the solubility of CO_2 in plasma, and PCO_2 the partial pressure of CO_2 in plasma.

If instead of pH one considers the H ion concentration, then the following modification of the Henderson-Hasselbalch equation can be used.

$$[H^+] = 24 \times \frac{PCO_3}{HCO_3} \text{ nanomoles/l}$$

Normally, $[H^+] = 24 \times 40/24 = 40$ nmoles/l (pH 7.4).

The Henderson-Hasselbalch equation expresses the relationship between three reactants—H^+, HCO_3^- and PCO_2, and can be used as an expression of acid-base balance within the body.

ROLE OF THE KIDNEYS IN ACID-BASE BALANCE

The kidneys play a crucial role in H ion regulation. They do so in the following ways:

(i) Regulating excretion and reabsorption of bicarbonate (HCO_3^-). Bicarbonate is filtered by the glomerulus, the quantity of bicarbonate in the filtrate being dependent on the plasma bicarbonate, and the glomerular filtration rate. The bicarbonate is then dealt with as follows:
  (a) Reabsorption of bicarbonate in the proximal renal tubules at a rate which is dependent on the PCO_2. The higher the PCO_2, the greater the degree of bicarbonate reabsorption; the lower the PCO_2, the lesser the degree of reabsorption of bicarbonate, and the greater its excretion. This enables respiratory acidosis (due to a high $PaCO_2$) to be compensated through retention of bicarbonate, and respiratory alkalosis (due to a low $PaCO_2$) to be compensated by an increased excretion of bicarbonate (see subsections on Respiratory Acidosis and Respiratory Alkalosis).
  (b) In metabolic acidosis, H ions are excreted into the urine. The enzyme carbonic anhydrase catalyses the reaction

$$H^+ + HCO_3^- \rightarrow H_2CO_3 \rightarrow H_2O + CO_2.$$

The CO_2 is reabsorbed and is excreted into the lungs. This is an important means by which the pH is controlled.

(ii) Use of Buffering Systems. H ions can be mopped up by phosphate buffers, thus tending to increase the pH, while at the same time conserving bicarbonate.
Thus under the influence of carbonic anhydrase,

$$H^+ + HCO_3^- = H_2CO_3 \text{ (in the tubular cells)}$$
$$H_2CO_3^- \rightarrow HCO_3^- + H^+$$

The bicarbonate ion is reabsorbed. The H ion is mopped up by $NaHPO_4$ thus—

$$H + NaHPO_4 \rightarrow NaH_2PO_4$$

which is excreted via the urine.
(iii) Ammonia. NH_4^+ is formed in the tubular cells by conversion of glutamine to glutamate. Thus,

$$CONH_2 \quad\quad COO^-$$
$$| \quad\quad\quad |$$
$$(CH_2)_2 \quad + H_2O \rightleftarrows NH_4^+ \quad (CH_2)_2$$
$$| \quad\quad\quad |$$
$$CHNH_3^+ \quad\quad CHNH_3^+$$
$$| \quad\quad\quad |$$
$$COO^- \quad\quad COO^-$$

GLUTAMINE   GLUTAMATE

NH_4^+ combines with chloride and is excreted via the urine, the reaction being controlled by the enzyme glutaminase. NH_4 excretion to be fully operative takes time. It is however an extremely important mechanism for pH control, as excretion of ammonia allows the excretion of a significantly large quantity of H ions via the kidney.
(iv) Reabsorption of Sodium. The active reabsorption of sodium from the filtrate into tubule cells causes a potential gradient across the cell membrane. The positively charged H ion within the tubule cell thus passes across the membrane into the filtrate, and is buffered within the filtrate by a phosphate buffer.

$$H + NaHPO_4 \rightarrow NaH_2PO_4$$

In summary, the kidneys help to maintain acid-base balance in the following ways:

(i) Retention of bicarbonate when the PCO_2 increases.
(ii) Excretion of bicarbonate when the PCO_2 falls.
(iii) Reabsorption of bicarbonate when there is accumulation of H ions in the blood.
(iv) Excretion of titratable acid and NH_4 to counter an increase of H ions in the blood.
(v) Excretion of H ions when there is a primary loss of bicarbonate.
(vi) Increased bicarbonate excretion in the urine, together with a loss of K^+ in the urine, when there is a primary increase in plasma bicarbonate.

DISTURBANCES IN ACID-BASE BALANCE

Terminology

Terms used: Acidaemia, alkalaemia, acidosis, alkalosis.
The normal pH of arterial blood is maintained within the range of 7.35 to 7.45.
Acidaemia exists when the pH of arterial blood is below the normal range i.e. less than 7.35.
Alkalaemia is the state in which pH of arterial blood is above the normal range i.e. greater than 7.45.
Acidosis is an abnormal state leading to an increase in the acid in the body.
Alkalosis is an abnormal state leading to a fall in acid or an increase in the alkali in the body.
When acidosis induces compensatory changes in the

body so that pH remains within the normal range, it is termed compensatory acidosis. When acidosis produces a fall in pH below 7.35, it is termed uncompensated acidosis. Uncompensated acidosis and acidaemia are thus synonymous.

Similarly, alkalosis can be compensated or uncompensated, and alaklaemia is synonymous with the latter.

Acidosis and alkalosis (as also acidaemia and alkalaemia) may result from primary respiratory or metabolic disturbances so that we have respiratory acidosis and metabolic acidosis, as also respiratory alkalosis and metabolic alkalosis.

Respiratory acidosis and respiratory acidaemia (uncompensated respiratory acidosis) result from alveolar hypoventilation which leads to hypercapnia.

Respiratory alkalosis and respiratory alkalaemia (uncompensated respiratory alkalosis) result from alveolar hyperventilation which causes hypocapnia.

Metabolic acidosis and metabolic acidaemia are caused by either accumulation of acid or loss of base from the body.

Metabolic alkalosis and metabolic alkalaemia are due to accumulation of base or loss of acid from the body.

Mixed acid-base disturbances are caused by a combination of respiratory and metabolic factors.

LABORATORY DIAGNOSIS OF DISTURBANCES IN ACID-BASE EQUILIBRIUM

Estimation of Serum Electrolytes

This is mandatory in every patient with acid-base disturbances, as electrolyte abnormalities are frequently seen and are often inseparable from changes in acid-base balance.

Interpretation of pH and Acid-Base Measurements by the Astrup Technique

In this technique, the pH and PCO_2 of the blood are measured by a sensitive instrument (radiometer). The values of standard bicarbonate, actual bicarbonate, CO_2 content, and base excess or deficit are then read from a standard nomogram. These concepts are briefly explained below.

The standard bicarbonate is the bicarbonate content in the plasma of blood which has been equilibrated at a PCO_2 of 40 mm Hg, as also with oxygen so as to saturate it with oxygen. The standard bicarbonate is a measure of the non-respiratory bicarbonate. It is the most active, mobile, rapidly reacting fraction of the total buffer potential, and its rate of excretion and retention is governed by the kidneys. A fall in the standard bicarbonate therefore indicates a metabolic acidosis; conversely a rise in the standard bicarbonate indicates a metabolic alkalosis. Normal standard bicarbonate indicates metabolic equilibrium.

The actual bicarbonate content is the bicarbonate concentration in mEq or mmoles/l in the plasma. It is not directly estimated; its value is derived from a nomogram in the Astrup technique, or from the CO_2 content of blood which can be estimated by the Van Slyke Apparatus.

The CO_2 content of plasma is the actual bicarbonate content + dissolved CO_2. As stated above, it can be estimated by gasometry (Van Slyke Apparatus), or is derived from a nomogram if the pH and $PaCO_2$ are known.

Base excess defines the presence in blood of excess or deficit of base, the physiological range being +/–2.3 mEq/l. It denotes the amount of strong acid or base per litre of blood, which has been added as a consequence of a metabolic disturbance. It is an *in vitro* concept, and is again derived from a nomogram if the pH and $PaCO_2$ are known.

Some of the terms described above are apt to prove confusing to the resident training in respiratory medicine. For purposes of simplification, acid-base changes are best interpreted by a consideration of the Henderson-Hasselbalch equation:

$$pH = pK + \log \frac{HCO_3}{PCO_2 \times 0.03}$$

In other words, pH is the 'balance' between the respiratory parameter represented by $PaCO_2$ (controlled by the lungs) and the metabolic parameter represented by bicarbonate (controlled by the kidneys). This is most simply illustrated in Figure 4.1. The PO_2 ($PaCO_2$) in this illustration and in subsequent illustrations is in mm Hg and the bicarbonate is in mEq/L.

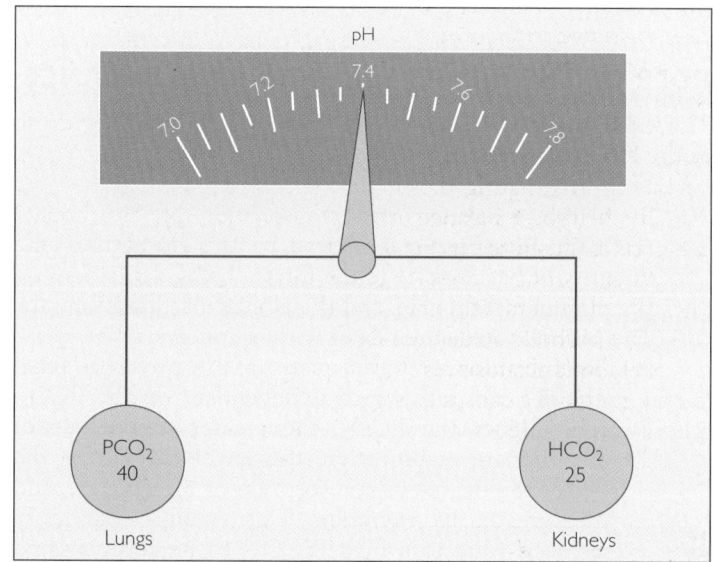

Fig 4.1: Normal acid-base balance.

A primary change in the respiratory parameter (partial pressure of carbon dioxide in arterial blood, $PaCO_2$) disturbs the 'balance' illustrated in Figure 4.1 to produce respiratory acid-base disturbances; a primary change in the metabolic parameter (bicarbonate) disturbs the balance and produces metabolic acid-base disturbances.

A rise in $PaCO_2$ primarily due to alveolar hypoventilation causes respiratory acidosis, and when this acidosis lowers the pH to < 7.35, respiratory acidaemia results. A fall in $PaCO_2$ produced by hyperventilation induces respiratory alkalosis and if the pH rises to > 7.45, respiratory alkalaemia results.

Homeostasis demands that primary changes in $PaCO_2$ lead to secondary changes in the plasma bicarbonate, so that the pH is kept within the normal range as far as possible. An acute rise in $PaCO_2$ (due to sudden hypoventilation following poisoning or a near respiratory arrest), will lead to a very small rise in the plasma bicarbonate (see earlier description on bicarbonate-carbonic acid reaction). The degree of retention of plasma bicarbonate is just 0.1 mmole or 0.1 mEq per 1 mm Hg rise in $PaCO_2$. The standard bicarbonate will remain unchanged. This can produce a gross imbalance between the respiratory and metabolic parameters, and can lead to a sharp and dangerous fall in pH. This is illustrated in Figure. 4.2

On the other hand, a slow or chronic rise in $PaCO_2$ (so frequently observed in patients with chronic airways obstruction) allows renal compensation to come into play. The kidneys retain bicarbonate—3–4 mEq or mmoles/l being retained for every 10 mm Hg rise in $PaCO_2$. Significant bicarbonate retention thus compensates for the chronic rise in $PaCO_2$, and helps to preserve the 'balance'. Retention of bicarbonate by the kidneys takes time; it probably starts 4–6 hours after the rise in $PaCO_2$, and is complete after one to three days. Compensation however can only occur up to a point—a rise in $PaCO_2 > 65$ to 70 mm Hg is generally associated with a fall in pH below normal in spite of bicarbonate retention. The degree of rise in bicarbonate enables one to determine whether in a given patient the respiratory acidosis is acute or chronic. Uncompensated respiratory acidosis and compensated respiratory acidosis (respiratory acidaemia) are illustrated in Figures. 4.2 and 4.3 respectively.

Comparison of degrees of rise in bicarbonate *in vivo* due to acute and chronic rise in $PaCO_2$ is illustrated in Figure. 4.4.

A fall in $PaCO_2$ primarily due to alveolar hyperventilation leads to a compensatory fall in plasma bicarbonate, the degree of fall approximating 0.1–0.3 mmoles/l for 1 mm Hg fall in $PaCO_2$. Acid-base balance in acute, uncompensated respiratory alkalosis is illustrated in Figure. 4.5.

When primary metabolic problems produce a fall in bicarbonate, metabolic acidosis results. When the pH falls to < 7.35, metabolic acidaemia results.

Metabolic alkalosis results following retention of bicarbonate due to metabolic causes; metabolic alkalaemia ensues when the pH rises to > 7.45.

Primary metabolic changes in bicarbonate result in secondary changes in $PaCO_2$, thus minimizing changes in the pH. Thus metabolic acidosis stimulates the respiratory centre, and the resulting hyperventilation reduces the $PaCO_2$. The degree of compensatory fall in $PaCO_2$ roughly equals 1.2 mm Hg for every 1 mmole or mEq/l fall in bicarbonate (or roughly equals 1.5 × bicarbonate content + 8). On the other hand, metabolic alkalosis depresses the respiratory centre and

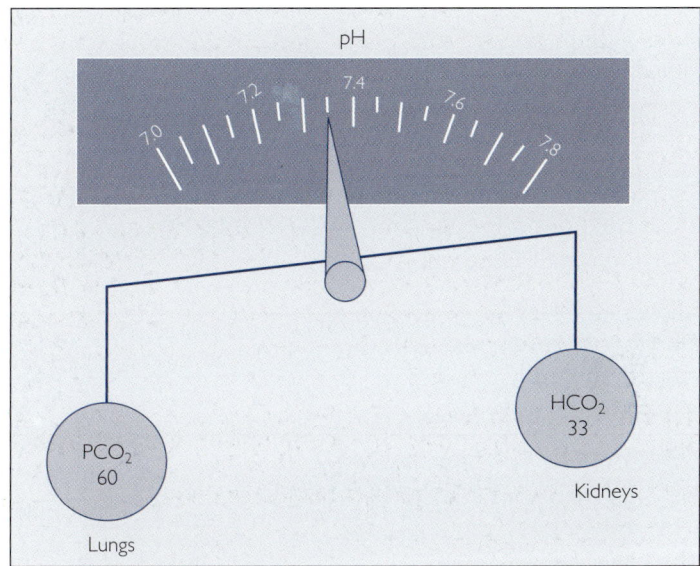

Fig 4.3: Compensated respiratory acidosis.

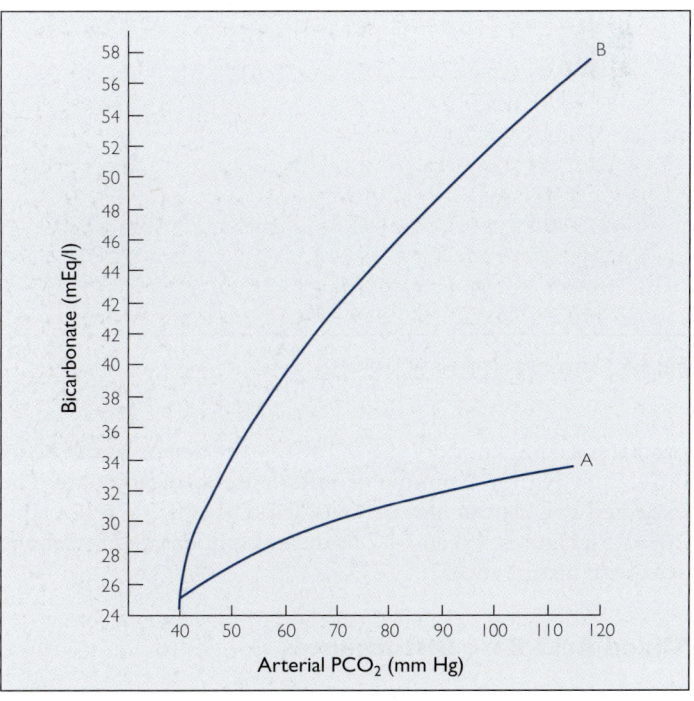

Fig 4.4: Comparison curves showing rise in bicarbonate levels in vivo chronic and acute hypercapnia. A = rise in acute hypercapnia. B = rise in chronic hypercapnia, because of retention of bicarbonate by the kidney.

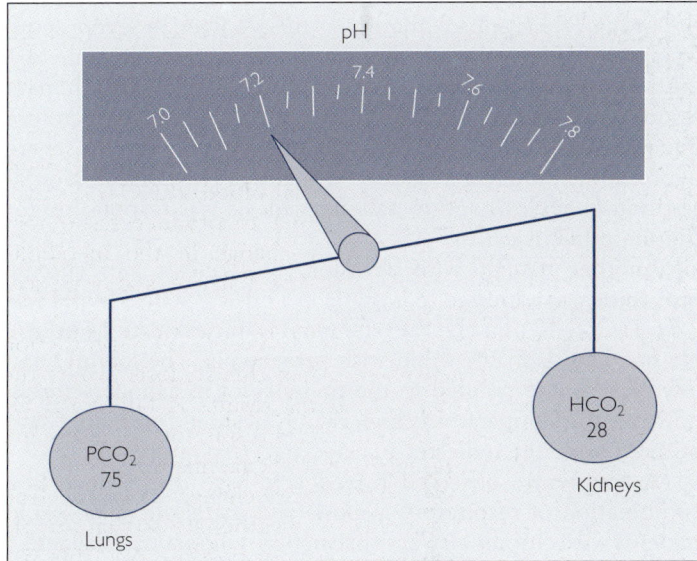

Fig 4.2: Uncompensated respiratory acidosis and acidaemia.

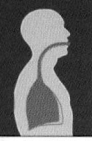

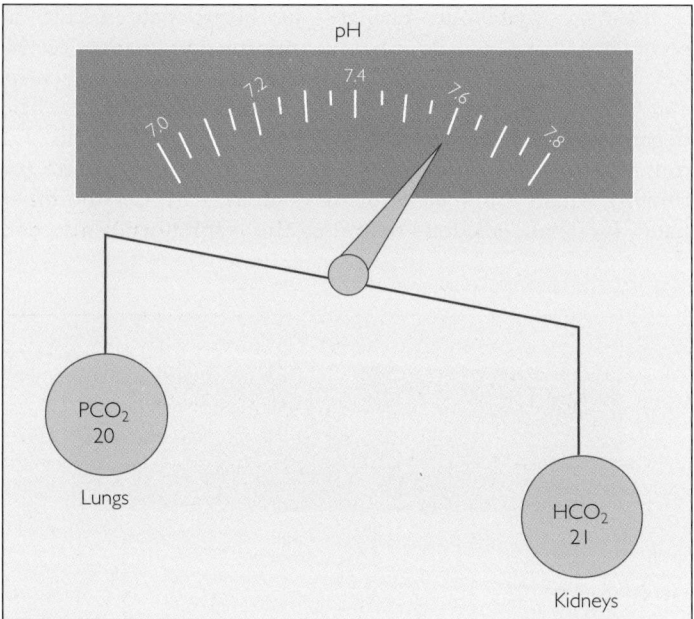

Fig 4.5: Acute uncompensated respiratory alkalosis.

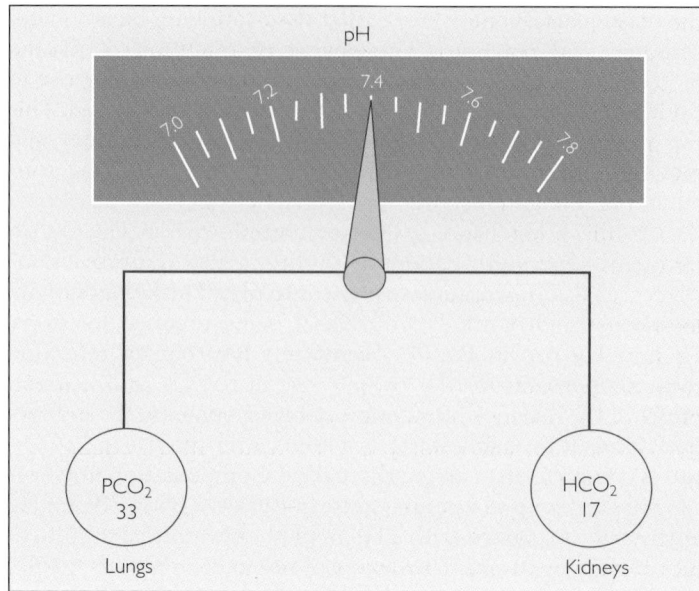

Fig 4.7: Compensated metabolic acidosis.

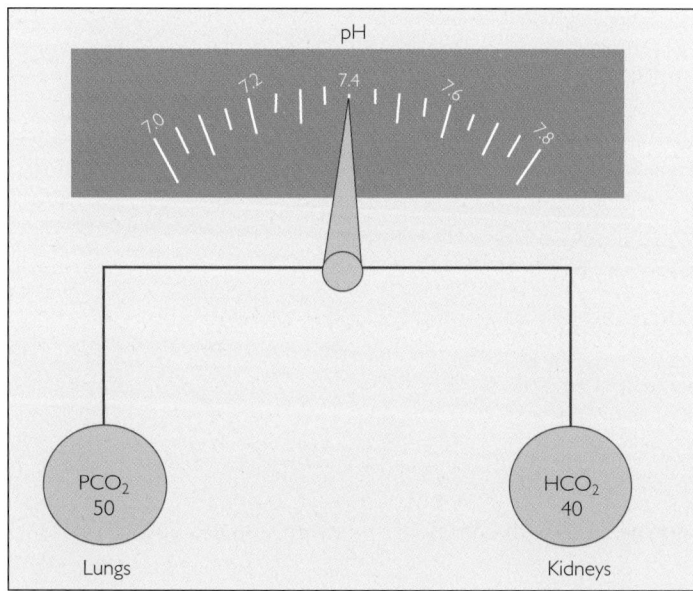

Fig 4.6: Compensated metabolic alkalosis.

produces a compensatory rise in PaCO₂, the degree of rise being 0.6–1 mm Hg for 1 mmole or mEq/l rise in bicarbonate. The expected PaCO₂ can also be considered as = 0.7 × [HCO₃] + 20(±1.5). Figures. 4.6 and 4.7 illustrate compensated metabolic acid-base disturbances.

Mixed Acid-Base Disturbances

Acid-base disturbances in critically ill patients are often due to both respiratory and metabolic problems occurring independently. They are often observed in patients with both acute and chronic respiratory failure. A consideration of the

clinical picture, the pH, PaCO₂ and bicarbonate, invariably clarifies the diagnosis. The degree of compensation present in relation to bicarbonate in primary respiratory disturbances, and the degree of compensation present in relation to PaCO₂ in primary metabolic problems, enables one to judge whether acid-base disturbances are due to mixed causes. The examples briefly quoted below help to give a more practical understanding of the problems involved.

A patient with chronic bronchitis emphysema deteriorated over a period of weeks, and was admitted to hospital in a critically ill condition with acute respiratory failure. The PaCO₂ was 82 mm Hg, PaO₂ 34 mm Hg, pH 7.15, bicarbonate 26 mEq/l. This patient obviously had respiratory acidosis (PaCO₂ 82 mm Hg). However, in a slowly deteriorating respiratory problem the rise in PaCO₂ should have been offset by a rise in plasma bicarbonate at a rate of 4 mEq/l for every 10 mm Hg rise in PaCO₂ i.e. approximately 40 mEq/l. Even in severe acute respiratory failure, the bicarbonate should increase at a rate of 1 mEq/l for every 10 mm Hg rise in PaCO₂. The low bicarbonate associated with the high PaCO₂ seen in this patient, is therefore due to an associated metabolic acidosis, possibly due to severe hypoxaemia inducing a lactic acid acidosis. The combination of respiratory acidosis and metabolic acidosis was responsible for the sharp fall in pH to 7.15.

Another patient with a history of diabetes and chronic bronchitis was admitted to hospital in a drowsy state. His pH was 7.21, PaCO₂ 42 mm Hg, PaO₂ 50 mm Hg, bicarbonate 14 mEq/l. He had ketosis in the urine with ketonaemia. The low pH and low bicarbonate pointed to the presence of metabolic acidosis; however, the comparatively high PaCO₂ (it should ordinarily have been 28 mm Hg), indicates an associated respiratory acidosis.

A frequently observed mixed acid-base disturbance is a combination of respiratory acidosis and metabolic alkalosis in patients with chronic airways obstruction, who are hypokalaemic due to the use of diuretics. The following example in a patient with the above problem is illustrative: pH 7.44; PaCO₂ 60

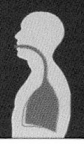

mm Hg; bicarbonate 38 mEq/l; serum K^+ 3mEq/l. A $PaCO_2$ of 60 mm Hg points to respiratory acidosis. However, the rise in the bicarbonate significantly exceeds the maximum of 0.4 mEq/mm Hg rise in the $PaCO_2$. This is due to a hypokalaemic metabolic alkalosis. The combination of respiratory acidosis and metabolic alkalosis allows the pH to be in the normal range.

A combination of respiratory acidosis and metabolic acidosis is often observed when respiratory failure due to alveolar hypoventilation, is combined with increasing hypoxia and poor tissue perfusion due to poor pump function. The following example is illustrative of this profile: pH 7.1; $PaCO_2$ 55 mm Hg; bicarbonate 15 mEq/l. Instead of the expected rise in bicarbonate due to a high $PaCO_2$, there is a fall in the bicarbonate because of metabolic lactic acid acidosis induced by hypotension and poor tissue perfusion in a patient with respiratory failure.

A combination of respiratory alkalosis and metabolic alkalosis is at times observed in hepatic failure. The latter causes tachypnoea with respiratory alkalosis. If there is associated vomiting, or there is aspiration of gastric contents through a nasogastric tube, the loss of H ions, K^+ and chloride leads to an associated metabolic alkalosis. The following example is illustrative: pH 7.61; $PaCO_2$ 25 mm Hg; bicarbonate 34 mEq/l.

A combination of respiratory alkalosis and metabolic acidosis may occur in septic shock and also in terminal acute liver cell failure. Both these conditions can cause tachypnoea with respiratory alkalosis. The metabolic (lactic acid) acidosis is related to shock and poor tissue perfusion. The same combination is often observed in patients who are hyperventilated on mechanical ventilation (with resulting respiratory alkalosis), and who are hypotensive from shock or poor pump function (which causes lactic acid acidosis).

Arterial pH of blood gases and bicarbonate levels should always be interpreted with reference to the history, clinical findings, and other investigations in every individual problem. Occasionally, the complexity of an acid-base disturbance is only apparent on a follow-up of the patient.

Clinical Features and Management of Acid-Base Disturbances

The clinical features and management of metabolic acidosis and metabolic alkalosis are not considered in this chapter. The respiratory physician should however be fully conversant with these metabolic disturbances.

Respiratory acidosis is discussed in the chapter on 'Acute Respiratory Failure in Adults'. Respiratory alkalosis results from alveolar hyperventilation causing a fall in the $PaCO_2$ and in the carbonic acid content of the plasma. It is observed in hysterical or functional states and in patients who are over-ventilated while on ventilator support. It can also occur in pulmonary embolism, cardiac failure in brainstem lesions and in some patients with hepatic failure. Purposeful or functional hyperventilation can lead to tingling, numbness of the hands, feet and circumoral area. Tetany manifested by carpopedal spasm may occur and the patient may faint. Fainting abolishes hyperventilation; $PaCO_2$ returns to normal and recovery ensues. Functional hyperventilation is best managed by asking the patients to rebreathe into a paper bag, and by reassurance.

CONTROL OF VENTILATION

The main function of the lung is to ensure efficient gas exchange of oxygen and carbon dioxide so as to maintain normal levels of PaO_2 and $PaCO_2$. This holds true not only with a subject at rest but in numerous conditions with varying demands of oxygen uptake and CO_2 output made by the body. The maintenance of gas exchange under varying conditions is only possible because of a fine control over ventilation.

Ventilation control has three elements:

1. A sensory system which feeds sensory inputs to a central controlling mechanism.
2. A central controlling mechanism in the brainstem which receives these sensory inputs and then sends out coordinated nervous impulses to the effector system.
3. Effector system   This system consists of respiratory muscles which effect ventilation.

CENTRAL CONTROLLING SYSTEM

The central controlling system is the respiratory centre in the brainstem. This centre consists of loosely arranged groups of neurones. It has three components i.e. three groups of neurons exerting ventilation control—the medullary centre, the apneustic centre in the lower pons and the pneumotaxic centre in the upper pons.

Medullary Respiratory Centre

This centre lies in the reticular formation of the brainstem, beneath the floor of the fourth ventricle. The dorsal group of neurones controls inspiration and the ventral group expiration. It is believed that the medullary respiratory centre has an inherent intrinsic rhythm which enables it to fire repetitive nervous impulses to the effector system (the diaphragm and inspiratory muscles). The medullary centre is responsible for the basic rhythm of ventilation and this rhythm persists even when all afferent stimuli to the centre are abolished.

The intrinsic rhythmicity of the medullary centre is characterized by a latent period followed by a progressive increase in the discharge of action potentials causing neuronal impulses to reach the muscle of inspiration. During this progressive increase in neuronal discharge from the centre, there follows a progressive increase in the strength of contraction of the inspiratory muscles. Then the action potential from the centre to the inspiratory muscles is turned off and expiration begins. In normal resting conditions, expiration consists of a passive relaxation of the chest wall to a position of equilibrium (which is at functional residual capacity (FRC) level). However, active expiration as for example in exercise is related to action potentials discharged from the ventral group of neucli beneath the floor of the fourth ventricles.

Apneustic Centre

The apneustic centre consists of loosely grouped neurones in the lower pons. The centre is so named because if a transection of the brain is made above this centre in experimental animals,

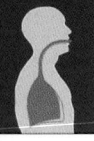

respiration is characterized by prolonged respiratory efforts or gasps (apneuses) interrupted by transient respiratory efforts. It appears that this centre influences the dorsal neurones in the medulla controlling inspiration, tending to prolong the progressively increasing action potentials arising in this medullary centre. It is uncertain whether the apneustic centre plays a role in control of ventilation. However, lesions in the pons are known to produce the breathing (apneustic breathing) described above.

Pneumotaxic Centre

Is in the upper pons. This centre has the ability to terminate the inspiratory action potential of the inspiratory medullary centre, thereby regulating the volume and rate of ventilation. It is believed to 'fine-tune' the inspiratory centre in the medulla.

Cortex

The cortex can exert voluntary control over ventilation to an extent, overriding the brainstem centres. This is evident when one considers voluntary hyperventilation which can be powerful enough to substantially reduce the $PaCO_2$. Voluntary hypoventilation is also possible though not to the same extent as hyperventilation, probably because of the effects of a lowered PaO_2 and an increased $PaCO_2$.

Influence of centres in the cerebrum other than the cortex is evinced by changes in ventilation produced by emotion, fear, rage which probably are related to the limbic system and the hypothalamus.

The Sensory System

Sensory receptors which on stimulation relay afferent nervous impulses to the regulating centre in the brainstem consist of central chemoreceptors, peripheral chemoreceptors and lung receptors.

CENTRAL CHEMORECEPTORS

Central chemoreceptors respond to changes in the chemical composition or the pH of the fluid or blood around them. They are situated below the ventral surface of the fourth ventricle in close proximity to the medullary respiratory centre and are of crucial importance in control of ventilation. The central chemoreceptors are bathed in the extracellular fluid of the brain, the composition of which is determined by local blood supply, local metabolism and the cerebrospinal fluid (CSF). The CSF is the most important governing factor. It is separated from the blood by the blood-brain barrier, which is comparatively impermeable to H^+ ions and HCO_3 ions but easily permeable to CO_2. When the PCO_2 rises, CO_2 diffuses through the blood-brain barrier into the CSF; H^+ ions are liberated and these H^+ ions stimulate the chemoreceptors. A rise in PCO_2 in the blood therefore chiefly stimulates ventilation through its effect on the H^+ ions and pH of the CSF. The increased ventilation serves to reduce the PCO_2 in the blood and thereby also reduce the CO_2 and H^+ ions' concentration in the CSF.

It should be noted that the change in CSF pH for a given increase in PCO_2 is much greater than the pH change in blood, because the CSF has much lower buffering capacity compared to blood. If pH in the CSF is lowered for a prolonged period,

compensation takes place by diffusion of HCO_3 through the blood-brain barrier into the CSF. The restoration of pH occurs far more promptly in the CSF as compared to restoration of the pH in the blood through renal compensation which may take over two days. Since CSF pH returns towards normal more quickly than blood pH, CSF pH exerts a more important effect in the control over ventilation.

PERIPHERAL CHEMORECEPTORS

Peripheral chemoreceptors are in the carotid bodies at the bifurcation of the common carotid artery and the aortic bodies above and below the aortic arch. The carotid body is the predominant chemoreceptor and consists of glomus cells which are of two types. Type I cells contain a store of dopamine and show an intense fluorescent stain. These cells are in close apposition to the nerve endings of the carotid sinus nerve. The Type II cells have a rich capillary supply. Changes in pH, PaO_2, $PaCO_2$ or other chemical changes in blood are sensed by glomus cells which are the site of chemoreceptors. This leads to release of neurotransmitters which influence the discharge rate of the afferent nerve fibres in the carotid body. Impulses reach the central nervous system through the carotid sinus nerve. The peripheral chemoreceptors in the carotid bodies are stimulated by a fall in arterial PaO_2, a rise in arterial $PaCO_2$ and a fall in pH. The carotid bodies have a large blood supply compared to their size as also a small arteriovenous oxygen difference. They respond to change in arterial PO_2 rather than venous PO_2. Their response to a fall in PaO_2 and a rise in $PaCO_2$ is extremely fast, even small cyclic changes in blood gases during breathing elicit a response from the carotid bodies.

Arterial hypoxemia therefore exerts a stimulant effect on the chemoreceptors within the carotid body leading to an increase in ventilation. In fact the increase in ventilation induced by hypoxemia is solely related to carotid body stimulation. Bilateral carotid body removal in an individual abolishes the increased ventilatory drive normally induced by hypoxemia. In fact in such patients arterial hypoxemia is noted to depress ventilation.

The response of the carotid body to change in $PaCO_2$ is less compared to change in PaO_2. Around 20% of the increased ventilatory response observed following a rise in $PaCO_2$ is believed to be related to stimulation of carotid body chemoreceptors. A lowered arterial pH also increases ventilation through stimulation of carotid body chemoreceptors. A combination of arterial hypoxemia, hypercapnia and a lowered pH has the maximal stimulatory effect on the central chemoreceptors.

LUNG RECEPTORS

1. Pulmonary Stretch Receptors   Pulmonary stretch receptors are slowly-adapting stretch receptors situated within airways smooth muscle. They are stimulated during lung inflation and their activity is sustained during inflation, showing little adaptation. The impulse from these stretch receptors travels via the vagus nerves to the medullary centre inhibiting inspiratory muscle activity. During deflation the opposite effect is observed, the lungs tending to initiate inspiration. This results in a self-regulating mechanism of negative feedback.

The reflex described through stimulation of the slow adaptive stretch receptors is termed the Hering Breuer inflation reflex. The stimulation of this reflex results in a slowing of the respiratory rate due to increase in expiratory time. The Hering Breuer reflex authenticated in animal experiments was believed to play a major role in humans as well, with regard to regulating the depth and rate of respiration. However, recent work suggests that this reflex plays little role in the control of ventilation unless the tidal volume is more than one litre, or in exercise.

2. Irritant Receptors   Irritant receptors are believed to be rapidly-adapting pulmonary stretch receptors situated between airways epithelial cells. They are stimulated by noxious stimuli like cigarette smoke, dust, and noxious gases as also by inhalation of cold air. Impulses from these receptors travel up the vagus nerve in myelinated fibres causing reflex bronchoconstriction and hyperpnoea. They are rapidly-adapting receptors and may play a role in the bronchoconstriction of asthma, through their response to noxious stimuli.

3. J Receptors   J Receptors were discovered by Prof. Paintal working at the Patel Chest Institute in New Delhi, first in the cat and then in the human being. These receptors are in the alveolar walls close to the capillaries. Impulses arising through stimulation of J receptors travel up the slow conducing unmyelinated fibres of the vagus nerves, resulting in reflex rapid shallow breathing. Interstitial oedema from any cause stimulates the J receptors. The rapid shallow breathing in patients with left ventricular failure is due to stimulation of J receptors. The tachypnoea associated with interstitial lung disease is also related to the stimulation of these receptors.

4. Bronchial C Fibres   These are close to the bronchial circulation. Their stimulation results in reflex rapid shallow breathing, bronchoconstriction and increased mucus secretion.

Besides central chemoreceptors, peripheral chemoreceptors and pulmonary receptors, ventilation can be reflexly influenced by other peripheral receptors. These are:

Nose and Upper Airways Receptors

Receptors present in the nose, nasopharynx, larynx, trachea respond to mechanical and chemical stimuli producing various reflex responses such as sneezing, coughing, bronchoconstriction and laryngeal spasm.

Receptors within Intercostal Muscles and Diaphragm

The intercostal muscles and diaphragm contain receptors in muscle spindles which sense muscle stretch. The stretch sensed by these receptors is used to reflexly control the strength of respiratory muscle contraction. Excessive stimulation of these receptors may be responsible for uncomfortable awareness of breathing that characterizes dyspnoea. This could be of particular relevance in patients with *chronic obstructive pulmonary disease* (COPD) who need extra respiratory muscle effort to meet the marked increase in resistive load.

Arterial Baroreceptors

An increase in arterial blood pressure particularly when sudden, can cause reflex hypoventilation through stimulation of the carotid and aortic baroreceptors. Conversely, hypotension can lead to hyperventilation. The reflex pathways involved in these reflexes are unknown.

Receptors in Muscles and Joints

Impulses arising through receptors in muscles and joints are believed to reflexly activate ventilation during exercise, particularly in the early phase.

An integrated response from the central controlling system in the medulla results following the processing of various sensory inputs mentioned above; the exact nature of this integration and its mechanism continues to be a subject of active research. It needs to be restressed that ventilation is most influenced by changes in $PaCO_2$, PaO_2 and pH of arterial blood. Experimental work shows that ventilation increases by as much as 1–2 L/min for each 1 mm Hg rise in $PaCO_2$. Lowering the PaO_2 results in even higher ventilation for a given $PaCO_2$. As mentioned earlier most of the increase in ventilation caused by an increased $PaCO_2$ is through central chemoreceptors but peripheral chemoreceptors also come into play with a faster response.

The ventilatory response to a rise in PCO_2 is reduced when the respiratory centre is depressed by various drugs such as narcotics and sedatives. Interestingly, the ventilator response to CO_2 is also decreased if the work of breathing is increased. Perhaps this may be one of the reasons for the reduced ventilatory response to CO_2 and for CO_2 retention in some patients of COPD. However the main reason for CO_2 retention in these patients is the inability of the respiratory muscles to produce the effort necessary to meet the markedly increased resistive load.

The PaO_2 exerts negligible control over ventilation under normoxic conditions. PaO_2 as seen in hypoxic conditions is however an important cause of increased ventilation. Only peripheral chemoreceptors are involved in causing reflex increase in ventilation.

A lowered pH as in any form of metabolic acidosis induces an increase in ventilation and this effect is independent of the $PaCO_2$. A fall in pH acts chiefly through peripheral chemoreceptors. Central chemoreceptors and the respiratory centre itself may to a lesser extent also be stimulated with a fall in pH.

VENTILATORY RESPONSE TO EXERCISE

Ventilation increases within some seconds of starting exercise. With maximal exercise, a fit young subject can increase the minute ventilation to 150 litres which is close to 16 times the minute ventilation at rest. There is a corresponding increase in oxygen consumption to 4 L/min and an increase in carbon dioxide output. The reason for this marked increase in ventilatory response to exercise is not understood.

The $PaCO_2$ does not change during exercise; in fact with a very high workload it may fall just a little. The PaO_2 remains constant; with maximal exercise there may be a slight fall but not at all enough to be responsible for the marked increase in minute ventilation. The pH of arterial blood remains constant except with very heavy workloads when there is a slight fall in the pH due to lactic acid production in the muscles and anaerobic glycolysis.

Several hypotheses have been put forward to explain the ventilatory response to exercise. Perhaps the very prompt rise

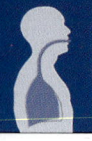

(within 10 to 15 seconds) in ventilation may be explained by stimulation of receptors in joints and muscles of the limbs which cause a reflex increase in ventilation. Evidently, changes in PaO_2, $PaCO_2$ and pH are not sufficient to explain the ventilatory response. One hypothesis states that it is the oscillation in arterial PaO_2 and $PaCO_2$ which stimulates peripheral chemoreceptors even though the mean PaO_2 and $PaCO_2$ remain unchanged. Another hypothesis is that the central chemoreceptors stimulate the respiratory centre to increase ventilation, so as to keep the $PaCO_2$ constant by a sort of servomechanism, acting very similar to a thermostat that keeps a constant temperature. A third hypothesis states that the increased ventilatory response is related to the high content of CO_2 presented to the lungs in the mixed venous blood. This has been shown to occur in animal experiments, ventilation increasing pari passu with increasing infusion of CO_2 into venous blood. Yet receptors which could initiate this increase in ventilation have not been found. Perhaps some increase in ventilation may be related to impulses from the cortex, the medullary respiratory centre, as also to a slight rise in body temperature during heavy exercise. None of the hypotheses stated above provide a satisfactory explanation for the ventilatory response during exercise.

SUGGESTED READING

Morgan TJ. Clinical review: The meaning of acid-base abnormalities in the intensive care—effects of fluid administration. *Crit Care*. 2005; 9: 204–11.

Story DA. Bench to bedside review: A brief history of clinical acid-base. *Crit Care*. 2004; 8:253–58.

Udwadia FE. Acid-base Disturbances in the Critically Ill. In *Principles of Critical Care*. 2005, second edition, Oxford University Press.

West JB. Control of ventilation. In *Respiratory Physiology The Essentials*. 2006, sixth edition Lippincott Williams and Wilkins.

CHAPTER 5

Pulmonary Circulation

The pulmonary artery arises from the right ventricle. It then divides into right and left branches. Each of these divides further and further into smaller branches. These vessels accompany the airways as far as the terminal bronchioles and then break up to form a vast capillary bed perfusing the millions of alveoli in the lungs. The capillary network is both profuse and rich; many physiologists regard the capillary bed as a sheet of blood to which oxygen is added from within the alveoli and from which carbon dioxide diffuses into the alveoli. The oxygenated blood is collected by small veins which merge to form four large veins (two on either side superior and inferior). These veins open into the left atrium thereby providing the left heart with oxygenated blood. The pulmonary circulation extends from the start of the pulmonary artery to the opening of the pulmonary veins into the left atrium.

HEMODYNAMICS OF THE PULMONARY CIRCULATION

The pulmonary circulation constitutes a low-pressure, high-flow, high-volume circuit. It carries a volume of blood equal to that carried by the systemic circulation but manages to do so with a far less driving pressure thus reducing the stress on the right ventricle. The right ventricle is not structured to handle 'load' (in contrast to the left ventricle), but fortunately can handle volume effectively. The systolic pressure of the pulmonary artery is 20–25 mm Hg and the diastolic 8 mm Hg with a mean pulmonary artery pressure of around 15 mm Hg. In contrast systolic and diastolic pressure in the systemic circulation are 120 mm Hg and 80 mm Hg respectively, the mean arterial blood pressure being about 100 mm Hg'—more than six times the mean pulmonary artery pressure. Pressures in the right atrium are around 2 to 5 mm Hg and in the left atrium 5 to 10 mm Hg. The pressure difference in the pulmonary circulation is 15 – 5 = 10 mm Hg. In the systemic circulation it is 100 – 2 mm Hg = 98 mm Hg; which is close to ten times that in the pulmonary circulation.

The walls of the pulmonary arteries and their branches are thin and contain relatively less smooth muscle, probably related to the low pressures within the whole system. The reason for the difference between the pulmonary and systemic circulation is largely related to much greater work required of the left ventricle to supply blood to various organ systems of the body, including structures above the level of the heart. In contrast, the right heart through the pulmonary circulation pumps the whole cardiac output solely to the lungs. It has less work to do and does so by maintaining lower pressure in the pulmonary circuit, enough however to allow efficient gas exchange within the lungs.

Though the mean pressure in the pulmonary artery is 15 mm Hg, the pressure in the pulmonary capillaries is uncertain. It is probably mid-way between the pressure in the pulmonary artery and veins. Studies suggest that there seems to be a gradual symmetrical drop of pressure in the pulmonary vessels towards the capillaries. In contrast, most of the pressure drop in the systemic circulation is just above the capillary level. However, it must be noted that the pressure within the pulmonary capillaries is not the same throughout the lung; it varies in different parts of the lung because of their exposure to different hydrostatic pressures. This aspect has been explained later in this chapter.

The thin-walled capillaries adjoin the alveoli which they perfuse. The blood in the capillaries is separated from the air in the alveoli by the thin endothelial lining of the capillary wall, the fused basement membrane of the capillary wall plus alveolar wall and the epithelial cells lining the alveoli. The pulmonary capillaries are therefore strongly influenced by the pressure within the alveoli and are likely to expand if alveolar pressure is low and collapse if the pressure is high. The alveolar pressure is atmospheric at end of expiration of a tidal volume breath. It is also atmospheric at end-inspiration with the mouth open. By and large therefore under ordinary circumstances, the pressure around pulmonary capillaries is close to the alveolar pressure. Over-inflation of alveoli compresses capillaries; under-inflation allows them to dilate.

The pressure around the larger pulmonary vessels and veins is, however, considerably less than alveolar pressure. This is because these vessels are kept open by the radial traction of the elastic lung parenchyma surrounding them, so that these vessels increase their calibre with lung expansion. Consequently, the effective pressure around them is low.

To summarize, whereas the calibre of the pulmonary capillaries (or alveolar vessels) is influenced by alveolar pressure and the intraluminal pressure within them, the calibre of the large vessels (extra-alveolar vessels) is influenced by lung volume rather than alveolar pressure. The large vessels at the hilum are outside the lung and are influenced by the intra-pleural pressure.

PULMONARY VASCULAR RESISTANCE

Vascular resistance in a vessel = Input pressure – output pressure/blood flow

Pulmonary vascular resistance = 15 – 5/5 to 6 = 1.7 to 2 mm Hg/L/min.

where 15 mm Hg is the mean pulmonary artery pressure, 5 mm Hg is the pressure in the left atrium and the pulmonary

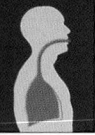

blood flow is 5 to 6 L/min. The pulmonary vascular resistance is thus markedly low, well nigh 10 times lower than the systemic vascular resistance. The high systemic vascular resistance is related to muscular arterioles regulating blood flow to various organ systems. The pulmonary vascular system has thin vessels walls with low resistance enabling a widespread distribution of a thin film of blood along the alveolar walls, ensuring efficient gas exchange.

Remarkably, this low pulmonary vascular resistance is capable of falling further if the pulmonary artery pressure is raised. There are two mechanisms responsible for this capability—

1. Recruitment. Normally (under resting conditions) some capillaries have no blood flowing through them. When pulmonary artery pressure is raised these vessels open up and have blood flowing through them thereby reducing overall pulmonary vascular resistance. This mechanism is termed recruitment.
2. Dilatation. A rise in pulmonary artery pressure leads to dilatation with a rounding of the normally flattened pulmonary capillaries, resulting again in a fall in pulmonary vascular resistance. The distension or dilatation of the capillaries is possible because of the very thin membrane separating the capillaries from the alveolar wall. Dilatation or distension is the chief mechanism for lowering pulmonary vascular resistance in the presence of significantly increased pulmonary vascular pressures. Both recruitment and distension may occur together to produce the same effect (Figure 5.1).

Lung volume is another important determinant of pulmonary vascular resistance. It has been mentioned earlier that the walls of the extra-alveolar vessels on inspiration are pulled apart thereby reducing their vascular resistance at large lung volumes. The walls of these extra-alveolar vessels contain smooth muscle which resists distension and tends to reduce their calibre. Therefore, when the lung volume is low, these vessels have an increased resistance. If a lobe or lung is completely atelectatic, the resistance of these extra-alveolar vessels is so high that the pulmonary artery pressure must be raised markedly above the normal before flow occurs at all. In other words the critical

opening pressure that enables blood to flow is significantly raised. Lung volumes also affect pulmonary capillary pressure. They do so in two ways—

1. If the intra-alveolar pressure is high as compared to the luminal pressure within the capillaries (i.e. an increase in transmural pressure) the capillaries are constricted and the pulmonary vascular resistance increases.
2. If the alveoli are distended for any reason even if there is no increase in intra-alveolar pressure, the distension of the alveoli squeezes the adjoining pulmonary capillaries and increases the pulmonary vascular resistance.

In summary both increase and decrease in lung volumes can increase pulmonary vascular resistance.

The extra-alveolar vessels have smooth muscle within their walls. Drugs which act on smooth muscle can thereby influence pulmonary vascular resistance. Norepinephrine and histamine contract smooth muscle and increase pulmonary vascular resistance. Isoproterenol is a drug which relaxes smooth muscle and this decreases pulmonary vascular resistance. Hypoxia is a strong constrictor of pulmonary capillaries and produces pulmonary hypertension. Hypercapnia normally causes vasodilatation of systemic vessels but constricts pulmonary vessels leading to pulmonary hypertension.

MEASUREMENT OF PULMONARY BLOOD FLOW

Pulmonary blood flow can be measured by the Fick Principle:

$$\dot{V}O_2 = Q\ (\ CaO_2 - CvO_2)$$
$$Q = \dot{V}O_2 / CaO_2 - CvO_2$$

where $\dot{V}O_2$ is the oxygen consumption per minute, CaO_2 is the arterial oxygen content, CvO_2 is the mixed venous oxygen content, and Q is the blood flow through the lungs.

$\dot{V}O_2$ is measured by collecting the expired gas in a large spirometer over a minute and measuring the oxygen concentration.

CaO_2 is estimated from blood withdrawn through the radial artery. CvO_2 is estimated by collecting a mixed venous blood sample from the pulmonary artery via a pulmonary artery catheter.

Pulmonary blood flow can also be measured by the indicator dilution technique in which a dye or other indicator is injected into the venous circulation and its concentration in the arterial blood is recorded.

DISTRIBUTION OF PULMONARY FLOW IN THE LUNG

Blood flow through the lungs is not uniformly distributed. In fact there is considerable inequality of blood flow in the human lung. In the upright standing posture, blood flow decreases from the bottom or base of the lung to the top or apex in an almost linear fashion. In the supine position, the blood flow at the apex increases but the basal flow is unchanged so that the blood flow is more uniformly distributed from the apex to the base. However, the flow in the posterior or dependent portion of the lung is more than in the anterior portion. On exercise both upper

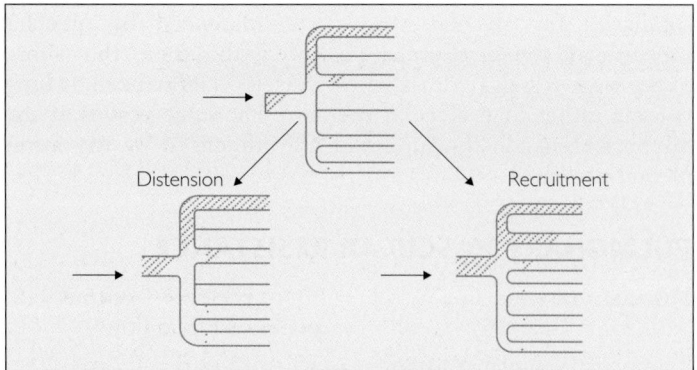

Fig 5.1: Recruitment and distension. These are the two mechanisms for the decrease in pulmonary vascular resistance that occurs as vascular pressures are raised. (Adapted from *Respiratory Physiology The Essentials* by John B. West, seventh edition, Lippincott Williams and Wilkins).

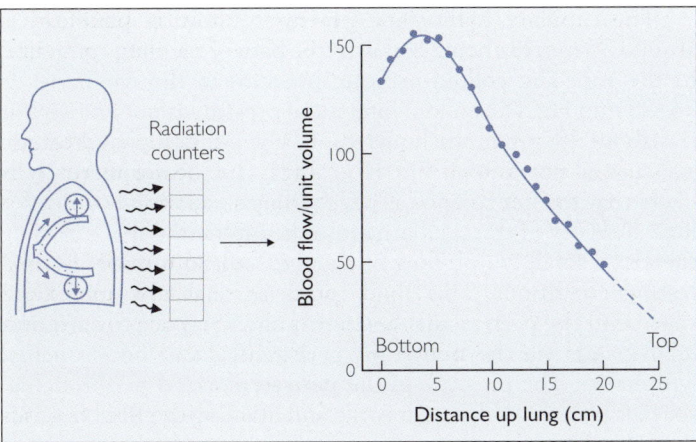

Fig 5.2: Measurement of the distribution of blood flow in the upright human lung using radioactive xenon. The dissolved xenon is evolved into alveolar gas from the pulmonary capillaries. The units of blood flow are such that if flow were uniform, all values would be 100. (With permission from *Respiratory Physiology The Essentials* by John B. West, seventh edition, Lippincott Williams and Wilkins).

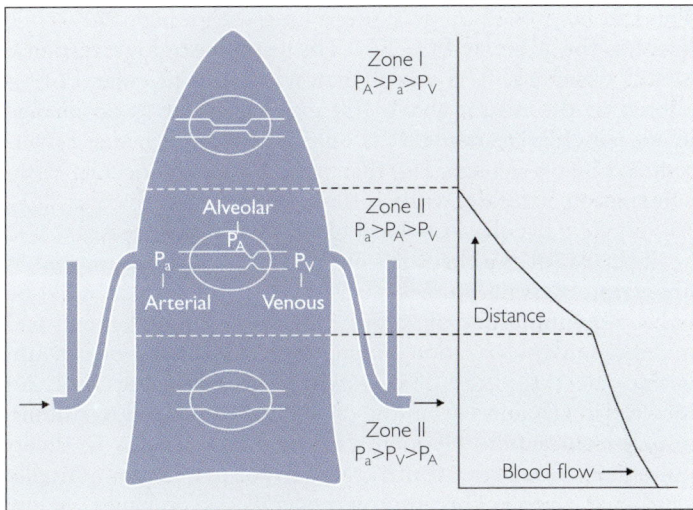

Fig 5.3: Uneven distribution of blood in the lung, based on the pressure affecting the capillaries. P_a is pulmonary artery pressure. P_A is alveolar pressure, P_V is venus pressure. (Adapted from *Respiratory Physiology The Essentials* by John B. West, seventh edition, Lippincott Williams and Wilkins).

and lower zones have an increased blood flow, the difference between the two being less marked than at rest (Figure 5.2).

The inequality in the distribution of blood flow within the lungs can be explained by differences in hydrostatic pressure from top to bottom. The difference in hydrostatic pressure from the apex of the lung to the bottom can be as high as 30 cm of H_2O. This large difference in hydrostatic pressure significantly affects regional blood flow in the existing low-pressure pulmonary circulation.

The lung can be looked upon as consisting of three zones (Figure 5.3). In the upper zone (Zone I), there may be regions where the pulmonary artery pressure falls well below the alveolar pressure (which is close to atmospheric pressure). If this does occur the pulmonary capillaries are squeezed shut and no blood flow occurs through them. This does not happen normally as the pulmonary artery pressure is just sufficient to raise blood right up to the apex of the lung. But it could well occur if the pulmonary artery pressure falls as after haemorrhage or hypovolemia from any cause, or if the intra-alveolar pressure in Zone I is increased as in a patient on positive pressure ventilator support. If this transpires, the alveolar pressure squeezes the capillaries shut and this portion of the lung cannot take part in gas exchange.

In Zone II (further down the lung), the hydrostatic effect causes an increase in the pulmonary artery pressure. The pulmonary artery pressure now is more than the alveolar pressure. The pulmonary venous pressure is however still low. The blood flow in this zone is not determined by the usual arterio-venous pressure difference but by the difference between the pulmonary arterial pressure and alveolar pressure. Venous pressure has no influence on blood flow unless it exceeds alveolar pressure.

In Zone III (which includes the base of the lung) there is increased blood flow and dilatation of capillaries due to hydrostatic forces. The venous pressure now exceeds alveolar pressure so that blood flow in Zone III is governed by the usual arterio-venous pressure difference. In this zone therefore the pulmonary artery pressure is greater than the pulmonary

venous pressure which in turn is greater than the pulmonary alveolar pressure. As one goes down towards the base of the lung, there is increased blood flow through the capillaries while the alveolar pressure remains constant. The transmural pressure (between capillary and alveolar pressure) rises and the capillaries are more dilated.

Finally, one must consider pulmonary flow at low lung volumes. At low volumes there is (as has been already explained) an increased resistance of the extra-alveolar vessels. This assumes importance as there is a resultant reduction in the regional blood flow starting first at the base of the lung which is less expanded. This region of reduced blood flow is sometimes termed Zone IV and results from a narrowing of the extra-alveolar vessels when the lung around them is partially atelectatic and poorly inflated.

West, in his excellent book on Respiratory Physiology, mentions other possible causes of inequality of blood flow. These include possible higher vascular resistance in some regions of the lung, perhaps a reduced blood flow to peripheral parts of the lung compared to the central areas. The random arrangements of blood vessels and capillaries may to some extent contribute to the inequality of pulmonary blood flow.

FACTORS INFLUENCING PULMONARY CIRCULATION

The hemodynamic factors determining blood flow, vascular resistance and pressure in the pulmonary circuit have already been discussed.

An extremely important influencing factor is a fall in the PO_2 of alveolar gas (a low P_AO_2). This results in hypoxic vasoconstriction of the pulmonary arterioles due to active contraction of smooth muscle within the pulmonary arteriolar walls. Almost certainly, it is the hypoxia itself which is responsible for this vasoconstrictive effect. Neurogenic factors are not involved. Equally important, experiments suggest that it is the low PO_2 of the alveolar gas and not a low PO_2 in the pulmonary arterial blood, which is responsible for this vasoconstrictive response.

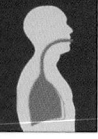

This can be proved by perfusing a lung with a high PO_2 while keeping the alveolar PO_2 low. The vasoconstrictive response is still observed. It is noted that when the alveolar PO_2 is altered in the region above 100 mm Hg, there is no change in the vascular response. It is only when the alveolar PO_2 is reduced below 70 mm Hg, that vasoconstriction occurs. Vasoconstriction increases with further lowering of alveolar PO_2. At very low alveolar PO_2, local blood flow almost ceases.

The exact mechanism of hypoxic vasoconstriction is unknown. Recent studies suggest that the effect may be induced by inhibition of voltage-gated potassium channels and membrane depolarization leading to accumulation of calcium within the cytoplasm of cells within the arteriolar wall. An increase in calcium within the cytoplasm could lead to smooth muscle contraction. Hypoxic vasoconstriction helps to divert pulmonary blood flow from hypoxic alveoli to better or normally ventilated alveoli. This improves overall gas exchange. A low alveolar PO_2 is found in hypoventilation from any cause, when a bronchus to an area of the lung is obstructed by secretions or by an intraluminal growth or from extrinsic obstruction.

At high altitude there is a generalized pulmonary vasoconstriction because of a low alveolar O_2 pressure throughout all alveoli in the lungs. The severe pulmonary hypertension is chiefly responsible for pulmonary oedema.

During foetal life, the pulmonary vascular resistance is very high because of hypoxic pulmonary vasoconstriction. When the baby is born, the first breath oxygenates the alveoli; the alveolar O_2 rises, the pulmonary vascular resistance falls and pulmonary blood flow (which in foetal life amounts only to 20% of the cardiac output) rises dramatically.

A rise in the $PaCO_2$ also causes pulmonary vasoconstriction though this is not as strong a stimulus as hypoxia. Remarkably, a rise in $PaCO_2$ causes vasodilatation in all vessels except the pulmonary vessels where it causes vasoconstriction. A fall in the pH, particularly in the presence of hypoxia also causes vasoconstriction. An increase in sympathetic vascular resistance probably also leads to some degree of increased pulmonary vascular resistance.

FLUID EXCHANGE ACROSS THE ALVEOLAR CAPILLARY MEMBRANE

The alveoli must be kept free of fluid if proper gas exchange is to be maintained, particularly so since just 0.3 μm of tissue separates capillary blood from alveolar air. Fluid exchange along the alveolar-capillary membrane obeys Starling's law. The filtration force tending to push fluid from the capillaries into the alveoli is the capillary hydrostatic pressure (P_C) minus the hydrostatic pressure in the interstitial fluid (P_I) i.e. $P_C - P_I$. The force tending to pull fluid into the capillaries is the osmotic pressure of the plasma protein in the blood (Π_C) minus the osmotic pressure of fluid in the interstitial space ($\Pi_C - \Pi_I$). This force is dependent on the coefficient α which indicates the efficiency of the capillary wall to prevent passage of proteins through it. Therefore fluid exchange across the alveolar capillary membrane is governed by the following equation

$$K\left[(P_C - P_I) - \alpha\,(\Pi_C - \Pi_I)\right]$$

where K is the constant called the filtration coefficient.

The capillary hydrostatic pressure (filtration pressure) is around 35 mm Hg being higher at the base of the lung compared to the top. The colloid osmotic pressure in the capillaries is 25–28 mm Hg. The colloid interstitial pressure is not known but it is about 20 mm in the lung lymph. The interstitial hydrostatic pressure is not known but is probably sub-atmospheric. It is likely that the net balance as per Starling's equation is to push a little fluid out of the capillaries into the interstitial space causing thereby a small lymph flow of about 20 ml/hour under normal resting conditions. This fluid tracks through the interstitial space into the perivascular and peribronchial space towards the hilar glands via the numerous perivascular and peribronchial lymphatics. The pressure in the perivascular and peribronchial space is low; this helps in drawing and draining the fluid towards the hilar glands.

Pulmonary oedema occurs when more fluid is filtered through the capillaries. Early pulmonary oedema is interstitial. Later the oedema fluid crosses the alveolar epithelium into the alveolar spaces. This probably occurs when the fluid filtered through the capillaries into the interstitium exceeds considerably the maximum drainage rate of the fluid within the interstitium. Fluid reaching the alveoli is actively pumped out by a sodium potassium ATPase pump in alveolar epithelial cells. But this is ineffective in the presence of significant alveolar oedema. Alveolar oedema interferes with gas exchange and leads to increasing hypoxia.

Pulmonary oedema in clinical medicine is related to one or more of the following three factors—increased capillary hydrostatic pressure as in left ventricular failure, a marked decrease in plasma osmotic pressure as is seen with any condition causing marked hypoproteinaemia and in particular hypoalbuminaemia, and finally increased capillary permeability, classically seen in the acute respiratory distress syndrome.

METABOLIC FUNCTION OF THE LUNG

Gas exchange is the prime and most important function of the lung. The lung also has a metabolic function. A brief account of the metabolic function of the lung is given below.

Like the heart, the lung is the only other organ to receive the whole circulatory output and therefore is aptly placed to metabolize or modify blood-borne substances. The lung is responsible for the biological activation of angiostensin I to angiostensin II. This conversion is catalyzed by the angiotensin-converting enzyme (ACE). Angiotensin II is 50 times more potent than angiotensin I and is unaffected by passage through the lung.

Many vasoactive substances are partially or completely inactivated after passage through the lungs. These include norepinephrine and prostaglandin E_1, E_2, E_3. Serotonin is removed through increased uptake and storage within platelets. Bradykinin is inactivated by ACE. Some vasoactive substances pass through the lung unchanged; these include epinephrine, vasopressin and prostaglandin A_1, A_2.

A few vasoactive substances are metabolized in the lung and are released into the circulation under certain circumstances. Good examples are the arachidonic acid metabolites. Arachidonic acid is derived from membrane-bound phospholipid through the action of phospholipase A_2. The further metabolism of arachidonic acid is along two pathways—one

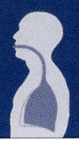

catalyzed by lipooxygenase and the other by cycloxygenase. The first catalytic reaction leads to the production of leukotreines. These cause airways obstruction and play a role in bronchial asthma. Other leukotreines are mediators of inflammatory processes. The second catalytic reaction leads to the production of prostaglandins and thromboxaneA$_2$. Prostaglandins are potent vasoconstrictors or vasodilators. Prostaglandins affect platelet aggregation and play an active role in the kallikrein-kinin clotting cascade. They also mediate bronchoconstriction in patients with bronchial asthma.

The lung has plenty of heparin-containing mast cells within the interstitium which may perhaps have a role in the clotting mechanism of blood. The lung also has an important immunological function because it secretes the immunoglobulin A$_2$ in the bronchial mucus. This immunoglobulin enhances the local immune response within the lung to infection.

Among the synthetic functions of the lung is the production of phospholipids such as dipalmitoyl phospho acetylcholine which is the important component of surfactant synthesized by alveolar Type II epithelial cells. Protein synthesis is probably important because collagen and elastin form the framework of the lung. Finally, the lung has a role in carbohydrate metabolism, as it elaborates mucopolysaccharides of bronchial mucous.

SUGGESTED READING

Cherniack NS, Widdicombe JG. Control of breathing. In *Handbook of Physiology. The Respiratory System*. 1986. Bethesda, MD, American Physiological Society, Vol. 2. Section 3.

Von Euler. Neural organization and rhythm generation in Crystal RG,

West JB, Barnes PJ, Weibel ER (eds). *The Lung Scientific Foundations*. 1997, second edition, Lippincott-Raven Press.

West JB. Control of ventilation. In *Respiratory Physiology The Essentials*. 2006, sixth edition, Lippincott Williams and Wilkins.

CHAPTER **6**

Respiratory Muscle Function Testing

When muscles contract they develop force and shorten. In the respiratory system the force of muscle contraction is estimated by measurement of the pressure and the shortening caused by contraction by change in volume. Quantifying pressure and volume changes is a measure of respiratory muscle function.

Respiratory muscle weakness is characterized by a fall in vital capacity (VC). A fall in VC is however not specific for respiratory muscle weakness. It is a fairly early feature in restrictive lung and chest wall disease and also occurs in well-marked obstructive airways disease. The clinician needs to take this into account and rule out the above mentioned diseases before attributing a fall in VC to respiratory muscle weakness. A marked fall (> 30%) in VC in the supine posture compared to the sitting or standing posture is indicative of severe bilateral diaphragmatic weakness.

MEASUREMENT OF STATIC MAXIMAL INSPIRATORY AND EXPIRATORY PRESSURES

Inspiratory and expiratory muscle strength can be estimated easily by measuring the maximum static inspiratory ($P_I$max) and expiratory ($P_E$max) pressure that a subject can generate at the mouth. The pressure is measured at the side port of a mouthpiece that is closed at one end. The maximum pressure sustained for one second is recorded (Figure 6.1). The pressure

recorded at the mouth in these tests is a measure of pressure developed in the respiratory muscles plus the elastic recoil pressure of the lung and chest wall. At residual volume (RV) where $P_I$max is usually measured the elastic recoil pressure of the lung and chest wall may be as high as 30 cm H_2O. Similarly, when $P_E$max is measured, which is at total lung capacity (TLC) the elastic recoil pressure of the lung and chest wall can be as high as 40 cm H_2O.

$P_I$max = Pressure generated by respiratory muscles + elastic recoil pressure of lung and chest wall.

$P_E$max = Pressure generated by respiratory muscles + elastic recoil pressure of lung and chest wall.

Clinical measurements of $P_I$max and $P_E$max do not consider elastic recoil pressure of lung and chest wall which ideally should be subtracted from the record of static maximum and expiratory pressure measured at the mouth to assess solely the pressure generated by the respiratory muscles.

The normal range of $P_I$max and $P_E$max is wide and therefore difficult in a particular individual to relate to the presence and degree of respiratory muscle weakness. Values less negative than the ones stated above are difficult to interpret. A low $P_I$max with a normal $P_E$max suggests diaphragmatic weakness. The predicted equations and lower limits of $P_I$max and $P_E$max are tabled below in Table 6.1.

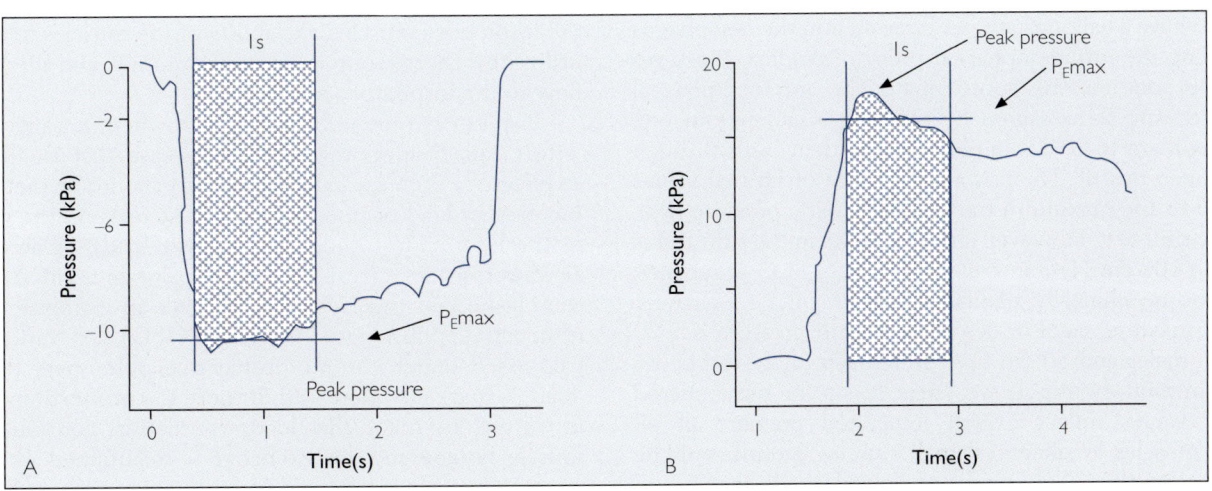

Fig 6.1: A. Pressure tracing from a subject performing a maximum inspiratory maneuver (P_{IMax}). A peak pressure is seen and the one second average is determined by calculating the shaded area. B. Typical pressure tracing from a subject performing a maximum expiratory maneuver (P_{Emax}). (Adapted from ATS/ERS: Statement on Respiratory Muscles Testing. *AM J Res Crit Care Med.* 2002; 166: 518–624).

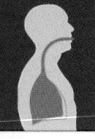

	P$_I$max cm H$_2$O		P$_E$max cm H$_2$O	
	Lower limit of normal	Predicted Mean	Lower limit of normal	Predicted Mean
Male	71	143 – (0.55 x age)	111	268 – (1.03 x age)
Female	39	104 – (0.51 x age)	88	170 – (0.53 x age)

Table 6.1:
Lower limits of normal and predicted equations for P$_I$max and P$_E$max

Source: Equations and lower of normal from Black LF, Hyatt RE: Maximal respiratory pressures: Normal values and relationship to age and sex. *Am Rev Respir Dis* 99: 696–702, 1969.

Transdiaphragmatic Pressure

If the previous test suggests inspiratory muscle weakness one needs to determine whether this is related to the diaphragm or not. The integrity and strength of the diaphragm is estimated by the measurement of the maximum transdiaphragmatic pressure (Pdia, max). The Pdia, max is the difference between the gastric pressure (which reflects intra-abdominal pressure) and the oesophageal pressure (which reflects intrapleural pressure) on a maximum inspiratory effort made from residual volume (RV). The gastric pressure is measured during this manoeuvre by a balloon catheter in the stomach and the oesophageal pressure by a balloon catheter in the oesophagus.

Sniff Pressure

A sniff is a short sharp inspiratory effort made from functional residual capacity (FRC) through one or both unoccluded nostrils with the mouth closed. It causes a rapid coordinated contraction of both the diaphragm and other inspiratory muscles. The transdiaphragmatic pressure measured during a short sniff reflects the strength of the diaphragm, and the pressure recorded by the balloon catheter in the oesophagus represents the overall combined pressure of the inspiratory muscles on the lungs. It is not necessary to have a balloon catheter inserted into the oesophagus for measuring the intraoesophageal pressure reading. Pressures measured in one nostril approximate the intraoesophageal pressure. Pressure is measured by wedging a catheter in one nostril using foam to hold it in place. The patient sniffs through the other open nostril. There is a wide range of normal values with regard to the maximum transdiaphragmatic pressure (Pdi, max) in the sniff test. However, if the Pdi, max in the sniff test is greater than 100 cm H$_2$O in males and 80 cm H$_2$O in females, there can be no clinically significant diaphragmatic weakness. Also, if the maximal nasal or oesophageal sniff pressure is > 70 cm H$_2$O in males and 60 cm H$_2$O in females, there can be no significant inspiratory muscle weakness. It is to be remembered that these values reflect overall integrated pressure of all inspiratory muscles. Weakness of small muscles' groups could be missed but again this would not be of clinical significance.

ELECTROPHYSIOLOGICAL TESTING

If the preceding test reveals weakness of the diaphragm, the next step would to be determine whether this is related to impaired transmission of nervous impulses in the nerve or neuromuscular junction or whether it is related to weakness of diaphragmatic muscle. Electrophysiological studies could determine this. However, in clinical practice this is indeed rarely necessary, because a good history, a careful clinical examination almost always will determine the correct issue. Electrophysiological testing is therefore of academic and research value to the clinician. The basic principles underlying this test will only be stated. The test involves measurement of Pdi following bilateral submaximal electric or magnetic stimulation of the phrenic nerves with simultaneous recording of the electromyography (EMG) of the diaphragm with either surface or oesophageal electrodes. If the phrenic nerve is stimulated, the diaphragm contracts and this contraction is termed as a *twitch*. For physiological and technical reasons, the transdiaphragmatic pressure developed in response to a single supramaximal phrenic nerve stimulation at 1 Hz called the twitch Pdi is measured. The result is independent of patient effort and also allows for the measurement of phrenic nerve conduction time. A prolonged conduction time points to phrenic nerve involvement.

THE CONCEPT OF LOAD VS. EFFORT, AND OF ENERGY DEMAND VS. ENERGY SUPPLY IN SPONTANEOUS BREATHING

In spontaneous breathing, the inspiratory muscles must generate force which is sufficient to overcome the elastic recoil of the lung and chest wall (elastic load), as also to overcome airway and tissue resistance (resistive load). To do so necessitates an intact neural discharge from the centre to the muscles of inspiration, normal neuromuscular transmission of nervous impulses, an intact chest wall and normal strength of the inspiratory muscles. We have therefore 'load' on the one hand and 'effort' of the neuromuscular apparatus to meet this load on the other. Ordinarily, not only does 'effort' meet the 'load' but there is sufficient reserve in the 'effort' that enables an upward adjustment of the minute ventilation in the event of an increased load, so as to maintain adequate gas exchange. 'Effort' as outlined above will be dependent on energy stores within the inspiratory muscles, the ability of the muscles to extract and utilize this energy source, oxygen saturation, and adequate blood flow to the inspiratory muscles.

Inspiratory muscle fatigue sets in when, for any reason, the 'effort' fails to meet the 'load'. In disease, this usually is due to an excessive increase in the 'load' that cannot be met by 'effort'. Increase in load occurs through an increase in 'the elastic load of the lung and/or chest wall (elastic load), or an increase in airways resistance (resistive load) or due to an increase in both the elastic and resistive load. To give an example, in chronic obstructive pulmonary disease (COPD) for various reasons (discussed under chronic obstructive pulmonary disease) the 'load' is markedly increased. If there is a proportionate increase in 'effort' to meet this load, ventilation continues without muscle fatigue and gas exchange is maintained. If however a stage comes when the 'load' is far too excessive and the 'effort' fails to meet it, gas exchange suffers and in due course of time muscle fatigue sets in. The question that needs an answer is the reason why effort of the inspiratory muscles cannot meet the excessive load. 'Effort' depends on energy supply to inspiratory muscles; it is when energy supplied to inspiratory muscles is less than the energy demand imposed by the excessive increase in load that effort fails to meet the load. One can therefore look upon load as being related to energy demand and 'effort' being related and dependent on energy supply. Inspiratory muscle fatigue occurs when energy demand exceeds energy supply.

There are certain respiratory parameters which enable us to assess increase in load which can be translated to mean an increase in energy demand. Load (i.e. energy demand) increases proportionately with the mean pressure developed by the inspiratory muscle per breath (P_I) expressed as a fraction of the maximum pressure developed by the respiratory muscles (P_I/P_{IMAX}); minute ventilation (V_E); V_T/T_I which is the mean inspiratory flow (Tidal volume/Inspiratory time); T_I/T_{TOT} i.e. inspiratory duty cycle (fraction of inspiration to total breathing cycle duration).

The product of T_I/T_{TOT} and the mean diaphragmatic pressure expressed as a fraction of maximal (Pdi/Pdimax) is defined as the 'tension-time index' (TTI_{di}) which is related to the endurance time (i.e. the time that the diaphragm can meet the load imposed on it). Whenever TTIdi is less than 0.15–0.18, the load can be sustained for a limited time i.e. the endurance time. The TTIdi is inversely related to the endurance time. The concept underlying tension time index is applicable not only to the diaphragm but to all inspiratory muscles, so that

$$TTI = P_I/P_{IMAX} \times T_I/T_{TOT}$$

Obviously, an increase in either P_I/P_{IMAX} or T_I/T_{TOT} will increase the TTI value which means an increase in load or an increase in energy demand.

To summarize, spontaneous breathing without respiratory muscle fatigue is possible when 'effort' required by the inspiratory muscles is adequate (in fact more than adequate) to meet the 'load' imposed on them. 'Effort' is related to energy supply and load dictates energy demand. Therefore when effort is inadequate for the load imposed (as when there is an excessive increase in load), or energy supply to inspiratory muscles does not meet their energy demands, both inadequate gas exchange and muscle fatigue set in. Parameters to assess increased load (whether increase in elastic load or resistive load) have been mentioned above. The concept of tension time index in relation to muscle fatigue is of considerable interest.

MUSCLE FATIGUE

'Fatigue is defined as the loss of capacity to develop force and/or velocity in response to a load that is reversible by rest'. Muscle fatigue should be distinguished from weakness in which the loss of capacity to develop force in response to a load is not reversed by rest. Where is the site of muscle fatigue located? Voluntary muscle contraction depends on a chain of events starting from the brain,'travelling through nerves, nerve endings, neuromuscular junctions, to the final contractile end organ—the muscle. Researchers in this field have classified fatigue into central fatigue, peripheral high-frequency fatigue and peripheral low-frequency fatigue.

Central Fatigue

Central muscle fatigue is said to exist when maximum voluntary contraction generates less force than that induced by maximal

electrical stimulation. If maximal electrical stimulation given during maximal voluntary contraction potentiates the force and strength of the muscle contraction, an element of central fatigue exists. A number of experiments suggest that when there is excessive load (increased energy demands) there occurs a form of central diaphragmatic fatigue. A significant part of the reduction of force during diaphragmatic contraction at such times is related to the failure of the central nervous system to fully activate the diaphragm. This could be related to a decrease in the central drive, decrease in motor units recruited by the central drive, or decrease in discharge rates of the motor units or a combination of the above factors. A decrease in discharge rate may well be an adaptive mechanism to help preserve for a longer time the strength of the diaphragmatic muscle.

Peripheral Fatigue

Peripheral fatigue exists when the force of muscle contraction falls in response to direct electrical stimulation. The fault may lie at the neuromuscular junction, the muscle surface membrane or may result from impaired excitation-contraction coupling or may be related to a defect within the muscle itself—perhaps an alteration in the contractile protein for unclear reasons.

Peripheral fatigue can be high-frequency fatigue which is a lowered force of contraction in response to high-frequency stimulation (50–100 Hz) and low-frequency fatigue which is characterized by reduction in force of contraction at low-frequency stimulation (1–20 Hz). The force of contraction in the latter situation is however not affected or reduced by high-frequency stimulation.

The site of high-frequency fatigue may be located pre-synaptically or post-synaptically. The block in transmission of the nerve impulses may again be an adaptive mechanism to prevent the muscle from using up all its stores of adenosine triphosphate (ATP).

The mechanism of low-frequency fatigue is not known. It is probably related either to the low availability of calcium, to lowered concentration of calcium in the muscle fibres or perhaps a lessened sensitivity of muscle fibres to calcium.

Whereas high-frequency fatigue resolves quickly when the work load is sharply reduced, low-frequency fatigue takes long to recover.

One must conclude by mentioning that respiratory muscle fatigue which has clinical relevance can be generally determined at the bedside by a careful clinical examination. The clinical features of respiratory muscle fatigue at the bedside have been detailed later in more than one section of the book. Admittedly the measurements required to objectively assess muscle fatigue are by and large not possible in critically ill patients where fatigue is most likely to arise or be actively present. Therefore the relevance of these measurements in respiratory medicine at this point in time is unfortunately poor.

INFLAMMATORY CHANGES IN RESPIRATORY MUSCLES

Strenuous diaphragmatic contraction over long periods of time against an increased 'load' as in COPD can excite an inflammatory reaction within the diaphragmatic muscle. The inflammation is related to cytokines produced within the

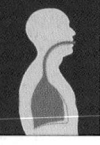

diaphragm itself due to excessive diaphragmatic activity. There results an ultrastructural injury to the diaphragmatic muscle. The exact mechanism of injury is not known. Besides cytokines induction, an influx of inflammatory cells, upregulation of adhesin molecules and formation of reactive oxygen radicals may all play a role.

ADAPTIVE CHANGES IN RESPIRATORY MUSCLES TO 'LOAD'

Compensatory adaptive changes occur in respiratory muscles when they are required to cope with increasing 'load' over long periods of time as for example in COPD. The main adaptation observed is a change in the type of muscle fibre of the respiratory muscles. Muscles fibres are classified either as Type I or Type II depending on the myosin heavy chain component of the myosin molecule. Myosin heavy chains exist in various isoforms. In increasing order of maximum shortening velocity there is myosin heavy chain (MHC) I, MHC II A and MHC II B; the MHC II B fibres show both maximum speed and maximum shortening during contraction. The diaphragm in healthy individuals consists of 50% Type I fibres, 25% II A and 25% II B fibres. The Type I fibres have a slower speed of contraction and are fatigue-resistant in comparison to Type II fibres. In COPD there is a transformation of Type II fibres into Type I fatigue-resistant fibres. This increases resistance to fatigue which is a decided advantage considering the increased load the respiratory muscles need to cope with. However, the transformation of Type II to Type I fibres also reduces the diaphragm's contractile strength and force-generating capacity.

Another adaptation of the respiratory muscles in COPD which is observed in animal models of COPD, and perhaps also occurs in COPD in humans, is a decrease in the number and length of sarcomeres. This adaptation results in a leftward shift of the length-tension curve, so that the muscle adapts to the shorter operating length caused by over-inflation of the lungs, as also to an increase in the AP diameter of the chest with more horizontally placed ribs. To an extent, this reduces the mechanical disadvantage of the diaphragm and the inspiratory muscles of the chest caused by hyper-inflated lungs.

The adaptation of respiratory muscles to increased load has as its counterpart a different form of adaptation when they are rendered inactive, as for example during prolonged mechanical ventilation. Inactivity and the unloading of work normally performed by the diaphragm can lead to atrophy of the diaphragmatic muscle and a reduction of its force-generating capacity. This ventilator-induced diaphragmatic dysfunction (VIDD) becomes apparent when the patient is weaned off ventilator support. VIDD is one reason for difficulty in weaning of some patients who have been on prolonged ventilator support. The reasons for diaphragmatic dysfunction following inactivity are unclear. Dysfunction could be partly related to muscle atrophy, structural injury and perhaps to muscle fibre remodelling.

SUGGESTED READING

American Thoracic Society/European Respiratory Society Task Force. Statement on Respiratory Muscle Testing. *Am J Respir Crit Care Med.* 2002; 166:518–624.

Black LF, Hyatt RE. Maximal static respiratory pressure in generalized neuromuscular disease. *Am Rev Respir Dis.* 1971; 103:641.

Black LF, Hyatt RE. Equations and lower of normal from: Maximal respiratory pressures: Normal values and relationship to age and sex. *Am Rev Respir Dis.* 1969; 99:696–702.

Laghi F, Tobin M. Disorders of respiratory muscles. *Am J Respir Crit Care Med.* 2003; 168:10-48.

Oro Levi M. Structure and function of the respiratory muscles in patients with COPD: impairment of adaptation?. *Eur Respir J.* 2003; 22:Suppl.46, 41s–51s.

Vincken GH, Cosio MG. Maximal static respiratory pressure in adults: normal values and their relationship to determines of respiratory function. *Bull Eur Physiopathol Respir.* 1987; 23:435.

CHAPTER **7**

Pulmonary Function Testing

Pulmonary function tests characterize respiratory physiology and therefore enable a physician to determine the nature of disturbance in lung function in a patient with respiratory complaints or respiratory disease. They provide an objective, quantitative assessment of altered lung physiology allowing a correlation with symptoms, clinical examination and radiography of the chest. The quantitative objective assessment of lung function done at periodic intervals helps to assess disease severity and the progress of disease in a given patient. This is particularly important when respiratory symptoms do not reflect disease severity or progression.

It must however be remembered that normal lung functions do not exclude lung disease. In fact, normal lung function can be associated with a serious lung pathology.

Disturbance in lung function often falls into specific patterns and recognition of these patterns by a clinician helps in the overall assessment of the patient. By themselves lung function tests do not provide a specific diagnosis because specific patterns of disturbance in lung function are common to a number of diseases and there is often an overlap between the two basic patterns arising from disturbed lung function. It is the triad of history cum clinical examination, radiography of the chest and lung function tests taken together and correlated that provides a specific diagnosis in most respiratory diseases.

OBJECTIVES OF PULMONARY FUNCTION TESTS

1. To assess objectively and quantitatively the nature and degree of altered physiology in a patient with respiratory disease.
2. To assess the effect of therapy on deranged lung function.
3. To keep a longitudinal follow-up of patients with respiratory disease and help in the assessment of the natural history of the respiratory disease in a given patient.
4. To allow surveillance in patients exposed to environmental insults, in patients who have received cytotoxic drugs or who have received radiotherapy to the lungs, mediastinum or chest wall.
5. To evaluate the effect of neuromuscular or cardiovascular disease on the respiratory system.
6. To identify presymptomatic lung disease in smokers.

The National Health and Nutrition Examination Survey and Lung Health Study confirmed through pulmonary function tests (PFTs) the presence of abnormal lung function in asymptomatic smokers. This study also provided data to show that the presence of abnormal PFT in this group prompted smokers to seek medical advice and attempt stopping to smoke. Based on the above findings, the study recommended office-based spirometry for current smokers 45 years of age and for any smoker with respiratory symptoms.

Spirometry

Spirometry allows basic lung function tests which can be performed in the office. Spirometry measures the volume of air exhaled or inhaled by a subject as a function of time, so that both volume and flow rates are available.

A basic and useful spirometry test is the measurement of a single forced expiration. This requires the subject to forcefully expel air from the point of maximum inspiration (i.e. total lung capacity, TLC) as hard and as completely as possible—i.e. to the point of maximal expiration (residual volume, RV). The total volume exhaled is termed the forced vital capacity (FVC) and the volume exhaled in the first second is termed the forced expiratory volume in the first second (FEV_1). Normally, the FEV_1 is 80% of the FVC i.e. FEV_1/FVC = 80%. The FVC and FEV_1/FVC are the most important values obtained from the forced expiration manoeuvre. When during the forced expiratory manoeuvre, expelled volume is charted against time, FEV_1 is easily obtained. A number of other functional measurements are provided if during the forced expiratory manoeuvre, volume expelled is charted against the flow rate. Table 7.1 lists the measurements possible when volume is charted against time and against the flow rate. Figure 7.1a shows expiratory volume plotted against time and Figure 7.1b is flow plotted against the volume.

Significant information can be derived from measurements of FVC and FEV_1. In pulmonary disease, two patterns are generally distinguished. In obstructive lung disease the FEV_1 is reduced giving a low FEV_1/FVC%. In restrictive lung disease as for example in pulmonary fibrosis both FVC and FEV_1 are reduced but the FEV_1/FVC% remains normal or is even increased. However, many respiratory diseases may be associated with mixed restrictive and obstructive patterns.

Though most laboratories measure VC through a forced expiratory manoeuvre, there are some who prefer to measure VC following a relaxed or slow expiration manoeuvre. This is because the VC determined by forced expiration or manoeuvre may result in increased airways resistance compared to airway pressures produced during a relaxed expiratory manoeuvre. The increased airways resistance associated with the forced expiratory manoeuvre can lead to decreased flows in some patients. This has prompted both the American Thoracic Society (ATS) and the European Respiratory Society (ERS) to recommend the use of a slow or relaxed VC relative to the FEV_1 to establish the diagnosis of obstructive airways disease. However, relaxed or slow VC measurements are often greater

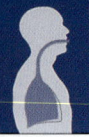

Table 7.1: Commonly used spirometry parameters		
Reported value	**Description**	**Interpretation**
VC	Vital capacity	Generally preserved in obstruction, but reduced in restriction
FVC	Forced vital capacity	Reduction in FVC is suggestive of restrictive lung disease or well marked airways obstruction, or a mixed pattern. Used to grade severity of restriction
FEV_1	Forced expiratory volume in one second	Reduced in restrictive as well as obstructive lung disease. Used to grade severity of obstruction
FEV_1/FVC	Ratio of FEV_1/FVC	Reduction is indicative of airways obstruction
$FEF_{25/75}$	Mean expiratory flow rate in the middle of half of FVC (mid expiratory flow rate)	Sensitive but non-specific indicator of small airways obstruction
PEF	Peak expiratory flow	Worsening correlate with severity of asthma; PEF is also effort dependent
MVV	Maximum voluntary ventilation	Disproportionate reduction relative to FEV_1 may indicate upper airways obstruction, muscle weakness or poor effort

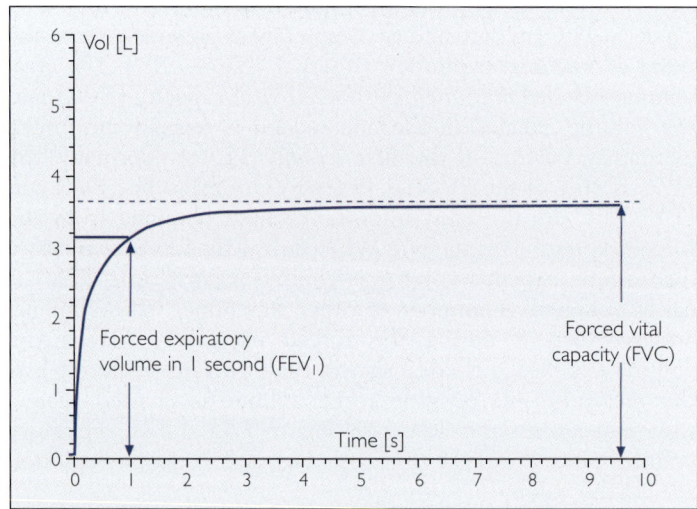

Fig 7.1a: Normal forced expiratory spirogram plotted as exhaled volume versus time. The forced expiratory volume at 1 sec (FEV_1) and forced vital capacity (FVC) are indicated by arrows. In above graph FVC = 3.6L, FEV_1 = 3.1 and FEV_1/FVC ratio = 86.1%.

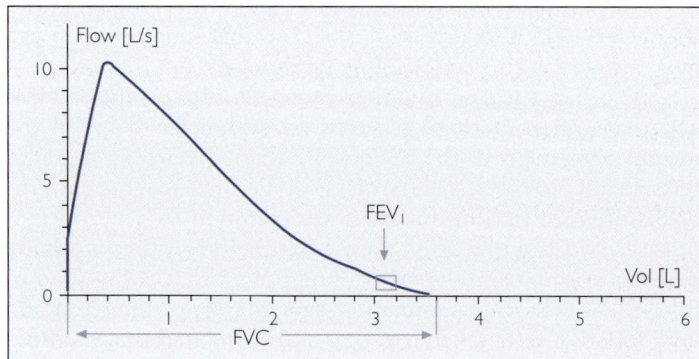

Fig 7.1b: Normal expiratory flow-volume curve. The same forced expiratory time volume maneuver shown in 7.1a is plotted as a flow volume curve. The airflow rate reaches a peak early in the exhalation, then decreases progressively until airflow ceases at residual volume.

than FVC measurements, so that FEV_1/VC may in this method overestimate the degree of airways obstruction.

In addition to FVC and FEV_1, a graphic representation of flow rate against forced expired volume gives expiratory flow rates between 25–75% of exhaled VC—the mid-expiratory flow rate. There are clinicians who believe that a reduction in mid-expiratory flow rate is indicative of small airways obstruction. The mid-expiratory flow rates show significant variability both within and between individuals. By and large they are not more sensitive in the detection of airflow limitation compared to the FEV_1/FVC ratio.

The peak expiratory flow rate is another measurement from a flow volume graph. The peak flow shows effort to effort variability even in the same individual. A peak flow

measurement can also be measured by a handheld peak flow meter, a device often used by asthmatic patients at home to assess the degree of airways obstruction.

BRONCHODILATOR RESPONSE

Spirometry is often done before and after the administration of an inhaled aerosolized bronchodilator like salbutmol. At times, particularly in patients with chronic obstructive pulmonary disease (COPD), bronchodilator response to ipratropium bromide or tiotropium is observed. For a bronchodilator response to be positive there should be an increase in either FEV_1 or FVC of 12% of the baseline value and an increase in the baseline value of FVC or FEV_1 > 200 ml. A change in the FEV_1 > 200 ml more closely relates to the reversibility of airways obstruction. At times a patient may experience symptomatic relief with bronchodilators without the expected change in FVC and FEV_1. This must not be dismissed; a reduction in

FRC and RV may be responsible for symptomatic relief in the absence of a change in FVC and FEV_1. Also, bronchodilator response can vary over time, a number of individuals (30–50%) changing over from positivity to negativity or vice versa.

A positive bronchodilator response as in asthma is an obvious indication for bronchodilator therapy. A negative response does not necessarily mean that sustained use of a bronchodilator will be of no benefit. This is with particular reference to COPD patients. Finally, in some patients the routine spirometry is normal yet there is significant increase in FVC and FEV_1 after use of an aerosolized bronchodilator, pointing to occult airflow limitation.

Bronchoprovocation Test

Spirometry performed before and after a bronchoprovocation challenge can help to identify bronchial hyperreactivity. Metacholine and histamine are generally used as bronchoprovocative agents. A positive bronchoprovocation test is characterized by a 15–20% fall in FEV_1 after aerosolized inhalation of either one of these agents. Bronchoprovocation test is chiefly used to identify patients with occult asthma who have symptoms of cough or complain of breathlessness and yet have normal spirometry. Bronchoprovocation tests can be positive in patients with allergic rhinitis, COPD and following viral upper respiratory tract infection. Patients with nasal allergy with no asthma may also show positive bronchoprovocation tests.

Flow Volume Loop

Current lung function machines have microprocessors which allow a flow volume loop incorporating both inspiration followed by a forced expiration recording both FVC and flow rates. Flow rates at 50% and 75% of the exhaled volumes are processed and reported. Flow rates at 75% of exhaled volumes mean really flow rates at remaining 25% of VC. Normal

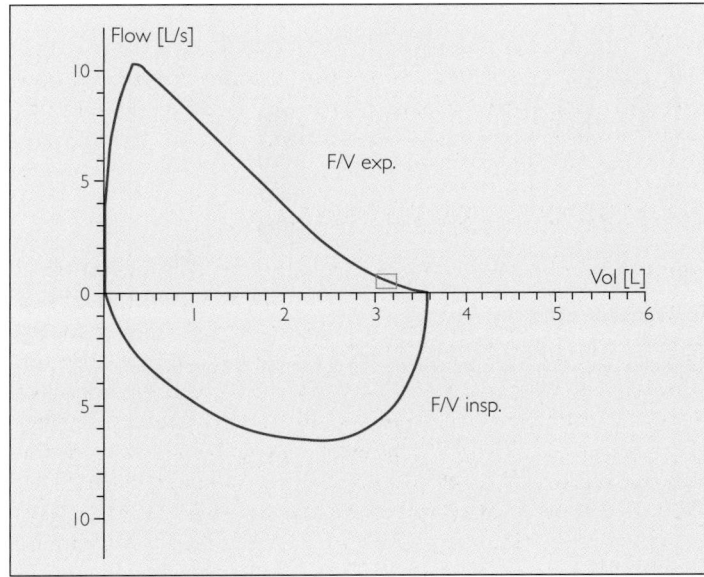

Fig 7.2a: Normal flow volume loop.

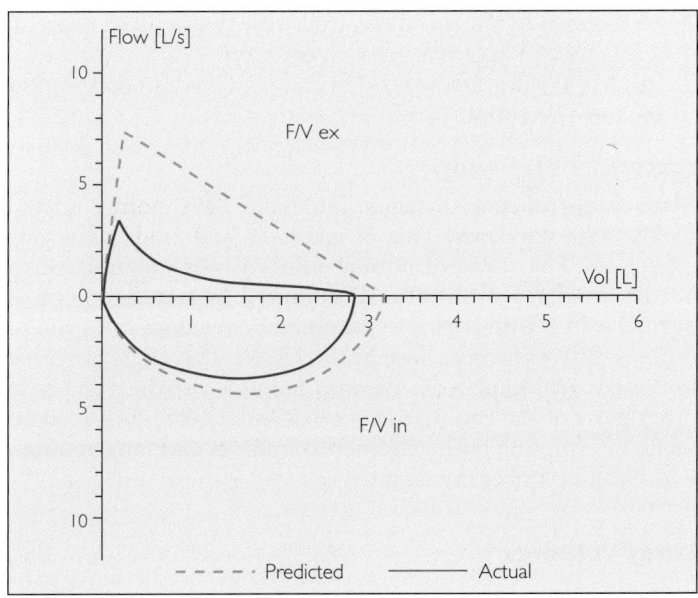

Fig 7.2b: Obstructive flow volume loop.

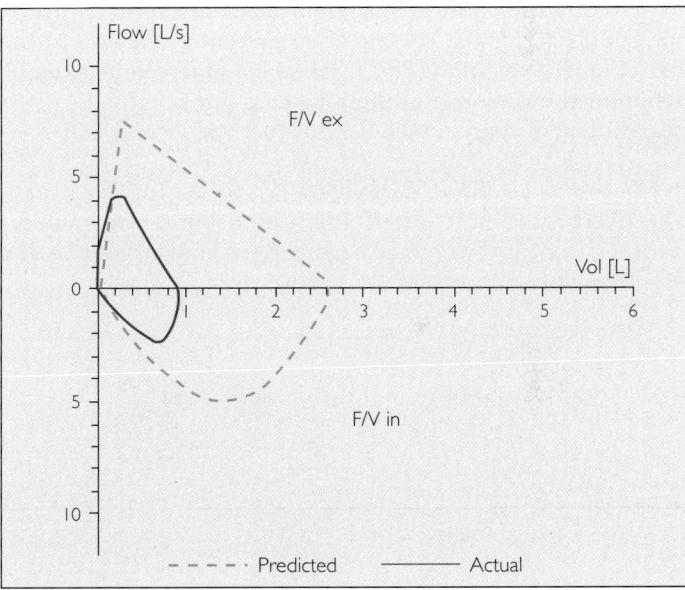

Fig 7.2c: Restrictive flow volume loop.

flow volume loop and flow volume loops in obstructive and restrictive lung disease are illustrated in Figure 7.2.

Maximum Voluntary Ventilation

Maximum Voluntary Ventilation (MVV) is measured through a manoeuvre that requires maximal inspiratory and expiratory effort over 12 to 15 seconds. This is extrapolated to one minute and is measured in litres. The MVV in any individual should be 30 to 40 times the baseline FEV_1. The MVV can be reduced in patients with COPD, upper airways obstruction, neuromuscular disease causing muscle weakness and when there is poor performance of the test. The MVV is a non-specific test but offers two valuable inferences—

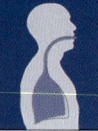

1. A reduced MVV correlates well with the reduced exercise capacity and breathlessness on exertion
2. An MVV value below 40–45 L/min is a contraindication for pneumonectomy.

REFERENCE STANDARDS

Many lung function machines in India have norms related to Western standards. This is incorrect and leads to wrong inferences. The range of normal values is not only related to height, gender, age but also to ethnicity. In fact the range of normal values with regard to spirometeric readings in Southern India is different from those in the North. The range observed in the city of Mumbai (in Western India) is not the same as in other parts of the country. This needs to be taken into account when interpreting both spirometric readings and lung volumes in different parts of the country.

Lung Volumes

Spirometry allows volume measurement of inhaled and exhaled air. It cannot determine the total amount of air in the lung (which is the sum of VC and RV); nor can spirometry give the volume of air left in the lung after maximal expiration (RV), nor can it provide the volume of air present in the lung at the end of quiet expiration (FRC). The static lung volumes can be determined by any one of the following three methods—inert gas dilution, nitrogen washout, body plethysmography.

INERT GAS DILUTION TECHNIQUE

The inert gas most often used is helium. The subject breathes from a spirometer containing a known volume and concentration of helium (10–15%). The breathing commences at the point of end-tidal expiration. Carbon dioxide is absorbed and oxygen is added during equilibration to make up for the oxygen consumed. The subject continues to breathe until a steady lower helium concentration is reached. The helium concentration in the spirometer and the lung are now the same. The unknown lung volume (FRC) which was added to the circuit (when the valve was turned allowing the patient to start breathing from the circuit) is calculated from the dilution of the initial helium concentration. FRC is thus calculated by direct measurement (Figure 7.3). TLC is determined as FRC plus inspiratory capacity, and RV as TLC–FRC.

Helium dilution technique assumes even distribution of helium throughout the lung. But this may not happen in patients with COPD and in patients with non-communicating air spaces or cavities. In such patients the FRC may be underestimated.

$$V_1 C_1 = C_2 (V_1 + V_2)$$
V_1 = volume of spirometer
C_1 = original concentration of helium
V_2 = FRC
C_2 = concentration of helium evenly distributed in the spirometer and lung

NITROGEN WASH-OUT TEST

The lung normally contains 80% nitrogen. Lung volumes are determined by washing out all nitrogen from the lungs. The subject is made to breathe 100% oxygen and the exhaled gas is collected by means of a one-way valve. The subject continues to breathe 100% oxygen till all the nitrogen from the lung is washed, the concentration of nitrogen reaching a fixed target value. The to-

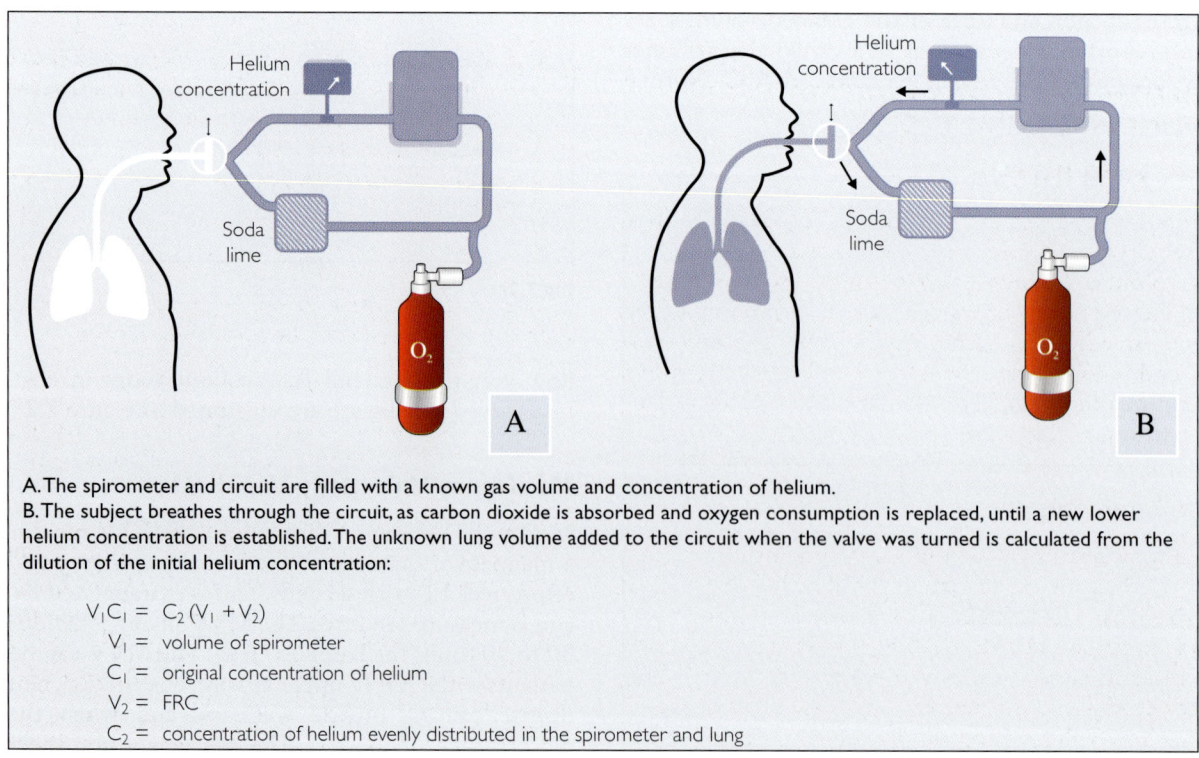

A. The spirometer and circuit are filled with a known gas volume and concentration of helium.
B. The subject breathes through the circuit, as carbon dioxide is absorbed and oxygen consumption is replaced, until a new lower helium concentration is established. The unknown lung volume added to the circuit when the valve was turned is calculated from the dilution of the initial helium concentration:

$$V_1 C_1 = C_2 (V_1 + V_2)$$
V_1 = volume of spirometer
C_1 = original concentration of helium
V_2 = FRC
C_2 = concentration of helium evenly distributed in the spirometer and lung

Fig 7.3: Lung volume measurement by helium dilution.

tal collected expired nitrogen is then analysed and knowledge of the original concentration is used to determine lung volume. This test has the same drawback as the helium dilution technique and is likely to underestimate FRC in patients with COPD. Nitrogen wash-out may need to be prolonged for a longer time—as long as 15 to 20 minutes. The normal wash-out time is 3 to 5 minutes.

BODY PLETHYSMOGRAPHY

Plethysmographic measurement of lung volumes is based on Boyle's law which states that at constant temperatures the product of pressure and volume of a gas remains constant $P_1V_1 = P_2V_2$.

Plethysmography measures mouth pressure changes during compression and rarefraction of intrathoracic air by a subject enclosed in a sealed box. This enables measurement of all static lung volumes. The patient in the box makes an inspiratory effort from end-tidal volume. If the pressure in the box before and after the inspiratory effort are P_1 and P_2 respectively and V_1 the volume of the box before inspiratory effort then $P_1V_1 = P_2 (V_1 - \Delta V)$ where ΔV is the change in the volume of the box. The value of ΔV is then obtained. Now Boyle's law is applied to the gas in the lung

$$P_3V_2 = P_4 (V_2 + \Delta V)$$

where P_3 is the mouth pressure measured before the inspiratory effort, P_4 is the mouth pressure after inspiratory effort and V_2 is the FRC (Figure 7.4).

Repeated measurements can be made quite easily unlike with the inert gas technique which requires recalibration before repeating the test. Plethysmographic measurements take all intrathoracic air into account, including air in bullae, in large air spaces and in non-communicating air spaces. Lung volumes are therefore far more accurate, particularly in patients with emphysema.

LUNG VOLUME CHANGES IN OBSTRUCTIVE AND RESTRICTIVE LUNG DISEASE

Obstructive Lung Disease

Airflow limitation and airflow obstruction during expiration causes early airway closure, so that expiration ceases at higher lung volumes. Loss of elastic recoil in emphysema is a contributing factor to early airway closure in expiration so that these patients breathe at a higher FRC. There is an increase in RV, FRC and a normal to high TLC. The RV increases to a greater extent than the TLC. The VC is lowered with increasing airways obstruction.

Restrictive Lung Disease

Parenchymal lung diseases which lower compliance rendering the lung more stiff cause a restrictive ventilatory pattern. This is characterized by a low TLC with a parallel reduction in FRC and RV. In some patients a fall in the RV in noted early because increase in elastic recoil (a feature of restrictive lung disease) leads to delayed closure of the small airways. Figure 7.5 illustrates flow volume loop in obstructive, restrictive and mixed patterns.

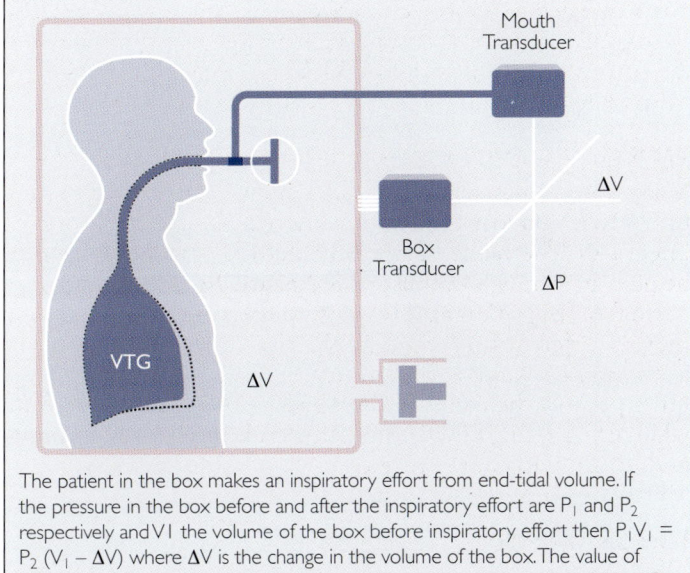

The patient in the box makes an inspiratory effort from end-tidal volume. If the pressure in the box before and after the inspiratory effort are P_1 and P_2 respectively and VI the volume of the box before inspiratory effort then $P_1V_1 = P_2 (V_1 - \Delta V)$ where ΔV is the change in the volume of the box. The value of ΔV is then obtained. Now Boyle's law is applied to the gas in the lung $P_3V_2 = P_4 (V_2 + \Delta V)$
Where P_3 is the mouth pressure measured before the inspiratory effort, P_4 is the mouth pressure after inspiratory effort and V_2 is the FRC.

Fig 7.4: Lung volume measurement by body plethysmography.

Diffusing Capacity

The transfer of carbon monoxide (CO) is limited solely by diffusion. Hence it is the gas ideally suited for measuring the diffusing capacity of the lungs. The equation for diffusion of CO across the alveolar capillary membrane can be written thus

$$V_{CO} = D_L \times (P_1 - P_2)$$

where V_{CO} is the gas transferred, D_L is the diffusion capacity of the lung which includes the area, thickness and diffusing properties of the alveolar capillary sheet and of the gas concerned, and where P_1 and P_2 are pressures of alveolar gas and capillary blood respectively. The diffusion capacity of the lung for CO is

$$D_L = V_{CO}/P_1 - P_2$$

However, the partial pressure of CO in capillary blood is extremely small and can be neglected. Hence,

$$D_L = V_{CO}/P_{ACO}$$

Thus the diffusion capacity of the lung for carbon monoxide is the volume of carbon monoxide transferred in ml per minute per mm Hg of alveolar partial pressure. The normal value of the diffusion capacity of CO at rest is about 25 ml/minute/mm Hg. This increases to three times the resting volume following exercise because of recruitment of blood-filled capillaries.

The usual method to measure the diffusing capacity of the lung is the single breath method. The subject exhales to RV and then takes a maximal inhalation (up to VC) of the test gas containing 0.3% CO and a diluent inert gas, 10% helium. The rate of disappearance of CO during 10-second breath hold is estimated by an infra-red analyser which measures the inspired

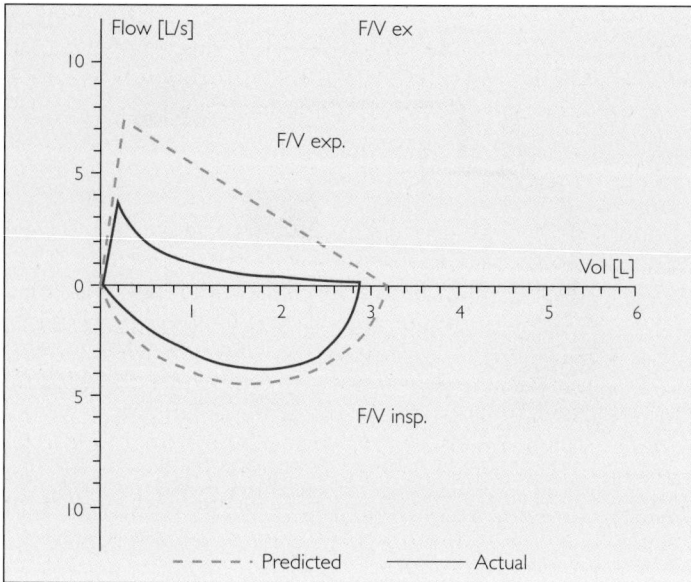

Fig 7.5a: Obstructive flow volume loop.

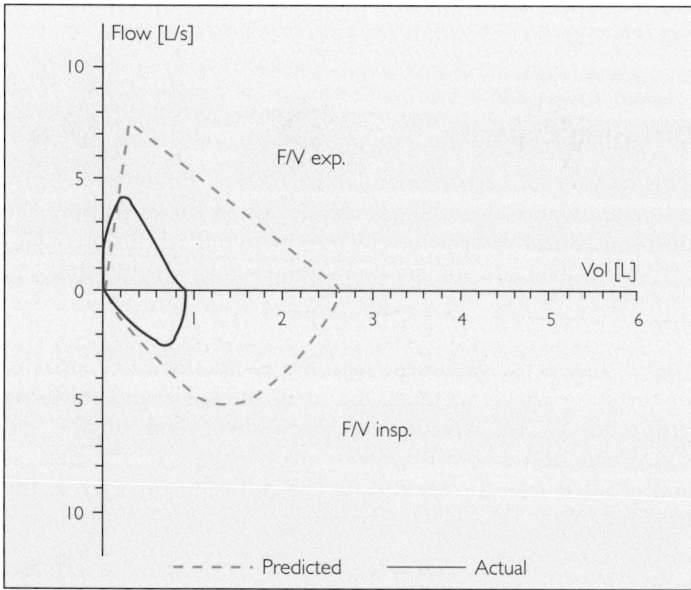

Fig 7.5b: Restrictive flow volume loop.

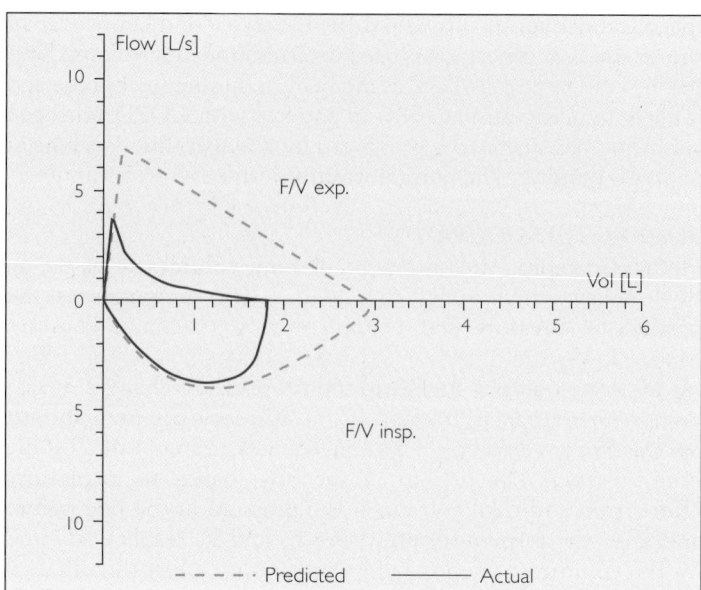

Fig 7.5c: Restrictive + Obstructive flow volume loop.

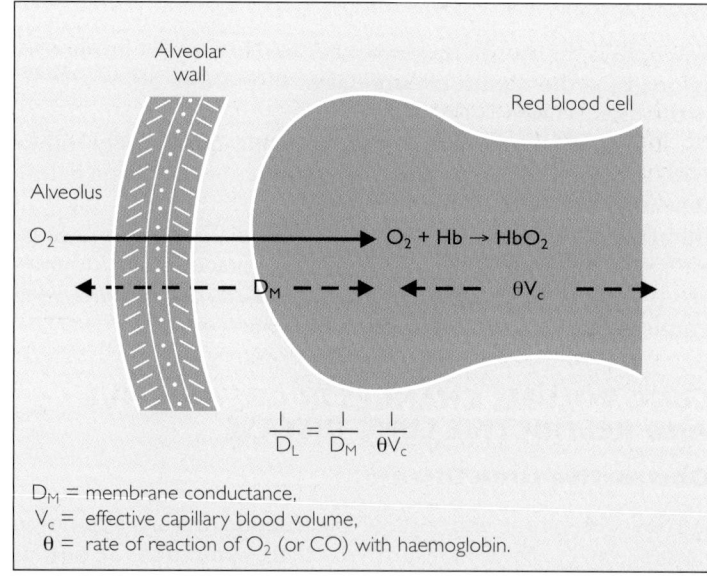

Fig 7.6: The diffusion capacity of the lung (D_L) is made up of two components, that due to diffusion process itself and that attributable to the time taken for O_2 (or CO) to react with haemoglobin.

D_M = membrane conductance,
V_c = effective capillary blood volume,
θ = rate of reaction of O_2 (or CO) with haemoglobin.

$$\frac{1}{D_L} = \frac{1}{D_M} \frac{1}{\theta V_c}$$

and expired concentration of CO. Allowance is made for the fact that concentration of CO is not constant during the breath-holding period.

A problem with the diffusing capacity measurement is that for various technical reasons the calculated values vary significantly, the published predicted values varying by 20% or more. It is therefore better for each laboratory to standardize its own values with the equipment it uses.

It is important to remember that diffusion is not just a measure of the thickness of the alveolar capillary membrane. A dominant factor is the capillary blood volume which influences the surface area available for gas exchange as also the haemoglobin available to accept the CO. Therefore, exercise, left to right shunts within the heart, as also any hyperdynamic

circulatory state that leads to an increased volume of blood in the capillaries of the lung wall increase the diffusing capacity. Extravasated blood as in pulmonary hematomas and intra-alveolar haemorrhage will also cause an increase in the diffusion capacity readings (Figure 7.6).

A fall in diffusing capacity is most consistently noted in patients with interstitial lung disease (particularly interstitial lung fibrosis) and in parenchymal lung disease.

It is however rare even in well-marked interstitial lung disease for the alveolar capillary wall to be so markedly thickened as to be solely responsible for a fall in diffusion capacity. Almost always, the main cause of a fall in CO diffusion is the ventilation perfusion inequality which is always present in patients with severe interstitial lung disease. The diffusion capacity is also reduced in emphysema, again because of ventilation perfusion inequalities which give rise to a considerable increase in dead space.

The diffusing capacity of the lung for CO as mentioned earlier is not just dependent on the area and thickness of the alveolar capillary membrane but is also affected by the distribution of diffusion properties, alveolar volume and volume of capillary blood. The term transfer factor is sometimes used to emphasize that the measurement is not solely related to the diffusing properties of the lung. Many laboratories also report the diffusing capacity as a ratio to the alveolar volume D_L/V_A, termed the transfer coefficient (KCO). This is to imply that a loss of lung volume for whatever reason is associated with a fall in the diffusing capacity. In early interstitial lung disease, the D_L is reduced more than the D_L/V_A which may even fall in the normal range. As the disease progresses both D_L and D_L/V_A are reduced. In emphysema, both D_L and D_L/V_A are low because of loss of capillary surface area. The D_L and D_L/V_A are also low in patients with pulmonary vasculitis, in recurrent pulmonary embolism and pulmonary hypertension.

LUNG COMPLIANCE

Lung compliance is the volume change per unit change of pressure. In the normal range of respiration (–5 to – 10 cm H_2O) the lung is remarkably compliant. The normal compliance is 200 ml per cm H_2O. At high expanding pressure, the compliance is reduced. In disease, low compliance is typically met with in interstitial lung disease, in particular interstitial pulmonary fibrosis. It is also reduced in diffuse bilateral inflammatory disease, in pulmonary oedema and in the adult respiratory distress syndrome. Lung compliance is increased in emphysema.

Measurement of compliance is technically difficult. A comparatively easy method of measuring compliance is to have a subject breathe out about 500 ml at a time from total lung capacity into a spirometer and to measure the oesophageal pressure through a balloon catheter within the oesophagus. The glottis should be open and the lung allowed to stabilize for a few seconds before a pressure reading is taken. After every 500 ml of air expired, oesophageal pressure readings are taken and a pressure volume curve plotted. This curve represents the compliance of the lung (Figure 7.7). It is noted from the curve that the lung compliance will vary depending on what lung volume is used. Compliance by convention is reported in relation to the slope over a litre above FRC measured during deflation.

AIRWAY RESISTANCE

Airway resistance is the pressure difference between the alveoli and the mouth per unit of airflow. It is best measured in a body plethysmograph. Before inspiration the box pressure is atmospheric. At inspiration the increase in alveolar volume by ΔV is associated with a fall in alveolar pressure. The increased ΔV in the volume of the alveolar gas compresses the air in the body box, and from this change in pressure ΔV can be calculated. If lung volume is known, ΔV can be converted into alveolar pressure using Boyle's law. Flow is simultaneously measured so that airways resistance is obtained. The same measurement can be made during expiration (Figure 7.8).

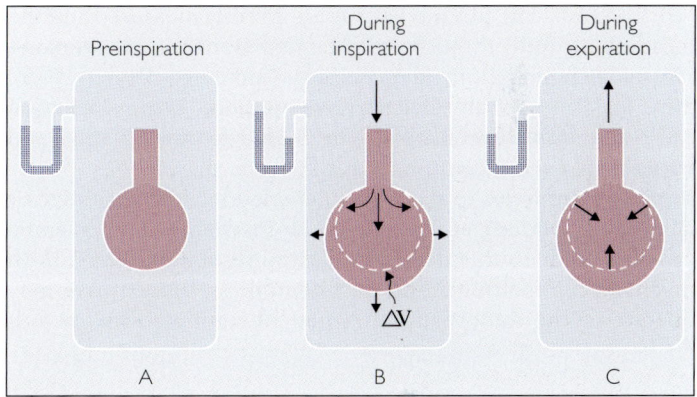

Fig 7.8: Measurement of airways resistance with the body plethysmograph. During inspiration, the lung is expanded, and the box pressure rises. From this, alveolar pressure can be calculated. The difference between alveolar and mouth pressure, divided by flow give airway resistance. (Adapted from *Respiratory Physiology The Essentials* by John B. West, seventh edition, Lippincott Williams and Wilkins).

Normal airway resistance is 2.5 cm $H_2O/L/s$. Factors influencing airways obstruction have been briefly discussed in the chapter 'Mechanics of Ventilation'.

CLOSING VOLUME

Early disease of small airways as for example in smokers can be brought out by using the single-breath nitrogen wash-out test. This test consists of the subject taking a full inspiratory (up to VC) breath of 100% oxygen. During the subsequent exhalation, the nitrogen concentration is measured at the lips through a nitrogen meter. Four phases are observed—

Phase I. In this phase only dead space air is exhaled
Phase II. This phase consists of a mixture of dead space gas and alveolar gas
Phase III. This phase consists of pure alveolar gas
Phase IV. Towards the end of expiration there is a sudden increase in nitrogen concentration.

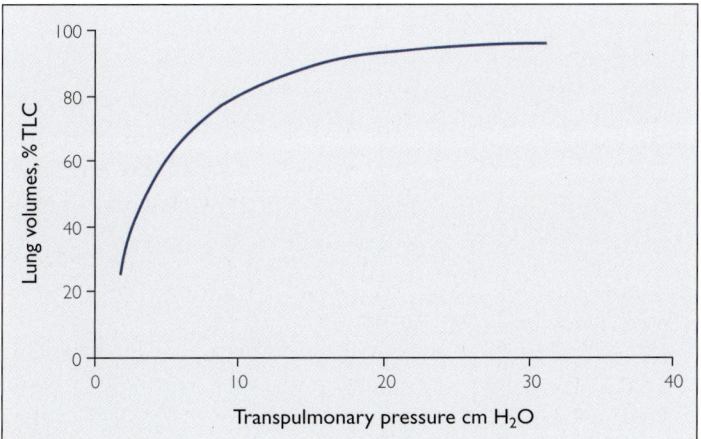

Fig 7.7: Pressure-volume curve of the lung during inspiration.

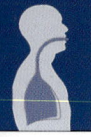

This signals the closure of small airways at the base of the lung. The abrupt increase in nitrogen concentration is due to emptying of the alveoli air at the lung apex which has a high nitrogen concentration. The reason for the higher concentration of nitrogen at the apex is because during maximum inspiration, the apex expands less (compared for example with mid-zones and bases) and is therefore less diluted with oxygen. The volume at which the small airways begin to close is the closing volume and is read off the nitrogen wash-out tracing. In a young healthy adult the closing volume is about 10% of the VC. The closing volume increases with age so that by the age of 70 years the closing volume in as high as 40% of VC. Disease of the small airways in cigarette smokers leads to earlier closure of the small airways with an increase in closing volume. Changes in closing volume may precede changes in the FVC, FEV_1 and FEV_1/FVC ratio in patients with early small airways disease (Figure 7.9).

ARTERIAL BLOOD GAS ESTIMATION

The arterial pH, PaO_2, $PaCO_2$ are measured as part of the lung function tests. The pH and $PaCO_2$ are directly measured and the bicarbonate concentration is calculated from the **Henderson–Hasselbalch** equation. Hypercapnia (increased $PaCO_2 \geq 50$ mm Hg) means alveolar hypoventilation. Hypoventilation can result from several causes. In COPD hypoventilation and hypercapnia most commonly result from the inability of the respiratory muscles to meet the increased load necessitated by changes in the lung and in chest wall mechanics. Hypercapnia can also occur from a decreased central respiratory drive. Both mechanical impairment and poor central respiratory drive may operate in the same patient. A patient with an $FEV_1 > 1$ L

rarely retains CO_2. The likelihood of CO_2 retention increases if the FEV_1 falls below 1 L, though amazingly some patients with FEV_1 close to 0.5 L still manage to breathe hard enough to prevent the CO_2 in the blood from unduly rising.

Most restrictive lung pathologies are associated with hyperventilation so that the $PaCO_2$ may be even less than normal. Advanced restrictive disease with few functioning alveoli is associated with hypercapnia.

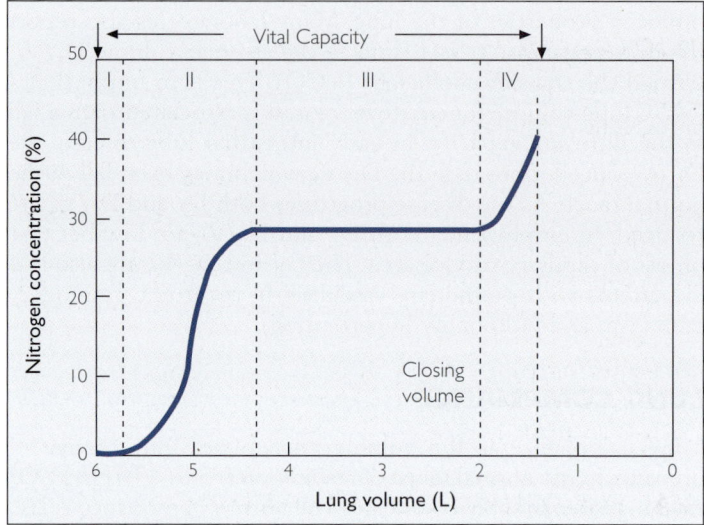

Fig 7.9: Measurement of the closing volume. If a maximal inspiration of 100% O_2 is followed by a full expiration, four phases in the N_2 concentration measured at the lips can be recognized (see text). The last is caused by preferential emptying of the apex of the lung after the lower zone airways have closed.

SUGGESTED READING

MacIntyre N, *et al.* Standardisation of the single-breath determination of carbon monoxide uptake in the lung. *Eur Respir J.* 2005; 26:720-35.

Miller MR, *et al.* General consideration for lung function testing. *Eur Respir J.* 2005; 26:153–61.

Miller MR, *et al.* Standardisation of spirometry. *Eur Respir J.* 2005; 26:319–38.

Pellengriino R, *et al.* Interpretative strategies for lung function tests. *Eur Respir J.* 2005; 26:948–68.

Wanger J, *et al.* Standardisation of the measurement of lung volumes. *Eur Respir J.* 2005; 26:511–22.

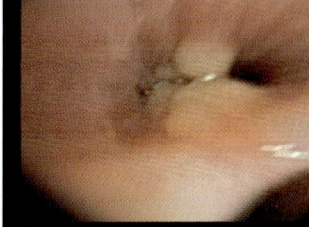

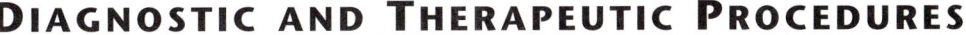

CHAPTER **8**

Diagnostic and Therapeutic Procedures

ENDOTRACHEAL INTUBATION

Endotracheal (ET) intubation can be performed orally or nasally through the larynx and into the trachea. The main indications for ET intubation are:

(i) relief of airway obstruction, e.g. facial burns, smoke inhalation, epiglottitis or vocal cord oedema
(ii) protection of airway, e.g. prevention of aspiration, incoordination of swallowing muscles, obtunded and comatose patients
(iii) ventilatory support, e.g. acute respiratory failure, during general anaesthesia, flail chest (also see chapter on 'Airway Management').

ORAL ENDOTRACHEAL INTUBATION

Intubation by mouth is preferred over nasal intubation as it allows a larger ET tube with less airflow resistance. However, oral intubation is less comfortable to the patient producing excessive secretions. Conscious patients find it difficult to tolerate the ET intubation and they may constantly gag or bite at the tube.

Instrument tray for oral ET intubation should include the following:

(i) Laryngoscope with both straight (Miller) and curved (MacIntosh) blades, ranging from size 0 (neonates) to 4 (adults). It is vital to check that the blades attach to the handles well and that both batteries and the bulb are in place, so that it lights sharply (brightly) on snapping open the blades of the laryngoscope.
(ii) Endotracheal tubes, which come in sizes ranging from 2 to 10. The size refers to the internal diameter (ID) of the tube in mm and it comes in 0.5-mm increments (see Table 8.1). Along the body of the tube, a radio-opaque line runs lengthwise for the proper verification of tube placement on X-ray. Markings in mm are also shown along the body for easy determination of the depth of insertion. The distal end of the tube has a cuff which is connected to a balloon at the proximal end which is used to regulate volume of air in the cuff via a 10 ml or larger syringe.

Portex tubes are the most commonly used tubes, but stiff rubber endotracheal tubes (Rush) should also be handy, as they may prove useful in difficult intubations.
(iii) Syringes, lubricants, securing tape, flexible guiding stylet, topical anaesthetic, McGill forceps, suction catheters and an AMBU bag with proper connections should also be provided.

Table 8.1: Estimation of size of ET	
Patient	Size
Neonates < 1,000 gm	2.5 mm
Neonates 1,000–3,000 gm	3.4 mm
Child 1–2 years	4–5 mm
Child 2–12 years	4.5 + (age/4) mm
Avg. adult female	7.5–8.5 mm
Avg. adult male	8–9 mm

Procedure for Oral Intubation

After assessing the patient, clearing the mouth of any foreign body such as dentures and checking the ET tray and laryngoscope, place the patient in sniffing position by tilting the

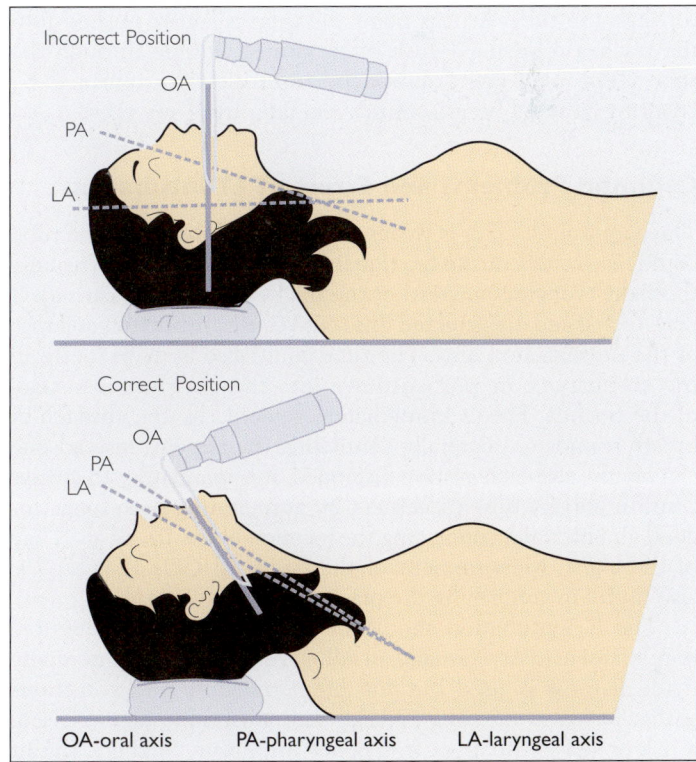

Fig 8.1: The position of the head and neck for endotracheal intubation.

head back so that the oral, pharyngeal and laryngeal axes are aligned. This is usually achieved by resting the head by about 10 cm with pads under the occiput while shoulders remain on the table (Figure 8.1). Always explain the procedure to the patient and reassure him if he is conscious. Next, lubricate the deflated cuff at the distal end of the ET. It is always best to ventilate and preoxygenate the patients with 100% O_2 using an AMBU bag and a face mask. If ET intubation is not successful in 30 sec, ventilate the patient once again using 100% O_2. Now hold the laryngoscope handle with the left hand (Figure 8.1) and insert the blade into the right side of the mouth, sliding the blade to the base of the tongue and simultaneously swapping the blade to the left. Manoeuvre the tip of the straight (Miller) blade underneath the epiglottis, or the tip of the curved McIntosh blade at the vallecula. Lift the handle and blade up anteriorly to display the tongue and attached soft tissues. You should be able to now locate the larynx and vocal cords and under direct vision insert the ET. Check for airflow at the proximal end and auscultate for breath sounds and then inflate the cuff. It is always best to confirm proper tube placement with X-ray chest.

NASAL INTUBATION

The initial preparations and head positioning are the same as for oral intubation. This is a blind technique and intubation is done by inserting the ET tube (size smaller than one would use for oral intubation) through a nostril. This should be advanced slowly and when the distal end can be seen through the mouth it is laryngoscopically guided by McGill forceps into the trachea. In a fully conscious and cooperative patient the tube may be advanced slowly during inspiratory efforts and when the distal end approaches the trachea air movement can be felt and heard through the tube. At this point the tube is gently pushed into the trachea releasing a gush of air almost audible through the tube. Tube placement should be immediately confirmed by ensuring bilateral breath sounds and later by X-ray chest.

Common Problems and Errors of ET Intubation

The commonest error is wrong placement of the tube. The tube could be wrongly pushed so that its tip lies in a bronchus (usually the right bronchus) instead of the trachea (above the carina). If undetected and uncorrected this could cause a disastrous collapse of the unventilated lung. The tube could also lie with its tip in the oropharynx, or pushed down into the oesophagus instead of the trachea. This is immediately detected by the absence of breath sounds on manually ventilating the patient. Instead one can see the stomach getting distended. It is mandatory to always confirm correct tube placement by auscultating both lungs for good air entry and confirming the location of the tip by an X-ray of the chest. Measurement of the end-tidal CO_2 ($ETCO_2$) is also useful in confirming the placement of the ET tube.

The ET intubation should be *secured* firmly to guarantee maximal sensitivity. Usually an adhesive tape or a commercially made harness is used but too often moisture and secretions gather between the tape and skin and loosen the tape creating a risk of self-extubation. It is hence important to check the fit frequently and to use adhesive tapes of good material.

Ischemic injury and tissue necrosis may occur if the *cuff pressure* is too high and exceeds the capillary perfusion pressure

in the trachea. The ET pressure should be less than 25 cm H_2O to allow adequate capillary pressure and for patients with hypotension, it should be kept even lower. To ensure and monitor proper cuff pressure, a Posey cufflator with an inbuilt manometer is available.

To avoid suction-induced hypoxia, the patient is pre-oxygenated and the suction time kept less than 15 sec.

Certain specific problems can be encountered when using the laryngoscope, especially in oral intubation. A common mishap is aspiration of dentures if one has forgotten to check and remove them. Trauma to the teeth and soft tissue can also occur. This can be avoided by being more gentle and careful during the procedure. Also, with experience, one can guide and manoeuvre the tube over the laryngoscope's blade with greater skill, especially in difficult intubations. Complications of ET intubation have been dealt with in the chapter on Airway Management.

The general criteria for extubation are listed in Table 8.2. For care of ET tube and extubation see chapter on 'Airway Management'.

Table 8.2: General criteria for extubation
I Rapid breathing test
f/VT < 100 min/l
(VT is tidal volume in litres)
II ABG
Acceptable blood gases on FiO_2 less than 0.4 and spontaneous minute ventilation < 10 l/mm
PaO_2/FiO_2 > 250 mm Hg
III Ventilatory pressure
Maximum inspiratory pressure > −20 cm H_2O
VC > 15 ml/kg
IV Cardiopulmonary assessment
Stable cardiac and pulmonary status

CRICOTHYROIDOTOMY

Cricothyroidotomy is a bedside surgical procedure which can be lifesaving when performed for the correct indication.

Indications

Surgical cricothyroidotomy is indicated in all patients who require immediate intubation which cannot be performed because of the following problems: (i) severe maxillofacial problems; (ii) poor visualization of vocal cords due to local oedema, blood or abnormal anatomy; (iii) cervical spine lesions requiring immobilization and where the neck cannot be manipulated.

Equipment

(i) Kelly or Crile clamp
(ii) Scalpel

(iii) Antiseptic solution and surgical gloves
(iv) Tracheostomy tube; No 6 size

Procedure

The most important part of the procedure is the correct identification of the cricothyroid membrane. The cricoid cartilage is the first small notch on sliding the index finger upwards in the midline from the sternal notch. The firm membrane between it and the thyroid cartilage (Adam's apple) is the cricothyroid membrane.

The patient should be supine with the neck in neutral position and the thumb and index finger of the non-operating hand should stabilize the tracheal laryngeal complex by firmly fixing the thyroid cartilage as shown in Figure 8.2. A 3 to 4-cm vertical or transverse incision should be made through the skin, dermis and cricothyroid membrane. This should identify the cricothyroid space which should be dissected and opened transversely by means of a sharp knife. In spontaneously breathing patients, a successful incision of the membrane should immediately be followed by a gush of air. The index finger should be immediately inserted in the space and a clamp is next inserted to spread the membrane and enlarge the space. Now by pulling the clamp upwards the trachea is elevated and a No. 6 tracheostomy tube is inserted under the clamp and the clamp is removed.

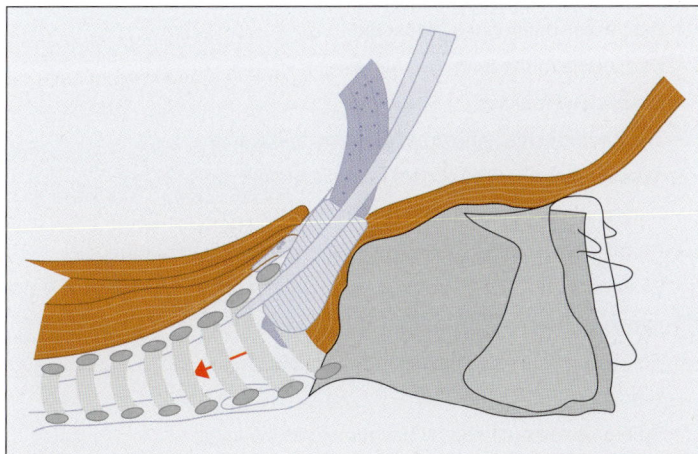

Fig 8.2: Procedure for cricothyroidotomy. Tracheostomy tube advanced behind the clamp and trachea pulled up by clamp.

Complications

(i) Laceration of the anterior jugular veins is a potential complication because of their paramedian and superficial location which is in close proximity to the incision. With a vertical incision the likelihood of injury to the veins is less. However, in the event they are injured the bleed can be stopped with manual pressure or at worse it may require suture ligation.
(ii) Oropharyngeal injury is a major complication and can occur if the scalpel penetrates the posterior wall of the trachea. This is avoided by dissecting the cricothyroid membrane with a finger or a blunt clamp but never by using

a sharp and penetrating instrument like a knife. Observing proper fixation of the thyro-laryngeal complex and taking an adequate incision enabling good visualization of the thyroid and cricoid cartilage is very important in avoiding this mishap.
(iii) Bleeding from adjacent structures is probably the most common problem but can be avoided or minimized by staying in the midline during the surgery.

PERCUTANEOUS DILATIONAL TRACHEOSTOMY

Indications

1. As an elective procedure when it is desirable to shift from ET intubation to a tracheostomy. In this situation, the ET tube is left in position and removed only at the appropriate time.
2. To secure an airway in an emergency, when ET intubation fails or when ET intubation is not considered feasible for technical or anatomical reasons.

It is to be noted that though percutaneous dilational tracheostomy (PDT) is perhaps more expedient than a formal tracheostomy in a dire emergency, it carries a greater risk of peri-operative cardiopulmonary complications and death. It requires not only expertise but also experience and should not be performed if these are not available. PDT should also be avoided in children and in obese patients.

Procedure

The two most commonly available kits for this procedure are:

(i) Cook kit or
(ii) Portex kit

In an elective PDT, the ET tube is left in place throughout the procedure and removed only at the appropriate time. The procedure begins with a small 2-cm vertical incision made mid-distance between the cricoid cartilage and sternal notch. After separating the pretracheal muscles the trachea is palpated through the incision. Next a needle attached to a 10-ml syringe filled with saline is digitally guided and inserted in the midline through the second and third tracheal rings, with constant suction on the syringe while inserting. On entering the trachea bubbles of air are aspirated into the syringe and at this point it is vital to hold the needle still and disconnect the syringe (Figure 8.3).

Once the needle is stabilized a guidewire is gently passed through its lumen and the needle then withdrawn. A dilator is next passed over the guidewire to dilate the existing tract. After removing the dilator a guiding catheter is passed over the guidewire and inserted into the trachea. Progressive dilatations are now done starting from 12 Fr dilator up to the largest 36 Fr and these are all done over the guidewire and the guiding catheter. Serial dilatations should be done at a correct angle and with minimal force to avoid injury to trachea or creating a false pretracheal passage. After the largest dilator is inserted and withdrawn a digit is inserted through the incision into the trachea for palpating the ET. An assistant is asked to withdraw

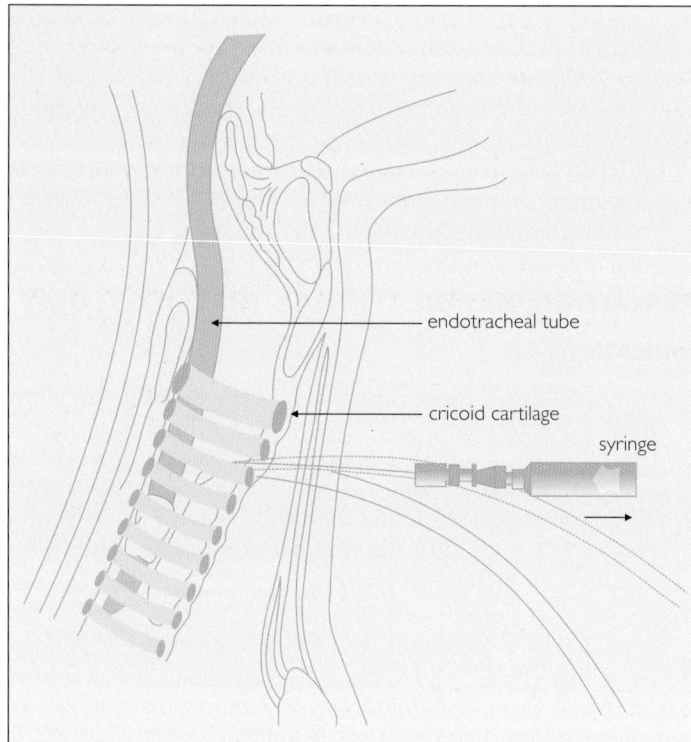

Fig 8.3: Procedure for percutaneous dilatational tracheostomy (PDT).

the ET slowly and stop withdrawal when the tip of the tube is right over the palpating finger. A No. 8 Shiley tracheostomy tube fitted snugly with a 28 Fr dilator is now introduced over the guidewire and guiding catheter complex into the trachea. Once the tracheostomy tube is in place the guidewire, the guiding catheter and the 28 Fr dilator are all withdrawn. The balloon of the tracheostomy tube is inflated and the tube placement is confirmed by auscultation and only then the ET is removed.

Complications

(i) Incorrect placement of needle. This may be avoided by introducing the needle under digital guidance.

(ii) Perforation of the posterior wall of the trachea by dilators. This can be avoided by not applying unnecessary force to the dilator while putting it into the trachea and placing the dilator at the correct angle.

(iii) Bleeding into the trachea. This can occur with a low placement of the tube causing injury to the thoracic inlet vessels; though rare the most lethal is an injury to the innominate artery. If such a complication should occur direct pressure should be applied until the patient is moved to the OT for surgical repair.

The sophistication, ease and safety of this technique have made it an increasingly popular approach which can be performed by a trained intensivist at the bedside. There is however an ongoing debate whether this is truly as safe as it was predicted and whether it is cost-effective. In any case, it is always an asset for an intensivist or the on-call surgeon to be familiar with the technique.

BRONCHOSCOPY

It was Gustav Killian who performed the first bronchoscopy when he removed a piece of pork bone from the right main bronchus of a patient in Germany in 1897. He is considered the 'father of bronchoscopy' and used a Mikulicz-Rosenheim oesophagoscope. Initially criticized for this pioneering procedure, the field has evolved at an amazing speed with dedicated bronchoscopy journals and conferences and several international and national bronchoscopy associations commonplace now. It is an essential tool in the armoury of the chest physician and is a field where technology continues to evolve at rapid pace.

Indications: The indications for bronchoscopy are both diagnostic and therapeutic and are listed in Table 8.3.

Table 8.3: Indications for bronchoscopy
Diagnostic
• Cough
• Unexplained wheeze and stridor
• Hoarseness and vocal cord palsy
• Hemoptysis
• Unresolved consolidation or collapse
• Chemical and thermal burns of the tracheobronchial tree
• Suspected pulmonary infections
• Carcinoma of the lung
• Mediastinal masses
• Tracheobronchial strictures, stenosis and fistula
• Assessment of endotracheal tube placement
• Diagnostic bronchoalveolar lavage
• Protected specimen brushing in ventilator acquired pneumonia
• Evaluation of ILD with transbronchial lung biopsy
Therapeutic
• Retained secretions, mucous plugs, clots
• Hemoptysis
• Strictures to be dilated by balloon bronchoplasty
• Obstructing tumours for bronchoscopic debulking
• Bronchopleural fistula
• Tracheoesophageal fistula
• Bronchogenic cysts
• Endotracheal intubation
• Therapeutic BAL in pulmonary alveolar proteinosis
Special procedures
• Brachytherapy
• Laser therapy
• Photodynamic therapy
• Electrocautery
• Argon plasma cauterization
• Cryotherapy
• Bronchial thermoplasty in ashtma

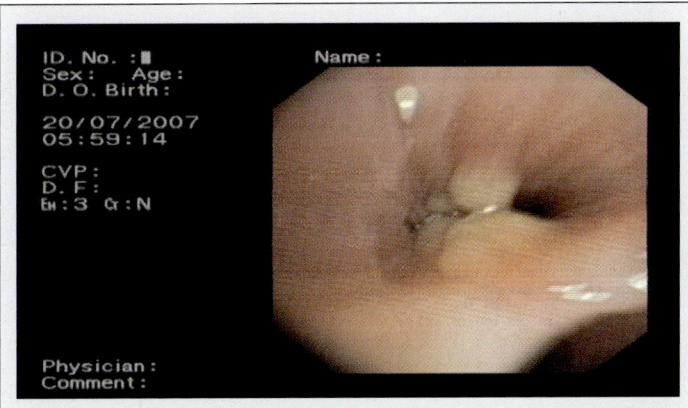

Fig 8.4: Bronchoscopic view of a left upper lobe tumour.

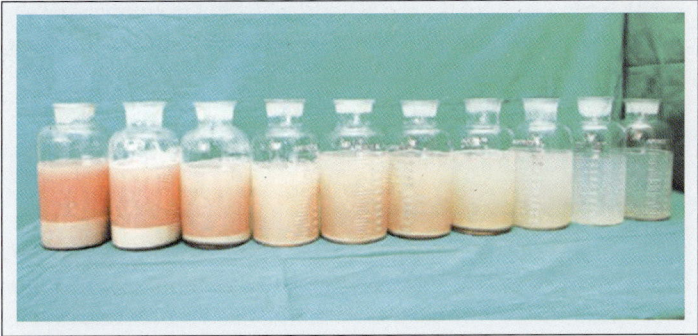

Fig 8.5: Therapeutic bronchoscopy to obtain bronchoalveolar lavage fluid in a patient of pulmonary alveolar proteinosis. Note the milky colour of the BAL fluid.

Safety and Contraindications

The safety of bronchoscopy has been documented by several earlier multicentre studies. Several recent surveys have confirmed very low rates of complications in experienced hands but this should not result in complacency because major complications do still occur mainly in improperly selected patients and in the hands of inexperienced bronchoscopists.

The contraindications to bronchoscopy are listed in Table 8.4.

Table 8.4: Contraindications to bronchoscopy
• Refractory hypoxemia which is likely to worsen during or after bronchoscopy
• Unstable cardiovascular status
• Bleeding diathesis: a low platelet count is a contraindication to biopsies but a BAL can still be safely performed.
• Uremia: a creatinine > 3 mg/dl is a relative contraindication to biopsy because of probable platelet dysfunction.

Procedure

The procedure is explained to the patient and informed consent taken. It is essential to explain the procedure and try and allay the anxieties of the patient at every step. A bronchoscopy should ideally be a painless, stress-free procedure for every patient. If badly performed however, it can be an extremely traumatic experience. We do not use any pre-medication except for a small dose of midazolam; 4% lignocaine sprayed at the back of the pharynx reduces cough during the procedure. We have also found transtracheal injection of 1–2 ml of 4% lignocaine to be very effective at suppressing cough during the procedure and permitting a smoother bronchoscopy. The nasal or the oral route can be used and it is important that the bronchoscopist be trained to introduce his scope via both routes. If the nasal approach is favoured, the nose must be inspected for any obvious septal deviation or obvious obstruction and some lignocaine jelly on a swab stick be used to numb the nasal mucosa. It should be noted that the blood concentration of lignocaine after topical administration may be up to 50% of that obtained after rapid intravenous administration. Lignocaine toxicity after over-liberal use of topical lignocaine at bronchoscopy has been reported hence the minimal dose should be used. If the upper airway has been well anesthetized it is quite easy to pass through the vocal cords after carefully inspecting their movements. A careful study of the tracheobronchial tree can then be performed and bronchoalveolar lavage (BAL), endobronchial biopsy and transbronchial biopsies be taken as indicated.

Bronchoalveolar Lavage

BAL is performed by wedging the tip of the bronchoscope in a segmental or sub-segmental bronchus, which has been anaesthetized by 2% lignocaine instilled through the bronchoscope. In the absence of local lung pathology the right middle lobe or lingual is recommended for this procedure because they are both readily accessible and give a good return of lavage fluid. Sterile saline is introduced in aliquots of 20–60 ml through the biopsy channel of the bronchoscope to a total of around 100–200 ml. In normal subjects BAL usually yields around 50% recovery of the instilled fluid. For diagnostic studies, instilling a total of 50–60 ml may be sufficient to obtain an adequate volume of returning fluid, which can then be sent for microbiological and cytological analysis. Larger BAL volumes are needed for research purposes when the yield of alveolar macrophages and lymphocytes needs to be higher. In normal volunteers BAL fluid comprises mainly of alveolar macrophages and a few lymphocytes. Neutrophils and eosinophils normally constitute less than 4% and 3% respectively. Finding BAL eosinophilia, neutrophilia and lymphocytosis may have value in a number of conditions but at present remains primarily a research tool.

The only condition where BAL has been proven to be of therapeutic value is pulmonary alveolar proteinosis where volumes of 12–13 litres may be instilled in one lung at a time.

Transbronchial Lung Biopsies

Both diffuse and localized lung lesions can be biopsied by passing the forceps beyond the visible bronchi into the adjacent alveolar tissue. We would recommend that this procedure always be performed with the aid of fluoroscopy so the exact position of the forceps is confirmed prior to taking the biopsy. The two main complications of the procedure are bleeding and pneumothorax. Biopsies taken too proximally can cause bleeding from the pulmonary vessels which are larger in this region. Those taken too peripherally can result in pneumothorax. To biopsy diffuse lung disease, the bronchoscope is wedged in the appropriate sub-segmental bronchus and the forceps advanced into the periphery of the lung under fluoroscopic guidance. The forceps are opened and then advanced after the patient is made to hold his breath at the end of expiration. The forceps are removed with the accompanying tissue with firm but not excessive pressure and withdrawn from the bronchoscope. The sample is shaken from the forceps in 10% formaldehyde. The diagnostic yield in diffuse lung disease increases when up to five specimens are taken, and if the patient tolerates the procedure, we would recommend taking this number of biopsies. The overall diagnostic rate in diffuse lung disease is 35–65%. The yield is higher in bronchocentric diseases like sarcoidosis and extrinsic allergic alveolitis where the yield in our hands has consistently been around 70–80%. The diagnostic yield in opportunistic infection is in the region of 76–88%.

TRANSBRONCHIAL AND OESOPHAGEAL ULTRASOUND-GUIDED BIOPSY OF THE MEDIASTINUM

Mediastinal lymphadenopathy is generally due to infective pathologies or mitotic lesions. The commonest infective pathology responsible for mediastinal adenopathy in our part of the world is tuberculosis. The commonest mitotic lesion causing mediastinal adenopathy is involvement of the mediastinal glands in lung cancer—chiefly a non-small-cell lung cancer (NSCLC) or a small-cell lung cancer (SCLC). Metastasis to mediastinal lymph glands from a cancer outside the chest is also an important consideration; finally, mediastinal adenopathy may be due to lymphoproliferative disease—chiefly Hodgkin's disease, non-Hodgkin's lymphoma or leukaemia. There are numerous ways of sampling mediastinal lymph nodes. These include a computed tomography (CT)-guided biopsy whenever this is feasible without danger to the patient, mediastinoscopy, thoracoscopy, mediastinotomy, a video-assisted thoracoscopy and biopsy through a formal thoracotomy. The last four procedures involve expense, hospitalization and carry a significant morbidity. Transbronchial and oesophageal ultrasound-guided biopsy of a mediastinal pathology is a minimally invasive procedure that has less morbidity and is less risky when compared to most of the procedures listed above.

Endoscopic ultrasound (EUS)-guided fine needle aspiration biopsy to start with was developed for gastrointestinal disease. It was soon realized that this technique could be adapted for sampling specific mediastinal pathologies as well. Today, both cytology and histology can be obtained by EUS guidance, thereby broadening the diagnostic scope of this procedure.

Two different systems are in use. The endobronchial miniprobes which can be used through the normal working channel of a fibreoptic bronchoscope and the endobronchial ultrasound-guided transbronchial needle-aspiration (EBUS-TBNA) bronchoscope which was introduced around 2005.

Indications for Transbronchial Ultrasound-Guided Biopsy of the Mediastinum

1. Diagnosis   This procedure helps to determine the cause of mediastinal adenopathy which is of uncertain aetiology.

2. Staging of NSCLC   This is probably the most important indication for a transbronchial ultrasound-guided biopsy. Sampling enlarged mediastinal glands in patients with NSCLC allows staging of the disease, which in turn allows planned treatment. In countries where tuberculosis is prevalent, one occasionally finds a patient with NSCLC who has a mediastinal adenopathy unrelated to cancer, but due to tuberculosis. Without sampling the mediastinal nodes, such a patient would have been deemed inoperable.

3. Diagnosis and staging of a wide range of other cancers originating outside the lungs.

4. Accurate differentiation between lymphadenopathy due to infection, cancer and lymphoma.

ENDOBRONCHIAL ULTRASOUND MINIPROBES

For use within the central airways, a flexible catheter for the probes with a balloon at the tip allows circular contact for the ultrasound, providing a 360° image of the parabronchial and paratracheal structures. Thereby, structures at a distance of up to 4.0 cm can be visualized. The probes can be used with a flexible bronchoscope that has a biopsy channel of at least 2.6 mm.

Use in Early Lung Cancer

Small radiologically invisible tumours are in some units managed by endoscopic therapeutic interventions. Tumours a few millimetres in diameter can be analyzed reliably by endobronchial ultrasound. They can be distinguished from benign lesions, and their extraluminal and intraluminal extent within the different layers of the bronchial wall determined. The use of EBUS with autoflorescence bronchoscopy has been evaluated in prospective studies and has become the basis for curative endobronchial treatment of very early malignancies in specialized institutions. Treatment involves the use of photodynamic therapy or brachytherapy or coagulation.

Use of EBUS in Advanced Cancer

1. EBUS allows a detailed analysis of intraluminal, submucosal and intramural tumour spread, features that are important for decisions on resection margins.

2. EBUS is useful to demonstrate the involvement of the great vessels such as the aorta or pulmonary artery, or involvement of the wall of the oesophagus by a mediastinal tumour. Studies have shown that EBUS is superior to CT in distinguishing compression of the tracheobronchial tree from infiltration of the tracheobronchial wall caused by a mediastinal tumour mass. The sensitivity of EBUS versus CT was 89 % vs. 25 % and the specificity 100 % vs. 89 % in this regard.

SCOPE OF THE EBUS-TBNA

The EBUS-TBNA can sample paratracheal nodes, as also nodes in the aortopulmonary window, pretracheal, subcarinal nodes and reachable hilar nodes.

The technique for fibreoptic bronchoscopy and the precautions during endoscopy have already been described. Images can be obtained by direct contact of the probe against the airway wall or by attaching a balloon to the probe tip and inflating it with saline. The balloon is designed not to over-inflate, so that the central airway remains unoccluded. When the lesion is clearly outlined, a 21-gauge full length steel needle is introduced through the biopsy channel of the bronchoscope. Doppler examination is used immediately before biopsy to avoid unintentional puncture and damage of vessels that may be present between the bronchus and the lesion. Under real-time ultrasound guidance the needle is then placed within the lesion. Suction is applied through a syringe attached to the needle while the needle is moved back and forth within the lesion. The biopsy obtained is sent for staining, histopathology.

A large trial reported results in 502 patients—572 lymph nodes were punctured and 94% yielded a diagnosis. Biopsies were taken from all reachable lymph nodes. Mean (SD) diameter of the lymph nodes was 1.6 cm and the range was 0.8 to 3.2 cm. Sensitivity was 92%,—and specificity was 100% in distinguishing benign from malignant lymph nodes. The positive predictive value was 93%. No complications were observed. A number of other studies have reported similar results, with no complications.

A study has also reported sampling of mediastinal nodes less than a centimetre in size. A positive diagnosis of malignancy was confirmed by surgical biopsy or exploratory thoracotomy. In this study, the sensitivity of EBUS-TBNA for detecting malignancy was 92% and the specificity 100%. Thus, EBUS-TBNA can sample even small nodes with safety and help in the final staging procedure before thoracotomy in patients with NSCLC.

ENDO-OESOPHAGEAL ULTRASOUND

Endo-oesophageal ultrasound enables the endoscopist to obtain a view of not only the lumen and wall of the oesophagus, but also of the surrounding structures. The target lesion outside the oesophagus is punctured through the oesophageal wall under ultrasound guidance. The material obtained in this way is available for cytological and polymerase chain reaction PCR analysis. For oesophageal ultrasound-guided fine needle biopsy, only a linear ultrasound probe is used.

Procedure

The patient is placed in the left lateral position, sedated with midazolam, and an endoscopy of the oesophagus performed. The ultrasound probe is passed into the distal part of the oesophagus until the left lobe of the liver is visualized. The left adrenal gland can also be visualized at this point of time.

The scope is then slowly withdrawn inch by inch while making circular movements to enable the endoscopist to view most parts of the mediastinum. Location, size and echo features of any surrounding lesion are noted. Suspicious lesions or lymph glands can be punctured through the wall of the oesophagus, a fine needle aspiration biopsy being performed under real-time ultrasound guidance.

In our part of the world, tuberculous caseous adenopathy due to tuberculous involvement of mediastinal glands posterior to the oesophagus is not an uncommon observation. These glands cause dysphagia. A fine needle puncture of these necrotic caseous glands under ultrasound guidance not only

gives a diagnosis but is of therapeutic value. The caseous contents are discharged into the oesophagus and the dysphagia is relieved.

CHEST TUBE DRAINAGE

Intercostal tubes are used to aspirate air or fluid from the intrapleural space. At times, as in a tension pneumothorax, intercostal drainage needs to be performed as an emergency procedure. This is basically a bedside procedure which can be performed easily and safely in the intensive care unit (ICU), and all senior resident doctors looking after ICU patients should familiarize themselves with the techniques of chest tube insertion.

Emergency Procedure

A tension pneumothorax can cause very rapid haemodynamic deterioration, leading to cardiopulmonary collapse and death, if not relieved immediately. Inserting a chest tube may be time-consuming, and a needle should be immediately inserted to relieve the pressure. A 16-gauge angiocath (catheter-over-needle device) is inserted in the second intercostal space, anteriorly in the mid-clavicular line. Once the pleural space is penetrated, the air under tension is immediately released and the pneumothorax is decompressed. At this point the needle is removed, leaving the catheter in the pleural space. The catheter hub is connected to a long tubing, the other end of which is placed underwater so that the air can bubble out in a more controlled manner. This is however a temporary procedure and preparation for an immediate chest tube placement must be made for more efficient decompression of the pnemothorax.

Drainage System

A conventional two or three-bottle system is commonly used for evacuation of intrapleural air and fluid as shown in Figure 8.6. Each bottle is placed in a series. The first is the trap bottle which collects the fluid from the pleural space and at the same time allows air to pass through to the next bottle i.e. the water seal bottle. This second bottle acts as a one-way valve, allowing air to escape from the pleural space, but preventing atmospheric air from entering the pleural space when negative pleural pressure is created during inspiration. The inlet tube in the second bottle is placed underwater, thereby creating a back pressure on the pleural space, which is equal to the submerged depth of the inlet tube. This back pressure, called the water seal pressure, is usually 1–2 cm of H_2O, and should ideally suffice to re-inflate the lung. Further negative pressure if required, can be provided by applying a central suction. However, for reasons of safety, a third bottle called the 'suction control bottle' is added in the series. This bottle has an underwater tube which is open to the atmosphere, as shown in Figure 8.6. The depth of this tube column determines the safety, by setting a limit on the negative pressure that is imposed on the pleural space. For example, if this column is 15 cm under water, any negative pressure > -15 cm H_2O from a central suction, will result in a constant bubbling of air into the third bottle, and prevent the sub-atmospheric pressure from exceeding –15 cm H_2O.

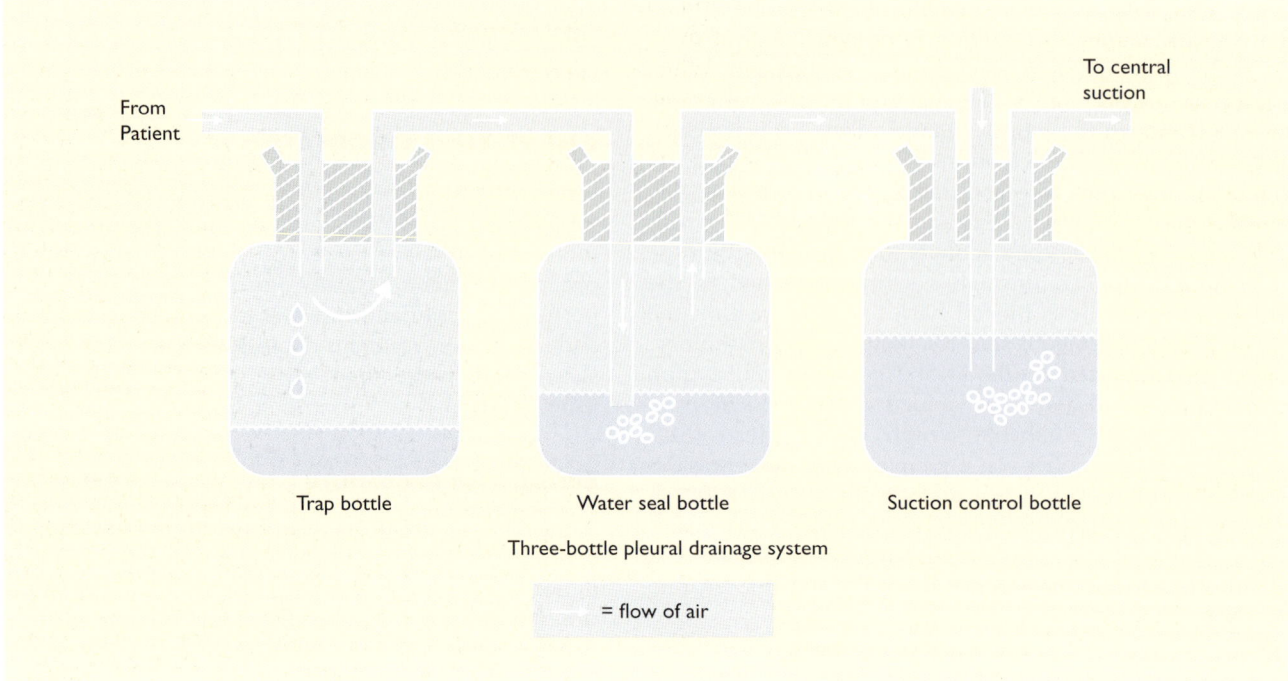

Fig 8.6: Three bottle pleural drainage system.

Procedure for Chest Tube Insertion

A chest tube tray containing sterile drapes, local anaesthetic, medium and large Kelly clamps, and other material such as sutures, antiseptic solution, and dressing materials should be kept ready. Chest tubes of various sizes are available from 12 Fr to 42 Fr. Larger sized tubes are used for traumatic haemothorax or haemopneumothorax, whereas smaller tubes ranging from 12 to 22 Fr may be used for spontaneous pneumothorax. The tube itself is made of a transparent material, with multiple side holes over the distal third of its length; there is also a radio-opaque strip at the distal end of the tube to mark its placement in the pleural space. These tubes are available in a trocar for tunnelling through the intercostal space. In case these special tubes are not available, a simple Malecot's catheter may be used.

The patient should lie flat with the involved side elevated by a pillow, and arms flexed over the head. After infiltrating the skin with lidocaine (1% or 2% solution), a skin incision is made at the appropriate site of tube insertion, which is usually in the fifth or sixth intercostal space in the anterior axillary line. Some operators prefer the second intercostal space in the mid-clavicular line, but the penetration of muscles and breast tissue is more difficult at this site. After incising the skin at the appropriate puncture site, the muscles and tissues are penetrated by either a blunt dissection using clamps and index finger to enter the pleural space or the tube is directly inserted with the help of a trocar. Rotating movements are used whilst advancing the tube with the trocar.

Once the pleural space is entered, the tube is advanced upward in the direction of the apex for treatment of a pneumothorax, and towards a post-basal position for drainage of fluid, with the last side hole inserted 2 or 3 mm into the chest to ensure dependent drainage. Prior to insertion, the approximate length of the tube that should lie within the thoracic cage is estimated, and the position where the tube should emerge from the chest wall is marked with a silk tie.

Once the tube is properly placed in the pleural space it is fastened to the skin with 1–0 or 2–0 silk sutures, using a mattress stitch. Before fixing the tube, ensure that the last side hole is in the pleural space. The ends of the suture are not cut, but are wrapped around the tube, and secured with a tape so that they can be used later to close the wound after the tube is removed.

Throughout the procedure the proximal end of the tube is kept clamped and is opened only when the tube is finally connected to the drainage system. The placement is confirmed by the drainage of fluid, or by the bubbling of air in the drainage bottle.

Precautions

There is no absolute contraindication for inserting a chest tube. Coagulation abnormalities however, should be corrected before insertion of the tube; in case of emergency, fresh frozen plasma or platelet transfusions may be given during the procedure.

A chest tube should never be inserted at the bedside for the purpose of draining a massive haemothorax. Accumulated blood in a massive haemothorax acts as a seal preventing further bleeding from the source, and insertion of a chest tube may precipitate catastrophic haemorrhage. Hence, a massive haemothorax should always be drained in the operation theatre where facilities for controlling such a bleed, if necessary with an open thoractomy, are available.

Complications

Common complications of chest tube drainage include improper positioning of the chest tube, inadequate drainage, bleeding, nerve damage, injury to the diaphragm, infection, surgical emphysema, and problems in the drainage system. Use of the correct technique of insertion and placement, and proper chest tube management while the tube is in place, will go a long way in preventing most of these complications.

Incessant pain may occur after re-expansion of the lung and may evoke a vasovagal response manifesting as bradycardia or hypotension. Intercostal nerve blocks or intrapleural lidocaine may help; parenteral analgesics may be needed if pain persists. Strong sedatives should however be avoided. Another major complication is re-expansion pulmonary oedema following rapid evacuation of a large, longstanding pleural collection. Symptoms usually occur within six hours after rapid drainage. This complication can be avoided by slow evacuation of large collections.

After Care of Chest Tube Drainage

(i) The bottle should never be raised above the chest level, as fluid may drain back into the pleural space and lead to infection, or cause a drowning disaster in the presence of a bronchopleural fistula. However if the kind of drainage system demonstrated in Figure 8.6 is used, this complication can be avoided, because the draining tube never comes in contact with the water in the bottle.

(ii) The fluid level in the tube should oscillate with each breath. Failure to oscillate may be due to blockage or a kink in the chest tube, or may be due to full expansion of the lung.

(iii) The intercostal tubes should always be clamped while changing the bottles.

(iv) The original level of water in the bottle should always be marked, so that hourly drainage can be measured.

(v) Very high negative suction via a suction pump should be avoided. Ideally, a suction control bottle should be added to the drainage system as a safety measure, as described earlier.

Chest Tube Removal

Chest tubes should be removed when there is minimal drainage (less than 100 ml/24 h), and the chest X-ray shows complete re-expansion of the lung after clamping the outside tube for 24 h. Check X-rays of the chest should be repeated after removal of the tube. Appearance of a small pneumothorax or minimal surgical emphysema is common, and often resolves by itself.

IMAGING-GUIDED BIOPSIES AND PROCEDURES

Imaging is very useful in acting as a guide to obtain material for microbiology as well as histopathology. The main contraindication relates to bleeding diathesis. An international normalized ratio (INR) beyond 1.4 and/or a platelet count less than 50,000 are generally considered contraindications. If the biopsy is necessary for further management, platelet transfusion and fresh frozen plasma may be used to minimize the risk of bleeding. Other relative contraindications are patient's inability to lie still, hold his or her breath or maintain a prone or decubitus position. Contralateral pneumonectomy, bulla, severe emphysema or vascular structures anticipated in the path of the biopsy needle are also relative contraindications.

Procedure

The first step is to obtain an informed consent. A detailed explanation of the risks and benefits of the procedure must be explained to the patient and accompanying relatives. The coagulation profile is checked. Patients on aspirin or antiplatelet agents should withdraw these drugs three to five days prior to any intervention. Images are obtained of the pathology and a biopsy path is planned. In planning the biopsy path care should be taken to avoid bullae, emphysematous areas and vessels. It is ideal to try and obtain access to the pathology via an extrapleural route if possible. Subcarinal lymph nodes can often be accessed via the paraspinal fat. Solid components of necrotic mass lesions should be sampled, as the necrotic component may not yield an adequate result. Once the access path has been decided, the entry point is marked on the skin. This area is thoroughly cleansed with povidine-iodine solution. The entry site is infiltrated with 2% lidocaine solution. Two types of needles may be used, fine needle aspiration cytology needles or core biopsy needles. It is believed that core biopsy needles have a higher complication rate than fine needles. However, a study of 5444 biopsies found no difference in the complication rate. The pneumothorax rate is related to the number of passes taken through the pleura. Unless the lesion is less than a centimetre in diameter core biopsies should preferably be obtained from all lesions. A coaxial system is used. This consists of a needle with a stylet which is introduced into the lesion. The stylet is then withdrawn and through this needle a trucut gun is introduced. The advantage of this is that multiple cores can be obtained with only one pass through the pleura. A 20-G coaxial is commonly used, but for mediastinal masses an 18-G coaxial may be used. It is important that the coaxial needle be placed within the lesion and not in the lung parenchyma. If this is correctly accomplished the incidence of pneumothorax is very low. After the biopsy is over, the stylet is reinserted and the coaxial assembly removed as it traverses the lung on its exit. If the lesion is less than 1 cm or fluid-filled, an aspiration is performed. A 22-G needle is adequate for fine needle aspiration cytology. To aspirate infected material a thicker gauge needle up to 16 G is used. If the lung is to be traversed, the same principle of reinserting the stylet and then removing the assembly should be adhered to; this reduces the incidence of pneumothorax.

Post-procedure, a check scan, preferably in expiration is obtained for any pneumothorax. The patient is then given oxygen and placed with the biopsy site dependant for an hour. These techniques help to reduce air leak, post-biopsy pneumothorax and transbronchial spread of biopsy-induced alveolar haemorrhage. A check scan is again obtained at the end of one hour; if there is no pneumothorax the patient is discharged. Ninety-eight per cent of all pneumothoraces requiring chest tube insertion develop in the first one hour.

The main complication is a pneumothorax. If the pneumothorax is small, it is treated with nasal oxygen to promote resorption of pleural air. If moderate or large, aspiration of air through a syringe and needle is often tried; if that fails a chest tube drain is placed ideally anteriorly through the second interspace. In most lung biopsies alveolar haemorrhage develops within the needle tract. These patients may experience minor haemoptysis. Significant haemoptysis requires observation and further management.

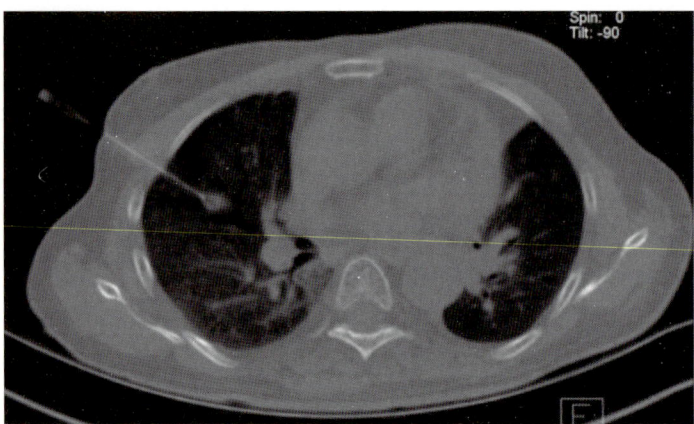

Fig 8.7: CT-guided FNAC. CT chest reveals a right upper lobe pulmonary nodule. A CT-guided FNAC has been performed; needle tip is seen in situ the pulmonary nodule.

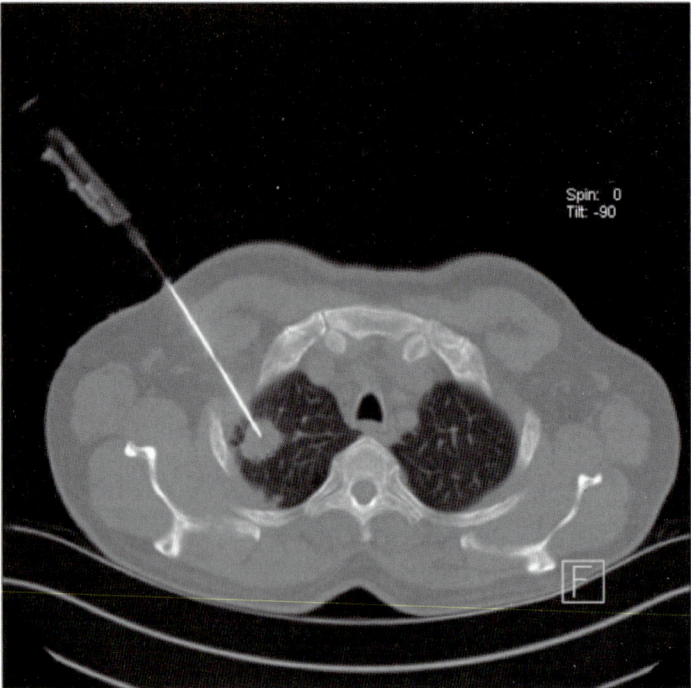

Fig 8.8: CT-guided biopsy. CT chest reveals a right upper lobe pulmonary nodule. Core biopsy of lesion was performed, note needle within lesion.

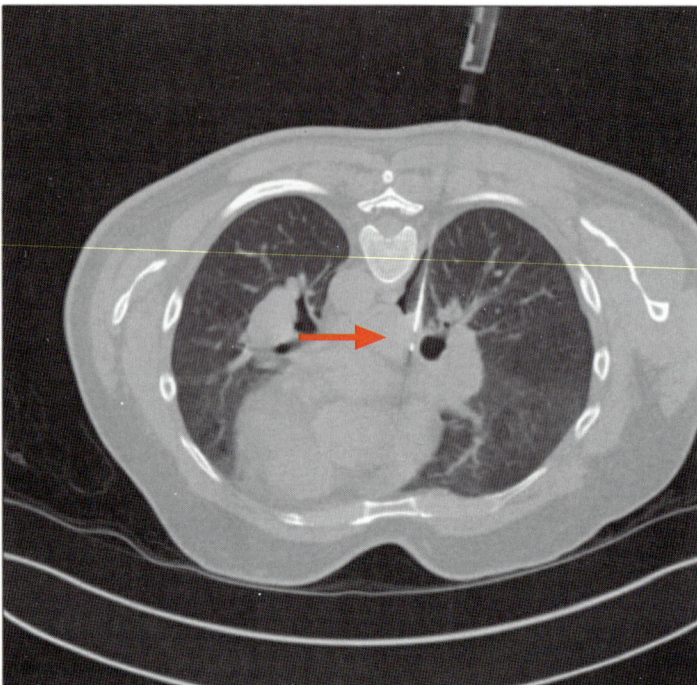

Fig 8.9: CT-guided core biopsy. CT chest reveals a core biopsy of subcarinal adenopathy. Note the open bevel of the trucut needle in the adenopathy. This demonstrates the site from where the sample will be obtained.

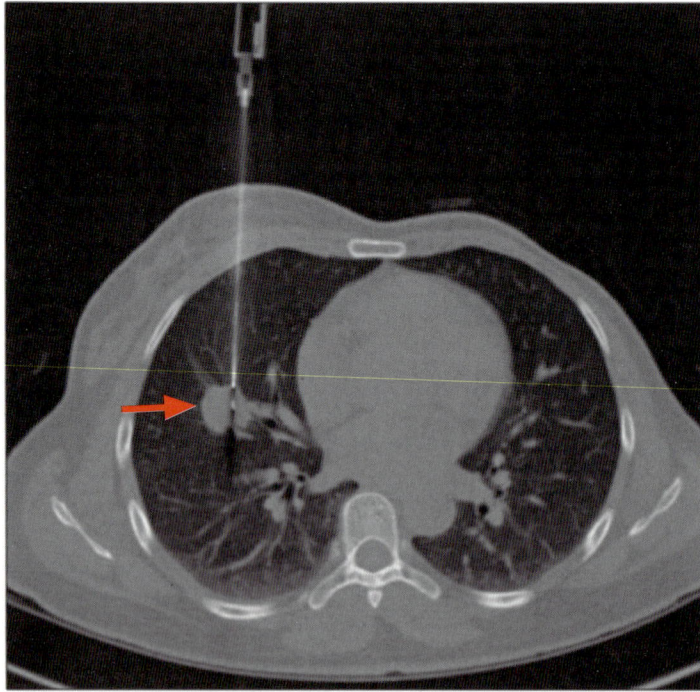

Fig 8.10: CT-guided biopsy. Core biopsy of right upper lobe pulmonary nodule. The open bevel of the needle is well visualized; this will be the site from where the sample will be obtained.

DRAINAGE

Imaging may be used as a guide to drain collection of air, fluid, blood or pus in the pleural space. Pigtail catheters or intercostal drains (ICD) may be used. Pigtail catheters are mounted on a needle and stylet. These are introduced into the fluid similar to a biopsy procedure. The stylet is withdrawn, fluid aspirated and sent for examination. The needle is then withdrawn and the pigtail deployed into the fluid collection. The pigtail is fastened to the skin by sutures. Pigtail catheters are available up to 14 Fr in size. They may get blocked by debris, necrotic tissue or thick pus. Intercostal drains have the advantage of being available from 16 FR and are excellent for drainage. Intercostal drains are introduced percutaneously under imaging guidance so that they are appropriately placed.

PLEURAL BIOPSY

Pleural thickening, pleural-based mass lesions on imaging are investigated by a CT-guided biopsy. If there is no pleural thickening and the pleural aspirate is non-diagnostic, a pleural biopsy is also warranted. The detection rate of granulomas in

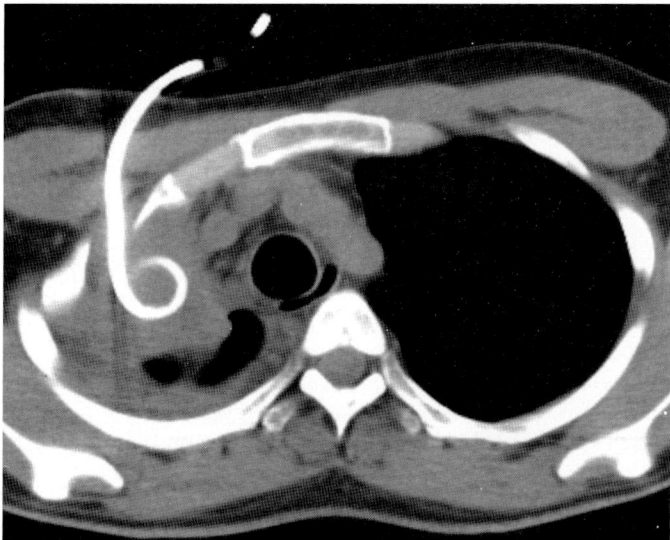

Fig 8.11: CT-guided pigtail drainage. Under CT guidance a pigtail catheter has been placed into a right upper zone loculated fluid collection. Fluid aspirate revealed pus.

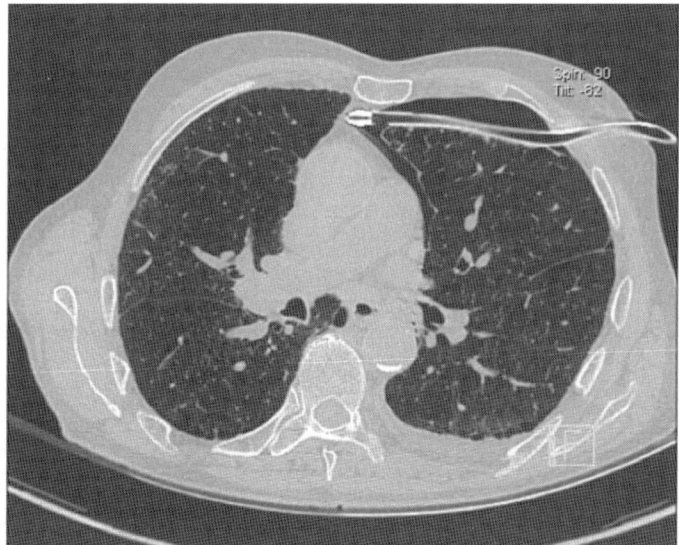

Fig 8.12: ICD Drainage. CT chest reveals a left pneumothorax with an ICD *in situ*.

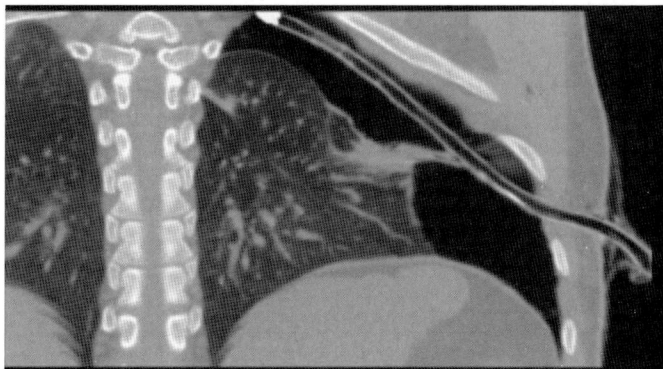

Fig 8.13: ICD drainage. Coronal CT reconstruction reveals a persistent pneumothorax on the left side. An ICD is seen *in situ*. The persistent pneumothorax is due to a pleural adhesion.

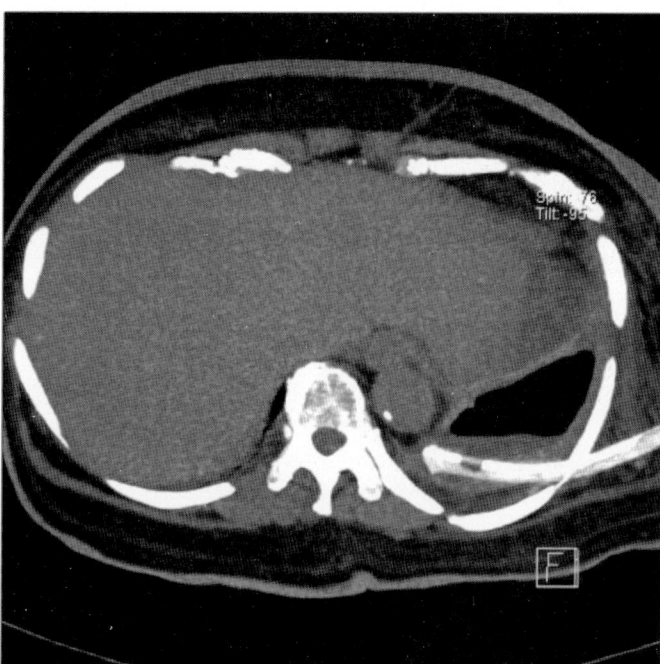

Fig 8.14: CT-guided ICD insertion. Under CT guidance, an ICD has been inserted into a left basal fluid collection which has an air/fluid level.

tuberculous pleural effusions is close to 50%. Another use of a pleural biopsy is in the detection of a mesothelioma. The most popular needle to perform a pleural biopsy is the Abrams needle. Other needles are the Cope and Raja needle. Pleural biopsies are performed similar to a pleural aspiration. The patient is seated leaning forward, with arms folded resting on a pillow. This helps as the scapula gets rotated forward. After preparation of the skin and instillation of local anaesthesia, a stab is made over the skin through a scalpel. The pleural needle is introduced; when the pleura is breached a sudden "give" occurs. Once the needle is in the pleural space the needle is opened by turning the ferrule, pleural fluid being aspirated and collected for examination. The needle is then withdrawn till the tug of the pleura is felt. When the needle is open, there is an aperture in the outer sheath which is open and which hooks with the pleura. Once hooked on to the pleura, the ferrule is closed. This closure of the aperture pushes a fragment of the pleura into the aperture. The needle is then pulled sharply out of the pleural cavity. This pulls the bit of pleural tissue in the aperture. The tissue is then put in formalin for histopathology or saline for microbiology. Multiple passes may be taken to obtain multiple bits of tissue. It is important that the aperture is not open between the 10 and 2 o'clock position, as in this position there may be danger of damaging the intercostal artery or nerve. A marker on the side of the needle indicates where the aperture is, thereby helping to avoid the 10 o'clock to 2 o'clock arc. Complications are similar to all pleural procedures, pneumothorax being most common, though this is rare when there is sufficient fluid in the pleural space.

RADIOFREQUENCY ABLATION

Inoperable neoplasms, metastases, may be ablated using radiofrequency. In this technique a radiofrequency probe is

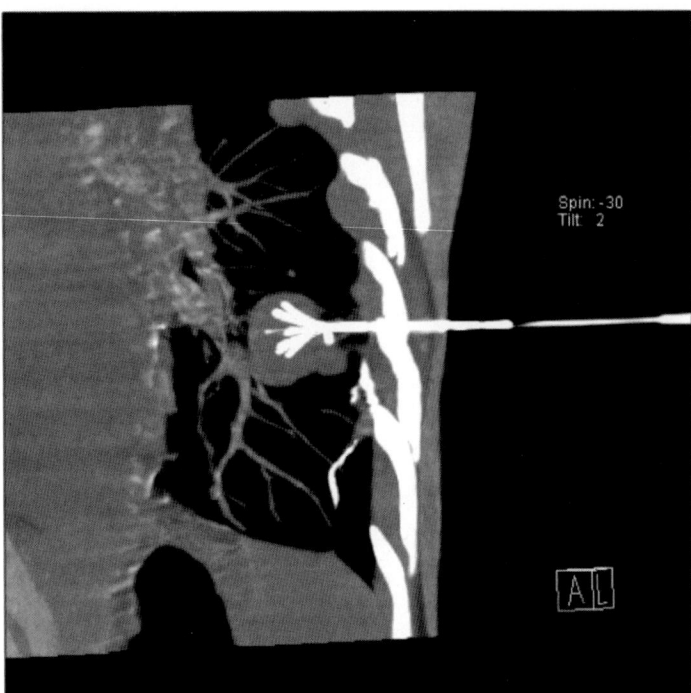

Fig 8.15: Radiofrequency ablation: CT chest coronal reconstruction reveals a nodular mass lesion with a radiofrequency probe inserted in the mass lesion percutaneously. The prongs are open. Each of these probes will pass an electrical current into the lesion to ablate the lesion.

inserted into the tumour, the tissues being heated to ablate the tumour. The technique is similar to performing a core biopsy. As the ablation time varies from 5 to 15 min depending on the size of the tumour, this procedure is generally performed under sedation or anaesthesia. Complications are similar to those of a core biopsy, and include pneumothorax and haemorrhage. The main advantage of radiofrequency ablation is that it is a relatively non-invasive procedure compared to surgery. The procedure may be repeated in the setting of multiple lesions or recurrences.

PERCUTANEOUS TECHNIQUES FOR CENTRAL VENOUS CATHETERIZATION

Presterilized sets of special catheters with associated devices are now available for percutaneous entry into larger veins e.g. the subclavian, internal jugular, femoral or brachial veins.

'Catheter-over-needle devices' are most commonly used, and are designed to eliminate the risk of the needle cutting through the catheter; the greatest danger of 'catheter-through-needle devices' is the shearing of the catheter if it is accidentally withdrawn through the needle. These devices consist of catheters of variable length which can be easily passed through the needle lumen, and can be advanced through the peripheral veins into the central veins.

Both these devices allow placement of a catheter in the central veins by direct puncturing of the vessel. However, if a Swan-Ganz or a pacing catheter needs to be passed through the vein, one may have to use special 'Introducer Sets'. These are usually expensive units consisting of a needle, guide-wire and a dilator over which a polythene sheath is tightly wrapped. These sets require use of the modified Seldinger technique for introduction of the wide-bore introducer sheath in the vein, through which the catheters can then be passed.

Modified Seldinger Technique (Figure 8.16)

The site of the puncture is infiltrated with 1% lidocaine. The vein is cannulated percutaneously with an 18-G thin-walled needle, following the appropriate landmarks and techniques for individual veins as described later. Blood is aspirated from the needle to confirm its entry into the vein, following which the soft end of a J-tip 0.035 inch guide-wire is inserted through the needle, and advanced into the superior vena cava (if the subclavian or internal jugular vein is used), or the inferior vena cava (if the femoral vein is used). The guide-wire should slide effortlessly through the vein, and should never be forced. After the guide-wire is satisfactorily inserted (check that it is not inserted too far in as it may produce ventricular ectopics), the introducer needle is removed, and a small nick is made near the puncture to facilitate the passage of the dilator. The tapered vein dilator carrying an introducer sheath is then advanced over the guide-wire with a twisting motion through the skin and subcutaneous tissue, into the vessel. Finally, the wire and dilator are removed, leaving the wide-bore introducer sheath in the vein, through which the Swan-Ganz or pacing catheter can be passed. The sheath should be secured well with sutures. Some of the introducer sheaths have a one-way valve at the proximal end to prevent backflow of blood, and a side port to allow continuous infusion of fluid to prevent clotting. Throughout this procedure, care should be taken to ensure that the proximal end of the guide-wire always remains outside, and does not migrate into the vein. If for any reason during the procedure the guide-wire needs to be removed and reinserted, the whole procedure should be repeated from the beginning; the needle should never be reintroduced over the guide-wire as it can shear the wire.

Techniques for Specific Veins

SUBCLAVIAN VEIN CATHETERIZATION

The patient lies flat or in a slight head-low position. Correct positioning is important; both arms should be stretched straight by the sides, and the patient should be lying on a firm flat surface so that both the shoulders are in the same plane. The site of puncture is a point just below the junction of the middle and inner thirds of the clavicle.

The skin is now punctured at the selected site, with the point of the needle directed towards the suprasternal notch; the plane of the needle should be horizontal to the ground and parallel to the parietal pleura (Figure 8.17). The needle is advanced with a gentle suction on the syringe until the subclavian vein is entered, often with a distinct give. It is sometimes necessary to slightly change the angle of the needle, in which case it is always essential that the needle is completely withdrawn before re-entering in a new direction. Once the needle is in the vein, depending on the catheter design, proceed either with the modified Seldinger technique, or directly introduce the catheter through the needle, or slide it from over the needle.

COMPLICATIONS

Pneumothorax is the commonest major complication of this procedure. The incidence of pneumothorax can be reduced

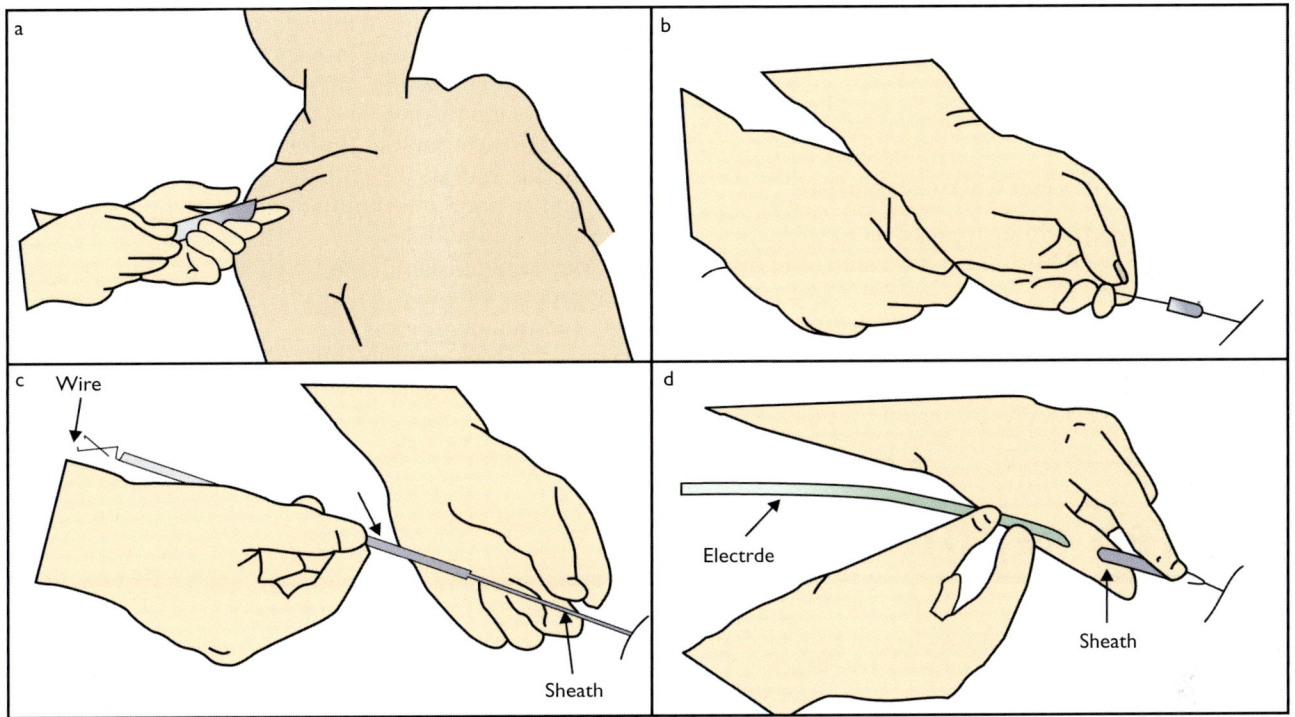

Fig 8.16: Modified Seldinger technique of inserting a guidewire and introducer set via subclaven vein puncture. (a) Direction of needle and site of puncture (b) Insertion of guidewire (c) the introducer sheath (with dilator) is first advanced over the guidewire. Next, with the sheath well in, the guidewire and dilator are removed (d) An electrode or catheter is inserted through the sheath. (From Vakil RJ and Udwadia FE. 1988. *Diagnosis and Management of Medical Emergencies,* third edition, Oxford University Press, Mumbai.)

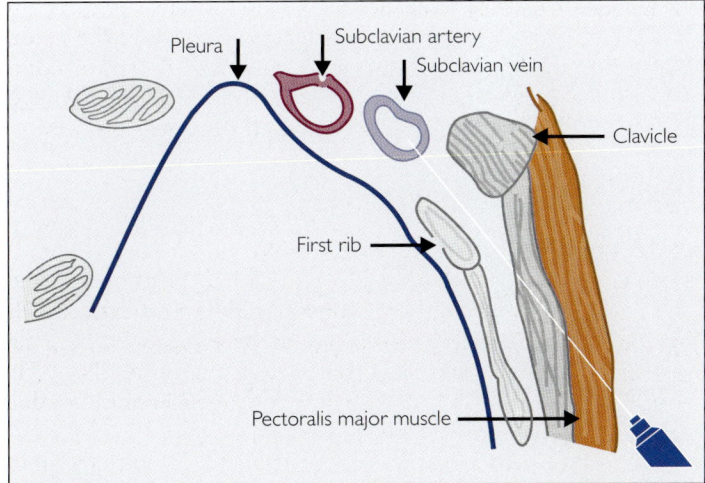

Fig 8.17: Percutaneous subclavian vein puncture: anatomical relationship of the subclavian vein. (From Vakil RJ and Udwadia FE. 1988. *Diagnosis and Management of Medical Emergencies,* third edition, Oxford University Press, Mumbai.)

by avoiding large-bore needles, multiple punctures, and by disconnecting the ventilator at the time of venepuncture. Other serious complications include air embolism, catheter-induced infection, perforation of the superior vena cava, and hemothorax (due to accidental puncture of the subclavian artery).

INTERNAL JUGULAR VENEPUNCTURE
The patient is placed in the Trendelenburg position, and the skin cleaned and carefully draped. The site of puncture is located two finger breadths above the clavicle at the outer border of the sternomastoid, with the patient's head rotated to the opposite side. The needle with the syringe attached, is directed towards the suprasternal notch. Aspiration of blood indicates entry into the vein. Air embolism and thrombophlebitis are the main complications encountered in this procedure. Accidental puncture of the internal carotid artery can also occur. Pneumothorax is rarely observed following this procedure.

FEMORAL VENEPUNCTURE
The femoral vein can also be entered percutaneously. The site of puncture is below the inguinal ligament, just medial to the point where the femoral artery pulse can be palpated. Wound infection is generally more common, and there is an increased risk of thrombophlebitis when the femoral vein is used.

ARTERIAL CATHETERIZATION

Except in unavoidable circumstances, it is wise to choose the radial artery for catheterization, as the risk of occlusion of a proximal artery such as the femoral or brachial could prove disastrous. It is vital to assess the patency of the ulnar artery by Allen's test prior to catheterization, as it is important to be sure that a competent ulnar artery is present. This is done as follows:

(i) The examiner compresses both arteries, when the patient makes a tight fist to squeeze all the blood out of the hand.
(ii) The patient then extends the fingers, and the examiner observes the blanched hand.

(iii) Compression on the ulnar artery is released, and the examiner observes the hand filling with blood. If filling does not occur, the ulnar artery is presumed to be non-functional.

Technique of Radial Artery Catheterization

The wrist is hyperextended and a small area over the radial artery is cleaned and prepared with alcohol and betadine solution. A small area on both sides of the artery is anaesthetized with 1% lidocaine solution. The artery is palpated with the forefinger and middle finger of one hand, and the needle (we prefer a 'catheter-over-needle device'), is now inserted percutaneously towards the artery. As the needle touches the vessel wall the arterial pulsations are 'damped'; the needle is now advanced further through the wall into the lumen of the artery. As soon as the blood gushes out, the catheter is advanced slowly over the needle, and the needle is then removed. The catheter hub is attached to a continuous flush system ('intraflo') via a pressure tubing. The hub of the catheter should be fixed firmly to the skin, and an antibiotic ointment dressing applied over the point of arterial puncture.

Maintaining tight compression over the puncture site, and proper attention to asepsis will go far in avoiding the two commonest complications of arterial puncture viz. local haematoma formation and infection. Clotting of the catheter can be prevented by using a low-dose continuous heparin infusion.

SUGGESTED READING

Clark VL, Kruse JA. Arterial Catheterization. In: *Critical Care Clinics, Procedures in the ICU*. 1992 (Guest Ed Kruse JA). 8(4), 687–97.

Denys BG, Uretsky BF. Anatomical variations of internal jugular vein location: Impact on central venous access. *Crit Care Med*. 1991; 19, 1516.

ED Brewis RAL, Gibson GJ, Geddes DM, Udaya B, Prakash S. *Respiratory Medicine*. 1994. *Bronchoscopy*. Raven Press, New York.

Goumas P, Kokkinis K, Petrocheilos J, *et al*. Cricothyroidotomy and the anatomy of the cricothyroid space. An autopsy study. *J Laryngol Otol*. 1997; 111: 354–6.

Halsted Residents of the John Hopkins Hospital, Baltimore. In: *Manual of Common Bedside Surgical Procedures*. 1996; (Eds Chen H, Sola J, Lillemoe K). p 20. Williams & Wilkins, USA.

Isaacs JH Jr, Pederson AD. Emergency cricothyroidotomy. *Am Surg*. 1999; 63: 346–9.

Miller KS, Sahn FA. Chest tubes: Indications, technique, management and complications. *Chest*. 1987; 91, 258.

Rosen M, Latto IP, Ng WS. *Handbook of Percutaneous Central Venous Catheterization*. 1981.

Swanson RS, Uhlig PN, Gross PL, *et al*. Emergency intravenous access through the femoral vein. *Ann Emerg Med*. 1984; 13, 244.

Slogoff S, Keats AS, Arlund C. On the safety of radial artery cannulation. *Anesthesiology*. 1983; 59, 42.

WB Saunders Company. London.

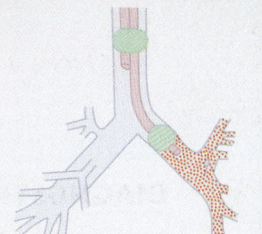

CHAPTER **9**

Cough

One of the commonest symptoms for which a patient seeks advice from the doctor is cough. Cough serves as a protective reflex that protects the lungs against aspiration. It also helps to clear secretions within the respiratory tract. Cough can be voluntary or involuntary. When involuntary it arises from the stimulation of a broad group of rapidly activating irritant receptors (RARs) found in the larynx and tracheobronchial tree. Cough receptors are also present in the pleura, oesophagus, stomach and the external auditory canal.

The RARs can be stimulated by diverse stimuli—mechanical, chemical and inflammatory. Inhalation of dust, smoke, or other irritants is an example of mechanical and chemical stimuli causing cough. A tumour in the airway or extrinsic pressure on the airways or distortion of airways due to pulmonary fibrosis causes mechanical stimulation of the RARs and cough. Mucosal inflammation, as for example in tracheobronchitis, is an example of inflammatory stimuli causing cough.

Another cough receptor present in the respiratory tract is the 'slowly adapting stretch receptor' (SAR) which terminates inspiration and starts expiration after lung inflation has reached an adequate level. These receptors also influence cough. In addition to the above, there exist thin unmyclinated vagal afferents not only in the mucosa of the respiratory tract but also in the alveolar walls. These receptors have been shown to be exquisitely sensitive to chemicals such as capsaicin sand bradykinin.

MECHANISM OF COUGH

Stimulation of cough receptors leads to afferent sensory impulses to the cough centre in the medulla via the vagus, glossopharyngeal, trigeminal and phrenic nerves. The vagus carries impulses from the larynx, trachea, bronchi, pleura, oesophagus and stomach. The glossopharyngeal nerve carries stimuli from the pharynx; the trigeminal from the nose and paranasal sinuses; the phrenic from the pericardium and diaphragm. The stimulated cough centre in the medulla sends impulses through the motor efferents in the cranial nerves, the phrenic nerve and through motor efferents supplying the muscles of the thoracic cage and the accessory muscles of respiration, thereby completing a reflex arc. Cough starts with a rapid inspiration, followed in quick sequence by closure of the glottis, contraction of the muscles of the rib cage and abdominal muscles that leads to a marked rise in pleural and intrapulmonary pressures. There is now a sudden opening of the glottis with a burst of air via the mouth to the outside. The intrathoracic pressure when the glottis is closed can be as high as 100 to 200 mm Hg so that the velocity of airflow through the airways when the glottis opens

is high, propelling secretions upwards to the throat and mouth. The vibrations of the tracheobronchial walls and of secretions present in the airways during the explosive forced expiratory effort are responsible for the sound of a cough.

The effectiveness of cough in propelling secretions depends on the lung volume at which the propulsive expiration is initiated. At high lung volumes (as in healthy individuals) when the 'equal pressure points' are located in the large airways, the propulsive force is large. In patients with small lung volumes the 'equal pressure points' are closer to the alveoli and the propulsive force 'downstream' towards the mouth is feeble. Small lung volumes are particularly observed in critically ill patients or postoperatively after thoracic, cardiovascular or upper abdominal surgery. Retained secretions because of a poor cough in these patients are a cause of atelectasis, which in turn further reduces lung volumes rendering cough even more ineffective.

The cough reflex can be impaired or interrupted at several levels in the reflex pathways. The receptors can be damaged by a lung pathology or their sensitivity diminished by anaesthesia or depressant drugs. The reflex may be dampened by a pathology involving the afferent pathways or through depression of the cough centre by drugs, disease, or raised intracranial pressure, or following involvement of motor efferents and the muscles supplied by the efferents in neuromuscular disease. At times, the nervous reflex arc is intact, but the effector muscles are weak because of a critical illness, electrolyte imbalance, age, debility or poor nutrition. Tracheostomy eliminates glottic closure, thereby leading to reduced intrapulmonary pressure and a comparatively feebler cough.

COMPLICATIONS OF COUGH

Cough when frequent, forceful and prolonged can result in fractures of the ribs, generally the sixth or seventh rib in the mid-axillary line. This can cause severe pain on breathing, more so on coughing. Small hairline fractures of a rib may not be evident on an X-ray of the chest or of the ribs but is always recognized on a computed tomography (CT) of the chest.

Post-tussive syncope is the result of a protracted bout of cough. The syncope ends without sequelae once the cough ceases. It is due to a poor return of blood to the right heart because of marked increase in intrathoracic pressure during the bout of cough. This leads to a sharp fall in cardiac output and syncope. The patients should be instructed to break up the cough into short bouts to prevent post-tussive syncopal attacks.

In older people, particularly in women, severe chronic cough can lead to urinary or even faecal incontinence which can be a source of great social embarrassment.

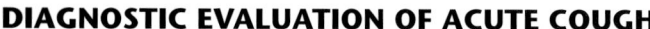

DIAGNOSTIC EVALUATION OF ACUTE COUGH

Diagnostic evaluation is helped by considering cough as acute or chronic. Acute cough starts abruptly and generally resolves within three to four weeks. The diagnosis is apparent from other clinical features associated with acute cough. The common causes are acute pharyngitis, laryngitis, tracheobronchitis either bacterial or viral in origin. Acute allergic rhinitis causing cough is easily recognized by the usual features of rhinitis. More serious causes of acute cough are pneumonia due to bacterial or other microbial infections. Mycoplasmal infection is an important cause of cough. Cough due to mycoplasmal infection is often paroxysmal, either dry or associated with scanty mucoid sputum, and accompanied by flu-like symptoms. Acute asthma may occasionally have cough as the predominant symptom. A careful physical examination will reveal the presence of airways obstruction. An acute exacerbation of chronic obstructive pulmonary disease (COPD) and an acutely evolving pleural effusion are conditions where cough is invariably accompanied by breathlessness and often by tachypnoea. Pulmonary infarction is associated with cough. Pleural pain, pleural effusion and dyspnoea are often associated features, together with a background of possible deep vein thrombosis.

Though acute cough generally ends by three to four weeks, occasionally cough caused by an acute viral infection may persist for a couple of months and is probably related to a temporary hyperreactivity of the airways resulting as a sequel to a viral infection.

Table 9.1:
Important common causes of acute cough

1. Acute upper respiratory tract infections
2. Acute rhinitis
3. Acute sinusitis
4. Asthma
5. Acute exacerbation of COPD
6. Pneumonia; mycoplasmal infection
7. Acute evolving pleural effusion
8. Pulmonary infarction

DIAGNOSTIC EVALUATION OF CHRONIC COUGH

Diagnostic evaluation of a patient with a chronic cough should include a careful history with regard to the nature of cough, whether dry, or productive of mucoid or purulent expectoration, whether there is presence or absence of breathlessness and of associated systemic features. A history of smoking and the number of cigarettes smoked is very important. Though cigarette smoking does often lead to a smoker's cough, a change in the character or intensity of cough always merits further investigation. A history of sinusitis or allergic rhinitis raises the possibility of a post-nasal drip being responsible for cough. Acid regurgitation, heartburn suggests cough related to gastro-oesophageal reflux. Chronic bronchial asthma is associated both with cough, wheeze and breathlessness. A history of haemoptysis warrants a thorough investigation. An easily and often forgotten cause of chronic cough is the use of angiotensin-converting enzyme (ACE) inhibitors. Cough may start soon after the use of these drugs or may commence after several months of use. The cough disappears when the drug is stopped, though it may take two or three weeks for it to disappear completely. An increased concentration of airways cough mediators such as bradykinin and prostaglandin are believed to be responsible for cough in patients who use ACE inhibitors.

The sudden onset of cough related to aspiration of a foreign body should never be forgotten, particularly in a child. Dyspnoea accompanies cough if there is obstruction to the large airways. If the foreign body is small and aspirated deep into the lung, cough is the main symptom. If foreign body aspiration is undiagnosed cough becomes chronic and persistent.

Persistent cough is often the first symptom in tuberculosis and in lung cancer. Cough with purulent expectoration is a feature of suppurative lung diseases such as lung abscess or bronchiectasis. A history of profuse watery or mucoid expectoration is occasionally a feature of alveolar cell carcinoma.

Clinical examination should be meticulous, physical signs pointing to airways obstruction due to asthma, COPD or restrictive lung disease need to be carefully looked out for. The easily recognized dry velcro crackles heard over lung bases are telltale features of interstitial pulmonary fibrosis. A monophonic wheeze suggests obstruction to a large airway. Coarse crackles over the bases in a patient having purulent expectoration suggest bronchiectasis. An examination of the ear, nose, throat and larynx is mandatory.

Investigations should include routine blood tests, an X-ray of the chest and sinuses, sputum examination, including microbiology and cytology, full lung function tests, serial peak flow measurements and if needs be an high-resolution computed tomography (HRCT) chest and bronchoscopy. *It should be remembered that any and every disease involving the lungs, pleura or mediastinum can cause chronic cough.* Almost always, any sinister pathology can ultimately be diagnosed by a careful history, a meticulous physical examination and relevant investigations.

It needs also to be remembered that chronic cough is an equally important symptom in diseases of the cardiovascular system. Chronic left ventricular failure or mitral valvular disease may present with cough, often worse in the sleeping posture, relieved when sitting up. It is generally associated with dyspnoea, but in some patients cough is the predominant symptom. A meticulous examination and investigation of the cardiovascular system is therefore as important as an assessment of the respiratory system if symptoms and clinical features so warrant.

The important and frequent causes of chronic cough almost always diagnosed by careful clinical assessment and relevant investigations are given in Table 9.2.

The diagnostic problem arises when the history and investigations (which include full imaging studies and bronchoscopy) are non-contributory in discovering the aetiology of chronic cough. The patient has generally visited several doctors with no relief. The causes that need special consideration (or reconsideration) are briefly described below.

Cough as a Variant of Asthma

Cough and not wheeze or breathlessness is the hallmark of cough-variant asthma. The airway inflammation in cough-

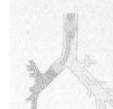

Table 9.2: Causes of chronic cough
Smoking
Asthma, COPD

Chronic pulmonary infection
  – Tuberculosis
  – Bronchitis
  – Bronchiectasis
  – Lung abscess
  – Fungal infections

Occupational lung diseases
  – Pneumoconiosis
  – Asbestosis
  – Byssinosis

Interstitial lung disease
  – Idiopathic interstitial pneumonia
  – Interstitial fibrosis from other causes
  – Infiltrative disorders of the lungs

Granulomatous lung disease   – Sarcoidosis
Foreign body aspiration

Tumours of the lung
  – Bronchogenic carcinoma
  – Alveolar cell carcinoma
  – Other tumours of the lung

Mediastinal pathology
  – Mediastinal tumour
  – Mediastinal lymphadenopathy

Pleural pathology
  – Chronic pleural effusion
  – Mesothelioma

Cardiovascular causes
  – Left ventricular failure
  – Mitral stenosis
  – Pulmonary infarction
  – Aortic aneurysm

Medication-related   – ACE inhibitors

Gastrointestinal causes
  – Gastro-oesophageal reflex
  – Large diaphragmatic hernia

Unexplained cough

Table 9.3: Diagnostic evaluation of chronic cough	
A careful history	Nature of cough, Expectoration, Breathlessness Smoking Sinusitis or allergic rhinitis Acid regurgitation, heartburn Chronic bronchial asthma Haemoptysis Use of ACE inhibitors
Examination	Clubbing ENT examination Physical signs pointing to airways obstruction (prolonged expiration, wheeze) or restrictive lung disease (like dry 'velcro' crackles) Careful assessment of CVS
Investigations	CBC, ESR Radiographic examination of the chest and sinuses Sputum examination Full lung function test Serial peak expiratory flow rates If needed: HRCT chest and bronchoscopy

supportive evidence of this variant of asthma. Finally, even if all diagnostic tests are negative, the diagnosis of cough-variant asthma is confirmed by the improvement of cough following the use of aerosolized bronchodilators and inhaled corticosteroids .

Eosinophilic Bronchitis

Eosinophilic bronchitis is an increasingly recognized entity characterized by heightened cough reflex, sputum eosinophilia, but with no evidence of either variable airflow obstruction or hyperreactive airways. The cough responds to corticosteroid therapy. The airways inflammation in eosinophilic bronchitis is similar to that in bronchial asthma, the difference being that eosinophilic infiltration in eosinophilic bronchitis is chiefly confined to the bronchial epithelium, whereas in asthma it is more concentrated in the bronchial wall and bronchial muscles. Eosinophils in the sputum (induced if necessary by hypertonic saline) are a pointer to the diagnosis. In the absence of any positive findings, a therapeutic trial with corticosteroids is always worthwhile.

Rhinitis—Post Nasal Drip

Many believe that this is perhaps the commonest cause of a chronic innocuous cough in an otherwise healthy individual, where all investigations are negative. Allergy or infection or both can cause a rhinitis with a post-nasal drip which causes an inflammation of the pharynx and larynx stimulating cough receptors which are concentrated in these areas.

Patients often report nasal congestion or 'stuffiness' and examination may reveal secretions dripping or trickling down an inflamed pharyngeal wall. Unfortunately, a drip is not always visible or present at the time of a clinical examination. Nasal polyps may be present together with tenderness over the sinuses. Investigations for rhinitis include nasal endoscopy, X-ray and CT of the paranasal sinuses which may show mucosal

variant asthma is similar to that occurring in patients with usual asthma but there is a markedly heightened cough reflex sensitivity in the former. The cough is generally dry or minimally productive; it may be more marked nocturnally, during stress or on exercise. None of these aggravating factors may however be present. Serial peak flow measurement may show variable airflow limitation or obstruction, but this again is not always elicitable. Spirometry with observed bronchodilator response to an aerosolized bronchodilator are routine tests but in most of these patients these tests are non-contributory. Demonstration of bronchial hypersensitivity by an appropriate bronchoprovocation test is both a sensitive and specific pointer to variable airflow obstruction and may be the only positive test in these patients. Eosinophilia and raised immunoglobulin E (IgE) levels are

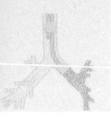

thickening and infected sinuses. An opinion from an ear-nose-throat specialist should always be considered.

Gastro-oesophageal Reflux

There is a bit of dispute as to the frequency of this aetiology in patients with chronic cough. The entity exists but perhaps it is often over-diagnosed when no other cause for cough appears plausible.

Gastro-oesophageal reflux cough is due to relaxation of the oesophageal sphincter with reflux of gastric contents into the oesophagus. Micro-aspiration of oesophageal contents into the tracheobronchial tree and stimulation of the oesophageo-tracheal-bronchial neural reflex are thought to be responsible for cough. Gastro-oesophageal reflux may occur during eating or after a meal, at night during sleep or even in waking hours. Typically, patients complain of heartburn, dysphagia, soreness of the throat or dysphonia but many patients with gastro-oesophageal reflux cough may have no such symptoms. Investigations for gastro-oesophageal reflux include a barium study in the Trendelenburg position which may demonstrate a reflux with or without the presence of a hiatus hernia. Twenty-four-hour oesophageal pH studies have a limited value in the investigation of cough believed to be due to gastro-oesophageal reflux because they are poor predictors of response to therapy. This test however needs to be done if surgery is decided upon to relieve cough believed to be related to the gastro-oesophageal reflux.

Chronic Bronchitis

Chronic bronchitis in a patient who is a cigarette smoker is easily recognized. Yet even if there is no history of smoking, chronic bronchitis causing cough with mucoid sputum is not uncommon in large heavily populated and dreadfully polluted cities of the world, including Mumbai, Delhi, Kolkata and Chennai in India. Exposure to combustion products of bio-fuels like wood and coal is an important cause of bronchitis and COPD in North India and should always be asked for in the history. Cough related to an occupational exposure is often missed if a careful occupational history is not taken.

Bronchiectasis

Some patients with bronchiectasis (generally cylindrical bronchiectasis) have cough but produce little or no sputum. There are generally no physical signs and a radiographic examination of the chest is normal. The diagnosis can be made on an HRCT of the chest.

Aspiration of a Foreign Body

A foreign body aspirated deep into the lung is an important cause of chronic cough. In India, aspiration of a 'supari' can lead to persistent cough with varying degree of inflammation generally in the lower lobe of a lung. A history of possible aspiration may only be given on direct questioning. Often the history is non-contributory. A bronchoscopy generally gives the correct diagnosis, but not always so.

Hyper-reactive Airways Following a Viral Infection

Recovery from acute viral infection can be followed by hyper-reactive airways causing persistent cough lasting for a couple of months. Recovery ensues spontaneously.

Psychogenic cough is often a diagnosis of desperation or despair. The diagnosis should be entertained when cough is markedly worse during periods of stress, when meticulous examination and investigations have excluded all organic disease, when empiric therapy for some of the important causes of chronic cough discussed above has failed and most importantly, when there is a clear background of emotional instability, or an obvious inability to cope with the ordinary or extraordinary stresses present in a patient's life. Even so, it is worth remembering that a patient's attitude and emotional responses may be conditioned by severe chronic persistent cough rather than being responsible for the cough.

Undiagnosed Chronic Cough

Chronic cough remains undiagnosed in 10–20% of patients in spite of full investigations. Various diagnostic labels are given to such patients. The cause of very heightened cough reflex

Table 9.4: Important common causes of chronic cough
Rhinitis with a post-nasal drip
Cough-variant asthma
Eosinophilic bronchitis
Gastro-oesophageal reflux
Post viral due to hyper-reactive airways
ACE inhibitor-related cough
Bronchiectasis (not associated with purulent sputum)
Bronchitis related to smoking, to atmospheric pollution or exposure to biofuels
Foreign body aspiration
Unexplained cough

Note: Any and almost every pulmonary pathology is capable of causing cough. The above causes need to be considered or reconsidered if history, clinical examination and routine investigations draw a blank.

Table 9.5: Specific treatment for chronic cough	
Causes	**Treatment**
Rhinitis	Nasal corticosteroids
GERD-related cough	Use of proton pump inhibitors Lifestyle modifications
ACE inhibitor-induced cough	Stop the drug
Asthma	Inhaled bronchodilators and corticosteroids Oral therapy as needed
Chronic bronchitis	Smoking cessation
Bronchiectasis	Antibiotics, postural drainage

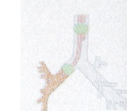

is not understood. Symptomatic treatment with codeine or related drugs or the use of nebulized lidocaine for symptomatic relief may be tried. Reassurance that the patient has no grave or dangerous disease often helps. A trial with inhaled steroids and aerosolized bronchodilators should be given to all patients with unexplained cough as cough-variant asthma responds to this therapy. Empiric treatment for a possible gastro-oesophageal reflux causing unexplained cough may also be tried but more often than not fails.

SUGGESTED READING

Bolser DC. Pharmacologic management of cough. *Otolaryngol Clin North Am.* 1 Feb. 2010; 43(1): 147–55, xi.

Holmes RL. Evaluation of the patient with chronic cough. *Am Fam Physician.* 1 May 2004; 69(9): 2159–66.

Irwin RS. Unexplained Cough in the Adult. *Otolaryngol Clin North Am.* Feb. 2010; 43(1); 167–180.

McGarvey LP. Future Directions in Treating Cough. *Otolaryngol Clin North Am.* Feb. 2010; 43(1); 199–211.

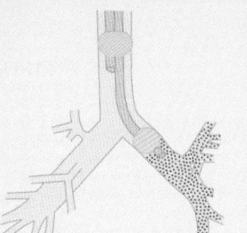

CHAPTER **10** **Haemoptysis**

Haemoptysis is the expectoration of blood, the source of bleeding being below the vocal cords either from the tracheobronchial tree or the lungs. In most cases haemoptysis though frightening to the patient is mild and self-limiting, requiring no treatment other than rest and sedation. In a few instances it is massive, exsanguinating and life-threatening. There is no generally accepted definition of what constitutes massive haemoptysis. Various reports in the literature use different criteria—haemoptysis varying from a mere 100 ml/24 hours to 1000 ml over a period of several days. From the practical point of view, *haemoptysis should be considered massive when it is life-threatening.*

Haemoptysis should be distinguished from blood originating in the nose or throat at or above the larynx. The patient has an urge to clear the throat and brings up blood when he does so. A careful history suggests the source of bleed and a careful examination of the nose and throat by a specialist will clear the diagnosis. Massive haemoptysis may be difficult to distinguish from severe haematemesis. A carefully taken history is again important. A patient can usually tell even when blood is aspirated and then coughed up, whether it originated in the respiratory tract or the upper gastrointestinal (GI) tract. Blood from the respiratory tract is generally bright red, frothy, mixed with sputum and has an alkaline pH. It may contain macrophages laden with hemosiderin. The bloody material brought up in haematemesis is more often dark rather than bright red; may contain food particles and has an acidic pH. In some cases both a bronchoscopy and an upper GI scopy are necessary to ascertain the source of the bleed.

A point worth noting is that the lung has two relatively important sources of blood supply—the pulmonary circulation and the bronchial circulation, so that bleeding with resultant haemoptysis can occur from either of these two vascular beds or from both. Generally speaking, bleeding and haemoptysis due to erosion or rupture of bronchial vessels is brisker and more profuse compared to bleeding from erosion and rupture of pulmonary vessels. This is because the bronchial circulation is part of the systemic vascular bed with a systemic blood pressure which is much higher than the pressure existing in the pulmonary vascular bed.

It is a cardinal principle in medicine that the cause of haemoptysis whether very mild (as with blood-streaked sputum), moderate or severe must be ascertained. At times the cause is evident as for example, haemoptysis in a patient with acute pneumonia or blood streaking of sputum in acute bronchitis. In other instances the cause is not apparent and deserves not only a good history and clinical examination but also more detailed investigations.

Numerous diseases involving the tracheobronchial tree or the lung can cause haemoptysis. There are however, some diseases which do so more commonly and which should therefore engage the clinician's attention. In the developing countries of the world, tuberculosis is by far the commonest cause of haemoptysis, the next most important common causes being bronchiectasis, lung cancer, pulmonary infarction and mitral stenosis. In the West, lung cancer would head the list if the patient was a smoker over the age of 40 to 45 years. Bronchiectasis and pulmonary infarction causing haemoptysis are still common in the West but haemoptysis due to mitral stenosis is decidedly rare.

Other pathologies that need to be kept in mind are pneumonia, lung abscess, aspergillomas, Wegener's granulomatosis and intraalveolar haemorrhage due to vasculitides or autoimmune diseases. It is also important to remember that haemoptysis can occur with acute left ventricular failure as also in coagulopathies or in patients with thrombocytopenia.

We will now briefly discuss the important causes of haemoptysis, followed by an approach to diagnosis and management. The few causes discussed below can be associated with mild, moderate or even life-threatening haemoptysis.

TUBERCULOSIS

Tuberculosis still remains the most important and most frequent cause of massive haemoptysis in India and other developing countries. Haemoptysis may occur in active tuberculous infection of the lung, or may be a sequel to burnt-out disease. Most patients with active tuberculosis who have severe haemoptysis, have cavitative lung disease with acid-fast bacilli present in the sputum. There are several mechanisms of haemoptysis in tuberculosis. These include:

(a) Bronchiolar ulceration with necrosis and rupture of the underlying bronchial vessels in tuberculous pneumonia. Rupture of pulmonary capillaries due to alveolar necrosis may also be an associated feature.

(b) Rupture of an aneurysmal portion of a branch of the pulmonary artery in cavitative tuberculosis. Rupture of a Rasmussen aneurysm is a well-accepted cause of massive haemoptysis in either active tuberculosis, or in patients with prior infection. Pulmonary arteries traversing thick≠-walled cavities develop aneurysmal dilatations due to local inflammation of the vessel wall. These aneurysms herniate and project into the cavity lumen. Sudden transient increase in pulmonary artery pressure, or continued inflammation of the vessel wall can cause rupture of the aneurysm with profuse haemorrhage and haemoptysis.

(c) A healed calcified lymph node at or near the hilum

can press on a bronchus, and erode through a bronchial vessel into the lumen of the airway, resulting in massive haemoptysis. The patient may cough up this calcified node in the form of a broncholith. This may immediately precede haemoptysis, or occur during a bout of haemoptysis.

(d) Haemoptysis can occur due to bronchiectasis which often occurs as a sequel to tuberculosis. Bleeding occurs due to erosion of tortuous, enlarged bronchial vessels, and a profuse anastomosis between the bronchial and pulmonary circulation.

(e) Chronic tuberculous cavities often predispose to the formation of aspergillomas. The latter can produce profuse bleeding.

BRONCHIECTASIS

Bronchiectasis is often associated with bronchial artery hypertrophy, expansion of the peribronchial and submucosal bronchial arterial network, and increased anastomosis between the bronchial and pulmonary circulations. Bleeding can originate from hypertrophied bronchial arteries (under high systemic pressure), or from the submucosal vascular plexus in the bronchiectatic segments.

CARDIOVASCULAR DISORDERS

Mitral stenosis is still an important cause of haemoptysis in developing countries, for rheumatic fever though not as frequent as it was four decades ago, still occurs.

Before the era of valvulotomy and mitral valve replacement, haemoptysis occurred in 9–18% of patients with mitral stenosis. Severe haemoptysis is generally due to rupture of engorged, tortuous, dilated varicose bronchial veins that result as a consequence of an elevated left atrial pressure and passive pulmonary hypertension. In these patients, haemoptysis may be precipitated by respiratory infection, by a bout of coughing, or by an increase in intravascular volume, as seen in pregnancy.

Left ventricular failure causes haemoptysis due to pulmonary congestion. Acute pulmonary oedema is associated with pink frothy sputum.

Pulmonary thromboembolic disease leading to pulmonary infarction often causes haemoptysis, associated with pleuritic pain together with a mild to moderate blood-stained effusion.

Rarely, rupture of an aortic aneurysm into the tracheobronchial tree leads to massive haemoptysis and death.

BRONCHOGENIC CARCINOMA AND OTHER TUMOURS

These very rarely cause massive or life-threatening haemoptysis. Haemoptysis in a smoker beyond 40–45 years should arouse suspicion of a bronchogenic carcinoma. Haemoptysis is rarely massive and is generally characterized by blood-tinged sputum or sputum mixed with blood. Haemoptysis may be the presenting symptom in 10% of patients or it may accompany or be preceded by cough and vague chest discomfort. Haemo-

ptysis in lung cancer can also be due to pneumonia distal to bronchial obstruction. Haemoptysis is an uncommon feature of metastatic carcinoma as these lesions generally do not involve the airways.

Carcinoids in the lung can cause haemoptysis which at times may be life-threatening and difficult to control.

LUNG ABSCESS

Bleeding occurs in 20–50% of patients with lung abscess. It is related to necrotizing inflammation of the lung parenchyma eroding bronchial and pulmonary vessels.

MYCETOMAS

Mycetomas are fungal balls occurring in patients with pre-existing cavitary lung disease. They are most frequently seen in tuberculous cavities, but have been reported in cavitary disease secondary to sarcoidosis, lung abscess, cavitary carcinoma, bronchiectasis, bullous emphysema, and pulmonary infarction. The most frequent mycetoma is an aspergilloma. The cause of massive bleeding in a mycetoma is disputed. Vascular injury by aspergillus-associated endotoxin, aspergillus-related proteolytic activity, and a Type III-related hypersensitivity reaction, have all been postulated.

TRAUMA

Blunt or penetrating injury to the chest can cause haemoptysis. Steering wheel injuries can cause a rupture of the tracheobronchial tree causing both haemoptysis and pneumothorax.

After a pneumonectomy, a large haemothorax may open into the tracheobronchial tree causing life-threatening haemoptysis. Drainage of the haemothorax with surgical repair of the tear in the bronchus is needed as an emergency measure.

AUTOIMMUNE DISEASES

Intraalveolar haemorrhage can result from Wegener's granulomatosis, other forms of vasculitides, Goodpasture's syndrome and autoimmune connective tissue disorders. The presenting features are haemoptysis, alveolar infiltrates on the X-ray, dyspnoea and hypoxemia. The degree of haemoptysis need not always be a guide to the severity of intraalveolar haemorrhage.

IATROGENIC HAEMOPTYSIS

This is a potential complication of bronchoscopy, transthoracic needle biopsy, or the use of a Swan-Ganz catheter.

Rupture of the pulmonary artery is the most catastrophic complication following the use of the Swan-Ganz catheter; it carries a mortality of 50% due to massive pulmonary haemorrhage. This complication is more frequently observed in patients with pulmonary hypertension.

VASCULAR ANOMALIES

Arteriovenous malformations may rarely cause fatal haemoptysis.

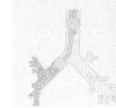

Table 10.1:
Important causes of life-threatening haemoptysis
• Tuberculosis
• Bronchiectasis
• Bronchogenic carcinoma , Carcinoid tumours
• Lung abscess
• Pulmonary infarction
• Cardiovascular diseases—Mitral stenosis, Left ventricular failure
• Mycetomas
• Trauma
• Iatrogenic haemoptysis—following bronchoscopy, Swan-Ganz catheterization or transthoracic needle biopsy
• Autoimmune disorders, Wegener's granulomatosis, Goodpasture's syndrome
• Vascular anomalies
• Cryptogenic haemoptysis

Table 10.2:
Investigations for haemoptysis
1. CBC, ESR, platelet count
2. Sputum examination—microbiological examination including culture for AFB
3. X-ray chest, if necessary HRCT chest
4. Bronchoscopy
5. Other relevant blood tests if there is a suspicion for vasculitides, autoimmune disease, connective tissue disease

Table 10.3:
Investigations for massive haemoptysis
1. X-ray chest
2. HRCT chest
3. Fiberoptic bronchoscopy
4. Angiography of the bronchial and pulmonary circulation to locate site of bleed

CRYPTOGENIC HAEMOPTYSIS

About 15% of patients with haemoptysis even after extensive investigation, have no detectable cause of their haemoptysis, and are labelled as cryptogenic haemoptysis. Patients with cryptogenic bleeds generally stop bleeding spontaneously, and require only supportive care. A periodic follow-up is mandatory in these patients.

DIAGNOSTIC EVALUATION

Diagnostic evaluation requires a careful history, a meticulous physical examination, routine blood counts and an X-ray of the chest. Sputum should be sent for microbiological examination and cytology. Culture for acid-fast bacilli should always be done.

When haemoptysis has been severe, blood may well have been aspirated into the opposite lung so that an X-ray of the chest may be misleading.

Brisk haemoptysis also warrants an urgent fiberoptic bronchoscopy to determine the site of the bleed and perhaps also help in management.

A high-resolution computed tomography (HRCT) of the chest is often rewarding though aspirated blood can cast ground-glass shadows in different parts of the same or opposite lung.

The presence of intraalveolar haemorrhage warrants tests for Goodpasture's syndrome, antineutrophilic cytoplasmic antibodies (ANCA) test for Wegener's granulomatosis and for microscopic polyarteritis. A suspicion of connective tissue disorders would dictate tests such as antinuclear antibody test and other relevant tests that may be deemed necessary. A suspicion of a coagulopathy would require a coagulation profile.

The intensity of the search for haemoptysis will depend on the circumstances and clinical probabilities in a given case. An obvious tuberculous lesion on an X-ray of the chest will require no test other than a complete sputum examination.

Haemoptysis due to a lobar pneumonia in a young adult needs no specific test. But if the cause is not determined by basic tests such as X-ray chest, and sputum examination, a thorough investigation is mandatory.

MANAGEMENT

Most often haemoptysis ceases on its own and all that is needed is rest and mild sedation. A fall in haemoglobin below 9 gm/dl and a fall in the haematocrit below 30% particularly in an older individual merits transfusion of packed RBCs. The problem therefore in most patients is not with management but with unravelling the cause when the cause is not apparent.

However, massive life-threatening haemoptysis is a difficult management problem. The first principle is to secure the airway, for death in the majority of patients with massive haemoptysis is not due to exsanguination but due to asphyxia produced by blood aspirated in both lungs. These patients invariably need ventilatory support. If the site of the bleeding is known, it is best to posture the patient so that the bleeding site is in the dependent position. This reduces the risk of aspiration. An urgent bronchoscopy is a must. More often than not, the bleeding site cannot be determined because of the blood in the tracheobronchial tree. If however the site of bleeding can be identified, therapeutic measures such as lavage with ice-cold saline, application of topical epinephrine, or the placement of a balloon catheter to isolate a segment or a lobe which is bleeding may be attempted.

If the bleeding site is not identified or if the bleed continues in spite of the measures stated above, it is best to do an angiography of both the brachial and pulmonary circulations to identify and embolize the bleeding vessel or vessels.

If this measure also fails the only option is surgical exploration to control the bleed. Obviously the mortality and morbidity in such desperate situations is extremely high.

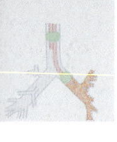

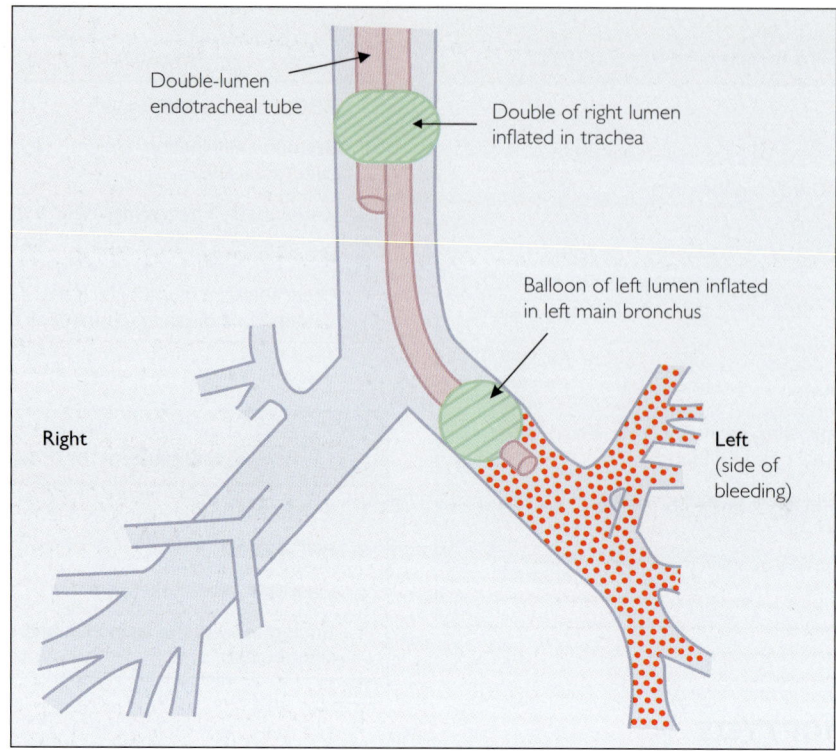

Fig 10.1: Schematic representation of proper placement of a left-sided double-lumen endotracheal tube. The inflated balloon in the trachea allows ventilation of the right lung. The inflated balloon in the left main bronchus prevents spill-over of blood from left into right side.

SUGGESTED READING

Bidwell JL. Hemoptysis: diagnosis and management. *Am Fam Physician*. 1 Oct. 2005; 72(7): 1253–60.

Corder R. Hemoptysis. *Emerg Med Clin North Am*. 1 May 2003; 21(2): 421–35.

Goh P, Lin M, *et al*. Embolization for hemoptysis: a six-year review. *Cardiovasc Intervent Radiool*. 2002; 17–25.

Udwadia FE. *Principles of Critical Care*. Second edition, Oxford University Press. pp 301–7.

CHAPTER **11** **Dyspnoea**

Dyspnoea is the uncomfortable awareness of the act of breathing. Dyspnoea is often referred to by the patient as 'breathlessness' or 'shortness of breath'. It is a worrying symptom, prompting the patient to seek medical attention. Dyspnoea may be accompanied by tachypnoea (faster rate of breathing than normal) but not necessarily so. Being subjective the sensation of discomfort associated with dyspnoea may be interpreted differently by different patients. Some, in particular asthmatics, interpret dyspnoea as a feeling of tightness in the chest; others complain of respiratory distress; still others interpret it as a feeling of suffocation. Despite this variability, dyspnoea invariably implies discomfort during breathing.

The physiological mechanism underlying dyspnoea is complex and not completely understood. The sensation of dyspnoea has two components—the first component is the sensory input to the cerebral cortex. The sensory input consists of information derived from several specialized sensory end-receptors. Specialized mechano-receptors are present in the respiratory tract—particularly in the trachea, larynx and large upper airways. Important receptors are also present in the lung parenchyma—the J receptors which are stimulated by stretch and which initiate sensory inputs carried by the vagus nerves to the brain. Sensory inputs are also received from respiratory muscles, the chest wall and from chemoreceptors sensitive to lack of oxygen (a low PaO_2) or to an increase in the $PaCO_2$. Additional sensory inputs not clearly understood may well arise following inadequate oxygen delivery or poor oxygen utilization. These numerous sensory inputs are processed at the spinal level and then at the supraspinal level before they reach the sensorimotor cortex. There is however no specific area in the sensorimotor cortex which is a special locus for dyspnoea. The second component is the perception and interpretation of these sensory inputs arriving at the sensorimotor cortex. The interpretation of perceived information in the sensorimotor cortex varies so that the subjective feeling of discomfort during breathing that constitutes dyspnoea may be interpreted and expressed in different ways and perhaps more importantly in different degrees by different patients.

In clinical practice one comes across some patients who complain of little or no dyspnoea even though they suffer from an underlying disease which if present in others invariably causes significant dyspnoea. The reason for this is unclear. Either for some reason they have a blunting or reduction of sensory inputs to the sensorimotor cortex of the brain, or the perception is inadequate so that the interpretation of what is perceived is not enough to produce the expected degree of discomfort on breathing. This is observed in some patients with severe asthma who may complain of little or no discomfort as also in some patients with significant left heart failure who do not (even on direct questioning) complain of dyspnoea.

CLINICAL OVERVIEW

When patients come with a history of breathlessness on exertion the two most likely causes are a disorder of the cardiovascular system or of the respiratory system. A good history is of immense help. Is the dyspnoea on exertion and if so what is the degree of exertion that causes dyspnoea? Does it occur at rest? Is there an associated wheeze and/cough? Is it related to posture? Is it accompanied by substernal or precordial discomfort? Are there any other associated symptoms? These are some of the many questions that need to be asked. A broad differential diagnosis of some important causes of dyspnoea is tabled below.

Table 11.1: Broad differential diagnosis of important causes of dyspnoea
1. Airways obstruction, airflow limitation Bronchial asthma, COPD, bronchiolitis, intrinsic or extrinsic obstruction to large airways
2. Restrictive lung pathology Interstitial lung diseases Parenchymal lung diseases; pulmonary oedema Diseases involving the pleura, chest wall
3. Airways obstruction + restrictive lung lesion
4. Cardiovascular causes Left heart failure, mitral stenosis Pulmonary hypertension Cardiomyopathies Pericardial effusion Congenital heart disease
5. Pulmonary thromboembolic disease
6. Non-cardiorespiratory causes Anaemia, thyrotoxicosis, neuromuscular disease, skeletal thoracic abnormalities, psychogenic

Pulmonary causes of dyspnoea broadly fall into three categories:
1. Diseases causing airways obstruction
2. Disease causing a restrictive lung lesion
3. A combination of both obstruction + restriction

DISEASES CAUSING AIRWAYS OBSTRUCTION

The two most frequent diseases causing dyspnoea related to airways obstruction are bronchial asthma and chronic obstructive pulmonary disease (COPD). The clinical description of these

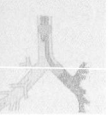

two diseases as also the detailed clinical features of airways obstruction are dealt with at length in separate chapters.

The diagnosis both from the history and physical examination is generally easy. Asthma at least in the early part of its natural history is episodic, though in late severe asthma dyspnoea may be present not only on exertion but even at rest so that it may resemble COPD. Very occasionally, asthma may present with dyspnoea on exertion with no obvious physical findings at rest. Bronchial hypersensitivity can however be demonstrated on appropriate testing. Also, in these patients there is a clear fall in peak flows if measured during the period of breathlessness perceived on exertion.

COPD is a chronic inflammatory progressive disease of the lung chiefly related to cigarette smoking. It is characterized by progressive airflow limitation with incomplete reversibility. Patients with COPD also have a disturbance in the mechanics of breathing, increased lung volumes and a disturbance in gas exchange.

An interesting observation is that some patients with well-marked COPD seem to breathe easily, not complaining of much dyspnoea. These patients (termed blue bloaters) retain carbon dioxide (CO_2) and suffer mainly from chronic bronchitis. Others with the same degree of COPD and with a similar disturbance in lung function are severely dyspnoec and manage to keep the $PaCO_2$ within normal limits. These patients suffer chiefly from emphysema and are termed pink puffers. It is now recognized that most patients with COPD have a mixture of bronchitis and emphysema in varying degrees. The pathogenesis of CO_2 retention has been discussed at length in the chapter on COPD.

One of the important signs of airways obstruction is the presence of a prolonged expiration associated with an expiratory wheeze. The tighter the airways obstruction, the more difficult it is to appreciate a wheeze. The wheeze may indeed be inaudible in patients with COPD obtunded as a result of CO_2 narcosis. It is important to ask the patient to make a forced expiratory manoeuvre to elicit a tight high-pitched expiratory wheeze. Similarly, the more severe an attack of acute asthma, the poorer the breath sounds with little or no wheeze.

Besides asthma and COPD, airways obstruction causing dyspnoea is seen in obstruction to the upper large airways (foreign body, tracheal stenosis, laryngeal stenosis, tumour partially obstructing a large airway, and extrinsic pressure on large airways).

Airways obstruction with dyspnoea is also seen in bronchiolitis, bronchiolitis obliterans, cystic fibrosis (rare in India but common in Western countries), bronchiectasis and some rare infiltrative and granulomatous diseases such as Langerhan's cell histiocytosis and pulmonary lymphangioleiomyomatosis. In children airways obstruction causing dyspnoea is more often due to epiglottitis, acute tracheolaryngitis, and foreign body inhalation. Asthma remains an important cause of dyspnoea in children and adults.

Restrictive Lung Disease

Restrictive lung lesions are typically exemplified by interstitial lung disease which indeed has many causes. The most classic is interstitial pneumonia of unknown aetiology. Increasing breathlessness with progressive hypoxia, at first on exertion and then even at rest is a feature of this disease. An early sign is the presence of end-inspiratory dry velcro crackles at the bases of both lungs which may precede the complaint of breathlessness on exertion. As the disease progresses and breathlessness increases, velcro crackles gradually extend upwards to ultimately involve the whole back and even the front of the chest. The lung functions are characterized by a restrictive defect—small lung volumes, a reduced total lung capacity, normal expiratory flow rates and a reduced diffusion capacity. The latter may be the first lung function defect to be observed in early interstitial lung disease.

Restrictive lung disease with dyspnoea can occur with any significant parenchymal pathology such as pneumonia, atelectasis, noncardiogenic pulmonary oedema or a pleural pathology such as pleural effusion or a pneumothorax.

Paralysis of both domes of the diaphragm whatever the aetiology can lead to marked dyspnoea. The patient is unable to lie flat for even a minute, becoming increasingly cyanosed and distressed. Breathing and oxygen saturation both improve when the patient is made to sit up at a right angle. The above complication is occasionally observed after major thoracic or cardiovascular surgery and is related to injury to the phrenic nerves.

A number of patients have a combination of airways obstruction + a restrictive lung lesion. Dyspnoea on exertion and in severe disease even at rest is a frequent complaint. Important diseases causing both airways obstruction and a restrictive lung lesion are listed in the accompanying table.

Table 11.2: Examples of obstructive + restrictive lung pathologies
1. Bronchiectasis
2. Extensive or burnt-out tuberculosis
3. Sarcoidosis
4. Tropical eosinophilia
5. Extrinsic allergic alveolitis (some patients)
6. Inhalation injuries to the lung involving injury to bronchioles and lung parenchyma
7. Interstitial lung disease associated with small airways obstruction
8. Langerhan's cell histiocytosis
9. Lymphangioleiomyomatosis

Cardiovascular Disease

Cardiovascular disease is an important cause of dyspnoea. Acute left ventricular failure causes acute pulmonary oedema and acute dyspnoea. Chronic left heart failure causes chronic pulmonary congestion and chronic dyspnoea.

Dyspnoea due to left heart disease can be equated to pulmonary congestion and for clinical understanding is best expressed thus:

Dyspnoea on exertion ≅ pulmonary congestion ≅ LV failure
on exertion on exertion

Dyspnoea at rest ≅ pulmonary congestion ≅ left ventricular
at rest failure at rest

Paroxysmal noctural ≅ sudden pulmonary ≅ acute LV failure
dyspnoea congestion at night at night

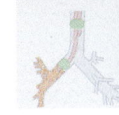

Orthopnoea ≅ pulmonary congestion ≅ Improved LV failure
relieved in sitting on sitting up;
posture, worse on aggravated on lying
lying down down

A good history and a good clinical examination should make a cardiac cause for dyspnoea apparent. A background of heart disease, an enlarged heart, diastolic gallop, relevant auscultatory murmurs and crackles at both bases of the lung are telltale features that allow a correct diagnosis. Congestive heart failure is manifested by increased jugular venous pressure, enlarged tender liver, pitting oedema of the feet. Pleural effusion (a transudate), generally right-sided may also be present. Relevant investigations may further give the nature of the cardiac ailment.

An important clinical observation is that in some patients, acute left ventricular failure presents with paroxysmal dyspnoea but instead of the usual crackles there are rhonchi and wheezes all over the chest. This presentation is rightly termed cardiac asthma and needs to be distinguished from bronchial asthma. The presence of background cardiac disease should always arouse suspicion of left ventricular failure. Left heart failure is also the diagnosis in the presence of an enlarged heart or abnormal auscultatory cardiac findings. It is of relevance that when a patient with bronchial asthma or COPD for any reason develops left heart disease and goes into acute left ventricular failure, the presentation is more often with rhonchi and wheezes over the chest than the usual pulmonary crackles. X-ray of the chest may reveal pulmonary oedema but this may not be easily detectable in a patient having large lungs due to longstanding asthma or COPD.

An extremely important cardiovascular condition that can present with breathlessness—generally of acute or subacute onset—is pulmonary thromboembolic disease. The only symptom may be dyspnoea and indeed there may be no physical signs whatsoever. A ghastly mistake of dubbing such a patient as functional is often made. A correct diagnosis always rests on an acute awareness of this entity. A background history such as a long flight or hours of travel in a car or train, or the use of oral contraceptives in a young female, should always arouse suspicion. Even a slight suspicion should prompt the physician to ask for a D-dimmer level, a Doppler of the lower limbs and an high-resolution computed tomography (HRCT) pulmonary angiography. The subject of pulmonary embolism is discussed at length in a separate chapter.

Pulmonary hypertension, in particular idiopathic pulmonary hypertension causing dyspnoea, is one other entity where the diagnosis is missed unless physical signs for pulmonary hypertension are sought and confirmed by 2D echocardiographic study.

Diseases other than cardiopulmonary pathologies producing dyspnoea should also be kept in mind. These include severe anaemia, neuromuscular disease causing weakness of the intercostals and/or diaphragm, myasthenia gravis, thyrotoxicosis, and skeletal abnormalities preventing proper expansion of the rib cage (ankylosing spondylitis, kyphoscolitic deformity). Dyspnoea on exertion is also complained by patients who are physically unfit through lack of activity and exercise and by obese individuals.

Dyspnoea due to anxiety (psychogenic dyspnoea) is typically characterized by sighing breathing, by hyperventilation which may lead to a washout of CO_2 causing carpopedal spasm and even a fainting episode. Tachycardia and inversion of T waves on electrocardiography (ECG) during the episode may lead to a wrong diagnosis of a cardiac disease.

Metabolic acidosis, either diabetic ketoacidosis or metabolic acidosis from any other cause produces deep breaths (Kussmaul's breathing) with or without an increase in the respiratory rate. Usually, the patient does not complain of any discomfort

Table 11.3: Diagnostic tests in the investigation of dyspnoea		
Tests	**Abnormalities detected**	**Possible diagnosis**
Basic blood tests	Leucocytosis; low haemoglobin	Infection, anaemia
ABG	Low pH; low PaO_2	Acidosis; respiratory alkalosis; hypoxia
BNP	Elevated BNP	Heart failure
X-ray chest	Abnormalities in lung fields, cardiac silhouette, pleura, mediastinum	COPD, interstitial lung disease, infiltrative lung disease; cardiac disease; mediastinal pathology, pleural disease, pneumothorax
Spirometry, lung volumes	Obstructive pattern Restrictive pattern	Airways obstruction; restrictive lung pathology
CO diffusion	Decreased	Interstitial lung disease, pulmonary vascular disease
	Increased	Alveolar haemorrhage
HRCT chest	Various abnormalities e.g. ground-glass shadows, alveolar shadows, interstitial shadows, centrilobular emphysema, mass lesions, obstruction to central airways	Depends on nature of abnormalities present
HRCT pulmonary angiography	Filling defects or defects in pulmonary arteries	Pulmonary embolism
Fiberoptic bronchoscopy	Obstruction to airways	Tumour, foreign body, extrinsic pressure
Biopsy-fibreoptic CT-guided video-assisted thoracoscopy		Biopsy results may confirm tumour and nature of lung disease

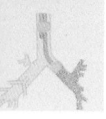

during breathing. Diabetic ketoacidosis has the typical smell of ketones in the breath, while uremic acidosis is associated with an ammonical smell in the breath.

In conclusion, the differential diagnosis and a final diagnosis of dyspnoea can be arrived at by a history, physical examination and relevant investigations which include blood tests, X-ray chest, lung function studies, HRCT of the chest and if the need arises fibreoptic bronchoscopy and biopsy to establish a histopathological diagnosis.

A clinical approach to the symptoms of dyspnoea in a patient is to determine whether it is acute or chronic. Acute onset dyspnoea has certain important likely aetiologies, chronic progressive dyspnoea is generally due to another group of causes. Causes of acute and chronic dyspnoea are listed below.

The important causes of acute dyspnoea in an adult are acute left ventricular failure, bronchial asthma, pneumothorax, acute pneumonia, and acute pulmonary thromboembolism. Atelectasis of a lobe or lung generally from secretions obstructing a bronchus is an important cause of acute dyspnoea frequently observed in the critical care unit.

In children acute dyspnoea is more often due to upper airways obstruction—acute viral epiglottitis, laryngitis, acute laryngotracheobronchitis, and foreign body obstructing a bron-chus. Acute bronchiolitis, pneumonia, bronchopneumonia are other important causes of dyspnoea in children.

Chronic progressive dyspnoea in adults is most often due to COPD, longstanding severe asthma, cardiac dysfunction leading to chronic left ventricular failure and interstitial lung disease. In the elderly there may well be both pulmonary and cardiac components to chronic progressive dyspnoea and the degree of contribution to dyspnoea by each of these components may be difficult to determine.

Pleural effusion if acute can cause acute dyspnoea; a slow accumulation of pleural fluid will cause progressive dyspnoea extending over a longer period of time. Progressively worsening anaemia is an important cause of gradually increasing dyspnoea.

Less common causes of chronic progressive dyspnoea are pulmonary hypertension and chronic pulmonary thromboembolic disease. Upper airways obstruction (e.g. tracheal stenosis) or subglottic stenosis or a tumour obstructing a large airway or extrinsic pressure on a large airway causing dyspnoea can be misdiagnosed as bronchial asthma.

Psychogenic dyspnoea has acute exacerbations but can become chronic if unrecognized and not appropriately managed. Thyrotoxicosis and neuromuscular disease are comparatively uncommon causes that should be kept in mind as they occasionally present with chronic progressive dyspnoea.

Table 11.4: Important causes of acute and chronic dyspnoea	
Acute dyspnoea **In adults**	**Chronic (often progressive) dyspnoea** **In adults**
Acute episodes of bronchial asthma Acute left ventricular failure Acute exacerbation of COPD Spontaneous pneumothorax Pneumonia Pulmonary embolism Massive atelectasis Acutely evolving pleural effusion Foreign body aspiration A partial obstruction to a large airway Intra-alveolar haemorrhage Trauma to the chest wall and intrathoracic structures	COPD Chronic left ventricular failure Asthma Interstitial pneumonia Interstitial fibrosis Slowly evolving pleural effusion Chronic pulmonary thromboembolic disease Pulmonary hypertension Slowly progressive upper airways obstruction (subglottic stenosis, tracheal stenosis, tumour obstructing a large airway, extrinsic pressure on a large airway) Anaemia Thyrotoxicosis Neuromuscular disease Psychogenic dyspnoea
In children	
Upper airways obstruction due to epiglottitis, laryngitis, tracheobronchitis, foreign body, pneumonia, bronchiolitis	

SUGGESTED READING

Karnani NG. Evaluation of chronic dyspnea. *Am Fam Physician.* 15 Apr. 2005; 71(8): 1529–37.

Mahler DA. Evaluation of dyspnea in the elderly. *Clin Geriatr Med.* 1 Feb. 2003; 19(1): 19–33, v.

Manning HL, Schwartzstein RM: Pathophysiology of dyspnoea. *NEJM.* 1995; 333:1547–53.

Thomas JR. Clinical management of dyspnoea. *Lancet Oncol.* 1 Apr. 2002; 3(4): 223–8.

CHAPTER **12** # Chest Pain or Discomfort

Thoracic pain or discomfort, a common complaint in patients with respiratory problems is equally common or perhaps even more common in several pathologies not involving the lungs, the pleura or the conducting airways. It is therefore vital for the chest physician to be also aware of the important causes of chest pain arising from sources outside the respiratory system. This section gives an overall perspective of some important causes of chest discomfort or pain.

CARDIOVASCULAR CAUSES

The first principle in the evaluation of chest pain, particularly precordial or substernal pain is to determine whether the pain is related to myocardial ischemia or infarction. Ischemic cardiac pain or the pain of myocardial infarction is often described as substernal heaviness, vicelike, crushing in character. It is the character rather than the severity which is more important for a correct diagnosis. Pricking pain, stabbing pain, pain localized at or below the nipple, pain associated with local tenderness is unlikely to be cardiac pain. Typically, cardiac pain radiates to the left shoulder and arm, sometimes to both shoulders and arms and often to the jaw and to the back. Clinical examination, serial electrocardiography (ECG) tracings and an estimation of cardiac enzymes help in diagnosis.

Pericarditis can cause precordial pain aggravated by breathing. The pain is generally accompanied by a pericardial rub and is often relieved on sitting up. Signs of a pericardial effusion may be evident on clinical examination, or on an X-ray of the chest and an echocardiography.

Aortic dissection is the cause of severe pain generally starting in the back, but is also felt in the front of the chest. Unequal pulses, reduced pulsations in the lower limbs, systolic murmur at the base often transmitted to the neck, an audible bruit over the back, are some of the important clinical findings. Patients generally are hypertensive to start with, yet appear to be in shock. The ECG is normal or shows non-specific changes; the diagnosis is confirmed by computed tomography (CT) or magnetic resonance imaging (MRI) of the chest.

PLEURITIC CHEST PAIN

Pleuritic chest pain is due to inflammation and oedema of the parietal pleura. It is worse on inspiration, coughing and is described as sharp or knife-like in character. It is generally localized but can be felt across the chest along the distribution of the intercostal nerves that supply the affected area of the pleura. Inflammation of the pleura over the central portion of the diaphragm leads to pain referred to the shoulder, while inflammation of the pleura over the lateral portion of the diaphragm is referred to the abdomen. Pleuritic pain is generally but not always associated with a pleural rub. Systemic features such as fever, malaise are generally present.

Pulmonary infarction can cause localized pleural pain. Systemic features may be absent and a pleural rub is not necessarily present.

SUBSTERNAL PAIN ASSOCIATED WITH ACUTE TRACHEOBRONCHITIS

Acute tracheobronchitis is often associated with a burning or a searing substernal soreness and pain, aggravated by coughing.

PULMONARY HYPERTENSION

Pulmonary hypertension can produce pain indistinguishable from angina on effort. In fact this pain is truly anginal, caused by ischemia to the right ventricle. Anginal pain can also be caused by a fixed very low cardiac output due to the severity of pulmonary hypertension.

Massive pulmonary embolism can cause substernal chest pain indistinguishable from myocardial infarction.

CHEST WALL PAIN

Chest wall pain which is not pleuritic and which does not arise from myocardial ischemia, infarction, or pericarditis, or any other cardiopulmonary problem, may have a musculoskeletal origin. Musculoskeletal pain like pleuritic pain is also aggravated on inspiration. The pain worsens on palpating the painful area.

Acute severe pain localized over one or more ribs in the mid-axillary line is most often seen following cough fractures of these ribs. A crepitus may be felt and imaging studies reveal the fracture.

More serious causes of chest pain are related to tumour deposits in the ribs or spine or local invasion of the thoracic cage from a lung cancer or from soft tissue tumours invading the thoracic cage.

Pancoast's tumour (superior sulcus tumour) described by Pancoast in 1932 causes pain localized to the ipsilateral shoulder radiating along the distribution of the eighth cervical and first thoracic nerves. The condition is often mistaken for shoulder arthritis or cervical spondylitis. The tumour causes Horner's syndrome due to involvement of the sympathetic trunk on the affected side and wasting of the small muscles of the hand if the first thoracic nerve root is infiltrated or compressed by the tumour. An X-ray of chest shows a circumscribed soft tissue shadow at the apex with destruction of C7, T1, T2 vertebrae together with their transverse processes.

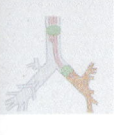

Vague chest discomfort or pain is a frequent complaint of patients with lung cancer and of patients with a mediastinal tumour or a mediastinal mass lesion.

MISCELLANEOUS CAUSES

Peptic oesophagitis with oesophageal spasm can cause substernal pain which may be difficult to distinguish from ischemic myocardial pain.

Cervical spondylitis can also cause pain over the precordium and in one or both upper limbs mimicking myocardial ischemia.

Tubercle of the spine, metastatic lesions in the spine, and spinal cord tumours can cause referred pain to the chest.

Severe unilateral chest pain over a localized area encircling the chest may precede the typical segmental vesicular rash of herpes zoster.

Chest pain is not an uncommon symptom of underlying anxiety. It may be associated with other features of an anxiety state, like hyperventilation, tachycardia, and sweating. The pain often shifts or if fixed is often located at or below the nipple. Clinical examination is normal and basic investigations reveal no abnormality.

Table 12.1: Important causes of chest discomfort /pain

Cardiovascular causes
    Ischemic cardiac pain
    Pericarditis
    Aortic dissection

Pulmonary embolism
Pleuritic chest pain, pulmonary infarction
Substernal pain associated with acute tracheobronchitis
Pulmonary Hypertension

Chest Wall Pain
    Musculoskeletal pain
    Fracture of ribs
    Tumour deposits in the ribs or spine
    Lung cancer, mediastinal mass lesions
    Pancoast's tumour

Miscellaneous Causes
    Peptic oesophagitis with oesophageal spasm
    Cervical spondylitis
    Tubercle of the spine, metastatic lesions in the spine, spinal chord tumours
    Herpes zoster
    Anxiety

SUGGESTED READING

Boie ET. Initial evaluation of chest pain. *Emerg Med Clin North Am.* 1 Nov. 2005; 23(4): 937–57.

Butler KH. Chest pain: a clinical assessment. *Radiol Clin North Am.* 1 Mar. 2006; 44(2): 165–79, vii.

Cayley WE Jr. Diagnosing the cause of chest pain. *Am Fam Physician.* 15 Nov. 2005; 72(10): 2012–21.

Eslick GD. Noncardiac chest pain: evaluation and treatment. *Gastroenterol Clin North Am.* 1 Jun. 2003; 32(2): 531–52.

Kelly BS. Evaluation of the elderly patient with acute chest pain. *Clin Geriatr Med.* 1 May 2007; 23(2): 327–49, vi.

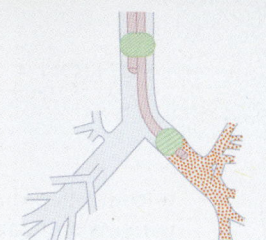

CHAPTER **13** **Clinical Examination of the Respiratory System**

A detailed history and a meticulous physical examination are vital for a thorough assessment of a patient with respiratory disease or for that matter any disease. Unfortunately, with the tremendous advance of science and technology and the advent of sophisticated gadgetry and gleaming machines, the art and science of history-taking and physical examination are sadly neglected. Instead of being in the forefront of a clinical approach, they are increasingly relegated to the background. An evaluation of a patient with symptoms pertaining to the respiratory system can never be complete and correct without a good history and a thorough physical examination. A radiographic examination of the chest is almost an extension of a physical examination in a patient with chest disease. This is because a radiographic examination of the chest can reveal serious disease when physical examination even by an experienced clinician draws a blank. Witness for example, the 'uncovering' of a tuberculous infiltrate or cavity or the presence of a lung cancer or mediastinal adenopathy by a radiographic examination of the chest in a patient who may essentially have no abnormal physical signs. Yet physical examination may uncover features which are not evident on a radiographic examination of the chest. For example, the presence of a pleural or pericardial rub heard on auscultation, or the presence of polyphonic wheezes signifying airways obstruction, or a monophonic wheeze signifying obstruction to a large airway are important clinical findings that cannot be detected by a radiographic examination of the chest. The history, physical examination and chest radiography complement each other to help arrive at a correct diagnosis. Though an X-ray of the chest is mandatory in most patients with persistent respiratory symptoms, its use as a screening procedure to uncover early disease which is treatable (for example, early cancer) has not been shown to improve mortality and is therefore of dubious value. Even so, a routine health check-up in almost all centres of the world includes an X-ray of the chest. The use of high-resolution computed tomography (HRCT) of the chest as a screening procedure is also of unproven benefit.

When the triad of history, physical examination and radiography of the chest fails to give a diagnosis, further sophisticated tests can be availed of. However, an approach that focuses primarily on these tests is bad medicine.

HISTORY

There is no substitute for a good history. Cough, and breathlessness or shortness of breath are the two most common symptoms in respiratory diseases. Less frequent complaints are haemoptysis and chest discomfort. A detailed history of each of these symptoms is rewarding. The association of systemic features like fever, weight loss, and joint pains is also of crucial importance and may be elicited only on direct questioning. An occupational history may give the clue to a diagnosis. For example, exposure to asbestos may have occurred several years back, yet the respiratory disease of the present may well be linked to this exposure. Improvement of symptoms over a weekend or on holidays may suggest symptoms related to an occupational exposure. Residence for a short period in India or in other tropical climes may suggest pulmonary problems endemic in these climes. For people living in India, history of temporary residence in a part of the United States where histoplasmosis or coccidiomycosis is common, may help to clarify the nature of an illness which resembles tuberculosis (TB) but which has not responded to anti-TB drugs and in which the sputum has no acid-fast bacilli.

A history of smoking cigarettes, bidis, and cigars is important. The duration a patient has smoked and the number of cigarettes smoked (pack years) is of equal importance.

A history of past or associated problems which produce symptoms outside the respiratory systems is important. Cough in a patient with scleroderma for example may be related to interstitial lung disease which is a pulmonary manifestation of scleroderma, or caused by aspiration pneumonia due to involvement of the oesophagus in scleroderma. A pleural effusion in a patient with a history of systemic lupus erythematosis (SLE) may well be due to this disease. A history of cancer of the breast, colon or kidney in the past may relate to respiratory symptoms caused by metastatic disease in the lungs.

It is important to inquire about symptoms unrelated to respiratory disease. Breathlessness and cough may be caused as much by heart disease as by respiratory disease. A history of anginal pains, pedal oedema, and a past history of myocardial infarction are all of great relevance. At times, particularly in older people, breathlessness and cough may be related both to respiratory and cardiac disease. Cancer of the lung may occasionally present with symptoms due to paraneoplastic syndromes. The significance of these symptoms in relation to the underlying diagnosis is often lost.

The possibility of HIV infection in relation to opportunistic infections causing pulmonary disease should always be kept in mind, particularly in parts of the world where HIV is highly prevalent. Other conditions where a patient is immunodeficient or immunosuppressed are following chemotherapy or the use of immunosuppressant drugs, haematological malignancies,

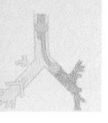

uncontrolled diabetes, chronic liver or renal disease, transplant patients and patients on corticosteroids.

A careful inquiry into personal habits is important. A history of drug abuse is not easily elicited, but if present, may give the answer to the cause of multiple abscesses in the lungs. The use of methotrexate for rheumatoid disease may be responsible for pneumonia of obscure origin. Bleomycin used as an anti-mitotic drug can cause crippling interstitial pulmonary fibrosis; Nitrofurantoin used for urinary infection can cause a hypersensitivity response in the lung and pleura with fever, cough and breathlessness.

A family history is also important as in bronchial asthma or cystic fibrosis. To give just one other example—a patient with repeated haemoptysis had visited one hospital after another with no diagnosis as to the cause in spite of full investigations. A careful family history revealed that his brother had recurrent epistaxis and had suffered from malena. The brother was asked to report to the clinic and he was found to have classical telengectasia on the lip and tongue. The diagnosis rested on the history!

PHYSICAL EXAMINATION

A good physical examination of the chest and heart in many hospitals, both here and abroad, unfortunately seems a practice of the past. Yet a meticulous physical examination not just of the respiratory system but also of all systems is crucial for full appraisal of a patient with chest complaints.

General Examination

A general examination even before going to an examination of the chest may present a clue to diagnosis. The presence of prolonged expiration, the use of accessory muscles of respiration, breathing through pursed lips is a feature of chronic airways obstruction. Flapping tremors or a slightly obtunded mental state point to CO_2 retention. Drowsiness in a patient with cancer lung may well relate to metastasis in the brain. Painful swelling of the ankles and knees together with lesions of erythema nodosum over the skin of the lower extremities is a feature of sarcoidosis, TB and fungal diseases such as histoplasmosis. Painful swelling of the ankles and painful swelling proximal to the wrists, when associated with clubbing is a feature of hypertrophic pulmonary osteoarthropathy.

The presence of iritis may be observed in sarcoidosis and in the vasculitides such as Wegener's granulomatosis. A unilateral miosis is a feature of Horner's syndrome. A puffy face with engorged non-pulsatile jugular veins is seen in the superior vena caval syndrome. In the majority of patients the syndrome is due to a lung cancer.

A firm gland between the two heads of the sternomastoid is always pathological and when biopsied gives the exact diagnosis. Cervical adenopathy when significant occurs in numerous diseases, in particular TB, other infectious diseases, sarcoidosis, lymphoma, and mitotic lesions.

Examination of the skin is of great importance. Erythema nodosum is a feature of TB, sarcoidosis, and drug reaction to name just a few conditions. Palpable purpura is a classical feature of vasculitides which could involve the lung as well. Sarcoidosis produces skin lesions some of which are fairly typi-

cal so that they provide a clue to the diagnosis of a patient who has cough and breathlessness.

Dilated veins over the skin of the upper chest and shoulders are observed with superior vena caval obstruction.

Raynaud's phenomena in a patient with respiratory symptoms suggest chiefly scleroderma or SLE. Clubbing of the nails occurs in various respiratory disorders—bronchiectasis, lung abscess, fibrosing alveolitis, lung cancer and in some patients with TB. Central cyanosis in respiratory disease points to well-marked hypoxia, ≤ 55 mm Hg. It points to severe hypoventilation or ventilation-perfusion inequality, or to a right to left shunt in the lungs. Diffusion defects contribute to hypoxia.

Pitting oedema can be due to heart failure—either primary or secondary to lung disease. Deep vein thrombosis is likely in the presence of a swollen painful lower extremity.

These are just a few of the many possible clues that can be unmasked on a general examination.

EXAMINATION OF THE CHEST

A careful count of the respiratory rate over a whole minute is of vital importance. A respiratory rate over 20 per minute, in particular over 25 per minute, is a cause for concern. The pulse: respiratory ratio is often reduced in acute lobar pneumonia. Movements of the chest are best judged from the foot end of the bed. Poor movement of one side of the chest compared to the other is seen with pleural effusion, pneumothorax, pneumonia, TB involving the upper lobe and in atelectasis of a lobe or lung. The pattern of breathing needs to be carefully observed. An indrawing of the upper abdomen during inspiration suggests a diaphragmatic paralysis.

Patients with bilateral diaphragmatic paralysis become breathless, hypoxic and cyanosed on lying flat. They are more comfortable on sitting or standing.

An indrawing of the lower intercostal spaces during inspiration is a sign of respiratory distress. It occurs in the acute respiratory distress syndrome (ARDS) and in severe airflow obstruction due to the high negative intrapleural pressure during inspiration. Paradoxical respiratory movements are also a sign of respiratory distress and respiratory muscle fatigue. Shallow breathing is seen in hypoventilating patients. Airflow obstruction is associated with prolonged expiration often with an audible wheeze. Restrictive diseases such as interstitial lung disease result in shallow rapid breathing. The same is observed in patients with acute left ventricular failure.

PALPATION OF THE CHEST AND NECK

One of the most important aspects of palpation is to determine whether the trachea is central or shifted to one side. A shift of the trachea to one side may arise because the trachea is pushed from the opposite side (as in a pleural effusion or pneumothorax) or is pulled towards the same side (as with an atelectasis of a lobe or a lung).

Palpation of the neck for lymph glands should never be forgotten if it has not already been done.

The apical impulse should be carefully located. A shift of the impulse is an indication of the shift of the lower mediastinum, either being pushed from the opposite side (as with pleural effusion) or pulled from the same side (as in atelectasis of a lobe or whole lung). The presence of dextrocardia in a patient with chronic cough with expectoration should suggest the possibility of Kartagener's syndrome.

Palpation to test movements of the chest may give the clue to the side of the disease. A lag in the movement of one side of the chest (either the lower, mid-upper or the whole chest) together with a diminished movement of the same side compared to the other, is seen with a pleural effusion, pneumothorax, thickened pleura, atelectasis, pneumonia or a large mass lesion in one lung.

Marked local tenderness and swelling over a rib suggests a fracture, a metastatic deposit or a myelomatous deposit at that site. Tuberculosis involving a rib can also cause local swelling, tenderness and pain.

Tactile fremitis (transmission of sound as a palpable vibration) is best felt with the ulnar border of the hand. It is increased over consolidation and decreased over a pleural effusion or over a pneumothorax.

Localized palpable pulsatile swelling over the chest may be felt in a patient with an empyema necessitans (there is an impulse over the localized swelling on coughing) and in an aneurysm of the arch of the aorta (in the second or third left intercostal space) and of the ascending aorta (second right intercostal space).

PERCUSSION

Auenbrugger discovered percussion when he realized that he could tell how full a beer barrel was by percussing it. The percussion note is normally resonant over an air-filled lung. It is impaired over an area of atelectasis or consolidation and is described as stony dull over a pleural effusion, a markedly thickened pleura or a large mass at the surface of the lung. A hyper-resonant note is obtained over large air-filled lungs that characterize emphysema. A localized hyper-resonant note is sometimes elicitable over a large-sized bulla. The liver dullness generally observed in the fifth intercostals space in the mid-clavicular line may be much lower or unelicitable in severe emphysema. The cardiac dullness may be absent in emphysema or in a left-sided pneumothorax.

An impaired note in the first and second left intercostal spaces is occasionally observed with pericardial effusion, aortic aneurysm and in mediastinal tumours.

AUSCULTATION

Even the art of auscultation is falling into disuse or perfunctory use. A resident (ignorant in auscultation) on a ward round in one of the teaching hospitals remarked (rather happily) that soon the stethoscope will be a museum piece allowed to rest on a hook in the wall! Auscultation to the experienced clinician is a guide to the state of the underlying lung.

Breath sounds are normally produced by the vibration of the vocal chords, of the movement of air in the trachea and large bronchi. The quality of these sounds can be determined by listening over the trachea. The breath sounds over the trachea are noted to be hollow with an expiration longer than inspiration and a pause between inspiration and expiration. These breath sounds are transmitted down several orders of bronchi and bronchioles. If one were to hear the sound over these breathing tubes, their character would be the same as over the trachea, only they would be not as loud because of the distance travelled by the sound waves. Once the respiratory

bronchioles open into the numerous open air spaces termed the alveoli, the character of the breath sounds changes. No longer do they have the 'bronchial' quality. The sound waves are dispersed within the alveoli, so that they now assume the character of normal vesicular breath sounds which are best heard rather than described. These sound vibrations go through the pleura and the chest wall to be heard by the clinician through the diaphragm of the stethoscope. Normal vesicular breath sounds have a rustling quality; the expiration is about one-third the duration of inspiration and there is no pause between inspiration and expiration.

ABNORMAL BREATH SOUNDS

Bronchial breathing is hollow breathing with prolonged expiration and a pause between inspiration and expiration. One promptly recognizes bronchial breathing most of all by its hollow character. It classically occurs over a consolidated lobe or an atelectatic lobe with a patent bronchus. The reason why bronchial breathing is heard over a consolidated lobe is easy to understand. The hollow bronchial sounds produced over the larynx and large airways go down the smaller breathing tubes but are not dispersed within the alveoli because the alveoli are solid and consolidated. These hollow breath sounds go unchanged through the consolidated lobe, through the chest wall to be heard by the listening clinician.

Bronchial breath sounds are termed as tubular, cavernous or amphoric. These all are typically hollow sounds, the difference between them being a difference in the timbre of the sound. Cavernous breath sounds occur over a cavity, the cavity acting as a resonator which emphasizes some overtones and suppresses others. Amphoric breath sounds may be heard over a pneumonthorax or a cavity and are likened to the sound heard when one blows over the top of an open bottle.

DECREASE IN BREATH SOUNDS

Decrease in breath sounds occurs over a pleural effusion, thickened pleura, pneumothorax and in atelectasis of a lobe or lung.

Diminished breath sounds are also observed in patients with emphysema, hypoventilating patients and in patients with paresis of the intercostal muscles or diaphragm.

Prolonged expiration is typically seen in airways obstruction as in chronic obstructive pulmonary disease (COPD) or bronchial asthma. Variation in the intensity of breath sounds over different areas over the lungs is frequent in patients with either COPD or asthma due to uneven distribution of ventilation related to uneven degree of airways obstruction over different parts of the lungs.

CHANGES IN VOCAL FREMITUS

Vocal fremitus as judged by the transmission of voice sounds when the patients says 'one two three' should be carefully elicited. Vocal fremitus is increased over consolidation and over an atelectatic lobe with patent bronchi. It is reduced over a pleural effusion, pleural thickening, pneumothorax and over a collapsed lobe with closed bronchi. When the vocal fremitus is loud and very clear, it is termed as bronchophony. At times the spoken words take on a nasal quality and this is termed as aegophony. This is heard most commonly when consolidated

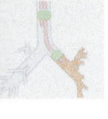

lung and pleural effusion coexist. Clear transmission of a whispered sound is termed as whispering pectoriloquy. It has the same significance as bronchophony.

ADVENTITIOUS SOUNDS

Adventitious sounds arising within the lung have been classified in various ways. The earlier classification (first proposed by René Laennec) considered adventitious sounds as—

Rhonchi (dry sounds), sibilant or high-pitched, sonorous or low-pitched

Râles (moist sounds)   Fine râles (as in consolidation)

Medium râles (as in a patient with airway secretions)

Coarse râles (as in patients with secretions within large airways such as the trachea or major bronchi)

The American Thoracic Society has given a classification based on the acoustic analysis of tape recordings and on the classification introduced by Forgac. This classification is as follows—

1. Continuous sounds (wheeze, rhonchi, stridor)
2. Discontinuous sound (crackles)

Wheeze, rhonchi and *stridor* are continuous musical sounds. Wheezes are high-pitched and originate in airways obstruction caused by spasm, mucosal oedema and secretions. Since airways obstruction is more marked during expiration they are more prominent in that phase of breathing, but they can also occur during inspiration. They are often polyphonic—i.e. vary in pitch and intensity over different areas of the lung in patients with asthma or COPD. A low-pitched monophonic wheeze is occasionally heard over a partially obstructed main bronchus or lobar bronchus (Chevalier Jackson's sign). Wheezes originate chiefly through vibration of the walls of the bronchi resulting from airflow limitation.

Rhonchi are due to the presence of mucus and secretions within airways. Rhonchi change in location and character on coughing because of movement of these secretions induced by coughing.

Stridor is an inspiratory noise that can be heard at a distance or by auscultation over the neck. It is caused by obstruction to the larynx or trachea or major bronchi.

Crackles Crackles (formerly called râles) are due to the explosive snapping opening of numerous small airways that close prematurely during expiration. Crackles are further classified as early inspiratory or late inspiratory. Crackles of interstitial lung disease (as in interstitial pulmonary fibrosis) occur typically in late inspiration. Crackles occurring in early inspiration are noted in patients with COPD. Crackles often heard all through the inspiratory phase are also heard over a consolidated lobe as in pneumonia, atelectasis and in pulmonary oedema.

Hypostatic congestion due to prolonged recumbency also gives rise to crackles. These crackles lessen or disappear on making the patient cough.

Crackles have also been classified as wet or dry. Wet crackles, for example, occur in pulmonary oedema (typically in left ventricular failure). Dry crackles also called 'velcro' crackles are easily recognized with a little practice and are typically heard in interstitial lung disease.

PLEURAL RUB

Pleural rub is a rough grating friction sound heard during inspiration and early expiration generally in the mid-axillary line and over the lung bases. The sound appears superficial and close to the ear. It signifies pleural inflammation. It is generally easily recognized except when brief in duration and faint; it may then be difficult to distinguish form localized crackles.

An examination of the cardiovascular system is as important as that of the respiratory system as many symptoms of respiratory disease are common to those of cardiovascular disease.

The question (impertinent in our opinion) often asked by students is why should one examine the chest in this detail when we have an X-ray chest at hand and numerous other sophisticated machines to give a diagnosis?

The answer is as follows:

1. A doctor who fails to use his eyes, ears and hands is a poor doctor or perhaps no doctor at all. A cultivated power of observation is the hallmark of a good physician.
2. If a doctor looks only or almost only at machines and their reports, he has no rapport with his patient. He fails to talk to him, fails to often touch him, and fails to empathize with him. The doctor-patient relationship which lies at the core of medicine stands eroded or broken and medicine is not even a shadow of what it should be.

SUGGESTED READING

Forgacs Paul. *Lung Sounds*. © 1978 Baillière Tindall, London.

Sarkar S. Evaluation of the dyspnoeic patient in the office. *Prim Care.* 1 Sep. 2006; 33(3): 643–57.

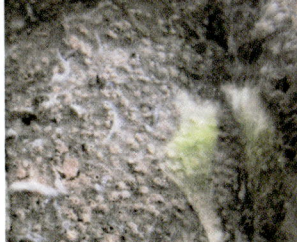

14   Introduction, History and Epidemiology

INTRODUCTION AND IMPACT IN INDIA

Tuberculosis (TB) is a disease that has existed since antiquity. It is a major threat to global health, being the second highest cause of death from an infectious disease after HIV/AIDS. In 2005 there were 9 million new cases and 1.6 million deaths from TB globally.

TB dominates medicine in India, being one of this country's major public health problems. It exists on an epic scale here with India accounting for a third of the world's entire TB burden and a fifth of all the smear-positive cases of the world. Three hundred million Indians are infected with TB, at least 14 million with active disease. Twenty-two per cent of the world's smear-positive cases reside here giving India the largest concentration of TB cases in the world. The incidence of smear-positive, infectious cases in India is 85 per 100,000. Readily transmitted in impoverished and crowded communities, TB impacts on lives in a manner no other disease can. TB is now the leading infectious cause of adult death in India. At a conservative estimate, each year, at least 500,000 people die of the disease. This works out to one death from TB every minute, a grim statistic that has sadly not changed over the decades. Once considered a disease of slums and ghettos and affecting the socially disadvantaged, TB has widened its reach in India affecting urban and rural communities and people from all walks of life.

TB exacts a great price economically as well. The World Economic Forum estimated in 2008 that India loses $3 billion per year from TB annually. Broken down to a personal level, TB causes suffering on an unparalleled scale in India. It devastates entire families by afflicting young bread-earners who lose employment, as a consequence taking on loans that can never be repaid so that eventually it causes incalculable human suffering.

HISTORY

Skeletal Data

Tuberculosis has probably been a human pathogen for millions of years. Skeletal remains are an important source of TB. The skeletal structure will be affected in about 5% of patients with TB and hence finding a destructive lesion like Pott's disease in the spine is the best evidence of TB for a palaeopathologist. The earliest evidence comes from a female skeleton aged 30 found in the cave of Arma dell' Aquila in Liguria, Italy, dating back to around 5800 BC. TB in mummified remains from Egypt was also noted from around 4500 BC with the most famous being that of the mummy Nesperhan in whom there is clear evidence of both spinal changes and a psoas abscess.

Disease in Asia appears later with the earliest evidence being from around 2700 BC. Skeletal evidence of TB from the Americas is more recent dating back to AD 1000 in North America and AD 700 in South America. In addition to traditional skeletal analysis, biomolecular evidence of TB opened up new insights in the origin and pathogenesis of this disease. Modern molecular and polymerase chain reaction (PCR) began to shed more information and it was now possible to establish the presence of TB even in human remains that had no obvious skeletal remains of TB. This is an exciting field and one that is only a few decades old.

Historical Data

By the 5th century BC, TB was mentioned in the great Hippocrates writings. In India, the ancient *Rig Veda* scriptures make reference to TB as early as 1500 BC. Further elaboration in the Ayurvedas (around 700 BC) make it clear that the symptoms of TB and its dreaded nature were evident even then: 'The physician who wants great fame cures a man attacked by consumption.' Ancient Chinese texts (2700 BC) and Egyptian papyrus gave vivid descriptions of glandular TB. TB was mentioned in the writings of non-medical giants like Homer (800 BC) and Pliny (1st century AD). TB also began to be featured in art sources and engravings; sculpture and paintings began to depict initially kyphotic spines and in the middle ages, emaciated, frail young women in melancholic poses.

By the beginning of the 17th century TB was becoming exceedingly common and The London Bill of Mortality records that 20% of deaths in England by the mid-1600s were from TB. In the 18th century John Bunyan famously referred to TB as 'Captain of all these men of death.' This was merely a reflection of the period, for by the beginning of the 19th century, TB was the main cause of death in most of Europe reaching 800 cases per 100,000 population. The Industrial Revolution in Europe and the poverty and overcrowding seen then, undoubtedly served to fuel the spread of TB in those days. India's current TB epidemic began in the mid-seventeenth century and rates in the community increased to reach their peak in the early years of the 20th century.

A famous catalogue of artists, writers and playwrights died of pulmonary TB adding to its mystique and perpetuating the myth that TB and genius were in some way related. At the height of the romantic era of TB, Alexander Dumas wrote, 'It was the fashion to suffer from the lungs; everybody was consumptive, poets especially; it was good form to spit blood after each emotion that was at all sensational, and to die before reaching the age

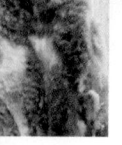

of thirty.' Indeed Elizabeth Barrett Browning was said to have remarked, 'Is it possible that genius is only scrofula?' The list of famous people down the ages who suffered from (and in most cases died of) TB is illuminating, and includes: Alexander Pope, Samuel Johnson, Jean-Jacques Rousseau, Johann Wolfgang von Goethe, Friedrich Schiller, Walter Scott, René Laennec, Niccolo Paganini, Percy Shelley, John Keats, Elizabeth Barrett Browning, Frederic Chopin, Charlotte, Emily and Anne Bronte, Fyodor Dostoyevsky, Anton Chekov, Walt Whitman, Mohammed Ali Jinnah, Franz Kafka, Eleanor Roosevelt, George Orwell, and Nelson Mandela to name a few.

The treatment in those ancient times was largely based on diet, hygiene, rest at high altitudes and sanatoriums, and avoidance of fatigue. In India too, the first sanatoria opened in the temperate hill stations.

The modern era of TB can be said to have begun in 1882 with Robert Koch's epic description of the tubercle bacillus. Three years later Conrad Roentgen with his discovery of the X-ray provided a new way to diagnose it. Chemotherapy of TB was only possible after the discovery of streptomycin by Waksman in 1944. Within a few years of the use of streptomycin it became obvious that resistance was going to emerge rapidly when this drug was used alone. This was perhaps a frightening precursor of the multi-drug-resistant'(MDR)-TB problem that was to leave its full impact only from the 1980s onward. Para-aminosalicylic acid (PAS) was introduced a few years later and added onto streptomycin. It became clear from these early days that combination therapy was the way to prevent resistance developing. The introduction of isoniazid in the 1950s and rifampicin in 1965 paved the way for modern short-course chemotherapy which was first introduced in the 1970s.

Coming back to India, initial efforts to combat TB only began at the start of the 20th century. These efforts were spearheaded by privately funded voluntary organizations, and though sporadic and inadequate, demonstrated the beginnings of the fight against TB in this country. The earliest sanatoria were set up in the temperate hill stations of India where those afflicted were provided rest and a healthy diet. It was not until India's independence in 1947 that the country took control of its own health and destiny and established two pioneering institutions: the Tuberculosis Chemotherapy Center in Chennai and the National Tuberculosis Institute in Bangalore. These were under the sponsorship of the Indian Council of Medical Research (ICMR) and the Government of India respectively. These two centres contributed truly pioneering research that helped shape India's and indeed the world's TB control policies. The famous Madras trials on domiciliary versus sanatorium treatment elegantly and scientifically established the efficacy of domiciliary treatment. Home-treated patients, despite their crowded living conditions and the absence of rest or a diet rich in proteins and vitamins, fared just as well over five years of follow-up. The resulting closure of sanatoria across the world that arose as an extension of this study probably saved the developed world millions of dollars.

Several intermittent chemotherapy regimens were also developed by the Madras and Bangalore centres, in close collaboration with the British Medical Research Council (BMRC). These served to establish the basis of many of the short-course regimens in use throughout the world. This was indeed the golden age of TB research in this country; an age that has sadly not been equalled by any subsequent generation of researchers.

India's National Tuberculosis Control Program (NTP) was born in 1962, geared at tackling the unique needs of TB control in India. The impact of the NTP will be discussed in the section on Epidemiology. Finally, India embraced DOTS in 1992, and the NTP was reborn as the Revised National Tuberculosis Control Program (RNTCP) which was modelled on the WHO-DOTS strategy.

DOTS in India

No account of the history of TB in India would be complete without discussing the impact of DOTS in this country. Starting with pilot studies in 1993 with coverage of 2.5 million population in just five states to 1996 when coverage of 20 million population was achieved, to 24 March 2006 when 100% DOTS coverage of more than a billion people was achieved, DOTS in India has been the fastest expanding programme in history and is a success story of epic proportions (Figure 14.1). The current DOTS programme claims 70% case detection rates and 85% success rates; a huge improvement from the earlier programme rates (Figure 14.2).

EPIDEMIOLOGY

Global

The natural history of TB epidemics is measured by epidemiologists in secular curves that span centuries. Compared to epidemics of infectious viral disease, TB epidemics progress very slowly through low transmission rates, weak immunity, and a long generation time. The standard TB epidemic runs over centuries and generates low TB incidence rates. One of the reasons for the slow speed is the immunological fact that only 10% of those infected go on to develop active disease. HIV and other risk factors, of course, dramatically change this equation as will be discussed later. Epidemic modelling shows that in the developed world, TB has been in decline ever since rates per capita peaked in industrialized countries in the early 19th century, interestingly, well before the advent of chemotherapy in the 1950s. The reasons for this 150-year natural decline have been debated by epidemiologists over the years. These include less overcrowding, improved living conditions, caseload shifts to older populations, and most intriguingly the possibility that genetic deletions over the decades have resulted in phenotypes of M. tuberculosis that are less virulent and less likely to cause cavitatory disease. Whatever the factor or combination of factors responsible, it is clear that there was a slow decline in the death rate of TB in Western Europe by 5% per year, starting well before the advent of chemotherapy.

This steady natural decline had ominously levelled off and in some parts of the world actually increased over the last 25 years. In the US, the annual steady 5% per annum decline in TB reduced to just 0.2% in 1985. The next year (1986), in a historic first, cases in the US actually increased for the first time in four

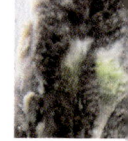

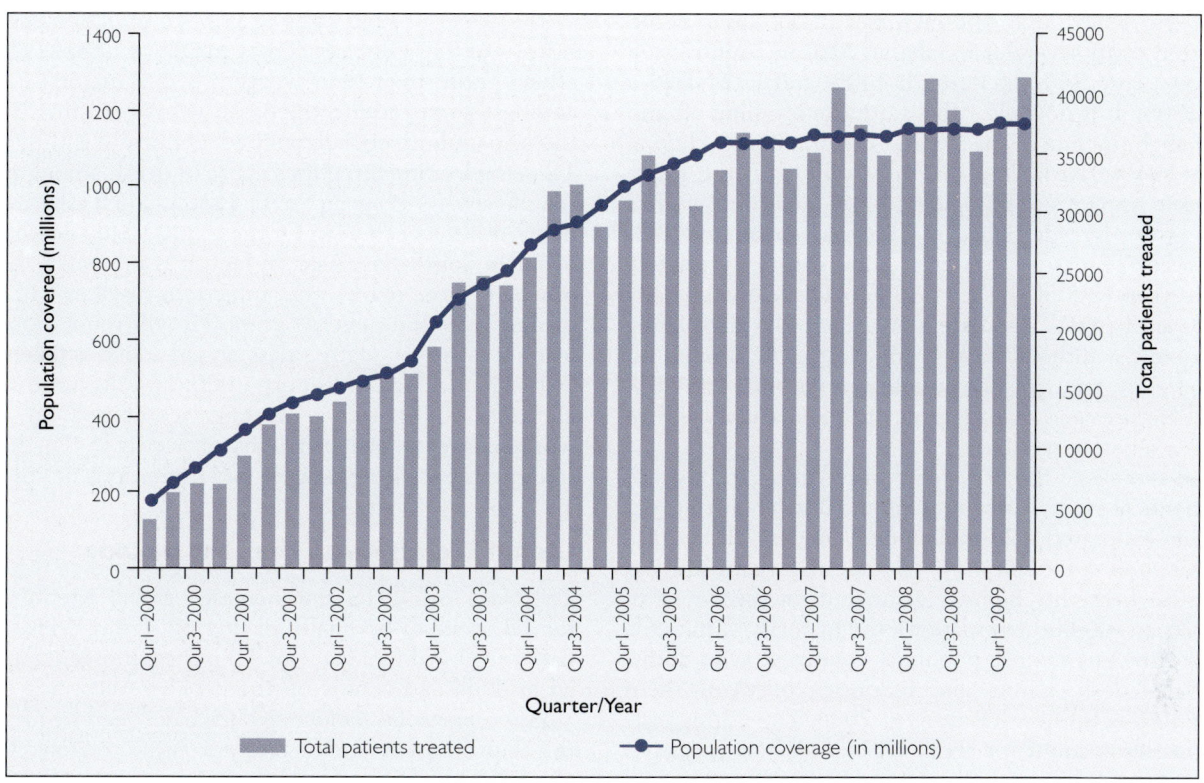

Fig 14.1: Population in India covered under DOTS and total tuberculosis patients put on treatment each quarter.

Source: Population in India covered under DOTS from 2000–9. (RNTCP performance report, India, 2nd quarter 2009, Central TB division, Ministry of Health and Family Welfare http://www.tbcindia.org).

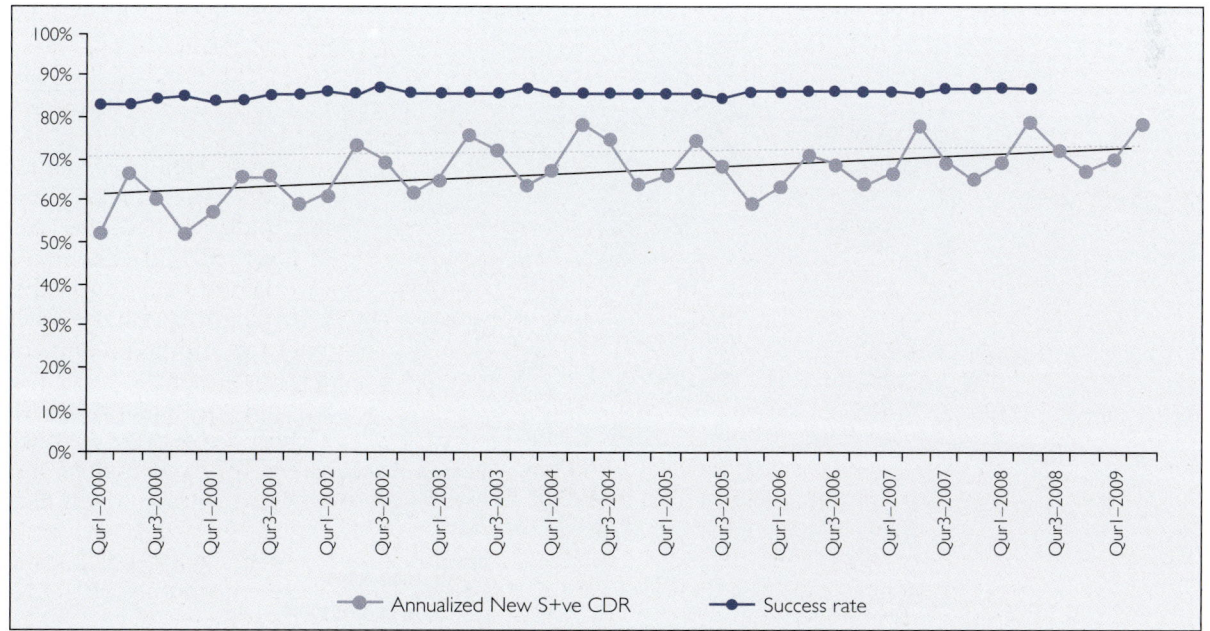

Fig 14.2: Annualized new smear-positive case detection rate and treatment success rate in DOTS areas, 2008–9.

Source: Annualized new smear case detection rates and treatment success rates. (RNTCP performance report, India, 2nd quarter 2009, Central TB division, Ministry of Health and Family Welfare http://www.tbcindia.org).

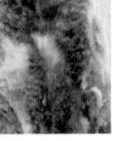

decades. In the 1990s, dramatic increases in TB cases began to be reported from several sub-Saharan African countries; in Tanzania cases rose 86%, in Burundi 140% and in Malawi a staggering 180%. It is now clear that both the levelling off and subsequent slight incline in the US and the dramatic incline in Africa were HIV-related. Thus this disease has had the single most dramatic impact on TB epidemiology since the world's first AIDS cases were described in 1981. An estimated 11% of all new adult TB cases in the year 2000 were HIV-related. In the same year 12% of the 1.84 million TB deaths globally were attributed to HIV. The extent to which HIV is fuelling the TB epidemic is difficult to ascertain. Currently, around 15 million people are known to be co-infected with TB and HIV. The clinical features and management of these patients will be discussed in a separate section.

Based on surveys of the prevalence of infection and disease and assessments of surveillance systems and death registrations, there were an estimated 9.27 million new cases of TB in 2007 with an estimated 4.1 million (44%) sputum smear positive. Whilst Africa had the highest estimated incidence rates (around 350 per 100,000 population), the majority of patients with TB live in Asia's most populous countries, with India, Pakistan, Bangladesh, China and Indonesia between them comprising 50% of all new TB cases in 2005. The 22 highest-burden countries account for about 80% of all new cases per year. India, China, Indonesia, Nigeria and South Africa ranked first to fifth in the total number of incident cases in 2007. Figure 14.1 gives the estimated number of new TB cases, by country, throughout the world. As can be readily appreciated, the estimated number of new TB cases in India at > 1000000, make it the country with the highest incident cases (Figure 14.3). Among the 15 countries with the highest estimated TB incidence rates, 13 are in Africa, almost certainly a reflection

of the effect of high rates of HIV co-infection on the natural history of TB. Globally, TB is mainly a disease of adults and affects more men than women. It is a major cause of death amongst young adults, the bread-winners of their families, and the impact both socially and economically is thus devastating. TB is the leading infectious cause of death among people more than five years of age in South-East Asia. TB kills 5000 people a day, 2 million each year. Of these 5000 daily deaths, over 2000 occur in South-East Asia. In fact, it is projected that although mortality from many other infectious diseases will continue to decline over the next 20 years, TB will remain one of the 10 leading causes of death unless urgent action is taken. According to the World Health Report, 2000, TB kills more women than all causes of maternal mortality combined. In some areas, women face special problems of access to TB diagnosis and treatment because of stigma and limitations on mobility.

Global Trends Over The Last Decade

The fruits of DOTS and increased global attention and funds for TB seem to be finally paying off. From WHO notification data the global incidence of TB per capita seems to have peaked in 2004 and is now on the decline. According to the latest WHO reports, TB incidence rates have been steady or falling in the South-East Asia and Western Pacific regions, Western and Central Europe, North and Latin America, and the Middle East. They have been increasing until most recently in Eastern Europe (mainly the former Soviet Union), and increasing in sub-Saharan Africa. These encouraging trends are best appreciated in Figure 14.4. While the rise in Africa is being fuelled by the HIV epidemic, in Eastern Europe it is political upheaval, economic decline and failure of TB control and health services that is responsible for the increasing TB incidence. These Eastern

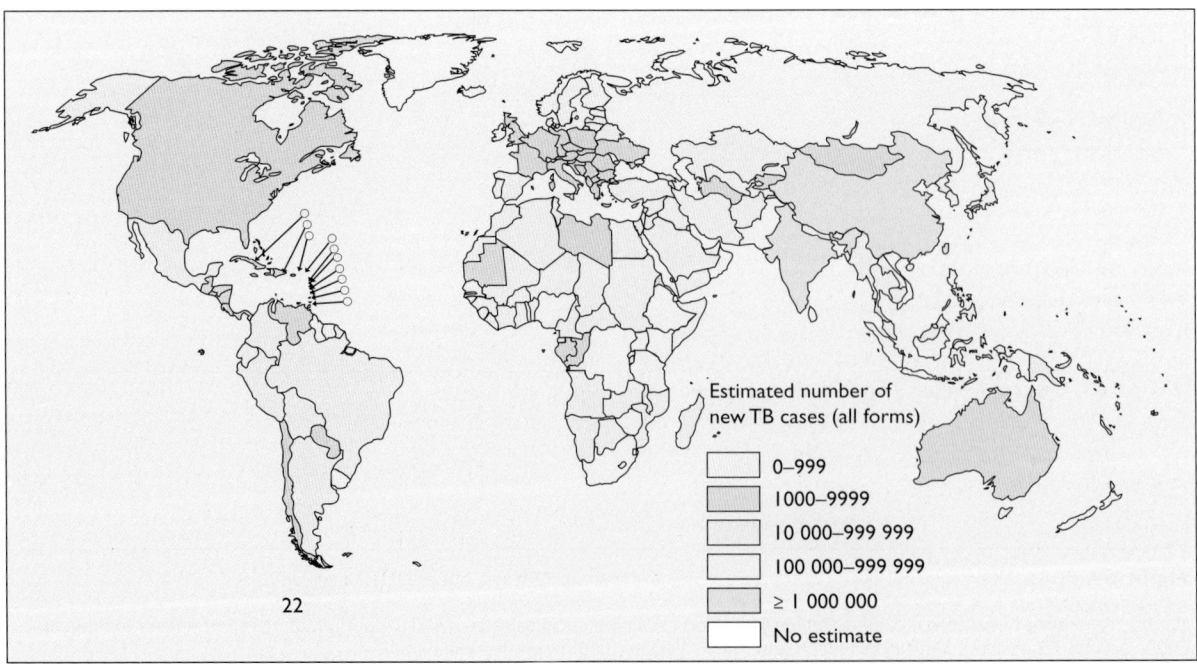

Fig 14.3: Estimated number of new TB cases, by country, 2007. (Global Tuberculosis Control, WHO report 2009).

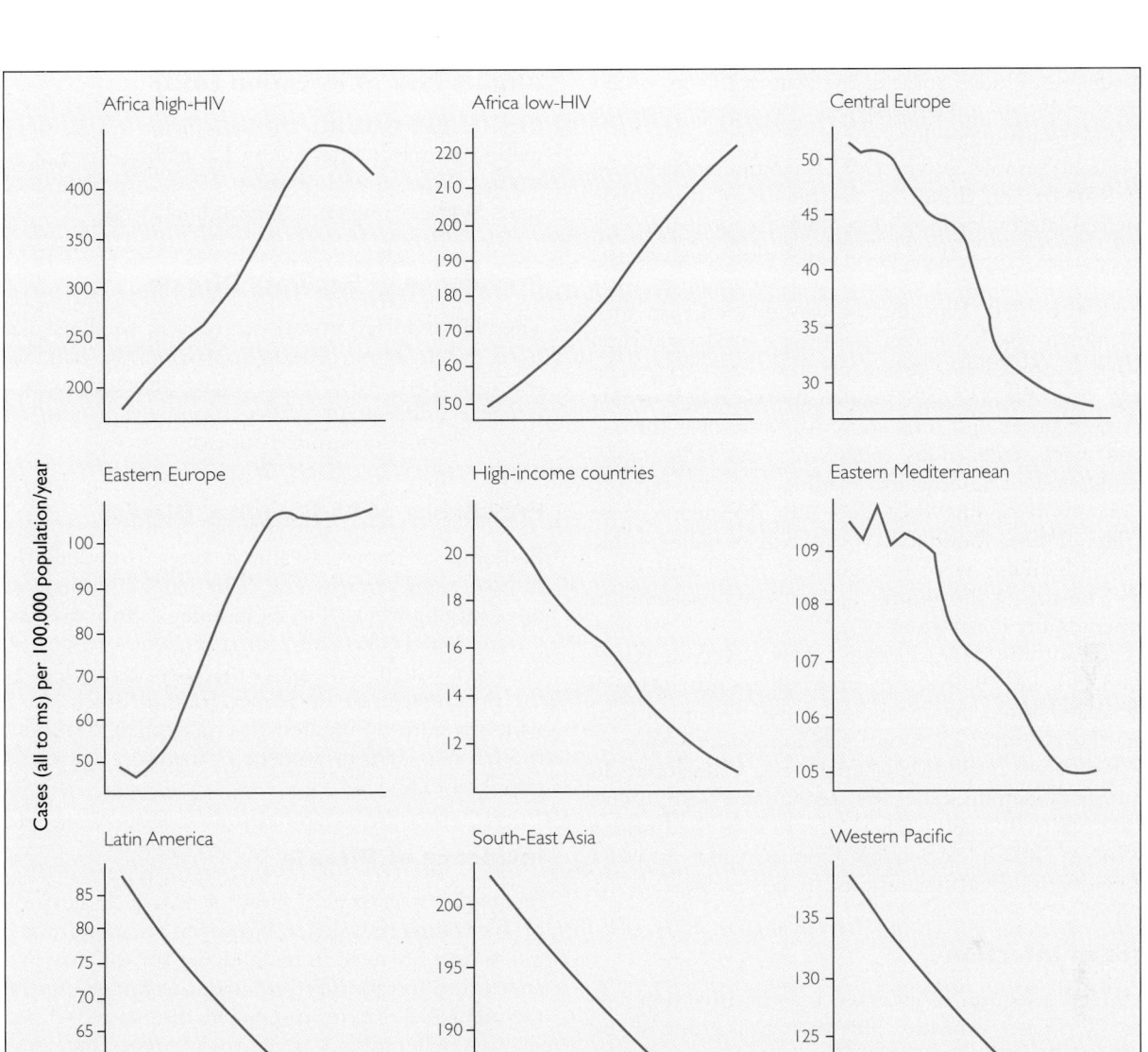

Fig 14.4: Trends in incidence in 9 epidemiological sub regions, 1990–2007. (Global Tuberculosis Control, WHO report 2009).

European states are also 'hotspots' for MDR-TB with more than 10% of new TB cases in Latvia, Estonia and parts of Russia being MDR-TB. Case reports suggest that over the most recent years there has been an encouraging trend; a slowing in the rate of increase of TB even in Eastern Europe and Africa. It must not be forgotten however, that because population growth was faster in 2005 (1.2% per year) than the decline in incidence, the total number of new TB cases arising each year was still increasing.

Epidemiology of TB in India

In India, some epidemiologists have expressed the opinion that the TB epidemic has also entered a phase of slow natural decline. The real situation belies these theoretical epidemiological models however. Indeed, because of India's rapid demographic

growth, continuing poverty and malnutrition, and the effects of HIV, the absolute numbers of cases with TB has actually increased.

Although developed countries have reliable notification systems that provide vital epidemiological data, notification for TB (at least from the private sector) is virtually non-existent in India. Thus the relevant facts regarding the current epidemiology of TB in India have not been fully elucidated. A number of studies and surveys over the last 50 years have shed some important light on the subject however. These epidemiological studies are of varying degrees of reliability and accuracy. Also, in a country as vast as India with its heterogeneous population, it is difficult to include a group representative of the country as a whole. Despite these limitations, enough data has accrued over the years to enable a reasonable estimate of the magnitude

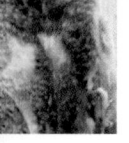

of the TB problem in India. Some of the historically important studies and the broad epidemiological conclusions reached from them shall be presented here.

The National Sample Survey (NSS), conducted between 1955 and 1958 by the ICMR at the behest of the Indian government, remains the main epidemiological source of the TB situation in India. It was on the basis of the findings highlighted by the NSS that the country's TB control programmes were structured by the NTP. The country was divided into four broad zones; north, south, east and west, with urban and rural representative samples being drawn up from each zone. The total sample size was 313,128 people, more or less evenly divided between urban and rural areas. All those over the age of five years were screened by miniature mass radiography with two independent radiologists reading each radiograph. Two sputum samples, one spot and one overnight, were collected from all those found to have any type of radiographic abnormality. Individuals were thus divided into bacillary or X-ray cases. The size of this sample has not been exceeded in any subsequent study in the country.

Four important longitudinal surveys done at varying stages between the 1950s and 1980s also deserve individual mention as they greatly added to our understanding of the epidemiological situation in the country. These are the longitudinal surveys from Bangalore, New Delhi, Madanapalle and Chingleput. In addition, further epidemiological information came from studies on tuberculin reactivity conducted as a prelude to the Bacillus Calmette-Guérin (BCG) vaccination. From all these studies a number of epidemiological conclusions can be reached:

Prevalence of Infection

Prevalence of TB infection, as reflected by a positive tuberculin skin test (TST) is a valuable epidemiological index of the burden of TB in a community. In a high-prevalence study like India, most of the population is infected at an early stage with 60–80% of the population being infected by age 25 and having a positive TST. The prevalence rates tended to be higher in males than females in most surveys. No differences were noted between different zones in the country or between urban and rural areas. This realization that rural villagers had similar prevalence rates to those residing in cities helped shape India's subsequent TB control policies. Two confounding factors have long been assumed to limit the diagnostic value of the TST in a country like India; the confounding effect of BCG (which is universally recommended at birth), and the effect of environmental mycobacteria. Hence, interestingly, when we conducted a similar survey using the new Interferon Gamma Release Assays (IGRAs) in healthy urban adult Indians attending a health check at the Hinduja Hospital in Mumbai, rates of around 80% were still seen. This demonstrates that the high rates of positive TSTs noted in earlier surveys were not false positives due to the effect of prior BCG or due to infection with environmental mycobacteria but represented true latent infection.

Incidence of Infection

Incidence of infection is a better indicator of the TB problem than the prevalence. Limited data are available, but it is estimated the overall incidence of infection is around 1.6%.

Annual Risk of Infection (ARI)

The TB ARI indicates the proportion of the population that will be primarily infected by TB in the course of a year. Indian studies show an ARI of about 1.5% with little decline over 15 years in the Chingleput longitudinal study.

Prevalence of Bacillary Disease

The NSS reported prevalence rates of bacillary disease ranging from 2.3 to 8 per 1000. Approximately half of these were smear-positive, with males being affected twice as often as females. Subsequent surveys done over three decades have shown essentially similar patterns.

Prevalence of Radiological Disease

Radiological disease is always more prevalent than bacillary disease in all surveys. The NSS and subsequent surveys show rates varying from 14 to 24 radiologically active cases per 1000 population. Pockets of high prevalence were noted in areas or zones which were particularly overcrowded. For example, the prevalence rate of 50 per 1000 in Block No. 8 in Kolkata which is slum-dominated was more than 20 times higher than the 2.5 per 1000 prevalence in the more affluent, less densely populated Block 34.

Incidence of Disease

Incidence is a much more sensitive indicator of the TB problem than prevalence. However, because of the expense and manpower involved in maintaining surveillance in even a small area, there are much fewer incidence studies. Available data put the incidence of sputum-positive disease at 1–3 per 1000, with slightly higher rates in males than females. Incidence figures are on the whole about a third of prevalence figures.

Mortality Rates

A study by Datta showed that case-fatality rates over an 18-month period were about 10% even in those who had completed chemotherapy. The mortality rose to 62% in those who had taken less than half the prescribed medications. Data from death surveys conducted by the Indian government as recently as 1992 showed that the estimated annual current mortality due to TB was around 400,000 deaths of which more than 75% were in the age group 15–45 years. Thus TB remains the single largest contributor to mortality in the productive years of adult life. Indeed, 37% of the world's deaths from TB are estimated to occur in India.

CURRENT EPIDEMIOLOGY IN INDIA

In terms of incidence, prevalence and mortality, the current Indian scenario is best clarified by looking at some data from the 2009 WHO report.

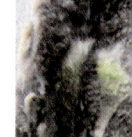

Table 14.1: Surveillance and epidemiology in India (Global Tuberculosis Control, WHO report 2009)		
Population (thousand)	1 169 016	
Estimates of epidemiological burden, 2007	ALL	in HIV + People
Incidence All forms of TB (thousands of new cases per year)	1 962	103
All forms of TB (new cases per 100 000 pop/year)	168	8.8
Rates of change in incidence rate (%), 2006–2007	**0**	**−4.1**
New ss + cases (thousands of new cases per year)	873	36
New ss + cases (per 100 000 pop/year)	75	3.1
HIV + incident TB cases (% of all TB cases)	5.3	–
Prevalence All forms of TB (thousands of cases)	3 305	52
All forms of TB (cases per 100 000 pop)	**283**	4.4
2015 target for prevalence (cases per 100 000 pop)	**293**	–
Mortality All forms of TB (thousands of deaths per year)	331	30
All forms of TB (deaths per 100 000 pop/year)	**28**	2.5
2015 target for mortality (deaths per 100 000 pop/year)	**21**	–

Source: Global tuberculosis control: epidemiology, strategy, financing: WHO report 2009.

SUGGESTED READING

Dubovsky H. Tuberculosis and art. *S. Afr Med J*. 1983; 64: 823–6.

Glaziou P. Global burden and epidemiology of tuberculosis. *Clin Chest Med*. 2009; 30(4): 621–36.

Iademarco MF. Epidemology of tuberculosis. *Semin Respir Infect*. 2003; 18(4): 225–40.

Toman K. *Tuberculosis case-finding and chemotherapy*. 1979, World Health Organization, Geneva.

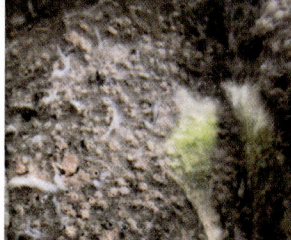
CHAPTER **15** | # Clinical Features, Diagnosis and Treatment

CLINICAL FEATURES

Primary Pulmonary Tuberculosis

When *Mycobacterium tuberculosis* first infects a non-immune individual it results in Primary tuberculosis (TB). This involves the combination of a small peripheral focus of infection in the lung parenchyma and affection of the draining regional lymph nodes. The lung lesion can affect any lobe but always affects the periphery of the lung. Pathologically, the lung lesion comprises caseating granulomas. Most often this remains walled off and heals with or without calcification. It is called the Gohn focus. In a quarter of cases there may be more than one primary focus.

Within a few days infection spreads to draining nodes so peri-bronchial, hilar or mediastinal nodes get enlarged either individually or in combination. Whereas right-sided lung lesions only result in right-sided adenopathy, a left-sided lung pulmonary focus may occasionally result in bilateral adenopathy. The combination of the peripheral lung lesion and the associated adenopathy is called a primary complex.

CLINICAL FEATURES

The majority of patients with primary tuberculous infections are asymptomatic. A strong immune response ensures the infection is overcome without the individual being aware of it. A few patients may have non-specific symptoms of an upper respiratory tract infection and some may run a short-lived fever. Some children, usually a minority, will be generally unwell, have anorexia and fail to thrive.

HYPERSENSITIVITY MANIFESTATIONS

Two less common but well-documented hypersensitivity manifestations of primary pulmonary tuberculosis are phlyctenular conjunctivitis and erythema nodosum. Phlyctenular conjunctivitis is usually seen within a few weeks of infection but can occur any time within the first year. Usually unilateral but occasionally bilateral, it is commoner in children and in African communities. Typically it appears as a small raised bleb at the limbus with a sheath of dilated vessels radiating outward. The reaction is self-limited and subsides within a week but recurrent lesions can occur over time. The presence of phlyctenular conjunctivitis should always raise the possibility of primary TB and such patients must have a tuberculin skin test (TST) and chest X-ray. Resolution once anti-TB chemotherapy is started is the rule but some patients may need local atropine or steroid drops to dampen the inflammation.

Erythema nodosum (EN) is another hypersensitivity manifestation and occurs in 1–15% of primary TB. EN usually occurs within a few days of tuberculin conversion. These lesions may however also occur in post-primary disease. Typically, EN lesions are tender, raised, bruise-like lesions better appreciated in Caucasians than in darker Indians. Joint pains and swelling of the ankle joints may accompany EN and the TST is invariably strongly positive. EN also occurs in sarcoidosis, but here the TST is invariably negative. Apart from TB and sarcoidosis a host of other infections and non-infectious conditions can be associated with EN.

A primary infection is most often detected when the contacts of an adult infectious case are being screened. A positive tuberculin skin test may be the sole manifestation of primary TB and a chest radiograph may then pick up a primary complex. In children with a primary complex auscultation is usually normal. On occasion, crackles may be heard over an extensive primary focus. Even less commonly, if the draining glands are markedly enlarged and obstruct a lobar bronchus (usually the middle lobe), a localized wheeze may be heard.

RADIOLOGICAL FEATURES

The primary complex is picked up at the time of tuberculin conversion in no more than a third of all individuals. The pulmonary component appears as a non-specific, peripheral consolidation. On occasion there may be a more extensive segmental or lobar consolidation. Atelectasis of a segment or lobe may be seen if the glands have obstructed a bronchus. The gland group most frequently affected are the hilar nodes. However, hilar and paratracheal gland enlargement on the same side and occasionally bilateral hilar enlargement may occur. Glandular enlargement has been noted to be much more frequent in Asian as opposed to Caucasian children. Mediastinal gland enlargement is also more common in HIV-infected individuals. The natural history of these lesions is that the lung and the glandular component both may calcify over the course of a year. In adults living in endemic areas, small calcific peripheral Gohn foci or calcified hilar glands may be observed on the chest radiographs of entirely asymptomatic individuals. These are the telltale signs of primary infection acquired in childhood and fought off without the patient having any recollection of a childhood infection.

Diagnosis

In children, the pulmonary component of a primary complex may mimic pneumonia and antibiotics are often first administered. However, if there is history of exposure to an adult with TB and if the TST is positive, the diagnosis of primary pulmonary TB becomes more clear. Since children rarely produce sputum, and gastric washings are considered invasive, a trial of anti-TB drugs

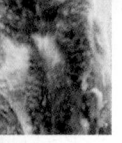

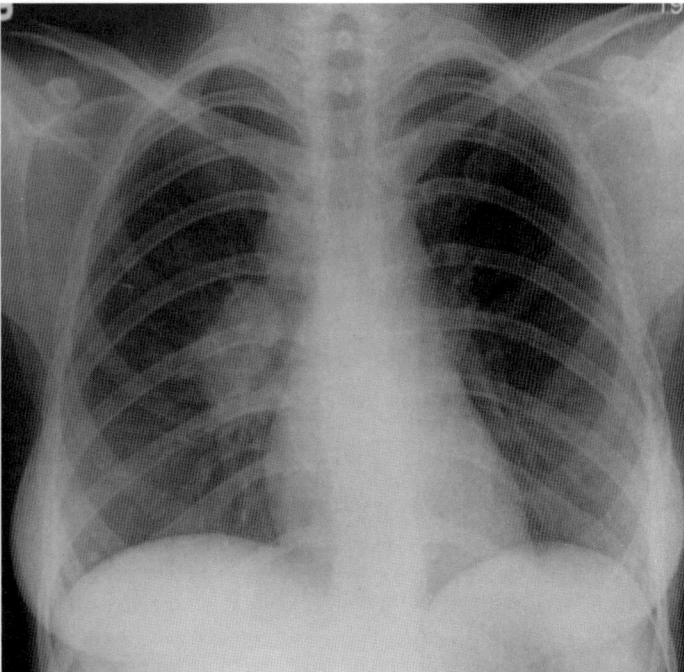

Fig 15.1: Primary complex: Chest X-ray demonstrates large mediastinal adenopathy in right paratracheal and hilar regions. Small subtle nodular opacities are seen in the right midzone representing a primary focus, the combination of both results in a primary complex.

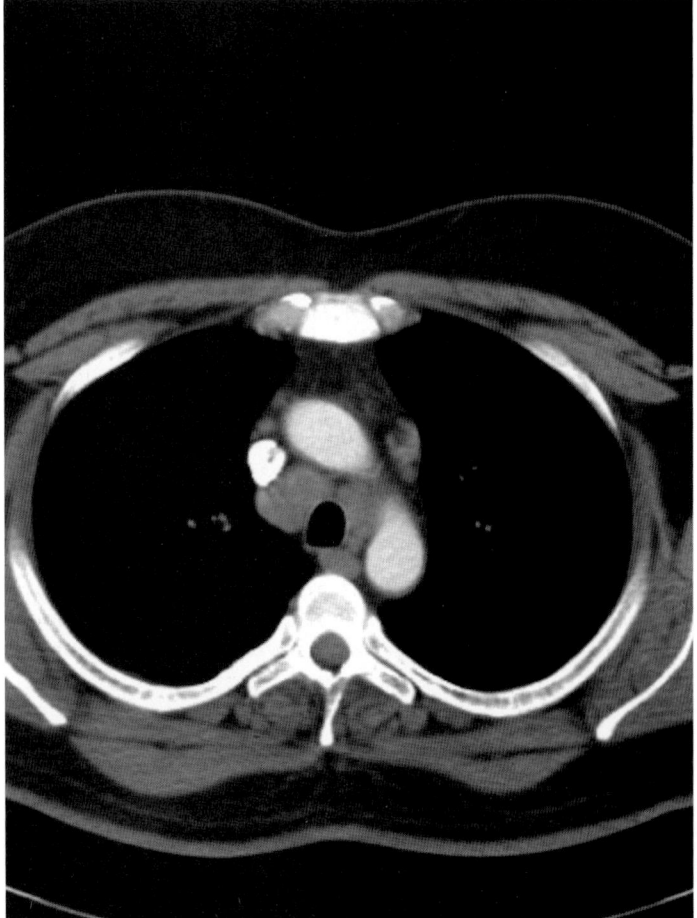

Fig 15.2: Primary complex: CT of chest demonstrates mediastinal adenopathy in right paratracheal, aorto-pulmonary window.

is often resorted to in a child who is unwell and has the above radiological findings with a positive TST.

COMPLICATIONS

1. The enlarged glands can cause subsegmental, segmental or even lobar atelectasis. This was formerly called epituberculosis. The middle lobe is most commonly affected as mentioned earlier.
2. Bronchiectasis occurs due to more permanent damage to the bronchi, most commonly after a lobar collapse.
3. Obstructive emphysema: Partial compression of a bronchus by a gland can lead to a situation where air enters a lobe on inspiration but is unable to escape on expiration. This results in an over-inflated, 'pseudo-emphysematous' lobe, often best appreciated on an expiratory chest'X-ray. This complication is more often seen in infants below the age of two years than in older children or adults.
4. Broncholith: This is a calcified node which protrudes into a bronchus and can rarely even be coughed out, often with accompanying haemoptysis.
5. Pleural effusions: may sometimes be associated with primary pulmonary TB. They are more common in children and usually resolve even without treatment.

NATURAL HISTORY AND LONG-TERM COURSE OF PRIMARY TB

Primary TB is the template from which all future forms of TB develop.

– Primary infection itself is usually asymptomatic and heals with no sequelae apart from tuberculin skin test conversion in 90% of those infected. Such patients are said to have latent TB infection (LTBI). It is believed that a third of the world's population (at least 2 billion) are latently infected.
– The local complications that can complicate primary TB have been discussed above.
– Post-primary pulmonary TB: is the form of TB which has the most global impact and is the major cause of morbidity and mortality from TB. Only 10% of patients with LTBI will go on to develop post-primary TB; half of these in the first year and the rest at any stage in the future, especially as their immune status weakens.
– Pleural effusions
– Miliary TB
– Meningeal TB
– Disseminated forms of TB affecting almost any and every part of the body but chiefly the skeletal system.

While post-primary pulmonary TB usually develops one to five years after the primary infection, pleural effusions and miliary TB usually develop within six to twelve months, while disseminated forms, like skeletal, central nervous system (CNS) and genitourinary TB develop several years after the primary infection.

POST-PRIMARY PULMONARY TUBERCULOSIS

Post-primary pulmonary tuberculosis is the form of TB that has the major impact globally. WHO estimated that in 2005, there were 9 million new cases and 1.6 million deaths from this form of TB. This form is also the infectious form and an average case infects about 10 contacts per year. This is therefore the form that has the greatest public health impact as well. It will be discussed in detail in this section.

Pathogenesis

Post-primary pulmonary TB may arise in one of three possible ways:

1. Direct progression of the Gohn focus to caseation and cavitation.
2. Reactivation of primary disease. Bacteria remain walled off and dormant for decades only to reactivate when host immunity is affected. Diabetes, malnutrition, chronic haemodialysis, steroids and other immunosuppressive therapies like infliximab, silicosis and HIV are some of the major risk factors that promote the conversion of latent TB to active disease. The degree of risk is outlined in the table below:

Table 15.1: Risk factors for conversion of latent TB to active disease	
Risk Factor	**Relative Risk**
Past history of TB	1–10
Diabetes	2–4
Malnourished	2–4
Hemodialysis	10
Immunosuppressive Rx	12
Silicosis	30
HIV/AIDS	100–170

3. Exogenous reinfection: molecular techniques have shown this to be far more common than previously believed, especially in endemic areas. This route is believed to be very important in the HIV-positive population.

Clinical Presentation

The common symptoms are:

FEVER

TB usually causes a temperature which is of low to moderate grade, characteristically has an evening rise and is often accompanied by drenching night sweats. Occasionally, the fever can be high-grade and even accompanied by chills and occasionally rigours. Fever can be the sole symptom of TB and TB (especially extra-pulmonary TB), remains one of the leading causes of pyrexia of unknown origin (PUO) in most series throughout the world. TB is especially likely to be the cause of PUO in certain populations like immunocompromised patients, diabetics or the elderly, though it remains an important cause of PUO in any patient. In a recent study, TB was found to be the cause of PUO in 12% of elderly patients compared to 2% of younger patients. In another study of elderly patients from Turkey, TB emerged as the most common cause of PUO prompting the investigators to recommend empiric anti-TB therapy in this population.

PUO secondary to TB is typically a low-grade fever with an evening rise, accompanied by drenching night sweats. Other temperature patterns associated with TB are intermittent, recurrent, and double quotidian fever (two temperature spikes in the day). The forms of TB most often linked to PUO are miliary TB and glandular TB. These are both pauci-bacillary forms, hence the sensitivity of both acid-fast bacilli (AFB) smear and culture is low. The utility of blood and skin tests is also very poor and CT scanning, bone marrow analysis, gland biopsy or liver biopsy may be needed. Bone marrow biopsy should be strongly considered in patients with PUO with no localizing organ-specific findings, especially if anaemia and leucopenia are also present. In this setting granulomas may be found in 50–80% of cases. Combined histopathology and TB culture seem to be more helpful than histopathology alone. Liver biopsy demonstrates granuloma in 80–90% of patients with miliary TB. About half the number of granulomas show caseation and half are AFB-positive on smear. Splenic biopsy has also been shown to be useful, especially in patients with PUO and splenomegaly or space-occupying lesions in the spleen. A study from India in 31 patients with PUO, diagnosed TB in 11 patients after splenic fine needle aspiration. Nearly two-thirds of the samples from patients diagnosed with TB were AFB-positive, with the highest rate of positivity in samples with inflammatory cells and necrosis without granuloma. The procedure was shown to have a very low rate of complications. Diagnostic laparoscopy may also be a useful procedure in PUO with suspected abdominal TB. Finally, in patients with PUO who are suspected to have TB and whose clinical condition is deteriorating, empiric, anti-TB trials may be considered. In a study by Onal published in 2006, empiric therapy established the diagnosis in 43% of their PUO cases that were caused by TB. A response to empiric therapy with a rifampicin-containing regimen may rarely result from this drug's anti-bacterial activity, but, as this is the most powerful anti-TB drug most clinicians would include it in an empiric trial. Fever may abate promptly following initiation of anti-TB treatment or may persist for several weeks.

COUGH

Cough is another cardinal symptom. Since the sensitivity of cough as a symptom of TB is very high, any individual with an otherwise unexplained cough of more than two weeks duration should be evaluated for TB. The specificity of cough as a symptom of TB is low as cough occurs in a wide range of conditions. The proportion of patients with TB being the underlying cause of chronic cough will depend on the prevalence of TB in the community. These are also the most infectious of all TB patients and inadequate evaluation of a patient with cough results in greater transmission of disease in the community. The cough is accompanied by sputum which is mucoid or purulent and often accompanied by haemoptysis. Sputum of copious quantities is produced when there is accompanying bronchiectasis. Cough may be dry and incessant in glandular TB when cough is secondary to pressure effects of glands on the bronchial tree. Endobronchial TB is characterized by cough with an accompanying wheeze which is often localized. This is usually misdiagnosed as asthma. Cough may be accompanied by hoarseness of voice in laryngeal TB.

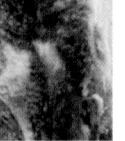
HAEMOPTYSIS

Haemoptysis is another key symptom of TB. The presence of haemoptysis should always raise the suspicion of TB, especially when it occurs in a non-smoker. It may be the presenting symptom of TB and a chest X-ray when done for the first time after a bout of haemoptysis may show extensive TB without any other accompanying symptoms. Haemoptysis is more common in cavitatory disease. Haemoptysis may vary from blood streaks in sputum to the sudden coughing up of large quantities of half to one litre of blood. This degree of massive haemoptysis is not uncommon, may be a presenting symptom, and can be a fatal complication of TB resulting in death by exsanguination. This degree of life-threatening haemoptysis is secondary to erosion of a TB focus into a bronchial artery and can be torrential because bleeding occurs at systemic pressures.

DYSPNOEA

Parenchymal lung involvement results in dyspnoea only if both lungs are extensively affected. Chronic dyspnoea may also be the result of the residual scarring and fibrosis that occur after TB is successfully treated. This may on occasion be severe enough to lead to respiratory failure.

GENERAL SYMPTOMS

Symptoms like malaise, fatigue, anorexia and weight loss are also common in TB. The weight loss can be profound, so that 10–20 kg weight reductions over a few months are not uncommon.

METABOLIC AND HAEMATOLOGICAL MANIFESTATIONS

A broad range of haematological and metabolic manifestations have also been reported in TB. Anaemia is not uncommon. This may be the anaemia of chronic disease with superimposed nutritional anaemia. In some cases anaemia or pancytopenia may result from direct involvement of the bone marrow. Mild leukocytosis occurs in about 10% of patients with TB. On occasion, leukemoid reactions may occur. Leukopenia has also been reported on occasion. Eosinophilia and an increase in monocyte counts may also occur with TB. Hyponatraemia is the commonest metabolic effect and is reported to occur in about 10% of patients due to inappropriate antidiuretic hormone (ADH) production (SIADH—Syndrome of inappropriate antidiuretic hormone secretion).

EVOLUTION OF SYMPTOMS

Symptoms are often mild at the onset and evolve gradually in a time course that spans weeks or months. On occasion however, TB runs a more acute course, and may mimic a bacterial pneumonia clinically and radiologically. Osler's famous dictum of TB being the sole differential diagnosis in a non-resolving pneumonia could equally apply to TB being the main differential diagnosis in what seems to be a lobar pneumonia. In a series of our patients presenting with community-acquired pneumonia (CAP) at the Hinduja Hospital, Mumbai, TB accounted for 7% of all presentations. In a similar study from the University Hospital, Singapore, TB accounted for 21% of all CAPs. In this study, TB was more often an etiological agent than S. pneumoniae.

PHYSICAL FINDINGS

Clinical examination is often normal in a patient with pulmonary TB, despite advanced radiological shadowing. General examina-tion may reveal clubbing in advanced suppurative disease and when there is secondary bronchiectasis. A careful general examination is also essential to pick out evidence of TB outside the lung; for example, cervical glands secondary to glandular TB. Scattered crackles are the most common respiratory finding. When there is upper airway stenosis a localized wheeze may be present. Upper lobe fibrosis may produce tracheal deviation and a flattening of the chest. A large cavity may produce amphoric breathing and this may also be heard over a bronchopleural fistula.

Diagnosis

Diagnosis of TB: depends on three rather antiquated tests: radiology, sputum and the tuberculin skin test. All these have several limitations, especially in the HIV co-infected population. It is estimated that the world spends a total of 1 billion US dollars on TB diagnostics annually. The cost of seeking a TB diagnosis represents 75% of the annual household income of the poorest socioeconomic classes.

Radiology

Reliance on the chest radiograph alone to diagnose TB results in both under-diagnosis and missed diagnosis. No X-ray pattern is absolutely typical of TB. In fact, 10% or more of the patients found to have TB may have normal-appearing X-rays. Furthermore, as indicated above, 40% or more of the patients who are considered to have TB on the basis of X-ray alone do not have the disease. Therefore, X-ray is an unreliable tool for both diagnosis and monitoring of pulmonary TB.

In an interesting Indian study which demonstrates the inherent flaws in chest radiography, over 2000 outpatients had chest radiography and 227 were diagnosed to have TB on radiographic grounds. Of the 227, 36% had negative sputum cultures and of the remaining 1773 patients, 1.5% had positive cultures. From these results, in terms of sensitivity of chest radiographs, 20% of 162 culture-positive cases would have been missed by radiography. Another study by Toman found there is great disagreement between radiologists when asked to read the same X-ray. The disagreement between radiologists on the question: 'Is there radiographic evidence of TB in this X-ray?' was as high as 45%. This sounds high but the disagreement index for a question as basic as: 'Is this X-ray abnormal?' was 34% and for 'Is a cavity present?' was as high as 28%.

A normal chest radiograph makes pulmonary TB less likely but as almost half the lung volume is obscured on a frontal chest radiograph by the mediastinum and diaphragm and subtle infiltrates at the apex of the lung are obscured by the clavicle and first rib, the X-ray may miss some patients with pulmonary TB and many with glandular TB. A lordotic X-ray may reveal apical TB with far greater clarity than a PA view. A high-resolution computed tomography (HRCT) for lung parenchyma and a contrast CT for the mediastinum may pick up lesions missed on chest radiography. A single X-ray is also often unable to accurately gauge the 'activity' of TB. Comparison with old X-rays, if available, is crucial for this distinction. Thus, even more than CT, there is no investigation as important as an old chest X-ray. If an old X-ray is not available, a lesion on an X-ray must not be assumed to be inactive without checking the sputum for AFB culture and confirming it is negative. The other classic, though rare situation where the X-ray (and indeed CT) may be normal but the patient has a positive sputum smear is endobronchial TB.

The following findings on an X-ray suggest TB: Opacities in the upper lobes or apical segments of the lower lobes, nodular opacities or infiltrates, presence of cavitation, consolidation that persists over several weeks, thus making pneumonia unlikely. Calcification and fibrosis suggest healed disease but as discussed earlier this is difficult to confirm on radiographic grounds alone. Other features outside the lung which may be pointers to TB include associated pleural or pericardial effusions or the presence of mediastinal adenopathy. CT features of TB include the 'tree in bud appearance' which though suggestive is not specific for TB.

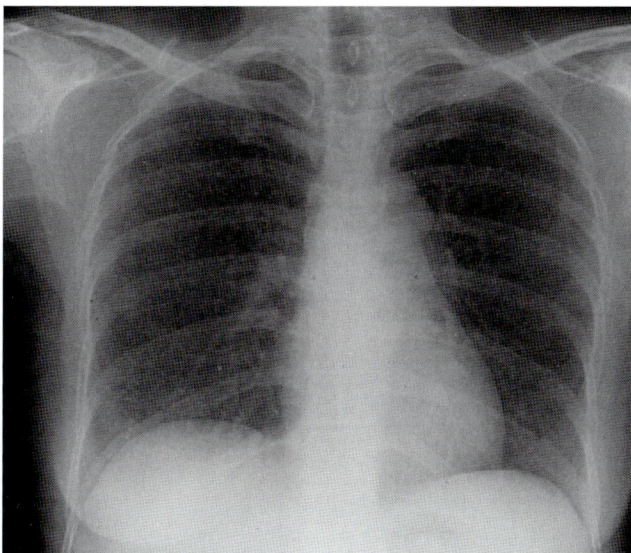

Fig 15.4: Miliary TB: X-ray chest demonstrates multiple miliary nodules in both lung fields.

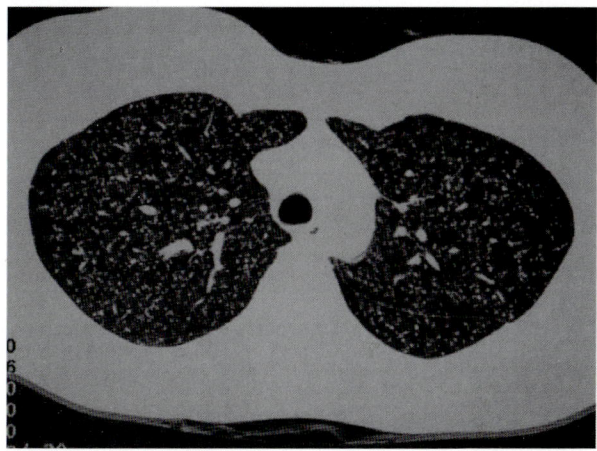

Fig 15.5: Miliary TB: HRCT demonstrates multiple small well-defined nodular lesions in both lung fields.

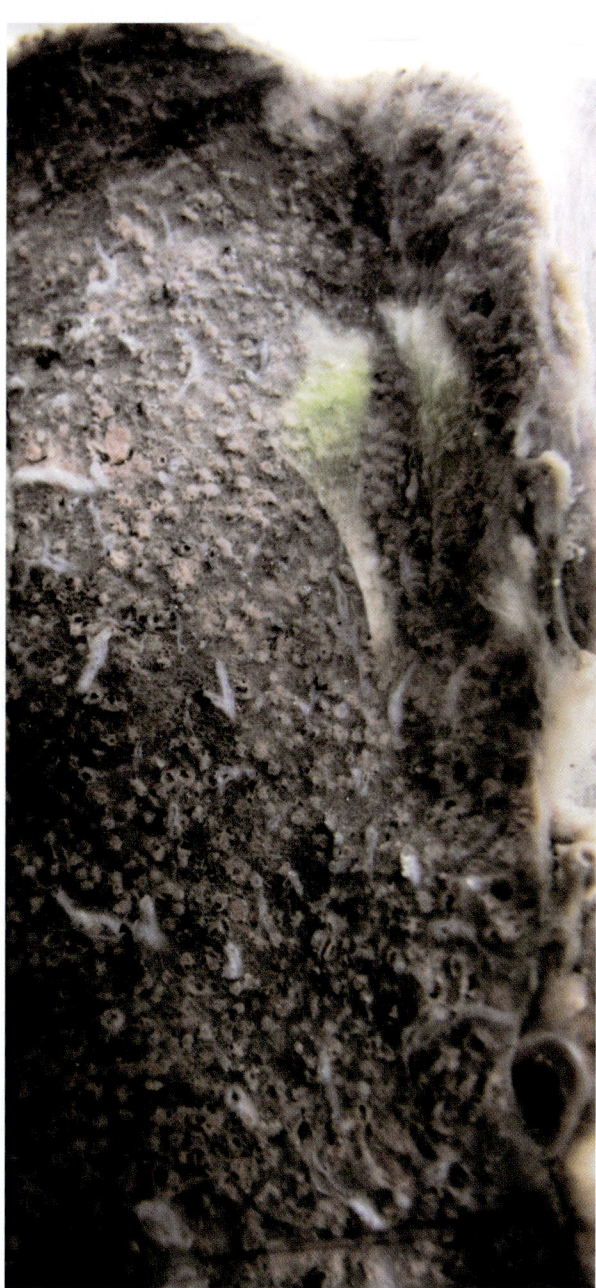

Fig 15.3: Miliary TB: Gross specimen of miliary TB with multiple small miliary lesions disseminated throughout the lungs.

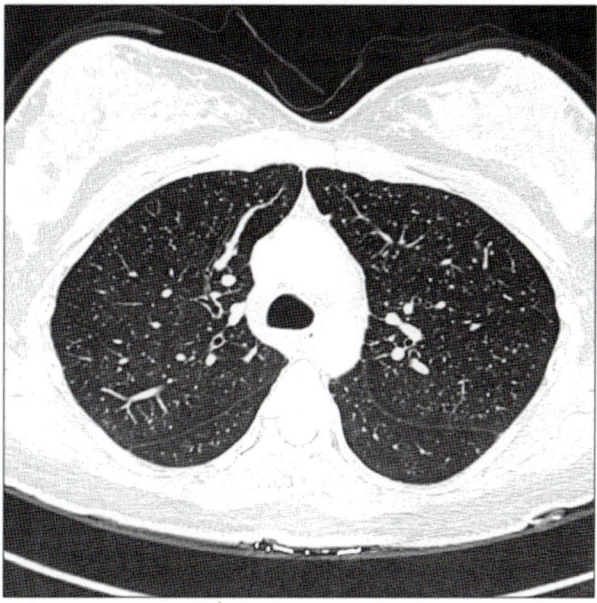

Fig 15.6: Miliary TB: HRCT chest demonstrates multiple small well-defined nodular lesions in both lung fields.

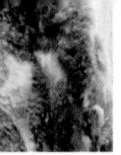

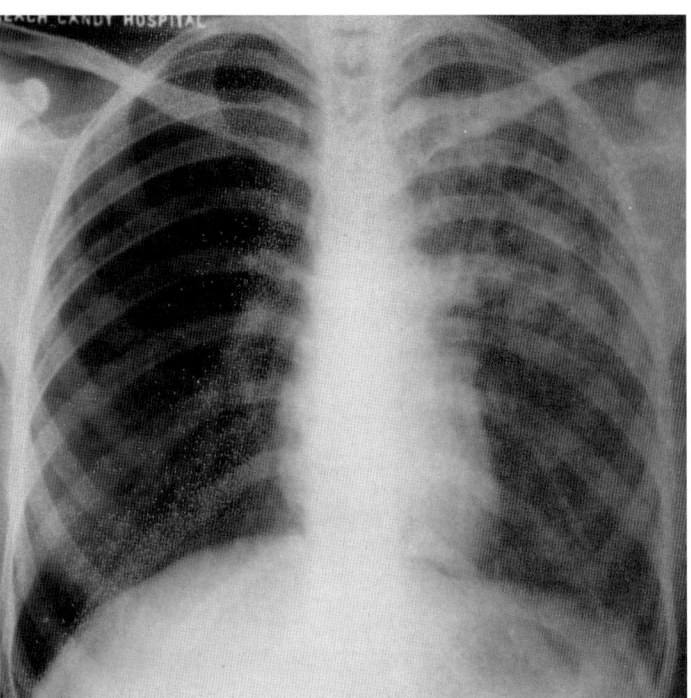

Fig 15.7: Pulmonary TB: Chest X-ray demonstrates ill-defined consolidations in the left upper lobe and mid zone with small cavities interspersed in the consolidation; these consolidations resembling cotton wool, location of the lesions and cavities are highly indicative of TB, sputum was positive for AFB.

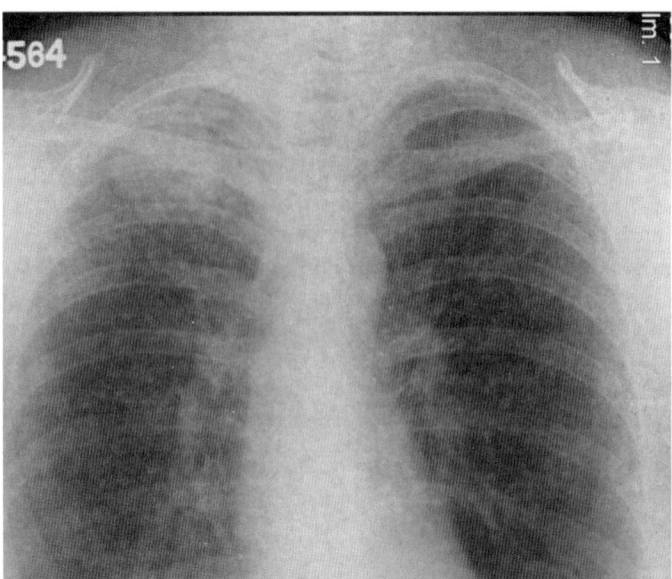

Fig 15.9: Pulmonary TB: X-ray chest demonstrates an ill-defined nodular lesion in the right apical region with internal cavitation and small peripheral nodules. The location of the lesion, presence of cavitation and small peripheral nodules are indicative of active Koch's infection.

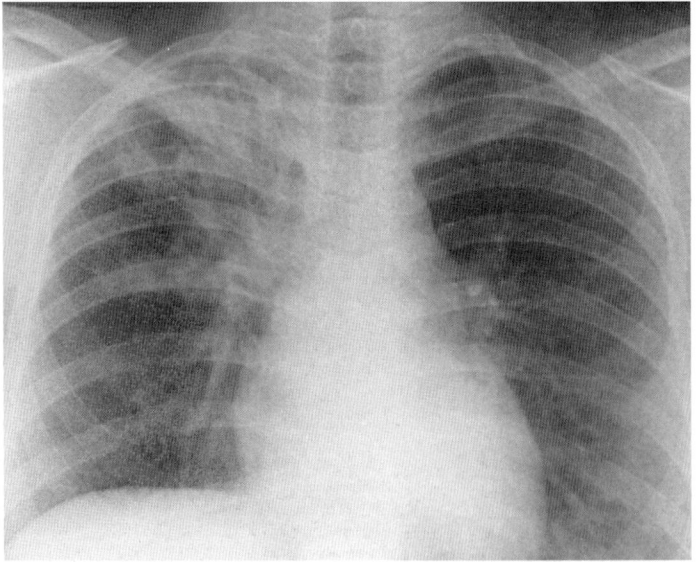

Fig 15.8: Pulmonary TB: Chest X-ray demonstrates ill-defined fluffy opacities with streaky opacities in the right upper zone and internal cavitation as a result of active TB.

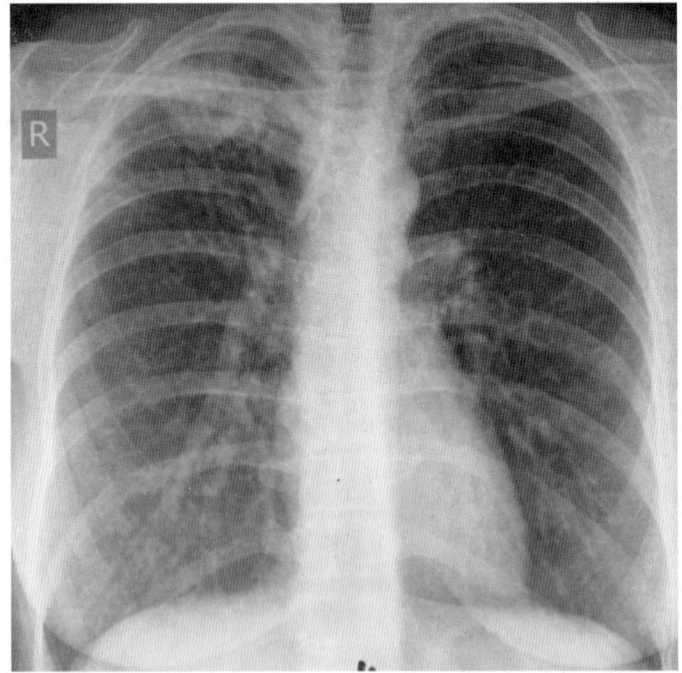

Fig 15.10: Pulmonary TB: Chest X-ray demonstrates a nodular lesion in the right apex with internal cavitation. The location as well as the cavitation are typical for pulmonary TB.

SPUTUM MICROSCOPY

When it comes to the sputum smear, little has changed since Robert Koch's time. Smear microscopy is the most basic and commonly used tool to diagnose TB worldwide. It has the advantage of being inexpensive and simple and operators can be trained easily and rapidly. Results can be provided to the physician within a few hours. A sample of each sputum is smeared on a slide, Ziehl-Neelsen stained and then air-dried. The presence of AFB is taken as evidence of TB. While a single smear of a respiratory specimen has a reported sensitivity of between 22–43%, when multiple specimens are examined, the detection rate improves considerably. The sensitivity of smears from other specimen sources is even poorer. Overall, sputum microscopy by traditional Ziehl-Neelsen (ZN) staining, may miss up to 50% of active pulmonary TB. Even the best laboratory will not pick up TB if < 10,000 bacilli are present /ml of sputum. Add

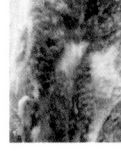

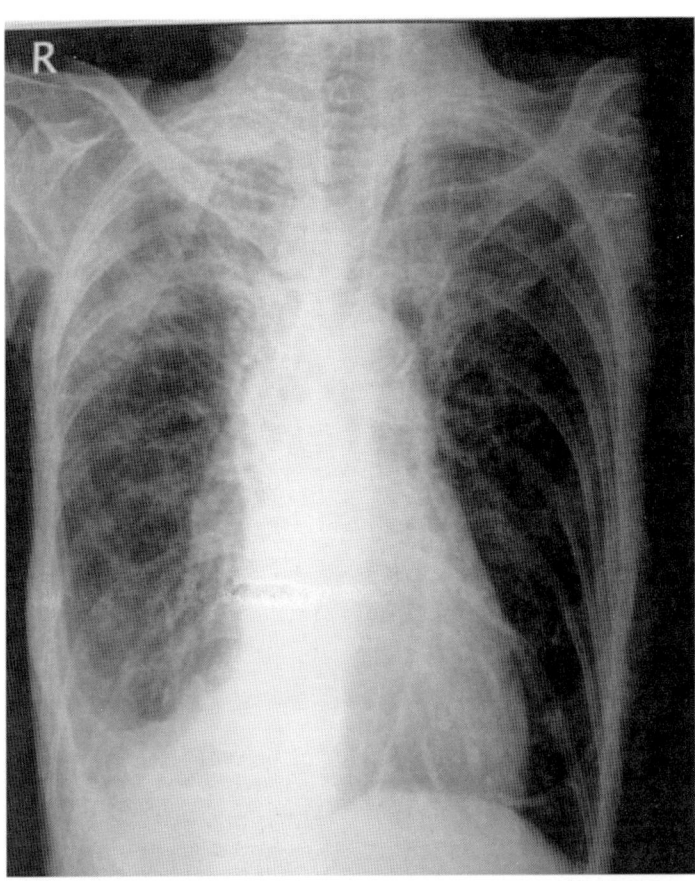

Fig 15.11: Pulmonary TB: Chest X-ray demonstrates ill-defined soft tissue areas in the right upper zone, also soft tissue in left upper zone with an associated right pleural effusion. Pleural fluid revealed a high adenosine deaminase (ADA) level.

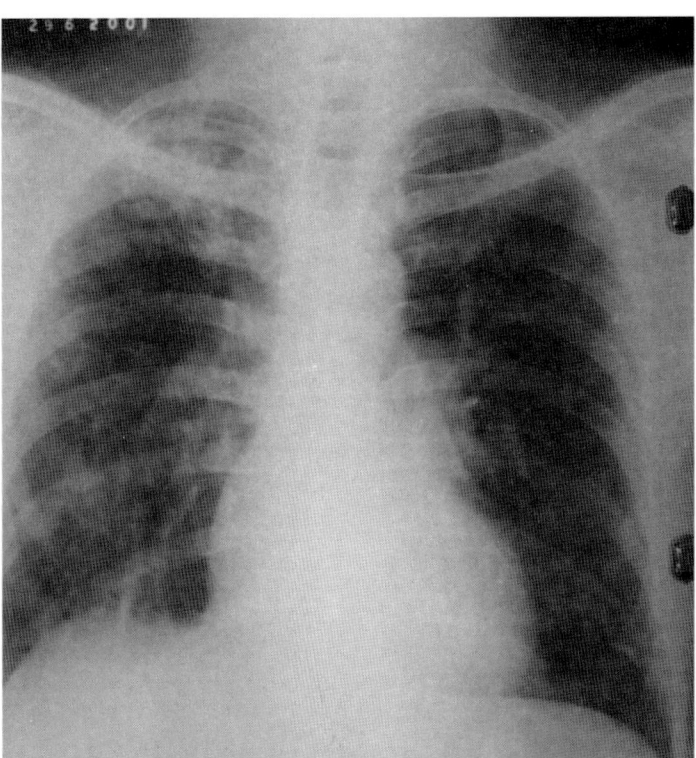

Fig 15.12b: Follow-up chest X-ray following eight weeks of anti-Koch's treatment.

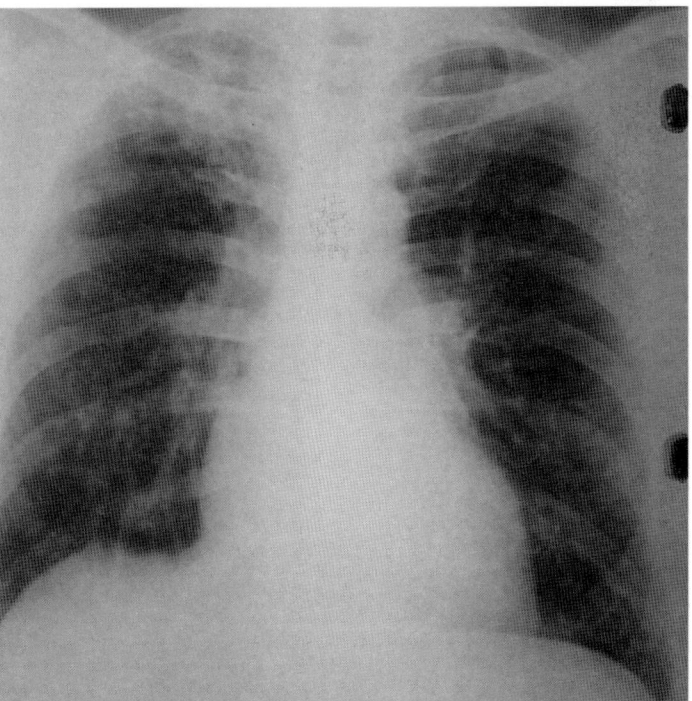

Fig 15.12c: Follow-up chest X-ray after five months of treatment demonstrates thin-walled cavity in right apex with associated fibrotic lesions and volume loss. Considerable resolution in pulmonary TB lesions.

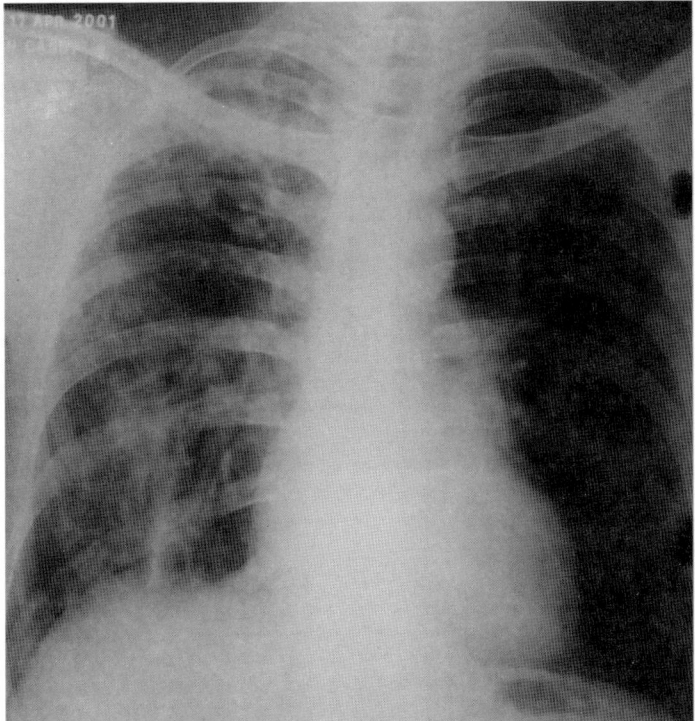

Fig 15.12a: Pulmonary TB: Chest X-ray demonstrates ill-defined fluffy opacities in the right apex with internal cavitations in the right apex. There are similar ill-defined opacities in the right mid and lower zones. Sputum AFB was positive.

to this the fact that some patients may be unable to produce an adequate sputum sample and that the sputum may not be correctly processed by the lab so that even more cases with TB may be missed. The current WHO recommendation, in their 2007 guidelines, is that the number of sputum sample

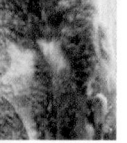

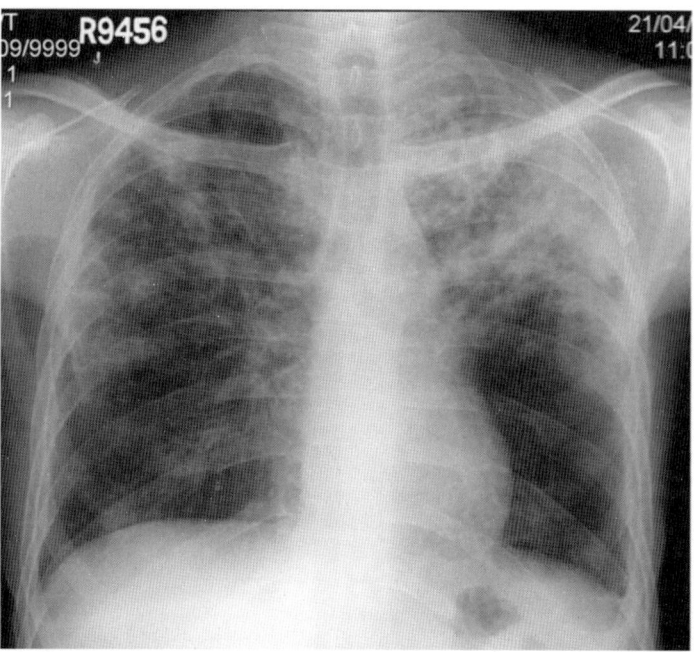

Fig 15.13: Pulmonary TB: Chest X-ray demonstrates ill-defined fluffy consolidations in both upper and mid zones which tend to conglomerate in the left upper zone. Sputum AFB was positive.

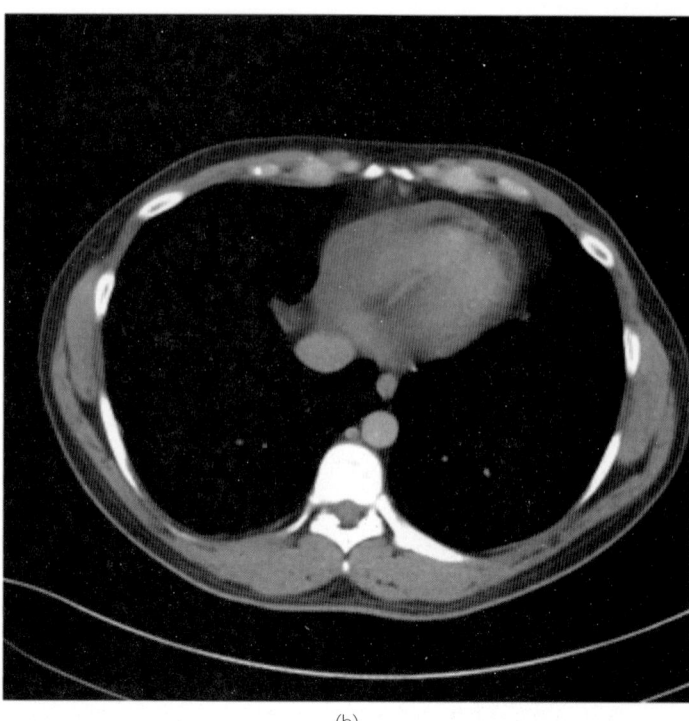

(b)

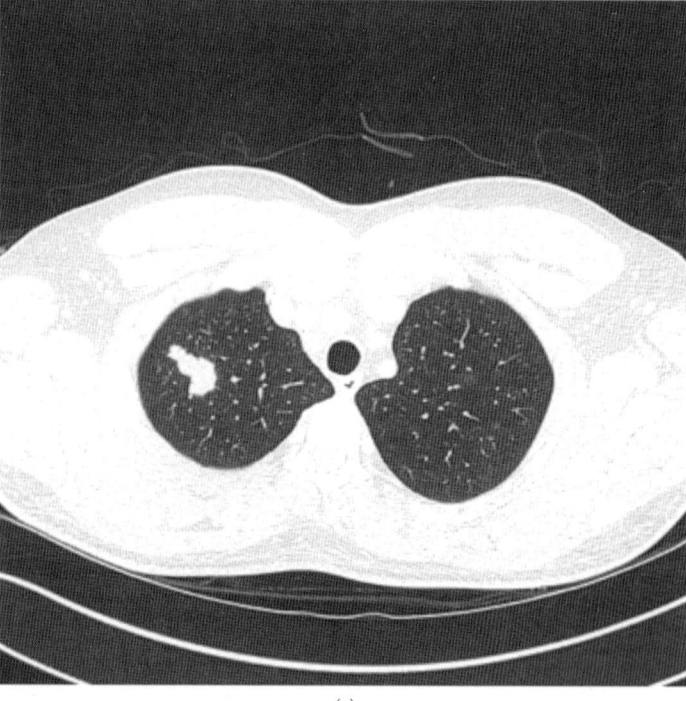

(a)

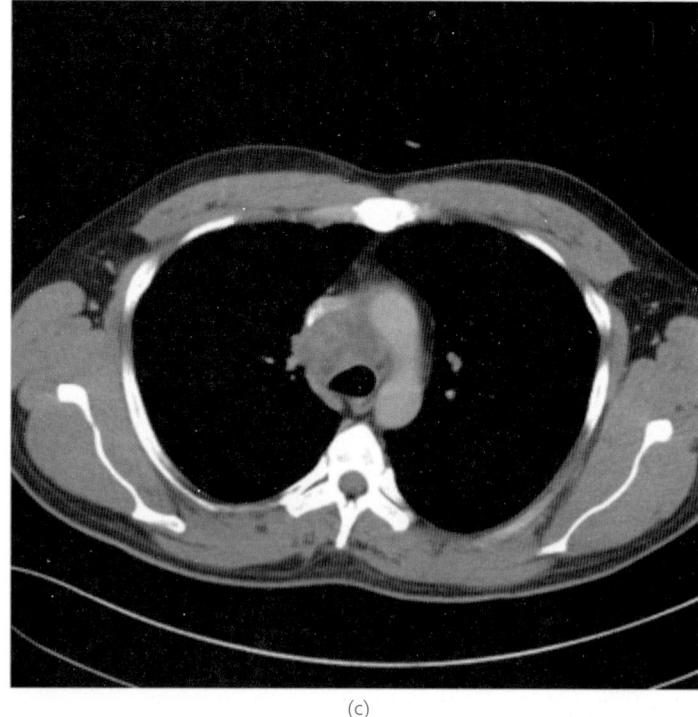

(c)

Fig 15.14: Pulmonary TB: Middle-aged male patient presented with fever, weight loss and a high erythrocyte sedimentation rate (ESR). Chest X-ray did not reveal any significant abnormality. (a) Chest CT demonstrates a nodular consolidation in the right apex (b) additionally there was a small pericardial effusion and (c) necrotic mediastinal adenopathy. A chest X-ray may miss small nodular consolidations in the apex as they are small in size and may be hidden behind the clavicle and first rib. The mediastinal adenopathy may also not be visualized, hidden by the mediastinal structures, as the adenopathy is retrocaval.

specimens can be reduced from three to two in countries where workload is high and resources are limited. This was based on the realization that the average incremental yield of the third smear was just 3%. This was confirmed in a recent study we performed at the Hinduja Hospital which looked at 400 consecutive

adult TB suspects and found that the incremental yield of the third sputum sample was 2.8% (seven additional patients). We found that analysis of 57 additional third smears was needed to diagnose one additional case of TB. This minimal additional yield of the third smear does not justify the burden it imposes

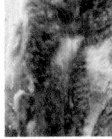

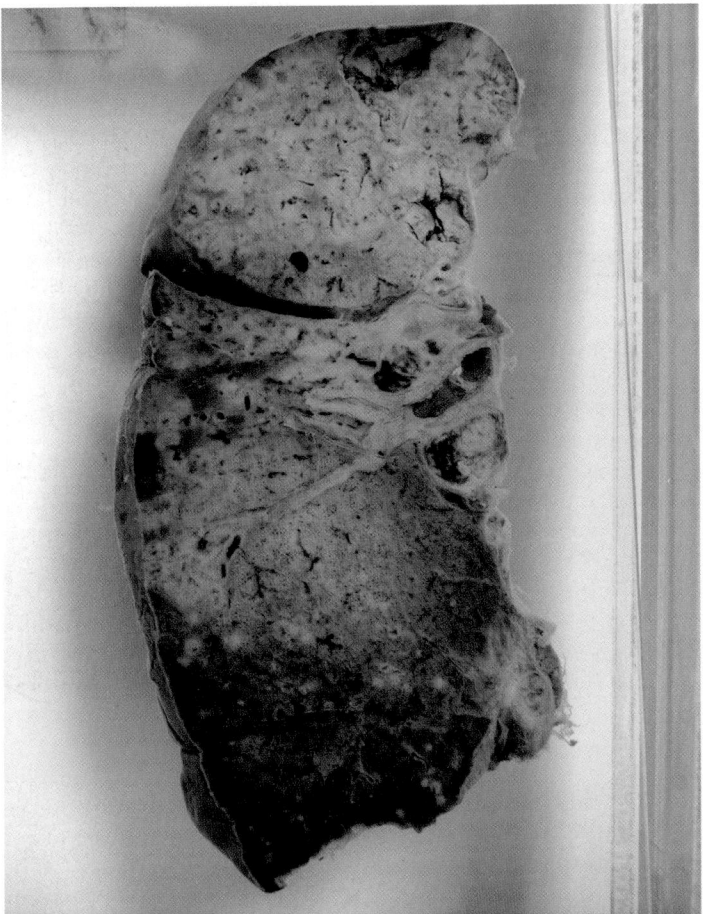

Fig 15.15: Cavitating TB: Gross specimen of cavitating TB, large cavity seen in the apex with tuberculous involvement in right upper lobe, apical segment of lower lobe as well as small tubercles in lower zones.

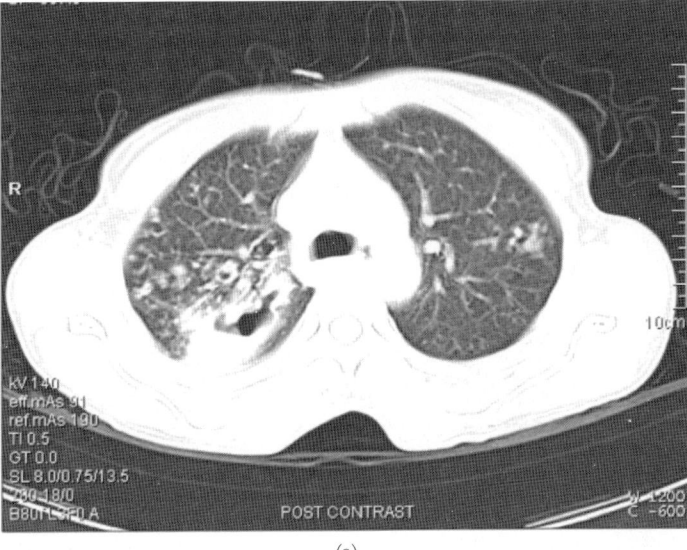

(a)

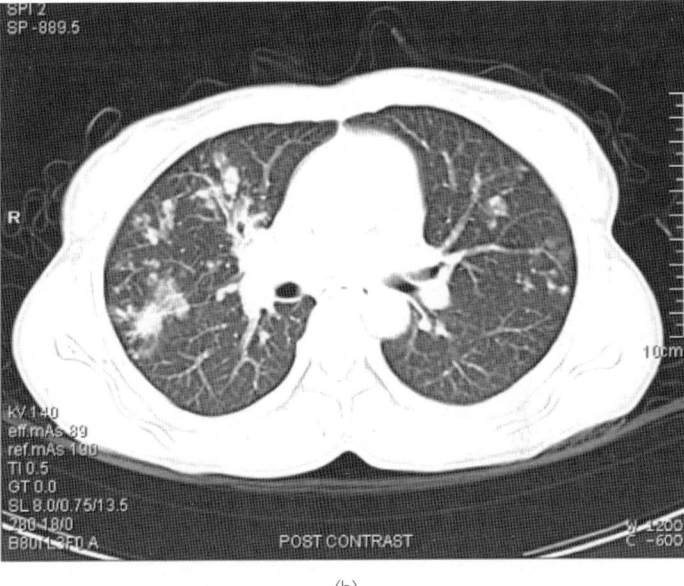

(b)

Fig 15.16: Pulmonary TB: (a, b) Chest CT demonstrates a thick-walled cavity in the right apex with associated nodular consolidations in the right upper lobe as well as left upper lobe.

on both the patient and the Indian healthcare system and the Revised National Tuberculosis Control Program (RNTCP) has rightly revised its guidelines to accept two sputum smears as adequate for diagnosing TB. Samples taken in the early morning are preferred since they are generally acknowledged to be more likely to be positive. For the 50% of patients who are simply unable to produce an adequate sputum sample, hypertonic saline nebulization to induce sputum, or where facilities exist, bronchoscopy with examination of bronchoalveolar lavage (BAL) fluid for AFB is done. In children, naso-gastric aspirates may be collected, preferably again in the morning.

Sputum examination, like all other tests, must be considered in the overall clinical context. Operator skill is a crucial variable, and even for experienced microscopists, accuracy has been shown to decline significantly if the number of slides to be processed is too large due to the physically demanding nature of scrutinizing multiple slides. Lab errors and non-tuberculous mycobacteria (NTM) are some of the causes of false-positive sputum smears.

Sadly, it is estimated that there are no more than 50,000 microscopy centres in the 22 high-burden countries which works out to one lab for every 75,000 people. Another paradox is that of the global network of 26 supranational reference laboratories (SRNL), only one is housed in India and two in the entire South East Asia region whilst 11 are concentrated in Europe.

SPUTUM CULTURE

Traditionally, mycobacteria have been cultured on either egg-based solid media or in liquid media and monitored for growth. The main drawback of traditional cultures is that due to the long division time of *M. tuberculosis*, 16–18 hours under optimal conditions, clinical samples take around four to six weeks to turn positive. Lowenstein-Jensen (LJ) medium is the solid culture medium most frequently used throughout the world. It is an egg-based formulation, with glycerol supplement for *M. tuberculosis*. Solid Middlebrook 7H10 and 7H11 containing agar are other culture media that are still in use in laboratories across the world. In the developed world, liquid culture media are more widely used. These have the advantages of faster recovery times and detection rates than conventional solid media. The two liquid systems most frequently used in the developed

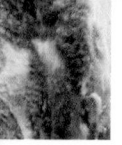

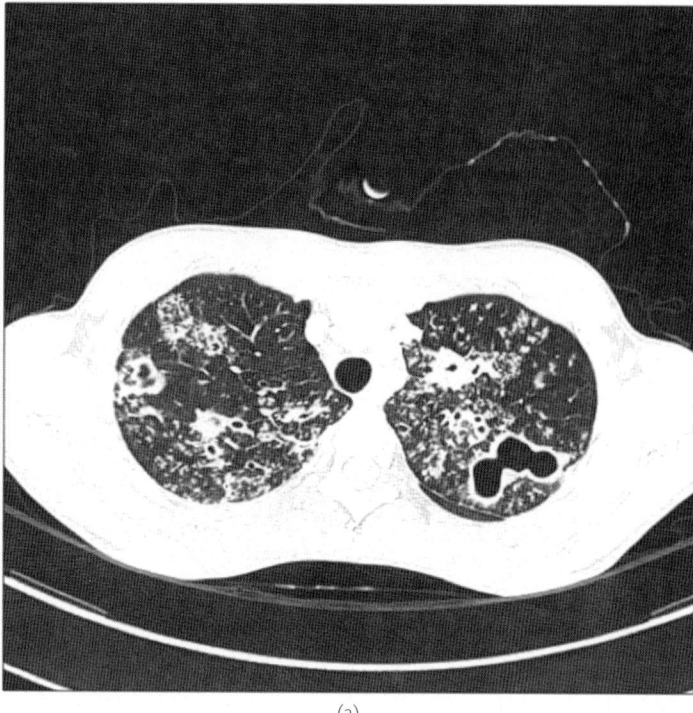

(a)

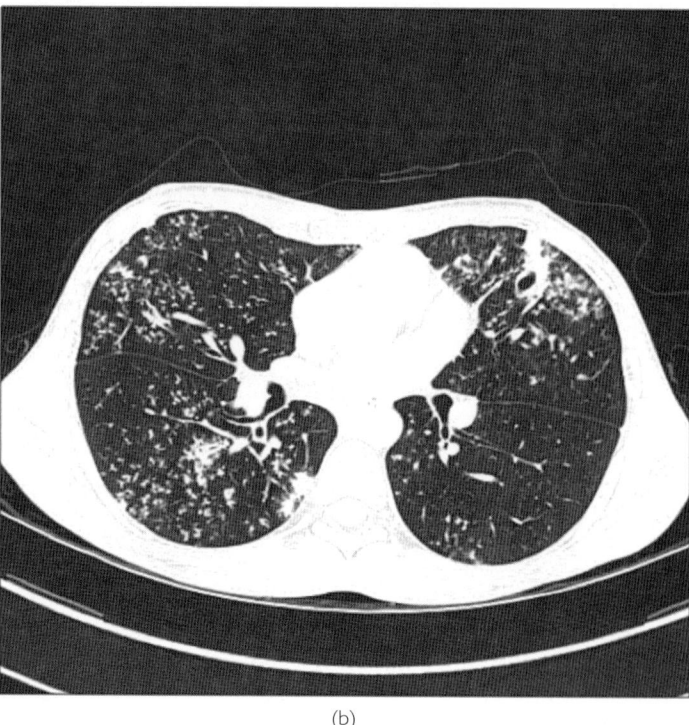

(b)

Fig 15.17: Pulmonary TB: (a, b) HRCT chest demonstrates thick-walled cavitating lesions and nodular consolidations in both apices, right middle lobe and left lingula.

world are the BACTEC 460 system and the MIGIT 960 system. Optimal recovery is achieved through a combination of rapid, automated liquid culture systems and solid LJ slopes. Our experience with both the BACTEC and the MIGIT system has been growing and we will discuss the advantages of these systems in the chapter on Newer Diagnostics.

SUSCEPTIBILITY TESTING

With the worldwide spread of multi-drug-resistant (MDR)-TB, susceptibility testing assumes great significance. In Mumbai, India, where we practice, an area of high prevalence of isoniazid and multi-drug resistance, we would recommend that ideally, sputum cultures and sensitivities should be requested in all patients when first seen. This may not be practical on a programmatic level but it was heartening to note that the new WHO 2009 guidelines have recommended that all patients who fail DOTS Category 1 treatment should have sputum cultures sent off and sensitivity performed on positive cultures instead of wasting a further eight months of treatment with Category 2 treatment.

The principles of *M. tuberculosis* testing were established by Canetti almost 50 years ago. Generally speaking, direct or indirect tests may be performed by either conventional or rapid methods. The inoculum for the direct tests is the processed clinical specimen in which AFB have been observed (i.e. smear-positive sputum). The advantage of this approach is that the results are obtained sooner and the inoculum is a true representative of bacterial population *in situ*. The inoculum for the indirect tests on the other hand is the primary isolate culture. This makes preparation of a uniform inoculum easier.

The conventional methods may be performed as direct or indirect tests by inoculating the microorganisms on to a solid medium that has a known concentration of the test drug. For each of the methods described, test concentration of drugs may be prepared in the medium by appropriate dilutions of stock solutions of antimicrobials. This is most easily done in the disc method by incorporating the necessary number of commercially available antimicrobial-containing elution

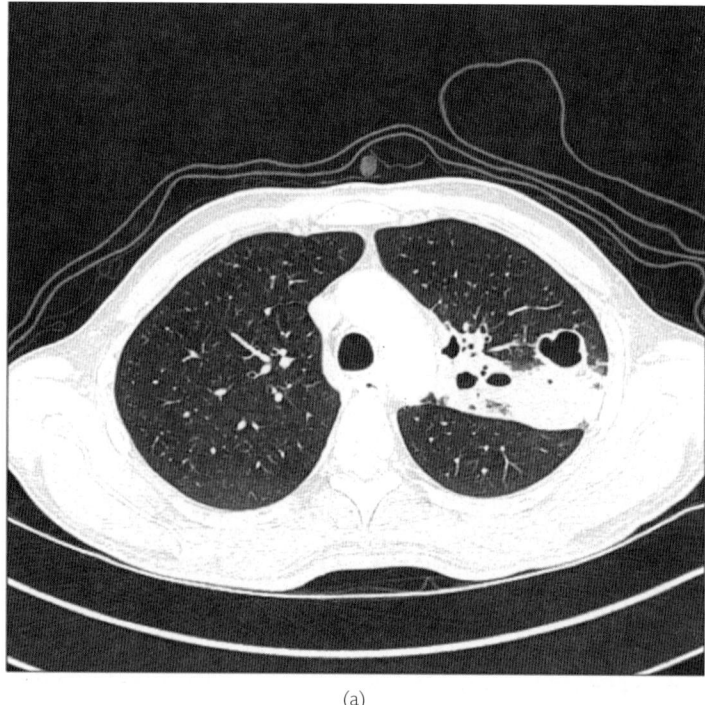

(a)

Fig 15.18a: Pulmonary TB: HRCT chest demonstrates left apico-posterior consolidation with internal cavitation.

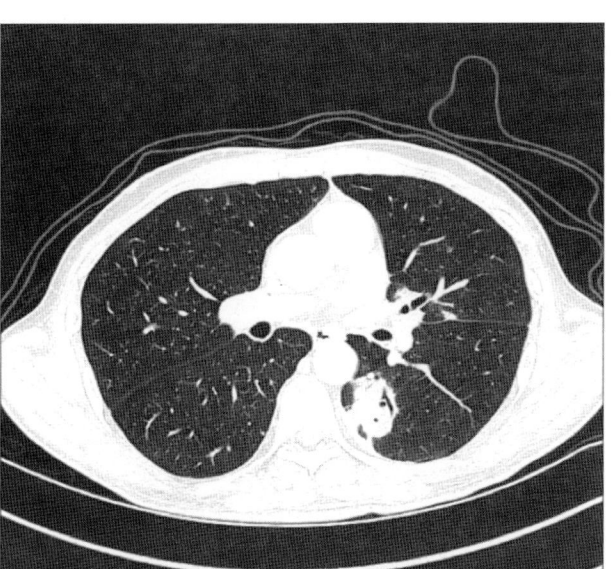

(b)

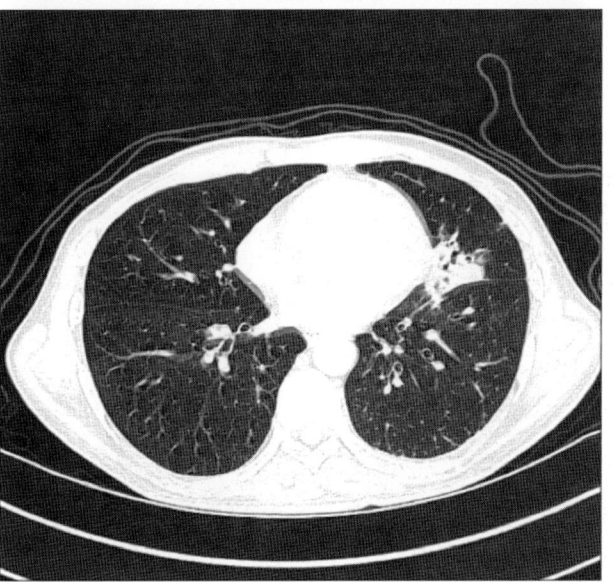

(c)

Fig 15.18b and c: Nodular consolidation in apical segment of left lower lobe and lingula. These are the typical areas of involvement of TB.

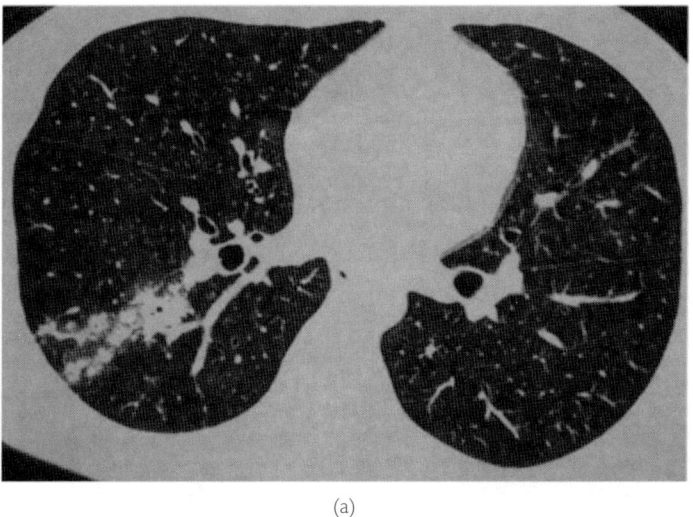

(a)

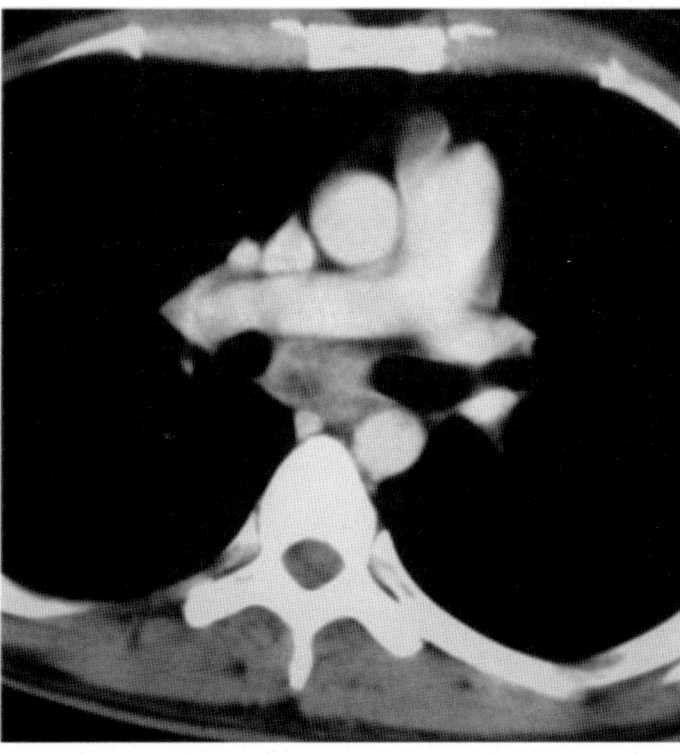

(b)

Fig 15.20a and b: Endobronchial spread of TB: HRCT demonstrates ill-defined nodular lesions in the right upper lobe posteriorly in a branching 'tree in bud' appearance indicative of endobronchial spread of infection. Mediastinal window demonstrates subcarinal adenopathy with internal hypodensity representing internal necrosis, a typical appearance of tuberculous adenopathy.

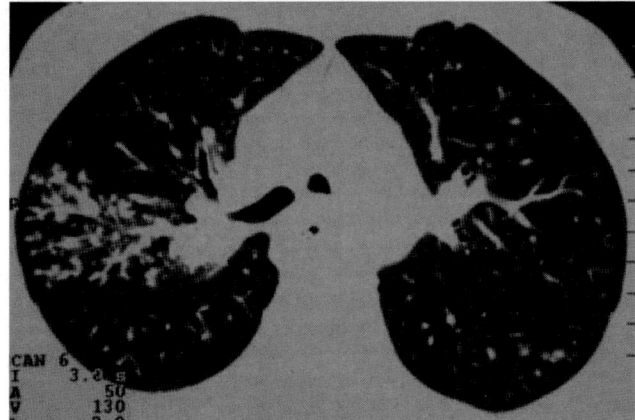

Fig 15.19: Endobronchial TB: HRCT chest demonstrates multiple small nodular lesions in a branching pattern extending from the hilum to the periphery of the lung. This appearance is termed 'tree in bud' appearance. The tree in bud appearance indicates endobronchial spread of infection.

discs in the medium. The three commonly used conventional methods are: the absolute concentration method, the resistance ratio method and the proportion method. The Centres for Disease Control (CDC) modification of the proportion method is generally considered the standard method in this diverse field. It should be noted that susceptibility tests for pyrazinamide can be performed in conventional media only at a reduced pH of about 5.5, a pH at which some strains will not grow. It is therefore recommended that pyrazinamide be

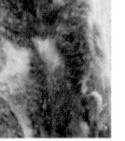

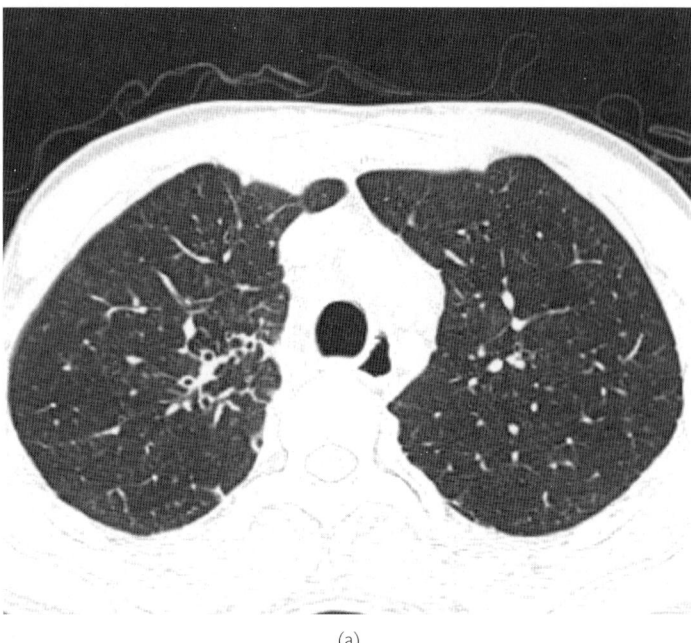

(a)

Fig 15.21a: Reactivation TB: HRCT chest demonstrates bronchiectasis and fibrosis in the right apex secondary to old healed TB.

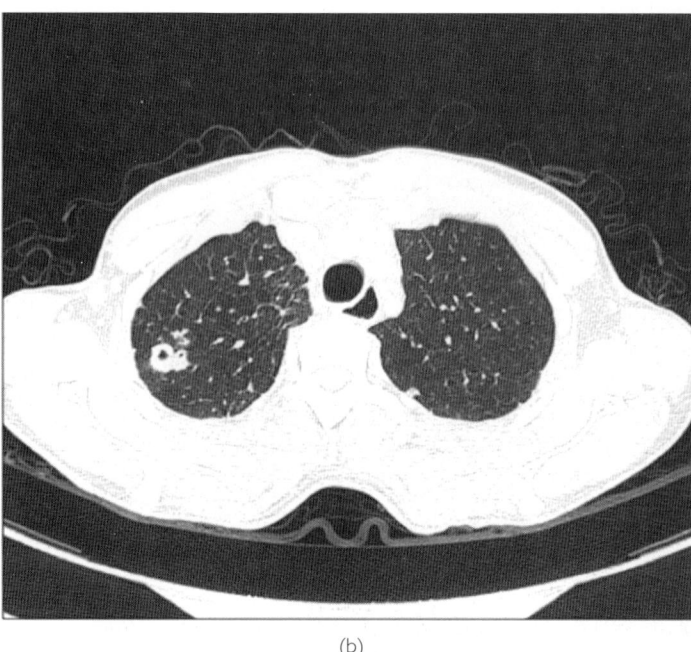

(b)

Fig 15.21b: Patient presented with low-grade fever, weight loss. HRCT chest revealed a nodular consolidation in the right apex with internal cavitation and small satellite nodular lesions in the apex.

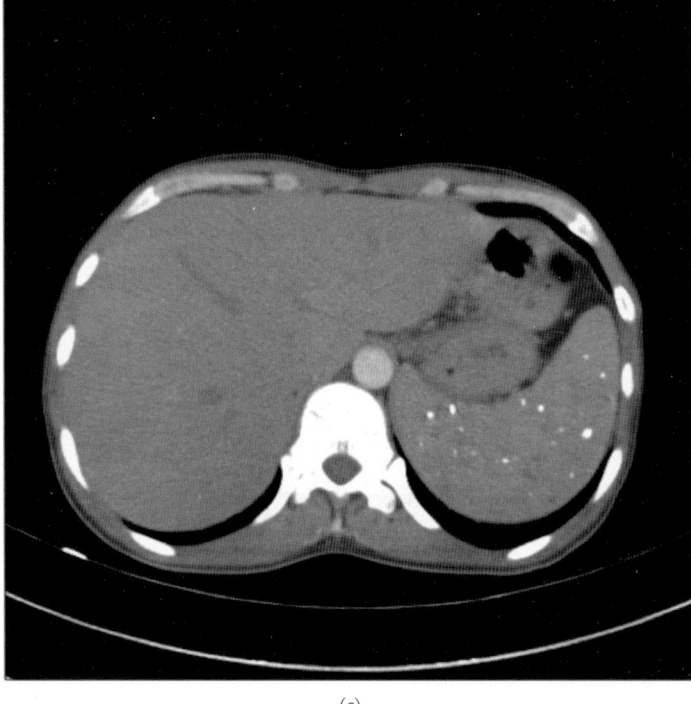

(c)

Fig 15.21c: CT abdomen demonstrates multiple calcified splenic granulomas, a residue from the previous TB infection.

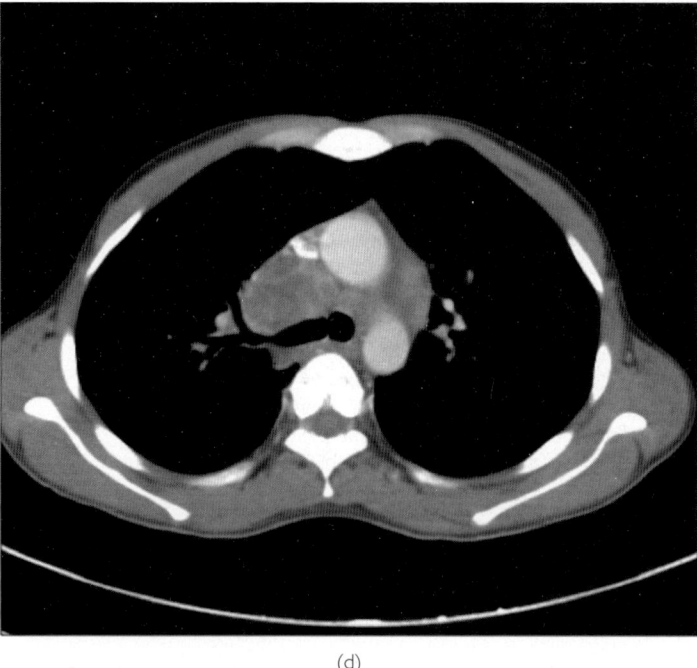

(d)

Fig 15.21d: CT chest with contrast revealed large necrotic mediastinal adenopathy in the right pre/paratracheal regions. The presence of nodular consolidations with cavitations and large necrotic mediastinal adenopathy is indicative of reactivation of pulmonary TB on a background of fibrosis, bronchiectasis and calcified granulomas.

tested by the BACTEC method. Essential to all susceptibility tests, regardless of method, are the critical concentration of drugs to be tested.

During the early 1980s the BACTEC radiometric system for primary isolation of mycobacteria was developed with a susceptibility test protocol. The use of this system increased the speed with which resistant strains were detected to just four to six days after inoculation. Another advantage of the BACTEC system is the ability to test for susceptibility to pyrazinamide. The MIGIT test has also been adapted to susceptibility testing and several studies have found high correlations between the BACTEC, MIGIT and proportion methods. The time to

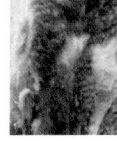

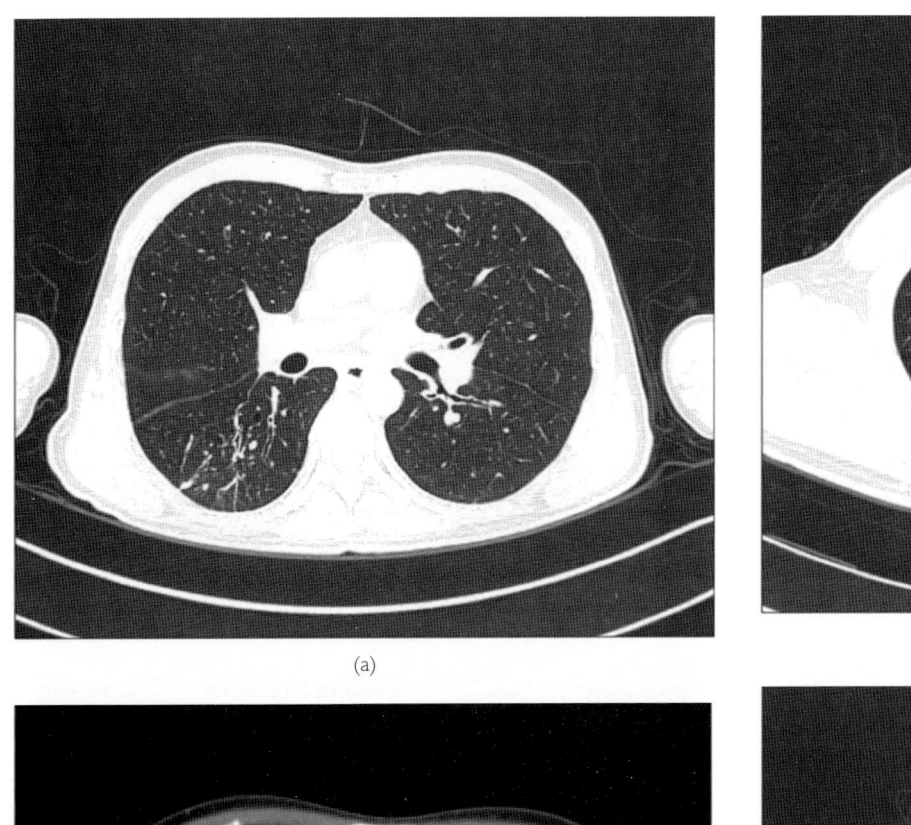

(a)

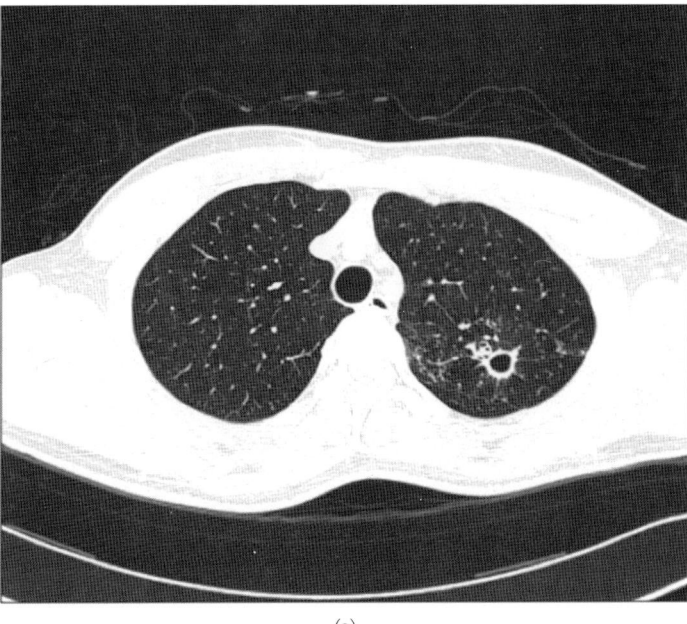

(a)

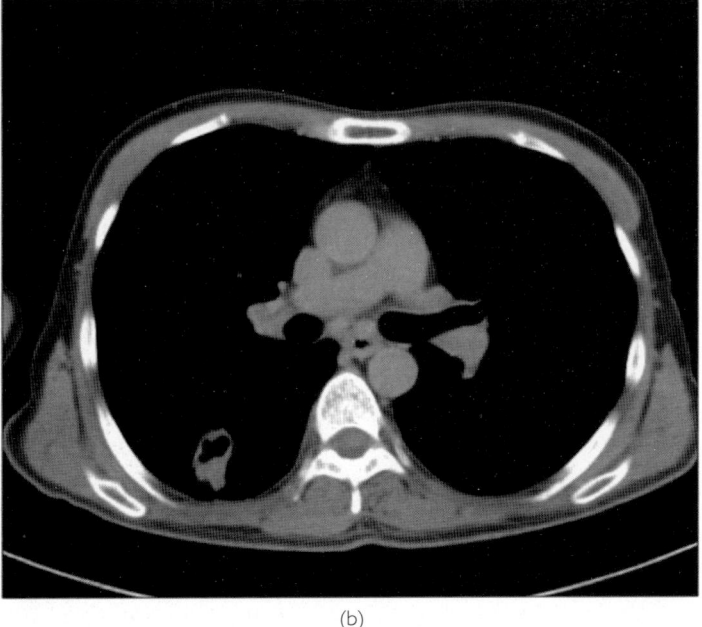

(b)

(b)

Fig 15.22: (a) Reactivation of pulmonary TB: Fibrotic lesions with associated bronchiectasis in the apical segment of the right lower lobe. These features are indicative of an old healed inflammatory process. The patient presented with fresh symptoms of fever and cough (b) Section lower to fibrosis demonstrated thick-walled cavity with air fluid level confirming reactivation of TB.

Fig 15.23: Cavitatory TB with haemoptysis: (a) thick-walled cavity with peripheral small nodular lesions in left apex as a result of pulmonary TB. The patient presented with haemoptysis (b) Sections through lingula demonstrate small ill-defined ground-glass densities in the left lingula.

detection of resistance with the MIGIT system is comparable to that for the BACTEC system. The newer liquid culture methods and molecular methods will be discussed in more detail in the chapter on Newer Diagnostics. The clinician needs to know more about the several available DST methods, both phenotypic and genotypic and these will be discussed in some detail here.

With the emergence of MDR and XDR–TB, the need for new, rapid and reliable DST is felt globally. Tests can be broadly divided into phenotypic and genotypic methods.

A) *Phenotypic methods* These methods rely on detection of the effects of the drugs on bacterial multiplication or metabolism, compared to controls not exposed to the drugs. The important phenotypic tests are: mycobacteria growth index (MGIT), microscopic observation broth-drug susceptibility assay (MODS), slide DST, microcolony method, colorimetric redox indicator methods, nitrate reductase methods (NRA), and mycobacteriophage based methods.

B) *Genotypic Methods* These methods are molecular methods based on identification of resistance conferring

5

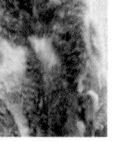

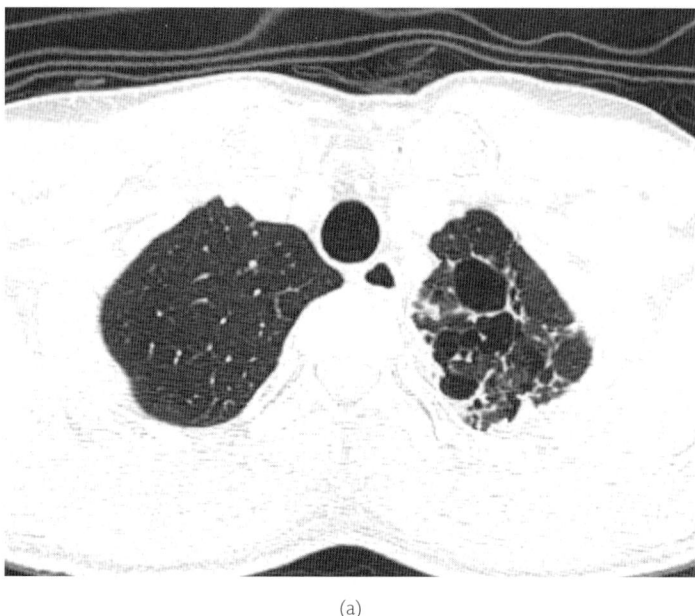

(a)

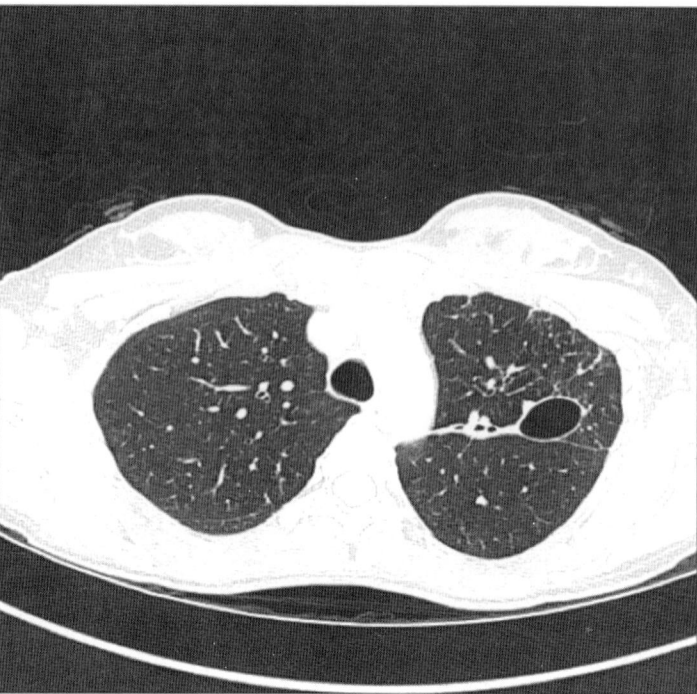

Fig 15.25: Old healed TB: Follow-up CT in a patient with left apical cavitatory TB demonstrates thin-walled cavity in left apex with associated fibrotic lesion and associated bronchiectasis. The thin-walled nature of the cavity, lack of surrounding inflammation, fibrosis and bronchiectasis are all indicative of old healed quiescent TB.

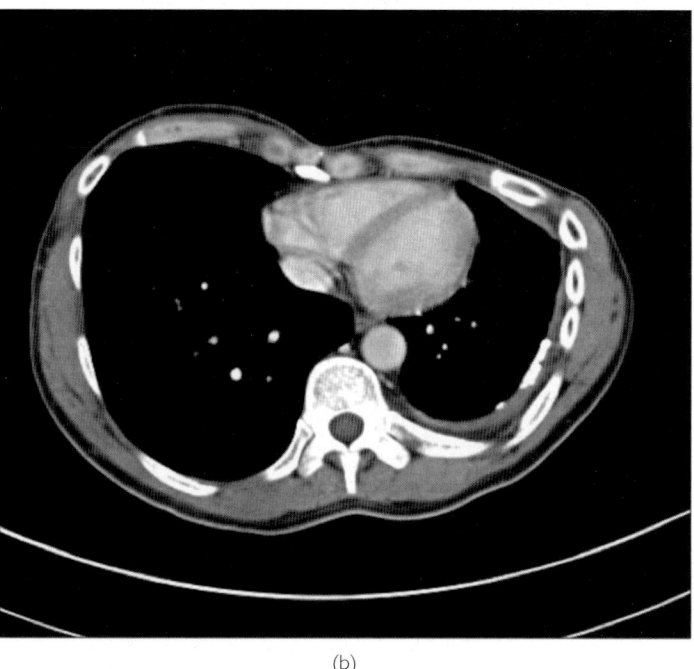

(b)

Fig 15.24: Old healed TB: (a) HRCT demonstrates fibrotic lesions with thin-walled air spaces in the left apex. There also appears to be loss of volume as the left apex is smaller in size than the right apex. The walls of the air spaces are not thick, there is no surrounding ill-defined soft tissue or satellite nodules to suggest active infection (b) Lower sections with mediastinal window demonstrate thickened pleura with calcification and loss of volume, small-sized left hemithorax indicative of old healed TB.

olutionize the future of DST. The notable advantage of all molecular tests is their rapid turnover time of 6-48 hours. This is likely to have major implications for patient management. The reader interested in further details is referred to the article by Van Deun which is a state of the art review on the subject. *(Ref: Van Deun A, Martin A, Palomino JC. Diagnosis of drug resistant tuberculosis: reliability and rapidity of detection. Int J Tuberc Lung Dis. 2010: 14; 131–40.)*

TUBERCULIN SKIN TEST (TST)

This is one of the oldest tests in medicine to still be widely used in current times. Tuberculin was first prepared by Robert Koch and wrongly assumed to be a cure for TB. The original preparation was purified by Seibert in the 1930s and was standardized a decade later in Denmark where it was labelled PPD-RT23. A final modification came when a small quantity of detergent (Tween 80) was added to the solution. This detergent prevented the absorption of the tuberculin by glass and plastic surfaces that resulted in occasional false-negative reactions. Two techniques may be used to perform the TST, the Mantoux test and the Heaf test. Of these, it is the Mantoux test that is widely used in India and in most of the developing world. This is performed by the intradermal injection of 0.1 ml of PPD containing 5 TU into the volar aspect of the forearm using a 27-gauge needle with a plastic or glass syringe. The injection must be made just beneath the surface of the skin so it raises a wheal of 6–10 mm in diameter. The test is read 48–72 hours later when the induration is measured in millimetres and reported. Depending on the size of the induration following a 5 TU Mantoux test,

mutations of the bacillary genome. Line probe assays based on reverse hybridization DNA strip technology have become a hot topic after they were endorsed by WHO for DST because of their combination of speed and accuracy, relatively low technical requirements and ease of sample transport. The INNOLIPA Rif TB, Geno Type MTBDR, and Genotype MTBDRsl assays are the tests poised to rev-

reactions should be considered significant and indicative of TB infection in the following categories of patients:

Indurations > 5 mm
HIV-infected person.
Close recent contact with an infectious case of TB.
Persons with chest radiographs consistent with old healed TB.

Indurations > 10 mm
All other persons with other risk factors for TB apart from those listed above.

Indurations > 15 mm
Considered positive in all persons (including those with prior BCG vaccine).

Limitations of the TST: The TST has a number of limitations which will be discussed here. It has a suboptimal sensitivity of only 70–90% in diagnosing active TB. Paradoxically, it is less sensitive in just the high-risk groups where accuracy is most needed like newborns and the immunosuppressed population. Its estimated specificity in healthy people with no known TB disease or exposure is also low at around 50–90%. This is because of its cross-reactivity with BCG and non-tuberculous mycobacteria (NTM). Another inherent flaw is the practical issue of patients needing to return 48–72 hours later to have the test read again. A study we conducted at the Hinduja Hospital in 2003 showed that a sizeable number of patients (around 40% of the 1028 tests done) simply do not show up to even have their induration read. No other test has such a high default rate. Technical problems also abound. Batches may be of poor quality, have a relatively short expiry date and require a cold chain for storage which is not practical in remote parts of the country. There is also frequent inter-reader variability. Technical issues like the boosting phenomenon and conversion and reversion may make the interpretation of a repeat test difficult. Thus, to state the obvious, the TST is an imperfect test.

The potential confounding effect of BCG on the TST requires special mention. A meta-analysis of the effects of BCG on the TST showed that prior administration of BCG increased the likelihood of a positive TST (Relative risk 2.1). This was less likely when BCG was administered in infancy and more likely when given after a year. Tests usually stayed positive up to 15 years of age. After this age, a strongly positive TST should not be attributed to prior BCG.

TREATMENT OF TUBERCULOSIS

The aims of treatment of TB are:

- To cure the patient and restore quality of life and productivity.
- To prevent death from active TB.
- To prevent relapse of TB.
- To reduce transmission of TB to others.
- To prevent the development and transmission of drug resistance.

The first-line drugs are isoniazid, rifampicin, ethambutol, pyrazinamide and streptomycin. The recommended dosing schedule as currently recommended by WHO is tabulated below for daily and intermittent (thrice-weekly) regimens:

DOTS is the accepted standard of care for administration of these first-line drugs. The components of DOTS are discussed here:

1. Uninterrupted, free, short-course chemotherapy supply: These days, each registered TB patient has a TB patient kit which contains the full course of treatment which ensures the treatment will be uninterrupted. The kit provides health workers with a container that has all the required medicines in the right quantities and doses. This helps limit confusion and wastage and makes it easier to monitor the regularity of treatment. It is hoped that the patient may feel a sense of ownership that helps ensure he actually keeps returning till he finishes his kit. The standardization that goes into each kit also avoids the chaotic situation that occurs in the private sector where there are a vast and bewildering number of drugs and kits in the market, many of poor quality and questionable bio-availability.

2. Quality microscopy: is the next tenet of DOTS. All patients suspected of having pulmonary TB should submit at least two sputum specimens for microscopic examination in a quality-assured lab. When possible, at least one of these should be an early morning sputum specimen as sputum collected at this time has been shown to have the highest yield. A case of pulmonary TB should be considered to be smear-positive if one or more sputum smear specimens at the start of treatment are positive for AFB.

3. Reporting and monitoring systems in place: Each patient must be properly registered and the site of TB (pulmonary or extra-pulmonary) recorded. Record must also be made of whether the patient is a new case (never had treatment for TB or has taken TB treatment for less than a month) or a previously treated patient (one who has received > one month of TB drugs in the past.) Patient outcomes must also be accurately recorded as: cured, treatment completed, treatment failed or defaulted. Such accurate data recording lends itself to thorough analysis of the results of the DOTS programme. Any deficiencies can be noted and corrective steps taken.

4. Direct observation: This is perhaps the most controversial of all the DOTS principles. A healthcare worker must supervise the actual act of swallowing. This is believed to be the most reliable way to ensure compliance. Opponents of direct observation maintain that the act of supervision can be costly and alienating and point to a Cochrane review of four trials that looked at direct observation versus self-treatment and concluded that there was no benefit of direct observation.

Criticisms of DOTS in the Indian Context

Just as we recognized the immense contribution of DOTS to TB control in India, it is equally important to be objective and critical when necessary. A number of criticisms can be raised regarding DOTS in India:

- A verifiable address is mandatory before a patient can be registered in a DOTS centre. The homeless, the slum dwellers (50% of Mumbai's population) and the large migrant population are thus automatically excluded. This immediately excludes the most vulnerable members of society,

	Recommended dose			
	Daily		**3 times per week**	
Drug	**Dose and range (mg/kg body weight)**	**Maximum (mg)**	**Dose and range (mg/kg body weight)**	**Daily maximum (mg)**
Isoniazid	5 (4–6)	300	10 (8–12)	900
Rifampicin	10 (8–12)	600	10 (8–12)	600
Pyrazinamide	25 (20–30)	–	35 (30–40)	–
Ethambutol	15 (15–20)	–	30 (25–35)	–
Streptomycin	15 (12–18)		15 (12–18)	1000

Table 15.2:
Recommended doses of first-line antituberculosis drugs for adults

those that would most benefit from being included in a DOTS programme.

- Women are even more reluctant to attend a DOTS programme as they are even more stigmatized. Thus there is a skewed male to female ratio of 3:1 in many DOTS centres.
- Indeed, DOTS may be generally too obtrusive for Indians. The disease sadly continues to carry a stigma and seen entering a DOTS clinic leaves no room for doubt that the patient is suffering from TB.
- There is a feeling that the difficult patients are weeded out of many DOTS centres perhaps so that the impressive end of term results are not spoilt. Thus, the marginalized members of society like alcoholics, the homeless and drug addicts, which DOTS programmes should be striving to include, are deliberately left out in the cold.
- Private patients are completely outside the purview of DOTS at present. Several studies have shown that as many as 50–80% of new TB patients will choose to go private at the start. Thus, this large TB patient population falls out of the confines of DOTS, and falls prey to private practitioners, the majority of whom prescribe drug regimens that are clearly inappropriate. In a landmark study published in Tubercle and Lung Disease by Uplekar in 1993, 143 private doctors practising in the Dharavi area of Mumbai were asked: 'What prescription would you give a sputum-positive patient with no history of prior TB?' The 102 respondents came up with 80 different regimens, the majority inappropriate and more expensive than the standard. Western doctors do not fare much better. In an audit by Iseman, of patients eventually referred to his unit in Denver, management errors had been made in 80%. There was an average of 3.93 errors per patient with the single commonest error being the addition of a single new drug to a failing regimen.
- DOTS clinic hours are rigid and do not suit daily wage earners who are faced with a choice of either getting their drugs or feeding their family on that day. Travelling the long journey to more distant DOTS centres in more remote parts of the country is especially difficult for the old, the sick, the invalid and the poor.
- The greatly extra workload imposed on the system by DOTS may eventually overwhelm the system unless far more is allocated in terms of funds and man-power.

- Finally, DOTS alone is clearly inadequate for the MDR-TB and HIV-TB co-infected populations unless DOTS programmes include second-line drugs (the so-called DOTS-plus) and antiretroviral drugs.

Despite these critiques the DOTS-based RNTCP has been remarkably successful in achieving the global targets of detecting 70% of the estimated TB cases and curing 85% of them. Attempts to integrate the private and public sectors and iron out the deficiencies in DOTS outlined above are clearly the way ahead.

CURRENT TREATMENT REGIMENS

The current standard regimens for new TB patients is two months of Isoniazid (H), Rifampicin (R), Ethambutol (E) and Pyrazinamide (Z) in the so-called intensive phase followed by four months of isoniazid (INH) and rifampicin in the continuation phase. This six-month regimen is associated with almost 100% bacteriological conversion by the end of treatment in those with drug-susceptible disease and has a relapse rate of roughly 3–5%. The total duration of treatment should be extended from six to nine months in those patients in whom cavitation is noted on the initial chest radiograph and in those whose sputum is still culture-positive despite two months of treatment. The standard six-month regimen can be administered as daily therapy throughout, as intermittent therapy throughout (three times weekly), or as a mix of approaches with a period of daily administration followed by a period of intermittent administration. In the HIV-positive patient co-infected with TB, daily treatment is to be preferred. The latest 2009 WHO guidelines permit the use of HR and E in the continuation phase as an acceptable alternative to HR in areas where high levels of INH resistance are known to prevent the inadvertent development of MDR-TB while on treatment. Another major and positive change in the latest WHO guidelines is that Category 2 has been phased out. Category 2, previously used in treatment failures, comprised of 2HRZES/1HRZE/5HRE. In our opinion, the majority of people who fail standard treatment have MDR-TB. Subjecting these patients to Category 2 treatment serves only to amplify their resistance and waste an additional eight months. The current recommendation is that all such treatment failures should undergo drug susceptibility testing (DST) and

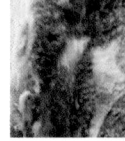

be started on an empiric MDR-TB regimen based on knowledge of local resistance patterns. This regimen can be modified and individualized once the DST is available. In countries which lack facilities for DST, the empiric MDR regimen should be continued throughout the duration of treatment.

FIRST-LINE DRUGS AND THEIR TOXICITIES

Isoniazid

Isoniazid has profound early bactericidal activity against rapidly dividing bacteria. Its major adverse effects are as follows:

- Asymptomatic elevation in transaminases: Aminotransferase elevations up to five times the upper limit of normal occur in up to 20% of persons receiving INH alone for treatment of latent TB infection. The enzyme levels usually return to normal even with continued administration of the drug.
- Clinical hepatitis: Data indicate that the incidence of clinical hepatitis is lower than was previously thought. Hepatitis occurred in only 0.1–0.15% of 11,141 persons receiving INH alone as treatment for latent TB infection in an urban TB control program. Prior studies suggested a higher rate, and a meta-analysis of six studies estimated the rate of clinical hepatitis in patients given isoniazid alone to be 0.6%. In this meta-analysis, the rate of clinical hepatitis was 1.6% when isoniazid was given with other agents, not including rifampicin. The risk was higher when the drug was combined with rifampicin, an average of 2.7% in 19 reports. For INH alone the risk increases with advancing age; it is uncommon in persons less than 20 years of age but is nearly 2% in persons aged 50–64 years. The risk may also be increased in persons with underlying liver disease, in those with a history of heavy alcohol consumption, and in the post-partum period. Acetylator status may be linked to hepatotoxicity but the link is controversial and screening for acetylator status is not of clinical value. The rate of fatal hepatitis with isoniazid is estimated to be 0.023 but recent studies suggest it may be substantially lower. Death has been associated with continued use of isoniazid despite evidence of hepatitis.
- Peripheral neuropathy: is an adverse effect of isoniazid that is dose-related. The risk is increased in patients with other risk factors for peripheral neuropathy like malnutrition, alcohol intake and diabetes, all common in the Indian context. Pyridoxine supplementation (20 mg/day) is essential to prevent this complication.
- CNS side-effects: seizures and psychosis have been rarely reported but the risk is difficult to quantify.
- Lupus-like syndrome: approximately 20% of patients receiving INH develop anti-nuclear antibodies. Less than 15% will develop a systemic lupus erythematosus (SLE)-like illness necessitating stoppage of the drug.

Rifampicin

Rifampicin has excellent activity against organisms that are dividing rapidly (early bactericidal activity) and against semi-dormant bacterial populations, thus accounting for its sterilizing activity.

- Hepatitis: Rifampicin interferes with the major bile salt exporter pump and may lead to a conjugated hyperbilirubinaemia. This is typically mild, asymptomatic, and of no clinical significance. On its own, rifampicin causes hepatitis (typically of a cholestatic pattern) much less frequently than isoniazid. When given in conjunction with isoniazid, rifampicin may potentiate isoniazid-induced liver injury, and one meta-analysis estimates the rate of hepatitis in patients taking both drugs to be as high as 2.55%.
- Cutaneous: Pruritis with or without rash is common, occurring in 6% of patients. It is generally limited and the drug can often be continued, but severe reactions necessitating stopping of the drug can occur in 0.1% of patients.
- Gastrointestinal (GI) symptoms: like nausea, gastritis and anorexia are frequent but rarely severe enough to necessitate stopping of the drug. Most can be treated symptomatically.
- Flu-like syndrome: occurs more frequently in those receiving intermittent rifampicin than in those on daily treatment with the drug.
- Severe immunological reactions: include thrombocytopenia, haemolytic anaemia, acute renal failure, and thrombotic thrombocytopenic purpura. These reactions are rare, occurring in less than 0.1% of patients and have an immune basis.
- Drug interactions: There are a number of drug interactions with potentially serious consequences. Of particular concern are reductions, often to ineffective levels, in the serum concentration of common drugs like warfarin, corticosteroids and oral contraceptives. Thus women using this form of birth control should be cautioned that contraceptives will lose efficacy while on rifampicin. In addition there are important bidirectional interactions between rifamycins and antiretroviral agents which will be discussed later.

Ethambutol

Ethambutol is a first-line drug for treating all forms of TB. It is included in initial treatment regimens primarily to prevent emergence of rifampicin resistance when primary resistance to isoniazid may be present. It is generally not recommended in children where visual acuity cannot be routinely monitored.

- Optic nerve toxicity: Retrobulbar neuritis is the main toxicity associated with ethambutol. This is manifested by decreased visual acuity or decreased red-green colour discrimination that may affect one or both eyes. The risk of optic toxicity is dose-dependent and is more common at doses of 30 mg/kg body weight or in patients with impaired renal function.

  Monitoring for ocular toxicity: Patients should have baseline visual acuity testing and testing of colour discrimination with Snellen charts and Ishara tests respectively. At each monthly visit, patients should be asked about blurred vision or scotomas. Monthly testing is recommended in those patients taking doses greater than 15–25 mg/kg for more than two months. Ethambutol should be immediately and permanently discontinued if there are any signs of visual toxicity.
- Cutaneous reactions and pruritis are not uncommon though reactions requiring discontinuation of the drug occur in 0.7% of patients.

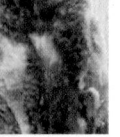

Pyrazinamide (PZA)

Pyrazinamide (PZA) is most effective against the population of dormant or semi-dormant bacteria contained within macrophages or in the acidic confines of caseous foci.

- Hepatotoxicity: Early studies using higher doses of 40–70 mg/kg per day reported hepatotoxicity at high rates. At the standard dose of 25 mg/kg hepatotoxicity occurs at a rate of 1%.
- Joint pains: Nongouty polyarthralgia may occur in up to 40% of patients receiving daily doses of PZA. This rarely requires discontinuation as it responds to nonsteroidal anti-inflammatory drugs (NSAIDs). Asymptomatic hyperuricaemia is an expected side-effect of the drug and does not usually require treatment. Acute gout attacks are rare except in patients with pre-existing gout in whom this drug should generally be avoided.

Streptomycin

Streptomycin is equivalent to ethambutol in the intensive phase of a six-month regimen.

Ototoxicity: which includes hearing and vestibular disturbances is the most important side-effect. The risk increases with age, concomitant use of loop diuretics, increasing single doses and cumulative doses > 120 g.

- Nephrotoxicity is less common with streptomycin than with amikacin or kanamycin. Renal insufficiency requiring discontinuation occurs in 2% of cases.

Symptom-based approach to management of side-effects of anti-TB drugs: The current WHO guidelines give a symptom-based approach to management of common side-effects. These side-effects may be classified as major and minor. In general, major effects necessitate stopping of treatment whilst minor effects should be treated symptomatically without discontinuation of drugs.

This approach is summarized in Table 15.3 below.

Managing individual side-effects: Only hepatitis, the most frequently described side-effect, will be discussed in detail here.

Hepatitis: Transient elevations of liver function during treatment are relatively common (20% of patients) and may not signify true hepatotoxicity. Drug-induced hepatitis, the most serious common adverse effect, is defined as a serum aspartate aminotransferase (AST) level more than three times the upper limit of normal in the presence of symptoms, or more than five

Table 15.3: Symptom-based approach to management of side-effects of TB drugs (WHO TB treatment guidelines 2010)		
Side-effects	**Drug(s) probably**	**Management**
Major		*Stop responsible drug(s) and refer to clinician urgently*
Skin rash with or without itching	Streptomycin, isoniazid, rifampicin, pyrazinamide	Stop anti-TB drugs
Deafness (no wax on otoscopy)	Streptomycin	Stop streptomycin
Dizziness (vertigo and nystagmus)	Streptomycin	Stop streptomycin
Jaundice (other causes excluded), hepatitis	Isoniazid, pyrazinamide, rifampicin	Stop anti-TB drugs
Confusion (suspect drug-induced acute liver failure if there is jaundice)	Most anti-TB drugs	Stop anti-TB drugs
Visual impairment (other causes excluded)	Ethambutol	Stop ethambutol
Shock, purpura, acute renal failure	Rifampicin	Stop rifampicin
Decreased urine output	Streptomycin	Stop streptomycin
Minor		*Continue anti-TB drugs, check drug doses*
Anorexia, nausea, abdominal pain	Pyrazinamide, rifampicin, isoniazid	Give drugs with small meals or just before bedtime, and advise patient to swallow pills slowly with small sips of water. If symptoms persist or worsen, or there is protracted vomiting or any sign of bleeding, consider the side-effect to be major and refer to clinician urgently.
Joint pains	Pyrazinamide	Aspirin or non-steroidal anti-inflammatory drug, or paracetamol
Burning, numbness or tingling sensation in the hands or feet	Isoniazid	Pyridoxine 50–75 mg daily
Drowsiness	Isoniazid	Reassurance. Give drugs before bedtime
Orange/red urine	Rifampicin	Reassurance. Patients should be told when starting treatment that this may happen and is normal
Flu syndrome (fever, chills, malaise, headache, bone pain)	Intermittent dosing of rifampicin	Change from intermittent to daily rifampicin administration

times the upper limit of normal in the absence of symptoms. Depending on the magnitude of the rise in transaminases, it may be graded as follows: if the AST level is less than five times the upper limit of normal, toxicity can be considered mild, an AST level 5–10 times normal defines moderate toxicity, and an AST level greater than 10 times normal (i.e., greater than 500 IU) is severe. In addition to AST elevation, occasionally there are disproportionate increases in bilirubin and alkaline phosphatase. This pattern is more consistent with rifampicin hepatotoxicity.

If hepatitis occurs, isoniazid, rifampicin, and pyrazinamide, all potential causes of hepatic injury, should be stopped immediately. Serologic testing for hepatitis viruses A, B, and C (if not done at baseline) should be performed and the patient questioned carefully regarding exposure to other possible hepatotoxins, especially alcohol.

Whilst waiting for liver function to normalize (generally a few weeks), a decision must be made whether to start a non-hepatotoxic regimen (if the TB is advanced and needs immediate treatment) or to keep the patient off all TB drugs till the liver function normalizes. This latter strategy is acceptable in patients with glandular TB or pleural TB who have a low bacillary load and are not too sick from their TB. On the other hand, if a delay of a few weeks is unacceptable due to the severity of the patient's TB (miliary, meningeal or cavitatory TB), three or more antituberculosis medications without hepatotoxicity, such as ethambutol, an aminoglycoside (streptomycin/amikacin/kanamycin/capreomycin), and a fluoroquinolone (levofloxacin or moxifloxacin), may be used until the hepatitis resolves.

Once the AST level decreases to less than two times the upper limit of normal and symptoms have significantly improved, the first-line medications should be restarted in sequential fashion.

The sequence outlined below is based on the current recommendations of the American Thoracic Society, CDC and Infectious Diseases Society of America. Because rifampicin is much less likely to cause hepatotoxicity than isoniazid or pyrazinamide and is the most effective agent, it should be restarted first. If there is no increase in AST after about one week, isoniazid may be restarted. Pyrazinamide can be started one week after isoniazid if AST does not increase. If symptoms recur, or AST increases, the last drug added should be stopped. If rifampicin and isoniazid are tolerated, and hepatitis was severe, pyrazinamide should be assumed to be responsible. In this situation it may be best to avoid the addition of this drug altogether. In this last circumstance, depending on the number of doses of pyrazinamide taken, severity of disease, and bacteriological status, therapy might be extended to nine months or a fluoroquinolone or aminoglycoside can take its place in the intensive phase.

Close monitoring, with repeat measurements of serum AST and bilirubin and symptom review, is essential in managing these patients.

TREATMENT OF TUBERCULOSIS IN SPECIAL SITUATIONS

1. Pregnancy and Lactation: All the first-line drugs except streptomycin may be safely used during pregnancy and lactation. Pyridoxine supplementation is essential in pregnant women receiving isoniazid. The safety profiles of the second-line drugs have not been ascertained, but they have been used in scattered case studies and small series with good maternal and foetal outcomes. Decisions about which drugs to continue must be individualized after a careful discussion of the possible teratogenic effects with the mother.

2. Renal failure: In a patient with a creatinine clearance < 30 ml/min or who is receiving dialysis, isoniazid and rifampicin may be given without any dose adjustment. Ethambutol and pyrazinamide must both be given in a three times a week frequency, with the actual dose in mg staying unaltered. All medications should be given post-dialysis on the day of the haemodialysis. All the aminoglycosides are best avoided, or, if they must be used, given no more than two or three times a week with serum concentration monitoring. Levofloxacin is also dependent on renal clearance and the frequency of administration must be reduced to three times a week.

SUGGESTED READING

Dedhia K, Udwadia ZF, Huggett JF, *et al.* Utility of the antigen-specific interferon-γ assay for the management of tuber009is. *Current Opinion in Pulmonary Medicine.* 2005; 11: 195–202.

Kobashi Y. Transitional change in the clinical features of pulmonary tuberculosis. *Respiration.* 1 Jan. 2008; 75(3): 304–9.

Lalvani A. Diagnosing tuberculosis infection in the 21st century. New tools to tackle an old enemy. *Chest.* 2007; 131:1898–1906.

Liebeschuetz S, Bamber S, Ewer K, Deeks J, Pathan AA, Lalvani A: Diagnosis of tuberculosis in South African children with a T-cell-based assay: a prospective cohort study. *Lancet.* 2004; 364: 2196–2203.

Pinto L, Udwadia ZF. The politics of TB: the politics, economics and impact of directly observed treatment in India. *Chronic Respiratory Disease.* 2007; 4(2): 101–6

Sharma SK. Miliary tuberculosis: new insights into an old disease. *Lancet Infect Dis.* 1 Jul. 2005; 5(7): 415–30.

Treatment of tuberculosis. *American Journal of Respiratory and Critical Care Medicine.* 2003; 167: 603–62.

Uplekar M, Shepard DS. Treatment of tuberculosis by private general practitioners in India. *Tubercle.* 1991; 72(4): 284–90.

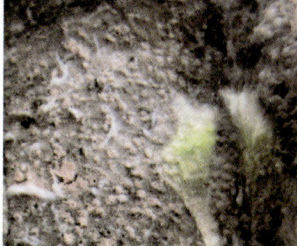

CHAPTER **16** | # MDR and XDR-Tuberculosis

MULTI-DRUG-RESISTANT TUBERCULOSIS

Terminology

Mono-resistant tuberculosis (TB) is resistance to only one drug. Included here are isolated isoniazid (INH) resistance and isolated rifampicin resistance.

Multi-drug-resistant (MDR)—TB is defined as a form of TB which is resistant to both INH and rifampicin.

A strict definition is necessary because resistance to both INH and rifampicin has a huge impact on the duration, cost and ultimately outcome of therapy.

Poly-resistant TB is a form of TB resistant to more than one drug but not the combination of INH and rifampicin.

Extensively drug-resistant (XDR)-TB is MDR-TB plus additional resistance to any fluoroquinolone and at least one of the second-line injectables (Amikacin, Kanamycin, Capreomycin).

Types of MDR-TB

Drug resistance amongst new cases (Primary): Drug resistance in a patient who has never been treated for TB or who has received less than one month of therapy.

Drug resistance amongst previously treated cases (Secondary or acquired): Drug resistance in a patient who has received at least one month of anti-TB drug therapy.

Pathogenesis

MDR-TB is an iatrogenic problem. It is caused by patients not taking the drugs as prescribed to them or by physicians not prescribing the correct drugs in the correct doses and/or for the correct duration. Soon after streptomycin was first introduced as a TB drug in 1947 it became apparent that resistance to individual drugs would develop at a predictable rate if the compounds were used as single agents. Resistance to an anti-TB drug is due to spontaneous chromosomal mutation at a frequency of 10^6 to 10^8 bacterial replications. These rates correspond to the average expected frequency of spontaneous mutation of chromosomes. As mutations resulting in resistance are unlinked, the probability of resistance to all three drugs used simultaneously is in the order of 10^{18} to 10^{20}. Even a large tuberculous cavity would be expected to contain no more than 1 million TB bacteria. Hence the chance of spontaneous drug resistance is almost impossible when three effective drugs are used in combination. This is the principle of modern short-course chemotherapy. MDR-TB is thus always a manmade or iatrogenic problem occurring when these drugs are prescribed in the wrong doses or taken irregularly.

The genetic basis of resistance to most of the commonly used anti-TB drugs has been recently elucidated.

Table 16.1: Mechanisms of drug resistance in *Mycobacterium tuberculosis*		
Anti-TB drug	**Genes involved in resistance**	**Frequency of mutations**
Isoniazid	1) katG 2) inhA	1) 47–58% 2) 21–34%
Rifampicin	rpoB	96–98%
Streptomycin	1) rpsL 2) rrs	1) 52–59% 2) 8–21%
Ethambutol	embAB	50%
Pyrazinamide	pcnA	Unknown
Fluoroquinolones	gyrA	75–94%

Epidemiology of MDR-TB

GLOBAL EPIDEMIOLOGY

A global surveillance study on drug resistance conducted by the WHO- International Union Against Tuberculosis and Lung Disease (IUATLD) working group on drug resistance between 1994–97 was published in the *New England Journal of Medicine* (NEJM) in 1998 and looked at data from 35 countries and covered an aggregate population of almost 20% of the globe. This study first put MDR-TB on the global map and demonstrated that MDR-TB was found in all countries surveyed. The overall median MDR-TB rate was as low at 2.2% (1.1–3.8%). It was this study however that established that there were 'hotspots' for transmission of MDR-TB and identified India, Soviet Union, Argentina, and The Dominican Republic as hotspots with the highest combined MDR-TB rate being in Latvia (22%). The latest global epidemiological update on MDR-TB comes from the 4th Anti-Tuberculosis Drug Resistance Report published jointly by the WHO and the IUATLD in 2008. This report included drug susceptibility results from 91,577 patients from 93 settings in 81 countries collected between 2002 and 2006. This data was even more reliable because it was only included if collected from National Reference Laboratories or Supranational Reference Laboratories. According to this, the latest WHO survey, it was estimated that in the year 2006, 489,139 MDR cases emerged. Thus MDR accounted for about 5.3% (95% CLs, 3.9–6.6) of the nine million new TB cases that emerged that year. The global distribution ranged from

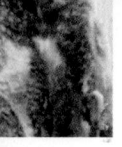

0% in some Western European countries to over 35% in some countries of the former Soviet Union. The three countries with the highest prevalence of MDR-TB among new cases were: Azerbaijan, Republic of Moldova, and Donetsk Oblast, Ukraine. The three countries with the highest prevalence of MDR-TB amongst retreated cases were: Uzbekistan, Azerbaijan, and Jordan. In terms of absolute numbers of MDR-TB cases in this study, China, India, and the Russian Federation were estimated to carry the highest number of MDR-TB cases. Between them, China and India accounted for approximately 50% of the global burden of MDR-TB.

INDIAN EPIDEMIOLOGY

The epidemiology of MDR-TB in India is bedeviled by a number of factors:

1. Lack of proper notification.
2. Lack of accurate recording of data.
3. Sampling of small, non-representative patient groups.
4. Very few laboratories are capable of performing reliable drug susceptibility testing (DST).
5. Non-standardized laboratory techniques, often with no quality control.
6. Failure in most studies to distinguish primary from secondary resistance.

Early small studies from different parts of India had put the primary MDR-TB rates at 1.6% (North Arcot), 0.7% (Pondicherry), and 0.9% (Jaipur). The problem with all these studies was that they included small, non-representative populations with considerable referral bias. Several studies from across the country in the 1980s and 1990s reported much higher rates of acquired resistance with rates of 49% from Gujarat (1986), 54% from Haryana (1992), 46% from Orissa (1994), and as high as 56% in Mumbai from patients we saw at the Hinduja Hospital in 1997.

A study from the Hinduja Hospital was also the first to point out the considerable urban-rural divide when it came to MDR-TB in India. Whilst the rural MDR-TB rates from a small district in Sakwar village, Maharashtra, were 3% of 150 samples, the urban MDR-TB rates from Mumbai over the same time period (1997–98) were much higher at 49% of 150 samples. The heterogeneous urban population and the unregulated and poor prescribing practice of the private sector in Mumbai was believed to be responsible for the vastly higher MDR-TB rates from a big metropolis like Mumbai.

In the 1994 report alluded to earlier, India had a combined MDR-TB rate of 13.3% which made it the second highest worldwide after Latvia. However, in our opinion, even this is a considerable underestimate. Indian data came only from New Delhi and included only 2240 isolates over a short period of six months. In addition no attempt was made to distinguish primary from acquired resistance.

In the more recent data from the fourth WHO report released in 2008 there were an estimated 110,132 MDR cases in India in 2006. Indian MDR-TB represented 20% of the global burden. MDR-TB accounted for 3% of new cases and 17% of retreated cases. In this report, the actual data came from four regions; Gujarat, Kerala, Bengal and Orissa. Despite the larger number of samples from different parts of the country,

in our opinion, this data too under-represents the scale of MDR-TB in India. MDR-TB seen in the Indian private sector remains unreported and hence even these figures are probably considerable underestimates of the scale of the problem.

Clinical Features of MDR-TB

MDR-TB is clinically indistinguishable from drug-sensitive TB. It remains essentially a microbiological diagnosis but must be suspected in certain settings. A cardinal rule is to suspect MDR-TB in any patient with a past history of TB treatment no matter how remote that history. MDR-TB must also be suspected in a patient with TB who gives a history of contact with a patient proven to have MDR-TB. HIV-positive patients are believed by some authorities to have a higher likelihood of developing MDR and XDR-TB but this link has never been proven. In Western countries, MDR-TB is much more common in immigrants from areas of known high prevalence of MDR-TB.

Homelessness, alcohol and substance abuse, and prison populations are also at higher risk of MDR-TB.

Diagnosis of MDR-TB

MDR-TB can only be diagnosed after culture and drug susceptibility testing is performed. Although culture and DST will never be practical or possible in all TB suspects in this country, it is important to identify patients at higher risk of drug resistance such as relapse, retreatment, and chronic cases, HIV co-infected patients, those with poor adherence to first-line drugs, and close contacts (including children) of drug-resistant source cases. In all the patient groups mentioned above a culture and DST should be mandatory.

Impact of MDR-TB in India

MDR-TB is particularly devastating in India because it is usually suspected and diagnosed late. Very few laboratories reliably perform DSTs in the country. There is no public provision for treating these patients who therefore are compelled to seek out multiple private practitioners of varying quality. Sadly, these patients are still stigmatized, and as second-line drugs are expensive, they end up being partially treated. This results in a huge pool of chronic MDR-TB patients who receive just enough treatment to keep them alive but not enough to cure them. Thus there is exponential spread of this deadly form of TB in crowded communities.

Reasons for the Spread of MDR-TB in India

MDR-TB took root in India as a result of a combination of the following factors:

1. A failing National Tuberculosis Programme (NTP): India's NTP which originated in 1962 was conceived on sound scientific and social grounds. It was, however, poorly implemented, and hence made no epidemiological impact over three decades. Indeed it begat and bred MDR-TB. Alarm bells were slow to ring and it was only in 1992 that the Indian government finally conceded that the NTP had failed. A joint panel of experts from WHO, SIDA, and the

Indian government concluded that it be abandoned in favour of the Revised National Tuberculosis Control Programme (RNTCP). This was funded by a soft loan of $142 million and based on the five DOTS principles we have discussed earlier.

2. Patient-related factors: TB is not an easy topic for an Indian patient to discuss. There is a large amount of secrecy, denial, and unfortunately even ostracism of Indian patients with MDR-TB. These attitudes are born out of ignorance. Compliance remains poor, with no more than a third of patients completing their treatment. 'Doctor shopping' is a peculiar Indian trait, with work by Uplekar showing that the average rural patient with TB visits 2.5 doctors and the average urban patient visits four before even commencing treatment. Indian patients switch doctors and systems of medicine with impunity so there is little continuity of care.

3. Doctor-related factors: India has a huge and unregulated private health sector. Seventy per cent of hospitals are privately run, and 76% of doctors engage in private practice. In addition, Indian doctors are a heterogeneous mix with around 50% being non-allopaths who practice a number of alternative forms of medicine including homeopathic, ayurvedic and unani systems. Besides these, an unknown number of 'doctors' practice without any qualification at all (hakims, tantriks, vaids). Unfortunately, even allopathic doctors in India are of greatly varying standards. They perform unnecessary tests, have little formal training in community health, do not keep adequate records, do not notify public health authorities about MDR-TB and seldom bother with contact tracing even in the homes of patients with MDR-TB. The poor prescribing practice of Indian doctors even when it comes to prescribing standard drugs has been exposed by Uplekar and been commented on in an earlier section of this chapter. We repeated Uplekar's study 20 years after the original, this time asking a group of 106 doctors in Dharavi how they would treat MDR-TB. While the majority would attempt to treat these difficult patients themselves, without referral to a specialist, only 3% were able to provide a correct prescription; 35% added a single second-line drug to a failing regimen (most commonly a fluoroquinolone). Without doubt irresponsible prescribing practices like these are the main factors fuelling MDR-TB in India.

4. Government factors: Many of India's health problems have arisen from policy failure and government callousness and bureaucratic short-sightedness. TB is no exception. Lack of funding and failure to grasp the scale and severity of India's TB crisis has allowed the TB epidemic to escalate to its current proportions. Even now, while DOTS caters admirably to the vast majority of patients with TB in the community, the large and expanding pool of MDR-TB is conveniently ignored. As a national strategy this has been justified over the years as acceptable public health realpolitick, as treatment of the individual MDR-TB patient is not cost-effective. Indeed, several hundred sensitive TB patients could be offered standard short-course chemotherapy for the cost of treating just one patient with MDR-TB. These patients have equal rights to treatment however, and it is only in the last two years that the situation seems to be changing with the setting up of DOTS-plus pilot projects in several states. This is clearly a huge step in the right direction for these desperately ill patients, but whether the RNTCP can

conjure up the large sums needed to treat all the MDR-TB patients in the country remains to be seen.

5. Social factors: The harsh fact that TB is a social disease is brought into sharp focus in a country like India which is plagued by seemingly insurmountable social and economic problems. The facts speak for themselves: a population well in excess of 1 billion with 46% below the poverty line, childhood malnutrition rates of 47% and among the highest infant mortality rates in the world at 46%. Despite this the 2009 budget allocated less than 1% of GDP to health in the public sector.

6. The HIV epidemic: India now has among the highest absolute numbers of HIV cases in the world (around 5 million). The HIV epidemic in this country is now established and mature: all ages, both sexes and all social strata are affected. Though the HIV prevalence in the general population remains relatively steady at 1%, there has been a frightening speed of escalation in high-risk populations, with HIV rates increasing from 1 to 51% amongst prostitutes in Mumbai and from 8 to 36% among STD clinic patients in a period of five years. Ignorance about AIDS remains profound with several polls showing that only a minority of Indian women of reproductive age had even heard about AIDS. A large dually infected population of TB-HIV patients is emerging, some with MDR strains. This will pose an enormous additional strain on the overstretched RNTCP programme in India.

XDR-TB

In March 2006 a report in MMWR (Morbidity and Mortality Weekly Report) by the CDC and WHO drew attention to the emergence of MDR-TB with additional extensive resistance

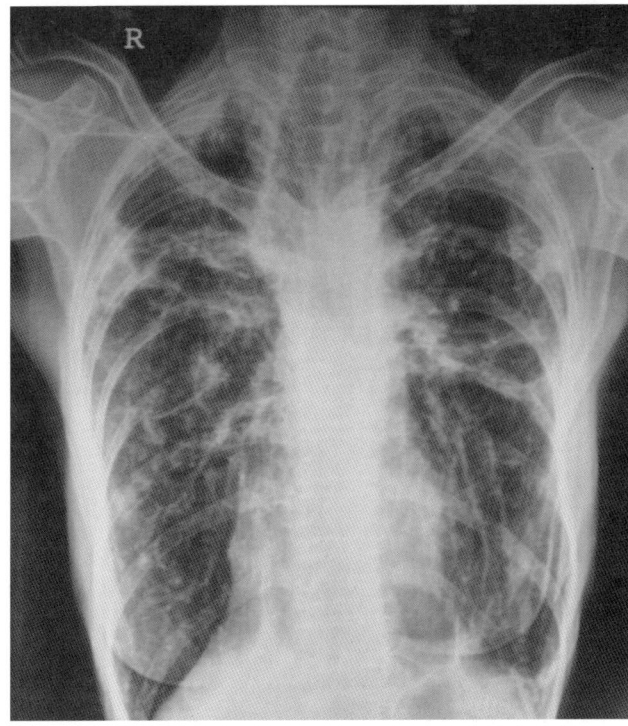

Fig 16.1: MDR-TB. Chest X-ray reveals extensive soft tissue infiltration, cavities in both upper and midzones with calcific and fibrotic lesions.

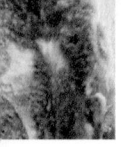

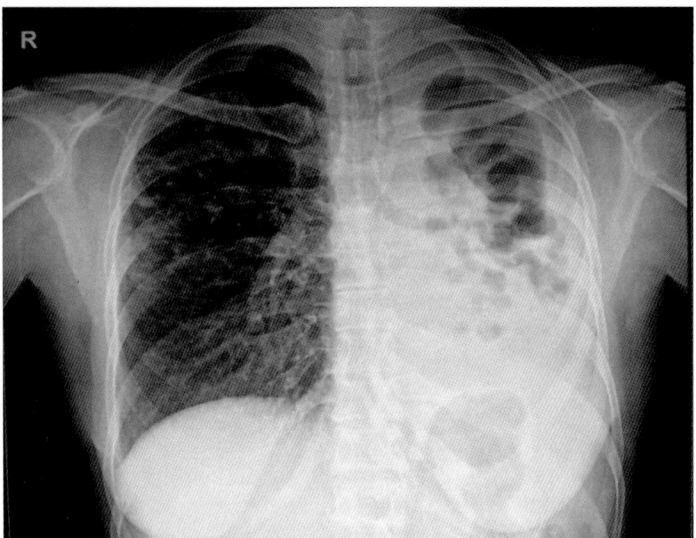

Fig 16.2: MDR-TB. Smear-positive despite DOTS 6 months cat 1, DOTS cat 2 8 months; subsequent smears confirm MDR-TB. Chest X-ray reveals destroyed left lower lobe with multiple cavities in left upper lobe, and right lung infiltration.

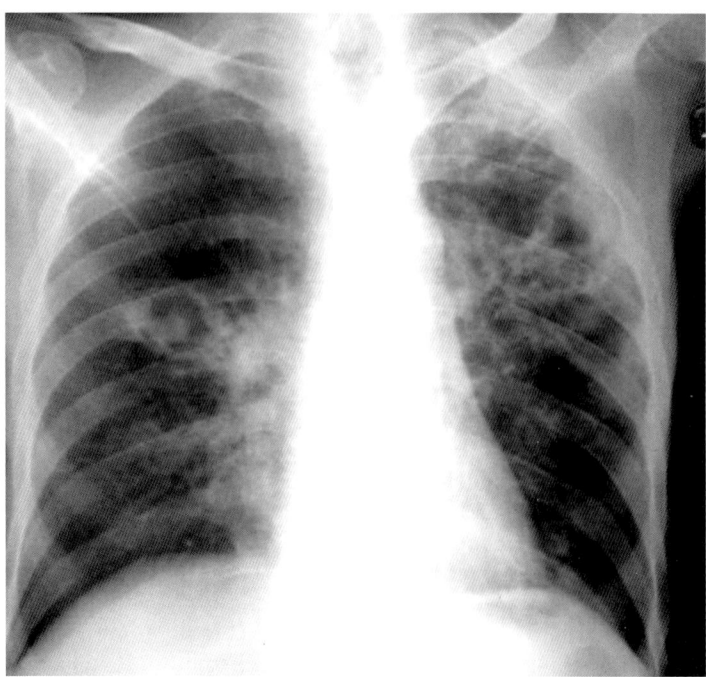

Fig 16.4: MDR TB. Chest X-ray demonstrates thick-walled cavitating lesions in the right midzone and left upper zone with associated ill-defined soft-tissue opacities.

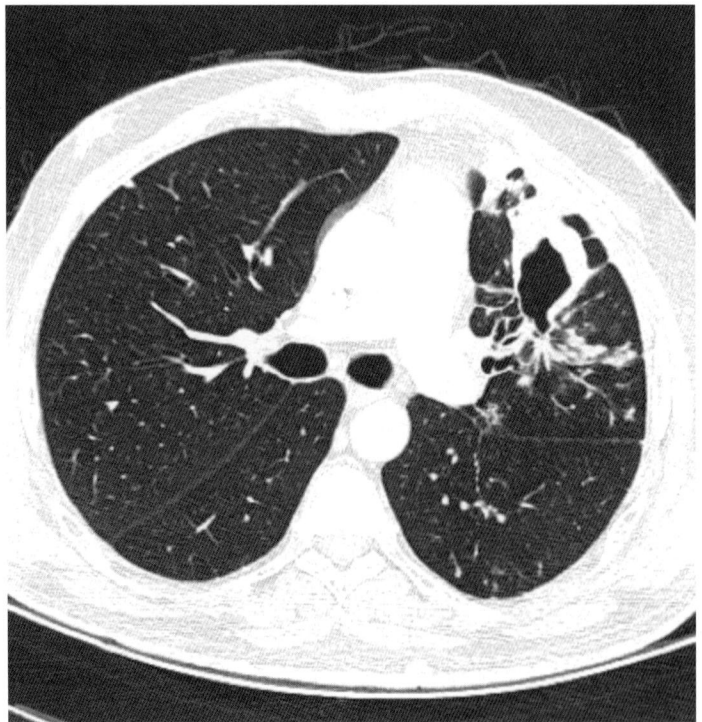

Fig 16.3: MDR-TB. CT chest demonstrates thick-walled cavitating lesions in the left lingula with peripheral fibrotic lesions and dilated bronchi.

to second-line drugs. Perversely, this report appeared on 24 March, world TB Day, exactly 124 years after Robert Koch had announced the discovery of the TB bacillus.

Definition

In the original MMWR report, XDR-TB was defined as a strain with INH and rifampicin resistance (MDR-TB) plus additional

resistance to at least three of the six classes of second-line drugs. These classes included the aminoglycosides, polypeptides, fluoroquinolones, thioamides, serine analogues, and para-amino salicylic acid. A few months later a revised taskforce of WHO met in Geneva, and modified the definition to its current version. XDR-TB is currently defined as resistance to INH and rifampicin plus additional resistance to any fluoroquinolone and at least one injectable second-line drug (amikacin, kanamycin or capreomycin).

The original report needs to be discussed in more detail since it brought XDR-TB to global attention. This retrospective survey looked at 17,690 isolates from 49 countries between 2000–04. To ensure microbiological authenticity, only strains tested from the 14 Supra National Reference laboratories were considered. The authors found that 20% of all isolates were MDR-TB and 10% of these MDR isolates met the original definition of XDR-TB. XDR-TB was present in 17 countries from all continents. The authors noted that the outcome of XDR-TB patients was far worse than of patients with MDR-TB strains. These patients were 50–64% more likely to die than those with MDR. Since the original CDC report, XDR-TB has been reported from across the globe. The current XDR-TB map of the world as of 2008 is shown in Fig 16.5 below. Recent data from Europe and America has confirmed this poor survival. From Europe (Russia, Italy, and Germany) data published by Migliori shows that XDR-TB has a significantly worse outcome than MDR-TB with these patients having a relative risk of 2.61 for unfavourable outcome compared to MDR-TB patients. From America, Iseman reported that the hazard ratio of death from XDR-TB in his cohort was 7.9 times that of MDR-TB.

The initial XDR-TB report generated huge public, media, lay-press and medical attention. It raised the profile of TB and drew global attention and funds towards TB. Eight months later, a leading article in the *Lancet* outlined the horrific clinical impact of XDR-TB. In this study, Gandhi and colleagues reported a cluster of cases from the Church Of Scotland Hospital in the Tugela Ferry township of rural KwaZulu Natal. Of 457 culture-positive patients at the hospital, 221 (41%) had MDR-TB and 53 of these (24%) had XDR-TB. They showed the strong link between XDR and HIV as all 44 patients of XDR-TB who were tested for HIV were positive. Molecular fingerprints for the South African XDR patients have been performed. The vast majority (nearly 90%) were found to have strains that were genetically similar (the F15/LAM4/KZN strain) which suggests patients were recently infected with the drug-resistant strain.

This study again gripped public and medical attention because of the high mortality reported; 52 of the 53 XDR-TB patients died, the median survival being just 16 days. Since then, survival data of small cohorts of patients with XDR-TB have been reported from all over the world. In general the survival is extremely poor in patients dually infected with XDR and HIV but better in patients with XDR-TB who are HIV-negative. However, even among non-HIV patients in industrialized countries, it is clear that XDR-TB is more difficult to treat and carries worse treatment outcomes than MDR-TB.

XDR-TB in India

The first series of XDR-TB cases from India emerged from the Hinduja Hospital, Mumbai. We retrospectively analyzed all samples sent for sputum culture at the mycobacterial laboratory of the hospital and noted that 11% of the 329 MDR-TB cases reported that year were in fact XDR-TB. Indeed, XDR-TB

has in all probability, existed for several years in India. India's unsupervised and chaotic MDR-TB programme is a recipe for further amplification of MDR-TB into XDR-TB strains. There are no public provisions for treating these patients apart from a few DOTS plus pilot projects and an unsupervised and chaotic private sector where second-line drugs are often added on singly and indiscriminately to clearly failing regimens. Special mention and condemnation must be made here of the indiscriminate use of fluoroquinolones. An ORG audit of a total of 318 million antibiotic prescriptions in 2004 showed ciprofloxacin was by far the most commonly prescribed antibiotic across the country. It was cheap, available off patent, and sold for a variety of nonspecific indications including viral infections and upper respiratory tract infections. Fluoroquinolone resistance to *M. tuberculosis* is a global phenomenon after its initial documentation from New York by Sullivan. At the Hinduja laboratory, Mumbai, fluoroquinolone resistance for *M. tuberculosis* increased from 6% in 1997 to 35% in 2004. Thus indiscriminate prior use has rendered a pivotal second-line drug near-worthless. MDR-TB plus fluoroquinolone resistance is sometimes called pre-XDR-TB. Treating this form of resistant TB is more difficult than MDR-TB. Resistance occurs by a single missense mutation in the gyrA region. Besides, it can occur rapidly; a single seven-day course of fluoroquinolone being sufficient to result in high-grade quinolone resistance for TB when used again a few days later.

Diagnosis

The high early mortality of patients with XDR-TB who are co-infected with HIV has made it even more essential to develop new faster tests for diagnosis of XDR-TB. Liquid cultures are

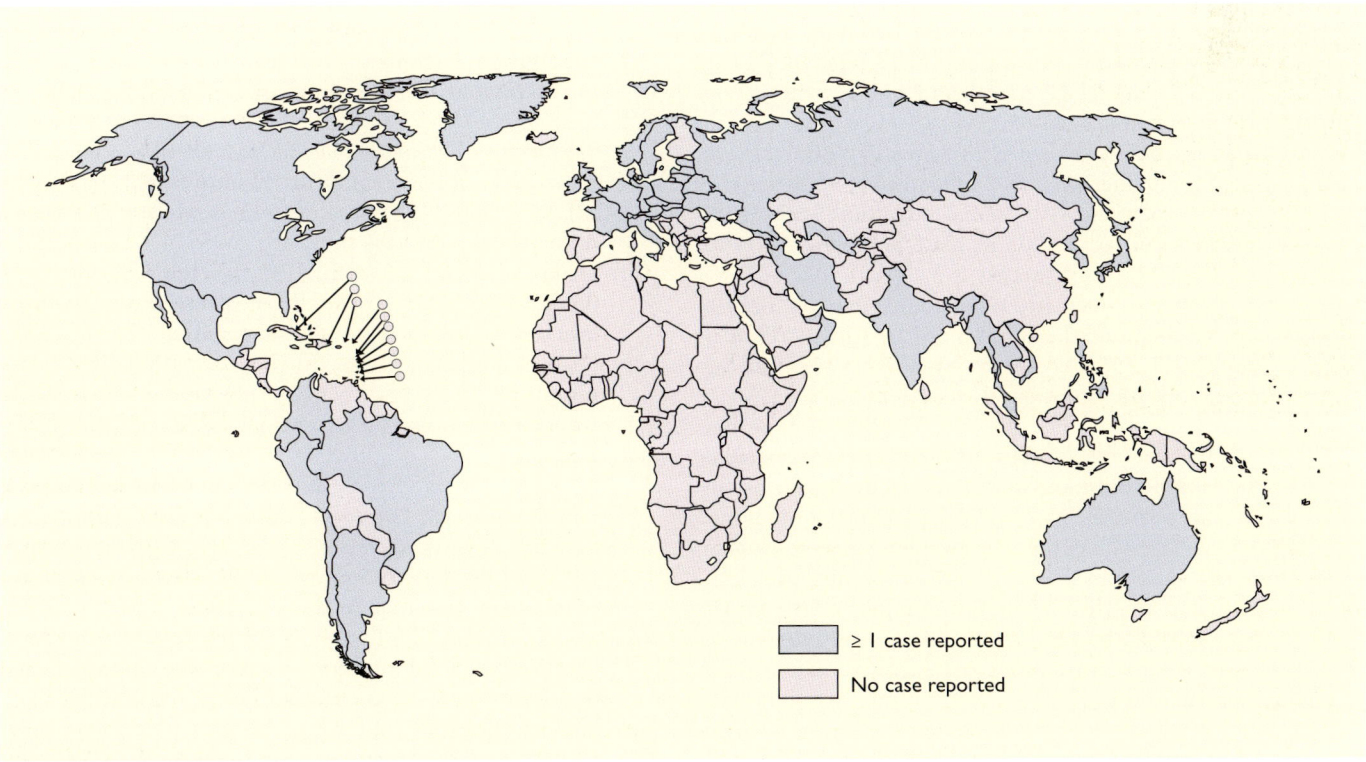

Fig 16.5: XDR-TB map of the world as of 2008 (Global Tuberculosis Control, WHO report 2009).

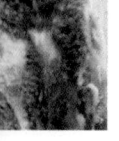

considerably faster than solid cultures as have been discussed but they are expensive and still take a minimum of two to four weeks. The NAATs are a major advance in rapid diagnosis of drug-resistant TB. Their major advantages are speed (results available in 48 hours for smear-positive specimens) and ease of interpretation. These newer tests are discussed in more detail in the chapter on Newer Diagnostics.

Treating MDR and XDR-TB

GROUPS OF DRUGS

Table 16.2: Groups of drugs	
Group 1 (1st line oral agents)	Isoniazid, Rifampicin, Ethambutol, Pyrazinamide
Group 2 (Injectables)	Streptomycin, Amikacin, Kanamycin, Capreomycin
Group 3 (Fluoroquinolones)	Ciprofloxacin, Ofloxacin, Levofloxacin, Moxifloxacin
Group 4 (2nd line oral agents)	Ethionamide, Prothionamide, Cycloserine, Para-aminosalicylic acid, Rifabutin, Thiacetazone
Group 5 (reserve drugs with uncertain anti-tuberculosis activity)	Clofazamine, Linezolid, Amoxicillin clavunate, Clarithromycin

PRINCIPLES OF TREATMENT

1. Be guided by sensitivity reports from a reliable lab bearing in mind that there are many inherent problems in the reliability of these tests for different first- and second-line drugs. If a reliable lab report is not forthcoming, as is the case in most parts of the developing world, a detailed drug history may be almost as useful and help in the initial formulation of a good regimen.

2. In terms of numbers of drugs in a successful regimen there are no fixed guidelines available. One needs to balance the efficacy of the regimen with the toxicity. Most authorities would recommend adding on at least four new drugs to maximize the chances of success.

3. Use any first-line drug to which the patient retains sensitivity, throughout the duration of treatment. Thus if the strain is still sensitive to pyrazinamide, it should be used throughout the duration of treatment.

4. Use a fluoroquinolone: The use of a fluoroquinolone has been shown in several studies to be a factor associated with a favourable outcome in MDR-TB. By definition, in XDR-TB there is resistance to any one fluoroquinolone. Whilst some experts feel there is complete cross-resistance amongst the quinolones as a group, others feel it might be worth using a higher generation quinolone like moxifloxacin (ideally if the lab demonstrates sensitivity) even if resistance to ciprofloxacin or ofloxacin has been demonstrated. This strategy may have been one of the factors behind the remarkable 60% success rates reported from an XDR-TB cohort in Peru by Carol Mitnick and colleagues in the *New England Journal of Medicine* in 2008.

5. Use an aminoglycoside: An injectable second-line drug is crucial to the success of an MDR or XDR-TB regimen. The choices of which aminoglycoside to use is unclear and no studies have compared different regimens. Streptomycin should be avoided in MDR-TB regimens because 50% of INH-resistant strains are also streptomycin-resistant. XDR-TB is by definition resistant to at least one aminoglycoside but even if the lab shows resistance to all three second-line injectables it is worth using one the patient has never been exposed to. The subject of cross-resistance amongst the aminoglycosides is complex.

   The duration of the aminoglycoside is again controversial. Current WHO recommendations are to use it for at least six months, especially if the other drugs in the regimen are weak and bacteriostatic.

6. Use as many Group 4 drugs as needed to make up a total of at least four new drugs in the regimen: When one runs out of all drug options one is increasingly compelled to turn to newer/experimental (so-called Group 5 drugs) to make up the numbers. One such example is being compelled to use a toxic and relatively untried Group 5 drug like linezolid. We have just published our experience from the Hinduja Hospital with this drug in 18 MDR and XDR-TB patients (*European Respiratory Journal*, 2010). In a dose of 600 mg/day we found it to be an effective but very toxic drug. The majority of patients developed a severe painful sensory peripheral neuropathy due to which the drug had to be discontinued.

7. Treatment duration: must be at least 18 to 24 months after cultures turn negative.

8. Treatment must ideally be supervised. Again this is ideal but it is often not practical or possible to supervise a regimen running into two or more years. Undoubtedly, one of the factors contributing to the excellent success rates in the Peruvian study mentioned earlier was the extent of the supervision. A trained healthcare worker gave each dose in the patient's house, under supervision throughout the long course.

9. Treatment must be daily or at least six days a week. There is no place for intermittent therapy in the treatment of MDR or XDR-TB. This of course adds to the cost and difficulty of supervision.

10. Drugs must be prescribed at the upper limit of their recommended dose. This attempts to make up for the inherent weakness of second-line drugs.

11. Second-line drugs are much more toxic and careful monitoring for side-effects is crucial when these drugs are used in large doses for extended periods of time.

12. Surgery whenever possible needs to be considered. In Iseman's series from Denver, surgery independently correlated with survival. Some generalizations about surgery can be made here; it should be reserved for patients with unilateral or predominantly unilateral disease. Patients must have reasonable lung function and respiratory reserve to successfully withstand major resection. Patients must have a good nutritional status. The timing of surgery is controversial; it is ideal to operate when the patient is smear-negative, but some patients may never achieve sputum negativity and hence in the face of highly resistant strains surgery is increasingly being offered to patients even

if still sputum-positive. The patient should have received at least three to four months of optimal chemotherapy before being subjected to surgery. Recent results of surgical resection even in XDR-TB cases have been encouraging. The surgery must be done in a specialized centre with a surgeon experienced in operating on these challenging cases. Surgical series from such special centres report good cure rates with acceptable morbidity and mortality. However, in inexperienced hands, these patients have a high incidence of postoperative complications including bronchopleural fistula and infected pleural and pneumonectomy spaces. It must be remembered that surgery is not a shortcut to therapy; the patient still needs to complete 18 to 24 months of drug treatment after cultures turn negative.

13. The nutritional status of the patient must not be ignored and every attempt made to ensure that the patient gains weight and gets a nutritious high-protein diet.

14. Finally, the emotional and social support the patient needs to overcome this long and difficult illness must never be underestimated. In the words of Julio Acha, from Peru, *'We work with people not with illnesses or mycobacteria.'*

Thus treating MDR and XDR-TB is amongst one of the most challenging problems in medicine. It is a lab and labour-intensive process but can be very satisfying.

SURVIVAL

A systematic review of MDR-TB treatment in 13 different studies reported in the *Lancet* in 2004 observed very diverse cure rates ranging from 38–100%. All studies except one had used individualized treatment regimens. More recent outcome data from Estonia, Latvia and the Russian Federation in 2007 showed cure rates as high as 75%.

Similar large series from XDR cohorts have not yet been reported but unlike the grim initial outcomes in the XDR-TB patients from South Africa who were also HIV-positive, the survival in XDR-TB patients who are HIV-negative is in the order of 40–60%. A recent systematic review on XDR-TB included two studies from North America and three from Europe. This review showed that XDR-TB can be successfully treated in more than 50% of patients. However, these patients had a higher probability of death, longer hospitalizations, longer treatment

durations, and delayed microbiological conversion compared with MDR-TB at reference centres in Italy and Germany.

Survival in our cohort of MDR-TB patients at the Hinduja Hospital runs at around 68% whilst it is around 40–50% in our XDR-TB patients.

COSTS

The cost of treating these patients varies in different series. Figures as high as US$180,000 per patient were quoted in Iseman's series in Denver, Colorado in 1993, where all patients were treated as in-patients. In the Indian private sector setting our costs run at $ 3600/patient treated on an outpatient basis and $ 4500 in surgically-treated patients. These costs are clearly beyond the reach of the average Indian patient and it is heartening to report that pilot DOTS-plus projects were initiated in the country in August 2007. Singla and colleagues have just reported their experience over seven years in a DOTS-plus project from New Delhi. All patients received a daily, standardized, fully supervised regimen of kanamycin, cycloserine, ofloxacin, ethionamide and pyrazinamide. Of the 126 patients enrolled, 61% were cured, 19% died, 18% defaulted and 3% failed treatment. These are encouraging results and the hundreds of thousands of MDR-TB patients in this country can only hope that the DOTS-plus programme will expand to a national level.

Predictors of outcome in MDR and XDR-TB:

The following factors correlate with outcome in MDR-TB.

Table 16.3: Predictors of outcome in MDR and XDR-TB	
SUCCESS	**FAILURE**
Use of PZA, ethambutol	Previous therapy
Use of quinolones	Number of drugs resistant
Use of sensitive injectables	Cavitary disease
Use of > 5 drugs	Low BMI
Surgical resection possible	HIV
Non cavitatory disease	Poor adherence
Sputum conversion at 2 months	Positive cultures at 2 months

SUGGESTED READING

Agrawal D, Udwadia ZF, Rodriguez C, *et al*. Increasing incidence of fluoroquinolone-resistant Mycobacterium tuberculosis in Mumbai, India. *Int J Tuberc Lung Dis*. 2009 Jan.; 13(1): 79–83.

Almeida D, Rodrigues C, Udwadia ZF, *et al*. Incidence of multidrug-resistant tuberculosis in urban and rural India and implications for prevention. *Clin Infect Dis*. 2003; 36: 152–4.

D'souza DT, Mistry NF, Vira TS, *et al*. High levels of multidrug resistant tuberculosis in new and treatment-failure patients from the Revised National Tuberculosis Control Programme in an urban metropolis (Mumbai) in Western India. *BMC Public Health*. 29 Jun. 2009; 9: 211.

Jain S, Rodrigues C, Mehta A, *et al*. High prevalence of XDR-TB from a tertiary hospital in India. American Thoracic Society 2007 International Conference; San Francisco, CA, USA; 18–23 May 2007, Abstract A510.

Rodrigues C, Shenai S, Sadani M, *et al*. Multi drug-resistant tuberculosis in Mumbai: it's only getting worse. *Int J Tuberc Lung Dis*. 2006; 10(12): 1421–1422.

Udwadia ZF. India's multi-drug resistant TB crisis. *Ann NY Academy of Sciences*. 2001; 953: 98–105.

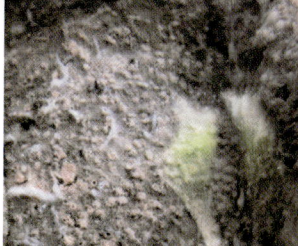
CHAPTER **17** **HIV-TB Co-infection**

One of the reasons for the great increase in the incidence of tuberculosis (TB) over the last two decades is because of the impact of HIV. Of the world's population of six billion, a third (two billion) are latently affected by TB and around 40 million are HIV-infected. About 15 million, globally, are HIV-TB dually infected; 70% of these reside in Africa and 20% in South East Asia. India which has long housed the world's largest TB population now has the dubious distinction of the largest TB-HIV dually infected population as well. The overlapping epidemics of TB and HIV have had disastrous consequences: about 10% of all TB globally is attributable to HIV and 12% of all the two million TB deaths were attributed to HIV.

In 1983 the initial cases of TB in Haitians first came to attention. Then, for the first time, in 1985, the usual annual steady decline (around 5%) in TB incidence in the US reduced to just 0.2% and then actually increased by 2.6% in 1986, the first time in 35 years that this trend had reversed. This was clear epidemiological evidence of a catastrophe ahead. In the decade that followed dramatic increases in TB incidence were noted in several sub-Saharan countries, especially those with the highest HIV prevalence. In the 1990s, reported TB cases went up by 87% in Tanzania, 140% in Burundi, 154% in Zambia and an unprecedented 180% in Malawi. This prompted the Centres for Disease Control (CDC) to list pulmonary TB as an AIDS-defining opportunistic infection (OI) in 1993 (extra-pulmonary TB had been recognized as AIDS-defining in 1987).

IMPORTANCE OF THE LINK

1. TB is the earliest HIV-related infection, occurring at CD4 counts averaging around 300/μl.
2. TB is also, globally, the commonest HIV-related OI.
3. TB is the commonest cause of mortality in HIV. Globally about a third of all AIDS deaths are due to TB. An autopsy study in Cote d'Ivorie detected TB in 54% of all autopsies.
4. TB is the only OI that is transmissible. This has great public health significance in crowded HIV clinics in the developing world.
5. HIV patients are more vulnerable to MDR and XDR-TB and have much higher mortality than their counterparts who are sero-negative.
6. Despite this, with early diagnosis and prompt initiation of treatment, the majority of these patients (especially those with sensitive strains) can be cured.
7. TB is preventable in HIV-positive populations and the important role of isoniazid preventive therapy will be discussed later.
8. Finally, TB accelerates the course of HIV.

The link between TB and HIV is strong and bidirectional. It is estimated that around 5–10% of HIV patients in the Western world will develop TB at some stage of their illness. In contrast, in Africa, India and South East Asia where large numbers of the population are latently affected, it is estimated that up to 75% of the HIV-positive population will go on to develop TB disease in the course of their HIV.

Looked at from the other side of the coin, the prevalence of HIV in the TB population of a country is also important. It is estimated that 9% and 12% of all TB patients in Mumbai and Manipur respectively were HIV-positive. Corresponding estimates for other countries are that 4% of all TB patients in the UK, 8% in the U.S, 66% in Uganda and 81% in Rwanda are HIV-positive.

It would be a missed opportunity not to check the HIV status in all newly diagnosed patients with TB. Sadly, countywide, WHO estimates that as recently as 2007, less than 5% of all TB patients in India were being screened for HIV.

Degree of Risk from HIV

HIV has emerged as the single most important risk factor for converting latent TB to active disease. The relative risk (RR) from HIV is 100 to 170, thus dwarfing the risk from more traditional factors like diabetes (2–4), haemodialysis (10), immunosuppressive treatment (12) and silicosis (30).

While the risk of latent TB activating in an immuno-competent person is no more than 10% per lifetime, in an HIV-positive individual that risk increases to 10% per year.

Mechanism of the synergy between TB and HIV: CD4-positive T-cells producing gamma interferon play a central role in the defence against TB. Interferon gamma activates macrophages to inhibit intracellular growth of M. tuberculosis. HIV causes selective depletion of the very same T-cells, thus decreasing the capacity of these cells to produce gamma interferon. Thus HIV markedly increases TB risk. At the cellular level elegant studies have shown that peripheral lymphocytes from HIV-positive patients with TB produce less gamma interferon compared with lymphocytes from HIV-negative patients with TB. Thus reduced T1 responses in patients with HIV contribute to their susceptibility to TB. Tuberculosis also has a negative impact on HIV; enhancing local HIV replication in the lung. This may help explain the reduced survival of those dually infected with HIV and TB.

Diagnosis

TB is much more difficult to diagnose in the HIV-positive individual for reasons that will be elaborated:

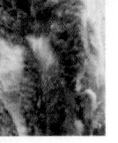

The tuberculin test is often falsely negative in the face of anergy and hence loses its value. Reactivity may be maintained in the early stages but declines as the CD4 count goes down and anergy sets in. The CDC recommends a 5 mm reaction after 5 TU as a positive reaction in an HIV-positive individual whilst others have recommended a 2 mm reaction or even a two-stage (boosted) test in these patients. The tuberculin test retains a vital role, and should be routinely done in all HIV-positive individuals, because a recent meta-analysis showed that those with a positive skin test had a 60% reduction in the incidence of TB when given preventive isoniazid therapy whilst this strategy was of no value in those who were tuberculin-negative. The newer interferon-gamma release assays (IGRAs) may retain their sensitivity in the HIV-positive population but more work is needed to determine their role in these patients. Of the two commercially available IGRAs, the ELISPOT is more accurate than the Quanti Gold in this patient population and is the preferred test.

Sputum microbiology is often negative in HIV-positive patients with TB. A study reported in the Lancet showed that almost 40–70% of all TB is smear-negative in the HIV-positive population. Thus, there is often a considerable diagnostic delay, and, if the clinical suspicion of TB is high, these patients should be commenced on empiric anti-TB therapy. Indeed, because HIV-TB is often pauci-bacillary and extra-pulmonary, cultures from diverse sites like urine, blood, bone marrow and gland aspirates are more likely to be positive than sputum.

Clinical Features

Early literature was replete with the so-called atypical features in patients with HIV who develop TB. We now know that the spectrum of clinical and radiological findings is no different from seronegative TB patients. The manifestations depend on the level of immunosuppression i.e. the CD4 load. Typical manifestations occur when the CD4 count is preserved, but as this drops so-called 'atypical' manifestations are noted. Atypical findings in advanced HIV include lower lobe infiltrates, the absence of cavitation and more focal or nodular consolidation. Normal X-rays may be seen in 7–14% of patients with TB and HIV hence a high index of suspicion is needed. Symptoms and signs cannot on their own distinguish TB from other OIs in the HIV-positive setting but note must be made of two clinical pointers: a prolonged fever (PUO) and excessive weight loss (> 11 kg). Whilst both these are nonspecific and can occur because of other OIs and HIV itself, TB remains the commonest cause of PUO in the HIV-infected.

Extra pulmonary TB is more common than pulmonary TB in the HIV-positive setting (odds ratio 2.3). This most frequently takes the form of glandular TB, though pleural effusions and ascites can also occur.

Timing of TB in HIV: Because of the virulence of TB, it can occur at any time in the course of HIV but often occurs early. It precedes other OIs by a few months to years and is often AIDS-defining. It occurs at a higher CD4 count (around 300–350) in most series. In a large Indian cohort of 594 HIV-positive patients followed up over five years by Kumarasamy in 2003, pulmonary TB was the commonest AIDS-defining illness (50% of all cases). It occurred at a lower median CD4 count of 111/ul and was independently associated with a higher risk of death (OR 3.52).

Treating TB in the HIV-Positive Patient

Treating patients who are dually infected is a complicated task. On the positive side, treating these patients with anti-TB therapy results in improvement in symptoms, radiology and sputum clearance, all at the same rate as in the HIV-negative TB patient.

Treatment can be divided into A) Treating the TB and B) Treating the HIV:

A) TB treatment: TB treatment must get precedence over HIV treatment. The drugs and regimen used to treat TB are no different in the HIV-positive from the HIV-negative patient. Standard short-course chemotherapy is used (HREZ) with all drugs being administered daily (ideally, under DOTS), there being no role for intermittent treatment in the context of HIV. The duration of treatment is a controversial issue. Both the American Thoracic Society (ATS) and the CDC recommend the standard duration of treatment (six months), though the CDC guidelines recommend prolongation of treatment to nine months in those with slow clinical or bacteriological response. A single study from Zaire showed that relapse rate could be reduced from 9% to 6% if duration of treatment was prolonged from six months to a year but even in this study, prolonging the treatment did not translate into improved survival. Hence, at present, six months remains the accepted duration of treatment. It must be remembered that significant numbers of patients labelled 'relapses', may in reality be 're-infections', and molecular studies will be the way to distinguish these two categories from each other.

Thus the TB paradox is that despite a number of studies having demonstrated the efficacy of the standard regimen for treating HIV-positive TB patients based on sputum conversion, resolution of radiographic abnormalities and time to clinical improvement, it has been consistently shown that co-infected patients have higher mortality rates. In several studies of TB-HIV co-infected patients from Africa, the risk of dying despite being on anti-TB treatment is 3 to 26 fold higher in the TB-HIV co-infected compared to TB patients who are not HIV-co-infected. A study in South African miners, which was the first to include autopsy data, showed that much of this excess mortality was from non-tuberculous AIDS-related conditions. This emphasizes the pivotal role of antiretrovirals (ARVs) in treating TB-HIV co-infected patients and makes a compelling case for their early introduction. Malabsorption of TB drugs must be considered in patients with HIV-related diarrhoea and monitoring of drug levels is ideally recommended in this setting. Drug toxicities, drug interactions and paradoxical reactions will be discussed later.

B) HIV treatment: There is no doubt that antiretroviral therapy (ART) has had a huge impact on survival in the TB-HIV co-infected patient. Controversy has raged on exactly when it should be introduced. Most experts feel that if the patient has a reasonably well preserved CD4 count, ART should be introduced after a delay of a few months of starting the anti-TB drugs. On the other hand, if the patient has a low CD4 count every attempt should be made to introduce ART earlier, even within two weeks

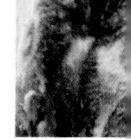

of starting anti-TB drugs. A study in 2010 from South Africa by Abdool Karim in the *New England Journal of Medicine* attempted to solve this issue. The authors showed that starting ART after completing the intensive phase significantly improved survival compared to commencing ART after completing anti-TB treatment.

Before starting ART, the physician should have a clear knowledge of the drug interactions between rifampicin and most of the PIs (protease inhibitors) and NNRTIs (non-nucleoside reverse transcriptase inhibitors).

Sadly, in India, according to the latest WHO estimates, only 2% of all the HIV-TB cases in the country in 2007 received ART.

C) Role of cotrimoxazole prophylaxis therapy (CPT): Every HIV-TB patient must be commenced on CPT with a daily trimethoprim-sulfamethoxazole tablet. This simple intervention significantly reduced the risk of death by as much as 46% in an African cohort of HIV-TB patients. This cheap and simple drug is greatly underutilized in the Indian context. Latest WHO estimates are that only 8% of HIV-positive TB cases received CPT in 2007.

D) Finally, isoniazid retains a vital role as primary prophylaxis in patients who are HIV-positive and have a positive tuberculin skin test. It is crucial to rule out active disease before offering isoniazid prophylaxis. This may be difficult as chest radiographs may be normal and sputum may not be produced. Once active disease has been excluded, isoniazid prophylaxis should be offered as this simple intervention has been shown to reduce the rate of reactivation of tuberculosis by almost 70%. Sadly, implementation is limited in the developing world by logistic deficiencies and poor health infrastructure.

E) Antiretroviral therapy (ART) as a means for control of TB in the HIV population: a number of observational cohort studies (12 in all), from countries across the globe, have demonstrated that the use of triple-drug ART is associated with a 50–92% reduction in TB incidence rates and a halving of the risk of TB recurrence. Most of this benefit occurs in the first two years of ART, the benefits being seen across a broad range of immunosuppression although the absolute reduction in TB rates is greatest in those with advanced HIV infection. Mathematical modelling suggests that if ART was implemented with high population coverage, at higher CD4 counts than currently used, it could have a significant impact on TB control at the community level.

Treatment-Related Problems

The following problems must be anticipated on treatment:

1. Increased incidence of drug toxicity. This includes more frequent hepatitis and peripheral neuropathy secondary to rifampicin and isoniazid respectively and potentially fatal Stevens Johnson syndrome in patients who receive thiacetazone. This drug, which is still commonly used in Africa, though rarely in India, must therefore never be used in the HIV-positive patient. A recent study showed that 34% of patients receiving both TB treatment and ART had to interrupt or discontinue their therapy because of drug-related toxicity.

2. Overlapping toxicity: The overlapping toxicity of ART and anti-TB drugs makes it difficult to ascertain which drug has caused the side-effect in question. For example, when hepatitis occurs, it can be caused not just by isoniazid, rifampicin or pyrazinamide but also with nevirapine. Drug rashes can be due to any of the anti-TB drugs but equally secondary to nevirapine, efavirenz or abacavir.

3. Drug interactions: Complex drug interactions occur in patients on anti-TB drugs and ART. All the PIs and some of the NNRTIs interact with rifampicin. The mechanism of this interaction is due to rifampicin being a potent inhibitor of the cytochrome P450–3A (CYPA) system. Thus when rifampicin is co-administered with PIs the consequence of this interaction is high levels of rifampicin (thus increasing the risk of rifampicin toxicity) and low levels of the PIs (thus reducing their efficacy). In fact when co-administered, the levels of all the commonly used PIs drop by almost 80–90% (except for ritonavir), thus compromising the efficacy of the ART regimen. This can be overcome, if a PI must be used, by substituting rifampicin with rifabutin, which is a less potent inhibitor of the CYPA system. Alternatively, it is best to use a non-PI-based regimen. Efavirenz has almost no interaction with rifampicin and hence this drug is to be favoured over the PIs when rifampicin is co-prescribed.

4. Paradoxical reactions: These are defined as transient worsening or appearance of new symptoms, signs or radiographic manifestations of TB occurring after initiation of treatment. They are more correctly referred to as Immune Reconstitution and Inflammation Syndrome (IRIS). It is important to distinguish a paradoxical reaction from treatment failure, drug-resistant TB, or a second/new OI. The clinical manifestations of IRIS may be as subtle as a persistent fever or new onset and rapidly expanding adenopathy or brain lesions which can sometimes prove life-threatening. They occur in about 36% of HIV-positives on anti-TB therapy plus ART as opposed to 7% on anti-TB treatment alone. Most occur within days to weeks of starting ART. The association between a shorter delay between TB treatment initiation and ART initiation is an area of debate. While some investigators have found no difference in time from TB therapy to initiation of ART between IRIS and non-IRIS subjects, others have reported significant differences between the groups, with IRIS generally occurring more often in subjects started on ART within two months of TB therapy initiation. In a recent study of 43 cases of *M. tuberculosis*-associated IRIS, the median onset of IRIS was 12–15 days with only four of these cases occurring more than four weeks after initiation of ART. They are more common and severe with increasing levels of immunosuppression and are thus more frequently seen when the CD4 count is low and the HIV RNA viral load is high. Other factors known to predispose HIV-positive patients in general to IRIS include: male sex, younger age and more rapid fall in viral load on ART. The frequency of IRIS has not been shown to be related to the type of antiviral used. In Gazzard's series of 55 patients with TB-HIV IRIS, patients who developed IRIS were more likely to present with disseminated TB, have a CD4 count <100 cells/mm3 and have a prompt rise in CD4 count in the initial three months of highly active antiretroviral therapy (HAART).

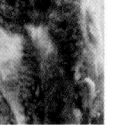

Types of IRIS

Two types of IRIS are recognized in TB-HIV. The first is Paradoxical TB-IRIS. This form occurs in patients whose TB has already been diagnosed and are already on anti-TB treatment prior to commencement of ART. In these patients, there is a paradoxical worsening of TB or TB occurring at a different site usually within three months of starting ART.

The second type of IRIS is called Unmasking TB-IRIS. This form occurs in patients not on TB treatment prior to starting ART. Active TB develops within three months of starting ART. A significant proportion of these cases are those who had pre-existing TB which had not been correctly diagnosed prior to starting ART because of the poor sensitivity of sputum smear and chest radiography in diagnosing TB in these patients.

Mechanism of IRIS

The mechanism is believed to be restoration of immunity towards mycobacterial antigen. After initiating ART, the CD4+ T lymphocyte count rises rapidly in the first month. This represents redistribution of memory cells from sites of immune activation, followed by a more gradual recovery of naive cells. Interestingly, the tuberculin skin test may turn from negative to positive again, evidence of improved CD4 number and function. Subsequent work showed purified protein derivative (PPD)-specific TH1 expansions as the cause of TB-IRIS. Treatment options include careful observation and symptomatic treatment in milder cases to administration of steroids in severe cases. Interruption of ART is rarely necessary but could be considered in life-threatening cases. Repeated aspiration may be needed for rapidly expanding lymph node masses. Table 17.1 gives features suggestive of Immune Reconstitution Inflammatory Syndrome in patients infected with Mycobacterium tuberculosis.

Table 17.2 gives the conditions to be considered in the differential diagnosis of IRIS.

Table 17.2: Differential diagnosis of IRIS
1. Progression of underlying disease
2. MDR or XDR-TB
3. Poor compliance with prescribed anti-TB drugs
4. Drug reactions
5. Association of TB with another OI (e.g. viral, fungal)
6. Association of TB with a malignant disease e.g. non-Hodgkin's lymphoma
7. Association of TB with a non-malignant, non-infective lung pathology

Table 17.1: Features of IRIS
1. Development of new features of the disease or exacerbation of the disease after starting HAART
a. New or exacerbation of an already present pulmonary lesion with or without increasing cough, dyspnoea
b. New or worsening radiological features of the disease
c. Fresh lymphadenopathy or worsening of lymphadenopathy already present; cold abscesses
d. New or worsening CNS disease
e. New or worsening systemic features such as fever, anaemia, weight loss, prostration
2. Immune Restoration: A rise in the CD4 count after HAART
3. A fall in the HIV viral load while on HAART

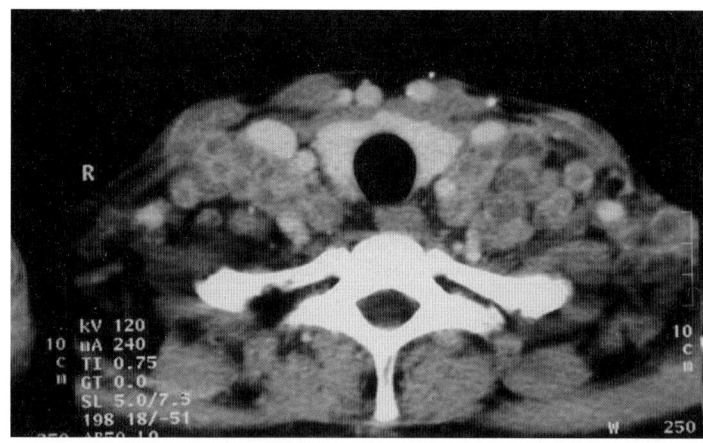

Fig 17.1: IRIS. Recently diagnosed sero-positive patient started on HAART developed large necrotic adenopathy in the neck. This was proven to be due to TB on a fine needle aspiration cytology (FNAC).

SUGGESTED READING

Getahun H. HIV infection-associated tuberculosis: the epidemiology and the response. *Clin Infect Dis.* 15 May 2010; 50 (Suppl 3): S201–7.

Goldfeld A. Pathogenesis and management of HIV/TB co-infection in Asia. *Tuberculosis (Edinb).* 1 Aug. 2007; 87 (Suppl 1): S26–30.

Gunneberg C. Global monitoring of collaborative TB-HIV activities. *Int J Tuberc Lung Dis.* 1 Mar. 2008; 12 (3 Suppl 1): 2–7.

Keshinro B. HIV-TB: epidemiology, clinical features and diagnosis of smear-negative TB. *Trop Doct.* 1 Apr. 2006; 36(2): 68–71.

Michailidis C, Pozniak AL, *et al.* Clinical characteristics of IRIS syndrome in patients with HIV and tuberculosis. *Antivir Ther.* 2005; 10(3): 417–22.

Nunn P. Tuberculosis control in the era of HIV. *Nat Rev Immunol.* 1 Oct. 2005; 5(10): 819–26.

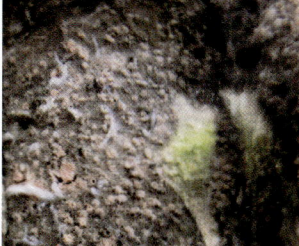

CHAPTER **18** **Newer Diagnostics and Future Needs**

NOVEL TECHNOLOGIES FOR TB DIAGNOSIS

The limitations of our current set of tests are apparent and have been discussed earlier. Indeed, these limitations have been exposed by the HIV epidemic and by the emergence of MDR and XDR-TB. We continue to rely on three antiquated tests: sputum microscopy, chest radiography and the tuberculin skin test which will collectively miss up to 50% of all cases with tuberculosis (TB).

In the past few years there has been resurgence in interest in developing new and modern tools for the diagnosis of TB. Thus groups like FIND (Foundation for Innovative New Diagnostics), GLI (Global Laboratory Initiative) and WHO have made the development of new diagnostics their priority. Funds from these ventures have come from the Bill and Melinda Gates Foundation, the Global Fund to Fight AIDS, TB and Malaria (GFATM) and UNITAID. With this influx of funding and political will, it is estimated that the world now spends a total of US$ 1 billion on TB diagnostics annually. No chapter on TB would be complete without a mention of some of these new tests:

1. Optimized smear microscopy: A recent advance includes the use of fluorescent LED-based microscopy which is 10–20% more sensitive than the traditional Ziehl–Neelsen (ZN) staining and as specific. The procedure is low-cost and uses ultra-bright, light-emitting diodes with an estimated bulb life of 15,000 hours. The LED system is currently being tested in field conditions and may represent an advance over traditional microscopy. Another advance that needs to be mentioned in the context of sputum is the realization that a number of processing tools can be used to increase the sensitivity of sputum microscopy. A meta-analysis of 83 studies found that centrifugation, sedimentation, and chemical modulation (bleach) were all effective ways to increase sensitivity of sputum microscopy.
2. Improved and newer culture methods: Liquid culture systems such as the BD BACTEC MGIT system and the fluorescent BACTEC 9000 are currently considered the gold standard for isolating mycobacteria. Both use an O2-quenched fluorescent dye and measure increasing fluorescence as O2 is depleted. Both are fully automated systems. Several meta-analyses have shown that these liquid systems are more sensitive for detection of mycobacteria and increase the case yield by at least 10% compared to the traditional media. Another huge advantage is that they reduce the delays in obtaining results to days rather than weeks. Finally, the same samples can be used to monitor drug sensitivity testing (DST) once a positive result is obtained, thus greatly reducing the time required to provide this information to

around 10 days compared to four weeks for conventional culture. Having said this, it must be remembered that they are more expensive, require greater investment, and are prone to contamination. They require stringent quality assurance systems and training standards. The current WHO policy is to recommend them as a part of a country-specific plan for strengthening laboratory capacity. Sadly, there are less than 40 installations of the BACTEC system throughout the country. The high initial investment (Rs 20 lakhs) and the higher cost of each culture (Rs 475 per patient versus Rs 40 for LJ medium) is probably a deterrent. Other concerns about the BACTEC system include the need for syringe and needle for inoculation and the use of radio-labelled products and their eventual safe disposal.

At our Level 2 mycobacterial laboratory at the Hinduja Hospital we have introduced the BACTEC system in 1998 and Rodriguez has recently published her experience with this system in a large and busy reference laboratory. Of the 12,726 specimens sent to the lab over six years, the overall recovery rate was 39% for the BACTEC system and 29% for the LJ medium. Thus the BACTEC system detected a total of 1455 (11.4%) additional positive cultures which is statistically highly significant. The average detection time for the BACTEC 460 system was also much faster at 13.3 days versus 31.2 for the LJ medium. The average reporting time for drug susceptibility results was just 6–10 days for the BACTEC system, a huge advantage for the physician keen to begin an individualized treatment regimen in an ill patient with suspected MDR-TB. More recently, our lab has begun using the automated MGIT 960 (Mycobacterial Growth Indicator Tube) system which has a number of advantages over the BACTEC 460 system. Rodrigues showed that the use of this system also greatly increased the rate of TB cultures. Of 6413 isolates positive for *M. tuberculosis*, 41% were positive by MGIT and just 24% by the conventional LJ medium. The mean turnaround time for mycobacterial growth in smear-positive specimens was nine days for smear-positive and 16 days for smear-negative specimens. The MGIT 960 TB system involves even greater initial investment than the BACTEC 460 (almost Rs 3.5 million) but a few sentinel referral centres could clearly use this new technology to great advantage. Higher culture rates and quicker result times are priceless for the individual patient and the physician struggling to treat these patients with resistant TB.

3. Phage amplification assays: have high specificity but lower and variable sensitivity. The prototype is the FASTplaque TB assay which has been field-tested in several parts of

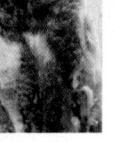

the developing world and is attracting great attention as a possible, cheaper alternative to automated systems in the developing world.

4. Molecular tests: Nucleic acid amplification tests (NAATs) have high specificity but modest and variable sensitivity. Commercial NAATs cannot be recommended to replace conventional tests to diagnose pulmonary TB.

Additionally, expense would make them even more unsuitable in the developing world. A test that is attracting great attention and holds great promise is the Xpert MTB/RIF assay which has been field-tested and marketed by FIND in high-burden countries. The Genexpert combines on board sample preparation with real time PCR amplification for rapid detection (2 hours) of M. tuberculosis as well as rifampicin resistance using on demand near patient technology.

Line probe assays (LPAs) have recently been introduced for molecular detection of drug resistance directly from smear-positive specimens. Two commercial LPAs that are most promising are the INNO-LIPA Rif.TB (Innogenetics) and the GenoType MTBDRplus (Hain Lifescience). The latter assay, in particular, has been shown to perform well for rapid detection of rifampicin resistance in smear-positive sputum specimens. Even more exciting was the introduction in 2009 of the newest assay, the GenoType MTBDRsl assay. This assay allows the simultaneous detection of the M. tuberculosis complex and resistance to fluoroquinolones, aminoglycosides and ethambutol. Thus, the combined use of GenoType MTBDRplus and the GenoType MTBDRsl assay allows the rapid detection of XDR-TB. These tests are clearly poised to revolutionize TB diagnostics. In 2008, WHO endorsed the use of LPAs for rapid detection of MDR-TB at the country level. In 2009, UNITAID approved funding for a program called EXPAND-TB that will supply MDR-TB diagnostics to high-burden countries.

5. Serological/Antibody-based tests are mentioned only to be condemned. They are used and abused in this country (TB IgG and IgM antibody tests) despite there being ample evidence that they are nearly worthless with suboptimal accuracy and highly inconsistent results.

6. Antigen-based tests: Antigen detection has the potential to overcome some of the well-recognized problems with antibody-based assays. The antigen test showing the most promise is urinary LAM (lipoarabinomannan), a heat-stable lipoglycan in the mycobacterial cell wall. The antigen-based assays have the added advantage of maintaining their accuracy even in the HIV-positive population.

7. Interferon-gamma release assays (IGRAs): Until recently, the diagnosis of latent TB infection (LTBI) rested solely on the tuberculin skin test (TST). The limitations of this test have been discussed in an earlier section. A recent advance has been the development of the T-cell-based IGRAs. The IGRAs are *in vitro* tests based on interferon gamma release after T-cell stimulation by antigens that are more specific to *M. tuberculosis* than the purified protein derivative used in the TST. These so-called 'Region of Difference' (RD) antigens such as ESAT-6 and CFP10, are encoded by genes deleted in all strains of the BCG vaccine during its attenuation process. They are also not found in most common non-tuberculous mycobacteria (NTM). Thus no false positives occur in patients who have received BCG

in the past or due to NTM. This makes the IGRAs much more specific than the TST. The sensitivity of IGRAs is not consistent across tests and populations but IGRAs seem to be at least as sensitive as the TST (estimated with active TB as the surrogate reference standard). It must be stressed that the IGRAs do not distinguish between latent and active disease hence a positive IGRA must not be construed to necessarily indicate active disease. Equally important, a negative IGRA cannot conclusively rule out active disease in an individual suspected to have TB.

Two IGRAs are currently available as commercial kits that are FDA-approved; the QuantiFERON-TB Gold assay (Celestis) and the T-SPOT.TB assay (Oxford Immunotech). The use of IGRAs is steadily increasing in the developed world and they are especially useful in these countries which have a low TB incidence. In Denmark, Switzerland and Germany the TST has been replaced completely by the IGRA. In the United States, France, Australia and Japan either the TST or IGRA is recommended. In the United Kingdom, Canada, Italy and Spain a two-step approach is currently recommended with the TST being performed first, followed by the IGRA to improve specificity and sensitivity.

Table 18.1: Novel technologies for TB diagnosis
1. Optimized smear microscopy
2. Improved and newer culture methods like Liquid culture systems—BD BACTEC MGIT system, Fluorescent BACTEC 9000
3. Phage amplification assays
4. Molecular tests e.g. Nucleic acid amplification tests (NAATs)
5. Antigen based tests e.g. Urinary LAM
6. Interferon gamma release assays

Role of the IGRAs in the Developing World

Whilst diagnosing and treating LTBI is an essential component of TB control in the developed world, it is clearly a less important strategy in the developing world. There are several reasons for this. Here, the high annual risk of infection and large paediatric burden imply substantial ongoing transmission; the priority of healthcare systems is thus the treatment of large numbers of active cases that promote ongoing spread. A substantial proportion of the population has LTBI and the lifetime risk of these patients developing active disease may be as low as 5–10%. In one of the first studies of its kind from India we showed that as many as 80% of healthy, asymptomatic adults attending the Hinduja Hospital for a health checkup, had a positive IGRA (T-spot TB test). In the face of such a high incidence of latent TB it is easy to understand why the IGRA has less value as a diagnostic test in high-burden countries than it does in the West. Having made these important provisos, the newer IFN-based assays probably do have applications in the developing world, especially since the TST is even less reliable here. BCG at birth, a universal practice in most developing countries, more than doubles the relative risk of a false-positive TST. Furthermore there is a high environmental mycobacterial burden and technical problems like the requirement for a cold chain, improper storage and shortages of syringes and needles are all more acutely felt. Consequently, the utility of the newer tests would be restricted to the following specific situations in the developing world: (i) epidemiological surveillance, (ii) HIV-TB co-infection, (iii) children with TB and (iv) malnourished TB patients.

(i) Epidemiological Surveillance: Accurate determination of the prevalence of latent infection in a community is essential for an improved understanding of the epidemiology of TB and to guide TB control strategies.

(ii) Diagnosing LTBI and TB in HIV-positives: HAART is inaccessible to much of the developing world. However, treatment of LTBI is one of the few interventions proven to reduce morbidity in the absence of ART. An IFN-γ assay utilising both ESAT-6 and CFP-10 antigens was more sensitive than the TST in a cohort of Zambian HIV-positive patients. Whether the IFN-γ assay can be used to accurately target preventive therapy with isoniazid to this group requires further study.

(iii) Children with TB: In the developing world, children carry a large proportion of the TB burden and rates of TB-HIV co-infection are increasing. Acquisition of sputum or other biological samples is challenging and treatment is often empiric. When exposed to an index case rates of infection with *M. tuberculosis* are high. LTBI has a high risk of progression to active disease (40% in infants under two years old and 24% in children under five years old), usually within 12 months of infection. This often takes the form of miliary TB or meningitis and therefore carries a high mortality. The IFN-γ assays may therefore be useful in this group where the TST has poor sensitivity and specificity.

In KwaZulu Natal, where TB is endemic and there is a high prevalence of malnutrition (28%) and HIV (30%), Liebeschuetz and co-workers found the IFN-γ assay more sensitive than the TST in 293 children with suspected TB. In children with culture-confirmed or highly probable TB the IFN-γ assay was more sensitive than TST (83% vs. 62%, n=133 in both groups and 81% vs. 35% if only culture-proven cases were considered, n=57). Significantly, the ELISPOT would have allowed an earlier diagnosis and commencement of treatment in the 52% of children who were smear-negative but culture-positive. Thus this assay proved to be a sensitive, relevant and robust new diagnostic test in the 'real world' setting.

(iv) Malnourished TB patients: Malnutrition is as potent a risk factor for reactivation of LTBI as diabetes and silicosis. In India, 50% of children under the age of four years are estimated to be malnourished; the TST is often non-reactive in this setting even in the face of active disease. Preliminary evidence suggests that the IFN-γ assay may overcome this problem. Considerably more malnourished children had a positive IFN-γ assay compared to the TST (78% vs. 44%).

Thus, to conclude, while current priorities of TB programmes, limited infrastructure and consideration of resistance patterns dictate that treatment of LTBI is not currently feasible in developing countries, in the special groups of patients referred to, this test would retain considerable value. Although concerns have been raised about laboratory expertise and infrastructure, the IGRAs have been performed by local doctors with no laboratory experience and only a week's training using microscope, centrifuge and incubator and further studies are underway in Vietnam, Southern India and Africa. Nevertheless, limited financial resources remain a major obstacle to the widespread use of this test in developing nations. Further studies are needed to establish the sensitivity and specificity of these tests at multiple geographic locations among patients of different ethnicities.

Table 18.2: Role of IGRA in the developing world
1. Epidemiological surveillance
2. HIV-TB co-infection
3. Children with TB
4. Malnourished TB patients

FUTURE NEEDS: WHAT'S NEEDED TO VANQUISH TB IN INDIA?

1. Social change: It is stating the obvious, but India will never claw itself out of its present TB crisis until the entire socioeconomic fabric of the country improves. The standard of living, housing conditions, grinding poverty, level of malnutrition, hygiene and wellbeing of the community as a whole, and education and literacy rates must improve if any TB programme is to make headway. It is sobering to recall that 50% of Indians live on less than US$1 a day and 50% of Indians still do not have access to safe drinking water. The synergy between health and development is clear; investments in health must be accompanied by investments in literacy and infrastructure for health in general to improve in this country.

2. Demographic control: India's vast and ever-expanding population is its strength and at the same time its greatest enemy. Unless some attempt is made at population control, the sheer numbers will overwhelm even the best conceived TB programme.

3. Adequate funding: Funds must be increased to keep pace with India's population explosion. TB control is one of the most cost-effective interventions known but the estimated funds needed to implement the revised TB programme alone run at a staggering US$200 million, a sum that exceeds India's entire health budget. If the Indian government is serious about its intentions to eradicate TB, it will have to allocate far more money than it presently does to tackle the problem. That India spends less than 1% of its GDP on health, yet spent US$10 billion on its recent nuclear weapon programme, is a sad reflection on the misplaced priorities of its politicians.

4. Global Aid: External aid from international health organizations and from the developed world is urgently needed. This may make the difference between success

and failure of the TB control programmes. Sadly, the containment of TB has for years been impeded by a global attitude of silent fatalism. The gross inequalities of wealth and healthcare must be addressed. Direct aid and debt relief are both needed from the developed world. Indeed, at present, just 0.1% of all external aid to developing countries is devoted to TB control. If even 5% of the domestic TB budget of the world's richest countries was diverted to Asia and Africa, the epidemic could be reversed.

5. Efficiency and accountability of District TB Centres (DTCs): It is people who run programmes, and unless the apathy and narrow vision of the people who implement the programme in each district are replaced by missionary zeal and a sense of purpose, any programme is doomed to failure. The activity of each DTC should be marshalled by programme managers with vision who can motivate their subordinates. Regular audits should be held to ensure that each DTC keeps its target in terms of case detection, case holding and cure.

6. DOTS, non-DOTS and NGOs: We need to build on the impressive gains of DOTS but strive to make DOTS more adaptive and less disruptive. DOTS should be integrated with the general health services of the country because ultimately the success or failure of DOTS will depend on these. In our quest to expand DOTS, we should not forget the paramount importance of ensuring quality of implementation. Private-public mixes where attempts are made to embrace and include the unwieldy private sector within the ambit of DOTS are essential. Finally, DOTS-plus is essential if our large population of MDR-TB patients is to have any hope of survival.

7. Educate the people: As India enters the 21st century, use must be made of every form of media available to educate its teeming masses. Even remote parts of the country have access to television and this would be the ideal medium for transmitting direct, simple and blunt messages educating people in their regional languages. TB must be demystified and destigmatized by bombarding people with messages they can understand on the spread of the disease, treatment options available and the vital importance of regular and prolonged treatment.

8. Involve and integrate the private sector: The glaring deficiencies of the private medical sector have already been highlighted in earlier sections of this chapter. No matter how well-structured the RNTCP, a large number of patients will slip through the net by choosing to first consult a private practitioner. There is ample evidence from several pilot projects that Private Public Mixes (PPMs), can be made to work. An applicable model is that private practitioners in these areas hold treatment boxes, undertake DOTS, assist in defaulter tracing and maintain essential records. Such projects have achieved more than 90% cure rates and serve as models of collaboration that can be adopted on a larger scale. The quality of medical education must also improve with doctors being forced to prescribe TB drugs as per standard guidelines. Audits should expose those with substandard prescribing practice. Finally, regular attempts at upgrading the knowledge of all private doctors should be made so that they realize they are crucial partners in the success of TB control programmes.

9. A new TB vaccine: BCG, the only licensed vaccine against TB was first administered almost a century ago. Since then it has been administered to over four billion people, more than 120 million doses annually. Despite this, its efficacy is limited. A recent meta-analysis showed the efficacy of BCG against infant TB was 74% and against TB meningitis was 64%. In spite of this, long-term use of BCG has failed to make a dent in the overall prevalence of TB infection. Research into a new TB vaccine is an intervention that could save millions of lives; a new vaccine offers the potential to change the epidemiology of TB. Sadly, the cost of developing such a vaccine would run at approximately US$1 billion and this has been the main deterrent for researchers. Hence it is heartening to report recent trials of a new MVA85A vaccine in Oxford. This was administered as a booster to BCG and on its own with encouraging initial results. Another Phase 11b proof-of-concept trial of the MVA85A candidate TB vaccine began in 2009 in 2800 four-month-old BCG-vaccinated infants in Worcester, Western Cape. Close behind MVA85A, in terms of clinical development, is the AERAS-402/Crucell Ad35 recombinant adenovirus vaccine. This non-replicating adenovirus expresses three mycobacterial antigens: Ag85A, Ag85B, and Tb10.4. Designed as a boost to BCG or recombinant BCG, it has already been tested in American and African adults and infants, and Phase IIB trials in South Africa are planned. Another trial of an M vaccae vaccine in a cohort of 2000 HIV-positive Tanzanians was also encouraging. These are the first new vaccine trials in 80 years and it is not inconceivable to hope that a new TB vaccine will finally emerge in the next decade.

10. The urgent need for new drugs: A physician struggling to treat a patient with XDR-TB acutely feels the need for new drugs. Last year a totally drug-resistant strain of tuberculosis (TDR-TB) was described from Tehran. It is not uncommon for patients referred to us at our centres to present with similar, almost totally drug-resistant, strains of TB. There is thus a desperate, unmet need for new drugs and new molecules. The primary reason why new molecules are not emerging faster is the huge cost of developing a new drug. At a conservative estimate it would cost US$ 500 million to develop such a molecule. To be profitable to the drug company that markets such a drug it would then need to be priced high. Yet, TB is overwhelmingly a disease of the poorer countries where patients and governments would not be able to pay these high rates. Of the nine million new cases of TB annually, only 1% occurred in the US and the European Union. There are several other reasons why there are so few new drugs in the pipeline. TB drug trials are among the most difficult to perform, as they need large sample sizes of several thousands of patients in Phase 3 studies. The long duration of trials is also a deterrent. The current gold standard for any drug in Phase 3 trials is two years after the study period, during which time the patient must be followed to ensure there is no relapse. Such trials are difficult, costly and require great organizational skills and infra-structure, often beyond the capabilities of a developing country where such trials need to be conducted. Happily, after years of neglect, the climate is slowly changing and global funds are being made

available. The most exciting of the new molecules waiting in the wings are the diarylquinolines (TMC207) and a nitro dihydro imidazooxazole (OPC-67683).

11. Integrate TB and HIV programmes: We need to accept that our current approaches to TB control are inadequate in the HIV era. Instead of pretending that these two epidemics exist in isolation, we need to integrate their control programmes. This includes more resources, enhanced surveillance, and a minimal package of care (isoniazid and co-trimoxazole prophylaxis) if not DOTS-TB and HAART for all patients.

12. Legislation: Finally, strict legislation should be enforced to ensure prescriptions are standardized according to guidelines with only allopathic doctors being allowed to prescribe TB drugs. Second-line drugs should be made available only on the prescription of a specialist. Only a few drugs and fixed drug combinations of proven quality and bioavailability should be allowed in the market.

Table 18.3: Future needs to vanquish TB in India
1. Social change
2. Demographic control
3. Adequate funding
4. Global aid
5. Efficiency and accountability of District TB Centres
6. DOTS, non-DOTS and NGO's
7. Education
8. Involve and integrate the private sector
9. A new TB vaccine
10. Need for newer drugs
11. Integrate TB and HIV programmes

SUGGESTED READING

Dorman SE. New diagnostic tests for tuberculosis: bench, bedside, and beyond. *Clin Infect Dis.* 15 May 2010; 50 (Suppl 3): S173–7.

Manuel O. QantiFERON-TB Gold assay for the diagnosis of latent tuberculosis infection. *Expert Rev Mol Diagn.* 1 May 2008; 8(3): 247–56.

Mori T. Usefulness of interferon-gamma release assays for diagnosis TB infection and problems with these assays. *J Infect Chemother.* 1 Jun. 2009; 15(3): 143–55.

Pai M, Minion J, Sohn H, *et al.* Novel and improved technologies for tuberculosis diagnosis: progress and challenges. *Clin Chest Med.* 2009; 701–16.

Piana F. Use of T-SPOT. TB in latent tuberculosis infection diagnosis in general and immunosuppressed populations. *New Microbiol.* 1 Jul. 2007; 30(3): 286–90.

CHAPTER **19** **Community Acquired Pneumonia**

DEFINITION

Pneumonia is defined as an inflammation and consolidation of the lung due to an infectious agent. Pneumonia that develops outside the hospital is considered community-acquired. Pneumonia developing 72 hours after admission to hospital is nosocomial or hospital-acquired. Pneumonitis is occasionally used as a synonym for pneumonia, particularly when inflammation of the lung has resulted from a non-infectious cause, such as a chemical or radiation injury.

AETIOLOGY AND EPIDEMIOLOGY

Pneumonia is a pulmonary infection caused by a variety of pathogens. Thus pneumonia is not a single disease but a group of specific infections, each with a different epidemiology, pathogenesis, clinical presentation and clinical course. The common organisms causing community-acquired pneumonia (CAP) are given in Table 19.1.

Pneumonia is a common disease. The attack rates are highest at the extremes of age. Pneumonia is the sixth leading

Table 19.1: Common organisms causing community acquired pneumonia
Aerobic bacteria
Streptococcus pneumoniae
Mycoplasma pneumoniae
Haemophilus influenzae
Chlamydia species
Legionella pneumophilia
Moraxella catarrhalis
Staphylococcus aureus
Nocardia spp
Mycobacterium tuberculosis
Anaerobic bacteria
Oral anaerobes
Actinomyces
Viruses
Influenza virus
Cytomegalovirus
Respiratory syncitial virus
Measles virus
Varicella-zoster virus
Fungi
Histoplasma capsulatum
Coccidioides immitis
Blastomyces spp

cause of death in the United States and the United Kingdom. Records from the early part of the twentieth century show a steady decline in the reported mortality from pneumonia that antedated the arrival of antibiotics. Around 1950, and coinciding with the beginning of the antibiotic era, the mortality rate levelled off and remained fairly constant. This mortality rate is heavily weighted against the elderly, so that the death rates were 35 and 21 per 100,000 for men and women respectively aged 55–64 years compared with 775 and 572 per 100,000 for those aged 75–84 years. This predilection of pneumonia for the elderly is not new and led William Osler in 1898 to describe the condition as 'the friend of the aged'.

The true incidence of pneumonia acquired in the community is unknown and undoubtedly many pneumonic episodes are treated by primary care physicians as 'lower respiratory tract infection' or 'bronchitis' without recourse to chest radiographs. Overall estimates of the annual incidence of CAP vary from 2 to 12 cases per 1000, being highest in infants and in the elderly. Estimates from the US run to 4 million cases annually with an attack rate of 12 per 1000 adults. The annual incidence of CAP in those aged over 65 years has been estimated to be between 25 and 44 cases per 1000, with a rate varying from two to eight times greater than this in subjects of similar age but living in institutions such as residential and nursing homes.

Pneumonia in children is a considerable problem, especially in poorer countries. About 15 million children worldwide die each year as a consequence of acute respiratory infections, one-third of them from pneumonia and 96% of these deaths occur in developing countries Although there may be large differences in the incidence of childhood pneumonia between communities in rich and poor countries, the huge differences in mortality rates alluded to are more likely to be explained by the lack of effective antimicrobial therapy and other supportive measures.

The global burden of disease study showed that lower respiratory tract infections would be the fourth commonest cause of death globally in the year 2010. In developing Asian countries the importance of pneumonia cannot be overestimated. In India pneumonia and respiratory infections are by far the commonest cause of morbidity in children accounting for about 30% of all child mortality. Datta from New Delhi obtained data suggesting that 38% of urban child deaths in India were caused by pneumonia. (*Ref: Datta Banik. Some observations on feeding programmes, nutrition and growth of pre-school children in an urban community. Indian Journal of Pediatrics 1977; 139–49*) This works out to a staggering 1.4 million child deaths/year caused by pneumonia in India alone.

Most series on the aetiology of CAP from the West list

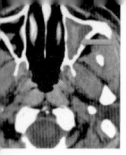

Streptococcus pneumoniae as the most commonly isolated pathogen. *S. pneumoniae* accounted for 55% of all pneumonia in Kauppinen's series of 125 cases from Finland, (Ref: Kauppinen MT, Herva E et al. The aetiology of community-acquired pneumonia among hospitalized patients during a Chlamydia pneumoniae epidemic in Finland. J Infect Dis. 1995 Nov; 172(5):1330–5.), 29% of the 268 hospitalized patients from the Netherlands, and 43% of patients hospitalized in Lieberman's series from Israel.

Other bacteria implicated commonly in most Western series include *Haemophilius influenzae* and *Mycoplasma pneumoniae*. Because of the lack of a gold standard it is difficult to compare the data on aetiology from different series because each uses different cultures and serological tests. However, Fine *et al.* performed a meta-analysis on 127 published pneumonia studies from across the globe and confirmed that in a total of 33,148 patients, *S. pneumoniae* ranked first being isolated in 4432 patients. *H. influenzae* and *Mycoplasma* were ranked second and third with 833 and 507 patients respectively (*Fine MJ, Smith MA, Carson CA, et al.: Prognosis and outcomes of patients with community-acquired pneumonia: a meta-analysis. Journal of the American Medical Association 1995; 274: 134–141*).

In many large series, however, no pathogen can be identified despite comprehensive bacteriological and serological testing. Thus in Bohte's series the aetiology of pneumonia remained undiagnosed in 40% of the 268 hospitalized patients with CAP. In the meta-analysis by Fine and Smith, referred to earlier, no aetiological agent could be identified in the overwhelming majority (11,229) of patients. It is believed that most of these patients without a specific identifiable pathogen probably represent *S. pneumoniae*. It is also possible that there are additional agents that have not yet been identified or recognized. Great interest has also focussed in the last decade on the prevalence of atypical pneumonia. This term was originally coined by Reinmann in 1938 to denote infection caused by a specific group of pathogens: *Mycoplasma pneumoniae, Chlamydia pneumoniae*, and *Legionella*. The relative prevalence of these atypical pathogens has been discussed in two large recent series. The first by Mundy *et al* found a prevalence rate of only 8% out of 385 CAP patients hospitalized over a year in the Johns Hopkins Hospital. (*Ref: Mundy LM, Auwaerter PG et al. Community-acquired pneumonia: impact of immune status. Am J Respir Crit Care Med. 1995 Oct; 152 (4 Pt 1): 1309–15.*)

At the other end of the prevalence spectrum, Lieberman's study of 346 hospitalized patients showed that one or more of these three atypical pathogens could be identified in no less than 63% of patients. (*Ref: D. Lieberman, F. Schlaeffer et al. Multiple pathogens in adult patients admitted with community-acquired pneumonia: a one year prospective study of 346 consecutive patients. Thorax. 1996 February; 51(2): 179–184.*)

There is much less data on the aetiology of pneumonia from developing countries in general and Asia in particular. The high cost of routinely performing microbiological and serological tests in all patients with CAP is probably the main reason for this. Besides, as discussed earlier the ability to determine the microbiological diagnosis of CAP remains poor even in the developed world. Moreover, the cost-effectiveness of making such an exact microbiological diagnosis has long been debated. At our hospital, a tertiary referral centre, a comprehensive pneumonia screen would cost Rs 6000 (i.e. around US $ 120). In a country where the per capita income currently stands at Rs 11,300, spending this sum of money would be an unjustifiable luxury outside of formal epidemiological studies. Empirical antibiotics started promptly, as per existing guidelines would be the preferred approach. However, the Asian region is very diverse and existing British and American guidelines cannot and should not be blindly transposed to this region without some idea of local prevalence. A detailed review of the available epidemiology from the Asian region is therefore outlined here.

Tuberculosis (TB) presenting as an acute pneumonia should never be forgotten in the Asian continent. Osler used to teach that TB should be the sole differential diagnosis in any pneumonia that failed to resolve appropriately and this axiom holds true even today in much of Asia which bears the burden of most of the world's TB. In Tan's series, 16% of patients had TB. Another prospective study of 96 consecutive adults hospitalized with CAP in a University hospital in Singapore found *Mycobacterium tuberculosis* to be the commonest pathogen. In this study *Mycobacterium tuberculosis* accounted for 21% of all cases of CAP, exceeding those caused by *S. pneumoniae* (12%) and *H. influenzae* (5.2%). A prospective study of CAP from Hong Kong enrolled 90 adults hospitalized at the Prince of Wales Hospital and found that TB presented as CAP in 12% of patients. The authors noted that it could not be differentiated from other causes of pneumonia on clinical or radiological grounds. In this study pneumococcal infection was diagnosed in only 12% of patients. A Japanese study of 188 cases of CAP found that *Mycobacterium tuberculosis* was the cause of 11% of all cases. These studies emphasize the role of pulmonary TB as an important cause of pneumonia in the Asian context.

Hospital-based surveillance of community-acquired infections can provide important data to inform health-policy decisions. A prospective multicentre hospital survey of S. pneumoniae disease from six major centres in India yielded important data. (*Ref: Invasive Bacterial Infection Surveillance (IBIS) Group. Prospective multicenter hospital surveillance of Streptococcus pneumoniae disease in India. Lancet 1999; 353:1216–20.*) The commonest pneumococcal serotype was Type 1, which accounted for 25% of Indian invasive serotypes. Similar studies from neighbouring Pakistan and Bangladesh, have revealed different serotypes in these countries and regional variations must be taken into account when vaccine formulations are recommended. Penicillin resistance was not encountered in the isolates in this Indian series but close surveillance is needed as neighbouring Pakistan reported that 9% of their invasive isolates were penicillin-resistant. By contrast, penicillin resistance is clearly an important problem in other parts of Asia like Japan. A study from Nagasaki noted that 50% of 49 cases of pneumococcal pneumonia were caused by penicillin-resistant pneumococci. The importance of such studies cannot be overemphasized. Vigilance and surveillance will go a long way in countering the spread of antibiotic resistance.

A large study on the aetiology of CAP from Mumbai has recently been completed. One hundred patients with CAP admitted to two hospitals in Mumbai (one private and one public hospital) over a period of one and a half years were prospectively studied. Despite a thorough search for the aetiological agent, no organism could be identified in 44% of the patients. *S. pneumoniae* was the commonest organism isolated, accounting for CAP in 22% patients followed by *Chlamydia* in 14% and *Haemophilus* in 9%. Overall, atypical organisms

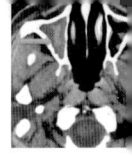

accounted for 19% of all cases. TB was an important cause of CAP accounting for 7% of the patients. This study demonstrates that when detailed aetiological tests are applied to patients with CAP in India, the aetiological pattern is very similar to that obtained from most Western series with *S. pneumoniae* heading all series. More such Indian studies from different parts of this vast subcontinent are needed to determine if there are regional variations in the aetiology of CAP. It is only then that rational antibiotic guidelines can be made.

Risk Factors

AGE
Age is an important independent risk factor in CAP, the incidence (as already mentioned), being highest in infants and the elderly. The frequency of hospitalization due to severe infection increases markedly with age, ranging from 1.6 per 1000 in adults between 55–64 years to 11.6 per 1000 after 75 years of age. Mortality in the elderly is significantly higher, 9 per 100,000 rising to 217 per 100,000 if there is one additional risk factor, such as congestive heart failure, diabetes, chronic obstructive pulmonary disease (COPD) and chronic renal failure.

ALCOHOLISM
The defence mechanisms of the respiratory tract are impaired by chronic alcohol consumption. Alcohol facilitates bacterial colonization of the respiratory tract, hinders mucociliary transport and facilitates aspiration due to impaired swallowing and cough reflexes. Alcoholism is also associated with impaired neutrophil, lymphocyte, monocyte and alveolar macrophage function contributing thereby to multiplication of bacterial organisms in the lower airways of these patients.

NUTRITION
Malnutrition impairs cellular immunity, impairs macrophage function and decreases the level of immunoglobulin A_2, thereby contributing to an increase in both the incidence and severity of pneumonia. Perhaps this is one reason for the increased frequency and mortality of pneumonia in children living in poor, developing countries.

SMOKING
Smoking impairs respiratory mechanisms. Mucociliary transport is adversely affected, as are humoral and cellular immune responses. Smoking is also believed to cause increased adherence of *S. pneumoniae* and *H. influenzae* to the oropharyngeal mucosal surface. Smokers, in particular heavy cigarette smokers, therefore are at increased risk of pneumonia.

ASPIRATION
Any background condition which promotes aspiration of infected oropharyngeal secretions or of gastric contents is a major risk factor for aspiration pneumonia. Aspiration pneumonia is therefore a grave complication in obtunded and comatose patients, in patients who have difficulty in swallowing (either neurogenic or mechanical) and in patients with periodontal disease.

Aspiration of acid gastric contents leads to chemical pneumonitis, the lower the pH of the gastric contents the more intense the inflammation. The chemical inflammation leads to a hemorrhagic bronchitis with well-marked bronchial spasm, alveolar damage, and damage to surfactant with resulting atelectasis.

Oropharyngeal secretions often contain anaerobes (anaerobic streptococci and Bacteroides species) as also Gram– negative organisms so that pneumonia resulting from aspiration is often due to these organisms.

ASSOCIATED CO-MORBID FACTORS
Associated co-morbid factors are common in patients with CAP, particularly in those requiring hospitalization. Perhaps the most frequent co-morbid factors are COPD and cardiovascular disease, in particular congestive heart failure. Other important co-morbid states associated with CAP are diabetes, chronic renal failure and immune deficiency as in HIV infection. Cardiac disease, in particular cardiac failure was associated with a four- to fivefold increase in mortality.

Table 19.2: Risk factors for CAP
1. Age (infancy and elderly)
2. Alcoholism
3. Poor nutrition
4. Smoking
5. Aspiration
6. Associated co-morbid factors like COPD and cardiovascular disease

PATHOPHYSIOLOGY

The pathogenesis varies with the infecting organism. Aspiration of the organisms residing in the nasopharynx or oropharynx is responsible for pneumococcal pneumonia, as also for pneumonia caused by other Gram-positive, Gram-negative and anaerobic organisms. Viral infections are due to inhalation of infected droplets from other patients. Inhalation of water droplets contaminated by Legionella produces a Legionella infection. Inhalation of infected particles from animals can lead to psittacosis, and Q fever.

Animal experiments performed several years ago showed that aspirated pneumococci (pneumococci introduced into the trachea) most often produce an initial infection around the hilum (parahilar). This infection then fans outwards towards the periphery. In some instances when the infection is mild and the body immune response is satisfactory, the infection may remain parahilar; at other times it extends for a variable distance towards the periphery, so that it may ultimately involve the whole lobe. The inflamed lung goes successively through the process of congestion, red hepatisation and finally grey hepatisation before resolution commences. The earliest to be involved parahilar area may be in a stage of red or grey hepatisation while the later involved periphery might still be in the stage of congestion. It is easy to understand why pneumonia confined to the parahilar region or extending just beyond it may show no physical signs other than perhaps a few crackles on auscultation, as there is a

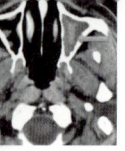

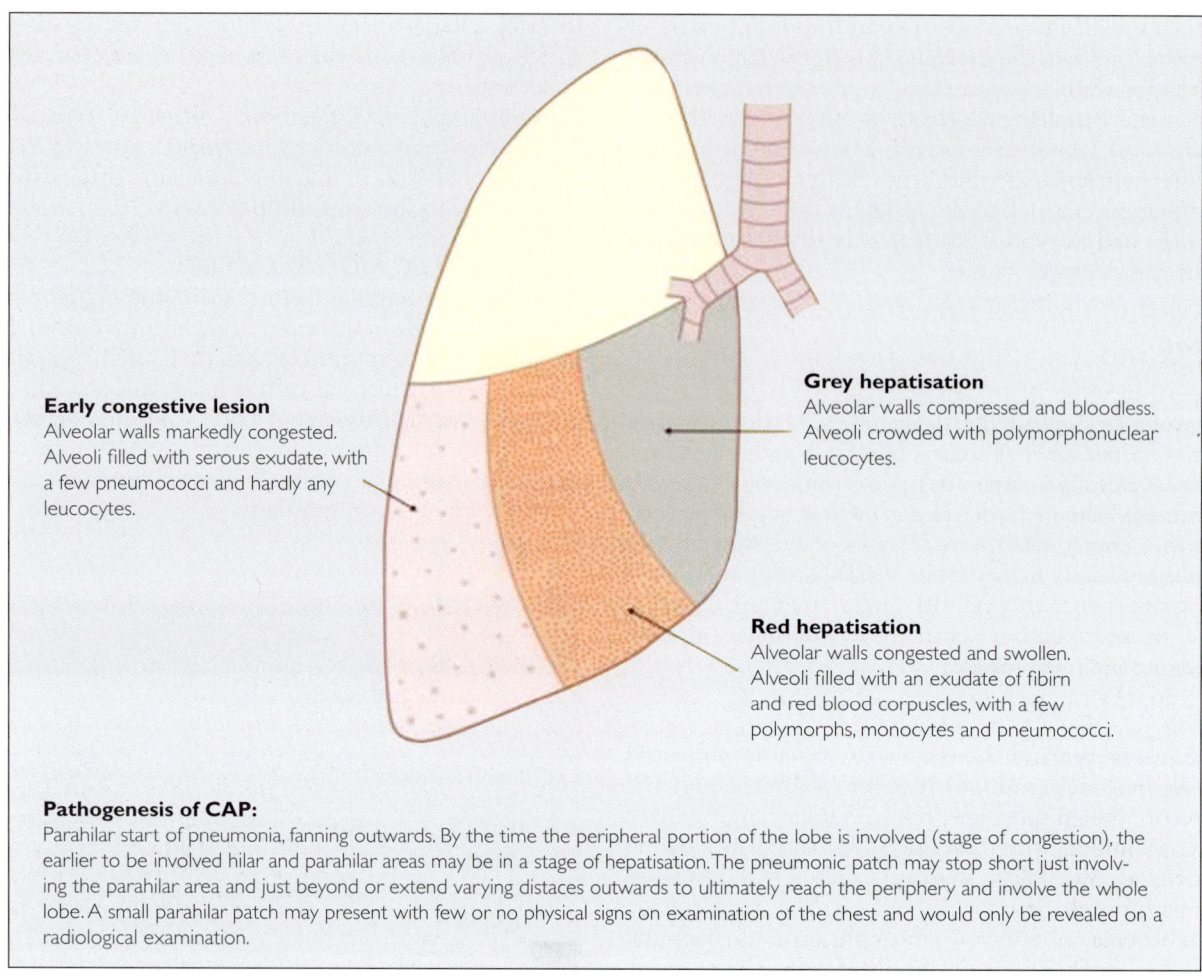

Early congestive lesion
Alveolar walls markedly congested.
Alveoli filled with serous exudate, with
a few pneumococci and hardly any
leucocytes.

Grey hepatisation
Alveolar walls compressed and bloodless.
Alveoli crowded with polymorphonuclear
leucocytes.

Red hepatisation
Alveolar walls congested and swollen.
Alveoli filled with an exudate of fibirn
and red blood corpuscles, with a few
polymorphs, monocytes and pneumococci.

Pathogenesis of CAP:
Parahilar start of pneumonia, fanning outwards. By the time the peripheral portion of the lobe is involved (stage of congestion), the earlier to be involved hilar and parahilar areas may be in a stage of hepatisation. The pneumonic patch may stop short just involving the parahilar area and just beyond or extend varying distaces outwards to ultimately reach the periphery and involve the whole lobe. A small parahilar patch may present with few or no physical signs on examination of the chest and would only be revealed on a radiological examination.

Fig 19.1: Pathogenesis of CAP.

fair depth of normal lung tissue beyond the pneumonic patch. In fulminant infections, infecting organisms were seen to spread quickly through the lung parenchyma to the pleura and spill into the bloodstream causing a bacteraemia.

Pneumonia, in particular staphylococcal infection and also Gram-negative infection may be caused by haematogenous spread. A single lobe may be involved. Multiple areas of consolidation are occasionally observed, often breaking down to form one or more abscesses as, for example, in staphylococcal pneumonia, as also in pneumonia due to Klebsiella and *P. pyocyaneus.*

CLINICAL MANIFESTATIONS

CAP has traditionally been thought to present as either of two syndromes: the typical presentation and the atypical presentation. Although recent data suggest that these two syndromes may be less distinct than was once thought, the characteristics of the clinical presentation may nevertheless have some diagnostic value.

The 'typical' pneumonia **syndrome** is characterized by the sudden onset of fever, chills, cough, pleuritic chest pain and breathlessness. The cough is usually productive; sputum may be rusty in colour and sometimes frankly bloody. In case of an anaerobic infection it may have a foul odour. Fever is usually

present, but some patients may be hypothermic (a poor prognostic sign) and some (20%) are afebrile at the time of presentation. General examination reveals a varying degree of tachycardia and tachypnoea. In severe infections, there may be central cyanosis and hypotension. On examination of the chest, crackles are heard over the affected area of the lung; physical findings of consolidation (dullness to percussion, increased tactile, and vocal fremitus, whispering pectoriliqui and bronchial breath sounds) are present in about 20% of patients with pneumonia. A pleural friction rub is heard in about 10% of cases.

Leucocytosis, at times marked, is generally present. However, in the elderly, in fulminant infections and in the immunocompromised there may be leucopenia. Blood cultures taken before antibiotic therapy are positive in about 10% of cases. Gram stain of a sputum specimen is generally positive for bacteria predominantly of a single type. Radiography shows lobar or segmental consolidation. Arterial blood gases show a low PaO_2, often low enough in serious infections to result in hypoxemic respiratory failure. In severe cases there is a combination of hypoxic and hypercapnic respiratory failure.

The typical pneumonia syndrome is usually caused by the most common bacterial pathogen in CAP, *S. pneumoniae*, but can also be due to other bacterial pathogens such as *H. influenzae, S. aureus, S. pyogenes*, other Gram-positive and Gram-

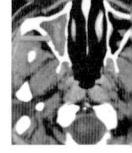

negative aerobes and anaerobes present in the oropharynx. Most importantly *Mycobacterium tuberculosis* infection can also cause a typical pneumonia syndrome.

Elderly patients usually present with fewer symptoms than younger patients. An interesting study on pneumonia in the elderly by Limthongkul and colleagues in Bangkok, Thailand showed that pneumonia in the elderly might present with no fever, no cough, and no signs of parenchymal infiltration but significant mental changes.

The 'atypical' pneumonia syndrome is characterized by a more gradual onset, a dry cough, a prominence of extrapulmonary symptoms (such as headache, myalgias, fatigue, sore throat, nausea, vomiting and diarrhoea) and abnormalities on chest radiographs despite minimal signs of pulmonary involvement (other than crackles) on physical examination. Atypical pneumonia is classically produced by *Mycoplasma*, *Legionella* and *Chlamydia* and the less frequently encountered pathogens *Coxiella burnetii*, *Francisella tularensis*, *H. capsulatum* and *Coccidoides immitis*.

Certain viruses also produce pneumonia that is usually characterized by an atypical presentation i.e. chills, fever, dry non-productive cough and predominance of extrapulmonary symptoms. Primary viral pneumonia can be caused by influenza virus infection (usually as part of a community outbreak in winter), respiratory syncitial virus infection (in children and immunocompromised individuals), measles and varicella-zoster infection (accompanied by the characteristic rash), and by cytomegalovirus infection (in patients immunocompromised by HIV infection or by immunosuppressive drugs). In addition, influenza, measles and varicella can predispose to secondary bacterial pneumonia as a result of the destruction of the mucociliary barrier of the airways. Viral infections and fungal infections are considered in the chapter on 'Non-Bacterial Pneumonia'.

PNEUMONIAS DUE TO SPECIFIC BACTERIAL INFECTIONS

Streptococcus Species

S. pneumoniae is the commonest cause of CAP, presenting generally with the 'typical' features described above. However, life-threatening community-acquired pneumococcal pneumonia may present with subtle manifestations. Tachycardia or increased respiratory rate, mental confusion and rapid deterioration in the clinical state leading to death may be observed.

S. pyogenes infection also can rarely cause 'typical pneumonia'. It generally follows viral infections such as measles, varicella in children and influenza in adults. Pleural effusions and empyema are frequent. Abscess formation with a bronchopleural fistula is more frequently observed.

Staphylococcal Species

Infection occurs by aspiration, inhalation or by haematogenous spread. Airborne inhalation or aspiration is the route of infection following a viral infection such as measles or influenza or in the presence of a co-morbid state such as COPD. Haematogenous spread is from an infective focus, such as within the skin, subcutaneous tissue, or as in endocarditis or following bacter-

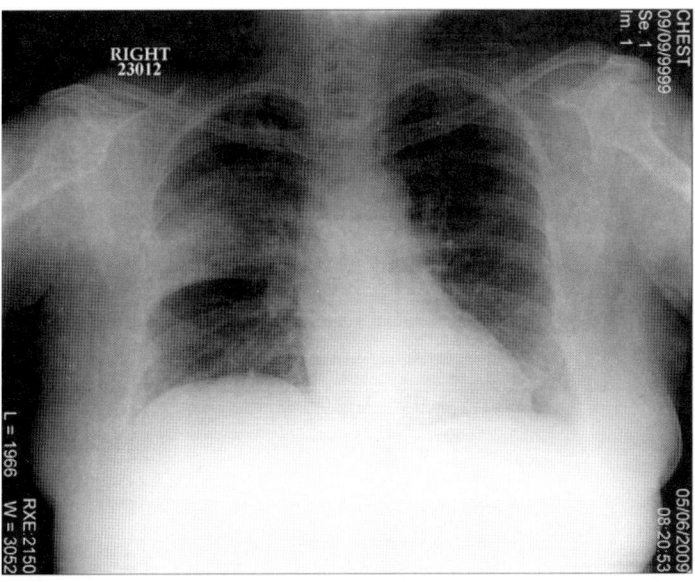

Fig 19.2: Pneumococcal pneumonia. Middle-aged female patient with cough and fever of five days' duration. Chest X-Ray demonstrates an ill-defined consolidation in the right upper lobe limited by the interlobar fissure representing a lobar pneumonia. The offending organism was the pneumococcus.

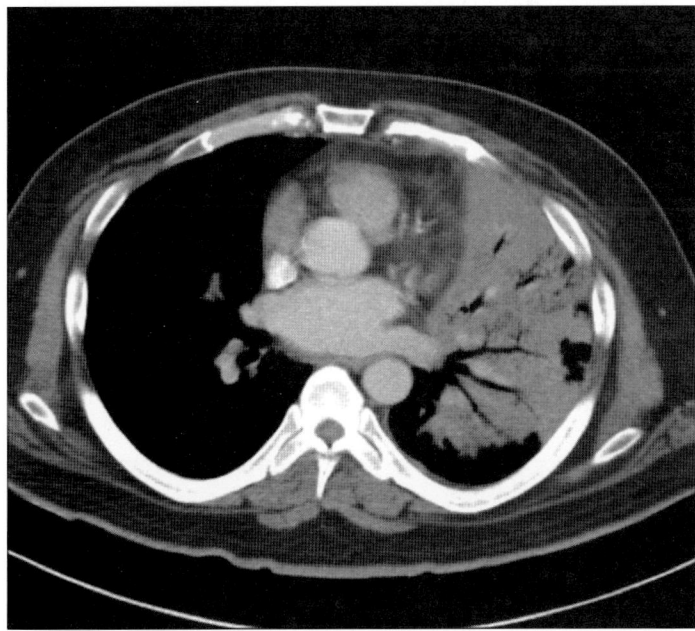

Fig 19.3: Middle-aged man presented with high fever, leucocytosis and haemoptysis. CT chest with contrast demonstrated a large ill-defined consolidation in the left upper lobe, and lingula with an air bronchogram.

aemia secondary to a septic focus anywhere within the body. Direct bloodstream infection can occur following intravenous drug abuse.

The clinical picture may resemble that described under 'typical pneumonia' with segmental or lobar consolidation. However, it may be different, because staphylococci frequently cause lysis of lung tissue. This can result (particularly in children) in rapidly expanding thin-walled pneumatoceles or bullae that may push the heart and mediastinum to the opposite side. At times the greater part of the lung may be occupied by one large

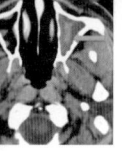

pneumatocele or bulla. Rupture of the bullae into the pleura can cause a pneumothorax or a pyopneumothorax. In adults, lysis of lung tissue leads to one or more abscess cavities. Nodular infiltrates may coalesce to form areas of consolidation with or without abscess formation. Pleural effusion, empyemas, bronchopleural fistula are frequent. Systemic features may be marked and sepsis with multiple organ dysfunction is observed in fulminant infections. The outcome of staphylococcal CAP depends on the virulence of the organism, the presence or absence of co-morbid factors, the age of the patient, presence of sepsis and pleural complications and the response to antibiotic therapy.

Though most community-acquired staphylococcal infections are methicillin-sensitive, there is an increasing incidence of *methicillin-resistant Staphylococcus aureus* (MRSA) infection

in the community, not just in the West but also in India and perhaps also in the other Asian countries. The MRSA infections in the community generally affect the skin and subcutaneous tissue but can also cause pneumonia, lung abscess and empyema. The MRSA in the community is a virulent organism usually containing the gene encoding Paton-Valentine leucocidin and the SCC mec Type IV element belonging to the USA 200 pulsed field. The Paton-Valentine leucocidin contains a toxin that creates lytic pores in the cell membrane of polymorphonuclear leucocytes thereby causing the release of chemotatic factors that promote inflammation and tissue destruction.

Mycoplasmal Infection

Mycoplasmal pneumonia may occur sporadically but is usually seen in small epidemics. A history of an immediate preceding upper respiratory infection is often present. The clinical features are as described under atypical pneumonia. However, extrapulmonary manifestations are varied and frequent. These commonly include arthralgias, cervical lymphadenopathy, bullous myringitis, nausea, vomiting, and diarrhoea. Immune haemolytic anaemia due to the presence of cold agglutinins in the blood is an aid to correct diagnosis. Myocarditis is a rare complication; precordial pain is at times related to pericarditis. Central nervous system involvement includes meningitis, meningoencephalopathy, and myelitis. Skin eruptions may be present, the most dreaded being erythema multiforme which may graduate into a full-blown Steven Johnson syndrome.

A clinical study of mycoplasma pneumonia by Hwang and colleagues in China *(Ref: Hwang JJ, Chen KL, Clinical study of Mycoplasma pneumoniae pneumonia. Gaoxiong Yi Xue Ke Xue Za Zhi.1993 Apr; 9 (4):204–11)* showed that all patients with *Mycoplasma pneumoniae* complained of fever and cough; 63% had dry cough, 37% had sputum production. Upper respiratory tract complaints such as rhinorrhoea, sore throat or earache were seen in 57% of patients, 55% has gastrointestinal symptoms of anorexia, nausea, vomiting, and diarrhoea. Other complaints included myalgia, arthralgia (29%), headache (30%), and general malaise (32%). Dyspnoea (17%) and chest pain (20%) were occasionally observed.

Radiological examination reveals diffuse infiltrates in one or both lungs, generally involving the lower lobes; these infiltrates clear slowly over four to six weeks.

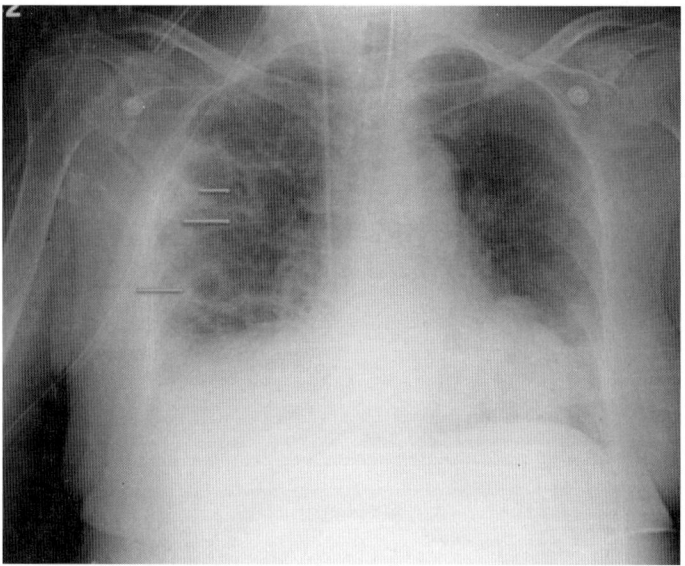

Fig 19.4: Staphylococcal pneumonia. Right lower lobe consolidation with multiple air-filled cysts in right upper and midzones representing pneumatoceles due to staphylococcal infection.

Mycobacterium tuberculosis

CAP due to *Mycobacterium tuberculosis* should always be kept in mind in developing countries. It may present acutely or subacutely, the upper lobe and the apical segment of the lower lobe being most frequently involved. The right middle lobe and the lingular segment of the left lung may also be sites of consolidation. The symptoms and signs may be indistinguishable from CAP due to other organisms. Diagnosis depends on demonstrating acid-fast bacilli in sputum and growing them on culture. It should be a rule that all patients with acute pneumonia in developing countries should have a Ziehl-Neelsen stain of a sputum specimen in addition to other microbiological tests deemed relevant. This would enable the clinician to avoid missing out on the diagnosis of tuberculous pneumonia.

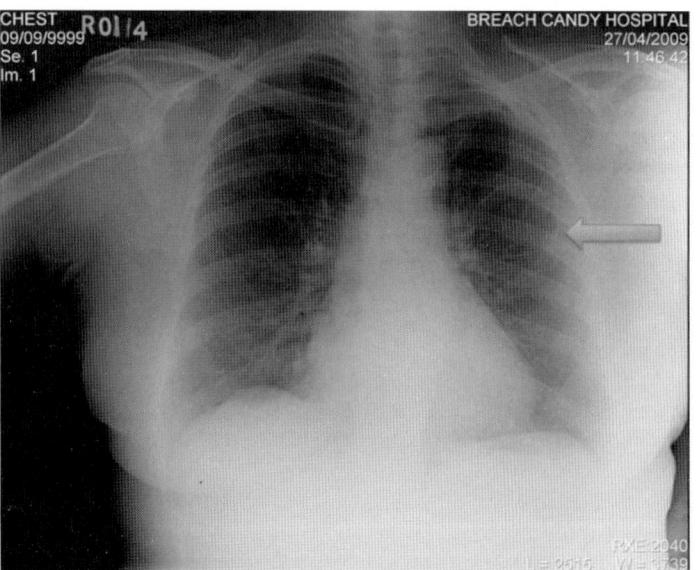

Fig 19.5: Staphylococcal pneumonia. Chest X-Ray demonstrates a thin-walled pneumatocele, a residue of a healed staphylococcal pneumonia.

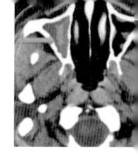

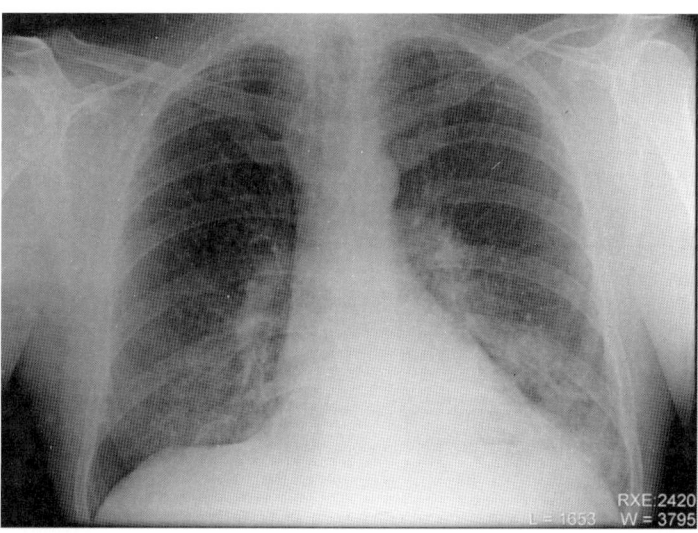

Fig 19.6: *Mycoplasma pneumonia.* A 47-year-old male patient presented with fever and cough, *white blood cells* (WBC) count was normal. Anti-mycoplasma titres were very high. Chest X-ray demonstrates streaky and conglomerated opacities in both lower zones, more so on the left side representing *Mycoplasma pneumoniae*.

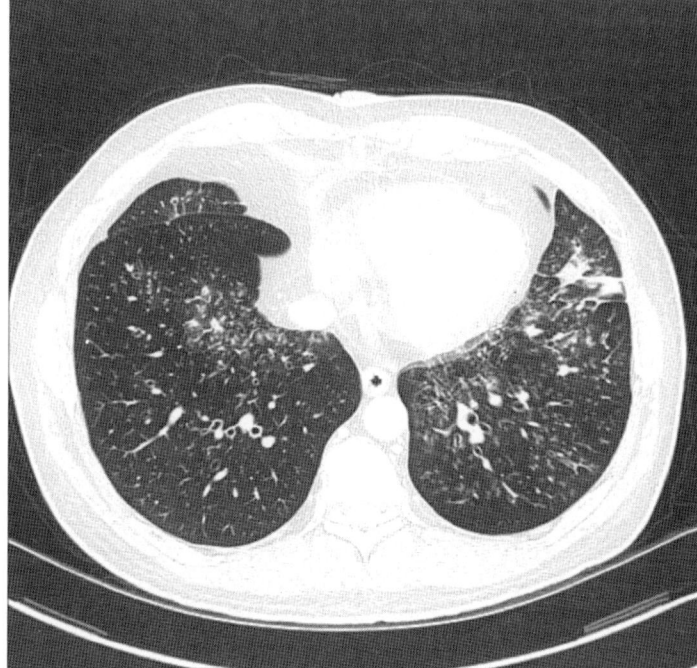

Fig 19.7: *Mycoplasma pneumoniae.* CT chest of a patient with mycoplasma pneumonia demonstrating bilateral linear and ill-defined lesions in the interstitial spaces.

Rarely, acute tuberculous pneumonia presents with bizarre manifestations. An unusual presentation is that of acute respiratory distress, tachycardia, tachypnoea, bilateral shadows in both lung fields, with respiratory crackles on auscultation (ARDS). There is cough but no sputum for examination. The patient can progress to acute respiratory failure with a low PaO$_2$ (< 60 mm Hg) even on supplemental oxygen. Multiorgan failure may be observed. The diagnosis is impossible without an examination of bronchoalveolar lavage (BAL) fluid, which shows acid-fast bacilli. A transbronchial biopsy

shows the presence of tubercles (caseating granulomas) on histopathological examination.

Chlamydia Species

The incidence of chlamydia pneumonia is uncertain. A study in Mumbai (mentioned earlier) showed that the organism was

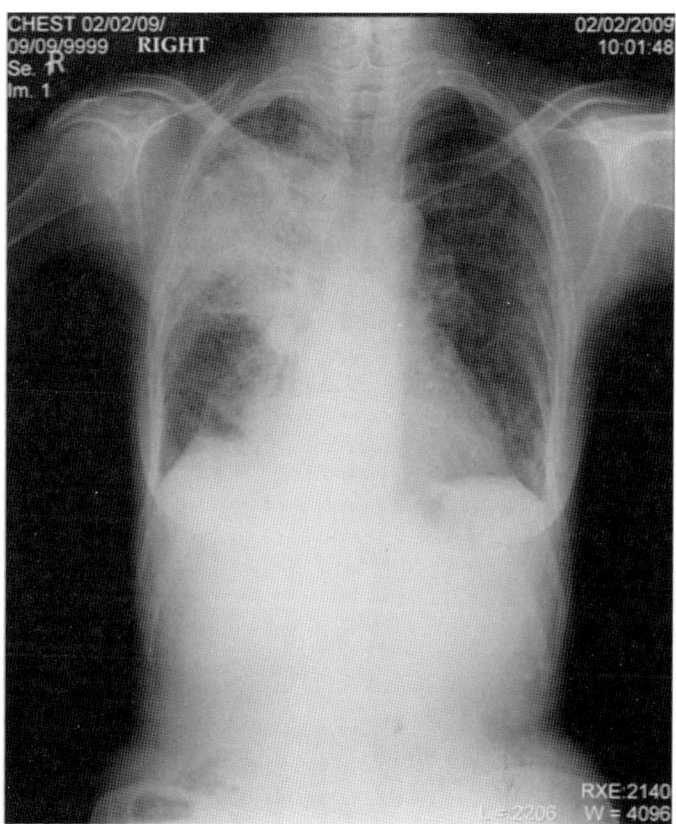

Fig 19.8: Acute tuberculous pneumonia. A 33-year-old male patient presented with high fever and chills and mild leucocytosis. Chest X-ray revealed a large lobar consolidation involving the right upper and mid-zone. Sputum revealed acid-fast bacilli (*Mycobacterium tuberculosis*).

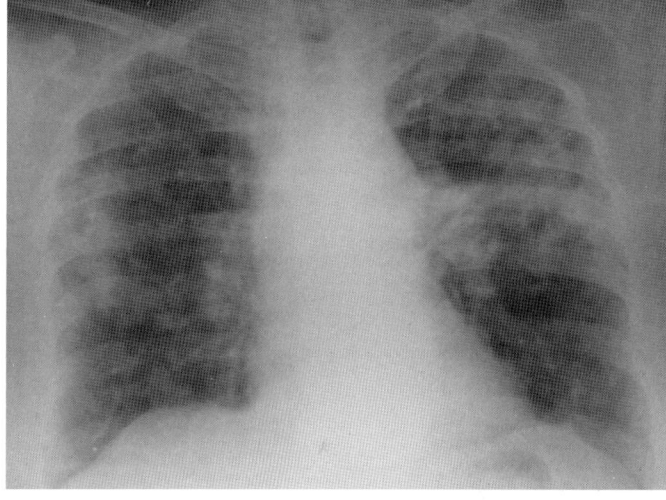

Fig 19.9: Tuberculous pneumonia. Chest X-ray reveals diffuse ill-defined reticular and soft tissue opacities in the upper and mid-zones. BAL revealed acid-fast bacilli.

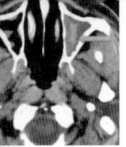

responsible for pneumonia in a significant number of patients. Sore throat may antedate the appearance of fever and cough and clinical features are as described under atypical pneumonia. The clinical course is generally mild though it may be severe in patients with co-morbid states such as COPD or congestive heart failure. Radiological examination shows unilateral or bilateral infiltrates that may take four weeks to resolve.

Legionella Pneumonia

Legionella species are intracellular aerobic organisms. Of the 30 species identified, *Legionella pneumophilia* is the most common. The organism exists in air-conditioning systems and in water. Spread of infection occurs by inhalation of air or droplets contaminated by the organism.

Infection may be asymptomatic, mild to severe. The incubation period is two to eight days. Severe infection is characterized by fever with chills, headache and myalgia followed within two to three days by a pneumonia. Cough with purulent sputum with or without haemoptysis is often present. Tachycardia, tachypnoea is observed. The presence of extrapulmonary features should suggest the possible diagnosis. These include involvement of many systems. Abdominal pain, diarrhoea, arthralgia are frequent. Headache and mental confusion may be prominent features. Hyponatraemia due to syndrome of inappropriate antidiuretic hormone hypersecretion (SIADH) is common and may be a diagnostic clue. Renal involvement may take the form of proteinuria, oliguria, azotemia and renal failure. Liver functions are often deranged and hepatosplenomegaly may be present. Pleural effusion, generally mild, may occur, but cavitation is not observed.

The greater and the more severe the extrapulmonary manifestations the more serious the prognosis. The presence of co-morbidities as always worsens the outcome. Legionella pneumonia is infrequently diagnosed in India, not necessarily because it is very rare, but because it is not carefully looked out for, largely due to lack of laboratory facilities.

Gram-negative Bacilli

Gram-negative bacteria chiefly include *Klebsiella pneumoniae*, *Escherichia coli*, *Pseudomonas aeruginosa* and Acinetobacter species. Gram-negative bacteria are most often responsible for nosocomial pneumonia but CAP attributed to these organisms may occur in old age or in association with co-morbid states. Co-morbid states include severe COPD, alcoholism, uncontrolled diabetes, neutropenia, immunosuppression or immune deficiency states.

Colonization of the oropharynx by Gram-negative bacteria in the above conditions is followed by aspiration into the lungs leading to pneumonia. In some instances pneumonia results from blood-borne Gram-negative bacterial infection. The clinical presentation is generally that of typical pneumonia. The prognosis, particularly when associated with co-morbidities is poor.

K. pneumoniae (Freidlander's pneumonia) generally occurs in older patients (> 60 years). Acute prostration, purulent sputum with haemoptysis and extensive involvement generally of one or at times both upper lobes is observed. The extensive consolidation may be associated with breakdown and abscess formation and often causes a downward bulging of the fissure. This is however not pathognomic of Klebsiella infection; it is also occasionally observed in pneumococcal pneumonia caused by *Streptococcus pneumoniae* Type III. Hypotension, respiratory failure, and severe sepsis with multi-organ failure characterize severe infection.

Pneumonia due to *P. aeruginosa* usually involves one or both lower lobes and occurs in the elderly and often chronically ill patients. Fever, tachycardia and quickly evolving acute respiratory failure may follow. Abscess formation and empyema are frequent. The prognosis is poor, death resulting from sepsis, acute respiratory failure or multi-organ dysfunction.

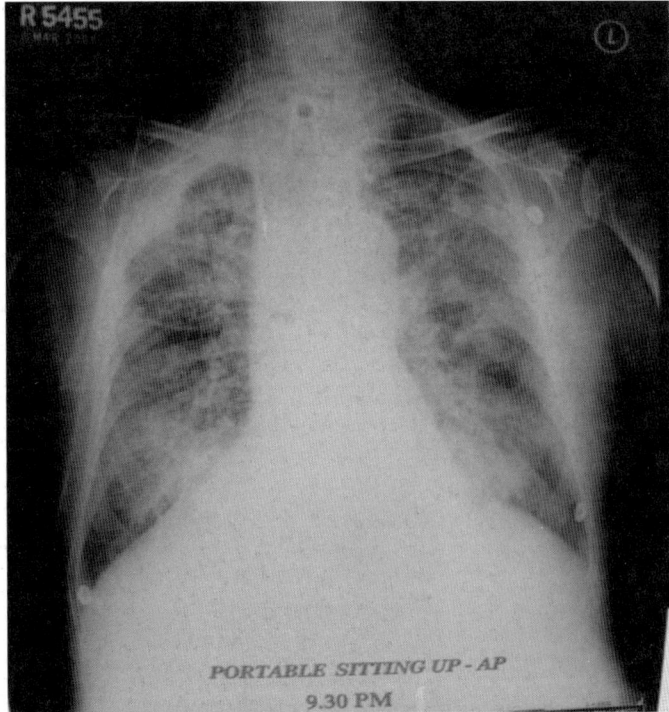

Fig 19.10: Legionella pneumonia. An 87-year-old male presented with dyspnoea, chest pain and fever. Chest X-ray demonstrates ill-defined areas of consolidation. Legionella antigen was detected on urine examination.

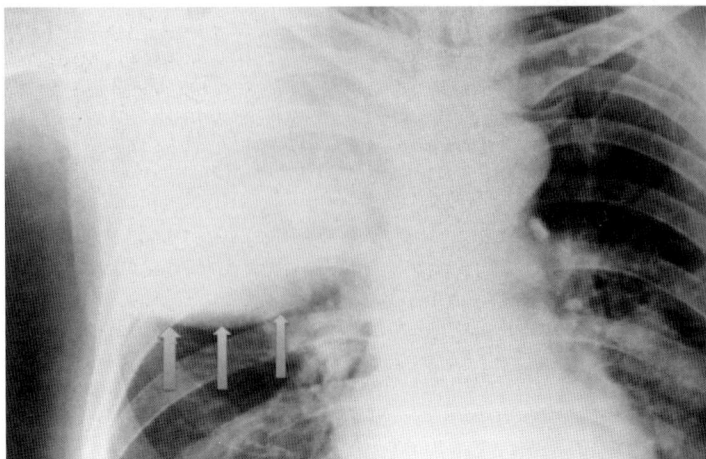

Fig 19.11: Klebsiella pneumonia. Chest X-ray demonstrates a large consolidation in the right upper lobe which is dense and homogenous; there is downward bulging of the fissure, a typical feature of Klebsiella pneumonia.

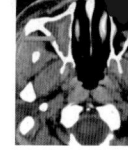

P. aeruginosa is a dangerous organism which is increasingly resistant to most antibiotics.

Pneumonia due to Acinetobacter is often bilateral, quickly progressive, often causes ARDS with severe hypoxemia. Abscess formation and empyema are frequent complications. Death can occur within a few days and is due to respiratory failure or sepsis.

Pneumonia due to *Pseudomonas pseudomallei* has been considered in the section on 'Tropical Infections Involving the Lung'.

Nocardia Species

Nocardia are Gram-positive aerobic bacilli chiefly present in soil. The commonest Nocardia species responsible for pulmonary infection is *Nocardia asteroides*. Most patients with nocardial pneumonia have underlying co-morbid states—COPD, malignancy, immunosuppression, long-term corticosteroid therapy. In 30–50% there may be no underlying disease. Fulminant nocardial pneumonia is uncommon but when present has a high fatality. In most patients the onset is subacute with mild to moderate fever, cough, increase in breathlessness in COPD patients and at times pleuritic chest pain. Imaging studies typically show nodules of varying size in one or both lungs, sometimes evident only on a CT scan. Infiltrates, lobar consolidation and abscess formation, either multiple small abscesses or a large abscess cavity, may be observed. Metastatic involvement leads to subcutaneous abscesses (presenting as pus discharging from inflamed nodules); metastatic abscesses in the brain lead to varying central nervous system (CNS) symptoms depending on the size and location of the abscess. Infection from the lung may involve the pleura causing an empyema, and at times the chest wall causing a fluctuant abscess within the parietes. In the absence of severe associated co-morbid states the prognosis is usually good, provided the diagnosis is made quickly and the patient receives appropriate therapy.

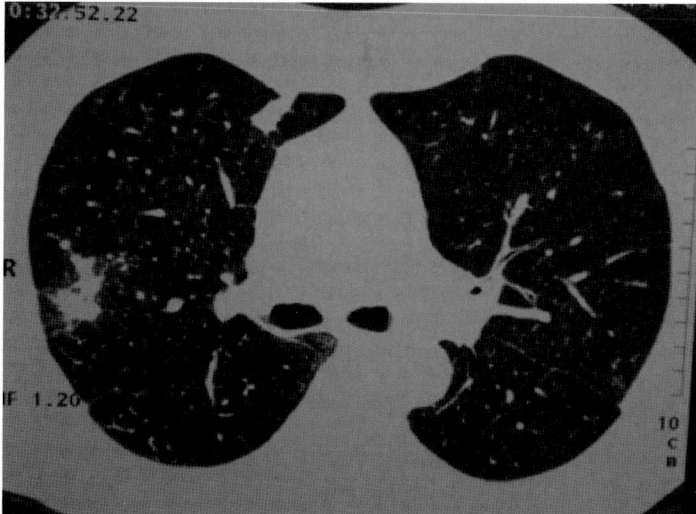

Fig 19.12: Norcardiosis. A 78-year-old male patient with a long history of COPD on long-term usage of inhaled and oral steroids (for an acute exacerbation), developed fever with cough and productive sputum with arterial desaturation. Microbiological examination of sputum demonstrated nocardia. HRCT chest demonstrates multiple conglomerated ill-defined nodules in the right upper and middle lobe.

Anaerobic Bacteria

Anaerobic bacterial pneumonia is due to aspiration of anaerobes from the oropharynx into the lungs. Alcoholism, obtunded patients, patients with an inability to protect the airway, prolonged seizures and bad oral/dental hygiene are background risk factors which are associated with aspiration pneumonia.

Pneumonia due to anaerobic organisms generally presents as a 'typical' pneumonia with fever, cough, dyspnoea, and pleuritic pain. Pneumonia generally involves the lower lobe or lobes. Aspiration in the supine posture leads to infiltrates involving the posterior segment of the upper lobe and/or the apical segment of the lower lobe. The sputum is purulent and often has a foetid odour. Necrotizing pneumonia with the formation of multiple abscesses may develop. Empyema is a frequent complication. Prognosis depends on prompt diagnosis and treatment with appropriate antibiotics.

Moraxella catarrhalis

Moraxella catarrhalis are Gram-negative diplococci commonly found in the oropharynx. On aspiration into the lungs they may cause pneumonia, particularly in patients with COPD, congestive heart failure and other co-morbid states. The clinical and radiological features are non-specific. Leucocytosis is common and the outcome generally favourable.

Actinomyces

Actinomyces israelii is a species consisting of Gram-positive filamentous branching bacilli. It was mistaken for a fungus for several years. These organisms are present in the oropharynx and may become pathogenic when aspirated into the lungs. Poor oropharyngeal hygiene, bad dental hygiene, COPD, bronchiectasis are underlying risk factors. The organism produces a subacute to chronic pneumonia (generally involving the lower lobe), which may extend by continuity and contiguity into the pleura and from the pleura to the chest wall, causing one or more sinuses that discharge pus through the chest wall. The clinical features suggest tuberculosis, a fungal infection or a bronchogenic carcinoma.

The presence of discharging sinuses in the chest wall particularly when they are multiple invariably points to actinomyces infection. The diagnosis is confirmed by examination of the pus which shows characteristic filamentous branching Gram-positive bacilli. Occasionally, thoracic actinomycosis is associated with cervico-facial actinomycosis. The discharging sinuses in the neck and face are often mistaken for tuberculosis. Actinomycosis can also present as an empyema and the aetiology may be missed if proper staining of pus and anaerobic cultures are not done.

Radiological features consist of areas of consolidation with small cavities involving a lobe or a segment. Infection may spread to involve the pleura causing an empyema and may also spread by contiguity to involve the ribs and the chest wall.

Infection due to *Yersenia pestis* and the Anthrax bacillus have been dealt within the section on 'Tropical Infections Involving the Lung'.

Table 19.3 gives a partial list of clues to the cause of pneumonia that may be obtained from the history and physical examination.

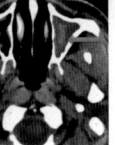

Table 19.3: Clues to the etiology of pneumonia from the history and physical examination	
Feature	**Organism**
Environmental	
Exposure to contaminated air-conditioning cooling towers, recent travel associated with a stay in hotel, exposure to a grocery store mist machine, visit or recent stay in hospital with contaminated potable water	*Legionella pneumophilia*
Pneumonia after windstorm in an endemic area	*Coccidioides immitis*
Outbreak of pneumonia in shelters for homeless men, jails, military training camps	*Strep. pneumoniae* *M. tuberculosis* *Chlamydia pneumoniae*
Exposure to contaminated bat caves, excavation in endemic areas	*Histoplasma capsulatum*
Animal contact	
Exposure to infected parturient cats, cattle, sheep or goats	*Coxiella burnetii*
Exposure to turkeys, chickens, ducks or birds	*Chlamydia psittaci*
Travel history	
Travel to Thailand or other countries in Southeast Asia	*Burkholderia (Pseudomonas) pseudomallei*
Pneumonia in immigrants from Asia or India	*M. tuberculosis*
Occupational history	
Pneumonia in healthcare workers in a large city with patients infected with HIV	*M. tuberculosis*
Host factors	
Diabetic ketoacidosis	*S. pneumoniae* *Staphylococcus aureus*
Alcoholism	*S. pneumoniae* *Klebsiella pneumoniae* *S. aureus*
COPD	*S pneumoniae* *H. influenzae* *Moraxella catarrhalis*
Solid organ transplant pneumonia (pneumonia occuring 3 months after transplant)	*S. pneumoniae* *H. influenzae* *Legionella spp* *Pneumocystis carinii* *Cytomegalovirus* *Strongyloides stercoralis*
Sickle cell disease	*S. pneumoniae*
HIV infection CD4 count < 200	*Pneumocystis carinii*
CD4 cell count > 200	*S. pneumoniae* *H. influenzae* *Cryptococcus neoformans* *M. tuberculosis* *Rhodococcus equi*
Physical findings	
Periodontal disease with foul-smelling sputum	Anaerobes
Bullous myringitis	*Mycoplasma pneumoniae*
Absent gag reflex, altered level of consciousness, or recent seizure	Oral aerobic and anaerobic bacteria due to aspiration
Encephalitis	*Mycoplasma pneumoniae* *Coxiella burnetii*
Cerebellar ataxia	*Legionella pneumophilia*
Erythema multiforme	*Mycoplasma Legionella*
Erythema nodosum	*Mycoplasma*
Erythema gangrenosum	*M. tuberculosis* *Chlamydia pneumoniae*
Cutaneous nodules (abscesses) and CNS findings	*Ps. aeruginosa* *Serratia marcescens* *Nocardia species*

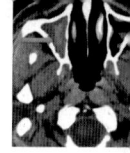

RECURRENT PNEUMONIA

Recurrent CAP is always a cause for concern. The commonest cause of recurrent pneumonia in the same lobe of a lung is bronchial obstruction. Bronchial obstruction is most often due to carcinoma of the bronchus particularly so in elderly patients. It could also be caused by a foreign body (a 'supari' in an adult) or following bronchial stenosis, which is generally a sequel of tuberculosis. An underlying unrecognized bronchiectasis may also be the cause of repeated pneumonia.

Recurrent pneumonia (not necessarily in the same lobe) in young adults may be due to congenital hypogammaglobulinemia. Serum protein estimation and a protein electrophoresis will prove the diagnosis.

Immunoglobulin G (IgG) deficiency in particular may underlie recurrent lower respiratory tract infections. Acquired human immune deficiency syndrome can also lead to recurrent attacks of pneumonia—to start with, infection is not due to opportunistic organisms. Asplenia, either congenital or following splenectomy predisposes to fulminant pneumococcal or *H. influenzae* infection which may recur. Sickle cell disease, neutropenia or a qualitative defect in neutrophils, T-cell defects or deficiency are other immune-related problems predisposing to recurrent infections.

Aspiration is an important cause of recurrent pneumonia. Achalasia of the cardia when mild, or a slowly increasing oesophageal stricture are causes which can be easily missed as the patient may not complain of any difficulty in swallowing unless specifically asked. Aspiration following a large hiatus hernia or well-marked gastro-oesophageal reflux is also occasionally responsible for recurrent episodes of aspiration pneumonia. Aspiration is also probably the underlying cause (together with impaired respiratory defence mechanisms) for recurrent pneumonia in chronic alcoholics. Recurrent pneumonia may occur in patients with pulmonary sequestration. Ciliary dyskinesia with impairment of mucociliary transport also causes frequent lower respiratory tract infections in young adults.

Finally, recurrent pneumonia also occurs in patients with cystic fibrosis—a common entity in the West but less common in the developing countries of the world.

INVESTIGATIONS

Routine blood count, erythrocyte sedimentation rate (ESR), urine examination, blood culture and blood biochemistry are necessary. The oxygen saturation should be promptly noted.

Chest Radiography

An abnormal chest radiograph is a *sine qua non* in pneumonia, providing an immediate visual impression of the extent of involvement. It can confirm the presence and location of a pulmonary infiltrate, assess the extent of the pulmonary infection; detect pleural involvement, pulmonary cavitation or hilar adenopathy and gauge the response to antimicrobial therapy. However, chest radiographs may be normal when the patient is unable to mount an inflammatory response (e.g. in agranulocytosis) or in the early stage of an infiltrative process (e.g. in haematogenous *S. aureus* pneumonia or in *Pneumocystis* pneumonia associated with AIDS).

It is emphasized that almost every causative agent can produce a wide variety of different radiographic appearances, so that it is unwise to assume that a confluent lobar pneumonia is bound to be caused by *S. pneumoniae* despite the probability that this is the case. Similarly, cavitation need not be due to *S. aureus* but may occur in necrotizing Gram-negative pneumonias, such as those caused by *Klebsiella pneumoniae*, or in pneumonia arising from the aspiration of anaerobic bacteria or even from infection with *S. Pneumoniae* when Serotype 3 is involved. A study from Shizuoka Hospital, Japan attempted to correlate radiological findings with aetiological agents. Whilst pleural fluid accumulation and cavitation occurred in tuberculosis mimicking an acute pneumonia, lobar, segmental and lobular shadows did not correlate with any particular pathogen. Thus whilst certain radiographic patterns are more commonly associated with some microbial agents than with others, it is difficult to predict the aetiology of pneumonia from the radiological appearance.

Radiographic response to treatment usually lags behind clinical improvement and pneumococcal pneumonia (especially bacteraemic forms) may take six weeks to clear on the chest film. *S. aureus* and *Legionella* are amongst the slowe-resolving pneumonias. Age is the single most important predictor of the speed of resolution. In patients who are elderly, pneumonia resolves at a much slower rate than in younger patients. Persistent, recurrent, worsening shadowing may indicate either inappropriate treatment or bronchial obstruction by a foreign body, or more commonly, tumour, particularly in patients over the age of 60 years. At times, computed tomography (CT) may be especially useful in distinguishing different processes—e.g. pleural effusion versus underlying pulmonary consolidation, hilar adenopathy versus pulmonary mass and pulmonary abscess versus empyema with an air-fluid level.

Table 19.4: Causes of recurrent pneumonia
1. Bronchial obstruction due to carcinoma bronchus, foreign body or bronchial stenosis
2. Bronchiectasis
3. Hypogammaglobulinemia; isolated IgG deficiency
4. Acquired human immune deficiency syndrome
5. Asplenia either congenital or following splenectomy
6. Sickle cell disease, neutropenia or qualitative defect in neutrophils, T-cell defects or deficiency
7. Aspiration Chronic alcoholics Achalasia of the cardia Oesophageal stricture Large hiatus hernia Well-marked gastro-oesophgeal reflux
8. Pulmonary sequestration
9. Cystic fibrosis

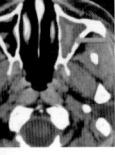
Laboratory Identification of Infecting Organisms

Laboratory investigation of a case of pneumonia should not delay treatment with antibiotics, the choice of which is based on a knowledge of the likely pathogens and an estimation of the severity of the infection. The lengths to which the clinician is prepared to investigate the microbiological cause of a case of pneumonia is likely to be determined by the severity of the illness at presentation, its response to initial treatment and the laboratory facilities available.

SPUTUM MICROSCOPY AND CULTURE

In poorer, developing Asian countries sputum examination is cheap, easy to perform and often the mainstay of diagnosis of CAP. Simple Gram staining of sputum which can be performed even at the bedside will give an immediate and accurate indication of the pathogen involved if large numbers of any one pathogen are seen. According to Macfarlane, such positive Gram stains have been shown to have a high specificity in the case of pneumococcal and staphylococcal pneumonia, though the sensitivity is low.

A few practical points about sputum testing need to be laboured here as they are particularly relevant in developing countries. First and foremost one must ensure the sample sent to the laboratory is a truly expectorated sample and not saliva. The presence of more than 25 squamous cells per high-power field indicates a sputum sample of poor quality and precious resources may be saved by requesting a repeat sample and not bothering to proceed with sputum culture. The second problem is that lower respiratory secretions are often contaminated by upper respiratory commensals during expectoration and the microbiologist reporting a potential pathogen should be aware that this may not reflect what is actually occurring in the lung. A laboratory trick to counter this is to wash or dilute the sputum so that only bacteria present in large numbers will grow on culture. The third problem is that even a single dose of an antibiotic can interfere with the culture of common pathogens like *S. pneumoniae* and *H. influenzae*. This is almost certainly the reason why so many hospital-based series of CAP from Asia and the West have no pathogen isolated in the majority of patients despite a careful search. The majority of patients hospitalized for pneumonia have already received one or more courses of antibiotics prior to hospitalization resulting in the sputum yield being very poor. Finally, in as many as a quarter of all patients with pneumonia, sputum is not produced. All these problems conspire to make sputum culture a relatively insensitive method of diagnosing bacterial pneumonia. Less than 50% of patients with bacteraemic pneumococcal pneumonia will have pneumococci isolated from their sputum.

A study from a public hospital in a poor part of India showed that attention to detail with bedside innoculation and dilution of the sputum specimen resulted in a higher yield (34%) of *S. pneumoniae*. If the sputum sample reached the laboratory late or did not undergo dilution the yield of S. pneumoniae and Gram-positive cocci was significantly reduced with higher numbers of Gram-negative rods indicating their overgrowth.

Because tuberculosis often mimics pneumonia in Asian countries it is worth doing acid-fast staining on sputum samples. It is the policy of our microbiology laboratory to perform Ziehl Neelsen staining on all sputum samples sent to the laboratory for routine culture. This has often helped clinicians make an early diagnosis of tuberculosis even when this has not been initially suspected.

Certain bacteria that can cause CAP are notoriously difficult to culture. *Legionella* is one such example and whilst occasional isolation on charcoal yeast extract medium may be possible, in the Asian context such a procedure would be expensive and time-consuming and perhaps best performed in only one or two central reference laboratories in each country.

SPUTUM IMMUNODETECTION

The diagnostic rate of pneumococcal pneumonia can be markedly increased by testing for pneumococcal polysaccharide capsular antigen in countercurrent immunoelectrophoresis or latex agglutination. This antigen can also be detected in blood and urine and an advantage of this test is that it is not affected by prior use of antibiotics. The sputum antigen is positive in about 80% of pneumococcal pneumonias, while urine and serum are positive in 36–45% and 9–23% of cases respectively. A study from Shanghai compared pneumococcal antigen detection by the coagglutination technique with sputum Gram stain and sputum culture. The positive yield was 46% by the coagglutination test, 27% by Gram staining and 17% by culture. Thus pneumococcal antigen detection by virtue of its speed, sensitivity, convenience and relative independence of antibiotic therapy provides a new dimension in the aetiological diagnosis of pneumococcal pneumonia. The antigen remains detectable for 7–14 days after bacteraemic pneumococcal pneumonia.

Other pathogens that may be detected by sputum immunodetection include *Legionella pneumophilia*, *Chlamydia pneumoniae* and *Pneumocystis carinii*.

BLOOD CULTURE

In the initial evaluation of a patient with pneumonia, at least two blood samples for culture should be obtained from different venepuncture sites. A positive culture may be obtained in 10–30% of cases, the higher percentage applying to pneumococcal pneumonia. This provides diagnostic proof (i.e. high specificity) of a pathogenic organism, often lacking where sputum culture and other tests are concerned. It is also of prognostic importance because bacteraemia is an indicator of more severe infection.

PLEURAL FLUID

If a pleural effusion is present in a patient suspected of having pneumonia, it should always be examined to exclude an empyema. Gram and acid-fast stains may be useful. The culture of pathogenic organisms is always significant and valuable. The fluid is always an exudate and some biochemical findings (low pH, high lactate dehydrogenase, low glucose) have been used to predict which parapneumonic effusions may develop into empyemas.

STANDARD ACUTE AND CONVALESCENT SEROLOGICAL TESTING

The usual serological tests involve the measurement of complement-fixing antibody levels in the blood, although the more sensitive enzyme-linked immunosorbent assay (ELISA) and immunofluorescent tests are tending to replace them. Serological tests may be used for infections caused by *Mycoplasma*

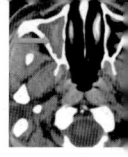

pneumoniae, Chlamydia spp., Coxiella burnetii and *Legionella spp.* By its nature, the complement-fixing test (CFT) is seldom of immediate value and when positive usually provides diagnostic information retrospectively, as two paired sera are required in order to demonstrate a fourfold rise in convalescent-phase antibody titre. It is usual to wait about 14 days between the two samples, although in some infections, such as *Mycoplasma*, a rise may be detected earlier; whilst in others, notably *Legionella*, the rise may take several weeks.

The problem with paired sampling is that the results are likely to come too late to be of clinical relevance.

Invasive Methods for Obtaining Respiratory Secretions

Other methods for obtaining respiratory secretions are more invasive and may be associated with morbidity. Their use is therefore confined to patients who are severely ill and in whom it is considered important to identify the organism rather than relying on an initial empirical antimicrobial approach or in whom such an approach has already been tried and failed.

FIBREOPTIC BRONCHOSCOPY

Fibreoptic bronchoscopy is usually safe, well-tolerated and has become the standard invasive procedure used to obtain lower respiratory tract secretion from seriously ill or immunocompromised patients with complex or progressive pneumonia and in selected patients with ventilator-associated pneumonia. It picks up oropharyngeal contaminants unless special precautions are taken using a protected specimen brush (PSB). The PSB can be combined with or used separately from BAL to obtain quantitative cultures in order to discriminate between the presence and absence of pneumonia, usually on ventilated patients in an intensive care setting. The diagnostic threshold for pneumonia, rather than airway colonization, has been reported as 10^3cfu/ml in respiratory secretions obtained by PSB. On the other hand, BAL subtends a wide area of tissue and lung secretions are diluted between 10 and 100fold, so that when interpreting results, a threshold of 10^4 cfu/ml may be taken. By combining PSB and BAL and by counting intracellular organisms, Chastre and colleagues claimed a sensitivity of 100% (compared with 86% for either technique alone) and a specificity of 96%. Bronchoscopy can therefore provide clues in a difficult case when other methods have failed, even when the picture has been clouded by almost inevitable prior use of antimicrobials. Infection with less usual organisms, such as *Legionalle spp.*, *M. tuberculosis*, *P. carinii*, other fungi or anaerobes may also be detected in such cases as well as the occasional unsuspected predisposing cause like the mechanical narrowing of a bronchus. On the other hand, negative results have to be treated with caution in patients already treated with antimicrobial therapy, since these may indicate either that the antibiotics are appropriate and that the organisms have been suppressed or that there was no infection there in the first place and the infiltrate was due to a non-infective cause.

In a study in China by Zhong and colleagues, secretions from the lower respiratory tract were taken for bacterial culture using Japanese-made single-sheath catheter (SSC) brush via fibreoptic bronchoscope in 53 cases with CAP. The results showed that bacteria were isolated in 42 out of 53 patients, the organism being pathogenic in 39 out of 53 (73.5%). Among the bacteria isolated from the 42 cases, Gram-negative bacilli accounted for the highest rate of 36% and pneumococcus was next with 31%. There were only three cases yielding contamination. Thus it showed that SSC has less chances of contamination and is convenient and practical.

PERCUTANEOUS TRANSTHORACIC NEEDLE PUNCTURE

This procedure employs a small-gauge needle that is advanced into the area of pulmonary consolidation with CT guidance. It requires the patient to cooperate, have good haemostasis and be able to tolerate a possible associated pulmonary haemorrhage or pneumothorax. Patients on mechanical ventilation cannot undergo lung puncture because of the high incidence of complicating pneumothorax. The diagnostic yield from this procedure ranges from 33 to 85%.

TRANSTRACHEAL ASPIRATION

Transtracheal aspiration may be carried out in patients who are unable to produce sputum or in whom the response to the chosen antibiotic is poor. The success of the procedure relies on the assumption that the tracheobronchial tree below the larynx is sterile, but false-positive results occur in patients with chronic lung disease because of tracheobronchial colonization. The technique has also been applied when anaerobic lung infection is suspected. A group from Japan performed this technique on 387 patients over an eight-year period from 1990–98 and isolated anaerobes in 20% of patients with CAP. Popular several decades ago, transtracheal aspiration is rarely carried out today.

Lung Biopsy

Transbronchial, thoracoscopic or open-lung biopsies tend to be reserved for diffuse pulmonary infiltrates of undetermined cause and in the context of suspected infection, are occasionally carried out in sick immunocompromised hosts in whom the presence of an unusual opportunistic pathogen is likely and in whom less invasive diagnostic approaches like BAL have failed to identify the cause.

Newer Microbiological Techniques

The tantalizing promise of new methods for the rapid detection and identification of specific organisms using molecular genetic technique seems close to being fulfilled but for most laboratories and clinicians has yet to be delivered, largely because of financial constraints. DNA probes have been developed for characterizing target organisms and minute amounts of target DNA can be amplified by the polymerase chain reaction (PCR) to improve the chance of their detection by the DNA probe so that the sensitivity of the test is increased. A PCR assay has recently been tested on the serum of patients with bacteraemic pneumococcal pneumonia and was found to have a sensitivity of 100% and specificity of 94%. Similar probes have been, or are being developed for a wide range of organisms including *Legionella pneumophilia, Mycoplasma pneumoniae, Neisseria meningitidis, Blastomyces dermatitidis, Histoplasma capsulatum, Coccidoides immitis, Mycobacterium tuberculosis, Mycobacterium avium, Mycobacterium intracellulare,* and *Mycobacterium scrofulaceum (MAIS group)* and

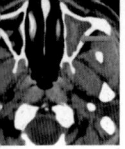

M. kansasi. Thus the identification of mycobacterial infection may take hours rather than weeks, although the organism still requires culture in order to allow antimicrobial sensitivities to be confirmed. These tests are generally outside the reach of all but a few referral laboratories in the developing Asian countries.

In a study done by Honda and colleagues in Japan, serologic data was compared with data obtained by capillary PCR to establish the efficacy of capillary PCR for the determination of *Mycoplasma* infection in samples obtained from throat swabs, BAL fluid and sputum of patients with *Mycoplasma* pneumonia. It was found that capillary PCR had a sensitivity of 80.6%.

Arterial Oxygen Saturation and Blood Gas Analysis

Oxygen saturation performed as a prompt screening procedure, should be followed by arterial blood gas analysis if desaturation is present. The degree of hypoxemia present is a measure of the severity of the infection and needs prompt correction. The need for inspired oxygen of 35% or more to maintain the oxygen saturation above 90% implies severe pneumonia as does a PaO_2 of 60 mm Hg or less, or a $PaCO_2$ of 50 mm Hg or more. These findings warn that assisted ventilation may become necessary.

Other Laboratory Findings

The white cell count is frequently raised in bacterial pneumonia, with a neutrophilia. Elderly patients are not always able to mount such a response. Sometimes when sepsis is overwhelming there may be leucopenia. A lymphocytosis may occur in viral infections or due to 'atypical' organisms. The white cell count may be normal in viral pneumonia. The presence of cold agglutinins in a patient's citrated blood is seen in over 50% of cases of *Mycoplasma pneumonia.*

Table 19.5: Diagnostic value of investigations in community-acquired pneumonia	
Tests	**Remarks**
Routine CBC and biochemistry	There may be leucocytosis, leucopenia or a normal count
Arterial oxygen saturation and blood gas analysis	Hypoxemia needs prompt correction. The greater the degree of hypoxemia, the more severe the infection
CXR	The etiology of a pneumonia cannot be definitely ascertained by the nature of the radiological shadows
Microbiological	
Sputum—Gram stain/culture	Check if sample satisfactory Collect sputum prior to starting antibiotics Oropharynegal contamination may be present Low sensitivity (10%), high specificity (70–80%) if positive Washing/diluting sample helpful
Blood Culture	Should be done prior to starting antibiotics Positive cultures rare in our set-up, but when present, identify the pathogen
Pleural Fluid-gram stain/culture	If positive, useful in establishing aetiological agent
Serological	
Antigen Detection:	
Pneumococcal (blood, urine)	Mainly useful for pneumococcal infection
Legionella (urine)	Accurate means of diagnosing Legionella infection
Cold Agglutinins	Positive in over 50% of patients with mycoplasmal pneumonia
Serological Tests	
Anti-mycoplasma	
Anti-chlamydia	
Anti-influenzae	Helps in diagnosis of Mycoplasma, Chlamydia, and viral pneumonias
Invasive Tests	
a) Examination of secretions, obtained from protected brush biopsies, broncho-alveolar lavage	Should be done in serious illness not responding to initial empiric antibiotic therapy
b) Percutaneus transthoracic needle puncture	Diagnostic yield 33–85%. Cannot be used in patients on mechanical ventilation due to the risk of pneumothorax
c) CT—guided biopsy of lesion	Helps in aetiological diagnosis
e) Transbronchial, thoracoscopic or open lung biopsy	Helps in diagnosis in the above situation if BAL, protected brush smears and CT guided biopsies are negative
Newer tests	
PCR assay	Serum of patients with bacteremic pneumococcal pneumonia: Sensitivity of 100% and specificity of 94%

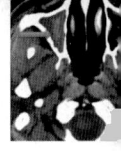

Numerous non-specific biochemical abnormalities have been noted, such as a raised blood urea, bilirubin, transaminases and alkaline phosphatase. Hyponatraemia due to inappropriate antidiuretic hormone secretion may occur in Legionella infection.

Urinanalysis may detect small amounts of protein and both red and white blood cells may be seen on microscopy. As mentioned above, pneumococcal antigen may be detected in urine more frequently than in blood but less frequently than in sputum. *Legionella* antigen may also be detected in urine by ELISA, indicating *L. pneumophilia* Type 1 infection (thought to account for about 80% of human legionellosis), and this test is well worth doing for a rapid answer in severely ill patients with pneumonia.

COMPLICATIONS

The most important complication is acute respiratory failure. There is often a large shunt from right to left in pneumonia, particularly when more than one lobe is involved. This leads to a marked fall in the PaO$_2$ even when the patient is on oxygen at 4–6 l/min. Acute respiratory failure can also occur because of the evolution of the acute respiratory distress syndrome following a fulminant lobar pneumonia. Multiple shadows in both lungs, with a large right to left shunt following a lobar consolidation are now invariably thought to be due to acute lung injury (ARDS), and not due to multilobar pneumonia as was earlier believed.

Acute life-threatening pneumonia is a source of sepsis. All the complications of the sepsis syndrome may be observed. These include hypotension, septic shock, tissue hypoperfusion with metabolic acidosis culminating in multiple organ failure.

Spread of infection to contiguous areas, or haematogenous spread, add to the gravity of the illness. Empyema is the commonest complication of CAP. It may be tucked away posteriorly in the paravertebral gutter and can be missed on a chest X-ray. It is clearly demonstrated on a CT of the chest. It may be responsible for the sepsis syndrome after the consolidation in the lung has resolved. Occasionally, CAP may break down to form a lung abscess; this can occur with infections caused by *Staphylococcus aureus*, *pneumococcus* Type III infection, anaerobic infection or following infections with Gram-negative organisms such as *Klebsiella pneumoniae*, and *P. pyocyaneus*. The abscess may communicate with the pleura causing an empyema and a bronchopleural fistula.

Acute purulent pericarditis is now a very rare complication. It is lethal if undiagnosed and not promptly treated. As little as 300 ml of pus in the pericardium can cause death from cardiac tamponade in a child. The diagnosis should be suspected when there is a sudden clinical deterioration in a patient with acute pneumonia, particularly in the presence of shock with a raised central venous pressure.

Acute pyogenic meningitis may be the presenting feature of an underlying pneumococcal lobar pneumonia. Neck stiffness and a positive Kernig's sign may however be present in acute lobar pneumonia even without acute meningitis. Meningism is more frequently observed with upper lobe pneumonia in young adults. A lumbar puncture is always mandatory as it is the only certain way of distinguishing meningism from meningitis.

A sharp deterioration in the clinical state with confusion, delirium, and severe prostration may also occur when infection from the lungs spreads haematogenously to produce one or more cerebral abscesses. Localizing signs may be present. A CT scan is invaluable in confirming the clinical diagnosis.

Acute left ventricular failure is rare except in patients with pre-existing left ventricular disease. Acute myocarditis can and does however occur in some patients with acute influenza. It is characterized by tachycardia, increase in breathlessness, hypotension, cardiac dilatation and a diastolic gallop. It may progress to an increasingly severe low output state and death from cardiogenic shock.

In the older age group, we have admitted to the ICU patients severely ill with acute pneumonia presenting with marked abdominal distension. Acute dilatation of the stomach is particularly dangerous as it compounds respiratory difficulties. Ileus may also occur due to toxaemia.

Femoral vein thrombosis is occasionally observed in patients critically ill with pneumonia. Sudden death in acute pneumonia could well be related to pulmonary embolism.

Severe lobar pneumonia may so damage the bronchi within the lobes as to lead to bronchiectasis as a permanent sequel.

Table 19.6: Complications of acute community-acquired pneumonia
1. Acute respiratory failure
2. Acute Lung Injury (ARDS)
3. Sepsis Syndrome/MODS
4. Acute circulatory failure
5. Spread of infection to contiguous areas or haematogenous spread e.g. empyema, acute meningitis, cerebral abscess, acute pericarditis
6. Acute left ventricular failure/acute myocarditis
7. Acute abdominal distension—acute dilatation of the stomach, ileus
8. Femoral vein thrombosis
9. Bronchiectasis (as a sequel)

DIFFERENTIAL DIAGNOSIS

A large pulmonary infarct is an important differential diagnosis of acute lobar pneumonia. The distinction at times is difficult. Acute extrinsic allergic alveolitis or acute cryptogenic fibrosing alveolitis may produce bilateral lower lobe shadows with increasing hypoxia. Acute eosinophilic pneumonia should be suspected on the fairly typical radiological features (peripheral shadows in both lung fields). Acute consolidation due to a vasculitis (e.g. Wegener's) may be indistinguishable from consolidation due to an infection. Pneumonia may occur as a presenting feature of bronchial obstruction produced by a tumour or a foreign body. Aspiration of betel nut *(supari)* can cause a life-threatening acute necrotizing pneumonia.

The possibility of an underlying amoebic liver abscess should always be considered in endemic areas in the presence of right lower lobe pathology. A subphrenic abscess may cause a pleural effusion, an empyema and/or a lower lobe consolidation.

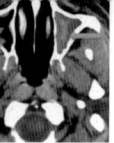

MANAGEMENT

When a patient with pneumonia first presents to a general practitioner or a hospital, the cause of pneumonia is generally not known. While sputum and blood culture should be collected at the outset, treatment must start on what are perforce empirical grounds. The first decision the doctor has to make is: 'Can this patient with CAP be successfully managed as an outpatient or should the patient be hospitalized?' The second and even more important question is 'What should my empirical choice of antibiotic be?'

Estimating severity of Pneumonia: A number of severity scores have emerged that attempt to determine the severity of a patient's pneumonia. These include:

1. **CURB index**: CURB stands for; Confusion, Urea > 7mmol/l, Respiratory rate > 30/min, Blood pressure systolic < 90 mm Hg, or diastolic < 60 mm Hg. Several elegant British Thoracic Society (BTS) studies have shown that the presence of two of these four denotes severe CAP with such patients having a 24fold higher risk of death.

2. **CURB-65**: includes all four core CURB variables with the addition of age > 65 years as the fifth variable. Three or more of these five variables are now needed to define severe CAP.

3. **PSI (Pneumonia Severity Index)**: uses 20 clinical variables to determine a score. These scores are then used to define five classes of increasing risk of mortality with Class 4 and 5 defining severe CAP.

4. **Modified BTS rule**: The BTS Rule is based on the presence or absence of three factors on admission—respiratory rate—≥ 30/min, diastolic blood pressure ≤ 60 mm Hg, and blood urea >7 mmol/L (blood urea done at any time after admission is also applicable). Patients with two or more of these features had a mortality of 19.4% compared with 0.9% in those with none or one of these features. The modified BTS Rule included mental confusion as the fourth factor. Those with two or more of the four features had a mortality of 22%.

5. **Revised American Thoracic Society (ATS) guidelines**: The presence of at least one major (need for mechanical ventilation or septic shock) or two minor criteria (PaO$_2$/FiO$_2$ < 250 kPa, multilobar shadowing on chest radiograph, or systolic blood pressure < 90 mm Hg) is used to define CAP severity.

All the scores are more or less comparable in terms of sensitivity, specificity and predictive value with the CURB score being most strongly recommended because of its simplicity and applicability at the bedside. *When the CURB score was applied to the Indian CAP series in one of our units, it was found to be robust with a PPV (positive predictive value) of 78% and an NPV (negative predictive value) of 94% in predicting who will die or require ICU transfer.*

Would considerations other than the CURB criteria or CURB–65 criteria, the modified BTS criteria or revised ATS guidelines influence the need for hospitalization? In most patients the CURB or CURB-65 criteria have a high sensitivity and specificity for recognizing patients serious enough to warrant hospitalization—but not always so. We would consider hospitalization if just one of the CURB criteria is present and the patient has any one or more of the following:

1. Multilobar involvement or cavitation or moderate-sized pleural effusion, or metastatic complications
2. PaO$_2$/FiO$_2$ < 250 or a PaO$_2$ < 60 mm Hg or an arterial blood pH < 7.3
3. Marked leucopenia or thrombocytopenia or anaemia (Hb—8.5 g%)
4. Hypothermia or hyperpyrexia
5. Tachycardia > 120/min
6. Presence of significant co-morbid disease—moderately severe COPD, cardiac disease, congestive heart failure, immunodeficiency states or immunosuppression from any cause
7. Home management impossible because of poverty, altered mentation, likelihood of poor compliance.

While Western countries have clear guidelines on the appropriate initial antibiotics for a patient with CAP, no similar guidelines are available for India or other countries of Asia.

Table 19.7: Estimating severity of pneumonia
1. CURB index
2. CURB-65
3. PSI (Pneumonia Severity Index)
4. Modified BTS rule
5. Revised ATS guidelines

Table 19.8: CURB Index
Confusion, **U**rea > 7 mmol/l, **R**espiratory rate > 30/min, **B**lood pressure systolic < 90 mm Hg, or diastolic < 60 mm Hg. The presence of 2 of these 4 denotes severe CAP with such patients having a 24 fold higher risk of death.

Table 19.9: CURB-65
Confusion, **U**rea > 7 mmol/l, **R**espiratory rate > 30/min, **B**lood pressure systolic < 90 mm Hg, or diastolic < 60 mm Hg. Age > 65 years as the fifth variable, 3 or more of these 5 variables are now needed to define severe CAP

Table 19.10: Revised ATS guidelines
The presence of any one of the following major or two minor criteria is used to assess the severity of the CAP.

Major Criteria	Minor Criteria—
1. Need for mechanical ventilation	1. PaO$_2$/FIO$_2$ < 250 kPa,
2. Septic shock	2. Multilobar shadowing on chest radiography
	3. Systolic blood pressure < 90 mm Hg

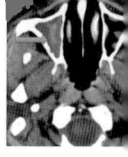

Table 19.11: Criteria for hospitalization			
Lack of response or further deterioration in condition at home	CURB Index CURB-65 PSI Modified BTS rule Revised ATS guidelines	Multilobar involvement Pleural effusions Metastatic complications Marked leucopenia or thrombocytopenia or anaemia Severe hypoxia	Poverty rendering home management impossible
A	B	C	D

Note: In our setup, all patients who come under category B or C would be cared for in a critical care unit to start with.

Indeed, because of the vastness and disparity of different parts of the Indian subcontinent, no guidelines could hope to be all-encompassing. Hence, as stressed in the section on 'aetiology', regional studies which should be carefully and prospectively performed, must first establish the local epidemiology. Thus, based on the firm knowledge of local epidemiology, patient population profile and economic issues, local guidelines can be individualized for regions of India or other different Asian countries. Blindly transposing Western guidelines to Asian countries would clearly be inappropriate. Worse still however would be empirical treatment given without knowledge or consideration of local epidemiological conditions. Furthermore, a mechanism for regular review at a regional level should ideally be in place to take account of changing patterns of disease such as the reduced susceptibility of common organisms to standard antibiotics and emergence of new or previously unknown pathogens. Such a review by Lim from Singapore noted that there had been a 60fold increase in the incidence of penicillin resistance in *S. pneumoniae* between 1987 and 1997. The review also made note of the small increase in the number of cases of Legionnaire's disease and the marked increase in the incidence of melioidosis. Similar reviews from Thailand show that melioidosis has become the commonest cause of CAP in this region (see 'Tropical Infections Involving the Lungs').

Choice of Antibiotics

1. Outpatient department (OPD)-treated patients
2. Hospitalized patients

OPD TREATMENT

For patients treated in the community in poorer countries, cost is often an important deciding factor. Cheap but reasonably effective antibiotic choices in India and the developing world would include oral amoxicillin or ampicillin, co-trimoxazole or a tetracycline derivative. A recent trial from one of the poorest areas of the developing world showed that co-trimoxazole was cheap and yet as effective as more expensive antibiotics in 134 Gambian children with pneumonia. It is important that general practitioners and rural healthcare providers are not seduced by the latest (and generally most costly) antibiotics. Responsible prescribing by this group of physicians will go a long way in preventing the emergence of antibiotic resistance. The impact that a rational antibiotic policy can make in reducing pneumonia mortality, even in the poorest part of rural India, can be seen from an inspiring study by Bang *et al*. This was a community-

based intervention trial to reduce childhood mortality from pneumonia in 6176 children in 58 villages in Gadchiroli, India. These interventions included mass education about childhood pneumonia and case management of pneumonia by trained paramedics and village health workers who were taught to recognize childhood pneumonia and treat it with co-trimoxazole. After a year of intervention, pneumonia-specific childhood mortality was significantly reduced in the intervention area as compared to a control area of 44 villages (8.1 vs. 17.5 deaths per 1000 children under five years). The difference in infant mortality (89 vs. 121 per 1000) and total under-five mortality (28.5 vs. 40.7 per 1000) was highly significant. The cost of co-trimoxazole was US $ 0.025 per child per year. This worked out to a mere $2.64 per child saved.

Another antibiotic which is a reasonable first choice and relatively inexpensive is erythromycin. In the many Asian regions where atypical pathogens are frequently encountered, this would be an appropriate initial choice. A study from Taiwan showed it to be as effective as the more expensive (but better tolerated) clarithromycin.

If cost is not a factor then oral antibiotics with a wider range include a β-lactamase stable antibiotic like co-amoxyclav or a second or third-generation oral cephalosporin like cefuroxime axetil. Other effective oral choices would be a newer macrolide like azithromycin or clarithromycin. While the newer quinolones are emerging as oral antibiotics for CAP in many parts of the world, it is our opinion that these drugs have a pivotal role as second-line drugs in multi-drug-resistant (MDR)-TB and should be reserved for this role in regions where TB is endemic.

HOSPITALIZED PATIENTS

These patients are likely to be more ill at the outset or have associated co-morbid conditions and should ideally receive intravenous antibiotics from the start. The initial choice of antibiotics is based on local epidemiology plus an assessment of how severe the pneumonia is.

In the ill, hospitalized patient all probable pathogens must be covered and an intravenous β-lactamase stable penicillin (e.g. co-amoxyclav) or a cephalosporin (e.g. cefuroxime or cefotaxime or ceftriaxone) together with a macrolide provides good initial cover for the majority of typical and atypical pathogens likely to be encountered.

Two situations which deserve separate mention are: (1) infection caused by *Staphylococcus* where flucloxacillin (supported by Rifampicin) or vancomycin may be considered and (2) infection caused by Gram-negative enteric bacilli

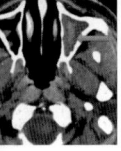

(including *Pseudomonas aeruginosa*). While the American Thoracic Guidelines recommend cover from the start for these organisms in all severely ill hospitalized CAPs we do not regard this approach necessary in the initial management of younger previously healthy patients.

In desperately ill individuals with life-threatening pneumonia, particularly in the elderly (in whom community-acquired Gram-negative infections are encountered with increasing frequency) it may be necessary to empirically cover all likely organisms—*Streptococcus pneumoniae*, Gram-negative bacteria, staphylococci, and atypical organisms. The antibiotic regime would include Amoxicillin to cover pneumococci, piperacillin-tazobactum or a carbapenem to cover Gram-negative bacteria, vancomycin if a staphylococcal infection is considered possible and a macrolide for atypical organisms. If an anaerobic infection is suspected one could add either metronidazole or clindamycin, or replace piperacillin-tazobactum with meropenem. This is indeed blunderbuss therapy but is at times unavoidable. Once a more definite diagnosis as to the nature of the infecting organism is available the antibiotic regime should be narrowed, restricted and de-escalated to one or two appropriate drugs.

The same empiric regime may need to be followed in younger individuals who fail to respond and appear to worsen after initial therapy with Amoxicillin (co-amoxyclav) and a macrolide or after initial therapy on a regime consisting of a second-generation cephalosporin and a macrolide.

Duration of Treatment

The antimicrobial treatment for uncomplicated pneumonias due to *S. pneumoniae*, anaerobes, *H. influenzae* and *M. catarrhalis* should be continued for seven to ten days. The duration of treatment for *Mycoplasma* and *Legionella* infection is two to three weeks. However, the presence of *S. aureus* or Gram-negative enteric bacilli or the development of suppurative

complications requires a more prolonged course of therapy (e.g. two weeks for non-bacteraemic staphylococcal pneumonia, four weeks for bacteraemic staphylococcal pneumonia and four to six weeks in case of an empyema). A recent study of 186 patients hospitalized for mild to moderate pneumonia in nine hospitals from 2000–03 in Netherlands showed three days of amoxicillin was as effective as eight days. Such a strategy if verified in larger trials would represent considerable savings in cost and curtail antibiotic resistance.

Assessment of Response to Initial Antimicrobial Therapy

Once antimicrobial treatment is initiated, it is important to monitor the patient for clinical response. Normally no change in antimicrobial treatment should be considered within the first 72 hours unless initial diagnostic studies identify a pathogen not covered by original empirical therapy (e.g. *M. tuberculosis*), a resistant pathogen is isolated from blood or another sterile site (i.e. pleural fluid), or there is clinical deterioration. Even when antimicrobial treatment is appropriate, clinical improvement may be delayed by several factors. The presence of coexisting illness and advanced age is associated with delays in improvement. Patients with structural abnormalities of the respiratory tract, particularly COPD, often do not respond as rapidly as previously healthy patients. Unrecognized immunosuppression, e.g. owing to AIDS or prior drug therapy, may also result in delays in clinical improvement. The virulence of the infectious agent may also delay response. Bacteraemic patients and patients with Gram-negative or staphylococcal pneumonias are generally slower to respond.

In appropriately treated patients, clinical response is often rapid, especially among patients without prior coexisting disease. In this population, fever usually disappears within two to four days, and the leucocytosis resolves by the fourth or fifth day of

Table 19.12: Antimicrobial therapy in CAP	
Types of patients	**Antibiotic used**
Ia. Hospitalized patients	β-lactamase penicillin—Co-amoxyclav: 1.2 gm 8 hourly iv or IV Cephalosporin like ceftriaxone: 2 gm 12 hourly iv + IV Macrolide like erythromycin 1 gm 6 hourly iv
Ib. Severely ill patients	IV Amoxicillin 500 mg QDS + Piperacillin-tazobactum—4.5 gm 8 hourly iv or a Carbapenem—Meropenem 1 gm 8 hourly iv + Vancomycin 500 mg 6 hourly iv (if MRSA suspected) Regime to be modified if infecting organism has been determined. Infection with Ps. aeruginosa requires a two-drug combination— Meropenem 1 gm 8 hourly + Aminoglycoside (Amikacin) 1 gm IV OD
II. OPD patients	β-lactamase penicillin—Amoxy-clav 625 BD orally or Cephalosporin—Cefuroxime 500 BD orally or Macrolide—Erythromycin 500 mg QDS or Levofloxacin 750 mg BD if atypical organism is suspected

Note: Quinolones should be used with great discrimination if at all in countries which have a high prevalence of tuberculosis. In poor rural parts of developing countries, the above drugs are difficult to use. Alternative therapy with amoxicillin 500 QDS or sulfamethoxazole and trimethoprim (Septran DS 1 tablet twice daily) can be effectively used.

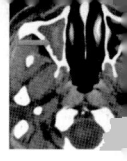

therapy. Physical findings remain abnormal in up to 40% of patients at Day 7. The chest radiograph may not normalize at four weeks even in young (<50 years old), previously healthy individuals and may not reach baseline for up to six months in the elderly patients with COPD, or in alcoholic patients. Chest radiographic abnormalities may worsen initially, but significant early (<48 hours) deterioration of chest radiograph, defined as a 50% or greater increase in the size of the infiltrate, progression to significant involvement of multiple lobes, or development of a large pleural effusion should raise concern that therapy is inadequate.

Supportive Treatment in Pneumonia

RESPIRATORY SUPPORT

Patients who are in obvious respiratory distress with tachypnoea are at increased risk of dying and need close monitoring, particularly if they are beginning to show evidence of exhaustion with drowsiness or confusion. The finding of a PaO_2 of less than 60 mm Hg when breathing oxygen at 2–4 L/min indicates a serious situation, as does hypercarbia. Many patients are already receiving supplemental oxygen; a PaO_2/FiO_2 ratio equal to or less than 300 mm Hg is a serious concern. A PaO_2 of 50 mm Hg or less in the presence of rising PCO_2 and acidosis are indications for mechanical ventilation. Sometimes improvement in oxygenation can be achieved by postural drainage so that the 'good lung' is dependent. Non-invasive ventilatory support using high-flow oxygen through a CPAP or BiPAP device may help tide over a crisis and relieve hypoxia provided the patient is sufficiently cooperative, not too tachypnoeic, haemodynamically stable and does not have excessive sputum production.

Inotropic agents such as dopamine or dobutamine may be required when severe pneumonia is complicated by hypotension. Pleuritic pain can be relieved by simple non-sedative analgesics. Physiotherapy is of no benefit and should be avoided in acutely ill patients who find cooperation difficult, who may easily become exhausted and even more hypoxic. It may however assist expectoration of sputum in less ill patients and in those who are recovering. Elderly or very feeble patients who have a great deal of sputum production which they cannot expectorate are aided by a bronchoscopic clearance of chest secretions.

Table below gives a list of factors that could be responsible for poor response of pneumonia to treatment.

Table: 19.13 Factors involved in poor response to empirical antimicrobial therapy
1. Incorrect microbiologic diagnosis
2. Inappropriate antimicrobial agent or dosing regimen.
3. Drug-resistant organism
4. Drug hypersensitivity or drug fever
5. Tuberculosis can mimic pyogenic pneumonia, also consider unusual organisms such as Actinomyces or Nocardia spp.
6. Infectious complication: empyema, metastatic spread, superinfection
7. Presence of endobronchial obstruction
8. Reconsider the pneumonia diagnosis: Could it be pulmonary embolism, malignancy, vasculitis, drug reaction, eosinophilic pneumonia or cryptogenic organising pneumonia

PROGNOSIS

The outcome of CAP depends on the early diagnosis and effective antimicrobial therapy along with the age of the patient, the severity of the disease along with the underlying associated co-morbid conditions. Pneumonia in the elderly is particularly dangerous due to frequent absence of classical symptoms and also due to the higher incidence of adverse effects to antibiotics.

In an interesting study by Chen and colleagues in Taiwan, the following variables were associated with a poor prognosis. They were:

1. The presence of septic shock
2. The use of ventilatory support
3. The presence of radiological spread
4. Treatment in an intensive care unit
5. Male gender
6. Development of acute respiratory distress syndrome
7. *Klebsiella* pneumonia in patients with alcohol habit
8. Patients with ultimately fatal underlying disease
9. An initial alveolar arterial gradient (A–a) O_2 > 200
10. An arterial pH< 7.25.

In a study by Dey and colleagues in Delhi it was found that old age, history of smoking, presence of chronic obstructive airways disease, late presentation to hospital, systolic and diastolic hypotension, high blood urea, low serum albumin and development of septic shock were associated with a poorer prognosis. In their study of 72 patients with CAP, 35% of elderly patients and 14% of young patients succumbed to fulminant sepsis or respiratory failure.

PREVENTION

The prevention of pneumonia aims at strengthening the host's responses once the pathogen is encountered. This includes the use of chemoprophylaxis or immunization for patients at risk. Chemoprophylaxis can be administered to patients who have encountered or are likely to encounter the pathogen before they become symptomatic (e.g. amantadine during a community outbreak of Influenza A, isoniazid for tuberculosis, or trimethoprim-sulfamethoxazole for pneumocystis). Vaccines are available for immunization against *S. pneumoniae, H. influenzae* Type b, influenza viruses A and B, and measles virus. Of these, the pneumococcal and influenza vaccines are found to be most effective and are indicated in patients over 65 years of age and in patients with cardiovascular diseases, pulmonary diseases, diabetes mellitus, alcoholism, liver cirrhosis and immunosuppression (HIV infection, chronic renal failure, organ transplant recipients, sickle cell disease, post-splenectomy state, haematological and lymphatic malignancies). The currently available 23-valent pneumococcal vaccine covers 88% of the serotypes causing systemic disease as well as 8% of related serotypes. The increasing prevalence of multiantibiotic resistance among pneumococci makes the pneumococcal immunization of high-risk individuals of utmost importance. The effect of pneumococcal vaccine lasts for 7–10 years after which it may be repeated. The influenza vaccine should be given yearly in high-risk individuals.

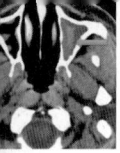
SUGGESTED READING

Apisarnthanarak A. Etiology of community-acquired pneumonia. *Clin Chest Med.* 1 Mar. 2005; 26(1): 47–55.

Bansal S, Kashyap S, Pal LS, Goel A. Clinical and Bacteriological profile of community acquired pneumonia in Shimla, Himachal Pradesh. *Indian J Chest Dis Allied Sci.* 2004; 46: 17–22.

Buising KL, Thursky KA, *et al.* A prospective comparison of severity scores for identifying patients with severe community-acquired pneumonia: reconsidering what is meant by severe pneumonia. *Thorax.* 2006 May; 61(5):419–24.

Datta Banik. Some observations on feeding programmes, nutrition and growth of pre-school childen urban community. *Indian Journal of Pediatrics.* 1977; 139–49.

Invasive Bacterial Infection Surveillance (IBIS) Group. Prospective multicenter hospital surveillance of streptococcus pneumoniae disease in India. *Lancet.* 1999; 353: 1216–20.

Ishida T, Hashimoto T, Aria M, Ito I, Osawa M. Etiology of community acquired pneumonia in hospitalized patients: A three year prospective study in Japan. *Chest.* 1998; 114: 1588–93.

Mandell LA. Epidemiology and etiology of community-acquired pneumonia. *Infect Dis Clin North Am.* 1 Dec. 2004; 18(4): 761–76, vii.

Niederman MS. Recent advances in community-acquired pneumonia: in patient and outpatient. *Chest.* 1 Apr. 2007; 131(4): 1205–15.

Tarver RD. Radiology of community-acquired pneumonia. *Radiol Clin North Am.* 1 May 2005; 43(3): 497–512, viii.

Woodhead M. Community-acquired pneumonia: severity of illness evaluation. *Infect Dis Clin North Am.* 1 Dec. 2004; 18(4): 791–807; viii.

Wunderink RG. Community-acquired pneumonia: pathophysiology and host factors with focus on possible new approaches to management of lower respiratory tract infections. *Infect Dis Clin North Am.* 1 Dec. 2004; 18(4): 743–59, vii.

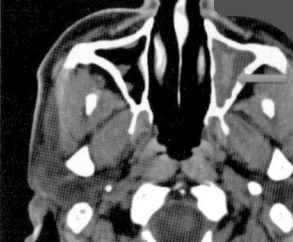

CHAPTER **20** **Non-Bacterial Pneumonia**

VIRAL PNEUMONIA

Epidemiology

Viral upper respiratory tract infections are common at all ages. Viral pneumonia however is uncommon in immunocompetent individuals, except in children and the elderly. The contribution of viral infection to community-acquired pneumonia (CAP) though uncertain is clearly underestimated. This is because reliable tests to confirm viral infections are difficult and outside the scope of the average hospital laboratory and also because of the relative lack of sensitivity of a number of these tests. This is particularly observed in India where there are just a few reference laboratories for virological studies which can claim a standard of excellence. The viral load in CAP in India is unknown though it undoubtedly does exist. In the West, in published series of adults, particularly the elderly, rates of viral pneumonia vary markedly depending on the type of tests, populations and the season in which the study was carried out. Viruses are identified in 0.3 to 30% of patients who have CAP, in studies using viral culture and serology for diagnosis. In a recent study on 105 patients with CAP in the West, respiratory viruses were detected in 14% of patients using conventional techniques compared to 56% by the reverse-transcriptase polymerized chain reaction (RT-PCR) technique. *(Ref: Templeton K.E., Scheltinga S.A., van den Eeden W.C., et al: Improved diagnosis of the etiology of community-acquired pneumonia with real-time polymerase chain reaction. Clin Infect Dis 41. 345–351.2005)* In all studies, regardless of diagnostic technique, Influenza A virus is the most common pathogen, responsible for 4–19% of cases. *(Ref: Flamaing J., Engelmann I., Joosten E., et al: Viral lower respiratory tract infection in the elderly: a prospective in-hospital study. Eur J Clin Microbiol Infect Dis 22. 720–725.2003)*

The large number of viruses known to cause lower respiratory infection and pneumonia are listed in the accompanying table:

Table 20.1: Viral causes of pneumonia	
Common respiratory viruses	**Other viruses**
Influenza viruses A and B	Measles virus
Respiratory syncitial virus (RSV)	Varicella zoster virus
Parainfluenza viruses	Cytomegalovirus
Adenovirus	Epstein Barr virus
Rhinovirus	Hanta virus
Coxsackie virus	

The important ones are Influenza A, B viruses, parainfluenza virus, respiratory syncitial virus (RSV), adenovirus, and the coronovirus. The measles virus (which like the parainfluenza and the RSV belongs to the paramyxoviridae family) as also the chicken pox virus can also cause pneumonia. The Hantavirus, a rare virus prevalent chiefly in North and South America can also cause serious pneumonic infection. Pneumonia due to the Hantavirus has also been reported from South India. *(Ref: Chandy S, Boorugu H, Chrispal A, Thomas K, Abraham P, Sridharan G. Hantavirus infection: A case report from India. Indian J Med Microbiol 2009; 27:267–70)*

SPECIFIC VIRAL PNEUMONIAS

Influenzal Pneumonia

THE INFLUENZA VIRUS

Three types of influenza virus have been identified—A, B, and C. Influenza A and B are responsible for close to 50% of all viral pneumonias in immunocompetent adults. Influenza C virus is a significant cause of respiratory infections in children under–six years of age. The majority of humans acquire immunity to Influenza C virus early in life so that subsequently clinical disease due to this virus is not generally encountered. The influenza A virus is the only type that can cause influenza to occur in large epidemic and pandemic forms.

Influenza A viruses are endemic gastrointestinal viruses of wild waterfowl, but have evolved elaborate mechanisms to jump species into domestic fowl, farm animals and humans. The major surface glycoprotein antigens on the virus envelope are the haemagglutinin and neuraminidase. The viral haemagglutinin binds to the host cell sialic acid-conjugated glycoprotein, an attachment necessary for viral entry into the cell. Neuraminidase is important for viral release and propagation. The 'naming' of the Influenza A virus depends on which of these proteins is present in a given virus. Thus the standard nomenclature is influenza A HxNx (where x is the number corresponding to the specific type of haemagglutinin and neuraminidase).

Periodic gene segment reassertments between human and animal viruses produce important antigenic changes referred to as 'shifts'. These can lead to explosive deadly pandemics as witnessed in 1888, 1918, 1957 and 1968. The influenza world pandemic of 1918 was responsible for 50 million deaths in the world. In intervening years these 'shifted' viruses undergo minor (i.e. less severe) antigenic changes called 'drifts' which allows the virus to escape human immune responses raised by previously circulating influenza viruses. The Influenza A virus has an amazingly inexhaustible range of mutational possibilities

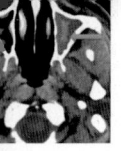

at several epitomes surrounding the viral haemagglutinin site that attaches to human cells. The mechanism as to how zoonotic influenza viruses mix with each other and with human strains to acquire extra properties of human virulence and human to human transmission, thereby causing an explosive outbreak is unknown.

Outbreaks of severe disease occur every 10 to 40 years. During outbreaks children are usually infected first, before adults, and morbidity and mortality are thus both high. The host immune response is chiefly directed towards the haemagglutinin antigen of the virus and involves both cellular and humoral antibody response. Secretory Immunoglobulin A also has a role in host defence. There is marked mucosal inflammation of the respiratory tract, characterized by mucosal oedema, hyperemia and in severe cases haemorrhage.

TRANSMISSION

Influenza is primarily transmitted from person to person by droplet infection (droplets > 5 μm) when an infected patient coughs or sneezes. Smaller droplets remain air-borne longer and thus spread further, being carried by air currents for varying distances (air-borne spread). Contact transmission may also play a role. Infected patients may touch mucus membranes (like nose or nasal secretions) and then touch (e.g. hand shake) other individuals (direct contact). There could also be indirect contact through touching objects or surfaces touched by other non-infected individuals. If either through direct or indirect contact, uninfected patients touch their own mucous membranes, the virus gets deposited and infection ensues.

SEASONAL INFLUENZA

Seasonal influenza is generally due to Virus A and occasionally due to Virus B. Epidemics generally occur in winter, anytime between November and April lasting six to eight weeks and varying in severity. In countries closer to the equator, the influenza season can be prolonged, being a multiphasic or year-round disease and is influenced in particular by the rainy season. Explosive epidemics are common in closed settings such as nursing homes, schools, dormitories. Rates of infection are high in those below 5 years of age, decline in those between 5 and 49 years of age and rise significantly in those aged 50 or over. Rates of hospitalization rise significantly with each decade over 60 years rising from 120 per 100,000 for ages 65 to 69 to 1195 per 100,00 for those over 85. Mortality rates increase even more dramatically rising from 19 to 358 per 100,000. These figures are from the United States.

The global impact of influenza on morbidity and mortality is considerable, there being one million deaths annually worldwide. Recent studies on the burden of influenza in East and South East Asia suggest that 11–20% of outpatient febrile illnesses and 6–14% of hospitalized pneumonia cases had laboratory-confirmed influenza infection.

Epidemiology in South East Asia and India

In temperate climates, influenza shows a marked peak in winter months. In tropical countries, seasonal incidence is less defined there being a high background influenza activity throughout the year in addition to epidemics that occur in intermediate months between the influenza seasons of the temperate countries of the Northern and Southern hemisphere. The reason why the seasonality of influenza varies with latitude is not clearly understood. Environmental factors do not appear to be linked with epidemics, except that the disease appears to be more prevalent in the rainy months of some tropical countries.

The impact of influenza in tropical countries is being increasingly recognized following epidemiological studies on influenza in Hong Kong. Hong Kong is a subtropical rich city located within the likely epicentre of pandemic influenza in South East Asia. It was shown that hospitalization related to influenza varied with age in a U-shaped curve where young infants and elderly patients were at a higher risk of pneumonia and poorer outcomes, a pattern similar to that observed in interpandemic influenza in temperate countries. The results of the epidemiological study of influenza in Hong Kong should not be equated with the likely impact of influenza in poor tropical countries where malnutrition, shortage of antibiotics to treat secondary bacterial infections and poor medical care may well influence the severity and outcome of influenzal infection.

There are two surveillance centres for influenza in India—National Institute of Virology (NIV), Pune and National Institute of Communicable Diseases (NICD), New Delhi. Three surveillance studies have been carried out at the NIV in Pune.

The salient features of the surveillance study extending from 1978 to 1990 showed that the highest number of cases occurred during the rainy months of July, August and September, the viruses isolated being H3N2, H1N1 and influenza Type B.

The surveillance study in 1980 showed three peaks—in the hot months of March, in the rainy season of July, August, September and a peak in the cool month of November. The viruses isolated were H3N2, H1N1 and influenza–Type B.

The third surveillance study in 2003 showed two peaks—one peak in March-April (H3N2), and another peak in July–August (H3N2). Type B was also prevalent in the rainy months. It was observed that the H3N2 was responsible for severe illness and for the highest hospitalization rate.

More research is needed on the epidemiology of influenza in the tropics. Modelling the influenza burden in tropical countries necessitates reliable surveillance data. Unfortunately, surveillance efforts were initiated very recently in tropical countries so that data on the influenza burden are of short duration. Laboratory surveillance needs to be strengthened if modelling of disease burden is to be feasible. Also, more studies

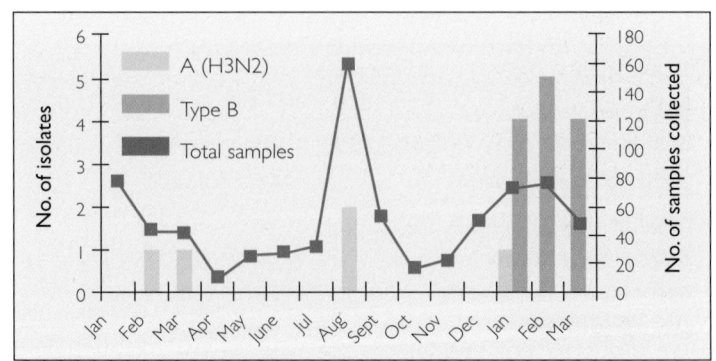

Fig 20.1: Monthly data of specimen collection and infuenza virus detection during the year 2004–05, NIV Pune.

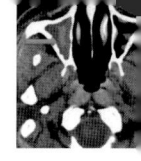

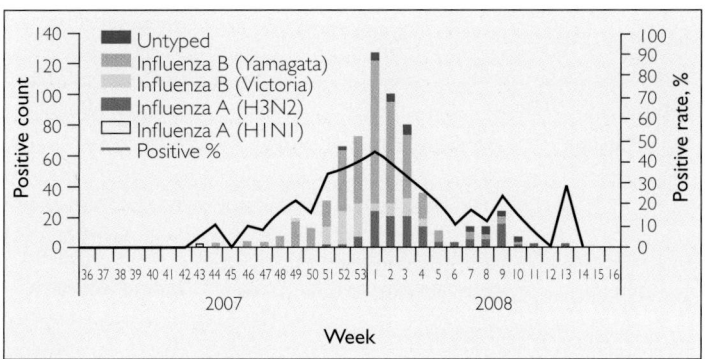

Fig 20.2: Weekly distribution of influenza isolates during the 2007–08 infuenza season, Beijing, People's Republic of China (Ref: Yang Peng, Duan Wei et al. Review of an Influenza Surveillance System, Beijing, People's Republic of China. Emerging Infectious Diseases. Vol. 15, No. 10 October 2009).

are needed to determine seasonal influenza patterns across a large range of latitudes, involving tropical countries in both hemispheres. Finally, further research is necessary to determine whether the influenza virus in temperate climes persists in a low-grade activity all through the year with exacerbations in winter or whether the virus is reintroduced from the tropics each year at the beginning of winter. Figure 20.1 shows the monthly data of specimens collected for influenza virus detection from 2004–05 at the National Institute of Virology, Pune.

Clinical Features

Typical clinical features include an acute onset of fever (ranging up to 102–103°F), myalgia, cough, usually dry but occasionally productive, sore throat, nasal discharge and congestion and headache. Conjuctival congestion may also be present. The occurrence of pneumonia is often heralded by worsening respiratory symptoms like tachypnoea, dyspnoea, respiratory distress and tachycardia. Hypotension is present in severe attacks.

Influenzal pneumonia may take the following forms—

1. Primary pneumonia caused by the virus itself.
2. Influenzal attack followed by a secondary bacterial pneumonia, the common bacterial organisms being *Staphylococcus aureus, Streptococcus pneumoniae* and *H. influenza*.
3. A combination of primary viral pneumonia together with a secondary bacterial pneumonia.

The radiological features of primary influenzal pneumonia are interstitial or patchy infiltrates. Secondary pneumonia due to bacterial infection is characterized by segmental or lobar consolidation. Primary and secondary pneumonia may occur in a patient at the same time. Occasionally, radiological shadowing pointing to pneumonia may be observed without any evidence of clinical deterioration.

In fulminant primary influenzal pneumonia, both lungs are extensively involved, death occurring within 48 to 72 hours. Acute respiratory distress syndrome is a feature of fulminant influenzal pneumonia.

It needs to be mentioned that primary pneumonia due to the influenza virus is rare outside pandemic settings, in non-immunocompromised patients. Age is an important risk

factor as are co-morbid conditions such as left heart failure, cardiovascular disease, chronic respiratory disease, diabetes, and well-marked hepatic or renal dysfunction.

Non-infectious pulmonary complications that can be induced by the influenza virus include bronchiolitis obliterans organizing pneumonia, usual interstitial pneumonia and transient Goodpasture's syndrome. The latter is reported to resolve with the cure of influenza.

Diagnosis

The diagnosis is based on clinical presentation at a time when viral activity causing respiratory infection is high in a community. The clinical features may however be indistinguishable from CAP due to other micro-organisms. A specific viral diagnosis can be made by—

1. Culture of respiratory secretions. Nasal secretions are believed to be better specimens compared to throat swabs to detect the influenza virus. Sputum, endotracheal secretions or bronchoalveolar lavage (BAL) specimens can also be used for culture. Cultures take two to three days to become positive and are thus of limited value for making therapeutic or isolation decisions.
2. Rapid antigen testing is available for Influenza A and B and offers prompt results. These tests have a sensitivity of 50–60% in children and of 90% in adults. False negative tests occur and treatment should not be withheld in these patients if there is a high index of suspicion.
3. Immunofluorescent or enzyme-linked immunosorbent assay (ELISA) techniques on nasal or pharyngeal cells obtained by brushing or washing can help in a quick diagnosis (within 15 minutes). This test again requires expertise and is not widely available, at least in developing countries.
4. Molecular testing such as RT-PCR offers the best sensitivity and specificity for the diagnosis of influenzal viral infection. It is technically demanding, expensive and available at only a few centres.
5. Serological test for antibodies is only useful for epidemiological purposes as it requires two serological assays 14 days apart. There needs to be a fourfold or greater rise in the influenza-specific antibody.

Table 20.2: Diagnostic tests for influenzal pneumonia		
Test	**Time to result**	**Noteworthy features**
Rapid antigen test	< 30 minutes	Fast, not technically defective
Immunofluorescent test	1–4 hours	Requires technical expertise
Culture	24 hours–5 days	Very sensitive—also detects other pathogens
Nucleic acid testing (RT-PCR)	4–24 hours	Very sensitive but requires technical advise
Antibody testing	Several weeks	Highly specific and sensitive

Treatment

Four antiviral drugs have been approved for the treatment of influenzal infection. These are amantadine, rimantadine,

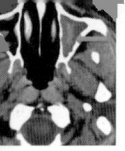

zanamivir, oseltamivir. Amantadine and rimantadine are effective against Influenza A, whereas zanamavir and oseltamivir are effective against Influenza A and B. These drugs are 70–90% effective for prophylaxis and reduce illness severity, duration of symptoms and virus shedding when given within 48 hours of onset of symptoms. Data on their efficacy in primary influenzal pneumonia is limited but they should unquestionably be used.

The Centre for Disease Control and Prevention–(CDC) recently reported that 92% of Influenza A (H3N2) and 25% of Influenza A (H1N1) were resistant to the amantadines. The CDC therefore does not recommend the use of this class of drugs at present. Zanamivir and oseltamivir are effective for Influenza A and B and are recommended as the current resistant rates are low. These recommendations are based on studies in the US. To what extent they apply to India and other South East Asian countries is not known.

It should be noted that each antiviral drug has side-effects that must be considered in treatment selection. Zanamivir can cause bronchospasm and should be avoided in patients with asthma or *chronic obstructive pulmonary disease* (COPD). Oseltamivir is well tolerated but may cause nausea and vomiting in 10% of patients.

Bacterial pneumonia is a fairly frequent complication (observational studies report 8–36%) of influenza infection. When present or strongly suspected, particularly in elderly patients, an appropriate antibiotic cover should be given. Blood and sputum cultures should help in the choice of antibiotics. Empiric antibiotic therapy may be necessary in critically ill patients and this should cover staphylococcal, pneumococcal and *H. influenzae*, the common bacterial pathogens that cause secondary pneumonias. Vancomycin or Linezolid is preferred for staphylococcal infection as *methicillin-resistant Staphylococcus aureus* (MRSA) strains have been reported to cause secondary bacterial pneumonia.

Supportive care is vital. This may necessitate appropriate ventilatory support as also cardiovascular support, since hypotension and dilated cardiomyopathy due to viral myocarditis may be other coexisting complications in patients with influenzal pneumonia. Not uncommonly, influenzal pneumonia precipitates heart failure in patients with a background of heart disease.

It is important to use paracetamol and to avoid aspirin or other salicylates (particularly in children) as symptomatic treatment for headache and fever. This is because salicylates used in this setting are known to be associated with Reye's syndrome. This syndrome is characterized by a non-inflammatory encephalopathy, cerebral oedema, fatty liver or liver cell dysfunction. This syndrome is associated with Influenza A and has a high mortality.

Non-respiratory complications of influenza may rarely be associated with influenzal pneumonia. These include myositis, rhabdomyolysis and central nervous system involvement which though rare include encephalomyelitis, transverse myelitis, aseptic meningitis, focal neurological disorders and the *Guillain-Barré* syndrome. If present, these merit special attention.

Prevention

ISOLATION

A patient diagnosed to be suffering from influenza needs to be isolated as promptly as possible, more so when there is an

Table 20.3: Antiviral drugs used in influenza		
Drugs	**Dose**	**Adverse effects**
Amantadine	100 mg twice daily for 5 days	
Zamamivir	10 mg (two inhalations thrice daily for 5 days) As chemoprophylaxis of 10 mg (two inhalations twice daily for 5 days)	Bronchospasm
Oseltamivir	75 mg twice daily orally for 5 days. As chemorophylaxis 75 mg once daily for 5 days	Nausea, vomiting

Note: The CDC advises the use of Zanamivir and Oseltamivir as therapy for influenza A as there is growing resistance of the virus to Amantadine and Ramantadine.

outbreak of this disease. Delay in isolation could easily result in spread from droplet infection caused by coughing or sneezing. In epidemics, contacts of infected person need to be traced, tested and if needs be isolated.

INFLUENZA VACCINE

Influenza poses both a health and economic burden to the community and is therefore a public health concern. Prevention rests on annual vaccination with trivalent killed virus vaccine. Recommendations are for early vaccinations in all adults over 50 years, children between six months to five years, patients of any age with chronic medical conditions (particularly those with COPD or chronic respiratory problems), pregnant women, immune suppressed patients, care-takers of high-risk patients and healthcare workers. Unfortunately, the awareness of the need for vaccination is extremely poor not only among patients in the large cities of India (leave aside smaller towns and rural India), but also among practising doctors.

There is however some conflicting evidence about vaccine efficacy in the elderly and high-risk patients. A Cochrane review of five randomized trials demonstrated a rate of 68% for vaccine effectiveness against influenza, and 43% against influenza-like illnesses. There were few participants beyond 70 years and there seemed to be little efficacy in this group. *(Ref: Rivetti D, Jefferson T, Thomas R, et al. Vaccines for preventing influenza in the elderly. Cochrane Database Syst Rev. 2006; 3:CD004876)*

Observational cohort studies have also shown conflicting results. In elderly patients vaccination failed to protect against influenza, influenza-like illness or pneumonia, but surprisingly was associated with 26% reduction in hospitalization from influenza and pneumonia, and 42% reduction in all-cause mortality.

Avian Influenza

In 1997 an H5N1 avian influenza virus emerged in Hong Kong, resulting in the death of six of the 18 affected patients, mainly young adults. The virus fortunately did not spread from human to human, and was controlled through massive culling of poultry. The H5N1 strain re-emerged in 2003, first in China, Japan, South Korea, then in Thailand, Vietnam, Indonesia, Cambodia, Malaysia leading to massive culling of poultry and attempts to curb the epidemic through vaccination of poultry. More than 60% of patients diagnosed with this viral strain died. In May 2005, a highly pathogenic H5N1 strain emerged in wild birds is Quinghai Lake, China, killing not only domestic poultry

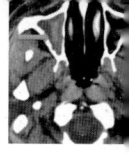

but wild aquatic birds. This highly pathogenic strain spread to many countries in Asia, Africa, Europe, and was the cause of multiple outbreaks in poultry.

Humans have been affected through close contact with birds and poultry but human to human contact has not been observed except rarely in very close contacts. The WHO states that till October 2008, a total of 387 confirmed cases from 15 countries with 245 deaths have occurred, of which more than 100 cases with 50 deaths have occurred in Vietnam.

This 'avian flu' differs from the usual seasonal influenza in that it is a serious severe illness with a mortality of 60%. The incubation period is three to eight days; the disease starts with high fever, cough with severe prostration and myalgia. Tachypnoea, dyspnoea, respiratory distress and hypoxia are noted within a week. The blood shows leucopenia, lymphopenia and thrombocytopenia. The X-ray chest shows patchy interstitial and alveolar infiltrates consistent with primary viral pneumonia rather than secondary bacterial pneumonia. Acute respiratory distress syndrome (ARDS) together with multi-organ failure are seen in patients with severe illness, generally resulting in death. Post-mortem studies show diffuse lung injury together with vascular congestion and hyaline membrane formation.

Patients with influenza-like symptoms who have been in contact with poultry afflicted by H5N1 virus should be isolated and tested for H5N1 infection. Diagnostic tests are the rapid antigen test, and direct fluorescent antibody tests which give quick results within two hours. Nasal discharge, throat swabs, BAL fluid can be tested by RT-PCR. This test offers the best sensitivity and specificity. Viral cultures are also done for the H5N1 virus. Most of these tests require sophisticated laboratories together with good expertise. Specimens thus need to be sent to accredited laboratories which give reliable results.

Patients with confirmed or suspected H5N1 should be treated with oseltamivir or zanamivir as this viral strain has been shown to be resistant to adamantadine and rimatadine. The current recommendation is a five-day course of oseltamivir in a dose of 75 mg twice daily. Antibacterial agents should be used to target the pneumoccocus and *S. aureus*, the two organisms chiefly responsible for secondary bacterial pneumonia.

Critical care is of vital importance. Ventilator support is essential in patients with respiratory failure or with ARDS. Support to all organ systems is crucial as multiple organ dysfunction is frequently observed.

Many virologists fear that the avian flu due to H5N1 infection has the potential to become an influenza pandemic. Though spread so far has been from infected poultry to man, the possibility of a slight genetic mutation of this virus, or a reassortment of its genetic material may not only enhance its virulence but could give it the property of spreading from human to human, a catastrophe that could well resemble the influenza pandemic of 1916–18. As yet this has not happened but the danger persists.

Swine Flu

The threat of a pandemic of Avian influenza still hangs like the sword of Damocles over the world. In the meanwhile in 2009 an H1N1 strain of the influenza virus A presented in swine-infected humans in Mexico. The H1N1 virus has the property of being transmitted from human to human through droplet infection following coughing or sneezing. There were a number of fatalities in Mexico. In a matter of months this H1N1 virus causing influenza spread to the United States and soon to Europe, Asia and the Far East. The WHO has alerted all countries and

Country	2003		2004		2005		2006		2007		Total	
	cases	deaths	cases	deaths	cases	deaths	cases	deaths	cases	deaths	cases	deaths
Azerbaijan	0	0	0	0	0	0	8	5	0	0	8	5
Cambodia	0	0	0	0	4	4	2	2	1	1	7	7
China	1	1	0	0	8	5	13	8	5	3	27	17
Djibouti	0	0	0	0	0	0	1	0	0	0	1	0
Egypt	0	0	0	0	0	0	18	10	20	5	38	15
Indonesia	0	0	0	0	20	13	55	45	40	34	115	92
Iraq	0	0	0	0	0	0	3	2	0	0	3	2
Lao People's Democratic Republic	0	0	0	0	0	0	0	0	2	2	2	2
Myanmar	0	0	0	0	0	0	0	0	1	0	1	0
Nigeria	0	0	0	0	0	0	0	0	1	1	1	1
Thailand	0	0	17	12	5	2	3	3	0	0	25	17
Turkey	0	0	0	0	0	0	12	4	0	0	12	4
Viet Nam	3	3	29	20	61	19	0	0	7	4	100	46
Total	4	4	46	32	98	43	115	79	77	50	340	208

Table 20.4:
Cumulative Number of Confirmed Human Cases of Avian Influenza A/(H5N1) Reported to WHO as of 14 December 2007

Note: Total number of cases includes number of deaths. WHO reports only laboratory-confirmed cases. All dates refer to onset of illness.
Source: World Health Organization. Cumulative number of confirmed human cases of avian influenza A/(H5N1) reported to WHO at http://www.who.int/csr/disease/avian_influenza/country/cases_table_2007_12_14/en/index.html.

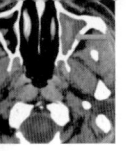
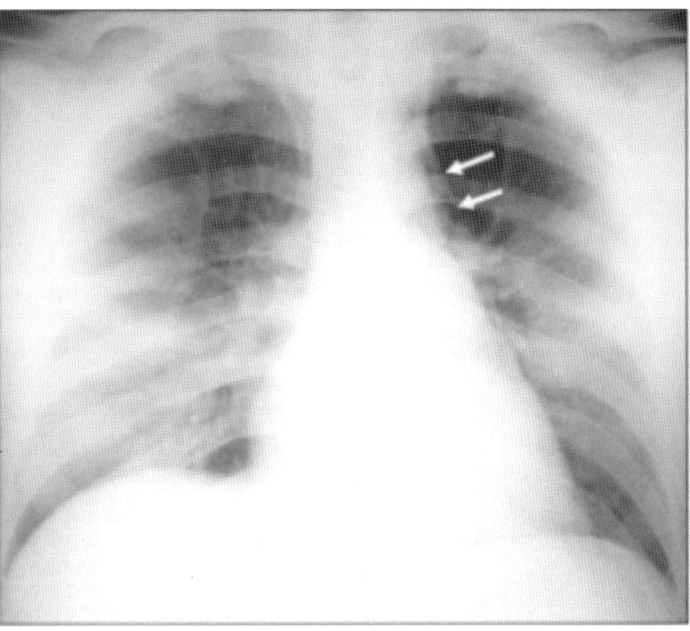

(a)

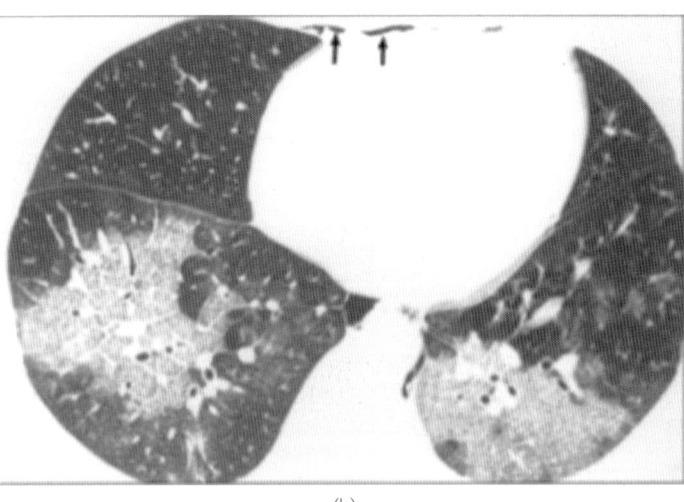

(b)

Fig 20.3: Severe Acute Respiratory Syndrome (SARS) (a) Chest X-ray demonstrates ill-defined consolidations in both lung fields in the mid- and lower zones. There is a thin paramediastinal air strip on the left side representing mediastinal emphysema (b) HRCT chest demonstrates ill-defined areas of ground-glass densities in both lower lobes with associated septal thickening interspersed in areas of ground-glass density.

pronounced this as a world pandemic. Till recently in a matter of months, 277607 patients have been afflicted with H1N1 virus all over the world; 3205 patients have died in this illness. Maximum deaths have occurred in Mexico; in other countries swine flu is by and large a mild though highly infectious illness. The danger again is the possibility of a further mutation in the virus or genetic reassortment that could enhance its virulence. If that indeed does transpire, the world may face a catastrophic pandemic.

Strict isolation of patients, tracing of contacts, testing them and if needs be isolating them is crucial for prevention. The pandemic is still active, though perhaps the hot summer months may see a decline in the activity of this virus. However, the rainy season in tropical countries and the winter months to come, hold a serious threat to the whole world.

CLINICAL FEATURES

The disease starts with usual flu-like symptoms—body ache, fever, prostration, sore throat and a persistent dry cough. A sore throat is invariably present. Running of the nose is not frequently observed. Some patients present with or later develop diarrhoea.

The major danger as with all severe influenzal attacks is involvement of the lungs characterized by pneumonia. This is often bilateral, the X-ray of the chest showing bilateral shadows chiefly involving the lower lobes. Tachypnoea and respiratory distress are warning signs of lung involvement. These patients often require ventilatory support and have a high morbidity and mortality. Death when it occurs is due to ARDS and multi-organ failure.

Rogelio Perez-Padilla *et al.* studied the outbreak of swine-origin Influenza A (H1N1) virus (S-OIV) from March 24 through April 24, 2009. A total of 18 cases of pneumonia with confirmed S-OIV infection were identified among 98 patients hospitalized for acute respiratory illness at the National Institute of Respiratory Diseases, Mexico. All patients had fever, cough, dyspnoea or respiratory distress, increased serum lactate dehydrogenase levels, and bilateral patchy pneumonia. Other common findings were an increased creatine kinase level (in 62% of patients) and lymphopenia (in 61%). Twelve patients required mechanical ventilation, and seven died. Death occurred from ARDS and multiple organ failure. *(Ref: Rogelio Perez-Padilla, Daniela de la Rosa-Zamboni et al. N Engl J Med. 2009 Aug 13;361(7):680–9. Epub 2009 Jun 29)*

TREATMENT

Oseltamivir 75 mg twice daily for five to seven days is the recommended specific therapy. Supportive treatment as outlined earlier is imperative in severe infection. A vaccine against the H1N1 virus is available and though the epidemic

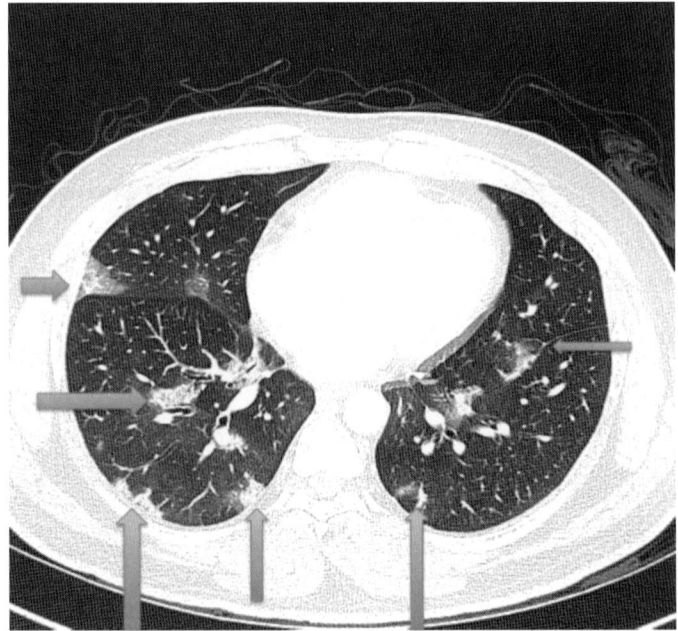

Fig 20.4a: A 33-year-old male patient presented with high-grade fever, cough and dyspnoea with ill-defined areas of increased lung attenuation in the subpleural and peribronchovascular regions marked by arrows. This pattern of areas of increased lung attenuation is seen in a number of patients with H1N1.

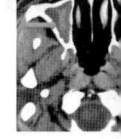

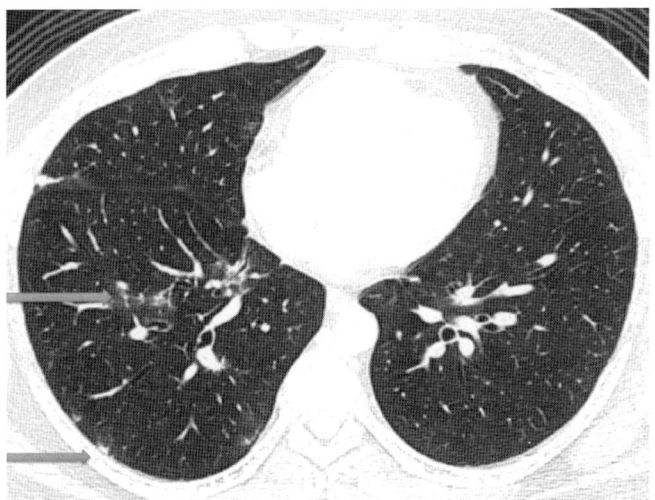

Fig 20.4b: Follow-up CT in patient demonstrates clearing of nearly all areas of increased lung attenuation.

has regressed significantly, this vaccine has come of use in many parts of the world.

DANGERS OF A WORLD INFLUENZA PANDEMIC

The WHO has predicted that a new influenza pandemic could lead to 1–2 billion cases of flu, 5–12 million cases of severe illness and 1.5 to 3 million deaths worldwide. It could result in 1 to 2.3 million hospitalizations, and 250,000 to 650,000 deaths in industrialized countries alone. Its impact on developing countries could be even more devastating. Nevertheless the WHO predicts that the expected pandemic would not be as horrendous as the 1918 pandemic which as stated earlier killed 50 million people, but on par with the 1957 and 1968 pandemics. Whether the present swine flu pandemic will fulfil such ghastly predictions stated above is to be seen. Again,

whether avian influenza graduates through a further mutational shift in the future to engulf the world in another dreadful pandemic remains uncertain. Fortunately, so far (mid-2010), the threat of a world pandemic is no longer there, both with regard to H1N1 infection which is on the decline as also with regard to Avian H5N1 infection.

Respiratory Syncytial Virus

Respiratory syncytial virus (RSV) infection is a common and important cause of lower respiratory tract infection in children. For many years it was considered to be a pathogen confined

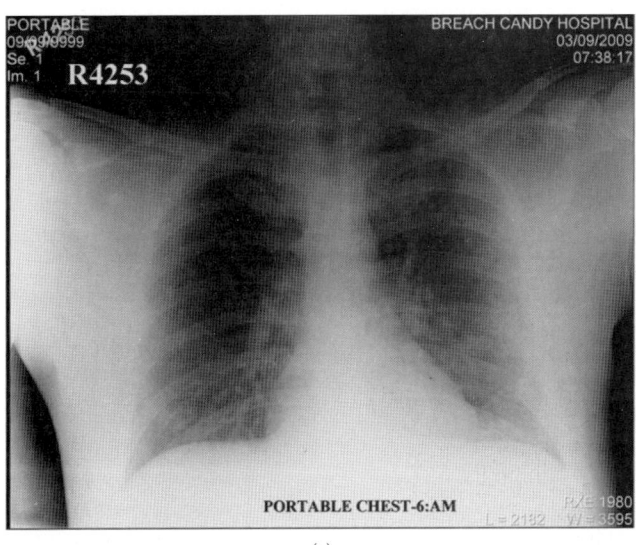

(a)

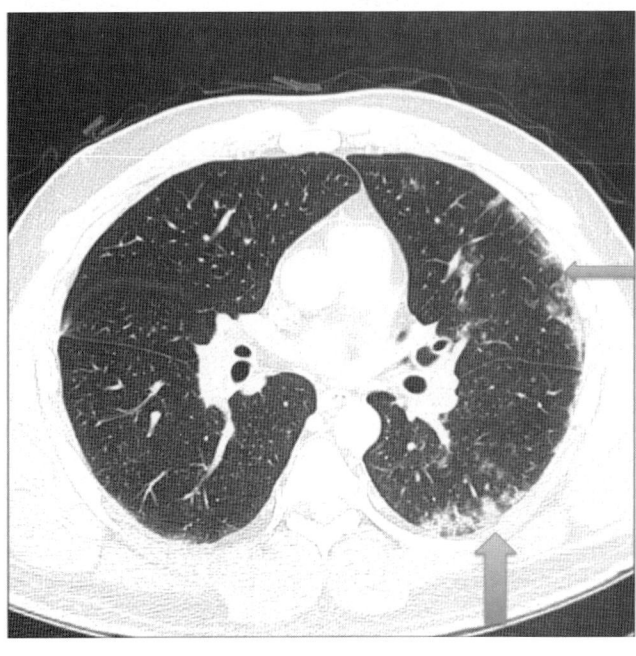

(b)

Fig 20.6: A 47-year-old executive presented with high-grade fever. (a) chest X-ray reveals diffuse bibasilar areas of haziness (b) CT reveals areas of air space opacification in subpleural regions of the left lower lobe, suggestive of H1N1.

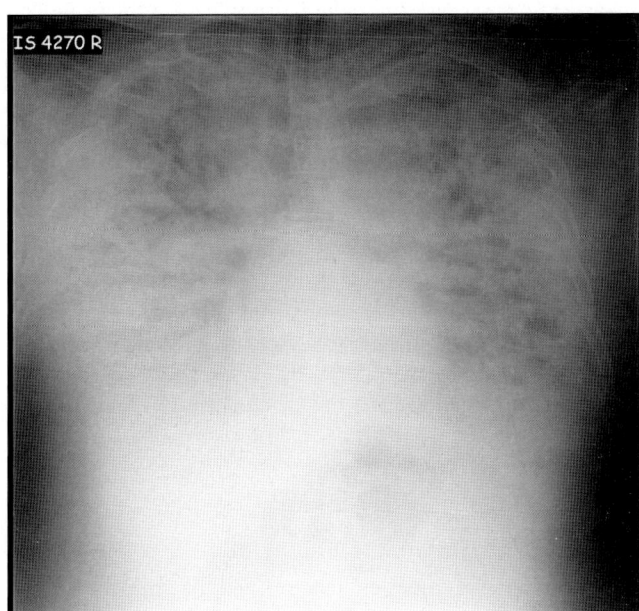

Fig 20.5: ARDS in H1N1. Chest x-ray demonstrates diffuse bilateral white out lungs in a case of H1N1 with ARDS.

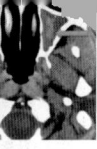
to paediatric practice; however, it is now being increasingly recognized as an important pathogen causing lower respiratory tract infection in adults. The incubation period is four to six days and epidemics occur in winter and early spring lasting one to five months. Several epidemiological studies in the West indicated that RSV is second to influenza as a cause of serious respiratory disease in adults. Its frequency as a cause of CAP in adults has been estimated at 3–5% over a year. Again there is no reliable epidemiological study to give an estimate of RSV pneumonia in India or for that matter in large metropolitan cities of the country.

Transmission of RSV is by droplet infection produced by coughing or sneezing as also by contaminated skin followed by autoinnoculation in the conjuctiva or nose. Infection leads to increased Immunoglobulin E (IgE) production; the degree of rise in IgE predicts the risk of wheezing episodes.

Clinical features include fever, nasal congestion, pharyngitis, cough which is often productive. Lower respiratory tract infection is frequent in 25–30% of infections and takes two forms—bronchiolitis and pneumonia. Clinically, these manifest as dyspnoea, tachypnoea, increasing cough, wheezing, rhonchi on auscultation and hypoxia. Although difficult to distinguish from influenza there are a few subtle clinical clues that may suggest RSV infection. Patients with RSV infection have more basal congestion with crackles on auscultation, wheezing, a productive cough and a comparatively low-grade fever compared to patients with influenza. Thus in elderly patients who give a history of a 'cold' followed by low-grade fever and wheezing, the diagnosis of RSV infection should be entertained.

The radiological features are characterized by interstitial infiltrates. Patchy segmental shadows and occasionally lobar consolidation have been reported. Bronchiolitis results in patchy atelectasis with areas of hyperinflation.

Diagnosis of RSV infection may be difficult to prove. Cultures of respiratory secretions—sputum, nasopharyngeal washing,–and throat swabs may take two to seven days to show positive results. Immunofluorescent techniques are frequently used on nasal washings; they allow a more reliable and rapid detection of the virus. Rapid antigen tests for RSV have poor sensitivity when compared to influenza. RT-PCR is more sensitive for detection of the virus in adult populations. Serological tests give a retrospective diagnosis if the antibody titre rises to fourfold or more after two weeks.

Treatment of RSV pneumonia in adults is supportive—antipyretics, fluids, oxygen when needed. Corticosteroids are useful in all age groups when there is wheezing, particularly if this is associated with hypoxia. Nebulization with β_2 agonists and budesonide offers symptomatic relief in patients with airways obstruction.

Aerosolized ribavarin improves the clinical course, particularly in severe disease and should be administered (60 mg/ml for two hours given by mask, three times a day). RSV-specific immunoglobulin is also approved therapy, particularly in high-risk infants.

Parainfluenza Viruses (PIV)

Four distinct serotypes are recognized 1, 2, 3, 4A, 4B. These viruses cause croup, bronchitis and pneumonia in children. PIV-3 is most often associated with pneumonia and is endemic the

year around. Pneumonia has also been reported in young adults and in the elderly though the burden of disease in the latter group is unclear. As with influenza, infection is transmitted by the droplet infection from respiratory secretions, the incubation period being two to seven days. Clinical features even when pneumonia occurs, are non-specific and are characterized by fever, nasal discharge, hoarseness and cough. Chest radiograph shows diffuse interstitial infiltrates as with any atypical or viral pneumonia.

Viral culture, RT-PCR and serological tests can be used to diagnose PIV infection. Ribavarin has *in vitro* activity against PIV; its use in patients with PIV infection has not proved curative.

Adenovirus

Adenoviruses are responsible for 5% of respiratory infections in children and less than 2% infections in adults. Epidemics have however been reported in military recruit populations. Infection occurs from inhalation of airborne droplet infection or by faeco-oral contamination. The incubation period is four to seven days. In children and young adults (particularly noticed in military recruits) adenovirus infection can result in bronchiolitis or pneumonia of variable severity. Diagnosis is by antigen detection or histopathological examination of nasal mucosal biopsy which shows intranuclear basophilic inclusions. Viral cultures may take several weeks to be positive. Serological diagnosis depends on a fourfold or more increase in antibodies after an interval of two weeks.

Coronaviruses

Coronaviruses are RNA viruses. Two groups of coronaviruses are identified and four strains are known to cause acute respiratory diseases ranging from cold to pneumonia. These include Group 1 (229E and NL63) and Group 2 (OC 43 and HKU 1). A new coronavirus, SARS-CoV which represents a split from Group 2 was identified as the cause of the severe acute respiratory syndrome (SARS) epidemic which originated in the Guangdong province in China and spread to different parts of the world.

The incubation period of SARS ranges from 2–10 days. It is a serious illness, the older age group being a significant risk factor for death. The clinical features are characterized by fever with chills, cough, and myalgia. Unlike other viral respiratory infections, rhinorrhoea and sore throat are uncommon symptoms. About two-thirds of infected patients develop prolonged fever, dyspnoea, tachypnoea, increasing hypoxia and diarrhoea. Chest radiographs show bilateral alveolar shadows which may be quickly progressive. Age and co-morbid medical conditions are independent risk factors and the mortality in those over 60 years is over 50%. Ribavarin, corticosteroids and intravenous gammaglobulins have been used as treatment but there is no proof of their efficacy. The disease fortunately is at present quiescent.

Measles Virus

Vaccination against measles has proved of immense benefit, particularly in poor developing countries. Yet there are many in developing countries who have not been vaccinated. In these patients measles still carries a significant mortality and morbidity.

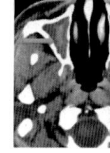

The measles virus belongs to the Paramyxoviridae family like the parainfluenza virus and RSV. The virus enters chiefly through the respiratory tract. Lower respiratory tract infections occur in close to 50% of patients and take the form of bronchitis, bronchiolitis and viral pneumonia. Measles pneumonia is the main cause of measles-related death in children. Radiographic appearances in measles virus pneumonia are characterized by widespread reticulo-nodular pulmonary infiltrates. Secondary bacterial pneumonia often occurs. Primary viral pneumonia and secondary bacterial pneumonia may coexist in the same patient.

Treatment is supportive; antibiotics are necessary for secondary bacterial infection. Fortunately, the measles vaccine has reduced the incidence of measles by 98%. If it still does occur, it occurs in the teenage years and is generally mild.

Varicella-Zoster Virus

Varicella hardly ever causes pneumonia in immunocompetent children. But the danger of pneumonia is ever present when varicella occurs in adults. When pneumonia occurs it generally occurs within four to five days of the start of the rash. Cough and pleuritic chest pain are frequently observed. A tell-tale warning sign is tachypnoea. Progressive dyspnoea, respiratory distress and hypoxia occur in critically ill patients. Radiographic appearances are characterized by nodular infiltrates diffusely spread over both the lungs. At times the X-ray appearance is of miliary mottling. Hilar adenopathy and small to moderate-sized pleural effusions may occur. The prognosis is grave and death occurs from respiratory failure. If the pneumonia resolves the nodules within the lung calcify; healed calcific nodules may persist for years or even lifelong.

The clinical picture of the characteristic varicella skin and mucosal rash is diagnostic. The virus may be cultured or detected by PCR technique. Serological tests include the fluorescent antibody test, the membrane antigen test and the ELISA test.

Treatment is with early administration of acyclovir (10 mg/kg) intravenously every eight hours for 10 days in all patients with varicella who develop pneumonia. Preventive administration of oral acyclovir in elderly patients, pregnant women, in patients with COPD or in patients who are immunocompromised is recommended in varicella, even in the absence of pneumonia.

Zoster immune globulin complements the use of acyclovir in patients with varicella pneumonia or in immunocompromised patients even in the absence of pneumonia.

Strict isolation is warranted until all skin lesions have crusted and the crusts have fallen off.

Hantavirus

The Hantavirus respiratory syndrome can result from several Hantaviruses. Almost all cases have been reported from North and South America. There has also been a report of proven Hantavirus infection from South India. Rodents serve as the reservoir and transmission to humans results from aerosolisation of the virus contained in their faeces.

Clinical features are those of a flu-like syndrome, with fever, myalgia, abdominal pain and diarrhoea. Respiratory involvement is characterized by dry cough, breathlessness, tachypnoea and increasing hypoxia. ARDS and shock are observed in severe infection. Haematological examination reveals leucocytosis, thrombocytopenia, haemoconcentration and circulating immunoblasts. Renal failure may complicate the overall clinical picture. Death is from respiratory failure, shock, and multi-organ dysfunction.

Diagnosis is made by serological and immunohistochemical techniques. Treatment is supportive. Ventilatory support is essential in severe forms of the disease. Intravenous ribavarine is being used in controlled trials; results are pending.

FUNGAL PNEUMONIA

Fungal infections of the lower respiratory tract (causing fungal pneumonia) that occur in normal hosts are histoplasmosis caused by *Histoplasma capsulatum*, blastomycosis caused by *Blastomyces dermatitides*, and coccidiomycosis caused by *Coccidiodes immitis* and *Paracoccidiosis braziliensus*. These diseases are seen in the north and south American continent and except for a few reported cases of blastomycosis, these are not observed in India and Southeast Asia. They will therefore merit a short description. Cryptococcal infections due to *Cryptococcus neoformans* and certain forms of aspergillus infection due to *Aspergillus fumigatus* can also occur in normal hosts and are observed all over the world including India. Fungal pneumonias that are chiefly restricted to severely immunocompromised patients have been dealt with in the chapter on 'Pneumonia in the Non-HIV Immunocompromised Patient'.

Aspergillosis

Aspergillus species are ubiquitous fungi. Airway colonization without infection is seen in patients with chronic lung disease such as bronchiectasis, and in burnt-out fibrotic tuberculosis. Invasive aspergillus is almost solely restricted to immunocompromised patients though there are very rare reports of its

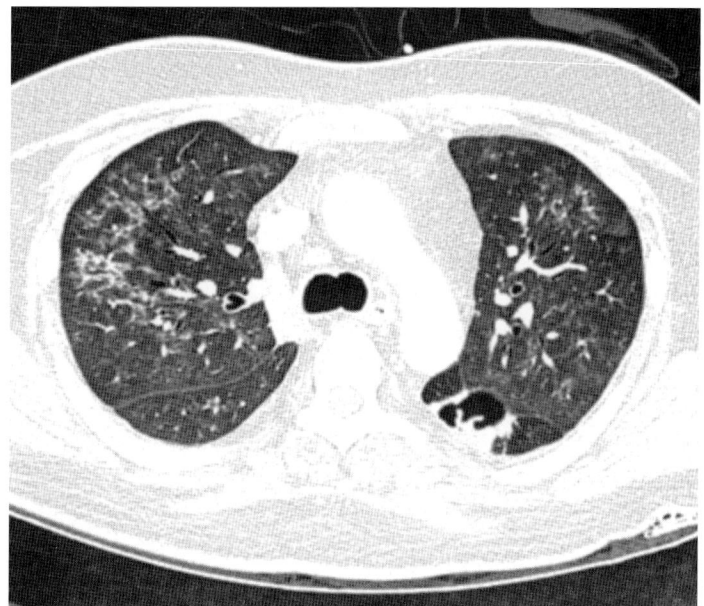

Fig 20.7: Aspergillus infection: HRCT chest demonstrates ill-defined nodular lesions in the upper lobes as well as a thin cavitating lesion in the apical segment of the left lower lobe representing an aspergilloma. There are multiple thin strands within the lesion representing hyphae.

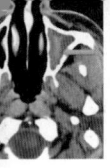
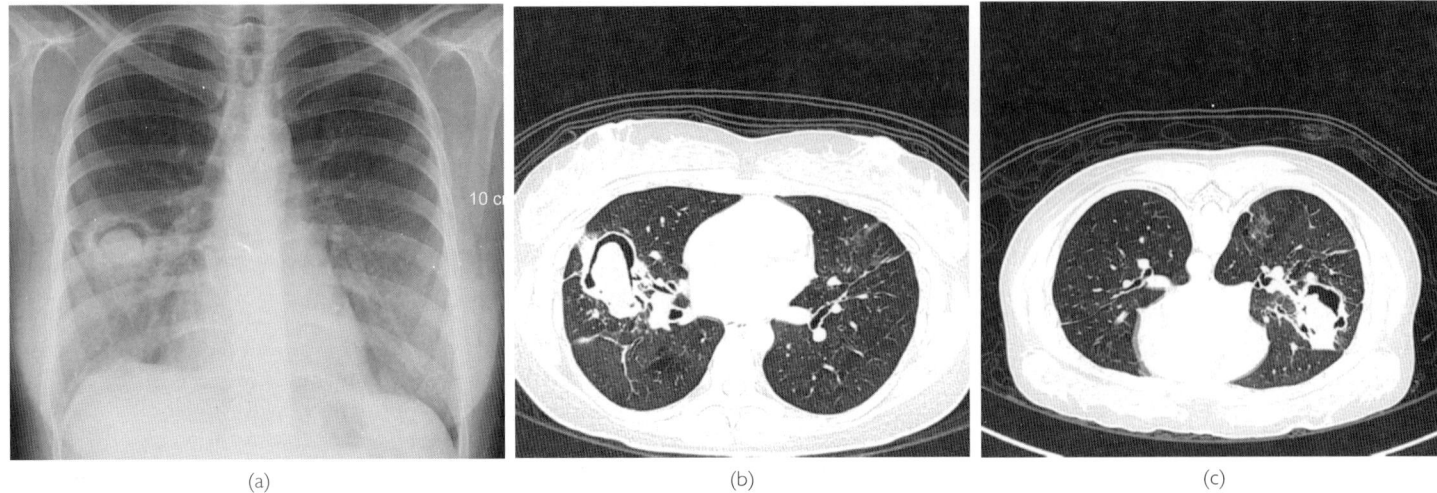

Fig 20.8a, b, c: A 23-year-old female with a past history of cavities due to Wegener's granulomatosis presented with fever and haemoptysis. (a) X-ray chest demonstrates a well-defined right mid-zone cavity with a fungal ball (b) HRCT chest demonstrates a thin-walled cavity in the right lower lobe with an internal mass lesion representing a fungal ball (c) On prone scans the fungal ball is seen to move.

occurrence in normal hosts as well. Invasive aspergillosis has been described elsewhere.

In normal hosts, *Aspergillus fumigatus* can cause extrinsic allergic alveolitis, allergic bronchopulmonary aspergillosis and aspergillomas. The first two of these conditions have been described in other chapters.

Aspergillomas are fungal balls containing *Aspergillus fumigatus*. These fungal balls exist in preformed cavities—most commonly in tuberculous cavities, but also in bronchiectatic cavities, in Stage IV sarcoid, healed lung abscess and in upper lobe cavities observed in patients with ankylosing spondylitis. Aspergillomas are often silent but occasionally cause haemoptysis which may be mild to moderate and self-limiting, or profuse and exsanguinating, causing death. Radiological appearances are characteristic, showing a solid shadow within a cavity with an airspace above. Computed tomography (CT) appearances at times allow a diagnosis of an aspergilloma which is missed on routine radiography.

Haemoptysis when severe is treated with embolization of the culprit bronchial vessel, revealed through angiographies. Both arterial and pulmonary angiographies need to be done so as not to miss out on identification of the culprit vessel. Intracavitatory instillation of Amphotericin B has also been tried. When bleeding persists or recurs, surgical resection if feasible should be undertaken.

Rarely, chronic necrotising pneumonia due to aspergillus infection has been recognized in non-neutropenic patients. It may occur on its own or at times appear adjacent to an aspergilloma.

Amphotericin B is the treatment of choice, though voriconazole and caspofungin are new additions to the therapeutic armamentarium. These drugs have been described in detail in the chapter 'Pneumonia in the Non-HIV Immunocompromised Patient'.

Histoplasmosis

Histoplasma capsulatum is found in soil contaminated by infected bird or bat faeces. The disease is chiefly restricted to the central United States, Mexico and Puerto Rico. Initially

restricted to rural societies it is now also found in urban sites, particularly in association with construction projects involving movement of contaminated soil.

The inhaled spores (2–5μm in diameter) reach the small airways and alveoli. The spores after inhalation are converted to yeasts which are ingested by macrophages. The yeast form proliferates in the macrophages and can disseminate to distant metastatic sites.

In the lung the fungus incites a cell-mediated immune response with the formation of a primary granulomatous focus with associated hilar and mediastinal lymphadenopathy very similar to what one observes with a primary complex in tuberculosis. The disease at this stage may be asymptomatic or may present with non-specific respiratory symptoms with perhaps a low-grade fever. The primary lung lesion may heal and calcify. If it does not heal, the caseous focus may cavitate causing fever, cough with expectoration and occasionally haemoptysis, very similar to the clinical features seen in tuberculosis. Yeast forms of histoplasma may be identified in the sputum on smear or grown on culture. The clinical and radiological picture may be indistinguishable from chronic fibrocaseous cavitative tuberculosis. If the disease is not contained, metastatic lesions may be observed in various organs of the body, particularly the liver and spleen. Mediastinal fibrosis is a well-known complication of histoplasma infection.

In patients who inhale a large number of spores, an acute syndrome develops generally after an incubation period of 14 days. This syndrome is abrupt in onset and resembles influenza or bacterial pneumonia or an acute form of tuberculosis. Miliary mottling on an X-ray chest indistinguishable from miliary tuberculosis can occur. Rarely, ARDS has been reported as a manifestation of a hyperacute infection.

DIAGNOSIS

Direct diagnosis is provided by culture of sputum or BAL specimens, though cultures may take several weeks to become positive. Tissue samples can demonstrate organisms with silver or acid schiff (PAS) staining. Bone-marrow smears may show *Histoplasma capsulatum* in severe metastatic infections.

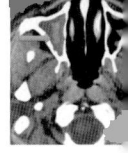

Indirect diagnosis can be provided by the complement fixation test, immunodiffusion or radioimmunoassay test, all of which take several weeks to become positive.

TREATMENT

Patients who have chronic progressive pulmonary disease or those with disseminated metastatic disease need to be treated with amphotericin B. The liposomal form of amphotericin B though expensive has less toxicity. Amphotericin B is given intravenously; the drug has many side-effects, notably renal toxicity. Ketoconazole is also effective but has frequent gastrointestinal and anti-testosterone effects. Fluconazole and Itraconazole (200–400 mg/day) are as effective as amphotericin B or ketoconazole in patients with mild illness.

Most primary infections are self-limiting, heal on their own and require no treatment. They however need a periodic follow-up to ensure that progressive pulmonary disease or dissemination has not occurred.

Blastomycosis

Blastomycosis is found in North America, Mexico, the Middle East, Africa and India. It is caused by the inhalation of spores of *Blastomyces dermatitides*. The fungus grows in the soil and the airborne spores are inhaled, reach the alveoli and are converted to the yeast form. Defence mechanisms involve polymorphonuclear leucocytes followed by a cell-mediated immune response that leads to the formation of granulomas. The disease can resemble an acute bacterial infection or mycobacterial infection, again indistinguishable from tuberculosis. Metastatic lesions can occur in the skin, bones, brain and other organs. Extrapulmonary infections can occur years after the primary infection.

Clinical features vary. In North America acute blastomycosis resembles an acute bacterial pneumonia, with fever with chills, cough with purulent sputum and pleuritic pain. In milder cases, the disease resembles tuberculosis with low-grade fever, cough, haemoptysis and weight loss. The radiological findings vary. Lobar consolidation is observed in acute cases. In the milder forms, infiltrates, cavities, rounded densities or even miliary shadowing may be observed. In the very severe forms of the disease, ARDS can occur even in immunocompetent hosts.

Skin lesions of blastomycosis may occur several years after a self-limiting pulmonary infection.

Diagnosis of blastomycosis is made by examination of respiratory secretions digested by potassium hydroxide. Cultures of respiratory secretions (sputum or BAL fluid) turn positive generally after a week. Silver or PAS staining of infected tissue may reveal the characteristic yeast forms of the fungus.

TREATMENT

Like histoplasmosis, in many patients blastomycosis is self-limiting and may require no treatment. Patients with acute disease or progressive disease are treated with amphotericin B. Itraconazole or ketoconazole are alternatives for less severe or slowly progressive disease.

Coccidiomycosis

Coccidiomycosis is due to infections with *Cocciodiodes immitis*, a fungus present in the soil. The disease is endemic in south

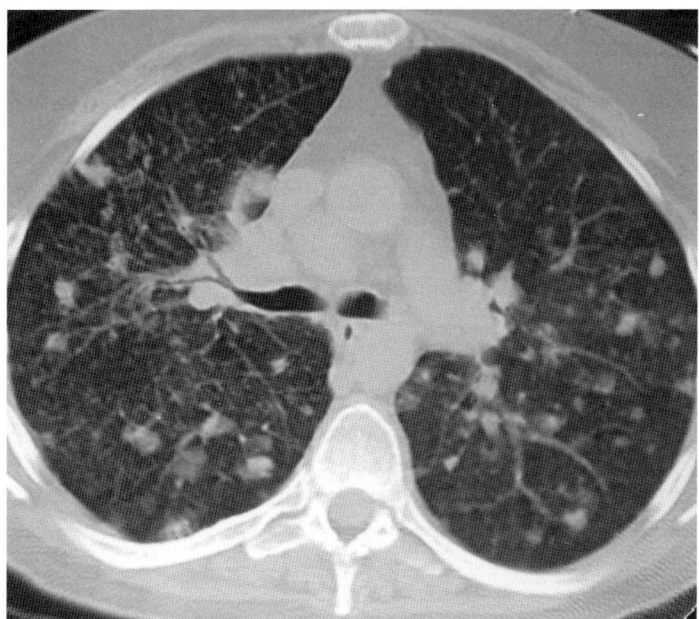

Fig 20.9: Intermediate-sized nodules from blastomycosis in a 40-year-old woman with persistent cough, chest pain, and intermittent fevers. The patient had experienced progression of symptoms over several months. CT scan shows multiple bilateral intermediate-sized nodules.

western United States and in Mexico, occurring mainly during hot dry summers. Inhalation of spores leads to both a suppurative lesion and to cell-mediated granulomatous disease within the lungs after an incubation period of about two weeks.

Clinical features include fever, chills, arthralgia, pleuritic chest pain, dyspnoea and haemoptysis. Physical examination may reveal signs of consolidation and/or cavitation. Pleural effusion may be present. On the other hand, primary infection may be silent, self-limiting and heal on its own.

Chest radiography initially shows one or more areas of consolidation which may cavitate. Hilar adenopathy is often present. The radiographical features as with histoplasmosis and blastomycosis may be indistinguishable from tuberculosis.

The primary lesion may heal as in tuberculosis or may continue to progress with fresh infiltrates, fresh consolidation and cavitation. Persistent fever, cough and weight loss occur. Disseminated coccidiomycosis may occur several months after the primary infection, involving the skin, bones, joints, meninges and the genitourinary system.

DIAGNOSIS

Diagnosis is made by microscopic examination of sputum after digestion with potassium hydroxide or by silver staining of infected tissues obtained through a tissue biopsy. Cultures of sputum or BAL fluid take almost a week to turn positive. Serological tests and skin tests are of great importance for epidemiological purposes.

TREATMENT

Many patients with coccidiomycosis have mild self-limiting disease and require no specific therapy. In progressive disease, fluconazole, itraconazole and ketoconazole are equally effective. In severe disease and in metastatic disease, amphotericin B is the drug of choice.

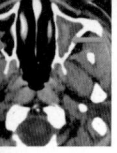

Cryptococcosis

Cryptococcosis is due to *Cryptococcus neoformans*, a fungus found throughout the world. Cryptococcosis is an uncommon infection and is usually self-limiting and asymptomatic. It may however cause lung infection or meningitis particularly in those with impaired cell-mediated immune responses.

Pulmonary infection can cause pneumonia, presenting with fever, cough, malaise and chest pain. The chest X-ray may show infiltration, consolidation or a mass-like shadow closely resembling a neoplasm. Hilar lymphadenopathy may be present.

Examination of the sputum especially using India Ink or sputum culture may show the presence of cryptococci.

However, it must be remembered that *C. neoformans* can colonize the airways of patients with chronic bronchitis or in immunocompromised patients without being responsible for disease. Hence positive sputum cultures do not necessarily denote disease. Examination of tissue obtained through a transbronchial, CT-guided or thoracoscopic biopsy is often necessary to confirm diagnosis. The presence of *C. neoformans* on staining or on tissue culture confirms the diagnosis with certainty.

Treatment Patients with progressive disease need treatment with amphotericin B. Ketoconazole, fluconazole and itraconazole are also effective.

SUGGESTED READING

Cao B, Li X-W, Mao Y, *et al.* Clinical features of the initial cases of 2009 pandemic influenza A (H1N1) virus infection in China. *N Engl J Med.* 2009; 361: 2507–17.

Chayakulkeeree M: Cryptococcosis. *Infect Dis Clin North Am.* 1 Sep. 2006; 20(3): 507–44, v–vi.

Falsey AR. Community-acquired viral pneumonia. *Clin Geriatr Med.* 1 Aug. 2007; 23(3): 535–52, vi.

Kauffman CA. Histoplasmosis: *Clin Chest Med.* 1 Jun. 2009; 30(2): 217–25, v.

Ksiazek TG, Erdman D, Goldsmith CS, Zaki Sr, Peret T, Emery S, Teng S, Urbani C, Comer JA, Lim W, Rollin PE, Dowell SF, Ling AE, Humphrey CD, Shieh WJ, Guarner J, Paddock CD, Rota P, Fields B, DeRisi J, Yang JY, Cox N, Hughes JM, LeDuc JW, Bellini WJ, Anderson LJ, *et al.* A novel coronavirus associated with severe acute respiratory syndrome. *N Engl J Med.* 2003; 348: 1953–66.

Lortholary O, Denning OW, Dupont B. Endemic mycosis: a treatment update. *J Antirnicrob Chemother.* 1999; 43: 321–31.

Mandell LA, Wunderink RG, Anzueto A, Bartlect JG, Campbell GD, Dean NC, Dowell SF, File TM Jr, Musher DM, Niederman

MS, Torres A, Whitney CG. Infectious Diseases Society of America/American Thoracic Society consensus guidelines on the management of community-acquired pneumonia in adults. *Clin Infec Dis.* 2007; 44: S27–S72.

Marr KA. Aspergillosis. Pathogenesis, clinical manifestations, and therapy. *Infect Dis Clin North Am.* 1 Dec. 2002; 16(4): 875–94, vi.

Riscili BP. Noninvasive pulmonary Aspergillus infections. *Clin Chest Med.* 1 Jun. 2009; 30(2): 315–35, vii.

Rothberg MB, Complications of viral influenza. *Am J Med.* 1 Apr. 2008; 121(4): 258–64.

Scalera NM and Mossad SB. The first pandemic of the 21st century: a review of the 2009 pandemic variant influenza A (H1N1) virus. *Postgrad Med.* 2009 Sep.; 121(5): 43–7.

Stamboulian D: Influenza. *Infect Dis Clin North Am.* 1 Mar. 2000; 14(1): 141–66.

Zimmer SM and Burke DS. Historical perspective—Emergence of influenza A (H1N1) viruses. *N Engl J Med.* 16 Jul. 2009; 361(3): 279–85.

Pneumonia in the Non-HIV Immunocompromised Patient

GENERAL CONSIDERATIONS

Pneumonia in the non-HIV immunocompromised patients carries a significant morbidity and mortality. Thus mortality rates for bone marrow transplant recipients who develop pneumonia and require ventilatory support is close to 90%. The morbidity and mortality are partly related to poor immune response to infection as also to the wide range of potential pathogens that can cause pulmonary infections in these unfortunate patients. Pneumonia can be caused not only by the usual organisms causing community-acquired pneumonia (CAP), but frequently by uncommon organisms and by opportunistic infections which are very rare in patients with a preserved immune response. Community acquired Gram-negative pulmonary infections are far more common in the immunocompromised when compared to the immunocompetent. Tuberculosis, particularly in countries like India where the disease has a high prevalence rate is also an extremely important consideration.

Atypical mycobacteria, nocardia, chlamydia are also more frequently observed as are fungal infections, in particular *Pneumocystis carinii*, aspergillus, candida and infection with rarer moulds. Viral infections, notably due to the cytomegalovirus (CMV) are both frequent and important. Protozoal (toxoplasmal) infection and rarely but importantly hyperinfection with *Stronglyloides stercoralis* also are to be considered. The list of potential pathogens is large and the important ones have been tabled below.

It is obvious that in view of this large range of possible infections, the diagnosis of the cause of pneumonia in the immunocompromised patient is difficult and its management complex. It is impossible in a given patient to cover such a wide range of possible organisms. An approach that narrows the potential pathogens to a basic minimum is to be aimed at. A specific aetiology should be sought and for this bronchoscopy, bronchoalveolar lavage (BAL) studies and transbronchial biopsies are often early investigational procedures. Bronchoscopy may yield a definite aetiological diagnosis in some patients, and even if the procedure is unrevealing it may enable the physician to exclude infectious agents as the cause of a pulmonary infiltrate or shadow. The early use of computed tomography (CT) scanning is imperative as lesions revealed on a CT may be masked or not evident on routine radiography. In spite of every diagnostic effort, in patients who are critically ill therapeutic intervention includes the empiric use of broad-spectrum antibiotics together with other anti-infective agents covering non-bacterial infections to ensure that the patients receive adequate therapy.

It is certain that with increased use of organ transplants and the associated increased use of immunosuppressants, the increasing incidence of cancer and the use of many new chemotherapeutic drugs in its treatment, the number of immunocompromised patients will increase tremendously in the years to come. This applies not just to the Western world but to developing and poor countries as well. Many of these will be young patients who will have undergone increasingly aggressive treatment in the hope of a cure. Improved outcomes in these patients necessitate better, quicker diagnosis and organized management protocols.

THE NON-HIV IMMUNOCOMPROMISED PATIENT

The immunocompromised patients considered in this chapter are patients with advanced malignancies, lymphomas, leukaemias, aplastic anaemia and severe neutropenia from any cause, and patients receiving organ transplants including bone-marrow transplant recipients. Chemotherapy, use of immunosuppressants, corticosteroid therapy and cytotoxic therapy (use of cyclophosphamide, mycophenolate mofetil) can also compromise immune function.

**Table 21.1:
Potential pathogens associated with pneumonia in the immunocompromised patients**

Bacteria—pyogenic bacteria

Gram-negative—Pseudomonas aeruginosa, Klebsiella pneumoniae, acinetobacter, E.coli, Proteus, Enterobacter, other gram negative organisms
Gram positive—Streptococcus pneumonia, Staphylococcus aureus, Enterobacter species
Mycobacterium tuberculosis
Other bacteria—Atypical mycobacteria, Nocardia, Mycoplasma, Legionella, anaerobes

Fungi

Pneumocystis carinii, Aspergillus species, Candida species, rarer fungi (Mucor, Penicillium, Fusarium), endemic fungi

Viruses

CMV virus, Herpes simplex, Varicella zoster, Respiratory viruses—Influenza, Parainfluenza, Adenovirus, Respiratory syncitial virus

Protozoa

Toxoplasma

Helminthes

S. stercoralis

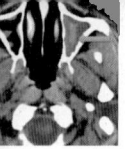

Table 21.2:
Immunocompromised Patients

Severely Immunocompromised

Acute Leukemias
Aplastic anemia
Severe neutropenia from any cause
Lymphoma
Solid Organ transplant recipients
Recent chemotherapy
Use of immunosuppresant drugs
Cytotoxic therapy
High dose of corticosteroid therapy (> 30 mg for > 3–4 weeks)

Lesser Degree of Immunocompromised

Uncontrolled diabetes
Chronic renal failure, particularly patients on dialysis
Liver cirrhosis
Multiple myeloma
Low dose cytotoxic therapy
Corticosteroids for long periods
Malnutrition
Extreme old age

Lesser degree of immunosuppression is also observed in patients with uncontrolled diabetes, in chronic renal failure, particularly in patients on dialysis, liver cirrhosis, multiple myeloma, low-dose cytotoxic therapy and in patients receiving a maintenance dose of corticosteroids for long periods. Many diseases in our country unfold against a background of poor nutrition which depresses the immune response to infection. Rarely, uncommon infections including opportunistic infections are observed due to poor immune response (in particular cell-mediated response) resulting from extreme old age.

Nature of Immunocompromised State

Immune defects can arise from the following causes—

1. Severe neutropenia (< 1500/ml)
2. A qualitative defect in neutrophil function (rare)
3. Cell-mediated immune deficiency (a T lymphocyte function)
4. Deficiency in antibody formation (a B lymphocyte function)
5. From a combination of two or more of these causes.

It needs to be stressed that cell-mediated immune response and humoral defence through antibody production are closely inter-related, interactive and interdependent.

CLINICAL APPROACH TO THE DIFFERENTIAL DIAGNOSIS OF PNEUMONIA IN AN IMMUNOCOMPROMISED PATIENT

It is of great importance to realize that fever, cough and even haemoptysis in an immunocompromised patient who has a focal or diffuse infiltrate in one or both lungs can be due not only to micro-organisms causing a true infective pneumonia, but could equally result from one or more of several non-infective causes. A distinction between the two is at times impossibly difficult. If determined to be of infective aetiology, a quick organized

attempt should be made to determine the specific or likely micro-organism responsible for the pneumonia.

A) *The initial approach in the differential diagnosis is to elicit a careful history.*

The nature of defects in the immune response that can lead to an immunocompromised state have been mentioned earlier. The history should therefore focus on the background disease responsible for the immunocompromised state as also on the current and prior immunosuppressive regimens. This enables the clinician to determine the likely nature of the immune defect as also on the degree of immune dysregulation likely to be present, both of which in turn could point to the likely causes of pneumonia in a particular patient. Thus patients with neutropenia or those with qualitative defects in neutrophil function are prone to pneumonia due to pyogenic bacteria (in particular Pseudomonas and Klebsiella), aspergillus infection, and infection with candida species. Those with defects in cell-mediated immune response are prone to pneumonia caused by *Mycobacterium tuberculosis*, *Pneumocystis carinii*, nocardia, atypical mycobacteria, herpes virus, respiratory viruses, Legionella, mycoplasma, toxoplasma and *S. stercoralis*. Patients who have a defect in antibody formation are prone to infection by *Streptococcus pneumoniae*, *H. influenzae* and herpes viruses. The morbidity and mortality of these infections is forbiddingly high in immunocompromised patients. In one large early study on renal transplant patients, pneumonia occurred in 20% of patients and accounted for 50% of deaths. Though such high

Table 21.3:
Nature of immune defects or compromise, causes of defect, related to likely pathogens causing pneumonia

Immune Defect	Cause of defect	Likely pathogens
Cell-mediated	HSCT Lymphoma Leukemia Graft vs. Host disease Azathioprine Mycophenolate Tacrolimus Corticosteroid therapy	Mycobacterium tuberculosis Pneumocystis carinii Nocardia Atypical mycobacteria Herpes virus Respiratory viruses Legionella Mycoplasma Toxoplasma S.stercoralis
Neutropenia	Acute leukemia Chemotherapy Aplastic anaemia HSCT (early phase) Diseases involving or infiltrating the marrow Cytotoxic drugs Immunosuppressants	Pyogenic bacteria—in particular gram negative infections Aspergillus Candida
Functional Neutrophil Defect	Corticosteroid therapy Azathioprine/mycophenolate	Same as above
Antibody Defect	CLL Lymphoma Myeloma HSCT Splenectomised patients	Streptococcus pneumoniae H.influenzae Herpes viruses

Note: HSCT—Hematogenous stem cell transplant.

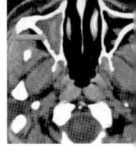

figures do not generally apply to current established centres in our country, they are a pointer to the possible morbidity and mortality in poor third world countries caring for renal transplant patients in comparatively less well-established transplant units. The table below gives the nature of the immune defect in relation to the underlying disease/treatment and relates these to the potential pathogens likely to cause infections, including pneumonia in these patients.

As mentioned earlier, fever and pulmonary shadows or infiltrates in an immunocompromised patient are not always related to infection. It is vital to be aware of this fact. Non-infective causes of pulmonary infiltrates or shadows include pulmonary oedema, intra-alveolar haemorrhage, pulmonary embolism, drug-induced pulmonary oedema, acute respiratory distress syndrome (ARDS), opportunistic neoplasms, and lymphoproliferative disease. Other non-infective lesions include recurrence of underlying tumours, recurrence of lymphoma or of leukaemia within the lungs, immune-mediated disorders (acute rejection after lung transplant, obliterative bronchiolitis after lung transplant or after an allogenic stem cell transplant, or graft vs. host reaction after an allogenic stem cell transplant), engraftment syndrome in haematogenous stem cell transplant and non-specific focal inflammation. Important non-infective causes of pulmonary infiltrates or shadows in the immunocompromised host are tabled below.

Table 21.4: Non-infectious causes that mimic infective pneumonia in the immunocompromised host
Pulmonary oedema
Inta-alveolar haemorrhage
Pulmonary infarction
Pulmonary atelectasis
Diffuse alveolar haemorrhage (DAH)
Diffuse alveolar damage
ARDS
Drug toxicity, Radiation toxicity
Progression of underlying mitotic disease
Engraftment syndrome in hematogenous stem cell transplant recipients (HSCT)
Transfusion related acute lung injury (TRALI)
Rejection of graft in graft vs host disease (GVHD)
Idiopathic pneumonia syndrome
Bronchiolitis obliterans organizing pneumonia
Posttransplantation lymphoproliferative disoders (PTLD)

The temporal relationship between the initiation of immunosuppression and the onset of pneumonia or a pulmonary infiltrate plays an important role in the differential diagnosis. In organ transplant and haematological stem cell transplant patients, pneumonia occurring within the first three or four weeks of the transplant is almost never due to an opportunistic infection but results from usual bacterial pathogens, in particular Gram-negative bacteria such as *Pseudomonas aeruginosa*, and Klebsiella. Severe neutropenia may also predispose to invasive fungal infections (aspergillus, other filamentous fungi, candida) in this time frame.

Cytomegalovirus pneumonia occurs one to four months after transplantation. Other opportunistic infections in this timeframe include pneumocystis, nocardial, fungal and viral infections. After four months, patients who have normally functioning grafts and who are on minimal immunosuppressants are more prone to the usual community-acquired infections, though opportunistic infections are possible. Those with poorly functioning grafts who require increased immunosuppressants remain susceptible to opportunistic infections. *Reactivation of latent tuberculous lung infection or a fresh pulmonary infection with M. tuberculosis is of great importance in our country and in countries with a high prevalence rate of tuberculosis. This is usually a late-onset infection.*

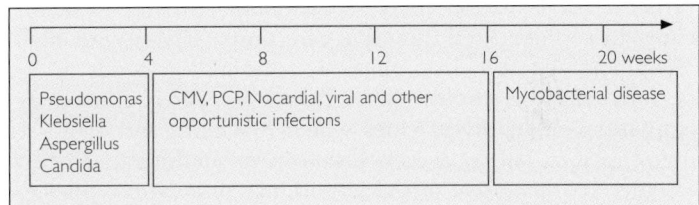

Fig 21.1: Various pulmonary infections in transplant recipients in relation to different time-frames.

Awareness of the presence of a positive serology for CMV antigen or of a strongly positive Mantoux test prior to immunosuppression may be of diagnostic help. Also, the specific use of prophylactic drugs or antibiotics may make infection with certain organisms unlikely. For example, trimethoprim-sulfamethoxazole has been proved to be very effective in the prevention of *P. carinii* infection. Therefore, a patient on this prophylaxis is unlikely to present with pneumonia due to *P. carinii*. On the other hand, the prophylactic use of flucanozole in single organ transplant (SOT) and hematopoietic stem cell transplantation (HSCT) in order to prevent candida infections is believed by some authorities to have increased the incidence of invasive aspergillosis. The overuse of flucanozole has also probably created selective pressure promoting the emergence of *Candida tropicalis, Candida glabrata* and *Candida kruezi*.

Epidemiological clues should always be sought. In our country and in other third world countries, depressed cell-mediated immunity is most likely to reactivate or cause fresh infection with *M. tuberculosis*. However exposure to fungi such as *Histoplasma capsulatum* or *Coccidiosis immitis* may predispose, particularly in endemic areas, to histoplasmosis or coccidiomycosis.

Symptoms are generally non-contributory—fever, cough, haemoptysis, and chest pain are common to many infections. In fact symptoms and signs may be absent, the presentation being an asymptomatic 'patch' or infiltrate within the lung. Yet at the same time some patients may present with a fulminant illness that may or may not be marked by high fever but is

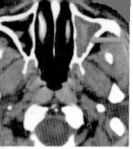
characterized by increasing tachypnoea, spreading pulmonary shadows, increasing hypoxia, cardiorespiratory and multiorgan failure.

B) Mode of Onset and Tempo of Progression

These often provide critical clues to a diagnosis. Their value is enhanced if the above features are considered with radiological and CT findings.

An acute onset over 24–48 hours is suggestive of a conventional bacterial infection or certain non-infective causes such as pulmonary oedema, pulmonary haemorrhage, pulmonary embolism, or a leukoagglutination reaction. A subacute onset over some days or weeks suggests possible tuberculosis, fungal infection, viral infection or nocardial infection. The same presentation may however also be observed with certain non-infectious causes such as drug-induced pneumonia, radiation pneumonitis or recurrence of a tumour against the background of a mitotic disease.

C) Physical Examination

Physical examination may occasionally provide valuable clues. In sophisticated intensive care units (ICUs) with high-technology equipments, physical examination tends to be perfunctory; this should never be so. Repeated clinical examination might reveal clues which machines and elaborate investigations fail to detect. The features enumerated below are merely illustrative of the importance of a careful physical examination.

(i) Tachypnoea in an immunocompromised patient, particularly in the absence of high fever is indicative of sepsis, pneumonia or acidosis. Physical signs in the chest may or may not be evident; an absence of signs on percussion or auscultation is often observed in these patients.

(ii) Skin lesions are occasionally present in cryptococcal, nocardial and candidal infections. They take the form of minimally painful or asymptomatic macules, papules or nodules, which on biopsy provide the correct diagnosis, thereby obviating the need for invasive diagnostic procedures. Erythema gangrenosum is occasionally observed in infections with *Pseudomonas aeruginosa*, and very rarely with other Gram-negative infections.

(iii) A careful search for enlarged lymph glands can be rewarding. Lymphadenopathy strongly suggests a tuberculous infection in our country due to *Mycobacterium tuberculosis*. An underlying lymphoma, presenting with an obscure pneumonia, has been occasionally diagnosed following the biopsy of a nondescript but clinically palpable lymph node.

(iv) Ocular examination is important, as ocular findings are common with disseminated CMV infection. The retina shows haemorrhages and yellowish-white exudates. Similar ocular findings have been noted in toxoplasmosis, and occasionally in candidiasis and aspergillosis.

(v) Examination of other systems is of crucial importance. Hepatosplenomegaly with lymphadenopathy may point to an underlying lymphoma or a myeloproliferative disorder. It is also commonly observed in disseminated haematogenous tuberculosis and toxoplasmosis.

(vi) Neurological examination may reveal subtle symptoms and signs suggesting meningitis or a focal neurological lesion. Brain abscess is common in nocardial infection, cryptococcal infection, and in disseminated disease due to *Mycobacterium tuberculosis*.

(D) Radiological Investigations.

Pulmonary infiltrates are never specific enough on a chest X-ray to allow a definitive aetiological diagnosis to be made. Nevertheless, a study of serial chest X-rays when combined with an analysis of the mode of onset and the progress of the disease often help in limiting the diagnostic possibilities. Focal or multifocal consolidation of short duration (< 48 hours) seen on a chest X-ray is invariably due to an acute bacterial infection. Slowly progressive consolidation with a subacute or chronic history favours tuberculosis, nocardial or fungal infections. Interstitial infiltrates spreading outwards from the hilar area and evolving in a subacute or chronic manner, suggest pneumocystis,

Table 21.5: Differential diagnosis of fever and pulmonary infiltrates in the immunocompromised patient, based on radiological signs and onset of symptoms		
Chest X-ray	Acute onset	Subacute/chronic onset
Consolidation	Bacterial Thromboembolic Haemorrage	Fungal Nocardial Tuberculous
Peribronchovascular	Pulmonary edema Leukoagglutinin reaction	Viral PCP Radiation Drug-induced
Nodular infiltrates	Bacterial Pulmonary edema	Tumour Fungal Nocardial Tuberculous

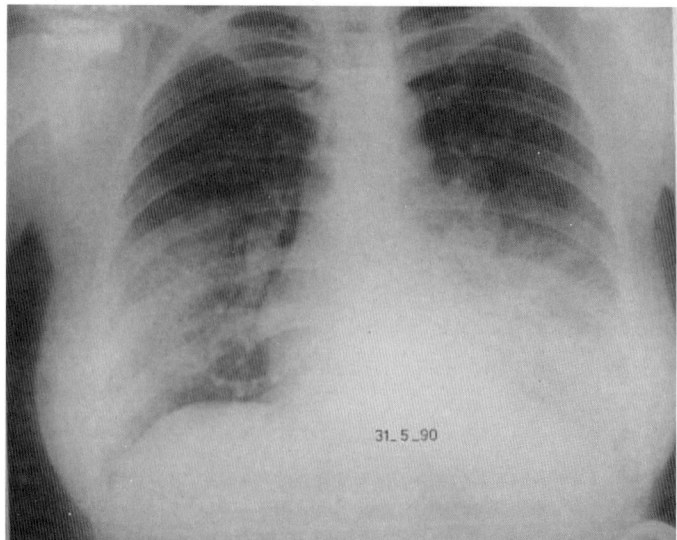

Fig 21.2: Chest X-ray reveals ill-defined consolidations in both mid and lower zones more so on the left side.

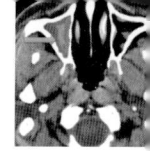

viral or drug-induced infiltration, or may be due to lymphangitis carcinomatosis. Acutely evolving interstitial infiltrates also occur in pulmonary oedema or in a leukoagglutination reaction.

Acute nodular localized alveolar consolidation or localized nodular infiltrates suggest pulmonary oedema or bacterial bronchopneumonia. Nodular infiltrates which are subacute or chronic and slow in evolving could be tuberculous, fungal or nocardial in aetiology. Such infiltrates could also be due to the recurrence or spread of an original tumour.

These radiological observations are not sacrosanct, and as mentioned at the outset, an exact diagnosis can never be made by the mere description of shadows on a chest radiograph. The overall picture has to be considered.

DIAGNOSTIC AND MANAGEMENT PROTOCOLS

Immunocompromised patients who are acutely and severely ill with pulmonary infection need critical care. Diagnostic and management protocols depend on facilities available in the ICU and the degree of sophistication of the pathology and micro-biology department of the hospital. Routine investigations include a blood count, erythrocyte sedimentation rate (ESR), C-reactive protein estimation, blood culture, sputum examination (if available) for Gram's stain, routine culture sensitivity, acid-fast bacilli (AFB) smear and culture, fungal cultures, and the examination of nasopharyngeal aspirates for viral studies. In some patients nebulization with hypertonic saline helps to obtain a satisfactory sputum sample.

A radiograph of the chest should be followed by CT of the chest. The latter is far more sensitive in evaluating the site, extent and nature of lung involvement. Arterial blood gases need to be done to determine the degree of hypoxia if present, and of hypocapnia or hypercapnia. Severe bacterial pneumonia, pneumocystis infection and CMV infections are associated with well-marked hypoxia. Invasive tests that may need to be performed are fibreoptic bronchoscopy with a study of BAL fluid

for all possible infections, and when necessary a transbronchial biopsy with staining, culture and histopathological examination of the biopsy material. The purpose is to establish a specific diagnosis that directs specific treatment. In acutely ill patients empiric therapy should be started without awaiting results of

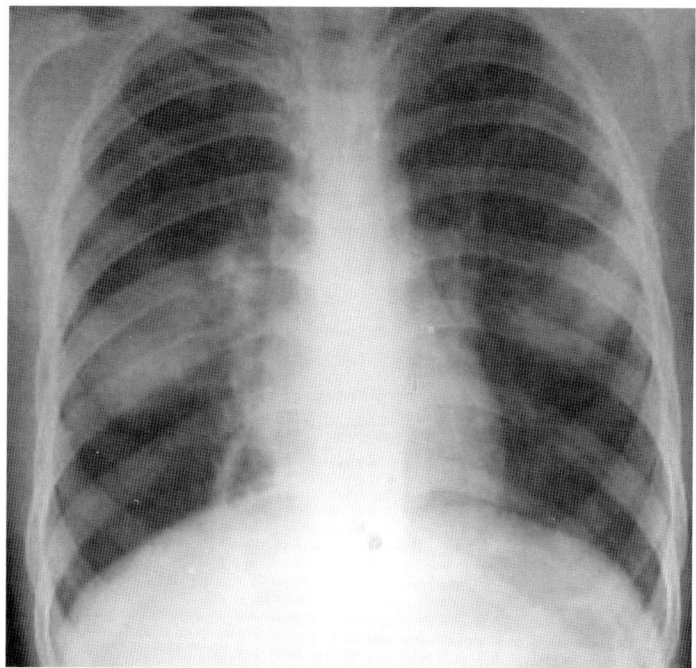

Fig 21.4: Chest X-ray reveals bilateral nodular lesions due to staphylococcal pneumonia.

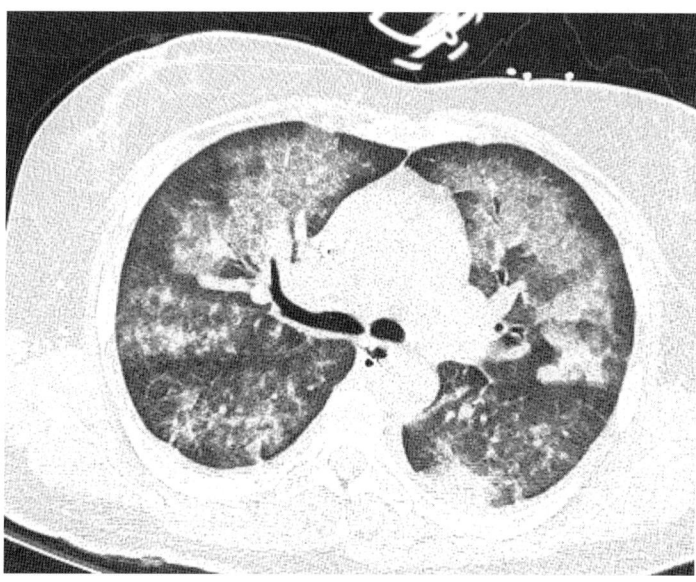

Fig 21.5: CMV infection. HRCT chest demonstrates ill-defined areas of increased lung attenuation in both lung fields representing ground-glass densities. These appearances are very similar to those seen in *Pneumocystis carinii* pneumonia. A BAL is required to differentiate between the two diseases.

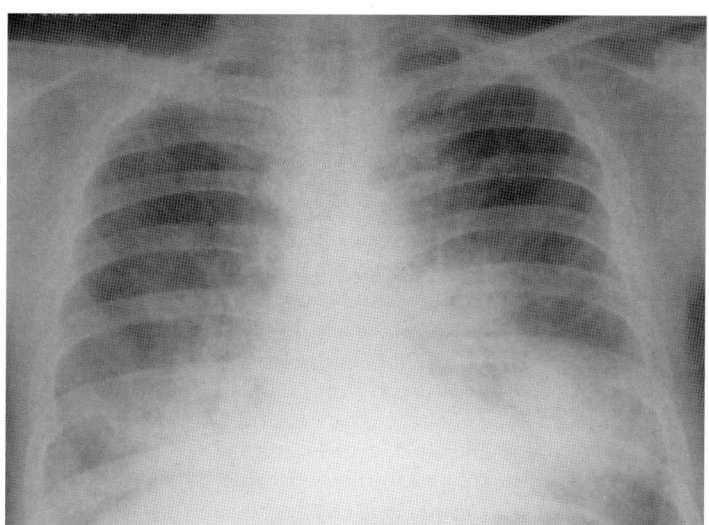

Fig 21.3: Chest X-ray reveals ill-defined fluffy opacities in both mid and lower zones. The opacities were secondary to a transfusion related acute lung injury (TRALI).

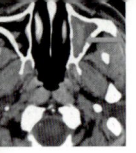

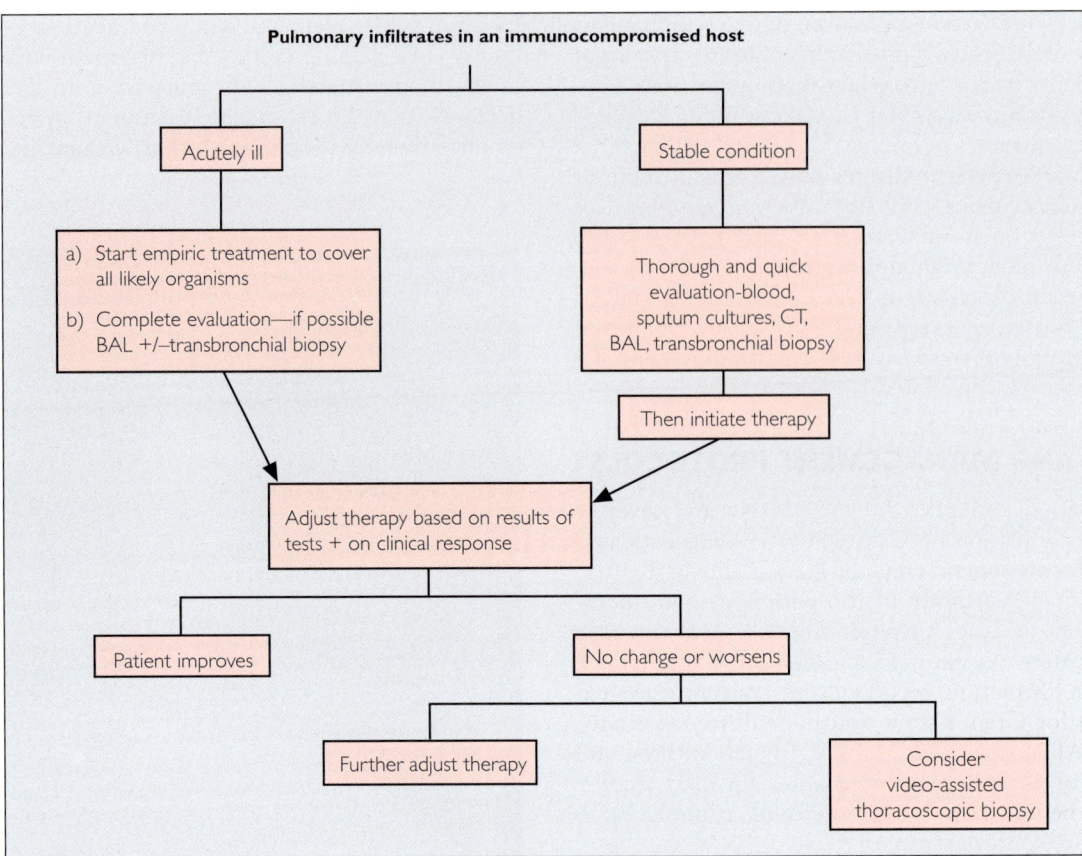

Fig 21.6: Algorithm showing an overall approach to pneumonia in an immunocompromised patient.

sputum and blood tests. Therapy could be changed later if the results so necessitate.

Diagnostic and management protocols and guidelines depend on the history, the background disease and/or treatment causing immunosuppression (which suggest the nature of organisms likely to cause pneumonia), the acuteness and severity of the illness, the physical signs and the nature of imaging findings. *It is unwise to follow protocols rigidly else they can cause more harm than good. They need to be modified for each individual according to prevailing circumstances.*

An overall approach to pneumonia in an immunocompromised patient is given in the algorithm below. Following this, five different clinical scenarios are discussed. It should be noted that a patient may not necessarily fit in any one of these five scenarios. Also, he or she could present with one scenario which shifts over time to another. Five clinical scenarios are discussed below.

1. An acutely ill patient with a lobar or focal consolidation or a focal alveolar infiltrate.

This is generally due to a bacterial infection and we advocate amoxicillin + piperacillin/tazobactum + a macrolide. This should cover gram positive, gram negative and atypical microorganisms. If there is a possibility of a staphylococcal infection, one may need to add flucloxacillin 1 gm QDS. In parts of the world or in units where methicillin-resistant staphylo-

coccal infection is prevalent IV vancomycin should be added to the regimen. Lack of response to the above regime should perhaps lead to a change of antibiotics—meropenem + vancomycin forming a potent effective combination. In pneumonia associated with severe neutropenia, particularly in those who have pleuritic pain, cough, haemoptysis and whose high-resolution CT (HRCT) is compatible with an Aspergillus infection one should add amphotericin B or voriconazole to the broad-spectrum antibiotics on an empiric basis. If the patient responds to this regime, the antibiotic course is continued for 10–14 days. A very prompt or dramatic response warrants de-escalation of the antibiotic regime within seven days of therapy.

If the patient does not respond within 48–72 hours one should opt to do a BAL with a careful examination of the BAL fluid. A transbronchial biopsy of the lesion if thought necessary could be done during the same procedure. A specific diagnosis would entail the use of specifically directed drugs towards the aetiological agent. If these procedures do not give a specific diagnosis or if the patient is too ill for BAL or transbronchial biopsy or if pathological and microbiological backing is poor as in several developing countries, further management should proceed on an empirical basis. Besides covering Gram-positive and Gram-negative infections, atypical organisms (e.g. Legionella, mycoplasma) should be covered with a macrolide given intravenously and a fungal infection (as already mentioned) by the use of amphotericin B.

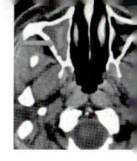

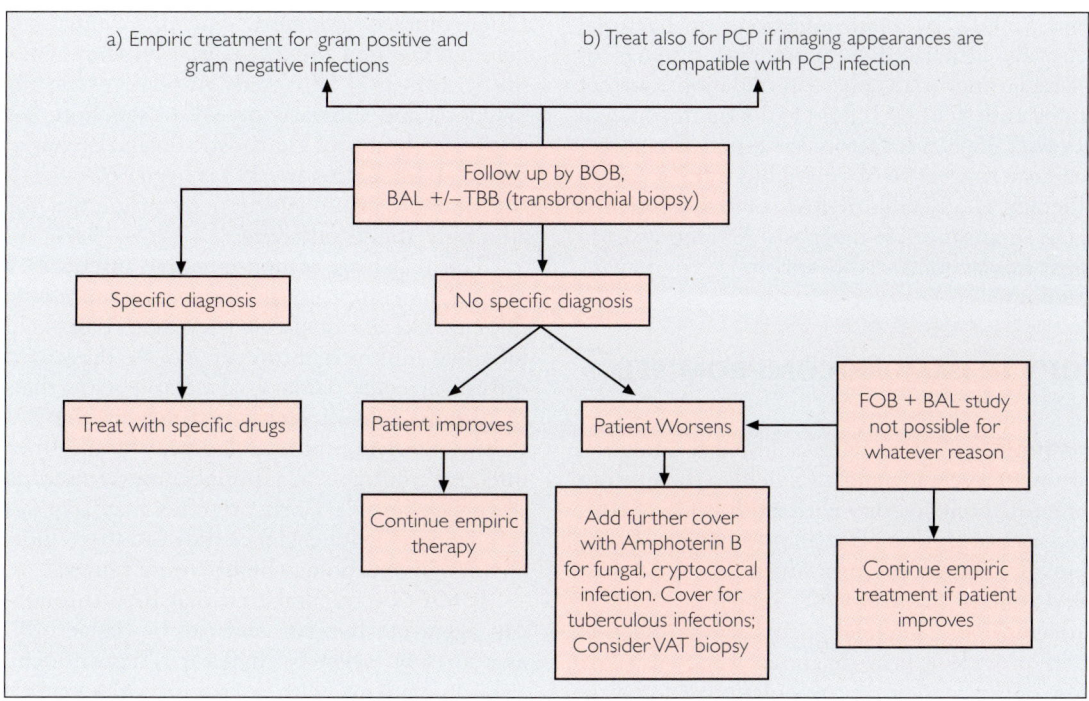

Fig 21.7: Algorithm showing an overall approach to pneumonia in an immunocompromised patient.

2. An acutely ill patient with diffuse bilateral alveolar infiltrates.

Bacterial infections are still possible and the patient needs empiric cover for Gram-positive and Gram-negative infections with intravenous amoxicillin + a third-generation cephalosporin or piperacillin/tazobactum + an aminoglycoside or a quinolone derivative. The sicker the patient the greater should be the cover for possible invading organisms. If the imaging appearances are compatible with a pneumocystis infection, a trimethoprim and sulfamethoxazole combination should be added to the regime. This is followed by bronchial lavage, and transbronchial biopsy for possible diagnostic help. If this is not possible for reasons stated above or if the diagnostic procedure fails to provide a clue, further treatment remains empiric. Deterioration of the patient should prompt the use of amphotericin B for cryptococcal, aspergillus or other rare fungal infections. If Legionnaire's disease is suspected as a clinical possibility a macrolide is added. Disseminated tuberculosis is invariably evident by the demonstration of AFB in the samples obtained through a bronchial lavage. Algorithm of the management protocol in the first two scenarios is given below.

3. Patient presenting with subacute or chronic focal consolidation on imaging.

If the sputum is unavailable, or is not diagnostic and if antibiotics used against Gram-positive and Gram-negative organisms are ineffective, a BAL study and a transbronchial biopsy should help in arriving at a specific diagnosis. If this fails and if the patient's condition allows, a video-assisted thoracoscopic biopsy should be done. This invariably gives the diagnosis. When the consolidated area is peripherally placed a CT-guided biopsy is

also of diagnostic help. Among other aetiologies, tuberculosis is an important cause of subacute focal areas of consolidation in one or both lungs.

4. Patients presenting with bilateral peri-hilar opacities fanning outwards on radiography with diffuse ground-glass opacities in both lungs.

Diffuse ground-glass opacities are met with chiefly in pneumocystis infection, CMV infection, viral pneumonitis, and occasionally with extensive bacterial pneumonias. If the patient is acutely ill or hypoxic as he or she may well be, empiric treatment should be prompt so as to cover organisms stated above. Investigations should follow. Though BAL may well give a specific diagnosis it is fraught with risk in severely hypoxic individuals. If done, it is best first to intubate the patient so that the patient if necessary can receive ventilator support with a high fraction of inspired oxygen (FIO_2). A transbronchial biopsy is best avoided particularly if the patient is on ventilator support (for fear of pneumothorax). In stable patients, investigations should include BAL and transbronchial biopsy. Empiric therapy is given or started simultaneously. Treatment is altered depending on the results of investigations and clinical response.

5. Patients Presenting with Nodular lesions

Nodular lesions are often caused by *Mycobacterium tuberculosis*, aspergillus and nocardial infections. Infected central line catheters or indwelling devices can cause metastatic bacterial or fungal nodules in one or both lungs. In the presence of positive blood cultures these metastatic bacterial or fungal pulmonary lesions should be treated with appropriate antibiotics without further need for invasive tests.

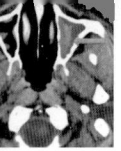
Nodular lesions caused by viral infections or bacterial infections are generally associated with imaging findings of ground-glass appearance and/or alveolar consolidation. Correct diagnosis necessitates a study of BAL fluid and a transbronchial biopsy. In patients with high-risk factors for aspergillus infection or a CT appearance suggestive of aspergillus infection, empiric antifungal therapy is advisable if BAL or transbronchial biopsy does not give an appropriate diagnosis. A video-assisted thoracoscopic biopsy however invariably enables a firm diagnosis of a fungal pathology.

BRONCHOSCOPY IN IMMUNOCOMPROMISED PATIENTS

Many immunocompromised hosts with pulmonary infection have either no sputum or a very low positive yield to the sputum they produce. Fibreoptic bonchoscopy with a full study of BAL fluid of the affected area of the lung (for all possible infections) remains a crucial invasive diagnostic procedure.

A study of BAL and a transbronchial biopsy are almost mandatory in the diagnosis of CMV and pneumocystis infection as these tests often provide a firm diagnosis. The sensitivity of BAL is however dependent on the population studied. In single organ transplant (SOT) patients, the sensitivity of BAL for CMV infection has been found to be between 20–60%. In immunocompromised cancer patients and in haematological stem cell transplant (HSCT) recipients the yield of BAL for CMV could increase to 95%. BAL remains a sensitive test for the diagnosis of pneumocystis infection in SOT patients, a positive yield being observed in 85–90%. The yield increases even more if transbronchial biopsy material is also studied. In HSCT patients the diagnostic yield with BAL and transbronchial biopsy for pneumocystis infection is in the range of 80–100%. Therefore unless an immunocompromised host is extremely ill and hypoxic, empiric treatment for CMV or pneumocystis infection based on clinical and radiological criteria alone is rarely justified, given the toxicities of the drugs used for these infections. In our experience BAL studies supplemented whenever possible by transbronchial biopsy have proved most useful in the diagnosis of tuberculosis (particularly when tuberculosis presents with widespread shadowing in both lungs or as a solid or nodular focal lesion), in nocardial infection and in determining the nature of Gram-negative infections in bacterial pneumonia. On the other hand, BAL with or without transbronchial biopsy is much less sensitive for fungal infections, a positive yield for Aspergillus being merely about 60%. We have also been unsuccessful with the diagnosis of Legionnaire's disease and viral infections (other than CMV) through the use of this procedure.

Rano and colleagues studied the use of bronchoscopy in immunocompromised patients with pulmonary infection (causing radiological shadows or infiltrates) and noted that there were three variables that independently predicted mortality—increasing severity of illness, need for mechanical ventilation and delay in diagnosis. The first two variables are understandable as patients in these categories must be very ill. The third variable is extremely important as in their study it was unrelated to the severity of illness. The risk of death in patients in whom there was a delay of > five days in the identification of pulmonary infection (infiltrate) was more than threefold in this study. (*Ref: A Rano, C Agusti et al. Pulmonary infiltrates in non-*

HIV immunocompromised patients: a diagnostic approach using non-invasive and bronchoscopic procedures Thorax. 2001 May; 56(5): 379–387). This study emphasizes the importance of early diagnosis and the early use of a bronchoscpic BAL to achieve a specific diagnosis. Diagnostic delay also has implications with regard to initial therapy. It has been observed several times over that inappropriate selection of antibiotics to initiate therapy adversely affects outcome.

The diagnosis of non-infective infiltrates within the lungs of immunocompromised patients (even after a BAL study) is difficult and almost always is a diagnosis of exclusion. Some non-infective infiltrates, however, can be diagnosed—these include diffuse alveolar damage, alveolar haemorrhage, and presence of tumour cells or lymphoma cells in the BAL fluid pointing to an underlying mitotic disease. The treatment of many non-infective infiltrates in immunocompromised patients is the use of corticosteroids. Corticosteroids may aggravate an underlying infection in the lung. Hence the need to exclude as far as possible any infective aetiology before using steroids.

It must be remembered that BAL through a bronchoscope can aggravate hypoxia and can be dangerous in patients who are already severely hypoxic. Transbronchial biopsies are risky in patients with a coagulopathy or in the presence of thrombocytopenia. Though a number of units in the West perform transbronchial biopsies in patients with a platelet count as low as 10,000/mm³, we would avoid transbronchial biopsies in patients with a platelet < 50,000/mm³ unless platelet infusions are given prior to the procedure.

Video-assisted Thoracoscopic (VAT) Biopsy

The advent of VAT biopsy has made open-lung biopsy for diagnostic procedures unnecessary. The procedure is safe in expert hands, can be performed under local anaesthesia and allows a specific diagnosis in appropriate circumstances.

The question that arises is that if all other tests (including BAL and transbronchial biopsy) are non-contributory, would a VAT yield a diagnosis amenable to treatment? We have found VAT biopsy useful (when other tests were negative) in the specific diagnosis of Aspergillus infection, tuberculous infection and infection with atypical mycobacteria. Reports from other units suggest that in fewer than half the patients subjected to VAT biopsy did results warrant a change in treatment. A positive yield was much lower in neutropenic patients and those on ventilator support.

Open-lung surgical biopsy is today hardly ever necessary to establish a diagnosis. Two questions need to be asked before this procedure is undertaken—-is the result of the open-lung biopsy likely to alter treatment? Is the patient fit enough to allow this procedure?

IMPORTANT SPECIFIC PNEUMONIA IN THE IMMUNOCOMPROMISED NON-HIV PATIENT

BACTERIAL PNEUMONIA

The commonest infection in immunocompromised patients is pneumonia caused by bacterial pathogens. Major risk factors are severe neutropenia and/or functional defect in neutrophils or phagocytes. Impaired cell-mediated immune response following

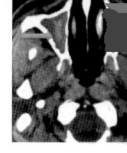

cytotoxic immunosuppressive therapy is also a risk factor for bacterial pneumonia. Patients with impaired B lymphocyte function as in lymphoproliferative disease, lymphomas, and multiple myeloma are prone to pneumonia caused by *Streptococcus pneumoniae* and *Haemophilus influenzae.*

Immunocompromised patients in hospital and particularly those in the intensive care unit (ICU) are at grave risk of pneumonia due to organisms such as *Pseudomonas aeruginosa*, Klebsiella, Acinetobacter, *E. coli* and other gram-negative bacteria. *Methicillin-resistant Staphylococcus aureus* (MRSA) infections also cause pneumonia in hospitals or units where this organism is prevalent. Immunocompromised patients treated in hospital and then living in the community are also far more prone to gram-negative bacterial infection when compared to those who are immunocompetent.

Clinical Features

The clinical features may be the same as in immunocompetent patients, with high fever, cough, rusty sputum, tachypnoea and physical and radiological signs of consolidations.

In patients with severe neutropenia, low-grade pyrexia is more frequent. In fact the patient may be afebrile, presenting with tachypnoea and a pulmonary infiltrate. Some patients may have a normal X-ray chest, pulmonary shadowing being revealed only on a *computed tomography* (CT) scan of the chest. Some of the other features of bacterial pneumonia in immunocompromised patients have been mentioned earlier in the section.

Diagnosis

Diagnosis is facilitated if a good sputum sample is available for examination (smear and culture). Blood cultures should always be sent. Patients who do not respond to conventional therapy should have a bronchoscopic bronchoalveolar lavage (BAL) study. This often gives a high positive yield. CT scans may reveal focal or dense lobar consolidation and help to distinguish bacterial from fungal or viral pneumonias. Test for *Legionella pneumophilia* antigen in the urine should be done if Legionella pneumonia is suspected.

Treatment

The nature of organisms that prevail and cause infection in a hospital or ICU and the antibiogram would help decide therapy in an immunocompromised patient who develops nosocomial pneumonia (NP). In critically ill immunocompromised patients with acute bacterial pneumonia, treatment should never await results of diagnostic tests. To give an example of just one regimen, one could use piperacillin tazobactum + an aminoglycoside as an immediate cover for gram-negative bacteria. If MRSA is prevalent in a unit, vancomycin should be added. If the patient fails to respond in 48 to 72 hours, the regime needs to be changed to another combination—for example, a carbapenem + vancomycin. One could add a macrolide if there is suspicion of Legionella or any other atypical organism. Immunocompromised patients admitted to a hospital for a community-acquired bacterial pneumonia need cover for both gram-positive and gram-negative organisms.

Severe bacterial pneumonia in immunocompromised patients is often complicated by the *acute respiratory distress syndrome* (ARDS) and by a pleural exudate that turns into an empyema.

Good oxygenation often with a high-flow oxygen mask is necessary. Ventilator support is frequently necessary in severe pneumonia. All organ systems must be given adequate support.

PNEUMOCYSTIS INFECTION

This has been dealt with in the chapter on 'Pneumonia in the Non-HIV Immunocompromised Patients'. Whereas in AIDS pneumocystis infection is subacute or even insidious in onset, in the immunocompromised non-HIV patient pneumocystis pneumonia is more often an acute opportunistic infection producing fever, breathlessness, tachypnoea, tachycardia and progressive hypoxia. Imaging features are those of perihilar shadows fanning out towards the periphery involving the greater part of both lungs. Other possible imaging features have been described in the chapter on 'HIV and the Lung'. The yield from BAL in these patients with conventional stains is 80% compared to HIV patients where the yield is over 95%. This is because fewer organisms are recovered in non-HIV patients. The sensitivity of BAL is therefore lowered in non-HIV patients with pneumocystis infection. Similarly, a positive yield (particularly in transplant patients) of induced sputum is low compared to HIV patients.

NOCARDIOSIS

Nocardia are gram-positive organisms that grow as branching filaments. Human infection is usually caused by *N. asteroids*. It is an important though a comparatively uncommon cause of pneumonia or pulmonary infiltrates in immunocompromised patients. An important setting for norcardial infection is patients with chronic airways obstruction who have received or continue to receive corticosteroid therapy. Nocardial infection may rarely occur as a community-acquired pneumonia (CAP) even in immunocompetent individuals. This has been briefly described in the chapter on 'Community Acquired Pneumonia'.

Clinical Presentation in the immunocompromised patient
1) The initial presentation often seen is that of an asymptomatic pulmonary shadow of uncertain aetiology. A radiograph shows one or more shadows often circumscribed, often varying in size and not infrequently cavitating.
2) A review of nocardial infection in 260 patients who had undergone heart transplant provides a useful outline of the clinical profile of this disease in the immunocompromised. Fever, dry cough are presenting features and the natural history is subacute, though at times nocardial infection in an immunocompromised host may resemble an acute bacterial pneumonia. Pleural involvement has been reported in a third of these patients. Nocardial infection can disseminate, particularly to the central nervous system (CNS). One or more abscess-like cavities in the lungs and in the brain should always suggest this diagnosis. Skin lesions may present as nodules which are positive for nocardia on a biopsy.

Diagnosis is difficult, as nocardia is rarely present in sputum samples and sputum cultures are frequently negative. If BAL studies and transbronchial biopsies are non-contributory, a thoracoscopic biopsy may help to establish a diagnosis. A CT-

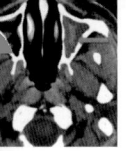
guided biopsy of a peripherally placed nodule or abscess has also proved successful in our rather limited experience.

MYCOBACTERIAL INFECTION

Mycobacterial infection chiefly occurs in patients with an impaired cell-mediated immune response. It is a frequent and important cause of focal or nodular shadows on radiography in immunocompromised patients in countries like India where the disease has a high prevalence. The likelihood of tuberculosis also depends on the reason for immunosuppression. Tuberculosis rarely complicates chemotherapy for acute leukaemia or haematological stem cell transplant (HSCT). The incidence is very significant in single organ transplant (SOT) recipients, being as high as 15–20% in countries where tuberculosis is endemic. Though the risk of tuberculosis is common to heart, lung and liver transplant, it is highest in renal transplant recipients. The disease generally occurs late in the time span after start of immunosuppression, the median time of occurrence being nine months after transplantation.

Clinical Features and Diagnosis

Clinically the patients present with pyrexia of unknown origin. Investigations reveal focal, segmental or lobar consolidation or infiltrates on radiography. CT scans may demonstrate lesions not observed on radiography. The posterior segment of the upper lobe or the dorsal segment of the lower is frequently involved. Miliary shadowing is observed in some cases. In countries where tuberculosis has a high prevalence rate, the radiological appearances are at times those of ARDS. In fact tuberculosis is an important cause of ARDS in tropical countries where the disease is endemic. Mediastinal and/or hilar adenopathy may be present. Atypical radiographic findings may well be present in immunocompromised patients.

If sputum is not available, a bronchoscopic BAL should be done, combined if possible with a transbronchial biopsy. These procedures are often rewarded by a definite diagnosis. If these tests are negative and there is strong suspicion of tuberculosis, or if there is progressive disease, a video-assisted thoracoscopic biopsy may provide a correct diagnosis.

Treatment is with standard chemotherapy regimen, though it must be kept in mind that infection may well be due to multi-drug-resistant strains of the mycobacterium.

INVASIVE PULMONARY ASPERGILLOSIS

Invasive pulmonary aspergillosis (IPA) appears to be an increasing cause of pulmonary infection in immunocompromised patients not only in the West but also in tertiary ICU centres in India. Aspergillus species are saprophytic filamentous fungi found in the environment. They propagate by producing spores which are 2–3 μm in diameter and which on inhalation reach the distal air spaces. Ordinarily, they are innocuous, but in immunocompromised patients with severe neutropenia or with impaired neutrophil or macrophage function these spores germinate into filamentous fungi and invade the lung tissue to cause IPA or invasive involvement of the paranasal sinuses. Metastatic spread to the brain, bones, skin and other organs may also occur. Aspergillus infection is generally due to *Aspergillus fumigatus*. *A. flavus*, *A. niger* and *A. terreus* may rarely also cause disease.

Risk Factors

The major risk factor is significant neutropenia or poor neutrophil function. The greater the degree of neutropenia and the greater its duration, the greater the risk. IPA is observed in 50% of patients where neutropenia persists > four weeks. Patients most at risk are those with haematological malignancies receiving chemotherapy, patients with aplastic anaemia and (in the early phase) in stem cell transplant recipients where severe neutropenia is an important complication. Patients who develop graft vs. host disease are also at risk, as are patients who receive liver, lung and heart transplants. Patients with acute leukaemia

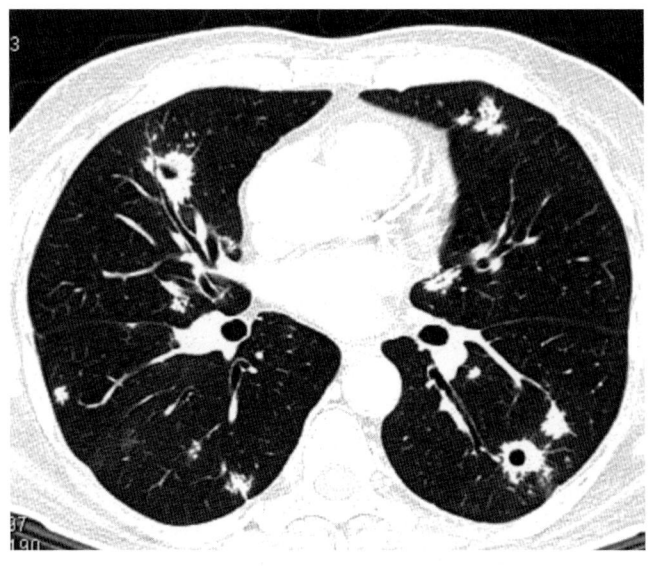

(a)

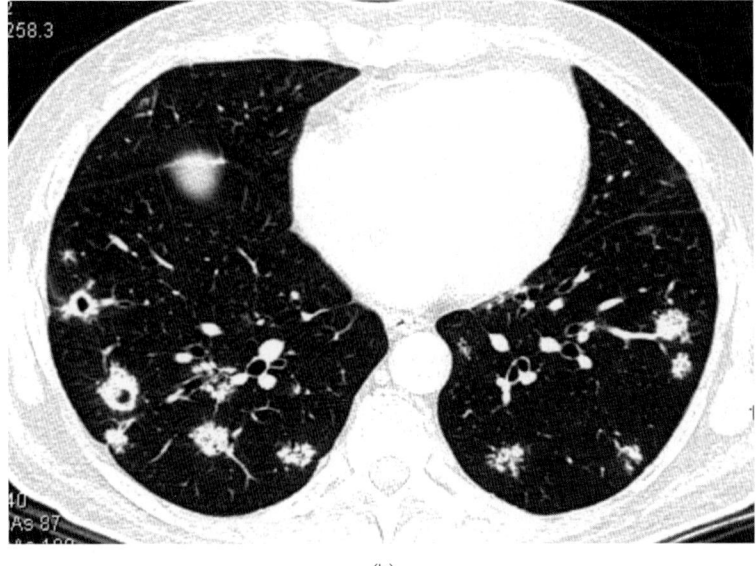

(b)

Fig 21.8a and b: Invasive Aspergillosis: HRCT demonstrates multiple ill-defined nodular lesions in a peribronchial location representing invasive aspergillosis.

develop IPA as a complication 20 times more frequently than patients with lymphoma or organ transplants. Patients on high-dose corticosteroids for prolonged periods are also at risk of developing this disease. The spectrum of background diseases predisposing to IPA includes patients with subacute hepatic necrosis receiving corticosteroids and intravenous antibiotics.

Perhaps the frequency and epidemiology of aspergillus infection is governed by the presence of airborne aspergillus in a particular eco-environment. Outbreaks of this infection have been related to the increased presence of the organism in the air around construction sites or due to inadequate air-conditioning systems.

Clinical Features

Fever, cough, pleuritic chest pain and haemoptysis may occur but these symptoms occur with other pulmonary infections as well. Persistent and severe haemoptysis should always raise suspicion of IPA as aspergilli grow into pulmonary vessels producing areas of pulmonary infarction. Massive fatal haemoptysis is known to occur. Chest radiographs may show areas of consolidation or nodules that may cavitate.

About 10% of immunosuppressed patients may present with pyrexia of unknown origin with a radiographic examination of the chest appearing normal. A CT of the chest in these patients may demonstrate nodular infiltrates compatible with IPA.

IPA is sometimes suspected on certain findings in CT studies. These include: a) a 'halo sign'—which is an area of lower attenuation shadowing surrounding a nodule or an area of consolidation; b) a 'crescent sign' which relates to a partially formed cavity due to infarcted lung tissue. The 'halo sign' is generally observed within a week of infection; the crescent sign is generally observed after some more weeks. The 'halo sign' is neither very sensitive nor specific, for many moulds other than aspergillus (e.g. fusarium) can cause a similar pattern on a CT scan. Radiographic appearances are varied. They may vary from nodular infiltrates to dense alveolar consolidation. Because of

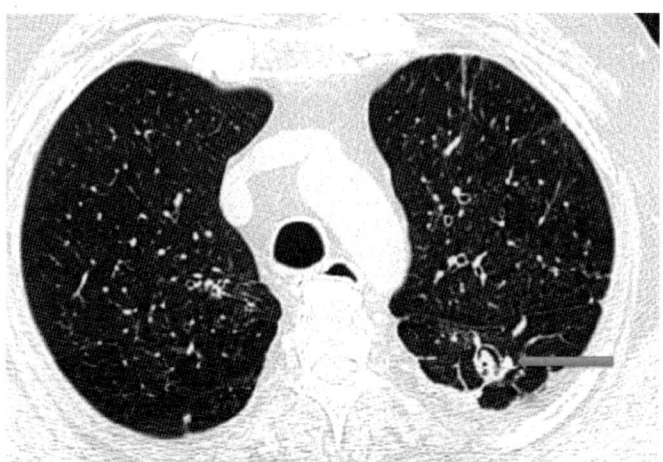

Fig 21.10: HRCT chest reveals a nodular lesion with a crescent of air along its superior aspect due to an aspergilloma.

the angioinvasive nature of the fungus, radiological appearances may resemble wedge-shaped pleural-based infarcts which may later cavitate. A CT is mandatory as it may reveal lesions not seen on an X-ray chest.

ASPERGILLUS TRACHEOBRONCHITIS

This form of aspergillus infection is localized to the tracheobronchial tree causing a tracheobronchitis characterized by dry cough and pyrexia. Though radiography of the chest is normal, CT scans may show focal areas of thickening of the bronchial walls.

CHRONIC NECROTIZING PULMONARY ASPERGILLOSIS

In milder forms of immunosuppression as in patients on cytotoxic drugs or in patients on a maintenance dose of corticosteroids, aspergillus infection takes the form of an indolent disease characterized by one or more patches of consolidation which may or may not cavitate. Cough, fever, weight loss are the presenting features. The course may remain indolent but slowly progressive, or may graduate to a more invasive form of the disease.

Diagnosis

In high-risk patients, the presence of clinical and imaging features compatible with IPA should prompt the use of specific therapy. Even so, a microbiological diagnosis is always to be preferred, because some species of aspergillus infection or infection with other rare filamentous fungi may be resistant to conventional treatment with amphotericin B. Sputum examination including sputum culture are poorly sensitive. Microbiological diagnosis is achieved by BAL study and/or by transbronchial biopsies. The presence of aspergillus in BAL fluid on smear and/or culture in an immunocompromised patient is highly predictive of IPA. However, isolation of aspergillus species by BAL culture can diagnose only 50% of cases of invasive infection. Transbronchial biopsy of affected areas may reveal fungal hyphae infiltrating lung parenchyma. If a transbronchial biopsy is unsuccessful in giving a diagnosis one should attempt a CT-guided biopsy or

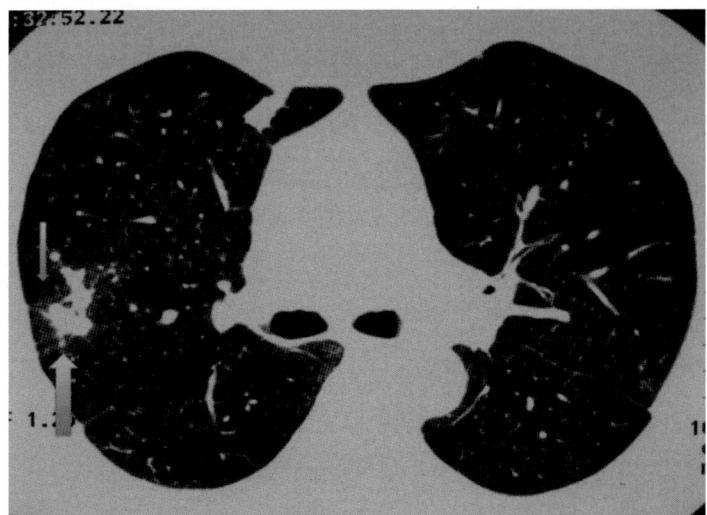

Fig 21.9: CT Chest reveals a nodular lesion in the right middle lobe with an ill-defined ground-glass appearance surrounding the consolidation representing a halo sign. This was due to aspergillus infection.

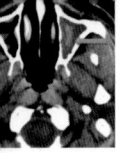

a video-assisted thoracoscopic biopsy which usually enables a firm diagnosis.

Non-Invasive Tests

Non-invasive tests include 1) Detection of galactomannan or glucan cell wall antigen on BAL specimens obtained through a fibreoptic bronchoscope or in the blood; 2) *polymerase chain reaction (*PCR) for aspergillus DNA from the blood.

Though highly sensitive, the galactomannan antigen test may give false positive results particularly in patients receiving piperacillin-tazobactam. Unfortunately, these tests are not available in India and developing countries as yet. It is believed that if performed routinely for surveillance in high-risk patients and if found positive, preemptive antifungal treatment could perhaps prevent overt disease.

The diagnosis of aspergillus tracheobronchitis can be made from positive cultures in bronchial washing as also from biopsy of tracheobronchial mucosa which show fungal invasion of bronchial mucosa.

The diagnosis of chronic necrotizing pulmonary aspergillosis often requires video-assisted thorascoscopic biopsy or in appropriate circumstances a CT-guided biopsy for confirmation of fungal aetiology.

Table 21.6: Diagnostic Tests for IPA
Microbiological Diagnosis: Culture of sputum, or bronchoalveolar lavage (BAL) fluid
Transbronchial biopsy
CT guided biopsy
Video-assisted thoracoscopic biopsy
Detection of galactomannan or glucan cell wall antigen in BAL specimens
PCR for aspergillus DNA from the blood.

Table 21.7: Diagnosis of aspergillus tracheobronchitis
Positive cultures in bronchial washing
Biopsy of tracheobronchial mucosa

Table 21.8: Diagnosis of chronic necrotizing pulmonary aspergillosis
Video-assisted thorascoscopic biopsy
CT guided biopsy in appropriate circumstances

Treatment

Till recently the only drug available for IPA was amphotericin B which has fairly serious toxic effects, particularly on the kidney. Treatment options are now much better because of two more anti-fungal drugs—a new azole voriconazole and a

new anti-fungal agent (an echinocandin) called caspofungin. Amphotericin B, voricanozole and caspofungin have by and large similar efficacy. Voriconazole and caspofungin are however to be preferred because of less side-effects. The role of combination therapy has not been evaluated but may well be promising as each of these three drugs has different mechanisms of action. Unfortunately, voriconazole and in particular caspofungin are very expensive for poor patients in poor countries. Duration of treatment should extend for at least two weeks.

Itraconazole is also effective against aspergillus but should be used orally only after systemic use of any one of the drugs mentioned above. Even in this context, oral voriconazole is preferable and more efficacious.

Chronic necrotizing pulmonary aspergillosis is an indolent disease. Oral voriconazole or itraconazole may need to be given for a prolonged period extending over months.

The role of surgery in the treatment of Aspergillus infection is limited to patients with a well-defined lesion causing massive haemoptysis, to localized lesions which fail to respond to medical therapy and to a focal lesion of IPA which is quiet but persists after full treatment. In the latter situation, removal may prevent recurrence of IPA following subsequent immunosuppression.

CANDIDA INFECTION

Pneumonia due to candida infection is rare but metastatic lung infection can occur in patients with candidemia or in patients with infected central venous catheters or other infected vascular indwelling devices. Pyrexia, accompanied by nodular lung shadows is observed. Metastatic lesions due to reasons stated above do not need an invasive workup. Fluconazole or Amphotericin B should be started promptly and an infected intravascular device should be promptly removed. The frequent use of fluconazole prophylaxis has led to an increased prevalence of strains resistant to usual antifungal drugs. These include *Candida tropicalis, Candida glabrata, Candida parapsilosis* and *Candida krusei.*

Table 21.9: Treatment of IPA
Amphotericin B: 0.5–1.5 mg/kg/d IV; lyopholized amphotericin B: 3–5 mg/kg/d IV
Caspofungin: 70 mg IV loading dose on day 1, followed by 50 mg/d IV; duration depends on response to therapy
Voriconazole: Loading dose: 6 mg/kg IV BD **Maintenance:** 4 mg/kg IV BD, once patient tolerates the drug, switch to 200 mg PO BD
Itaconazole: 200–400 mg daily orally
Surgery in selected circumstances

NON-ASPERGILLUS FILAMENTOUS FUNGAL INFECTIONS

These include infections with zygomycetes, fusarium and Penicillium. Infection with these filamentous fungi is indistinguishable from IPA. The diagnosis needs to be considered

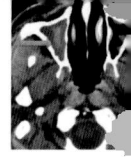

in patients with IPA who do not respond to adequate therapy. Diagnosis can be made from culture of BAL fluid and invasive biopsies. The mortality is extremely high. Infection with *Penicilliosis marneffei* is very rare in India, though a few HIV patients suffering from the infection have been reported from Manipur in Northeast India. It is however fairly common in Southeast Asia, particularly in Thailand, and has been reported also in non-immunocompromised patients. This infection has been briefly dealt with in the section on 'Tropical Infections Involving the Lung'.

CRYPTOCOCCAL AND ENDEMIC FUNGI

Cryptococcal infection is comparatively rare in immunocompromised non-HIV patients. The presentation may be with low-grade pyrexia with focal and multifocal consolidation. In patients with marked suppression of cell-mediated immunity, lobar consolidation may occur. Diagnosis is through staining and culture of sputum and BAL fluid for *Cryptococcus neoformans*. Treatment is with Amphotericin B. This may be combined with flucytosine. Oral fluconazole may then need to be continued for prophylaxis.

Infection with histoplasma and coccidiodes need not be seriously considered in India, but they remain important considerations in countries where these fungal infections are endemic.

CYTOMEGALOVIRUS INFECTION

Cytomegalovirus (CMV) infection is common in the general population occurring usually in children or adults. The infection is asymptomatic or causes a self-limiting mild disease. Latent infection can be detected by serological testing. In patients with markedly depressed cell-mediated immunity (CD4 counts well below 200) CMV is reactivated and produces CMV disease, infecting the lungs and at times several other organs. Patients with impaired cell-mediated immunity who are serologically CMV-negative are extremely prone to fulminant CMV infection if given blood products or a transplant organ containing leucocytes from CMV-positive donors. Though most frequently observed in HIV-infected patients with very low CD4 counts, CMV infection can occur occasionally in non-HIV immunocompromised patients.

Clinical Features

CMV pneumonia is usually insidious in onset presenting with fever, cough, tachypnoea, dyspnoea and progressive hypoxia. At the start, chest radiography may be normal; later it shows parahilar shadows fanning out into the periphery, very similar to the radiological appearances in pneumocystis infection.

CT scans are far more sensitive in detecting infection. They invariably show symmetrical diffuse ground-glass opacities (again similar to pneumocystis infection) with multiple small centrilobular nodules. Rarely, the radiological and CT changes are asymmetrical.

Severe infection is associated with the involvement of other organs. Leucopenia is always present. Liver function can be deranged with a significant rise in liver enzymes and gastrointestinal symptoms can occur from involvement of the colon and the gastrointestinal tract. A telltale feature is the occurrence of CMV chorioretinitis which is quite distinctive in its appearance.

The differential diagnosis of CMV pneumonia is from other viral infections, from *Pneumocystis carinii* pneumonia (PCP) infection, from drug-induced pneumonitis, ARDS and intra-alveolar haemorrhage.

Diagnosis

1. The surest way of proving CMV infection in CMV pneumonia is through a BAL study and a transbronchial biopsy. Intranuclear 'owl's eye' inclusion bodies in cytology studies on BAL fluid are confirmatory as are inclusion bodies present in histopathological studies of transbronchial biopsies.
2. Cytology on BAL fluid is however not a very sensitive test for CMV pneumonia. The main diagnostic techniques in use today are based on probing BAL fluid directly for the presence of CMV antigen or by probing cell cultures inoculated with BAL fluid after 48 hours' incubation.
3. Positive viral cultures of BAL fluid or biopsy specimens are the gold standard in diagnosis but the sensitivity of viral cultures is not as good as is desired. Also, cultures take long to give results.

CMV pneumonia does not occur in the absence of CMV reactivation. CMV reactivation is tested by the presence of CMV antigenemia and by determining the viral load through PCR techniques. A large and increasing viral load substantiates to a great extent the diagnosis of CMV pneumonia.

Table 21.10: Diagnosis of CMV		
I) BAL study	a)	Intranuclear 'owl's eye' inclusion bodies on cytology studies
	b)	Presence of CMV antigen
	c)	Positive viral cultures of BAL fluid
II) Transbronchial biopsy		
III) Positive viral cultures of biopsy specimens		
IV) Serum for PCR and viral load		

Treatment

The treatment of choice is the use of ganciclovir. Foscarnet and cidofovir are second-line drugs.

Ganciclovir is phosphorylated within infected cells and inhibits viral DNA polymerase. It is given intravenously in a dose of 2.5–5 mg/kg BD or TDS. It has a strong myelosuppressive effect and may prove too toxic in patients who have just received stem cell transplants. An oral formulation of ganciclovir, called valganciclovir has recently been introduced.

The second-line drug foscarnet has a mechanism of action similar to ganciclovir but has renal toxicity which limits its use. The dosage is 60 mg/kg TDS given intravenously. Cidofovir also has a similar action to ganciclovir but has both myelosuppresive toxic effects as also renal toxicity. Patients need to be well-

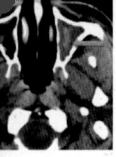

hydrated and given probenicid before therapy. Treatment with any one of these drugs is for two to three weeks.

Patient with CMV disease are also given intravenous immunoglobulin as a form of passive vaccination against CMV.

Some centres prefer to use one or the other of the three drugs prophylactically in severely immunocompromised patients whenever there is evidence of increasing CMV reactivation. It is hoped that if such patients do develop CMV infection, the outcome is better, because of the early initiation of therapy.

OTHER VIRAL INFECTIONS

HERPES VIRUSES

Rarely herpes simplex virus (HSV) or herpes zoster virus (HZV) causes pulmonary infection in immunocompromised patients. Presentation is similar to CMV infection. Skin lesions present in herpetic infections afford the right clue. The virus can be isolated from BAL fluid. Acyclovir is given intravenously in full doses.

RESPIRATORY VIRUSES

Respiratory viruses can cause lower respiratory tract infection in immunocompromised patients. Infection occurs through inhalation of infected droplets. The common responsible viruses are Influenza A, parainfluenza virus, respiratory syncitial virus. Infection with adenovirus and rhinovirus has also been reported. There is a woeful lack of appropriate facilities for detecting viral infections in our country and in most countries in the tropical belt.

Respiratory viral infections are generally a late complication of immunosuppressed patients, reflecting persistent poor cell-mediated immune response in transplant patients and in patients on immunosuppressive drug therapy.

Clinical features are those of bronchiolitis—cough, fever and end inspiratory high-pitched squeaks. X-ray chest is invariably normal but a CT chest may show evidence of inflammation of small airways with 'tree and bud' changes. Some degree of alveolar shadowing may also be present. The main differential diagnosis is from mycoplasmal and chlamydia infection. The diagnosis in well-equipped laboratories is confirmed by identifying viral antigen in nasopharyngeal aspirates or in BAL fluid samples by the use of an immunofluorescent test. Viral cultures if positive are the gold standard for diagnosis. PCR techniques may perhaps have greater sensitivity. The prognosis of viral infections in the absence of actual pneumonia is good. Obliterative bronchiolitis may however occur as a sequel. Treatment with antiviral agents is generally ineffective.

SUGGESTED READING

Belleza WG. Pulmonary considerations in the immunocompromised patient. *Emerg Med Clin North Am.* 1 May 2003; 21(2): 499–531, x–xi.

Cunha BA. Pneumonias in the compromised host. *Infect Dis Clin North Am.* 1 Jun. 2001; 15(2): 591–612.

Shorr AF. Pulmonary infiltrates in the non-HIV-infected immunocompromised patient: etiologies, diagnostic strategies and outcome. *Chest.* 1 Jan. 2004; 125(1): 260–71.

Tamm M. Pulmonary cytomegalovirus infection in immunocompromised patients. *Chest.* 1 Mar. 2001; 119(3): 838–43.

Vento S. Lung infections after cancer chemotherapy. *Lancet Oncol.* 1 Oct. 2008; 9(10): 982–92.

Waite S. Acute lung infections in normal and immunocompromised hosts. *Radiol Clin North Am.* 1 Mar. 2006; 44(2): 295–315, ix.

Wheat LJ. Approach to the diagnosis of invasive aspergillosis and candidiasis. *Clin Chest Med.* 1 Jun. 2009; 30(2): 367–77, viii.

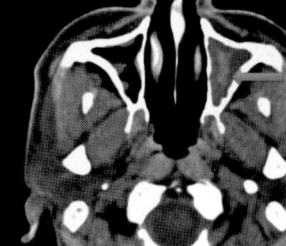

CHAPTER **22** Nosocomial Pneumonia

GENERAL CONSIDERATIONS

Nosocomial pneumonia is a frequent, important and dreaded complication in hospitalized patients. Its morbidity and mortality continues to remain high in spite of advances in microbiological therapy, improving critical care and the use of a wide range of preventive measures. Nosocomial pneumonia chiefly afflicts the most critically ill patients in a hospital. Impairment of defence mechanisms of an ill patient and easy access of dangerous pathogens to the lower respiratory tract are both equally responsible for nosocomial pneumonia. An intensive care unit (ICU) milieu is therefore ideal for this major complication.

Nosocomial pneumonia all over the world is much more frequent in patients who are intubated and require ventilator support. In fact ventilator-associated pneumonia is the most common nosocomial infection in the ICU, comprising roughly one-third or more of the total nosocomial infections. Over 90% of ICU-acquired nosocomial pneumonias occur during mechanical ventilation (ventilator-associated pneumonia, VAP), 50% occurring in the first four days after ventilation. Ten to twenty per cent of patients who require mechanical ventilatory support for > 48 h will acquire VAP with a mortality of 15–50%. Patients who have VAP have worse outcomes and longer hospital and ICU stays. VAP appears to be an independent risk in critically ill patients with a doubling of the mortality rate directly attributable to VAP. The discussion in this chapter is therefore with special reference to VAP though this discussion can be extrapolated to the other forms of nosocomial pneumonia as well.

The clinical diagnosis of nosocomial pneumonia as will be discussed later is unfortunately imprecise and its treatment difficult. A microbiological diagnosis is necessary through a careful examination of lower respiratory secretions. Treatment guidelines in relation to antibiotic therapy should be dictated by knowledge of the bacteriology in each hospital and critical care unit. Two principles emerge—

1. The prompt empiric use of the most appropriate antibiotic or antibiotic combination in the correct dosage in a critically ill patient reduces morbidity and mortality.
2. The de-escalation of antibiotic therapy based on the clinical response and on the microbiological results of the examination of respiratory secretions prevents the development of bacterial resistance.

DEFINITIONS

Nosocomial pneumonia (NP) is pneumonia due to pathogenic organisms, which occurs 48 hours or more after hospitalization and which was not incubating at the time of admission. Nosocomial pneumonia includes hospital-acquired pneumonia (HAP), ventilator-associated pneumonia (VAP) and healthcare-acquired pneumonia (HCAP). HAP can be managed in the ward, or in the ICU if the illness is severe.

VAP is pneumonia due to pathogenic organisms, which occurs 48–72 hours after intubation and mechanical ventilator support.

Healthcare-associated pneumonia (HCAP) according to the American Thoracic Society guidelines (for the diagnosis and treatment of NP) has the following epidemiological features:

a) a patient who was hospitalized for two or more days within 90 days of the present infection;
b) resided in a nursing home or long-term facility;
c) received recent intravenous antibiotic therapy, chemotherapy or wound care within the past 30 days of the current infection or attended a hospital or haemodialysis clinic.

These patients in a way are similar to hospitalized patients, in that they are susceptible to colonization with drug-resistant organisms.

Though the discussion in this chapter centres on HAP and even more on VAP, the same principles can be extrapolated to HCAP.

PATHOGENESIS

Aspiration Pneumonia

Almost always, NP is due to aspiration of infected secretions or particulate matter from the mouth and pharynx into the lower respiratory tract. Retained infected secretions within the large and small airways can also produce NPs. In most sick patients in the ICU, the oropharynx is colonized by aerobic Gram-negative bacteria within 5 to 10 days, whereas in healthy adults the normal organisms are anaerobic bacteria, and harmless commensals like *Neisseria pharyngitidis*. The severity of the illness plays an important role in perpetuating this colonization. Invasive diagnostic and therapeutic procedures further promote the aspiration and transfer of infected, colonized oropharyngeal contents into the lower respiratory tract. The upper airway is usually colonized before the lower airway, but organisms such as *P. aeruginosa* can colonize the lower airway as a primary event. The reason for colonization of the mouth, oropharynx and airways by pathogenic bacteria and in particular by Gram-negative organisms, is the subject of research. In healthy individuals a film of fibronectin covers the epithelium lining the mucosa of the mouth and oropharynx, and prevents the

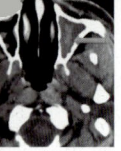
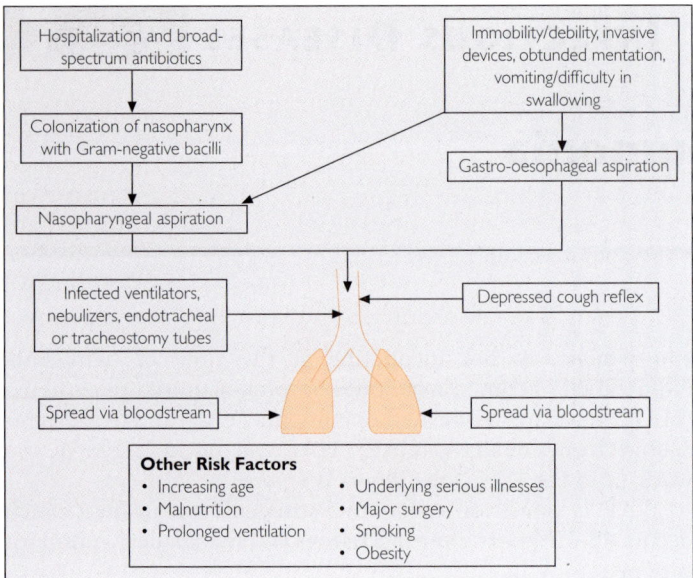

Fig 22.1: Pathogenesis of nosocomial pneumonia.

Gram-negative bacteria from adhering to the epithelial cells. This protective coating is lost in very ill individuals, so that pathogenic Gram-negative organisms adhere to receptors present on epithelial cells of the mucosa and soon colonize it. The number of these bacterial receptors on both upper and lower airway epithelial cells is increased in many illnesses. This change is associated with increased colonization at these sites. Risk factors for increased colonization due to enhanced adherence of bacteria to mucosal cells in the airways include serious illnesses, smoking, azotaemia, surgery and malnutrition.

Gastric Colonization

The acid within the stomach serves as a major deterrent to bacteria swallowed in the saliva. If gastric acidity is suppressed by the use of antacids and H_2 antagonists, the bacteria within the stomach survive, multiply, and soon colonize the upper gastrointestinal (GI) tract. Gastric contents laden with Gram-negative bacteria could easily regurgitate and be aspirated into the lungs, causing aspiration pneumonia. This is particularly frequent in obtunded or sedated patients or following a large vomit. Prophylaxis and treatment of bleeding stress ulcers with sucralfate which does not significantly increase gastric pH in most patients, has resulted in a reduced incidence of NP.

Haematogenous Pneumonia

Rarely, infected emboli from a septic thrombophlebitis can lead to septic infarcts within the lung. Catheter-related sepsis or any other source of sepsis can cause bacteraemia with haematogenous spread of infection into the lungs, causing pneumonia.

Inhalation Pneumonia

Contaminated respiratory equipment (nebulizers, humidifiers, ventilator tubing etc) is a source of infected aerosols. Infected particles 3–5 microns in size can be deposited into the terminal bronchioles and alveoli, thereby causing a lower respiratory tract infection.

Iatrogenic Causes

Lack of aseptic precaution during suction of tracheobronchial secretions, either through an endotracheal tube or tracheostomy is an important cause of lower respiratory tract infection.

FACTORS PREDISPOSING TO NOSOCOMIAL PNEUMONIAS

These can be divided into:

(A) *Host Factors* in which defence mechanisms are suppressed by (i) overwhelming infections, serious illnesses e.g. severe sepsis, extrapulmonary infections, prolonged shock, burns or severe trauma, or following major surgery; (ii) background factors which are associated with a greater propensity to infection. These include underlying chronic lung disease (chronic bronchitis), diabetes mellitus, cardiac disease, renal failure, liver cell dysfunction, underlying malignancy, advanced age, malnutrition prior to the onset of a critical illness or occurring acutely during the course of an illness, and total parenteral nutrition.

(B) *Therapeutic Interventions.* The most important of these are endotracheal intubation, tracheostomy and mechanical ventilation. Nasogastric tubes encourage gastric colonization with pathogens, and perhaps provide a scaffolding or conduit for these pathogens to reach the pharynx; aspiration of these pathogens or of infected particulate matter results in pneumonia. Corticosteroids/antimitotic agents are immunosuppressants, and their use both encourages and masks infection. As mentioned earlier, there is evidence that excessive neutralization of acid to treat upper GI bleeds by antacids and H_2-antagonists also facilitates upper GI tract colonization with Gram-negative bacteria, and predisposes to pulmonary infection. The use of very high oxygen concentrations in mechanical ventilation over prolonged periods of time may also be detrimental to lung morphology and physiology, and may predispose to infection. Prolonged antibiotic therapy can induce a superinfection by organisms resistant to conventional therapy, and lead to NP resistant to the usual antibiotics.

(C) *Environmental Factors* like overcrowding, an overall unclean environment (which unfortunately is frequently seen in developing countries), increased prevalence of multiple, resistant organisms, and *transmission chiefly through the contaminated hands of ICU personnel*, all predispose to the development of nosocomial infections.

CLINICAL DIAGNOSIS

The clinical diagnosis of NP, including VAP, is difficult and often erroneous. This is proven by a post-mortem study showing that the clinical diagnosis of pneumonia was incorrect in 60 per cent of cases. The diagnosis of NP requires the presence of the following important features:

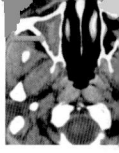

Table 22.1:
Factors predisposing to nosocomial pneumonia

A. Host Factors

Overwhelming infections/serious illnesses e.g. severe sepsis, prolonged shock, burns, severe trauma or following major surgery

Background factors e.g. chronic lung diseases, diabetes mellitus, cardiac, renal or hepatic dysfunction, advanced age, underlying malignancy, malnutrition

Total parenteral nutrition

B. Therapeutic Interventions

Endotracheal intubation/tracheostomy with mechanical ventilator support

Use of invasive procedures (including central lines)

Nasogastric tube

Use of corticosteroids/chemotherapy

Prolonged use of antibiotics

Colonization of upper GI tract with Gram-negative bacteria following use of antacids/H_2-antagonists

Use of high FIO_2 whilst on mechanical ventilation

C. Environmental Factors

Overcrowding

Overall unclean environment (unfortunately so frequently seen in developing countries)

Transmission chiefly through contaminated hands of ICU personnel.

Increased prevalence of multiple, resistant organims

(i) A chest X-ray which shows a new or progressive alveolar infiltrate or fresh appearance of a cavity.

(ii) Fever > 38.3°C or hypothermia < 36°C.

(iii) Leucocytosis > 12,000/mm^3 or leucopenia < 4000/mm^3.

(iv) Purulent sputum or in the case of VAP, purulent tracheal secretions.

The presence of an abnormal radiographic infiltrate together with at least two of the other three clinical criteria stated above has a high degree of sensitivity but a low specificity. When all three clinical criteria are present in a patient with a fresh alveolar infiltrate on an X-ray chest, the specificity improves but the sensitivity falls to an unacceptable level (< 50 per cent).

Table 22.2:
Clinical Diagnosis of nosocomial pneumonia

i) Chest X-ray which shows a new or progressive alveolar infiltrate

ii) Fever

iii) Leucocytosis > 12000/mm^3 or leucopenia < 4000/mm^3

iv) Purulent sputum, or in the case of VAP, purulent tracheal secretions

Note: The presence of an abnormal radiographic infiltrate together with at least two of three clinical criteria stated above has a high degree of sensitivity but a low specificity.

Diagnostic problems in an individual patient can be formidable for the following reasons:

(i) A systemic inflammatory response characterized by fever and leucocytosis may be present, but its absence does not exclude the diagnosis of pneumonia. Also, fever and leucocytosis can occur in infections other than pneumonia and in non-infective pathologies in a critically ill patient.

(ii) Absence of sputum or of significant lower respiratory tract secretions in patients with a tracheostomy (with or without ventilator support), does not necessarily exclude pneumonia in the presence of a recent infiltrate on an X-ray chest in a critically ill patient.

(iii) A 'shadow' on a chest X-ray is not necessarily inflammatory. Localized shadows in one or both lung fields can be due to pulmonary oedema, pulmonary haemorrhage, pulmonary infarction, acute respiratory distress syndrome (ARDS), and other non-inflammatory causes. Atelectasis is often mistaken for pneumonia in a critically ill patient. A clearing of the shadow after vigorous physiotherapy differentiates infiltrates caused by atelectasis from those due to infection.

(iv) NP in a patient with ARDS may be impossibly difficult to diagnose on a chest X-ray. A number of pathologies can cause asymmetric consolidation in patients with ARDS. An air bronchogram on a chest X-ray in a patient with ARDS is not necessarily predictive of NP.

In a study of autopsy-proven VAP, no single radiographic sign had a diagnostic accuracy > 68 per cent. The presence of an air bronchogram was the only sign that corresponded best with pneumonia, predicting 64 per cent of pneumonias in this study.

In another study by Wanderink, it was noted that when VAP was diagnosed on any combination of clinical + radiological findings, the actual incidence of pneumonia on post-mortem examination was only 30–40%.

In an attempt to improve sensitivity and specificity, the National Nosocomial Infection Surveillance System (NNIS) laid down criteria for the diagnosis of NP. These criteria are given in Table 22.4.

In recent years the Clinical Pulmonary Infection Score validated by Pugin and colleagues has been frequently used. This score combines different clinical, laboratory, physiological,

Table 22.3:
Shadows on X-ray chest which may mimic nosocomial pneumonia

Atelectasis

Pulmonary oedema

Pulmonary infarction

Haemorrhage

Lung injury (ARDS)

Drug reaction

Recurrence or spread of mitotic disease

TRALI (Transfusion related acute lung injury)

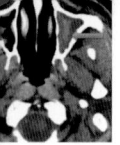
Table 22.4: **National Nosocomial Infecton Surveillance System (NNIS)** **criteria for the diagnosis of pneumonia**		
Clinical: One of the following:		
Fever 38°C with no other recognised cause		
WBC count < 4,000 or > 12,000/mm³		
For adults < 70 years old, altered mental status with no other recognzed cause		
And at least two of the following:		
New-onset purulent sputum or change in character of sputum, or increase in respiratory secretions or suctioning requirements		
New-onset or worsening cough, dyspnoea or tachypnoea		
Râles or bronchial breath sounds		
Worsening gas exchange, increased oxygen requirements, increased ventilatory support		
Microbiological (optional) Positive culture result (one): blood (unrelated to other source), pleural fluid, quantitative culture of BAL or PSB; > 5% BAL obtained cells contain intracellular bacteria		

Table 22.5: **Clinical Pulmonary Infection Score (CPIS)—Clinical criteria** **for the diagnosis of pneumonia**			
Variables	0	1	2
Temperature, °C	≥ 36.1 to ≤ 38.4	≥ 38.5 to ≤ 38.9	≥ 39 to ≤ 36
WBC count,/μL	≥ 4,000 to ≤ 11,000	< 4,000 to > 11,000	
Secretions:	Absent	Present, nonpurulent	Present, purulent
P$_a$o$_2$/fraction of inspired oxygen > 240 or ARDS	> 240 or ARDS		≤ 240 and no ARDS
Chest radioghaphy	No infiltrate	Diffuse or patchy infiltrate	Localized infiltrate
Microbiology	No or light growth	Moderate or heavy growth: add 1 point for same organism on Gram stain	

radiological and microbiological parameters to enable the clinician to improve on the specificity of the clinical diagnosis. A score of greater than 6 is believed to correlate well with the diagnosis of pneumonia. However, some studies suggest that the sensitivity and specificity was only 77% and 66 % respectively. More recent studies have tried to improve on both sensitivity and specificity by also considering Gram staining of lower respiratory tract secretions.

The above discussion suggests that clinical features combined with radiographic findings are of help, but lack sufficient specificity in the diagnosis of NP. Bacteriological evidence of pulmonary parenchymal infection is therefore also considered necessary to make a firm diagnosis. The cost-effectiveness of different methods used to obtain this bacteriological evidence

and the relation of the evidence obtained to ultimate patient management and patient outcome are matters of continued discussion. These methods are briefly discussed below.

CLINICAL FEATURES OF SEVERE NOSOCOMIAL PNEUMONIA

Nosocomial pneumonia can at times be fulminant, particularly when caused by Gram-negative organisms such as *P. aeruginosa*

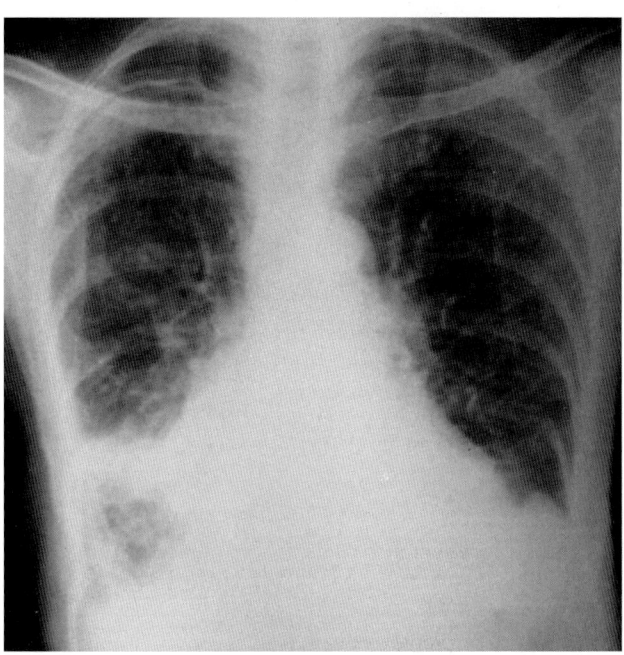

Fig 22.2: Nosocomial pneumonia. A 73-year-old man admitted for hernia surgery, developed fever and leukocytosis on Day 3 postoperatively. Patient had vomited post anaesthesia and developed aspiration pneumonia. Chest X-ray reveals an ill-defined consolidation in the right lower lobe with evidence of loss of volume; the right hemithorax is slightly smaller in size than the left. These appearances of a consolidation and loss of volume are very suggestive of aspiration pneumonia.

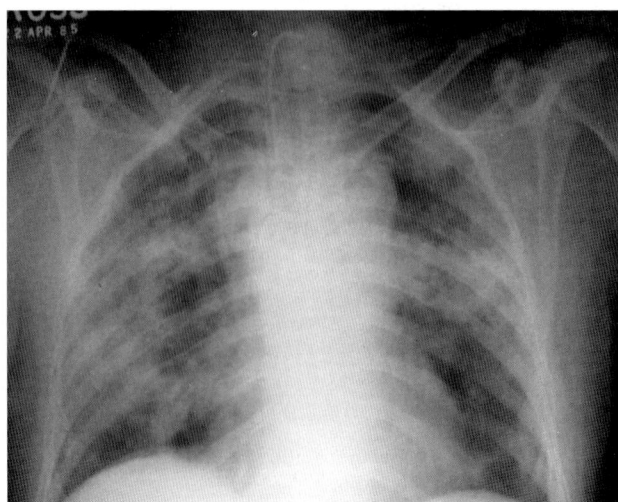

Fig 22.3: Ventilator-associated pneumonia. Elderly gentleman was admitted to the ICU and required ventilator support. Within three days he developed fresh and increasing shadows in both lungs suggesting ventilator-associated pneumonia.

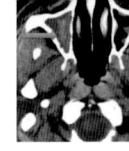

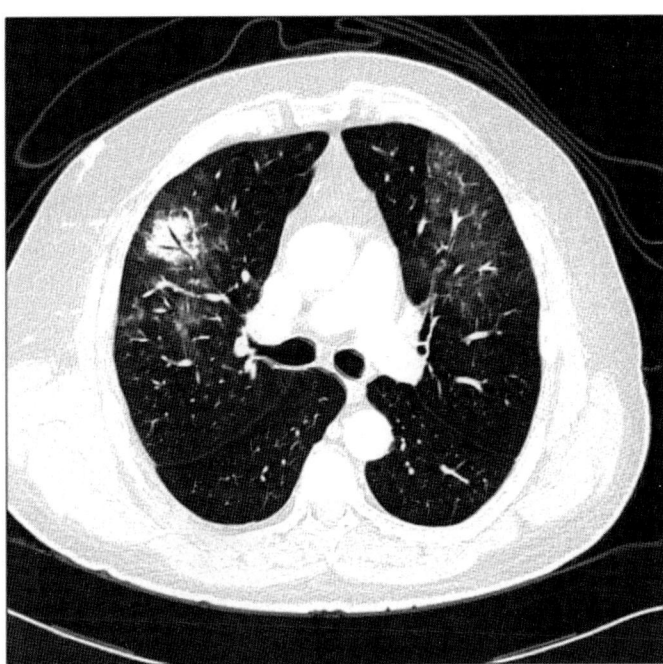

Fig 22.4: Nosocomial pneumonia. CT chest in a patient admitted for hip replacement surgery. Patient developed fever on the fifth postoperative day. CT chest reveals an ill-defined area of consolidation in the right middle lobe with an air bronchogram, patchy pneumonitis is seen in the left lingula.

Table 22.6: Severe nosocomial pneumonia
Respiratory failure, with increasing hypoxia
Rapid radiographic progression
Severe sepsis with hypotension and/or MOF
Acute renal failure requiring dialysis

or Acinetobacter. The clinical features are increasing respiratory failure with persistent hypoxia in spite of high FiO_2, PEEP and good ventilator support. There is a rapid progression of radiographic shadowing, severe sepsis, with hypotension and/or multi-organ failure (MOF). The patient soon develops renal failure necessitating dialysis. The mortality is spite of appropriate antibiotics is well over 80%.

BACTERIOLOGICAL EXAMINATION OF RESPIRATORY SECRETIONS

Non-invasive Approach

Examination of the sputum in a patient breathing spontaneously can be informative. The sputum sample must however be representative of lower respiratory tract secretions if staining with Gram's stain and cultures for organisms are performed.

The presence of flattened epithelial cells from the oral cavity in a sputum sample serves as a marker of mouth and upper airways secretions. If the sputum contains more than 10 epithelial cells per field it is not suitable for further examination or culture. On the other hand alveolar macrophages inhabit only

distal airways so that their presence denotes that at least part of the specimen being examined is from the lower respiratory tract. The presence of elastin fibres in a sputum specimen is often taken as evidence of necrotizing pneumonia.

In intubated or tracheostomised patients, respiratory secretions can be obtained by tracheal aspiration. The aspirate is stained with Gram's stain and cultures of the aspirate could either be just qualitative or quantitative. Qualitative cultures of aspirates have a high sensitivity (perhaps close to 90%) but a poor specificity (0–33%) because of contamination with bacteria present in the upper respiratory secretions. A negative culture is however of considerable value; in that it makes the diagnosis of NP highly unlikely. The use of quantitative cultures with a cut-off point at 10^6 cfu/ml increases the specificity of the non-invasive method.

Interestingly, there are a number of studies that show no significant difference between non-invasive quantitative culture of tracheal aspirate and. the use of invasive methods to culture lower respiratory secretions with regard to overall mortality or morbidity.

Invasive Diagnostic Tests

ROLE OF PSB SAMPLING

Samples of lower respiratory tract secretions can be collected by special protected brushes through a fibreoptic bronchoscope (PSB sampling). The brush is housed in a catheter that is plugged at the distal end. The protective housing allows the catheter to be advanced through a bronchoscope without coming into contact with the upper airways. Brushing should be obtained from the area of abnormal radiological shadows observed on the X-ray chest. The material should be stained by Gram's stain and cultured qualitatively and quantitatively. A culture yielding 10^3 cfu /ml or greater concentration of organisms supports the diagnosis of NP and identifies the pathogens. The sensitivity of PSB tests ranges from 33–100%, with a median of 67%, and the specificity ranges from 50–100% with a median of 95%. PSB sampling therefore offers greater specificity and lesser sensitivity in the diagnosis of NP.

Bronchoscopic procedures even when performed expertly carry a risk to critically ill patients on ventilator support. The main complication is hypoxia during the procedure; this could lead to hypotension, arrhythmias and even death. Hypoxia may persist for several hours after the procedure, particularly in patients with ARDS.

ROLE OF BRONCHOSCOPIC ALVEOLAR LAVAGE

Bronchoscopic alveolar lavage (BAL) has also been used in the diagnosis of VAP. The sensitivity of quantitative BAL fluid cultures ranges from 42–93% with a mean of 73%. For quantitative cultures a CFU (colony-forming units) count/ml of 10^3 to 10^5 is considered a positive result. The specificity ranges from 45–100% with a mean of 82%.

ROLE OF BLINDED INVASIVE PROCEDURES

The risk and expense entailed in bronchoscopic procedures has led to the development of other tests requiring less expense, expertise and risk. These tests include the following non-bronchoscopic techniques: blinded bronchial sampling (BBS), mini-BAL, blinded sampling with PSB (BPSB). The sensitivity

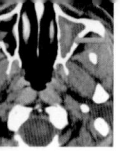

and specificity are reported to be similar to bronchoscopic techniques.

The merits and de-merits of the different non-invasive and invasive methods used to establish a bacteriological diagnosis are tabled below.

Table 22.7: Bacteriological diagnosis strategies			
Non-invasive	**Sensitivity**	**Specificity**	**Comments**
Tracheal aspirate			
Qualitative	> 90%	0–33%	
Quantitative 10^5–10^6 CFU/ml	76%	Better specificity than qualitative method	Increased specificity
Invasive			
PSB			
Quantitative 10^3 CFU/ml	67%	85.90%	Unreliable if specimen obtained after starting antibiotics
BAL			
Quantitative 10^4–10^5 CFU/ml	73%	82%	Highest accuracy for diagnosing VAP. Poor specificity in patients who are heavily colonized

Positive Blood Culture, Positive Culture of a Pleural Exudate

In a patient with clinical and radiological features compatible with NP, a positive blood culture may or may not be a pointer to the nature of the organism causing the infection. However, cultures of an organism from a tapped pleural exudate are certain bacteriological evidence of NP. Unfortunately, pleural effusions or empyemas are infrequent and blood cultures are positive only in a small minority of patients with NP.

In conclusion, the diagnosis of NP should be based on an overall perspective of clinical, radiological and bacteriological findings. There is no diagnostic criterion or procedure that serves as gold standard for the diagnosis of nosocomial (including VAP) pneumonia.

Does the use of invasive methods to establish a specific bacteriological diagnosis help in management so as to improve ultimate patient outcome, with regard to mortality and morbidity? Most studies suggest that the use of invasive methods do not influence ultimate outcome. There is however one large randomized study which showed that the use of PSB in the management of NP was associated with a lower mortality on Day 14 but not on Day 28; also this invasive diagnostic technique was associated with more antibiotic-free days on Day 28. However, a recent Canadian trial suggests that invasive techniques (PSB or BAL studies) do not influence mortality and morbidity in NP when compared to non-invasive techniques. (*Ref: The Canadian Critical Care Trials Group. A randomized*

trial of diagnostic techniques for ventilator-associated pneumonia. New Engl J Med 2006;355:2619–2629). Another meta-analysis of five *randomized controlled trials* (RCTs) studying a total of 1367 patients showed that quantitative cultures did not score over qualitative cultures to reduce mortality among patients with VAP. Neither did quantitative cultures reduce ICU stay nor reduce time on mechanical ventilation compared to use of qualitative cultures. It emphasized that mortality was reduced by the use of appropriate antimicrobial agents from the beginning of therapy. (*Ref: Quantitative versus Qualitative cultures of respiratory secretions for clinical outcomes in patients with Ventilator associated pneumonia, Berton et al, Cochrane Database of Systematic Reviews 2008 Issue 4.*)

Therefore in our present state of knowledge it can be concluded that there is no scientific evidence, nor for that matter expert consensus to show that antibiotic treatment based on bacteriological examination and culture of lower respiratory tract secretions via special bronchoscopic procedures is superior to empiric treatment aided by culture sensitivity reports on sputum or on tracheal secretions aspirated through a tracheostomy or an endotracheal tube. The only concession in favour of bronchoscopic diagnostic procedures is that specificity in diagnosis is improved, and perhaps the unnecessary use of antibiotics is avoided for clinically insignificant organisms, or in situations where smears and cultures are negative. However, since patient outcome has not been altered for the better by the use of invasive diagnostic bronchoscopic procedures, it is justifiable in poor developing countries to treat NP (suspected on clinical and radiological evidence) empirically with a suitable planned antibiotic regime.

We would recommend invasive techniques to obtain lower respiratory secretions (particularly a BAL study) under two circumstances:

1. To help identify specific organisms in NP occurring in an immunocompromised patient, since opportunistic organisms may well be responsible for the pneumonia.
2. In instances when a patient with NP fails to respond within 48–72 hours to empiric antibiotic therapy. Before changing the antibiotic regime, an attempt at a more specific diagnosis through use of invasive diagnostic procedures (PSB or BAL) may perhaps be of help.

TREATMENT
Antibiotic Therapy

Early prompt empiric antibiotic therapy is of critical importance in patients suspected to be suffering from NP or VAP. Respiratory secretions should be quickly sent for microbiological tests. Empiric therapy should however not be delayed by procedures for collection of respiratory secretions nor should it await the result of laboratory tests. Many studies have demonstrated the critical importance of early and appropriate antibiotic therapy. By appropriate is meant:

a) The correct choice of one or more antibiotics—at least one chosen antibiotic should act on the causative organism.
b) The antibiotic is given in the correct dose, by the correct route and at correct intervals.
c) Treatment is initiated at the earliest.

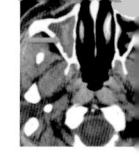

Studies have also shown that when the initial antibiotic therapy is incorrect or inadequate (either in its choice or dosage schedule) then changing the antibiotic as per the result of culture sensitivity makes little difference to the high morbidity and mortality.

The optimal selection of antibiotics depends on several factors—

1. A knowledge and awareness of the prevalence of core organisms in a hospital and in a particular ICU setup. Core organisms responsible for NP in units all over the world are predominately Gram-negative bacteria. In many units, particularly in the West, m*ethicillin-resistant Staphylococcus aureus* (MRSA) also features prominently. It is the exact prevalence of different Gram-negative organisms and their varying sensitivity to antibiotics that is important. This prevalence and sensitivity to antibiotics may vary from unit to unit. Also prevalence and sensitivity patterns may vary in the same units from time to time. A bacteriological surveillance in each hospital and in every ICU is therefore of crucial importance. An awareness of the nature of organisms responsible for NP and VAP in a unit as also the sensitivity profile helps in the choice of correct antibiotic therapy.
2. Clinical Background. According to the American Thoracic Society guidelines, the two most important factors determining the choice of antibiotics are—a) The presence of risk factors for infection with multi-resistant organisms; b) The time onset of pneumonia—early ≤ 4 days or late > 4 days.

In patients who have an early NP or VAP and who have no risk factors for infection with multi-resistant organisms, monotherapy suffices either with ceftriaxone, a fluoroquinolone or amoxicillin-clavulinic acid.

Patients with late onset NP or VAP or those with risk factors for infection with multi-resistant organism should be treated with an antibiotic regime which covers a resistant *P. aeruginosa*, a resistant Acinetobacter and other Gram-negative bacteria prevalent in a unit. Polymicrobial infections are also found. The choice of antibiotics could be a third or fourth generation cephalosporin + an aminoglycoside, or piperacillin-tazobactum + an aminoglycoside, or meropenam + an aminoglycoside.

The exact choice would depend on the antibiogram prevailing in a particular unit at that point in time. In units where MRSA is prevalent, besides using any one of the above covers for *P. aeruginosa* and other Gram-negative bacteria, vancomycin should be added to cover possible MRSA infection. In units where a resistant Acinetobacter (resistant to carbapenams, piperacillin-tazobactum, third and fourth generation cephalosporins) is prevalent, colistin needs to be incorporated into the antibiotic regime.

It is important for the clinician to be aware of the pharmacokinetics of the antibiotics in use. Antibiotics such as aminoglycosides and quinolones are bactericidal in a concentration-dependent fashion, so that they are most lethal to bacteria at high concentrations. Also, they have a 'post-antibiotic effect' (PAE) which means that these antibiotics can suppress bacterial growth even after the antibiotic level falls below the minimum inhibitory concentration (MIC) of the organism. Therefore for both aminoglycosides and quinolones, combining a whole day's regime into a single daily dose (every 24 hours) can take advantage of both the concentration-dependent killing of Gram-negative bacteria as also suppression of bacterial growth due to the PAE.

On the other hand, other antibiotics such as vancomycin and the beta-lactams are bactericidal in a time-dependent fashion, the degree of killing being dependent on the time that the serum concentration of the drug is above the MIC. These antibiotics also have no post-antibiotic suppression effect on the infecting organism. These antibiotics therefore need to be dosed more frequently through the day or even given as continuous IV infusions so as to keep drug levels above the MIC of the infecting organism as long as possible.

Finally, mention must be made of the possible use of aerosolized antibiotics in the treatment of severe Gram-negative VAP. Aminoglycosides, colistin, polymyxin B are the antibiotics that have been used. A side-effect of aerosolized antibiotics has been bronchospasm, induced either by the antibiotic or the diluent present in the preparation.

DURATION OF ANTIBIOTIC THERAPY

Many intensivists and clinicians would continue the antibiotic regime for 10 to 14 days or even more, till clinical and radiological resolution ensue. However, a randomized controlled trial has shown that patients receiving treatment for only eight days had no greater mortality nor an increased rate of recurrence. Not withstanding the above study, the length of treatment should be individualized for each patient. Mild to moderate NP or VAP may require just an eight-day treatment. Severe NP, particularly when due to resistant *P. aeruginosa* or resistant Acinetobacter, often requires a prolonged regime extending to two or more weeks.

DE-ESCALATION OF ANTIBIOTIC THERAPY

A strategy which is being investigated in several studies is the de-escalation of antibiotic therapy after three days depending on the result of microbial cultures. A single antibiotic might thus replace an earlier combination of two antibiotics or there could be a step-down from a carbapenam to a third or second-generation cephalosporin if the clinical condition has improved and the microbiological cultures so dictate. Studies have shown that this strategy reduces the use of antimicrobials without increasing mortality or recurrence. It would also help to reduce the danger of emerging antibiotic resistance. Here again one should consider each patient on his or her own merit and not blindly follow statistically validated studies involving many patients. It would be wrong to deescalate patients with severe NP or VAP or to deescalate in critically ill patients with multiple problems who show no significant features of clinical resolution.

RESPONSE OR LACK OF RESPONSE TO THERAPY

Response of NP or VAP is generally observed within 48 to 72 hours. The response is both clinical, radiological and in relation to gas exchange. Even after VAP responds, ventilator support may be necessary in critically ill patients for several other reasons. In some patients with resistant *P. aeruginosa* infection, Acinetobacter infection or with other resistant Gram-negative infection, response may take longer, at times as long as three to four weeks. The longer the time for resolution to occur, the worse the ultimate outcome, particularly in the elderly and in those with other co-morbid factors.

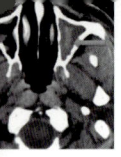

Thirty to fifty per cent of NPs, in particular VAP may not respond to antibiotic therapy. There could be several causes for a lack of response. These include a wrong diagnosis of pneumonia or a lack of appropriate antibiotic coverage against the causative organism. At times, though the choice of antibiotic therapy is correct, persistence of the aetiological agent leads to a persistent or worsening pneumonia. Persistence of the offending organism may be due to several factors; an important cause is an inappropriate dosing regime.

Superinfection pneumonia is a serious problem that often causes death. Superinfection follows prolonged antibiotic therapy. Organisms causing superinfection are generally drug-resistant and therefore lethal. They include resistant strains of Pseudomonas, Acinetobacter, other Gram-negative bacteria, MRSA, Enterococci, fungi and multi-drug-resistant Enterobacteriaceae.

Table 22.8:
Possible causes of non-resolution of VAP on antibiotic therapy

1. Wrong diagnosis—a non-infective pathology, rather than an infective one.
2. Inappropriate antibiotic regime
3. Inappropriate dosing of antibiotic
4. Persistent respiratory failure; prolonged ventilatory support
5. An underlying fatal pathology e.g. cancer
6. Severe gram-negative infection which persists
7. Underlying unsuspected immunosuppression
8. Acquired resistance to the antibiotic
9. Recurrent infection
10. Superinfection
11. An unexpected pathogen—Mycobacterium tuberculosis, fungi, respiratory viruses, mycoplasma

Support to all Organ Systems Many patients with NP and particularly patients with VAP are critically ill. Support to the cardiovascular system, maintenance of effective gas exchange and support to all other organ systems is absolutely necessary.

Table 22.9:
Principles in treatment strategy

i) Prompt, early use of appropriate antibiotic/antibiotics preferably after collecting lower respiratory secretions (which ever method followed) for culture and sensitivity.
ii) Empiric therapy should however not be delayed by procedures for collection of respiratory secretions
iii) Subsequent modification of antibiotics regime as per culture + sensitivity reports
iv) Avoid repeating the same antibiotic class if patient has received it in the past 2 weeks
v) Avoid prolonged use of antibiotics
vi) Consider de-escalation of therapy in appropriate cases

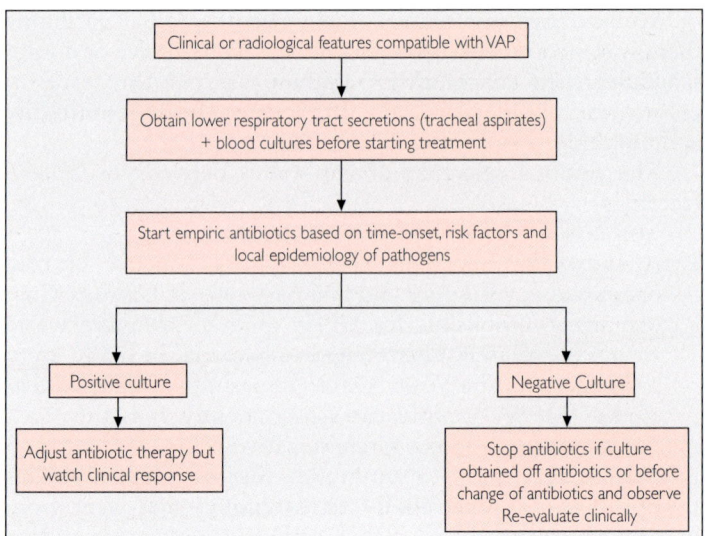

Fig 22.5: Algorithm showing strategy for treatment of VAP.

PROGNOSIS

Nosocomial pneumonia is the leading cause of death due to hospital-acquired infections. The mortality rate ranges from 20—70%. High-risk organisms that lead to increased mortality include *Pseudomonas aeruginosa*, Acinetobacter, Enterobacter, other Gram-negative organisms, *S. faecalis*, *S. aureus*, Candida species, Aspergillus and polymicrobial infections. It must be however remembered that NP is more common in patients who are critically ill with multiple problems. To what extent death can be attributable to NP per se may be impossible to judge. It is likely that many critically ill patients die with pneumonia rather than die of pneumonia.

Death in NP can result from any one or more of the following—septic shock, respiratory failure, multiple organ dysfunction, ARDS, cardiovascular instability, GI bleed. In VAP it could also be occasionally related to barotrauma.

PREVENTION

Prevention of NP is of great importance, both to reduce mortality and morbidity as also to reduce hospital cost. Prevention of aspiration, particularly in the aspiration-prone patient is crucial. Patients on ventilator support and patients fed via a nasogastric tube should have the head end of the bed elevated at 45°. Feeds should be withheld if the earlier feed is retained within the stomach.

Enteral feeding is always preferable to parenteral feeds as the latter predisposes to nosocomial infection.

Sucralfate should be preferred to H_2 antagonists or proton pump inhibitors as prophylactics for GI bleed, as the latter increase the pH of the stomach contents and thereby permit the growth of Gram-negative organisms which may contribute to nosocomial infections including NP. Use of H_2 antagonists or proton pump inhibitors is best reserved for an active GI bleed.

There is divided opinion on the role of decontamination of the upper GI tract in prevention of nososcomial infection, including NP. Decontamination, if practiced, is achieved by the

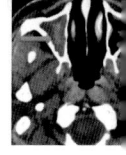

oral use of a combination of non-absorbable antibiotics against Gram-negative bacteria plus an anti-fungal agent.

Patients should be turned frequently; physiotherapy to the chest, deep breathing, increasing mobility in bed all help to prevent atelectasis and infection.

Meticulous asepsis should be observed during suction of tracheal secretions.

Hand-washing before and after examining a patient is an important prophylaxis against transmitted infection. Humidifiers, nebulizers, and all other respiratory equipment should be disinfected or sterilized as necessary.

Oral hygiene is also of crucial importance and may reduce or perhaps prevent the growth of Gram-negative organisms within the oropharynx of critically ill patients.

An infection control team which organizes surveillance of infection, puts into effect measures that prevent and control infection is of crucial importance. A periodic survey and knowledge of the nature of organisms responsible for NP in the wards and in the ICU together with knowledge of the antibiogram is a vital duty of the infection control team.

Table 22.10: PREVENTION—modifying risk factors to reduce incidence of VAP
Non-invasive ventilation in patients with respiratory failure if possible (Level I)
Orotracheal intubation preferred over nasotracheal intubation (Level II)
Continuous aspiration of subglottic secretions if available (Level I)
Condensate collecting in the ventilator circuit should be prevented
Endotracheal tube pressure maintained at 20 cms H_2O (Level II)
Reduce the number of ventilator days (Level II)
Patients should be kept in semi-recumbent position as far as possible (Level I)
Enternal nutrition preferred over parenteral nutrition (Level I)
Oropharyngeal hygiene (Level I)
Avoid or minimize use of paralytic agents and also avoid constant heavy sedation (Level II)
Does prophylactic antibiotic therapy reduce the incidence of VAP? (Level I)
Sucralfate or H_2 antagonist for bleeding prophylaxis? (Level I)

Note: Level I (high)—Evidence comes from at least 1 randomized well-designed, controlled trial. Level II—Evidence obtained from at least one well-designed controlled study without randomization. Level II studies also include any large case series in which systematic analysis of disease patterns and/or microbial etiology was conducted, as well as reports of new therapies that were not collected in a randomized fashion.

SUGGESTED READING

Berton, *et al.* Quantitative versus Qualitative cultures of respiratory secretions for clinical outcomes in patients with Ventilator associated pneumonia. *Cochrane Database of Systematic Reviews.* 2008, Issue 4.

Fagon JY. Hospital-acquired pneumonia: diagnostic strategies: lessons from clinical trials. *Infect Dis Clin North Am.* 1 Dec. 2003; 17(4): 717–26.

Kieninger AN. Hospital-acquired pneumonia: pathophysiology, diagnosis, and treatment. *Surg Clin North Am.* 1 Apr. 2009; 89(2): 439–61, ix.

Kollef MH. Prevention of hospital-associated pneumonia and ventilator-associated pneumonia. *Crit Care Med.* 1 Jun. 2004; 32(6): 1396–405.

Porzecanski I. Diagnosis and treatment of ventilator-associated pneumonia. *Chest.* 1 Aug. 2006; 130(2): 597–604.

Udwadia FE. *Principles of Critical Care Medicine*, second edition. 2005. Oxford University Press, New Delhi.

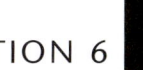
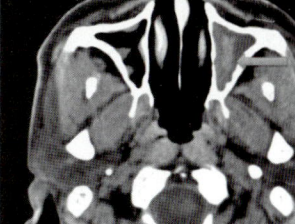
CHAPTER **23**

Non-tuberculous Mycobacterial Infections

GENERAL CONSIDERATIONS

Pulmonary tuberculosis which is endemic in many countries of the world is caused by the *Mycobacterium tuberculosis* complex, which comprises *Mycobacterium tuberculosis* and its geographical variants, *Mycobacterium bovis*, *Mycobacterium africanum*, *Bacillus Calmette-Guérin* (BCG) and *Mycobacterium microti*. This chapter deals with lung disease caused by non-tuberculous mycobacteria (NTM). These mycobacteria were previously called by various names, atypical, anonymous, environmental, opportunistic, potentially pathogenic environmental mycobacteria. At present the terminology of non-tuberculous mycobacteria given by the International Working Group on Mycobacterial Taxonomy is universally accepted.

These 'other mycobacteria' are ubiquitous in the environment, found primarily in both natural and tap water, in soil, dust, animals and food. Exposure to these organisms is therefore unavoidable. However, unlike *M. tuberculosis* and *M. leprae*, NTM are not obligate pathogens. They do not ordinarily cause disease in humans, nor is there evidence of human to human transmission. They are opportunistic organisms which generally cause disease in immunocompromised individuals or if the skin or mucosal barriers are breached. Infections caused by NTM result in pulmonary disease, skin, soft tissue infections and lymphadenitis.

Disseminated infection may occur in patients with AIDS and in patients with interleukin (IL)-12 and interferon (IFN)-γ receptor abnormalities. The confusing aspect is that NTM can exist as contaminants and also as non-infective colonies in the sputum of a significant number of patients with chronic lung disease, including pulmonary tuberculosis due to the *Mycobacterium tuberculosis* complex. The question that often arises in a particular patient with pulmonary disease is whether these mycobacteria are colonizers or infectious agents producing pulmonary disease? Pulmonary infections caused by NTM are clinically and radiologically indistinguishable from tuberculosis caused by *M. tuberculosis*. Therefore it is only when the microbiologist has identified the organism on culture and from other characteristics that a clinician becomes aware that he may well be dealing with infection due to NTM rather than from classic tuberculosis. It needs to be noted that the identification of acid-fast bacilli in a Ziehl-Neelsen-stained sputum specimen cannot reliably distinguish *Mycobacterium tuberculosis* from NTM which may be contaminants or colonizers rather than agents responsible for actual infection. The question that arises in a patient with pulmonary disease who has NTM isolated on culture is—should one start treatment and when does one do so?

Infections caused by the *Mycobacterium avium* complex (MAC) have been increasingly reported from Western countries and recently have also been observed in India. The opportunistic NTM that most commonly cause lung disease are the MAC, *M. kansasii*, *M. scroflulaceum*, *M. xenopi*, and *M. malmoense*. A very small number of pulmonary infections have also been reported due to *M. fortuitum*, *M. chelonae*, *M. simiae*, and *M. szulgai*. There are many other NTM that exist in man's environment. In fact lipid profile and molecular-based techniques have helped in identifying 127 species. Those NTM not mentioned above are saprophytic and for all practical purposes do not produce disease.

EPIDEMIOLOGY

The Developed World

The prevalence of classic tuberculosis shows an overall decline in the developed world. Remarkably, the proportion of non-tuberculous mycobacterial lung disease has shown an increasing trend.

The Centre for Disease Control and Prevention (CDC) reported that one-third of mycobacterial isolates in the United States were NTM in 1979 and 1980. The ratio of TB to NTM isolates declined from 3.2:1 between 1976 and 1981 to 1:1.6 between 1988 and 1991 in a community hospital in the United States. The proportion of NTM to classic *M. tuberculosis* in isolates varies in different geographical areas of the world as also in different parts of the same country. There is however a reported increase in the prevalence of NTM lung disease not just in the United States but in other countries as well.

It is unclear whether this increasing prevalence of NTM lung disease is genuine, or is related to better recognition because of the introduction of quicker and more sensitive laboratory techniques and also because of many more sputum specimens being received for culture and exact identification of mycobacterial growth. In the West, the known association of NTM with diseases such as cystic fibrosis, fibronodular bronchiectasis, and pulmonary disease in post-transplant patients and following iatrogenic immunosuppression has led to a greater awareness of the presence of NTM in these situations leading to a reported increase in prevalence. Other reasons offered to explain the increased prevalence of NTM disease in the West in immunocompetent individuals include a reduced immunity to mycobacteria due to the reduced prevalence of tuberculosis, to the well-nigh universal use of BCG vaccine and the use of 'showering' during bathing. NTM are frequent in tap water; these organisms are aerosolized and concentrated

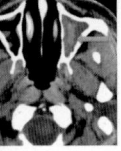

in shower heads leading to greater concentrated exposure with perhaps greater risk of pulmonary infection.

MAC is considered to be the most frequent organism causing NTM lung disease. Other pathogens isolated in NTM lung disease include *M. kansasi, M. malmoense, M. xenopi* and the rapid growing mycobacteria, *M. abscessus* and *M. fortuitum.*

A genuine reason for an increase in the prevalence of NTM lung disease is the great AIDS pandemic. The great degree of immune suppression observed in this disease has led to over a million hosts with AIDS rendered susceptible to infections with opportunistic infections, including infection by NTM.

India and the Developing World

There is a great paucity of reports of NTM disease from India and the developing world. This is for two reasons—(1) Except in well-equipped laboratories of tertiary hospitals in the large cities of India and in a few research centres, mycobacterial specimens positive for AFB on a Ziehl-Neelsen stain are presumed to be related to tuberculosis and are not routinely cultured. (2) There is no paucity of AIDS patients in India and the developing countries and these constitute ready hosts for opportunistic infections. However, tuberculosis is widely prevalent in the developing world and AIDS patients die of tuberculosis or other infections before the CD4 count falls low enough for NTM disease to occur. There is now increasing evidence to show that NTM are present in our environment. Paramasivan and colleagues from the Tuberculosis Research Centre in Chennai in 1985 *(Ref: Paramasivan CN, Govindan D et al—Species level identification of NTM from South Indin BCG trial area during 1981.Tubercle 1985:66:9–15)* reported *M. avium intracellulare* (MAI) to be the most frequent isolated species (22.6% of all NTM), followed by *M. terrae* (12.5%) and *M. scrofulaceum* (10.5%). In 1994 Kamala and colleagues *(Kamala T, Paramasivan CN et al Evaluation of procedures for isolation of NTM from soil and water samples obtained in Northern India. Appl Environ. Microbiology 2004;70 (6): 3751–53)* showed that MAI and *M. scrofulaceum* were present in water and dust and could be isolated from sputum samples of individuals. In 2004, a similar study demonstrated *M. avium, M. terrae, M. fortuitum* and *M. chelonae* in water and *M. avium, M. terrae* and *M. chelonae* in soil.

In 2007, a study from Wardha collected soil and water samples from the environment of those patients from whom NTM were isolated in clinical samples. Though *M. avium* was isolated in four of the soil isolates, molecular typing did not show the strain to be the same as that isolated from a patient.

The data on the pathogenicity of NTM in India is scarce. In 2005, NTM bacteraemia was reported by Narang and colleagues in HIV-seropositive patients *(Ref: Narang P, Narang R, Mendiratta DK, Roy D, Deotale V, Yakrus MA, et al. Isolation of Mycobacterium avium complex and M. simiae from blood of AIDS patients from Sevagram, Maharashtra. Indian J Tuberc 2005;52: 21–6).* This was the first report demonstrating dissemination of NTM infection in India. Similar cases have been reported and many more await recognition in our part of the world.

The rate of NTM bacteraemia in AIDS patients in the Mahatma Gandhi Institute of Medical Sciences, Wardha, in 2002 was 8.5%. In 2007 it had fallen to 5.3%, probably due to anti-retroviral therapy (ART) given to AIDS patients at an AIDS centre close to the hospital.

We have seen proven NTM pulmonary disease in a few immunocompetent patients in our unit. Greater awareness and better laboratory facilities will uncover the slowly increasing role of NTM infection in both immunocompetent and immunocompromised hosts.

CLINICAL FEATURES

There is very little or no data from developing countries with regard to pulmonary disease produced by NTM. In the West the four species of NTM most frequently responsible for lung disease are *M. avium-intracellulare-scrofulaceum* (MAIS), *M. kansasii, M. malmoense,* and *M. xenopi.* The clinical and radiological features do not differ among these four species. The following clinical profiles have been reported from the West:

Cavitatory Lung Disease

Over half the patients have pre-existing lung disease, chiefly chronic obstructive pulmonary disease (COPD); some have old healed tuberculosis. The clinical features are indistinguishable from pulmonary tuberculosis and include fever, cough, sputum, haemoptysis, weight loss and increasing breathlessness. At least 10% are asymptomatic. There are often added features of chronic obstructive lung disease. The X-ray and CT appearances are indistinguishable from pulmonary tuberculosis and consist of infiltrates with cavitation in either one or both lungs chiefly involving the upper lobes.

Fibronodular Bronchiectasis

In Western studies, 12% of patients with MAC demonstrated a reticular fibrotic radiographic pattern rather than cavitatory disease. Sputum cultures showed either *M. kansasii* or MAC. Fibronodular bronchiectasis was observed in the absence of cavitation and in patients without pre-existing lung disease or immunosuppression. Cough and sputum production are the most common symptoms; haemoptysis may also occur. Fibronodular bronchiectasis has been termed Lady Windemere's syndrome after the play by Oscar Wilde. It is believed to occur in elderly women who suppress their cough so that infected secretions are retained in the middle lobe and lingula. It is suggested that MAC induces peribronchial inflammation and thickening that can progress to severe cystic bronchiectasis.

Hypersensitivity Pneumonitis

A syndrome indistinguishable from hypersensitivity pneumonitis has been described in the West in patients exposed to solutions that contain NTM. Granulomatous disease has thus been reported after exposure to hot tub baths that contain MAC.

CONDITIONS ASSOCIATED WITH NTM LUNG DISEASE

It is now increasingly recognized that NTM can perhaps contribute to disease progression and may be present in a number of

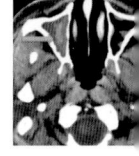

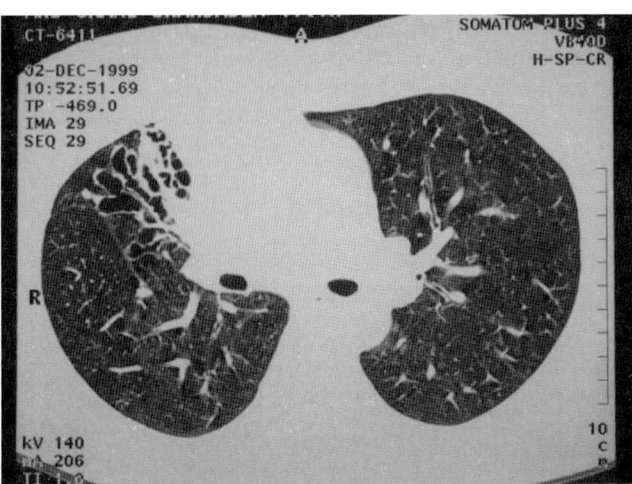

Fig 23.1: HRCT chest reveals cystic bronchiectasis in the right middle lobe with atelectasis; BAL revealed atypical mycobacteria. This is an example of Lady Windemere's syndrome.

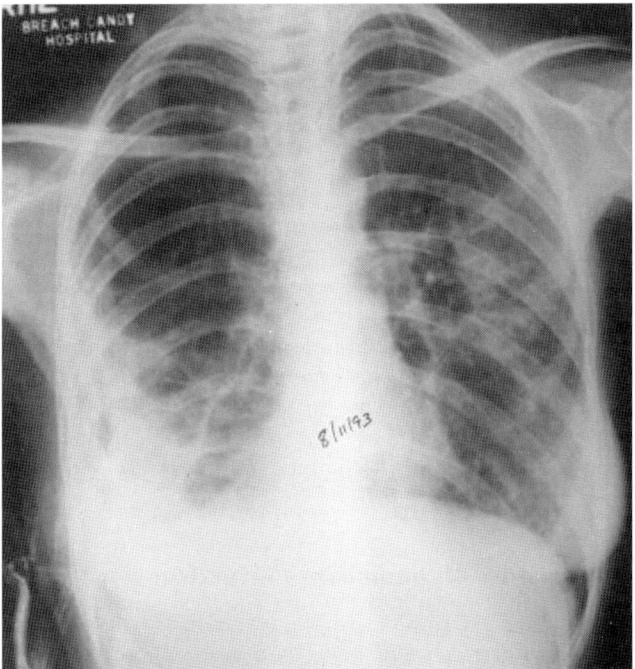

Fig 23.2: X-ray chest reveals ill-defined consolidations with associated fibrosis and cavitation in the left mid-zone and right lung bases. BAL revealed MAC.

pulmonary pathologies—COPD, cystic fibrosis, old healed tuberculosis, silicosis, bronchiectasis and pulmonary alveolar proteinosis. It must be accepted that in a given patient it may indeed be difficult to determine whether the presence of NTM constitutes colonization or actually contributes directly to the disease.

NTM Pulmonary Disease in The Immunocompromised Patient

NTM are opportunistic organisms and are more likely to cause disease in immunosuppressed patients as compared to immunocompetent patients.

NTM disease has been reported after solid organ transplants and in haemopoietic stem cell transplants. NTM pulmonary disease is reported to be relatively uncommon after renal transplants.

The use of tumour necrosis factor antagonists—infliximab and etanercept in rheumatoid disease, Crohn's disease and several other inflammatory conditions has also led to infections with NTM though unquestionably infection due to tuberculosis is more frequent.

Finally, a background of HIV infection with low CD_4 counts (< 100 cells/ uL) is the ideal breeding ground for several opportunistic infections including NTM. Disseminated NTM disease occurs when the CD_4 count is < 50 cells/ uL. *M. avium* is the most common cause of disseminated disease in HIV patients. Paradoxically, patients with disseminated disease rarely have pulmonary disease, though the sputum may be positive on culture for *M. avium-intracellulare*.

The other NTM associated with HIV infection is *M. kansasii*. Pulmonary disease due to infection with *M. kansasii* generally occurs without dissemination. This probably reflects the fact that *M. kansasii* is more pathogenic than MAC and that it causes disease in patients who are less immunosuppressed.

LABORATORY IDENTIFICATION

The details of microbiological identification of NTM are beyond the scope of this chapter. The species of most clinically relevant NTM can be established by cultural and basic biochemical tests. These involve pigment production, temperature range in which growth occurs, oxygen preference and the ability to hydrolyse tween 80.

Amplification techniques targeting specific DNA sequences are being used in special reference laboratories for quicker identification. Thus commercial DNA probes that target ribosomal RNA allow rapid identification of *M. tuberculosis*, MAC, *M. avium*, and *M. intracellulare*. Other techniques to identify NTM include high-performance liquid chromatography (HPLC) and genetic techniques directed to 65 kd heat shock protein genes and the 16S ribosomal RNA. These genetic techniques include amplification as in the polymerized chain reaction (PCR), probe hybridization, restriction fragment length polymorphism (RFLP) and DNA sequencing.

SUSCEPTIBILITY

The drug sensitivity patterns of clinically relevant NTM are shown below. The *in vitro* sensitivity of *M. kansasii* to rifampicin and ethambutol corresponds to the clinical effectiveness against the mycobacterium. However, with respect to the other NTMs there seems to be a lack of correlation between *in vitro* sensitivity and clinical response to treatment. A recent prospective trial by the British Thoracic Society has confirmed this *(Ref: BTS research Committee. First randomized trial of treatments for pulmonary disease caused by M avium intracellulare, M malmoense, and M xenopi in HIV negative patients: rifampicin, ethambutol and isoniazid versus rifampicin and ethambutol. Thorax 2001; 56:167–172 doi:10.1136/thorax.56.3.167).* There is also a degree of synergy between rifampicin and ethambutol, in that each drug individually may be ineffective but when combined becomes effective. This is with specific reference to strains of MAIS (*M. scrofulaceum* and *M. avium-intracellulare*), *M. xenopi*

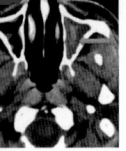

Table 23.1: Sensitivity of opportunistic mycobacteria to individual anti-tuberculosis drugs in vitro						
Species	INH	Rifampicin	Ethambutol	Streptomycin	Cipro	Ethio
M.kansasii	R	S	S	B	V	S
MAIS complex	R	R	R	R	R	S
M.malmoense	R	V	V	R	S	S
M.xenopi	R	V	R	S	S	S

Note: INH: Isoniazed; Cipro: Ciprofloxacin; Ethio: Ethionamide R-Resistant, S-Sensitive, B-Borderline, V-Variable.

and *M. malmoense*. The significance of *in vitro* sensitivity tests of the newer drugs (quinolones, clarithromycin, azithromycin, rifabutin) in relation to actual clinical response against NTM infection is not yet known. It is however recommended that in *M. kansasii* infection reported to be resistant to rifampicin, sensitivity tests to all other first-line and newer drugs may help in management.

DIAGNOSIS

Certain principles must be kept in mind if NTM pulmonary infection is to be diagnosed with a fair degree of accuracy once these organisms have been identified by the microbiological laboratory.

1. NTM are ubiquitous, may be present in the water used in the laboratory and contaminate respiratory secretions. Contaminations must be distinguished from infection.
2. NTM may colonize the respiratory tract, particularly in patients with chronic respiratory disease and may not be actually responsible for infection. Colonization should be distinguished from infection. Admittedly, this may at times be impossibly difficult.
3. Persistent or progressive symptoms with repeated isolation of the same species of NTM, coupled with progressive radiological changes for which there is no other explanation suggests infection rather than colonization.

The American Thoracic Society has published the following guidelines as diagnostic criteria before starting long-term therapy:

1. NTM must be cultured a minimum of three times in the preceding years or twice if one of the specimens is positive for mycobacterium in patients presenting with features compatible with NTM pulmonary disease. It is however mandatory by proper testing to exclude infection by *M. tuberculosis*.
2. The diagnosis of NTM can also be confirmed if NTM are in greater than 1+ density on stained smear or on culture of bronchoalveolar lavage (BAL).
3. The diagnosis of NTM is also confirmed if a lung biopsy shows characteristic features of granulomatous infection together with a sputum or BAL that contain NTM on smear or culture.

Some researchers are of the opinion that recommending repeated positive cultures is too stringent a requirement,

in particular for *M. kansasii* infection. Perhaps even a single positive culture when combined with compatible clinical features should warrant start of therapy.

TREATMENT

Treatment of *M. kansasii*

Recommendations given below are based on a prospective study of ethambutol and rifampicin carried out by the British Thoracic Society (BTS). *(Ref: Mycobacterium kansasii pulmonary infection: a prospective study of the results of nine months of treatment with rifampicin and ethambutol. Research Committee, British Thoracic Society.)*

Nine months' treatment with rifampicin and ethambutol was associated with a 10% relapse/re-infection rate. Perhaps chemotherapy should be given to patients for 15–24 months.

Treatment of MAIS complex

In a prospective BTS study, rifampicin and ethambutol or rifampicin, isoniazid and ethambutol were given for two years. At the end of five years, 36% of 75 patients had died, but in only three patients was death directly attributable to infection with MAIS complex.

Considering the result of this study as also other studies, an appropriate recommendation would be to use rifampicin and ethambutol for two years adding empirically one or more of the following drugs—isoniazid, clarithromycin, ciprofloxacin, streptomycin, rifabutin if the patient fails to respond. The ongoing BTS study will give further information on the role of clarithromycin, quinolones and immunotherapy in *Mycobacterium vaccae*. *(Ref: Treatment of Pulmonary Disease Caused by MAIS, M. Xenopi or M. Malmoense: A Comparison of Two Triple-Drug Regimens and an Assessment of the Value of Immunotherapy With M. Vaccae, Research Committee of the British Thoracic Society.)*

Treatment of *M. malmoense* Infection

Ethambutol and rifampicin are the two main drugs in treatment; the duration of treatment being two years. A randomized trial of two regimens—ethambutol and rifampicin and rifampicin, ethambutol, and isoniazid for two years showed no differences in the outcome between the two groups. After five years, 34% had died, 42% were still alive and cured, and 10% had failed to become culture-negative or had relapsed. *(Ref: First randomized trial of treatments for pulmonary disease caused by M. avium-intracellulare, M. malmoense, and M. xenopi in HIV-negative patients: rifampicin, ethambutol and isoniazid versus rifampicin and ethambutol, Research Committee of the British Thoracic Society.)*

Ciprofloxacin and clarithromycin are often reported to be effective *in vitro* but their clinical efficacy has not been proven.

Treatment of *M. xenopi* Infection

In the BTS study, the death rate was higher than that reported for *M. kansasii*, MAIS and *M. malmoense*, though only a small minority died because of the mycobacterial disease.

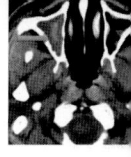

The present recommendation is to use ethambutol and rifampicin or rifampicin, ethambutol, and isoniazid for two years. Streptomycin may be added if the response is inadequate. The efficacy of ciprofloxacin and clarithromycin is undetermined.

TREATMENT OF NTM PULMONARY INFECTION IN INDIA AND DEVELOPING COUNTRIES

The identification of the exact species of NTM causing pulmonary infection is a luxury given to very few research laboratories in developing countries. If a diagnosis of NTM infection is made on the basis of clinical features and by laboratory investigations through basic culture and biochemical tests, how does one proceed if species identification is not available. Results of the BTS study show that rifampicin, ethambutol, together with isoniazid are the key drugs in treating these infections. If the response is inadequate, our present state of knowledge dictates that additional drugs should be used empirically. These could include a quinolone or clarithromycin or streptomycin or ethionamide. Two of these may perhaps be added to the basic regime. The simpler the combination of drugs the less toxic the effects and greater the compliance.

The Role of Surgery

If a NTM pulmonary infection fails to respond, surgery should be considered if the disease is localized, if the patient is fit for surgery and if lung functions render surgical treatment feasible. Very often, the presence of bilateral disease or crippling background disease in the form of COPD renders surgery impossible. If surgery is performed successfully for localized disease, chemotherapy should be continued for a further period of 18 months to two years.

TREATMENT OF NTM INFECTION IN AIDS

Response to therapy depends not so much on antimicrobial therapy as on the degree of immunocompromise.

In AIDS the infection may not be confined to the lungs but may be systemic with persistent bacteraemia. In these patients the prognosis is poor. The use of highly active antiretroviral therapy (HAART) has considerably improved prognosis in NTM infection with AIDS. The recommended treatment for MAIS complex, *M. malmoense* or *M. xenopi* is rifampicin, ethambutol and clarithromycin. Therapy should be continued indefinitely as discontinuation leads to either relapse or recurrence. In poor developing countries where species identification is not possible the above regime should be promptly started as it covers the management of all major NTM species causing pulmonary infection including *M. kansasii*.

It should be noted that drug interaction between rifampicin, macrolides and protease inhibitors may render the choice of antimicrobial regimens difficult.

SUGGESTED READING

BTS research committee. First randomised trial of treatments for pulmonary disease caused by M avium intracellulare, M malmoeuse, and M venopi in HIV negative patients: rifampicin, ethambutol and isoniazid versus rifampicin and ethambutol. *Thorax.* 2001; 56: 167–172 doi:10.1136/thorax.56.3.167.

Field SK. Lung disease due to the more common nontuberculous mycobacteria. *Chest.* 1 Jun. 2006; 129(6): 1653–72.

Glassroth J. Pulmonary disease due to nontuberculous mycobacteria. *Chest.* 1 Jan. 2008; 133(1): 243–51.

Griffith DE. Diagnosing nontuberculous mycobacterial lung disease. A process in evolution. *Infect Dis Clin North Am.* 1 Mar. 2002; 16(1): 235–49.

Kamala T, Paramasivan CN, Herbert D, Venkatesan P, Prabhakar R. Evaluation of procedures for isolation of NTM from soil and water samples obtained in Northern India. *Appl Environ. Microbiology.* 2004; 70(6): 3751–3.

Narang P, Narang R, Mendiratta DK, Roy D, Deotale V, Yakrus MA, *et al.* Isolation of Mycobacterium avium complex and M. simiae from blood of AIDS patients from Sevagram; Maharashtra. *Indian J Tuberc.* 2005; 52: 21–6.

Piersimoni C. Pulmonary infections associated with non-tuberculous mycobacteria in immunocompetent patients. *Lancet Infect Dis.* 1 May 2008; 8(5): 323–34.

Schluger NW. Tuberculosis and nontuberculous mycobacterial infections in older adults. *Clin Chest Med.* 1 Dec. 2007; 28(4): 773–81, vi.

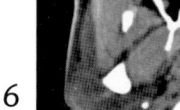

DEFINITION

Bronchiectasis (bronchus-tube; ectasis-to stretch) is a chronic respiratory disease characterized by a permanent abnormal dilatation of bronchi. This structural abnormality of the bronchi predisposes to retention of respiratory secretions and to bronchial infection. Chronic bronchial suppuration results and is characterized by cough with expectorating of mucopurulent sputum which in many patients is copious in quantity.

TYPES OF BRONCHIECTASIS

The dilatation of bronchi may take several forms:

1. Cystic or saccular bronchiectasis is observed when there is severe damage to the bronchial wall so that balloon-like dilatation of the bronchial wall is observed. Though this form of bronchiectasis is now uncommon in the developed world because of vaccination against childhood illnesses, improved socioeconomic conditions and access to good healthcare; it still persists in India and poor countries of the world. Cystic bronchiectasis is generally a result of severe viral (e.g. measles) or bacterial infection in childhood and is characterized by finger clubbing and by the production of large quantities of sputum.
2. Cylindrical bronchiectasis results from a lesser degree of damage to the bronchial wall and is characterized by cylindrical dilatation of the bronchi. It is often diffuse, the lower lobes being more frequently involved.
3. Varicose bronchiectasis features focal areas of bronchial constrictions, a stenosis in the cylindrically dilated bronchi.
4. Traction bronchiectasis occurs in patients with well-marked pulmonary fibrosis, the fibrosis pulling the bronchial walls apart.

EPIDEMIOLOGY

The prevalence of bronchiectasis is difficult to ascertain as published reports even in the West are based mainly on study of chest radiographs which are not sensitive in diagnosing bronchiectasis. The prevalence is certainly underestimated as the advent of high-resolution computed tomography (HRCT) scans has revealed bronchiectasis in patients who would have otherwise remained undiagnosed. CT scans have also uncovered milder forms of bronchiectasis as in patients with chronic obstructive pulmonary disease (COPD), chronic asthma and in smokers with chronic bronchitis. A high incidence of bronchiectasis has been reported in certain ethnic groups e.g.

native Americans in North America, Maoris in New Zealand and Western Samorians. It is uncertain whether this increased prevalence is related to genetic factors or to environmental influences. Population surveys to determine the prevalence of bronchiectasis will only be accurate if cheap, widely applicable yet accurate imaging techniques are developed in the future.

AETIOLOGY

There are a number of known causes that are briefly discussed below. Yet in a number of patients (perhaps close to a half), the cause remains unknown.

Post-Infective

A lower respiratory tract infection may damage the bronchial walls leading to bronchiectasis. In India, childhood illnesses, in particular measles, other viral infections, and whooping cough are the main culprits. Tuberculosis is another important aetiological factor in countries where the prevalence rate of this disease is high. Bronchiectasis related to tuberculosis is generally seen in the upper lobes. However, in lungs severely damaged by extensive tuberculosis, bronchiectasis is often extensive and diffuse. Bacterial infection causing pneumonia could also damage bronchi sufficiently to result in localized bronchiectasis but the cause and effect in many instances remains uncertain. Bronchiectasis is often observed in Mcleod's syndrome, a form of obliterative bronchiolitis due to infection occurring in childhood. The insult to the developing lung results in the radiological finding of a unilateral hypovascular, hyperlucent lung with increased air-trapping clearly demonstrated in expiratory film.

Mechanical Obstruction

Mechanical bronchial obstruction, either luminal (foreign body, growth) or due to a bronchial stenosis or due to extrinsic pressure (e.g. from lymphadenopathy) can cause bronchiectasis. Two mechanisms operate: (a) The occurrence of atelectasis causing a pull on the bronchial walls due to negative intrapleural pressure; (b) poor drainage of bronchial secretions with resulting infection and damage to the bronchial wall. The second mechanism is probably the main reason for bronchiectasis in these situations.

Brock syndrome or the middle lobe syndrome is characterized by shrinkage of the middle lobe together with bronchiectasis of this lobe, caused by extrinsic pressure on the middle lobe bronchus, usually due to tuberculous lymphadenopathy. The middle lobe is more prone to atelectasis

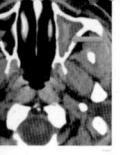

with subsequent bronchiectasis because it is long, narrow, acutely angulated and surrounded by a cuff of lymph glands. The narrow acutely angulated middle lobe bronchus may also be predisposed to bronchiectatic changes in conditions associated with poor mucus clearance as in primary ciliary dyskinesia. Non-tuberculous adenopathy can also occasionally lead to this syndrome. A stenosis of the middle lobe bronchus, again generally tuberculous in nature, also produces the middle lobe syndrome. Lady Windemere's syndrome is encountered in middle-aged ladies with ineffective cough. It is characterized by middle lobe bronchiectasis with infection caused by non-tuberculous mycobacteria.

Non-infective Inflammatory Obliterative Bronchiolitis and Pneumonitis

Inhalation of toxic gases like chlorine, ammonia or smoke can inflame bronchial mucosa and damage bronchial walls leading to bronchiectasis. The basic pathology due to inhalation of toxic gases is an obliterative bronchiolitis; however, damage to walls of the larger bronchi leads to cylindrical bronchiectasis. Acid reflux with aspiration into the lung can cause episodes of airways' obstruction. Whether chronic aspiration could ultimately lead to bronchiectatic changes is purely speculative.

Immune-Mediated Causes

This is classically observed in allergic bronchopulmonary aspergillosis which results over time to well-marked proximal bronchiectasis chiefly involving the upper lobes. Bronchiectasis is due to two main factors: a) atelectasis caused by inspissated plugs of mucus, containing fungal hyphae; (b) Type I and III immune-mediated responses to the *Aspergillus fumigatus* colonizing the airways leading to damage to the bronchial wall. A fuller description of allergic bronchopulmonary aspergillosis is given in a separate chapter.

Conditions causing obliterative bronchiolitis can also damage large airways leading to cylindrical bronchiectasis. This is observed in chronic graft vs. host disease, lung transplant rejection, rheumatoid arthritis and rarely, following the use of drugs such as penicillamine.

Immune Deficiency

Immune deficiency should always be suspected in patients with recurrent acute pulmonary infection rather than in those with persistent chronic infection. Agammoglobulinaemia or hypogammaglobulinaemia is the commonest immune deficiency detected in these patients. It leads to repeated episodes of lower respiratory tract infections including pneumonia. Bronchiectasis often results. Immunoglobulin G (IgG) subclass deficiency (deficiency in IgG$_2$) is in particular associated with pneumonia due to pneumococcus. Repeated infections can lead to bronchiectasis. IgA deficiency or absence occurs in 0.1–0.2% of the population. In some patients, particularly when associated with IgG$_2$ deficiency, repeated respiratory infections occur resulting in bronchiectasis.

An acquired immunodeficient state exists in patients with multiple myeloma, lymphoma and lymphatic leukaemia.

Recurrent respiratory infections can occur, leading to some degree of cylindrical bronchiectasis. Bronchiectasis can also complicate HIV infection following frequent respiratory infections.

Impaired Mucociliary Clearance

Impaired mucociliary clearance results in chronic or recurrent bronchial infection and inflammation leading to damage to bronchial walls and bronchiectasis. The three conditions causing impaired mucociliary clearance are primary ciliary dyskinesia, Young's syndrome and cystic fibrosis (CF).

Primary ciliary dyskinesia is a rare autosomal recessive condition with incomplete penetration, characterized by ultrastructural abnormalities in the cilia. The abnormalities consist of absence of one or both of the dyenin arms, or an abnormality of the microtubules or radial spokes. As a result the cilia are either immotile, beat slowly or beat in a disorderly fashion or in different directions, thereby impairing mucus clearance.

Cilia line not just the bronchi (right up to the respiratory bronchiole) but the nose, paranasal sinuses, the middle ear and eustachian tubes and the tail of spermatozoa. Poor ciliary function is present in all these sites, so that bronchiectasis is often associated with chronic sinusitis, middle ear disease and infertility. Impaired ciliary function may present in the neonatal period with mucus plugging, atelectasis and pneumonia. More frequently, symptoms of recurrent infection are observed in childhood and adolescence. In 50% of patients with primary ciliary dyskinesia, there is a dextrocardia and some of these patients also have a situs inversus. The triad of bronchiectasis, dextrocardia with or without situs inversus and chronic sinusitis together with infertility in adult males constitute the Kartegener's syndrome, named after the paediatrician who first described it. This syndrome is related to a genetic abnormality characterized by the presence of XXY.

Young's syndrome is rare and is characterized by the triad of bronchiectasis, sinusitis and azoospermia due to functional (i.e. non-obstructive) blockage in the head of the epididymis which is usually enlarged on palpation. The respiratory secretions are viscid, leading to prolonged, delayed mucociliary transport. The cause of Young's syndrome is not known though it has been linked to mercury poisoning in childhood.

Cystic fibrosis (CF) is the most important cause of impaired mucociliary transport. The disease though common in the West has a comparatively low prevalence in India.

The overall outlook and prognosis is much worse in CF when compared to primary ciliary dyskinesia, despite absent mucociliary clearance in the latter condition. The poor mucociliary clearance in CF is because of reduced hydration and increased viscosity of airway secretions due to abnormal ion transport. Early infection of bronchi is often due to *S. aureus* and *H. influenzae* but ultimately chronic recurrent infection at a young age is due to *P. aeruginosa*. The host-bacteria interaction is probably related to the basic genetic defect in CF. An antimicrobial peptide β deficiency which normally protects the bronchial epithelium from infection has been shown to be inactivated by the increased salt content of the airway secretion in CF. It has also been shown that *P. aeruginosa* adheres more strongly and in greater numbers to CF epithelial bronchial cells.

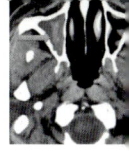

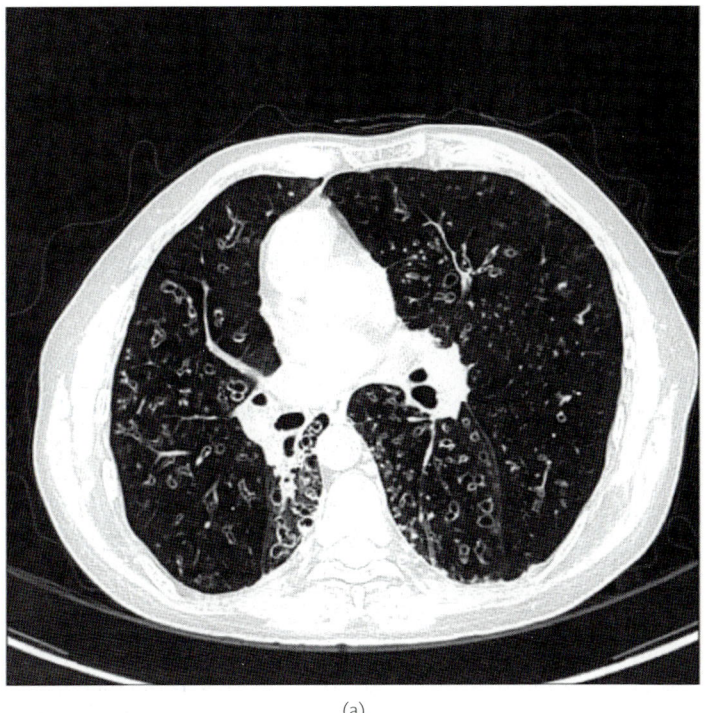

(a)

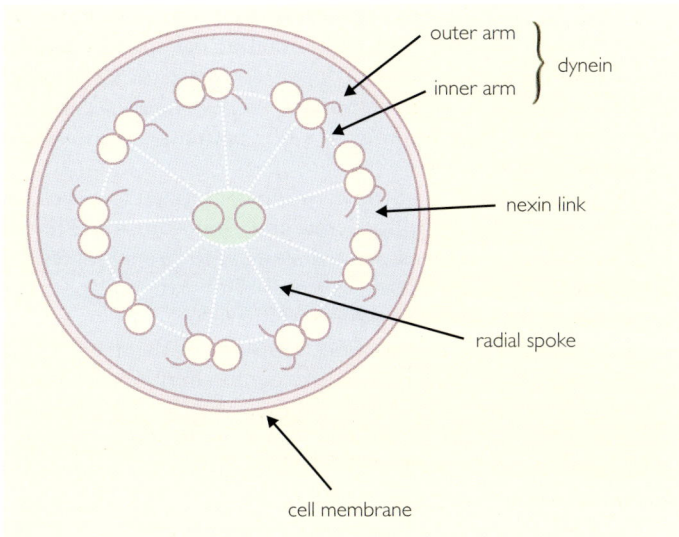

Fig 24.2: Normal cilia. Schematic cross-sectional sketch of a normal ciliary shaft showing the '9-2' arrangement of microtubules, small amount of matrix, and ciliary membrane. In ciliary dyskenisia, there is an absence of one or both dynein arms or an abnormality of the radial spokes. The cilia are therefore immotile, beat slowly or in a disorderly fashion leading to poor mucociliary clearance.

Pulmonary Fibrosis

Fibrosis from any cause (cryptogenic fibrosing alveolitis, sarcoidosis, tuberculosis, radiation effect) if severe enough, can lead to traction bronchiectasis.

Inflammatory Bowel Disease

Ulcerative colitis is a known association of bronchiectasis. To a lesser extent bronchiectasis is also associated in some patients with Crohn's disease and coeliac disease. Two kinds of presentation are observed in ulcerative colitis. The first is after total colectomy in patients with severe ulcerative colitis. Cough and purulent sputum occur soon after, due to bronchiectasis. The second presentation is when patients with one condition develop the other several years later.

Other Causes and Conditions

1. Congenital bronchiectasis can result because of absence or diminished amounts of cartilage in the bronchi (William Campbell syndrome). Bronchial dilatation results because of disruption of the bronchial architecture. Bronchiectasis also occurs in congenital tracheomalacia, in Ehlers-Danlos syndrome and Marfan's syndrome due to atrophy or lack of elastic or muscular elements in the bronchi. Intralobar sequestrations have dead-end bronchi which retain secretions and can get repeatedly infected leading to bronchiectasis.

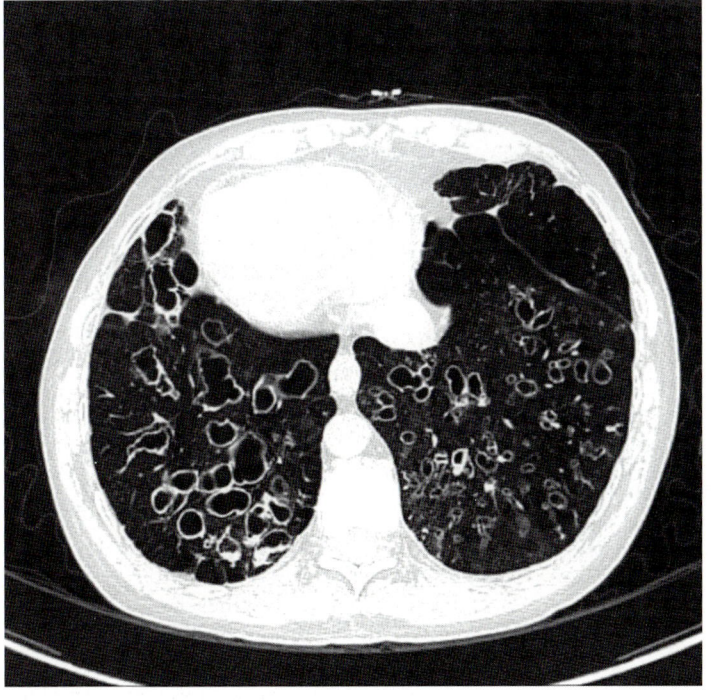

(b)

Fig 24.1a and b: Kartegener's syndrome. HRCT chest reveals cystic bronchiectasis in both lung fields with dextrocardia.

This again is probably related to the basic genetic mutational defect in the long arm of Chromosome 7 in patients with CF, which leads to abnormalities in the CF transmembrane conductance regulator.

2. Pulmonary involvement in the form of obliterative bronchiolitis and/or bronchiectasis is an important manifestation of rheumatoid arthritis, Sjogren's syndrome and other connective tissue disorders.

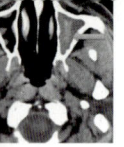

3. Panbronchiolitis characterized by dyspnoea, cough with productive sputum and inflammation of the bronchial walls was first described in Japan and then in China and Korea. It is less recognized outside these countries. We have encountered this pathology in a few patients. It can lead to bronchiectasis.

4. The yellow nail syndrome is characterized by yellow dystrophic nails, lymphoedema and rhinosinusitis. Pleural effusion may also be associated along with bronchiectasis.

5. Idiopathic bronchiectasis A number of patients (perhaps close to 50%) with bronchiectasis have no definite attributable cause. There is at times a history of recurrent colds and cough associated with wheezing in childhood. A latent period of good health is then followed by the development of bronchiectasis between the age of 20–30 years. At times the features of bronchiectasis seem to be the result of a viral infection which did not completely resolve. Whether there is any relation between cause and effect in these situations and if so the mechanism of initiation and perpetuation of the disease is unclear.

6. Non-tuberculous mycobacteria (NTM) and bronchiectasis: NTMs known to be associated with bronchiectasis include *Mycobacterium avium-intracellulare* complex (MAC) and *M. Kansasii*. These cause a progressive bronchiectasis usually restricted to the middle lobe and lingula. This affects otherwise healthy, non-smoking, older women of slender build and the resulting syndrome is called Lady Windermere syndrome.

Table 24.1: Causes of bronchiectasis	
Post-infective	Measles, other viral infection, whooping cough, tuberculosis, bacterial infection
Mechanical obstruction	Intraluminal (foreign body, tumour) and external compression (lymphadenopathy)
Non-infective inflammation	Inhalation of toxic gases
Immune-mediated causes	Allergic bronchopulmonary aspergillosis, chronic graft vs host disease, rejection of lung transplant
Impaired mucociliary clearance	Primary ciliary dyskinesia, Young's syndrome, Cystic fibrosis
Immune deficiency	Hypogammaglobulinemia, IgG deficiency, IgA deficiency, HIV infection
Pulmonary fibrosis	Tuberculosis, sarcoidosis, cryptogenic fibrosing alveolitis
Congenital	Intralobar pulmonary sequestration; defects in bronchial wall
Miscellaneous	Inflammatory bowel disease, connective tissue disease (Rheumatoid arthritis)

PATHOPHYSIOLOGY

The development of bronchiectasis depends on an infectious insult leading to mucosal inflammation and tissue damage and/or an impairment of host defences. These factors interact to form a self-perpetuating vicious cycle. Thus tissue damage resulting

from mucosal inflammation predisposes to recurrent or chronic mucosal infection. Also, tissue damage will impair local host defences which in turn predisposes to recurrent or chronic mucosal infection. The initiation of this vicious cycle may be either through an infectious mucosal insult or an impairment of host defence either congenital or acquired, the former being more common than the latter. Bronchial obstruction, whatever the aetiology, is one other factor which could induce bronchiectasis through impairment of mucociliary drainage which invites infection distal to the obstructed bronchus.

Inflammation results in destruction of the mucosa, the elastin layer of the bronchial wall, as also the muscle and cartilaginous elements of the bronchus which show varying degrees of destruction. The bronchial architecture is lost and the bronchi permanently dilate. Neutrophils are drawn to the lumen of the bronchi; the bronchial wall shows well-marked lymphocytic infiltration resembling the follicular type of bronchiectasis described several years ago. Copious secretions may block these dilated bronchi as it becomes difficult to clear the viscid mucus through cough or ciliary movement. Bacteria adhere to and multiply within the mucus perpetuating both infection and inflammation. The inflammation extends into the bronchioles and in longstanding cases there results obstruction of the small airways through fibrosis. There is therefore invariably some degree of airways obstruction in patients with bronchiectasis.

The host response to infection is through both B lymphocyte activity and cell-mediated T-cell response. Tissue injury is mediated by neutrophils (attracted to the lumen of inflamed bronchi through chemotaxis) which liberate proteases and oxidants, and through cytokines such as Interleukin 8 and other mediators from host cells. Serum levels of adhesin molecules

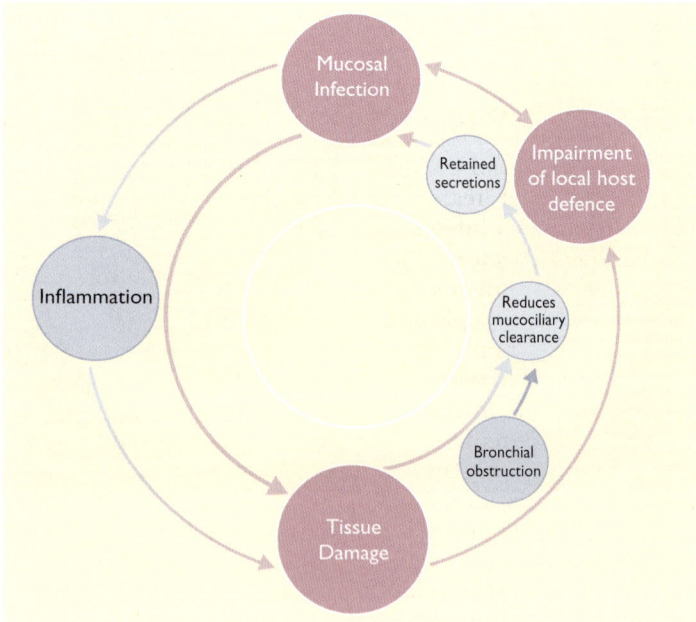

Fig 24.3: Pathophysiology of bronchiectasis. Mucosal inflammation and impairment of host defences result in an interactive self perpetuating viscious cycle leading to bronchiectasis. The initation of the cycle may predominantly be due to mucosal infection or primarily due to impairment of host defence. Occasionally bronchial obstruction is the initiating cause; it acts by impairing mucociliary clearance, and thereby promoting mucosal infection. Mucosal infection spreads to involvement of the bronchial walls as well.

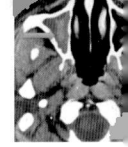

are elevated suggesting endothelial activation, probably within the lungs.

Unfortunately, the inflammatory response fails to eradicate infection in patients with well-marked established bronchiectasis. This is partly due to impaired host defences, the large bacterial population within the bronchi and perhaps due to certain properties of the infecting bacteria.

Commonly found pathogens in patients with bronchiectasis in our units are Gram-negative organisms like *Klebsiella pneumoniae, H. influenzae, Pseudmonas aeruginosa* and Gram-positive organisms like *Staphylococcus aureus* and *Streptococcus pneumoniae*.

A study of 100 patients with bronchiectasis in Hong Kong showed that P. aeruginosa was the most frequent pathogen found in the sputum sample with *H. influenzae* being the second most frequent.

Table 24.2:
Sputum pathogen amongst 100 bronchiectasis patients in Hong Kong

Pathogen	% of frequency
Pseudomonas aeruginosa	33
H.influenzae	10
Streptococcus pneumoniae	6
S. aureus	5
Other gram-negative bacilli	5
NTM	3
Moraxella catarrhalis	2
Yeast	1

Source: Ho PL, Lam WK et al. The effects of Pseudomonas aeruginosa infection in clinical parameters in steady state bronchiectasis. *Chest.* 1998; 114: 1623–9.

CLINICAL FEATURES

Chronic cough and expectoration of mucopurulent sputum are the cardinal features of bronchiectasis. Patients with chronic persistent infection expectorate purulent sputum daily. Those with recurrent episodes of infection bring up large quantities of purulent sputum during periods of exacerbation. In between acute episodes, some degree of cough with expectoration generally persists. At times acute exacerbations may be associated with a marked decrease in sputum production because the infected sputum is very viscid and difficult to expectorate. Acute exacerbations are often associated with low-grade fever, pleuritic chest pain and general malaise. High temperatures are unusual and should suggest the likelihood of a complicating pneumonia. Haemoptysis is often observed. Generally there is just blood-streaking of sputum or the haemoptysis is slight in quantity. Rarely, there is massive haemoptysis (>300 ml) which requires active intervention to avoid a fatal outcome.

Bilateral extensive bronchiectasis or bronchiectasis associated with well-marked airways obstruction leads to dyspnoea on exertion or even at rest.

Two unusual presentations of bronchiectasis need to be kept in mind. The first is the patient who comes with recurrent pneumonia. An underlying bronchiectatic lobe is one of the causes of recurrent pneumonia. The second is the patient who has what has been termed 'dry bronchiectasis' and who presents with repeated episodes of haemoptysis very often with no abnormality on routine radiography.

Physical Signs

Clubbing is invariably present in bilateral extensive cystic or saccular bronchiectasis. It is however uncommon in the generally observed cylindrical bronchiectasis affecting both lower lobes. Crackles over the bronchiectatic lung are usually heard mostly over one or both bases. Rhonchi are often present as airways obstruction is a very frequent feature in bronchiectasis. A mistaken diagnosis of asthma is therefore occasionally made. During episodes of acute exacerbation, a pleural rub may be heard and there may be signs of a complicating pneumonia.

Lung functions show a normal or more often reduced forced vital capacity (FVC), a reduced forced expiratory volume in one second (FEV_1) and a reduced FEV_1/FVC. In our experience at least half the patients show significant improvement in the FVC, FEV_1 and FEV_1/FVC after the use of an aerosolized bronchodilator or after nebulization with salbutamol. In extensive severe disease, the total lung capacity (TLC) is decreased as is the transfer factor of the lung for carbon monoxide (TLCO).

IMAGING STUDIES

A chest X-ray may be normal in close to 50% of patients with bronchiectasis. Peribronchial fibrosis and mucosal hypertrophy lead to thickened bronchial walls which may be evident as 'tram lines' in the lower lobes. Dilated bronchi running perpendicular to the X-ray beam appear as small thick-walled rings. Cystic bronchiectasis is evident as multiple thin-walled ring shadows; when these ring shadows overlap they may give a honeycombed appearance to the lung. Dilated bronchi filled with secretions give rise to a tubular glove-finger appearance or to opacities that may be mistaken for consolidation. These appearances are particularly observed in bronchiectasis caused by allergic bronchopulmonary aspergillosis.

High-resolution thin section (1–2 mm) CT scans have completely replaced bronchography for the definitive diagnosis of bronchiectasis. Occasionally, the CT scan will not only diagnose bronchiectasis but also give the likely diagnosis as in allergic bronchopulmonary aspergillosis, tuberculosis, sarcoidosis, obstruction of a bronchus, and panbronchiolitis. CT findings are related to dilated air-filled bronchi, or to dilated fluid-filled bronchi and to crowding of dilated bronchi due to volume loss of the lung in the affected area. Dilated bronchi that are perpendicular to the scanning plane have a circular signet ring appearance because of the smaller pulmonary artery in comparison to the circular dilated bronchus. Dilated bronchi parallel to the scanning plane appear as 'tramlines' which do not decrease in diameter as they progress to the periphery. Mucus-filled bronchi appear as branching tubes or nodules; there may be a tree-in-bud appearance. Air trapping due to associated small airways obstruction can be demonstrated by scans taken during expiration; there is increased translucency in areas of air-trapping.

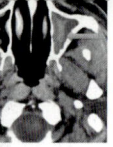

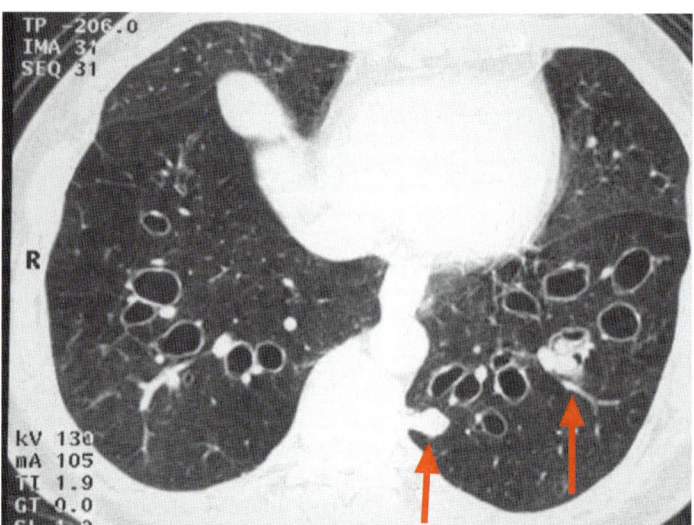

Fig 24.4: Bronchiectasis. HRCT reveals dilated bronchi in both lower lobes. The accompanying pulmonary arterial branch is of much smaller diameter as compared to the dilated bronchus. Normally the ratio is 1:1. Also, there is soft tissue in the dilated bronchi in the left lower lobe representing mucoid impaction.

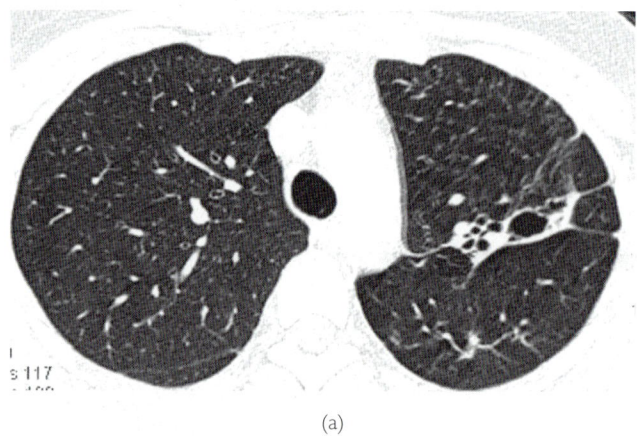

(a)

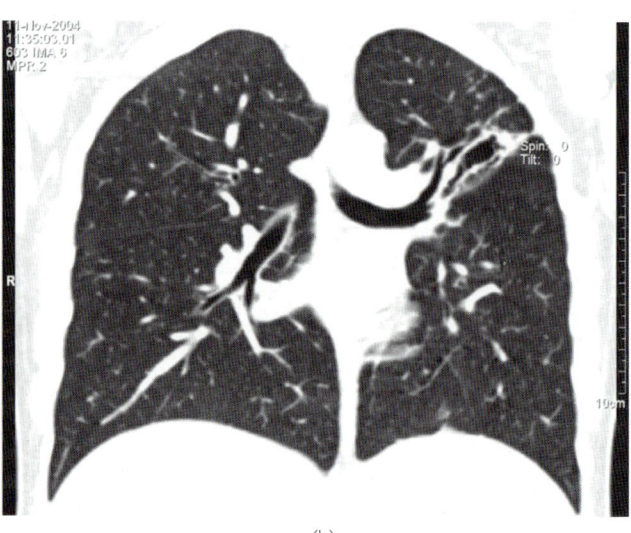

(b)

Fig 24.5: Traction bronchiectasis. (a) Axial and (b) coronal scans reveal: fibrotic lesions in the left apex with associated dilated bronchi as a result cicatricial bronchiectasis.

Patchy obstruction to the small airways may also give a mosaic appearance in the affected area on the CT scan.

INVESTIGATIONS

The diagnosis of bronchiectasis is made on the history, clinical examination and imaging findings, particularly on an HRCT of the chest. Further investigations include a blood count, erythrocyte sedimentation rate (ESR), and C-reactive protein (CRP). Both the ESR and CRP are simple but important markers of the degree of inflammation within the lungs. Serial readings at periodic intervals form a rough guide to the increase or decrease of the inflammatory process within the bronchiectatic lung. A sputum examination for smear, culture and antibiotic sensitivity is essential as it guides antibiotic selection in treatment. Sputum culture for *Mycobacterium tuberculosis* and atypical mycobacteria should be asked for as well.

Further investigations are directed to determine the cause of bronchiectasis. They are tabled below. In younger patients with associated sinusitis, tests for ciliary dysfunction are important. The saccharine test is a good screening test for ciliary dysfunction. A particle of saccharine is placed 1 cm behind the front edge of the inferior turbinate. The patient is requested to sit quietly with the head looking down and report when a sweet taste is felt. If sweetness is felt in less than 30 seconds it is normal. Sniffing during the test or looking upwards will give a false quick recording. If the saccharine test is positive, ciliary integrity and function need to be tested by submitting a sample of the nasal epithelium to light microscopy and electron microscopy. Young patients or even patients between 30 and 40 years who have recurrent lower respiratory infections or who have recurrent pneumonia should be tested for hypogammaglobulinaemia and for deficiency in a subclass of IgG or a deficiency in IgA. It may

Table 24.3: Protocol for investigation for bronchiectasis
CBC. ESR, C-reative protein (CRP)
Sputum examination—routine smear, culture, AFB smear, culture
Pulmonary function tests
X-ray chest
HRCT chest
Skin test for aspergillus sensitivity
Saccharine screening test for nasal mucociliary clearance—if positive more detailed test for ciliary function
Sweat NaCl for suspected cystic fibrosis
Serum protein electrophoresis for hypogammaglobulinemia particularly in young patients
In selected patients—
Fibroptic bronchoscopy
IgM, IgA, IgG subclass
Precipitin test for aspergillus infection
Semen analysis
Tests for associated conditions

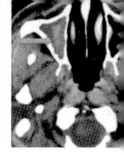

not be necessary to do all tests tabled below in every patient. Investigations may perhaps be tailored depending on the cause or causes likely to operate in a particular patient.

COMPLICATIONS

1. Extensive bilateral bronchiectasis besides leading to deteriorating health and weight loss can lead to respiratory disability, hypoxia and chronic hypercapnic respiratory failure, particularly when associated with well-marked airways obstruction. In some instances cor pulmonale results.
2. Pneumonia may complicate bronchiectasis. Occurrence of recurrent attacks of pneumonia is well known. Pleural effusion and empyema may result from contamination of the pleural space.
3. In earlier years, when the wide range of antibiotics available today was non-existent, suppurative bronchial disease was occasionally complicated by the occurrence of a metastatic brain abscess.
4. Chronic suppurative bronchiectasis in poor countries where healthcare is unavailable or hopelessly inadequate still remains a cause of amyloid disease.
5. Massive life-threatening haemoptysis in an occasional complication.

CLINICAL COURSE

At one time it was believed that once bronchiectasis occurred in a lobe of the lung it would remain so and was unlikely to involve other lobes and neighbouring areas of the lung. This is no longer true. Bronchiectasis may remain localized to one portion of the lung in some patients. In other patients a follow-up shows involvement of not only the neighbouring area of the

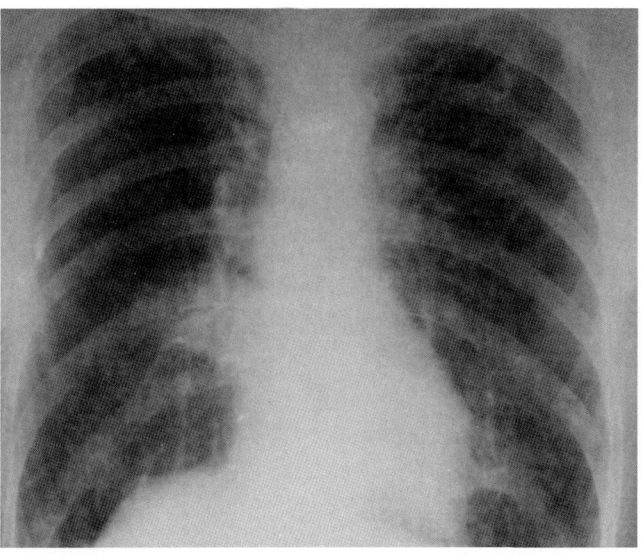

(a)

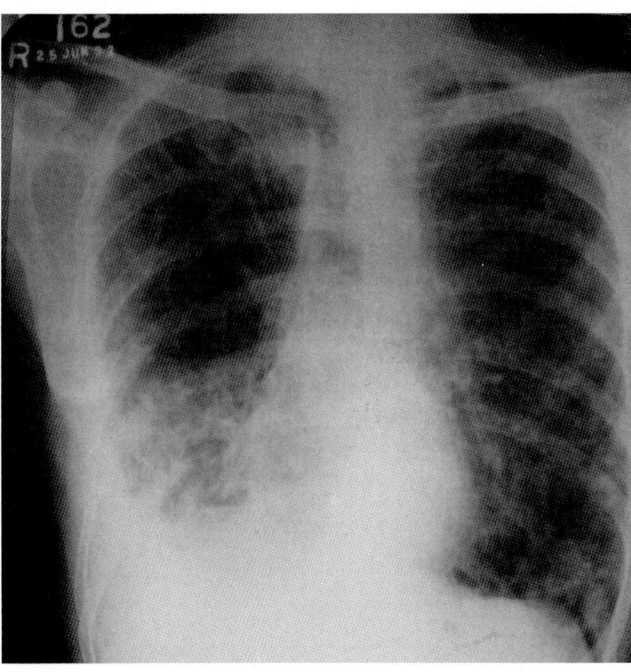

(b)

Fig 24.7: (a) A 57-year-old male patient with history of repeated episodes of chest infection in the past ten years. Chest X-ray demonstrates multiple cystic lesions with associated nodular and fibrotic lesions. These would be as a result of cystic bronchiectasis (b) Six months later patient developed high fever and productive cough. Chest X-ray reveals ill-defined consolidation with pleural effusion in right lower lobe, as well as nodular consolidations in left lower lobe. These changes were due to secondary pleuropulmonary infection.

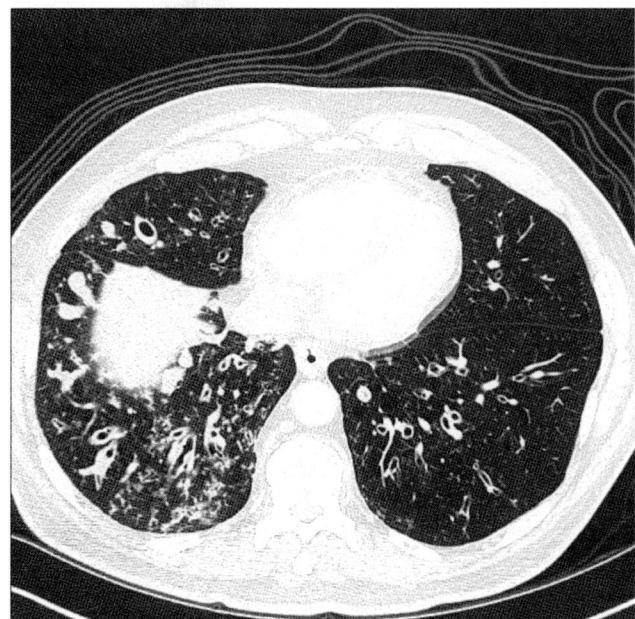

Fig 24.6: HRCT reveals dilated bronchi in both lower lobes. On the right side there is bronchial wall thickening, peribronchial nodules as well as soft tissue in the bronchial lumen. These features are a result of secondary infection.

lung but involvement of the other lung as well. In some patients the rapidity of involvement is frightening, diffuse bilateral bronchiectasis being observed in a matter of a few years.

If causes known to lead to progressive spread of bronchiectasis (such as primary ciliary dyskinesia) have been excluded, rapid spread of bronchiectasis may well be due to abnormalities in the immune response of the host and/or the number and virulence of micro-organisms responsible for bronchial inflammation and suppuration.

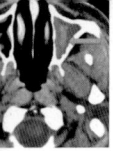

TREATMENT

Treatment is directed to alleviating symptoms and preventing as far as possible further progression of the disease.

Medical Treatment

POSTURAL DRAINAGE

Retained secretions within dilated bronchi lead to bacterial infection. Infection leads to tissue injury as a result of inflammatory mediators and noxious bacterial products. Neutrophils attracted to the bronchial lumen through chemotaxis add to the tissue injury by liberating proteases and oxidants. Retained secretions thus ultimately cause further damage to the bronchial wall with further disruption of bronchial architecture. The cornerstone of treatment is physiotherapy and postural drainage to help keep the dilated bronchi as dry as possible. Postural drainage should be preceded by steam inhalation to help liquefy thick mucopus. Inhaled steam is a far better mucolytic than any other mucolytic agent available today. Postural drainage should be accompanied by percussion and vibration over the affected areas of the lung to help dislodge secretions from the diseased bronchi. Breathing exercises and in particular Yogic breathing exercises also help. Postural drainage should be done at least once daily and during exacerbations at least two to three times in the day. The patient should be told to watch the colour of his or her expectoration. Once the bronchiectatic area is drained adequately, the expectoration during and after drainage is often mucoid denoting control of infection. It is important to instil discipline in patients so that they practice postural drainage religiously. Stopping postural drainage just because there is very little sputum during drainage is always a mistake.

Besides physiotherapy and postural drainage, airway clearance measures include cough-assist devices of various kinds e.g. flutter valves, low-frequency acoustic vibrators, and high-frequency chest wall oscillators. These of course are not available in most poor developing countries. What is more, they are only of marginal assistance and use when compared to time-tested physiotherapy and postural drainage.

Nebulization with hypertonic saline is also useful to help the patient expectorate extra-viscid sputum as in cystic fibrosis.

rhDNase has been used to reduce viscosity and improve transport capacity of purulent respiratory secretions particularly in cystic fibrosis. It is however far too expensive and unavailable in poor developing countries.

ANTIBIOTIC THERAPY

This is the second cornerstone in the management of bronchiectasis. Antibiotics are tailored as per the organisms grown on culture and their sensitivity tests. It must be remembered that in bronchial infections bacteria are present in the mucus, on the epithelial surface, often invading the mucosa and bronchial wall.

Therefore the antibiotic used has to reach the site of infection—the bronchial mucosa and bronchial wall. This consideration is important in the choice of an antibiotic. Quinolones and macrolides when administered reach effective concentrations within the lung and the bronchial mucosa, whereas aminoglycosides and betalactams do not.

In severe acute exacerbations, antibiotics are given intravenously in appropriate doses and at appropriate intervals for a period of 7–10 days or even longer.

In milder exacerbations, oral antibiotics generally suffice. Infection with *Pseudomonas aeruginosa* is particularly nasty and difficult to eradicate. An anti-pseudomonal third-generation cephalosporin like ceftazidime, or piperacillin/tazobactum or a carbapenem should be given intravenously. Resistant strains of *Pseudomonas aeruginosa* might require the use of intravenous colistin. When infection is due to other Gram-positive/negative organisms the choice of antibiotics is guided by sensitivity tests. Antibiotics often used are cefuroxime, ceftriaxone, and amoxicillin-clavulinic acid in the appropriate doses.

The problem arises in patients who get recurrent relapses with severe exacerbations in spite of intravenous antibiotics. Many units consider the use of long-term prophylactic antibiotic therapy in these patients. Before embarking on this regime it is important to ascertain that postural drainage is being correctly and religiously done. Prophylactic antibiotic therapy gives rise to many concerns—chiefly the occurrence of resistant organisms

Table 24.4: Antibiotics in bronchiectasis			
Route	**Antibiotics**	**Dose and duration**	**Ps aeruginosa**
Oral	Amoxicillin/clavulinic acid	625 mg BD for 10 days orally	Ciprofloxicin 750 mg for 10–14 days
	Quinolone (ciprofloxacin)	750 mg BD for 7 to 10 days	
	Azithromycin	500 mg OD for 7 to 10 days	
	Doxycycline	100 mg BD for 10 days	
Intravenous	Cefuroxime	750 mg TDS for 10 days	
	Ceftriaxone	2 g BD for 7 to 10 days	
	Amoxicillin/clavulinic acid	1.2 g TDS for 8 to 10 days	
		4.5 g TDS for 10–14 days	Piperacillin/Tazobactum
		2 g BD for 10–14 days	Ceftazidime
		1 G TDS for 10–14 days	Meropenam + an aminoglycoside (dose as per weight)—Gentamycin or amikacin given once daily infusion

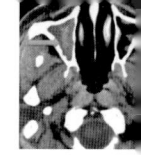

that render antibiotics ineffective, as also the side-effects and toxicity associated with prolonged use of antibiotics. Three approaches have been recommended.

1. Regular pulsed courses of intravenous antibiotics
2. Prolonged oral antibiotics
3 Inhaled antibiotics given as an isotonic solution via a nebulizer.

Nebulized antibiotics are best administered as prophylaxis to prevent or delay relapses following a course of intravenous antibiotics. Nebulized antibiotics are less effective as treatment for acute exacerbations, perhaps because they do not reach the site of infection due to excessive bronchial secretions and bronchospasm. Antibiotics used via nebulizations include beta lactams, aminoglycosides (gentamycin, tobramycin) and colistin sulphate. The greatest experience with nebulized antibiotics is in cystic fibrosis for the treatment of *Pseudomonas aeruginosa* infection. Nebulized gentamycin improved lung functions, reduced airway inflammation and mucous secretion, decreased frequency of exacerbations and hospital admission in these patients. For resistant *Pseudomonas aeruginosa* strains, nebulization with colistin is to be preferred. Nebulization with antibiotics occasionally causes bronchospasm severe enough to prevent the use of this approach.

Prolonged oral antibiotic therapy has also been shown to be beneficial in the group of patients which frequently suffer repeated exacerbations of infection. This approach is limited by the side-effects of prolonged therapy and by the development of bacterial resistance. Ciprofloxacin or any quinolone therapy is most often used for prolonged oral therapy as quinolones attain satisfactory concentrations in the lung and within bronchi.

Regular pulsed courses of intravenous antibiotics have been advocated, particularly in bronchiectasis associated with cystic fibrosis and benefits have been claimed in five-year survival. The course is administered before full relapse occurs to keep the bacterial load suppressed and thereby reduce inflammation. The length of time between courses is arbitrarily decided, varying from 6–10 weeks. Regular pulsed therapy with intravenous antibiotics has also been used for bronchiectasis due to causes other than cystic fibrosis, when there are frequently recurring acute infective episodes. The choice of antibiotics is guided by the nature and sensitivity of the infecting organisms. Piperacillin-tazobactum or a carbapenem is often chosen for Gram-negative infections.

Anti-inflammatory Therapy in Bronchiectasis

The goals of therapy in bronchiectasis include not just the control of infection but also suppressing inflammation. Recent work on suppressing inflammation in bronchiectasis has looked at:

1. Macrolides
2. Inhaled corticosteroids

MACROLIDES

Erythromycin given continuously is the treatment of choice in panbronchiolitis in Japan even when bronchial infection is due to *P. aeruginosa*. A similar approach has recently been used in bronchiectasis. Perhaps the benefits of prolonged erythromycin use may be related to reduced exotoxin production by *P. aeruginosa* at concentrations that do not inhibit bacterial growth. Macrolide antibiotics also exert anti-inflammatory effects by reducing tumour necrosis factor alpha (TNF-α), IL-1β and IL-6. Two small studies on bronchiectasis in cystic fibrosis have shown good results with modest improvement in FEV$_1$ and lower rates of exacerbations. There have also been a few studies on the effect of macrolides in bronchiectasis not related to cystic fibrosis. Modest improvement in FEV$_1$, and reduction in the exacerbation rate have again been reported. More work on a larger number of bronchiectatic patients needs to be done before the efficacy of macrolides in this disease can be established.

INHALED CORTICOSTEROIDS IN BRONCHIECTASIS

Inhaled beclomethasone in a dose of 750 ug bid or inhaled fluticasone in a dose of 500 ug bd has been shown to exert an anti-inflammatory effect. This is evinced by a reduction in sputum volume, reduced sputum leukocyte density, reduced IL8, reduced leukotrine B4 and in one study an improvement in FEV$_1$. Again more work requires to be done on a larger number of patients before conclusions can be drawn on the anti-inflammatory benefits of inhaled corticosteroids in bronchiectasis.

Anti-inflammatory therapy should be considered in the following conditions:

a. Symptomatic patients
b. High sputum volumes
c. Frequent exacerbations
d. Pseudomonas colonization

The impact of anti-inflammatory measures in bronchiectasis is summarized in the following table:

Table 24.5: Impact of anti-inflammatory therapy		
	IC	**MACROLIDES**
Symptoms	Maybe	Maybe
Sputum volume	Yes	Yes
Exacerbations	No	Maybe
PFT	No	No
QOL	Maybe	??
Microbiology	??	??

Note: IC—Inhaled corticosteroids, QOL—Quality of life.

Airways Obstruction in Bronchiectasis

Some degree of airways obstruction invariably occurs in bronchiectasis. Aerosolized bronchodilators (salmeterol and fluticasone) often give symptomatic relief when there is a degree of reversibility in the airways obstruction. When bronchospasm is marked during acute exacerbations, nebulization with salbutamol, tiotropium, and budesonide may be of help. Inhaled steroids may reduce inflammation within the bronchi. Oral

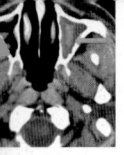
or even intravenous corticosteroids in a short course of 10–12 days may be of use during acute exacerbations, but prolonged use of oral corticosteroids should be avoided because of side-effects and the absence of proven benefit.

Other Medical Treatment

Bronchiectasis caused by or associated with hypogammaglobulinaemia or selective immunoglobulin deficiencies responds well to regular replacement therapy with intravenous immunoglobulin. The interval between infusions depends on the clinical response. A period of three to four weeks between infusions is generally chosen at the outset. Selective antibody deficiencies including IgG subclass deficiency can also be treated by replacement. It must be noted that patients with IgG sub-class deficiency and complete absence of IgA may develop IgA antibodies after transfusion of blood products or infusion of immunoglobulins containing IgA. This leads to severe anaphylaxis if immunoglobulins are given. IgA-free infusions should be given to these patients. Massive haemoptysis is a frequent occurrence and complication of bronchiectasis. It is managed by bronchoscopic techniques, bronchial artery embolization and sometimes by emergency surgery.

Surgical Treatment

Surgical resection of a bronchiectatic lobe is curative. Surgery should only be advised in patients where the bronchiectasis is localized and there is no underlying condition which predisposes in the future to generalized bronchiectasis, as for example in primary ciliary dyskinesia. Good results are obtained after surgical resection of severe localized bronchiectasis. There is an improvement in general health, and freedom from fever, malaise and infective episodes. Lung function is not significantly reduced as the diseased lobe contributes very little to lung function.

Every patient with localized bronchiectasis does not require surgery. Patients with mild or even moderately severe bronchiectasis do well with medical therapy—in the main, postural drainage plus the use of appropriate antibiotics during infective episodes. If, however, episodes of recurrent infection are frequent or if bronchiectasis clearly disturbs the patient's lifestyle, surgery is indicated. Surgery is also indicated if there is repeated haemoptysis as the fear of possible massive haemoptysis in the future always exists. Massive haemoptysis is preferably treated with embolization of the culprit bronchial artery and/or of the pulmonary artery vessel if that is responsible for the bleed. Surgical resection may be necessary as an emergency procedure if embolization fails.

Surgery is inadvisable when the disease is not localized and involves both lungs as in cylindrical bronchiectasis which generally involves both lower lobes. However, in patients where the disease is more generalized, surgery may still be performed as a palliative measure on a grossly diseased local area of the lung which has not responded to medical treatment and which may act as a source for further spread of the disease.

In our opinion a contraindication for surgery even in patients with localized bronchiectasis is the presence of significant airways' obstruction unrelieved by aerosolized or nebulized bronchodilators. These patients continue to remain symptomatic after surgery.

Lung transplantation (single-lung, double-lungs, heart-lung) should be considered in severe bilateral bronchiectasis not responding to medical therapy, particularly if there is chronic respiratory failure. Single-lung transplantation is considered unadvisable for fear of developing bronchiectasis in the transplant lung from the opposite bronchiectatic lung and for fear of dissemination of infection (present in the opposite bronchiectatic lung) following the use of immunosuppressants.

Outcome

A study by Keistinen *et al.* in the European Respiratory Journal in 1997 presented the follow-up data from the National Finnish Registry of 842 adult patients with bronchiectasis matched (age and sex) with asthmatics, COPD and followed up for 8–12 years. There were 1–51 hospitalizations (mean 2.2) and a 28% death rate in the group with bronchiectasis (239 deaths) compared to a 20% death rate in asthma and 38% death rate for COPD. There is unfortunately no reliable reported follow-up of patients with bronchiectasis in India.

SUGGESTED READING

Barker Alan F. Bronchiectasis. *N Engl J Med.* 2 May 2002; 346(18): 1383–93.

Bronchiectasis. *Chest.* Volume 134, Issue 4 (October 2008). Copyright © 2008. The American College of Chest Physicians.

Bronchiectasis. Javidan-Nejad C. *Radiol Clin North Am.* 1 Mar. 2009; 47(2): 289–306.

Cohen M, Sahn SA. Bronchiectasis in systemic diseases. *Chest.* 1999; 116: 1063–74.

King PT, Holdsworth SR, Freezer NJ, Villanueva E, Holmes PW. Characterization of the onset and presenting clinical features of adult bronchiectasis. *Respir Med.* 2006; 100: 2183.

Lavery K, O'Neill B, Elborn JS, Reilly J, Bradley JM. Self-management

in bronchiectasis: the patients' perspective. *Eur Respir J.* Mar. 2007; 29(3): 541–7.

Pasteur MC, Helliwell SM, Houghton SJ, Webb SC, Foweraker JE, Coulden RA, Flower CD, Bilton D, Keogan MT. An investigation into causative factors in patients with bronchiectasis. *Am J Resp Crit Care Med.* 2000; 162: 1277–84.

Schneiter D, Meyer N, Lardinois D, Korom S, Kestenholz P, Weder W. Surgery for non-localized bronchiectasis. *Br J Surg.* 2005; 92: 836.

Tsang KW, Ho PL, Lam WK, Ip MS, Chan KN, Ho CS, Ooi CC, Yuen KY. Inhaled fluticasone reduces sputum inflammatory indices in severe bronchiectasis. *Am J Respir Crit Care Med.* Sep. 1998; 158(3): 723–27.

CHAPTER **25** **Lung Abscess**

A lung abscess is a localized area of infection causing suppurative parenchymal necrosis. A lung abscess is generally single, or may occur as multiple discrete lesions. A tuberculous cavity is excluded from the definition of a lung abscess. However, tuberculosis is an important differential diagnosis particularly in areas where this disease is highly prevalent.

AETIOLOGY

1. **Aspiration** of anaerobic, anaerobic plus aerobic or occasionally only aerobic organisms, colonizing the mouth and upper respiratory tract is perhaps the commonest cause of a lung abscess. Periodontal disease and bad mouth hygiene are often present in these patients. Any condition which predisposes to aspiration, e.g. obtundation from any cause, inability to protect the airway, difficulty in swallowing, will also predispose to either an aspiration pneumonia or a lung abscess. The more frequent the aspiration and the more infected and greater the volume of the aspirate, the greater the chances of pulmonary complications. Rarely, superinfection of a pulmonary infarct or of damaged lung tissue (as after chemical inhalation injury) by aspirated anaerobes or aerobes can also result in a lung abscess.

2. **Suppurative Pneumonia**   Progression of pneumonic consolidation to suppurative necrosis is often associated with cavitation. Organisms which have a potential to cause a suppurative necrosis of a consolidated lobe are *Streptococcus pneumoniae* Type III, *Staphylococcus aureus*, *H. influenzae* and Gram-negative organisms such as *K. pneumoniae*, *Ps. pyocyaneus*, and *E. coli*. A lung abscess due to *Entamoeba histolytica* (generally caused by a liver abscess rupturing into the lower lobe of the right or rarely the left lung) is an important cause of a lung abscess in the tropics. In immunosuppressed individuals, *Nocardia asteroides* and fungal infections, in particular infection due to Aspergillus species can cause a lung abscess. Chronic primary pulmonary fungal infection (histoplasmosis, coccidiomycosis, blastomycosis) can cause one or more cavitatory lesions in patients living in areas where these fungal infections are endemic.

3. **Bacteraemic Spread**   Organisms may reach the lung from a septic focus anywhere within the body. Bloodstream infections from any cause (e.g. an infected central venous catheter) may lead to seeding of the lungs with microorganisms and lead to one or more lung abscesses. Drug addicts who inject heroin or other drugs via the peripheral veins are particularly prone to one or more lung abscesses.

4. **Septic Pulmonary Emboli**   Septic pulmonary emboli originating from septic thrombophlebitis anywhere within the body or septic emboli arising from vegetations on the tricuspid valve (as seen in drug addicts who use drugs through intravenous injections) in subacute bacterial endocarditis are other causes to be reckoned with.

5. **Penetrating trauma** to the chest and rarely even blunt trauma to the chest can cause a lung abscess. In the former instance infection is directly introduced into the lung; in the latter a contusion caused by the blunt trauma may become secondarily infected.

PATHOLOGY

Infection from whatever route causes either a large area of consolidation or causes smaller areas of consolidation which coalesce to form larger areas. Superadded necrosis of the involved areas is often associated with suppuration. More often than not, this consolidated, necrotic, suppurative area opens into a draining bronchus. The patient then has purulent expectoration which may be profuse in quantity. The abscess now communicating with a bronchus has an air-fluid level. The abscess cavity which contains necrotic pus is lined by inflammatory granulation tissue and is surrounded by a ring of consolidated lung tissue. If it does not heal the abscess becomes chronic. If the abscess is close to the pleura it may cause an empyema or may open into the pleural space causing a pyopneumothorax and a bronchopleural fistula. Metastatic spread of infection to other sites—notably the brain (causing a cerebral abscess) is today a rare complication.

A lung abscess heals with fibrosis which may obliterate the abscess cavity. Occasionally, a thin-walled sterile cavity remains as a sequel, the inner lining of the cavity being epithelialized or lined by fibrous tissue.

Since aspiration is the most important predisposing factor associated with a lung abscess, the abscess is most frequently situated in the posterior segment of the upper lobe, the apical segment of the lower lobes and occasionally the posterior segment of the lower lobe.

A lung abscess is considered acute if four to six weeks old and chronic if it persists for a longer period.

CLINICAL FEATURES

An acute pyogenic lung abscess in its formative period will cause high fever with chills, severe prostration and lassitude. A dry cough is generally present. Pleuritic pain may occur if the abscess is close to the pleura. Once the abscess communicates with the bronchus so that the purulent necrotic secretions are coughed up, the systemic toxicity is reduced. Fever may be low-

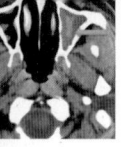

grade or even absent; the patient continues to cough up dirty, purulent, often foetid sputum. Anaerobic infection is often associated with a foetid smell in the breath and in the sputum that can be perceived from a distance.

Clinical examination reveals tachypnoea of varying degree; there may be diminished movement of the chest wall overlying the abscess, and an impaired percussion note because of the surrounding consolidation. Breath sounds could be normal, diminished or bronchial in character. Bronchial breath sounds when present are related to the surrounding consolidation. At times the bronchial breath sounds may have a cavernous or amphoric character. Crepitations may be heard over the involved area of the lung.

The abscess may heal if properly treated or it may become chronic if diagnosed late or not correctly treated. A chronic lung abscess is often associated with well-marked clubbing and sometimes with pulmonary osteoarthropathy.

A lung abscess may not always be acute in onset. Over half to two-thirds have a subacute or even chronic presentation. Small frequent aspiration of infected material into the lung may lead to small areas of infective necrosis. These may slowly coalesce to form a larger area of infection plus necrosis. The onset in these patients may be insidious with low-grade fever and cough which to start with is dry and is only later associated with purulent expectoration. As the areas of involved lung tissue increase, symptoms may become more pronounced. A lung abscess in such patients may be diagnosed late in the natural history of the disease, the diagnosis being established by imaging studies, particularly by high-resolution computed tomography (HRCT) of the chest.

Metastatic seeding of the lung from bacteraemia or from septic emboli can cause multiple areas of consolidation, with cavitation. Staphylococcal lung infection of bacteraemic or embolic origin often causes multiple abscesses.

Gangrene of the lung

Gangrene of a segment or lobe of the lung is a rare complication of fulminating necrotizing pneumonia with suppuration. Gangrene is characterized by sloughing of the involved segment or lobe due to thrombosis of both pulmonary and bronchial vessels with resulting infarction. The organisms most commonly involved are *K. pneumoniae*; other organisms implicated include *E. coli*, anaerobes, *Streptococcus pneumoniae*, *H. inluenzae* and *S. aureus*.

Besides the severity of the illness, the striking feature is the dreadful odour that permeates the whole ward. Though increasingly rare, pulmonary gangrene is still observed in patients with fulminant infection who have not received adequate and timely antibiotic therapy.

COMPLICATIONS

Complications include empyema, pyopneumothorax with a bronchopleural fistula; very rarely, there is metastatic spread of infection. Overwhelming sepsis with multi-organ failure can occur in fulminant infection, particularly in immunocompromised patients. In earlier years (five to six decades ago) a chronic lung abscess was an important cause of secondary amyloidosis. This is only rarely observed in present times.

IMAGING FEATURES

The chest radiograph to start with shows infiltrates which coalesce in parts or areas of consolidation most often in segments of the lung mentioned earlier. Cavitation may occur soon or may be observed after a week or even later.

A chronic lung abscess appears as an irregular-shaped cavity surrounded by a ring of consolidated lung. The graduation from a 'pneumonia' to a 'necrotizing pneumonia' and finally to a necrotizing pneumonia communicating with a bronchus so as to produce a cavity (often with an air-fluid level) may take days or weeks.

An empyema may be observed as an associated complication in one-third of the patients. A pyopneumothorax with a bronchopleural fistula may be the presenting radiological appearance in some patients.

An HRCT of the chest may reveal one or more abscesses in a consolidated area well before these become apparent on a radiographic examination of the chest.

DIAGNOSIS

Clinical features combined with imaging features enable a quick diagnosis. The organisms responsible are generally obtained through routine microscopy with Gram stain together with aerobic culture and anaerobic cultures of sputum. With a patient coughing up frank purulent sputum it is generally not necessary to perform invasive procedures to obtain lower respiratory secretions. When there is little or no sputum microbiological diagnosis based on sputum examination may be

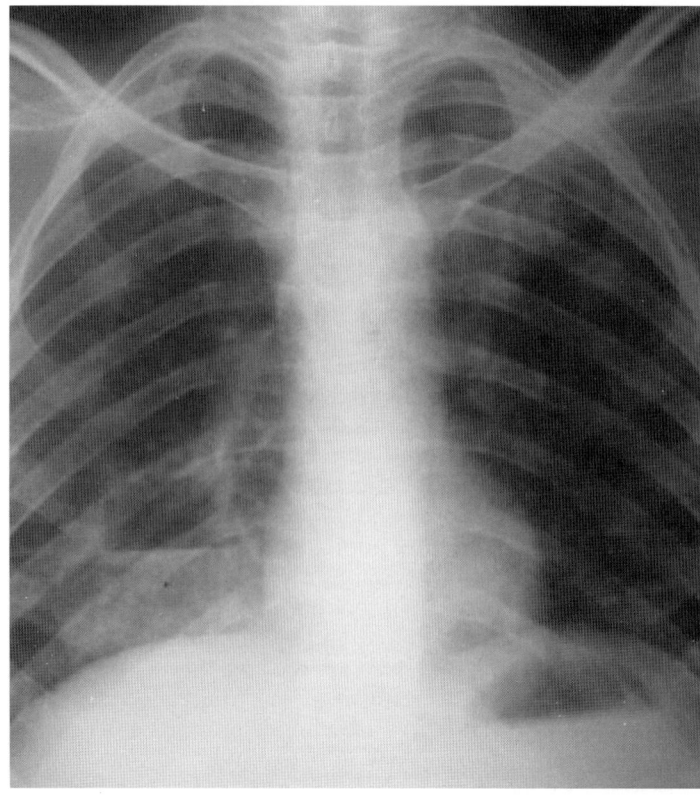

Fig 25.1: Chest X-ray reveals an air-fluid level in a well-defined cavity in the paracardiac region of the right lower lobe. This represents a lung abscess.

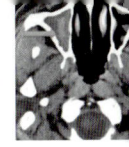

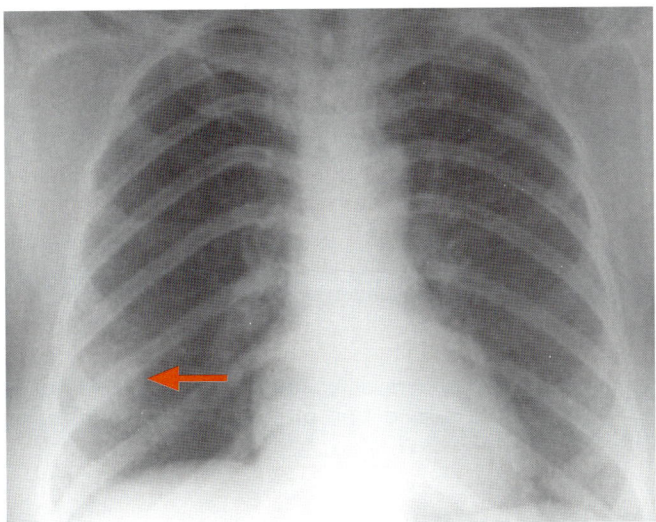

Fig 25.2: Chest X-ray reveals a well-defined round nodular lesion in the right lower lobe, HRCT revealed an air-fluid level in the lesion. CT-guided aspiration revealed pus indicating a lung abscess.

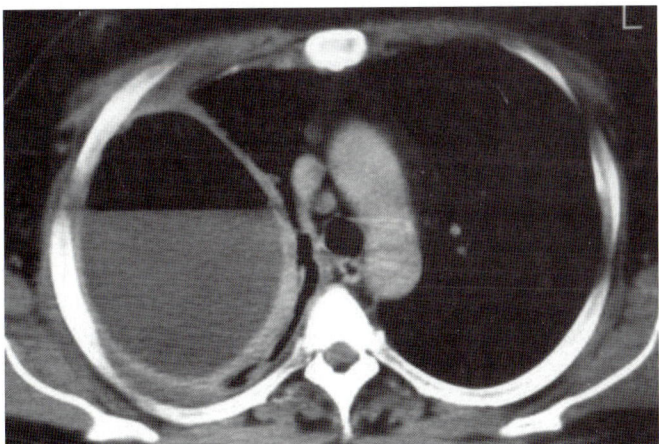

Fig 25.3: CT Chest demonstrates a large lesion with an air-fluid level in the right hemithorax. The lesion has acute margins with the chest wall representing a large abscess.

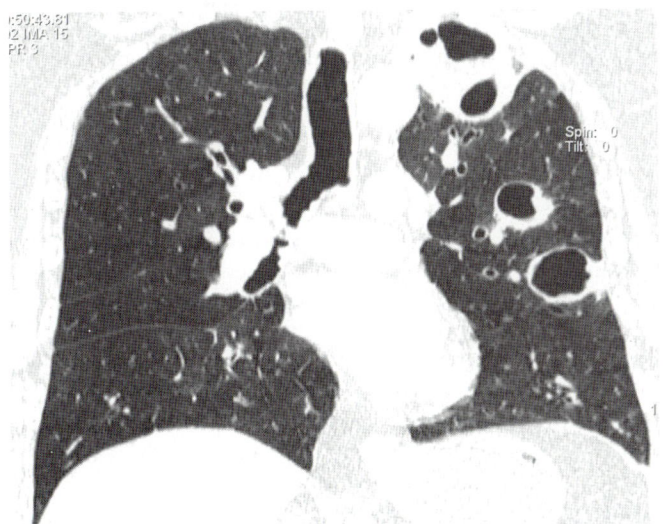

Fig 25.4: HRCT chest coronal reconstruction demonstrates multiple well-defined cavities in the left lung representing multiple abscesses. These were staphylococcal in aetiology and totally responded to postural drainage and antibiotics.

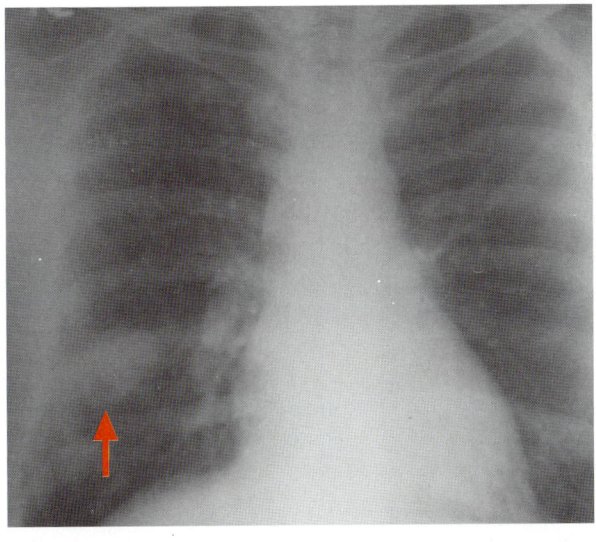

(a)

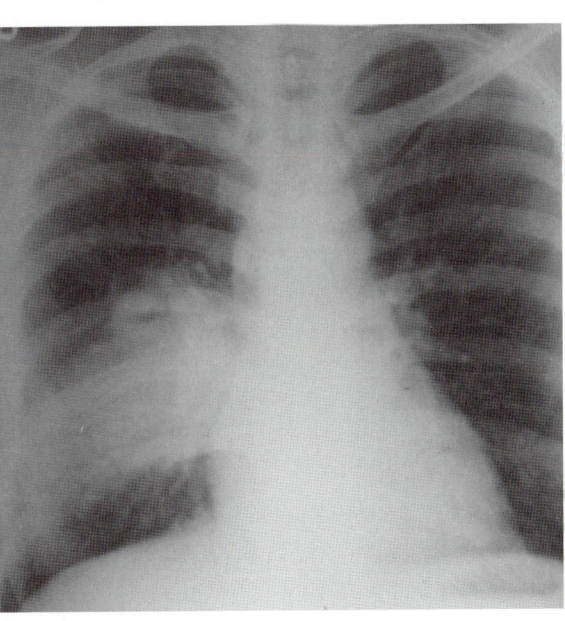

(b)

Fig 25.5: Cryptococcal lung abscess (a) Chest X-ray demonstrates a small well-defined nodular lesion in the right lower lobe with internal cavitation (b) this lesion progressed in a short time to become a large consolidation with a small nodular lesion along its superior aspect with an air-fluid level. At surgery this was a cryptococcal lung abscess.

misleading as the organisms grown are often colonizers from the upper respiratory tract. In severe nosocomial infection causing pneumonia or lung abscess, prompt treatment with appropriate antibiotics should be started after collecting a sputum specimen for examination or after collecting an aspirated sampled through the endotracheal tube in an intubated patient. Treatment in these patients should never await a microbiological diagnosis based on sputum examination. Most studies show that invasive methods to obtain lower respiratory tract secretions for a bacteriological diagnosis in nosocomial pulmonary infection do not favourably influence morbidity or mortality. Two points are further worth noting—

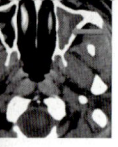

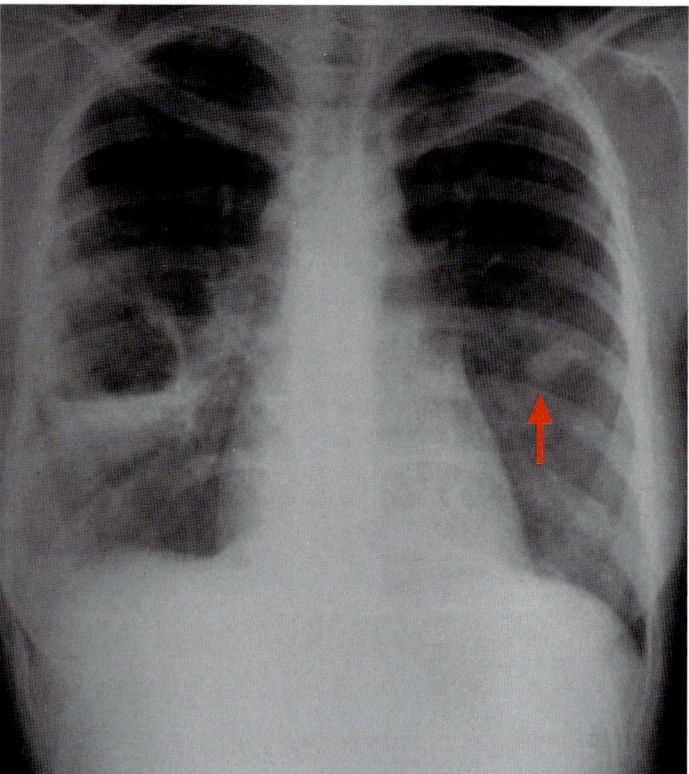

Fig 25.6: Chest X-ray reveals a thick-walled cavity with an air-fluid level in the right mid-zone. Nodular lesions are seen in the left mid-zone. The chest X-ray appearances are indicative of an abscess. This patient was febrile, had a very high ESR and was ANCA-positive. This was due to Wegener's granulomatosis. Not all air-fluid levels on a chest X-ray are lung abscesses.

1. Cultures of sputum or endotracheal aspirates should be preferably done at the bedside. This is a necessity for anaerobic culture.
2. Sputum staining and culture for acid-fast bacilli should always be done for any cavitatory lesion in the lung.

Sputum cultures in lung abscess often grow anaerobes or both anaerobes and aerobes. Among anaerobes *Fusobacterium nucleatum* or *Peptostreptococcus* species cause more virulent infection. Among aerobes *K. pneumoniae*, *P. aeruginosa*, *S. aureus* and *Streptococcus pyogenes* are most frequently involved in a necrotizing suppurative pneumonia. *B. pseudomallei* is an important cause of lung abscess in Southeast Asia, particularly Thailand. It is an uncommon but important cause of lung abscess in India (particularly south India) as well.

A fibreoptic bronchoscopy is indicated as a diagnostic procedure for the following reasons:

1. To exclude bronchial obstruction either from a tumour or foreign body as an underlying cause of a lung abscess distal to the obstruction.
2. To determine whether a cavitating lesion is a carcinoma of the lung or an infective lung abscess. In such patients a CT-guided biopsy may also be done or could be an alternative to bronchoscopy and a transbronchial biopsy.
3. To determine the microbiology of a lung abscess which persists in spite of treatment. A bronchoalveolar lavage

(BAL) study through a fibreoptic bronchoscope may reveal uncommon organisms such as Nocardia, fungi, actinomycetes, *Burkholderia pseudomallei*.

When a lung abscess is felt to be related to bacteraemia, blood cultures should be done; the cause of bacteraemia should be determined and if possible removed. Multiple lung abscesses point to septic emboli often related to septic thrombophlebitis. Drug addicts who mainline drugs like heroin or cocaine intravenously can develop bacterial endocarditis on the tricuspid valve. They present with fever, tricuspid incompetence and pulmonary symptoms like cough, breathlessness and occasionally haemoptysis. Radiological examination of the chest reveals multiple areas of consolidation often breaking down to form multiple lung abscesses.

DIFFERENTIAL DIAGNOSIS

In the early phase before cavitation occurs a formative lung abscess will appear as a pneumonia—either as aspiration pneumonia or a 'bronchogenic' lobar or segmental consolidation.

Once a cavity appears the differential diagnosis is from other cavitating lung pathologies. Pulmonary tuberculosis is an important differential diagnosis particularly in countries where tuberculosis has a high prevalence. Repeated negative sputum for acid-fact bacilli on smear and culture in a patient coughing up frank purulent sputum, generally excludes tuberculosis.

An important differential diagnosis of a large lung abscess is a loculated empyema with an air-fluid level (see section on Diseases of the Pleura).

A carcinoma of the lung may present as a cavitating lesion indistinguishable from a pyogenic lung abscess. Sputum cytology should always be done particularly in a smoker. Other relevant investigations include CT-guided biopsy or a fibreoptic bronchoscopy only if thought necessary.

A subphrenic pathology, in particular an amoebic abscess should always be considered in the differential diagnosis of a lung abscess in the right lower lobe.

A pyogenic lung abscess due to the usual Gram-positive or Gram–negative infections needs to be differentiated from an abscess due to *Nocardia asteroides*, *Rhodococcus equi* infections and cavitatory lesions caused by fungi such as histoplasma or rarely by cocccidiomycosis or blastomycosis in patients living in endemic zones.

Actinomyces infection of the lung is rare and difficult to diagnose. The appearance of chest wall sinuses discharging 'sulphur granules' containing actinomyces in a patient with a chronic lung abscess (often associated with an empyema) allows a definite diagnosis. A BAL study may help to make a diagnosis when actinomyces presents as a chronic lung abscess or a chronic pneumonia.

Burkholderia pseudomallei should be suspected and looked for even in India. Paragonimiasis as a cause of a cavitatory lesion is an important differential diagnosis in Southeast Asia, particularly in Thailand.

Among non-infective lesions (other than lung cancer), the single most important differential diagnosis is Wegener's granulomatosis. A cavitatory lesion which spontaneously changes its appearance or disappears to again appear at the same or

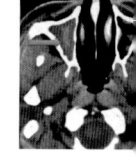

another site in the lung is strongly indicative of Wegener's granulomatosis.

Other causes of non-infectious cavitatory disease include lymphomas and intra-pulmonary nodules of rheumatoid lung disease and advanced Stage IV sarcoidosis.

TREATMENT

Conservative treatment in the management of a lung abscess is based on the appropriate use of antibiotics and on postural drainage to help evacuate the purulent secretions within the abscess. Postural drainage should be supplemented by efficient physiotherapy.

In an acute lung abscess presenting with severe systemic symptoms it is important to cover for Gram-positive, Gram-negative organisms and for anaerobes. A penicillin derivative—ampicillin or amoxicillin clavulinate covers Gram-positive infection and a third-generation cephalosporin covers most Gram-negative infections. Antibiotics should not be withheld pending result of microbiological studies on sputum or lower respiratory secretions. The choice of antibiotics might need to be however altered once culture sensitivity reports are available. It is always wise to cover for anaerobic organisms even if none are grown on culture. For this reason, treatment should also include either metronidazole or clindamycin. The mortality of lung abscess in the pre-antibiotic era was 30–40%. Following the introduction of penicillin and other antibiotics 90% of lung abscesses resolve, provided diagnosis is early and treatment with antibiotics and postural drainage is adequate. Antibiotic therapy may need to be continued for three to four weeks for full resolution to occur.

The role of surgery depends on serial clinical and radiological evaluation of the patient. If the patient is unable to cough up infected purulent necrotic material within the abscess cavity, bronchoscopic drainage if carefully done may help. Bronchscopic drainage poses the grave danger of spillage of infected material into other lung segments or into the opposite lung leading at times to a serious respiratory crisis. However, in critically ill patients or in patients who develop a lung abscess distal to a partial bronchial obstruction bronchoscopic drainage could be lifesaving.

Bronchoscopy and CT of the chest play an important role in evaluating a patient who fails to respond adequately to routine conservative management. Response both in systemic features and the quantity and nature of purulent secretions is generally observed within 7 to 10 days. Failure to respond should suggest the following possibilities:

a. Incorrect choice of antibiotics
b. Bronchial obstruction
c. Resistant organisms or unsuspected organisms like fungi, parasites, Legionella, *Burkholderia pseudomallei*
d. Tuberculosis
e. Thick loculated pus within the abscess cavity which has not communicated with a bronchus
f. Poor penetration of antibiotics into infected lung tissue and into an area of suppuration which has a low pH.
g. Presence of a complicating empyema which is not evident on radiographic examination but which is visualized on a CT chest.

Rarely, metastatic septic spread of the disease may cause failure to respond adequately to treatment.

Surgical Intervention

Surgery is indicated—

a. If response to conservative management is poor and if the clinical condition worsens.
b. In a large abscess. However, it is indeed surprising how even a very large abscess can heal on conservative management alone.
c. If bronchial obstruction from a tumour or a foreign body prevents drainage of abscess contents.

In patients who are very poor surgical risks, percutaneous drainage via a catheter with a sufficiently large bore may serve as a temporary measure. Spillage of the abscess contents into the pleura during the above procedure may however prove disastrous.

Ultimate outcome depends on the resistance and immune response of the host and the nature of the infection—a battle between the seed and the soil. It also depends on the susceptibility of the infecting organism to the antibiotics used. In eldery patients, in co-morbid diseases like diabetes, *chronic obstructive pulmonary disease* (COPD), and ischemic heart disease and in immunocompromised patients there is an increased mortality.

SUGGESTED READING

Kerlan RK Jr. Abscess drainage in LaBerge JM, ed. *Interventional radiology essentials*. Philadelphia: Lippincott Williams & Wilkins, 2000; 317–29.

Mansharamani N and Balachandran D. Lung abscess in adults: clinical comparison of immunocompromised to non-immunocompromised patients. *Respir Med*. Mar. 2002; 96(3): 178–85.

Mueller PR and Berlin L. Complications of lung abscess aspiration and drainage. *AJR Am J Roentgenol*. 2002; 178: 1083–86.

Pfitzner J and Peacock MJ. Lobectomy for cavitating lung abscess with haemoptysis: strategy for protecting the contralateral lung and also non-involved lobe of the ipsilateral lung. *Br J Anaesth*. Nov. 2000; 85(5): 791–4.

Podbielski FJ, Rodriguez HE, Wiesman IM, *et al*. Pulmonary parenchymal abscess: VATS approach to diagnosis and treatment'. *Asian Cardiovasc Thorac Ann*. 2001; 9:339–341.

Takayanagi N, Kagiyama N, Takashi Ishiguro, Daidou Tokunaga, Yutaka Sugita. Etiology and outcome of community-acquired lung abscess. *Respiration*. 2010; 80(2): 98–105.

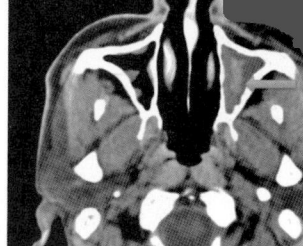
CHAPTER 26   Upper Respiratory Tract Infections

SINUSITIS

The paranasal sinuses include the maxillary, frontal, ethmoidal and sphenoidal sinuses. The sinuses are lined by respiratory ciliated epithelium and mucous-producing goblet cells. The ciliated cells move the mucus towards the sinus ostia and from there to the nasopharynx.

ACUTE SINUSITIS

The commonest cause of an acute sinusitis is a viral infection (e.g. a common cold) which inflames the ciliated epithelium, damages cilia and ciliary movement, obstructs sinus ostia thereby preventing drainage and promoting infection.

Acute allergic rhinitis can also cause sinusitis through mucosal oedema with ostial obstruction from oedema or from nasal polyps.

Any pathology in the nose or the paranasal sinus or sinuses that blocks ostial drainage can do likewise e.g. deviated nasal septum, tumour, granulomas, nasogastric or nasotracheal tubes. The organisms causing sinusitis in the above instances are generally bacteria—the–*H. influenzae*, *Streptococcus pneumoniae* and occasionally Gram-negative bacteria. Acute maxillary sinusitis can also occur as a result of spread of infection from infected second bicuspid premolar tooth or infected first, or second molars.

Community-acquired bacterial sinusitis is generally due to *H. influenzae* infection or *Streptococcus pneumoniae* and occasionally *Staphylococcus aureus*. *M. cattarhalis* infection is reported to be more common in children.

Clinical Features

Clinical features consist of nasal congestion, purulent nasal discharge, postnasal drip often causing cough, and sinus pain. The location of pain depends on the sinus involved. Maxillary sinusitis produces pain over the cheek and upper teeth with tenderness on pressure over the maxilla. Frontal sinusitis produces pain over the frontal area and the supraorbital ridges which may be tender on pressure. Infection of the ethmoids causes pain over the bridge of the nose on either side; sphenoidal sinusitis causes retroorbital pain, occipital pain or pain over the vertex of the head. Purulent sinusitis can produce fever, malaise and leucocytosis.

A differential diagnosis from an acute viral upper respiratory infection is difficult as identical symptoms may occur in the latter.

An X-ray of the paranasal sinuses is helpful only if there is well-nigh complete sinus opacification or mucosal thickening of at least 4 mm. Sinusitis may be present without these findings. A *computed tomography* (CT) of the sinuses is far more sensitive than routine radiography and is essential for diagnosis of sphenoidal or ethmoidal sinusitis.

Nasal endoscopy (done by an otolaryngologist) reveals purulent secretions from the sinus ostia.

Treatment

Amoxicillin clavulanate or cefuroxime given orally for eight to 10 days generally controls infection. Steam inhalation and decongestant nasal drops help sinus drainage. If thick pus is formed within a sinus, surgical drainage is necessary. Surgical attention is also necessary when orbital cellulitis occurs as a complication of sinusitis.

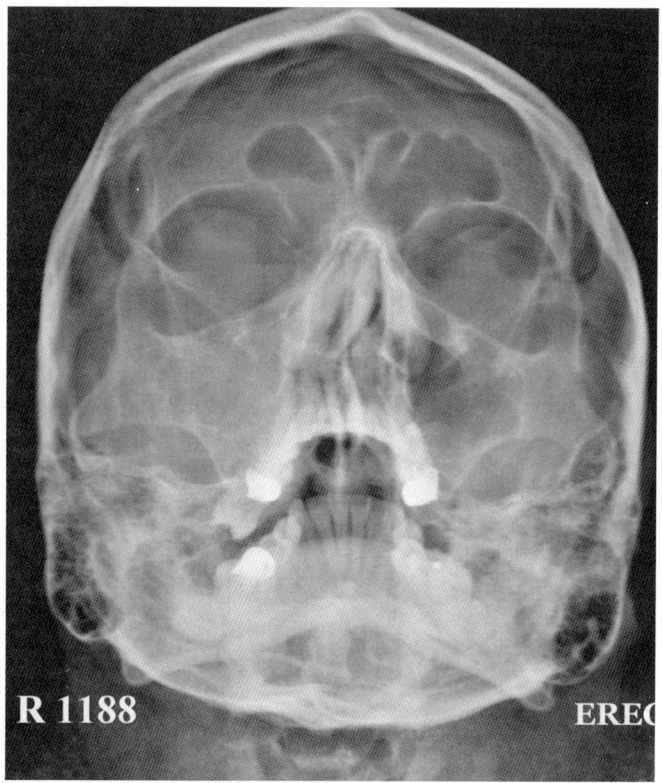

Fig 26.1: Sinusitis. Plain X-ray of sinuses; total opacification of the right maxillary sinus due to sinusitis.

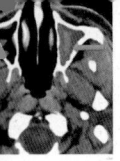
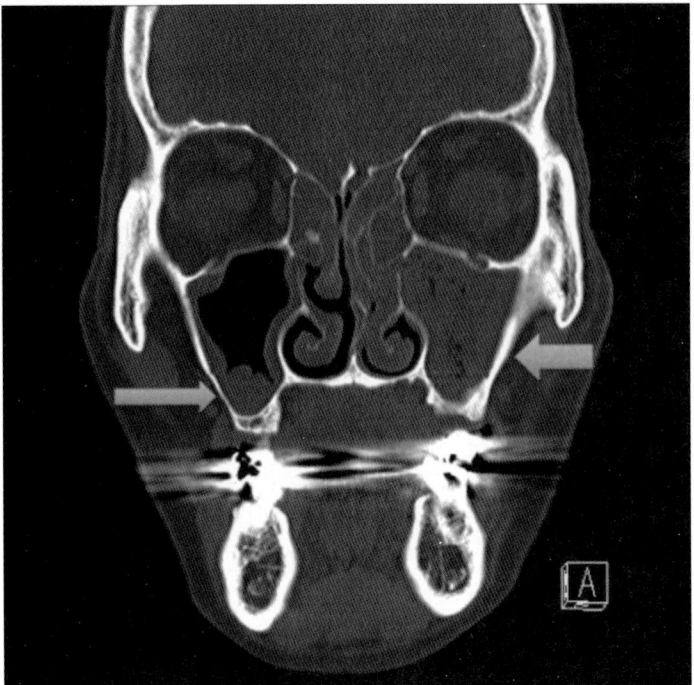

Fig 26.2: Coronal CT scan reveals mucosal thickening of the right maxillary sinus, soft tissue opacifying ethmoid, frontal, and left maxillary sinuses. Specks of air are seen in the left maxillary sinus. These changes are due to acute sinusitis.

CHRONIC BACTERIAL SINUSITIS

Chronic bacterial sinusitis is characterized by pain, fullness and heaviness over the sinuses (at the sites mentioned) for days, weeks, or months. There is purulent discharge which may occur intermittingly from the nose, a post-nasal drip causing an inflamed pharynx and larynx, a foul odour and taste and a feeling of malaise and fatigability. A low-grade evening rise of fever may be present. The above features may occur episodically or persist in a smouldering form with periodic exacerbations.

A CT of the sinuses is important not just to define the sinus or sinuses involved but to define the extent of the disease and to determine if there is any organic pathology blocking the sinus ostia and causing a chronic sinusitis. The patient should also be evaluated by an ear-nose-throat (ENT) specialist with the same objectives. Obstruction to the sinus ostia can result from a deviated septum, large nasal polyps, granulomas such as sarcoid or Wegener's granulomatosis and cancers in the region of the nose and sinuses. Impaired mucociliary clearance from whatever cause results in chronic or recurrent sinusitis and recurrent or chronic bronchial infection. Primary ciliary dyskinesia (described under bronchiectasis) is a rare autosomal recessive condition with incomplete penetration which causes both sinusitis and bronchiectasis. Cystic fibrosis is generally associated with chronic sinusitis. Kartegener's syndrome (dextrocardia, sinusitis, bronchiectasis, infertility, with or without situs inversus) has been mentioned under bronchiectasis.

Culture of pus discharged from the nose may identify pathogens. Blind nasal swabs may grow organisms which may be colonizers. Fungal culture, in particular for aspergillus, must always be asked for in chronic or recurrent sinusitis. Treatment is the same as for acute sinusitis. Drainage of pus may be necessary. A specialist ENT opinion must be sought.

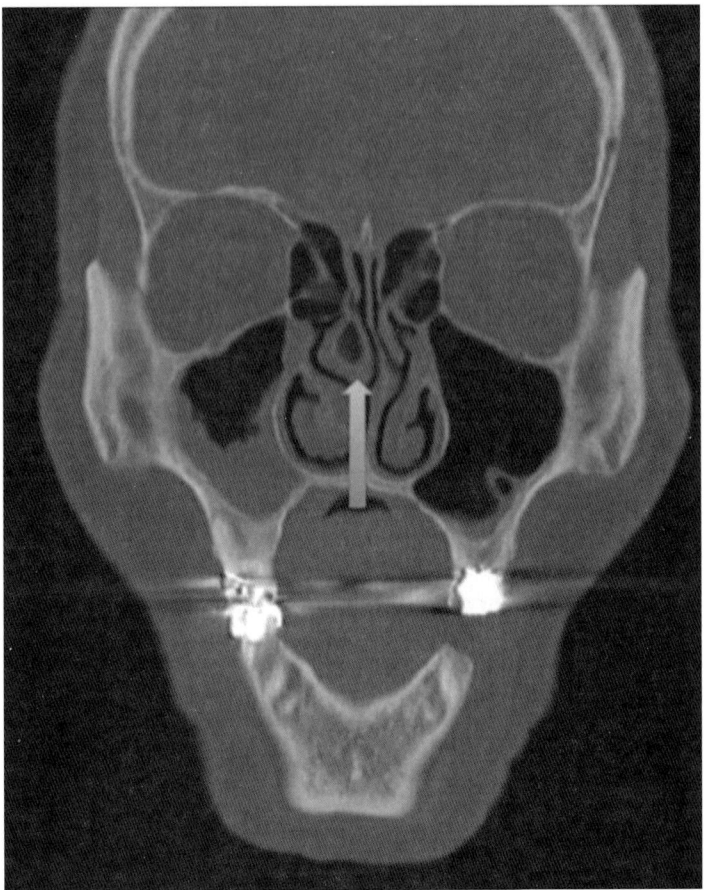

Fig 26.3: Chronic sinusitis. Coronal CT reveals pnuematization of the right middle turbinate (arrow) causing narrowing of the right maxillary ostium with resultant right maxillary mucosal thickening in the right maxillary sinus.

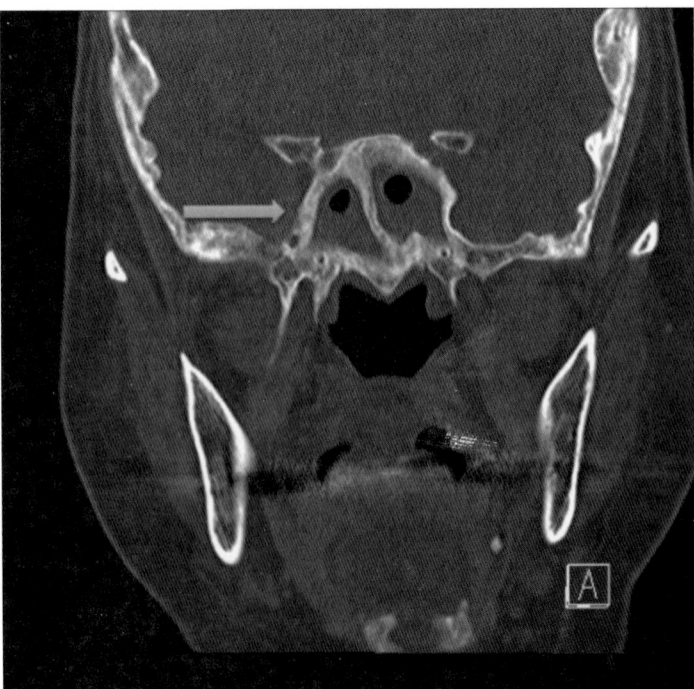

Fig 26.4: Coronal CT demonstrates soft tissue in sphenoid sinus with thickening of sphenoid sinus walls. The bony thickening is secondary to chronic sinusitis.

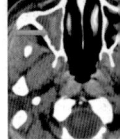

COMPLICATIONS OF BACTERIAL SINUSITIS

The most important complications are preseptal cellulitis and deeper orbital infections both grouped under orbital cellulitis. They both generally occur following ethmoidal sinusitis since the ethmoids are separated from the orbit by just a thin plate of bone. Preseptal cellulitis only involves the eyelids and surrounding structures. The eyelid appears swollen but there is no restriction of eye movements nor any orbital signs. Orbital cellulitis may go on to graduate into an orbital abscess, causing proptosis, chemosis of the conjuctiva and disturbed vision. When it follows upon an ethmoidal sinusitis, the eye is deviated downwards and outward. If treatment is delayed, vision is invariably lost.

Organisms involved are generally *S. pneumoniae*, Group A streptococcus and *H. influenzae*. Antibiotics should be given intravenously, providing a broad cover for these organisms.

A CT scan should be done in the presence of even suspicious orbital findings. An orbital abscess necessitates urgent surgical drainage.

Frontal and sphenoidal sinusitis can lead to intracranial complications. These include epidural abscess, subdural abscess, and dural vein thrombosis. Sphenoidal sinusitis can occasionally lead to thrombophlebitis of the cavernous sinus because of the proximity of the latter to the sphenoid sinus.

FUNGAL SINUSITIS

Fungal sinusitis can occur in three forms: sinus aspergilloma, allergic fungal sinusitis, and invasive fungal sinusitis.

Sinus aspergilloma is a non-invasive fungal disease occurring as a fungal ball in the maxillary sinus. It causes the usual features of chronic sinusitis often affecting the maxillary sinus. Surgical removal of the aspergilloma ball is curative.

Allergic fungal aspergillosis is characterized by a hypersensitivity reaction to fungi ubiquitous in the environment and in nasal mucosa where the fungus is trapped following inhalation. The condition is characterized by all the features of chronic sinusitis, nasal discharge, blocked nose and sinus pain. There is often a background history of nasal polyps and bronchial asthma. A CT shows inhomogeneous opacification of one or more sinuses. Bone erosion may be present but this is due to pressure necrosis and not actual invasion. Allergic fungal sinusitis is on par with allergic bronchopulmonary aspergillosis; the former is a hypersensitivity reaction within the sinus and the latter a hypersensitivity reaction in the conducting airways and the lung. The incriminating fungus is invariably *Aspergillus fumigatus*.

The condition is often diagnosed at surgery because sinus secretions are characteristically thick, sticky and brownish (likened to anchovy sauce). Fungal hyphae may be present but there is no evidence of tissue invasion. Fungal cultures most frequently grow Aspergillus species. A short course of corticosteroids given over 15 days often serves to clear the allergic fungal sinusitis just as a similar course relieves the clinical features of allergic bronchopulmonary aspergillosis.

Invasive Fungal Sinusitis

Invasive fungal sinusitis carries a high risk of mortality. Mortality is even further increased if the immune state of the patient is impaired and if the ethmoids or sphenoid sinuses are involved

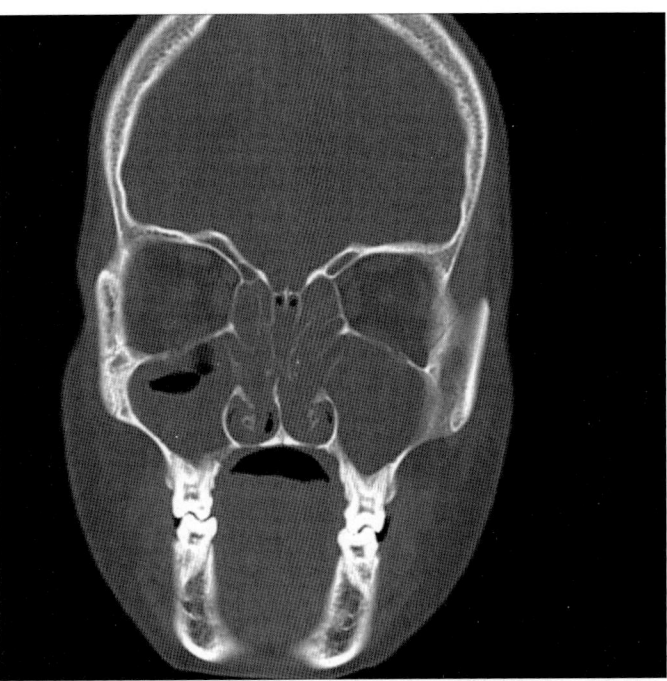

Fig 26.5: Extensive soft tissue in the paranasal sinuses, especially ethmoids with extension into nasal cavity, disruption of ethmoidal bones causing obstruction to maxillary ostii and resultant soft tissue in maxillary sinuses. These appearances of soft tissue involving all sinuses, disrupting ethmoidal bones and extending into nasal cavity are typical of aspergillus infection.

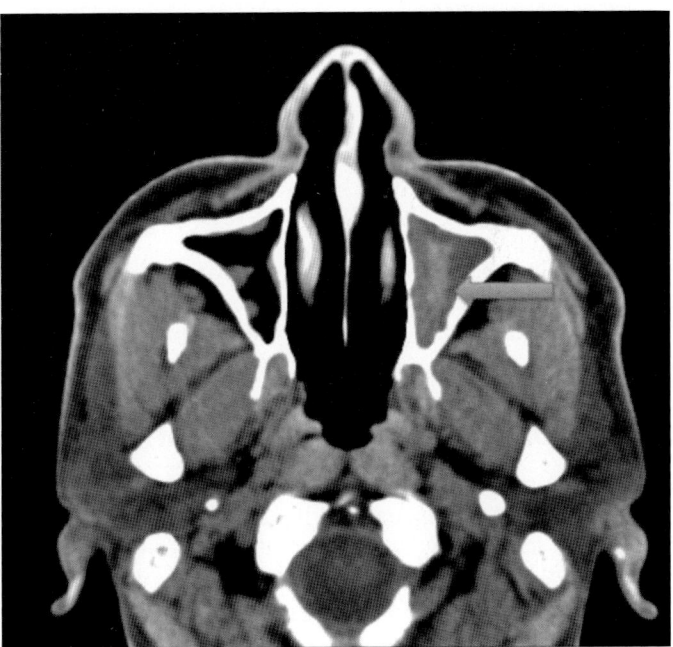

Fig 26.6: Axial scan of paranasal sinuses reveals soft tissue in left maxillary sinus with internal hyperdensity. The internal hyperdensity is indicative of aspergillus infection.

because of the proximity of the latter to the orbit, the cavernous sinus and intracranial structures.

RHINO-CEREBRAL MUCORMYCOSIS

Invasion of the nasal mucosa and of one or more paranasal sinuses by the moulds of the order mucorles (mucor, rhizopes)

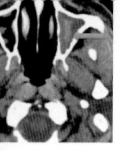

is the most devastating invasive fungal infection. Seventy per cent of infections occur in diabetics. Other risk factors are immunocompromised patients, the use of immunosuppressants, oral corticosteroids, haematological malignancies and organ transplant patients.

Clinical Features

Early clinical features consist of a swelling around both eyelids of one eye, conjuctival injection and pain over the frontal and temporal areas. The clinical features very quickly progress to resemble those of orbital cellulitis. There is proptosis of the eye, limitation of eye movements, diminished vision in the eye that may progress to blindness. Hypoaesthesia may be present in the distribution of ophthalmic and maxillary divisions of the trigeminal nerve. Necrotic blisters or eschars may be present over the skin of the eyelid and over the site of the alae nasi, also involving the mucosa of the external nares.

Nasal endoscopy shows friable mucosa with black eschars which signifies infarction of the mucosa of the nose and sinuses. Biopsy of the eschars and surrounding friable mucosa shows non-septal hyphae invading tissue, blood vessels and nerves.

A CT of the paranasal sinuses shows sinusitis with bone erosion and destruction and with varying degree of invasion of the orbit. Absence of eschar does not exclude the diagnosis; biopsy of the mucosa may still reveal the typical non-septal hyphae of mucor.

Treatment

Treatment consists of extensive surgical debridement of all infected tissue. Amphotericin or lyophilized amphotericin 5–7.5 mg/kg/d over 2 hours intravenously for 10–15 days is the treatment of choice. Voriconazole is of no use against mucor. Posaconazole is a new antifungal that has been used in patients not responding to amphotericin.

Unless diagnosed very early in the natural history of the disease, the prognosis is indeed very grim. Death invariably occurs (with few exceptions), particularly in immunocompromised patients.

OTHER FUNGI CAUSING INVASIVE SINUSITIS

Other fungi may also cause invasive fungal sinusitis. The most important and the most frequent fungus to do so belongs to the Aspergillus species. Again it is the immunocompromsied host who is most frequently infected where the onset and course is acute and is as described above. Rarely, invasive aspergillus infection of the nasal mucosa and of the sinuses can occur in normal hosts. Symptoms of orbital cellulitis as described above may evolve subacutely over weeks.

Involvement of the ethmoidal or sphenoidal sinuses by either mucor or aspergillus or other fungi carries the highest mortality. Invasive fungal inflammation spreads quickly to the apex of the orbit with involvement of the second, third, fifth, and sixth nerves. Severe pain, proptosis, and diminished vision quickly leading to blindness is observed. There is ptosis, restricted eye movements and hypoaesthesia over the ophthalmic and maxillary divisions of the fifth nerve. Spread to the cavernous sinus is common because of close proximity to the sphenoid and ethmoid sinuses. Fungal invasion of the meninges and the neuraxis is also observed. Death invariably results.

CT and magnetic resonance imaging show invasion of the sinuses with involvement of the orbit, particularly at the apex. Diagnosis is made by demonstrating fungal invasion of tissue by biopsy.

Treatment

Voriconazole given intravenously is useful for invasive aspergillus infection. It should be given for over three weeks and then continued orally. Extensive surgical debridement should be done early in immunocompromised patients. Medical treatment may alone suffice in immunocompetent patients if the disease is diagnosed early.

TRACHEOBRONCHITIS

Acute tracheobronchitis is characterized by inflammation of the mucosa of the trachea and bronchi. Mucosal inflammation of the trachea alone is termed tracheitis and of the bronchi is called bronchitis.

Tracheobronchitis is most often due to a viral infection. The viruses most frequently involved being the rhinovirus, coronovirus, influenza virus and adenovirus. Secondary bacterial infection may follow in the wake of a viral infection and is generally due to *H. influenza* or *Streptococcus pneumoniae*. Mycoplasmal infection can be a primary cause of a tracheobronchitis; occasionally, infection is due to *Bordetella pertussis*.

Clinical features consist of fever, cough which may be dry or productive of mucoid sputum. Tracheitis when severe causes substernal tightness and soreness; coughing produces a sharp burning discomfort in the chest. Rhonchi are generally audible on auscultation. Secondary bacterial infection causes the sputum to turn purulent.

Acute viral tracheobronchitis is self-limiting and requires no specific therapy. Symptomatic relief is provided by steam inhalation and oral paracetamol. The presence of secondary bacterial infection may require the use of an antibiotic, particularly in the presence of high fever and other systemic manifestations. Amoxicillin clavulanate is usually the drug of choice. Severe tracheobronchitis due to a mycoplasmal infection is best treated with a quinolone or a macrolide. Culture of tracheobronchial secretions for *Bordetella pertussis* is necessary if the cough is persistent, paroxysmal or has a clear whoop often followed by vomiting.

LARYNGITIS

Laryngitis may be associated with rhinitis or with tracheobronchitis. It is generally due to a viral infection. Cough which causes pain in the throat and over the pharynx and is accompanied by a hoarse sound points to the diagnosis. Dysphonia or total loss of voice may be present. Systemic features in the form of mild fever may also be noted. A codeine linctus offers symptomatic relief of cough.

Rest to the voice, steam inhalation, lozenges to soothe the throat, warm salt water gargles and symptomatic use of paracetamol offers relief.

Laryngitis that persists needs a careful laryngoscopic examination. Tuberculosis is an important cause. Besides

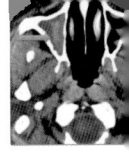

hoarseness of the voice, there is pain over the larynx on swallowing. Tuberculous laryngitis is usually but not always associated with pulmonary tuberculosis. A laryngeal swab is invariably positive for acid-fast bacilli both on staining and culture.

Hoarseness of the voice with discomfort in the throat put down to laryngitis may be the first symptom of a laryngeal cancer involving the vocal cord or the arytenoid region.

Hoarseness of the voice wrongly diagnosed as laryngitis can also result from paralysis of the recurrent laryngeal nerve from various causes. Myxoedema may cause a hoarse voice with throat discomfort and may be mistaken as laryngitis. Syphilis as a cause of laryngitis is now very rarely seen.

The dictum should be that a 'laryngitis' that persists or is chronic needs an overall review and a laryngoscopic examination.

CROUP

'Croup' is the term given to an acute laryngotracheobronchitis characterized by subglottic oedema. It occurs in children between three months to four years of age generally in the winter months and in early spring. The disease is most often due to the parainfluenza type 1 virus. Other viruses known to cause croup are the influenza virus, adenovirus, rhinovirus, enterovirus. Rarely it is due to M. pneumoniae.

Clinical features include fever, a persistent cough which has the timbre of a 'bark' and a stridor due to subglottic oedema. The stridor is inspiratory or both inspiratory and expiratory. The course of the illness is often fluctuating with periods of worsening alternating, within hours, with periods of improvement.

The diagnosis is based on clinical grounds. A viral etiology can be proven by using one of the rapid viral antigen detection techniques on nasopharyngeal swabs. The most important differential diagnosis is from acute epiglottitis. The latter is not associated with a 'barking' cough. Children with acute epiglottitis are more toxic and ill and worsen rapidly.

Treatment

Treatment consists of nebulizing racemic epinephrine which gives prompt relief. Rebound subglottic oedema needs to be carefully watched for. Corticosteroids are also of use. Nebulization of humidified air has also been tried but is of doubtful use.

ACUTE EPIGLOTTITIS

Acute epiglottitis is a life-threatening respiratory emergency as it can cause quick upper airways obstruction and death unless promptly recognized and treated. The condition chiefly seen in children is characterized by a cellulitis at the base of the tongue and the base of the epiglottis. It then involves the epiglottis itself which is swollen, pushed backwards so that it quickly obstructs the airways. The disease is rare in children vaccinated against H. influenzae Type b. In poor developing countries vaccination against H. influenzae is the exception rather than the rule. It therefore still occurs; its prevalence though uncommon is not determined. Epiglottitis can also occur in adults, the commonest cause being infection due to H. influenzae. Other infectious agents known to cause epiglottitis are Streptococcus pneumoniae, Group A streptococci, Staphylococcus aureus, and H. parainfluenzae.

Clinical Features

Symptoms evolve rapidly within 6 to 12 hours and in children is characterized by fever, toxemia, sore throat, cough (which lacks the barking character of croup), difficulty in swallowing with drooling of saliva. Upper airways obstruction causes difficulty in breathing so that the child prefers to sit up, is tachypnoeic with an inspiratory stridor.

Adolescents and adults have a less fulminant course, symptoms being present for 2 to 4 days. Fever, sore throat, cough, dysphagia, and difficulty in breathing due to an obstructed airway are the usual symptoms. A flexible fiberoptic nasopharyngoscopy reveals a swollen erythematous epiglottis. A throat swab culture should be obtained to identify the infecting organism.

Treatment

The airway must necessarily be secured and maintained. This is done by immediate insertion of an endotracheal or nasotracheal tube after the child is promptly transported (in a sitting position) to the operation theatre of a hospital. If intubation is not possible a tracheostomy needs to be urgently performed.

Adults who have no impending obstruction should be carefully observed. Broad spectrum antibiotics (amoxicillin-clavalunate) should be given intravenously for H. influenzae infection.

If epiglottitis is due to or is suspected to be caused by H. influenzae infection, the patient and all members of the family should be given rifampicin prophylaxis to eradicate carriage of the organism.

SUGGESTED READING

Ames WA, Ward VM, Tranter RM and Street M. Adult epiglottitis: an under-recognized, life-threatening condition. *Br J Anaesth.* Nov. 2000; 85(5): 795–7.

Brook I. Acute and chronic bacterial sinusitis. *Infect Dis Clin North Am.* Jun. 2007; 21(2):427–48, vii.

deShazo Richard D, Chapin Kimberle and Swain Ronnie E. Fungal Sinusitis. *N Engl J Med.* 1997; 337: 254–9.

Frantz TD, Rasgon BM and Quesenberry CP Jr. Acute epiglottitis in adults. Analysis of 129 cases. *JAMA.* 1994; 272: 1358–60.

Piccirillo Jay F. Acute Bacterial Sinusitis. *N Engl J Med.* 2004; 351: 902–10.

Reveiz L, Cardona AF and Ospina EG. Antibiotics for acute laryngitis in adults. *Cochrane Database of Systematic Reviews.* 2007, Issue 2.

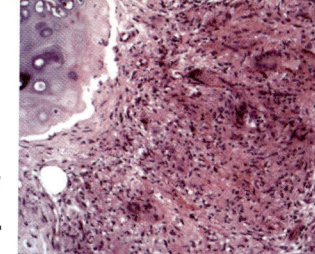

ANTIBIOTIC RESISTANCE AND ITS MANAGEMENT

CHAPTER **27** **Antibiotic Resistance and its Management**

Antibiotic resistance is increasing at a dizzying pace today—a remarkable testimony to the ability of bacteria to collect and exchange resistance genes with unimaginable efficiency. The basic mechanisms of bacterial resistance are well known. These encompass four general mechanisms, namely drug inactivation, altered target, decreased permeability, and multidrug efflux. The earlier challenges that bacterial resistance posed, were well matched by the discovery of newer molecules by the pharmaceutical industry. Critical new aspects with major implications for emergence, dissemination and maintenance of resistance include hypermutability, integrons and plasmid addiction. Globally, today, the situation has changed and with far fewer therapeutic alternatives for effective treatment, antimicrobial resistance is becoming a major concern. Resistant organisms are associated with greater morbidity and mortality and are certainly impacting the current practice of medicine. Traditionally, infections are different in both hospitals and in the community as they represent different ecosystems and different operational antibiotic selective pressures. This distinction is now becoming blurred. Infections caused by the 'ESKAPE' pathogens (*Enterococcus faecium*, *Staphylococcus aureus*, *Klebsiella pneumoniae* *Acinetobacter baumannii*, *Pseudomonas aeruginosa*, *and Enterobacter spps.*) effectively 'escape' antibacterial drugs both in hospitals and the community.

From a community perspective, upper respiratory tract infections (URTIs) are probably the most inappropriately treated group of infections. Partly due to the unavailability of cost-effective diagnostic tests to differentiate common viral infections from *Streptococcus pyogenes*, physicians would rather 'cover for bacterial infection' with broad-spectrum antibiotics. Similarly, the leading cause of lower respiratory tract infections (LRTIs) is *Streptococcus pneumoniae* and despite reassuring data that pneumoccocal resistance in the Indian subcontinent is not alarming at all, broad-spectrum cephalosporin antibiotics rather than oral amoxicillin are prescribed for a variety of reasons.

RESISTANCE IN SPECIFIC RESPIRATORY COMMUNITY PATHOGENS

Streptococcus pneumoniae

Penicillin resistance in *S. pneumoniae* is caused by reduced affinity binding by the beta lactams to the penicillin-binding proteins (PBP). Pneumococcal resistance can occur by homologous recombination of the six PBP genes. PBP2b is the primary resistance determinant for penicillin resistance whereas PBP2x is the primary determinant for cephalosporin resistance. Oral streptococci have been postulated to be the major reservoir for the novel DNA required to create the mosaic genetic sequences demonstrated by the altered pneumococcal PBP genes. Penicillin-resistant strains are resistant to penicillin derivatives, such as ampicillin and the ureidopenicillins, and are generally resistant to first- and second-generation cephalosporins. Cefotaxime and ceftriaxone are often effective because of their high levels of activity and because of the high tissue levels attained. At present, in India, penicillin, macrolide and fluoroquinolone resistance is reassuringly low, but resistance to cotrimoxazole is alarming. This is in stark contrast to other parts of the world including India's immediate neighbours, where alarming rates of resistance are reported. A debate is ongoing as to whether infections caused by resistant strains are really associated with poorer outcomes than infections caused by susceptible strains. As a consequence, the Clinical and Laboratory Standards Institute (CLSI) in 2008 revised the parenteral penicillin breakpoints with separate categories for meningeal isolates (S <0.06 µg/ml and raised the breakpoints for non-meningeal isolates (S < 2 µg/ml and R >8 µg/ml). With this change in interpretive standards, *in vitro* penicillin resistance decreased and does not seem to be a major problem in non-meningeal isolates. However, penicillin-resistant strains are frequently resistant to non-β-lactam antimicrobial agents and are often multidrug resistant. Resistance to erythromycin, tetracycline, co-trimoxazole, and chloramphenicol are the most common. Macrolide resistance is the most prominent example of pneumococcal resistance with regard to prevalence rate and the level of resistance. A recent

Table 27.1: Penicillin-Non-Susceptible *S. pneumoniae*—India				
Year	Carriage		Invasive		Study
	Pen I	Pen R	Pen I	Pen R	
1993-7	–		1.3	–	*Lancet* 1999, 353:1216
1996-2000	–		7.3	–	*Ind J Med Res* 2001, 114:127
1998-9	12.8		3.8	–	*Clin Infect Dis* 2001, 32:1463
2000-1	–		7.8	–	*Antimicrob Agents Chemother* 2004, 2101
1999-2002	16		18.3	–	*Ind J Med Microbiol* 2007, 25:256
2004	15.4		–	–	*Ind J Ped* 2007, 74:19
2000-6	–		18	1	SAPNA

Note: Pen I refers to MIC 0.12–1 µg/ml.
Pen R refers to MIC >2 µg/ml.
These values are based on the CLSI 2004 criteria.

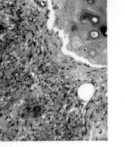

surveillance study in the United States shows that prevalence of macrolide resistance in *S. pneumoniae* is approximately 26%. The most common mechanism of macrolide resistance in *S. pneumoniae* is caused by target-site modification encoded by erythromycin ribosome methylation (erm) genes that provide inducible cross-resistance to all macrolides, lincosamides, and streptogramin B. Two other mechanisms of resistance to macrolides include active efflux pump encoded by efflux genes (*mef*A, *mef*E) that result in resistance to macrolides alone (M phenotype); and ribosomal mutations in the 23S rRNA gene.

Fluoroquinolone resistance has developed during therapy, especially in patients with prior fluoroquinolone exposures, leading to clinical failure. The older fluoroquinolones (for example, ciprofloxacin) lack reliable activity against pneumococci. Newer fluoroquinolones, such as levofloxacin, moxifloxacin, and gemifloxacin, inhibit most strains at achievable levels. The mechanism of decreased susceptibility to the newer fluoroquinolones is primarily due to mutations in the *par*C gene of topoisomerase IV and the *gyr*A gene of DNA gyrase.

Haemophilus influenzae

H. influenzae-related respiratory infections are on the rise the world over. Recognition of non-encapsulated strains as causative agents in acute exacerbations of chronic obstructive pulmonary disease is compelling. In India, *H. influenzae* is not often isolated by microbiological laboratories and thus resistance rates are not clearly defined. In a multicentre study in India, the incidence of β lactamase production in Haemophilus spps. in LRTIs was noted to be 17.2%. Approximately 90% of β lactamase-producing *H. influenzae* possess the constitutive plasmid TEM-1 enzyme. These isolates are resistant to amoxicillin but remain fully susceptible to the β lactam/β lactamase inhibitor combinations. The cephalosporins vary in their activity against the β lactamase-producing strains. The third-generation cephalosporins are most active and some second-generation cephalosporins such as cefaclor and cefprozil are the least active. Non-β lactamase-producing strains with altered PBPs are infrequently isolated. *H. influenzae* is usually resistant to erythromycin but susceptible *in vitro* to azithromycin; the 14-OH metabolite of clarithromycin continues to be fairly active.

Moraxella catarrhalis and Streptococcus pyogenes

In the US, more than 95% of all *M. catarrhalis* produce a chromosomal, constitutive β lactamase called the Brovasio enzyme (BRO-1 and BRO-2) which may compromise treatment with amoxicillin. However, most strains are susceptible to cephalosporins, β lactamase inhibitor combinations and macrolides. In contrast, *S. pyogenes* continues to be susceptible to penicillin but resistance to macrolides and tetracyclines ranges up to 40% in both classes.

Staphylococcus aureus and Community Acquired Methicillin-Resistant Staphylococcus aureus (CA MRSA)

Staphylococcus aureus has developed resistance to newer antibiotics over the years. Usually, in complicated post-viral respiratory infections such as influenza, today the world over, more than 90% *S. aureus* produce β lactamase, rendering penicillin and its derivatives ineffective. Methicillin resistance is also frequent and may exceed 50% in some tertiary care centres. MRSA evolved through the acquisition of the staphylococcus casette chromosome *mec* (SCCmec). Resistance to methicillin and other β lactam antibiotics is mediated by the *mec*A gene, which encodes for an additional PBP (PBP2a) that has low affinity for β lactams. To date, eight types of SCC*mec* (I–VIII) have been reported. CA MRSA are both phenotypically and genotypically distinct from Healthcare Associated MRSA (HA MRSA) and are genotypically SCC*mec* IV and SCC*mec*V types. They are susceptible to multiple classes of antibiotics other than the β lactams such as clindamycin, co-trimoxazole, tetracyclines etc. In a recent study in Mumbai, of the SCC*mec* IV strains, 83% were susceptible to many antimicrobial classes and the rest were susceptible to three classes, none being MDR.

The emergence of CA MRSA especially in skin and soft tissue infections in the community has abolished the belief that resistant organisms bear a fitness cost in the presence of antibiotic stress. These highly competent clones are capable of spreading locally and internationally. Known to cause severe necrotizing multilobar pneumonia in young healthy adults and children, these strains usually produce the Panton Valentine Leucocidin (PVL) that enhances their toxigenicity.

RESISTANCE IN NOSOCOMIAL ISOLATES

Enterobacteriaceae and Non Fermenters Gram-negative Bacilli

Hospitals today are facing an unprecedented crisis due to the increasingly rapid emergence and dissemination of antibiotic-resistance genes. As hospitals concentrate vulnerable patients, it is an accepted fact that antibiotic resistance is far more prevalent.

Today infections with Extended Spectrum β Lactamases (ESBLs) are posing an immense threat to clinical therapeutics. ESBLs are clavulanate-inhibited transferable enzymes that hydrolyse all penicillins, ampicillin, amoxicillin, as also all cephalosporins with an oxyimino side chain (cefotaxime, ceftriaxone, ceftazidime, cefepime etc.), as well as monobactam, and aztreonam. They are inactive against carbapenems and cephamycins. ESBLs are mainly encountered in organisms like *E. coli*, *Klebsiella* spps, *Proteus mirabilis*, *Enterobacter* spps, *Citrobacter* spps etc. ESBLs are frequently plasmid encoded and may also carry genes encoding resistance to other drug classes like aminoglycosides, quinolones, co-trimoxazole. Nosocomial infections, ESBLs as well as *AmpC* production by Enterobacteriaceae are posing a huge threat to clinical therapeutics. In most Indian city hospitals, the overall prevalence of ESBLs is more than 60%. Though organisms such as *E. coli*, *Proteus* spps, *Enterobacter* spps, *Citrobacter* spps etc., are not traditional respiratory pathogens, *Klebsiella pneumoniae* is known to cause pneumonia in certain risk groups. Risk factors for nosocomial infection with ESBL producers include prolonged hospital stay, use of invasive medical devices, therapy with second or third-generation cephalosporins, penicillins and fluoroquinolones, administration of total parenteral nutrition (TPN), recent surgery, and haemodialysis.

In patients with late-onset ventilator-associated pneumonia (VAP), *Pseudomonas aeruginosa* and *Acinetobacter baumannii* are established pathogens. In India, with high rates of ESBLs,

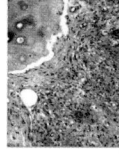

empiric therapy with carbapenems is the standard of care in seriously ill patients. Predictably, in patients on carbapenem antibiotics, or in situations with poor infection control practices, the carbapenemases tend to get selected out and easily spread. Carbapenemase-producing Gram-negative organisms can hydrolyze all penicillins, cephalosporins, and carbapenems and they have been reported in several large outbreaks in hospitalized patients. *Klebsiella pneumoniae* carbapenemase (KPC) is classically associated with *K. pneumoniae*.

Metallo-β lactamases are β lacta-hydrolyzing enzymes that contain a zinc moiety and are known to cause several extended outbreaks of nosocomial infections and are commonly found in Pseudomonas and Acinetobacter species. There are two major groups of metallo-β lactamases: the IMP-type carbapenemases and the Verona integron-encoded metallo-β lactamase (VIM) carbapenemases. The emergence of the New Delhi Metallo beta lactamase (NDM)-1 in Enterobacteriaceae that have the potential to spread, is a worrying development; the risk of a wider international spread cannot be ignored.

Additional mechanisms augmenting β lactamase activity involve loss of porin channels in the outer cellular membrane, upregulation of efflux pumps, decreasing antibiotic concentrations in the periplasmic space and facilitating hydrolysis by β-lactamases.

Unfortunately, the emerging threat of pan-resistant Gram-negative bacilli with their remarkable resilience and environmental versatility epitomize the opportunistic infections that we will now have to contend with.

PREVENTING AND REDUCING RESISTANCE

Antibiotic resistance poses an ever-increasing threat to public health. We propose the following '10 commandments' to reduce overall antibiotic resistance.

1. Establish an aetiological diagnosis using rapid diagnostic tests wherever possible.
2. Draw up rational guidelines in the form of an antibiotic policy by the hospital infection control committee core group (infectious disease physician, clinical microbiologist, and clinical pharmacologist) with input from chest physicians for specific lung infections to help curtail unnecessary use. Empiric antibiotic therapy should be based on the knowledge of common causative pathogens for a particular infection (Table 27.2), known local susceptibility surveillance data, and host factors with special regard to patient co-morbidities and specific risk factors. Antibiotic history is also becoming an important consideration in choosing the right drug. From the perspective of the community, knowing the epidemiology of prevalence of organisms with the likely antibiotic resistance pattern of specific pathogens is vital.

3. Deescalate from broad-spectrum empiric therapy to narrow spectrum as soon as susceptibilities are available. From the perspective of serious infections in the hospital, there is also an urgent requirement to focus on culture and susceptibility before empiric therapy, so that once this has been initiated, streamlining of antibiotics to a narrower spectrum, and to efficacious and more cost-effective options can be quickly instituted.

4. Choosing appropriate dosing for the right duration is an important aspect of antibiotic regimens. Pharmacokinetic (PK) and pharmacodynamic (PD) principles which optimize Time above MIC specifically for the β lactams, Area under the Curve (AUC)/MIC ratios for the fluoroquinolones, and Peak to MIC ratios (C max/MIC) for aminoglycosides, should be followed. We need to identify antibiotic exposures that prevent amplification of resistant subpopulations of bacteria.

5. Do not treat undrained abscesses or foreign body infections with antibiotics. Abscesses require drainage and infected foreign bodies require to be removed.

6. Distinguish colonization from true infection, especially in the interpretation of positive cultures from non-sterile sites such as sputum or endotracheal aspirates. Within limitations, quantitative cultures may help to delineate true infection.

7. Do not continue to treat only leucocytosis or fever with antibiotics in the intensive care setting, without determining their cause.

8. Methods to detect outbreaks in hospitals, especially those with resistant organisms must be in place.

9. Education and training of doctors helps to ensure appropriate usage. Education alone is the foundation that will enhance and influence prescribing behaviour. Strategies that inform rather than dictate work better in curtailing use.

10. Demand compliance with good infection control practices including hand hygiene, barrier precautions and environmental disinfection. Guidelines for Infection Control certainly serve to stem the tide of dissemination of resistant determinants in the hospital.

MANAGING ANTIBIOTIC RESISTANCE

Preserving the effectiveness of the current antibiotics by reducing resistance and improving outcomes is the goal of antimicrobial stewardship. Raising awareness about the escalating problem of antimicrobial resistance with interventional programmes is required. Recently, the Infectious Disease Society of America (IDSA) and the Society of Healthcare Epidemiology of America (SHEA) published guidelines for developing an institutional antimicrobial stewardship programme. The goals include optimizing clinical outcomes while minimizing the unintended consequences of antimicrobial use by focusing on two evidence-based principles, namely prospective drug use audit

Table 27.2: Per cent Aetiology of Community-Acquired Pneumonia (CAP) in a study in Mumbai	
Streptococcus pneumoniae	30
Chlamydia pneumoniae	13
Haemophilus influenzae	7
Moraxella catarrhalis	6
Mycoplasma pneumoniae	4
Legionella pneumophila	2
Klebsiella pneumoniae	2
Staph aureus	1

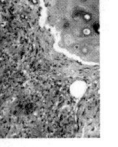

with intervention/feedback, and formulary restriction with preauthorization requirements for specific agents. Comprehensive programmes are cost-effective with dose optimization, parenteral to oral switches etc. Indeed, planning and implementing such stewardship programmes in a well-orchestrated and well-designed manner is a huge challenge. Most practising physicians are not overly concerned about the long-term ecologic effects of antibiotics on microbes. Resistance to antibiotics is unavoidable from an evolutionary perspective, and the simple truth about antibiotics is—the more you use them, the more you will lose them! With the Gram-negative antibiotic pipeline practically drying up for the next 10–15 years, it is time to dispel our misplaced optimism that some new drug is bound to arrive.

The 10 × 20 initiative promises a global commitment to develop ten new antibacterials by 2020. However, we must remember that antibiotic prescribing is the main driver of resistance, and resistance is clearly a function of the volume consumed. No single strategy to combat this burgeoning problem of antibiotic resistance seems to be working effectively. Lastly, we must appreciate that we are indeed fortunate to belong to a generation of physicians who have been able to treat and cure infections in this golden era of antibiotics. If we have to pass on this antibiotic legacy to our future generations there is an urgent need for introspection. After all, resistance in bacteria is not a matter of 'if' but of 'when'.

SUGGESTED READING

Boucher Helen W, Talbot George H, Bradley John S, Edwards Jr John E, Gilbert David, Rice Louis B, Sheld Michael, Spellberg Brad, Bartlett John. Bad bugs, No drugs: No ESKAPE! An update from the Infectious Disease Society America. *Clin Infect Dis*. 2009; 48:1–12.

D'Souza Namita, Rodrigues Camilla, Mehta Ajita. Molecular characterization of Methicillin-Resistant Staphylococcus aureus (MRSA) with emergence of epidemic clones of Sequence Type ST 22 and ST 772 in Mumbai, India. *J Clin Microbiol*. 2010; 48(5) in press.

Deshpande Payal, Rodrigues Camilla, Shetty Anjali, Kapadia Farhad, Hegde Ashit, Soman Rajeev. New Delhi Metallo beta lactamase (NDM)—1 in Enterobacteriaceae; Treatment options with carbapenems compromised. *JAPI*. 2010: 58; 147–9.

Jae-Hoon S, Sook-In J, Kwan SK, Na YK, Jun SS, Hyun-ha C, Hyun KK, Won SO, *et al*. High prevalence of antimicrobial resistance among clinical *Streptococcus pneumoniae* isolates in Asia (an ANSORP) study; *Antimicrob Agents Chemother*. 2004; 48: 2101–7.

Lakshmi V. Need for National/regional guidelines and policies in India to combat antibiotic resistance. *Ind J Med. Microbiol*. 2008; 26(2):105–7.

Lalitha MK, Kurien Thomas. Antibiotic resistance among *Streptococcus pneumonia*: in Antibiotic resistance—the modern epidemic: Current status and research issues—proceedings of the 9th Sir Dorabji Tata Symposium (eds), Raghunath D, Nagaraja V, Durga Rao C. 2009; 147–52.

Mehta A, Rodrigues C, Kumar R, Rattan A, Sridhar H, Gunde V, Mattoo V. A Pilot programme of Haemophilus Surveillance in India. *Ind J Clin Pract*. 1997; 7(10): 81–4.

Raghunath D. Emerging antibiotic resistance in bacteria with special reference to India. *J Biosc*. 2008; 33(4): 593–603.

Shanthi M, Sekar Uma. Multi-drug Resistant *Pseudomonas aeruginosa* and *Acinetobacter baumannii* Infections among Hospitalized Patients: Risk Factors and Outcomes. *JAPI*. 2009; 57: 636–40.

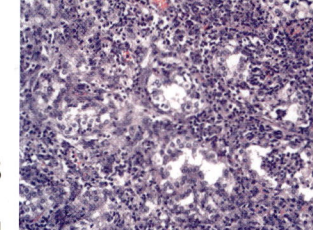

CHAPTER 28

HIV and the Lung

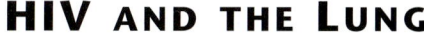

The lungs have been at the forefront of the HIV epidemic ever since its first description. The seemingly innocuous first description of what was to become HIV came from the initial historic Morbidity and Mortality Weekly Report (MMWR) report on 5 June 1981 with the title 'Pneumocystis pneumonia—Los Angeles'. Not even the most pessimistic reader of that initial account could ever have guessed the scale of the subsequent pandemic less than three decades later with almost 50 million people affected worldwide. Recent data shows that more than 80% of HIV infections in Asia are in Thailand and India, and that the mode of disease transmission was primarily unprotected sexual intercourse with female sex workers.

The reader is referred to a separate text for a thorough understanding of HIV infection and its natural history. The

Table 28.1:
Prevalence of HIV/AIDS world-wide

Region	Adults & children living with HIV/AIDS	Adults & children newly infected	Adult prevalence*	Deaths of adults & children
Sub-Saharan Africa	22.4 million	1.9 million	5.2%	1.4 million
North Africa & Middle East	310,000	35,000	0.2%	20,000
South and South-East Asia	3.8 million	280,000	0.3%	270,000
East Asia	850,000	75,000	<0.1%	59,000
Eastern Europe & Central Asia	1.5 million	110,000	0.7%	87,000
North America	1.4 million	55,000	0.4%	25,000
Western & Central Europe	850,000	30,000	0.3%	13,000
Global Total	33.4 million	2.7 million	0.8%	2.0 million

Source: Adapted from AVERT, Link-www.AVERT.org

Table 28.2:
China AIDS Statistics

Estimated total population, July 2008	1,330,045,000
Estimated number of people living with HIV/AIDS, end 2007	700,000
Proportion of adults with HIV/AIDS who are women, end 2007	29%
Estimated adult prevalence of HIV/AIDS, end 2007	0.1%
Estimated number of AIDS deaths in 2007	39,000

Source: Adapted from AVERT, Link-www.AVERT.org

Table 28.3:
Thailand AIDS Statistics

Estimated total population, July 2008	65,493,000
Estimated number of people living with HIV/AIDS, end 2007	610,000
Proportion of adults with HIV/AIDS who are women, end 2007	42%
Children (0–15) living with HIV/AIDS, end 2007	14,000
Estimated adult prevalence of HIV/AIDS, end 2007	1.4%
Estimated number of AIDS deaths in 2007	31,000

Source: Adapted from AVERT, Link-www.AVERT.org

table given below shows the extent of the HIV pandemic with special reference to Thailand and China. The Indian data on pulmonary infections in HIV patients is considered separately.

This chapter discusses the pulmonary involvement in AIDS, the lung being the single most common involved organ both on autopsy and clinical studies. An autopsy study from 1985 showed that there was pulmonary involvement in 90% of AIDS patients with a wide spectrum of infectious and non-infectious complications being encountered. Both HIV-1 and HIV-2 have been isolated from the lung and it is clear that the lung is an important organ of viral replication. The spectrum of pulmonary problems encountered in HIV is given in Tables 28.4 and 28.5.

PULMONARY IMMUNE RESPONSE IN AIDS

HIV infection besides severely impairing the overall general immune response of the body also impairs the local immune response within the lung. The mechanism underlying the dysregulation of the pulmonary immune response continues to be the subject of research. Immune dysregulation is probably a result of the interaction between the human immunodeficiency virus circulating through the lung capillaries, other circulating antigens with a potential to cause disease, airborne inhaled antigens and local immune cells responsible for local immune responses. This local battle within the lungs takes place under the shadow of an overall generalized depressed immune response (in particular cell-mediated immunity) of the immune system of the body.

Attempts to study the dysregulation of the local pulmonary response to HIV infection include the use of *in vitro* cell cultures to mimic the actual pulmonary environment and the study of cells recovered from bronchoalveolar lavage (BAL) fluid through bronchoscopy in infected patients. In the latter form of study, most patients have advanced disease, many are on antiretroviral drugs and most have more than one pathogen

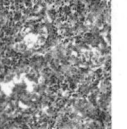

Table 28.4: Pulmonary Infections in HIV
Bacterial Infections:
M. tuberculosis
Strep pneumoniae
H. influenzae
Non-tuberculous mycobacteria (MAC)
Staphylococcus aureus
Nocardia, Listeria
Klebsiella spp
Rhodococcus equi
Parasitic Infections:
Toxoplasma gondii
Cryptosporidium spp
Microsporidium spp
Leishmania spp
Strongyloides spp
Fungal infections:
Pneumocystis carinii pneumonia (PCP)
Cryptococus neoformans
Histoplasma capsulatum
Candida albicans
Coccidioides immitis
Aspergillus spp
Viral Infections:
Cytomegalovirus
Herpes simplex
Varicella zoster
EB virus
HHV-6
JC virus
RSV
HHV-8 (KSAHV)

Table 28.5: Non-infectious Pulmonary Manifestations
Malignancy:
Kaposi sarcoma
B cell lymphoma
Primary effusion Lymphoma (Body-Cavity Associated Lymphomas)
Castleman's diseases
Bronchogenic carcinoma
Idiopathic:
ILD: LIP, NSIP
Airway disease: bronchiolitis, emphysema
Diffuse infiltrative CD8 lymphocytosis
Sarcoidosis
BOOP
Primary pulmonary hypertension
Alveolar haemorrhage

causing pulmonary disease. Each of these features can influence results of immune studies so performed. An unsettled question is the site or sites of local immune response to HIV infection within the lung and whether the cells within BAL fluid are representative of the immune response arising from one or more of these sites.

RISK FACTORS FOR RESPIRATORY DISEASES

Risk factors depend on the following:

Geography

Geography, socioeconomic factors associated with certain geographical areas of the world influence the nature of pulmonary infections, notably with reference to mycobacterial and fungal disease. Pulmonary tuberculosis is the commonest pulmonary infection in HIV patients in India.

Severity of Immunocompromise

The lower the CD4 count and the higher the plasma RNA viral load, the greater the risk of pulmonary infection. HIV patients with CD4 counts below 200 cells/uL are far more prone to recurrent attacks of bacterial pneumonia, and to infection by exotic opportunistic organisms such as *Pneumocystis carinii*, other fungi such as the Aspergillus species and *Penicillium marneffei* or opportunistic bacteria such as *Nocardia asteroids* and *Rhodococcus equi*. Opportunistic viral infections also make their appearance with very low CD4 counts. These exotic infections are merely a reflection of marked T-cell depletion causing markedly lowered cell-mediated immune response coupled with macrophage dysfunction.

Drug Addiction

Intravenous use of drugs by drug addicts is a great risk factor for the development of pulmonary infection, in particular bacterial pneumonias and mycobacterial infection.

History of Previous Infections

HIV patients with a previous history of bacterial pneumonia or an episode of Pneumocystis carinii pneumonia (PCP) in the past are at greater risk of recurrence of these infections. This is perhaps chiefly related to the underlying poor host immune response but may also be influenced by environmental factors. Since HIV-infected smokers seem to have a higher rate of pneumonia than non-smokers, background structural and functional damage to the lungs (as in smokers) may well be an additional risk factor. Recent studies suggest that chronic obstructive pulmonary disease (COPD) and lung cancer occur more frequently among

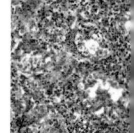

HIV-infected individuals compared to the general population. This emphasizes the added urgency of stopping smoking in HIV-infected individuals.

Use of PCP Prophylaxis

Numerous studies have shown that the use of trimethoprim + sulfamethoxazole in all patients with a CD4 below 200 cells/uL has clearly reduced the incidence of PCP. This subject is discussed later in the chapter.

Use of Highly Active Antiretroviral Therapy (HAART)

The use of specific antiretroviral therapy to combat HIV by controlling and reducing its replication has been shown to clearly reduce the incidence of pulmonary infections and slow the tempo of the natural history of the disease. In the richer countries of the world where HAART is readily available, opportunistic infections associated with very low CD4 counts (i.e. cytomegalovirus (CMV) infection, infection by mycobacterium avium intracellulare) are much less frequent. Malignant diseases such as Non-Hodgkin's lymphoma are being more frequently observed.

INDIAN DATA

Data from India is limited but an early autopsy study by Lanjewar and Duggal in 2001, (*Ref: N Lanjewar and R Duggal Pulmonary pathology in patients with AIDS: an autopsy study from Mumbai. HIV Med. 2001 October; 2(4): 266–271*) showed tuberculosis accounted for 61% of all pulmonary disease with bacterial pneumonias featuring second in terms of frequency at 18%. A more recent study by one of the authors (*Ref: Udwadia ZF, Doshi AV, et al. Pneumocystis carinii pneumonia in HIV-infected patients from Mumbai. J Assoc Physicians India. 2005 May; 53: 437–40*) was a prospective study of all hospitalizations for HIV in a tertiary centre in Mumbai over two years (2002–03). In this study, which looked at 300 consecutive HIV +ve admissions, the lungs were the single most common organ system affected (120 of 300 admissions, 40%). In this study, tuberculosis (pulmonary and extra-pulmonary) was the most common pulmonary cause of admissions (46/120, 40%). The novel information that emerged from this study was that PCP, previously considered rare in the Indian context, ranked second in importance (34 admissions, 30%). Bacterial infections (pneumonia) ranked third with 30 cases (25%). Malignancies and miscellaneous conditions accounted for 4% each. A more recent study from Chennai (*Ref: S. Rajasekaran, A. Mahilmaran Manifestation of tuberculosis in patients with human immunodeficiency virus: A large Indian study. Ann Thorac Med. 2007 Apr–Jun; 2(2): 58–60*) showed that of 12, 750 HIV-confirmed patients visiting the hospital, 4, 383 (34.4%) patients had tuberculosis. Among them, 2, 448 (55.9%) had pulmonary tuberculosis, and the remaining 1, 935 (44.1%) had either disseminated or extra-pulmonary tuberculosis.

PULMONARY INFECTIONS IN HIV DISEASE

Co-infection with tuberculosis and HIV has been comprehensively covered in the section on 'Pulmonary Tuberculosis'. Opportunistic infections, both bacterial and non-bacterial have been dealt with in an earlier chapter titled 'Pneumonia in the

Non-HIV Immunocompromised Patient'. *The clinical features and treatment of different pneumonias including pneumonia caused by opportunistic infections in immunocompromised HIV-infected patients and in non-HIV immunocompromised patients are very much the same.* The reader is therefore referred to the chapter on 'Pneumonia in the Non-HIV Immunocompromised Patient' as also to the chapter on 'Non-Bacterial Pneumonia'. However, the following features in relation to pulmonary infections in HIV-infected patients need to be stressed.

1. Tuberculosis is the commonest pulmonary infection encountered in HIV patients in India, Africa and Southeast Asia.
2. Severe advanced HIV disease can result in the suppression of cell-mediated immune response with CD4 counts falling to < 50 cells/uL. As a result, the range of exotic opportunistic pulmonary infections in HIV is generally greater than in non-HIV conditions causing immunosuppression.
3. Symptoms and signs of pulmonary infection in HIV-infected patients with very low CD4 counts are meagre or even absent, rendering diagnosis of various pulmonary infections difficult.
4. Multiple infections due to multiple organisms (including opportunistic microorganisms) are to be expected in AIDS patients with very low CD4 counts. As an example pneumocystis pneumonia is often associated with cytomegalovirus infection and at times with infections caused by mycobacterium avium intracellulare.
5. Response to therapy even when this is specific is perhaps poorest when pulmonary infections occur in severe HIV disease with very low CD4 counts (<50 cells/uL).
6. Specific therapy in relation to both opportunistic and non-opportunistic infections in HIV patients needs to be combined with antiretroviral therapy. Specific treatment has been mentioned in the chapter on 'Pneumonia in the Non-HIV Immunocompromised Patient'. For details on combined antiretroviral therapy the reader should consult another text.
7. Immune Reconstitution Inflammatory Syndrome (IRIS) Before the era of antiretroviral therapy for HIV infection, it was observed that patients with tuberculosis on anti-TB drugs who appeared to be responding to therapy, could occasionally develop for a short while, clinical deterioration with exacerbation both in the clinical and radiological features of the disease. Yet the overall patient response to continued medical therapy was good. This 'paradoxical reaction' was believed to have an immunological basis.

Following the widespread use of HAART, similar 'paradoxical reactions', often of marked severity, have been observed in HIV-infected patients. These 'reactions' in the context of HIV-infected individuals have been termed the *Immune Reconstitution Inflammatory Syndrome (IRIS)*. The syndrome has a varied clinical presentation, and has been observed in a wide range of opportunistic infections in HIV patients, treated with both antiretroviral drugs as also with therapy directed against the prevailing opportunistic infection. Typically and most commonly this 'reaction' is observed after the initiation of antiretroviral therapy in a patient being treated for pulmonary tuberculosis. There is observed a return or exacerbation of tuberculosis, together with systemic features such as fever, dyspnoea and a radiological worsening of the lesion. This may

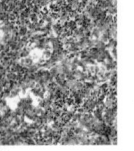

be associated with the development of new lesions at different sites. Though IRIS is most commonly observed in infections due to *Mycobacterium tuberculosis*, it is also seen with other opportunistic infections due to *Mycobacterium avium intracellulare*, fungi (cryptococcal infection in particular), and viruses (hepatitis, herpes viridae).

IRIS has been more fully discussed in the chapter on 'HIV-TB Co-infection' (see section on 'Pulmonary Tuberculosis') to which the reader should refer.

The rest of this chapter focuses chiefly on PCP, offers a few pertinent remarks on community-acquired pneumonia (CAP) and briefly discusses malignancies in relation to HIV infection and idiopathic non-infective non-malignant disorders associated with HIV infection.

Pneumocystis carinii Pneumonia

INTRODUCTION AND EPIDEMIOLOGY

Globally, PCP accounted for almost two-thirds of the AIDS index diagnoses in the first decade of the HIV pandemic. It remains the most prevalent opportunistic infection (OI) in patients with HIV even today. Considered rare in the Indian, Asian and African context, our letter in the *New England Journal of Medicine* in 2004 pointed out that in the developing world it was probably being under-diagnosed due to lack of special diagnostic facilities like high-resolution computed tomography (HRCT) scanning, bronchoscopy and BAL studies and special immunofluorescence stains. Our study not only showed it to be common when diligently searched for but also revealed that almost half of all our cases (49%) would have been missed without access to sophisticated diagnostic techniques. Earlier deaths from tuberculosis and more pathogenic organisms may also have been partly responsible for less PCP being reported from Africa and India. In our series, PCP occurred at a mean CD4 count of just 96 cells/µl.

In the developed world while PCP remains one of the commonest OIs, there is little doubt that its incidence is declining in the West. There are two reasons for this decline; firstly, effective trimethoprim-sulfamethoxazole (TMP-SMX) is used in almost all patients with CD 4 counts < 200 as such patients are almost nine times more likely to develop PCP. The second reason behind the decline is the widespread availability of antiretroviral (ARV) therapy. PCP will always retain its importance in HIV and sadly, continue to develop in patients unaware of their HIV status, those with no access to care, those unwilling or unable to adhere to therapy and non-responders or failures with ARV therapy.

TAXONOMY

The longstanding controversy about whether to place PCP in the parasitic or fungal families has finally been settled by elegant gene sequencing studies by Edman reported in Nature, incontrovertibly linking PCP to the FUNGAL family. Pneumocystis jiroveci (PCJ) is the proposed new name after the Czech parasitologist Otto Jirovec. This new name first proposed by Frenkel has now been accepted by Centers for Disease Control and Prevention (CDC) and the National Institutes of Health (NIH) from 2002.

CLINICAL FEATURES

The commonest symptoms are dyspnoea and cough. The single commonest sign is tachypnoea. A study from Zimbabwe established that a respiratory rate > 40/min is the single best clinical predictor of PCP in HIV-positive patients. Crackles and ronchi are infrequent and while hypoxia is common, it is by no means universal. In one of our units, 50% of patients had a normal SaO_2 at rest and 15% had a completely normal clinical examination. The mean duration from onset of symptoms to final diagnosis averaged as long as 30 days in our series. In fact, rapid onset of symptoms, high fever and rigours are all rare in PCP and are much more commonly encountered in pyogenic infections.

RADIOLOGY

In the early stages, bilateral mid-zone interstitial shadows are seen. These are often subtle and normal chest radiographs have been reported in 5–34% of series. In our Hinduja Hospital series 10% of patients had normal radiographs. HRCT greatly increases the diagnostic yield, with bilateral patchy areas of centrally located ground-glass density being the commonest CT pattern. In approximately 10% of cases air-filled cysts or pneumatoceles may be seen in the upper lobes. A variety of atypical radiographic features have been reported. These include: upper lobe infiltrates (especially in patients on nebulized pentamidine prophylaxis), cystic changes, pneumothorax, pleural effusions, focal nodular lesions, cavitation and adenopathy. It must be pointed out that effusions, upper lobe infiltrates and adenopathy are all much more likely to be secondary to TB than PCP, especially in the Indian context. Of importance is the fact that while the evolution of the shadows is often rapid, they are slow to resolve. A study by DeLorenzo in Chest in 1987 of 104 PCP patients showed that at three weeks only 35% of patients' radiographs had actually improved and at five months complete resolution had occurred in only 43%.

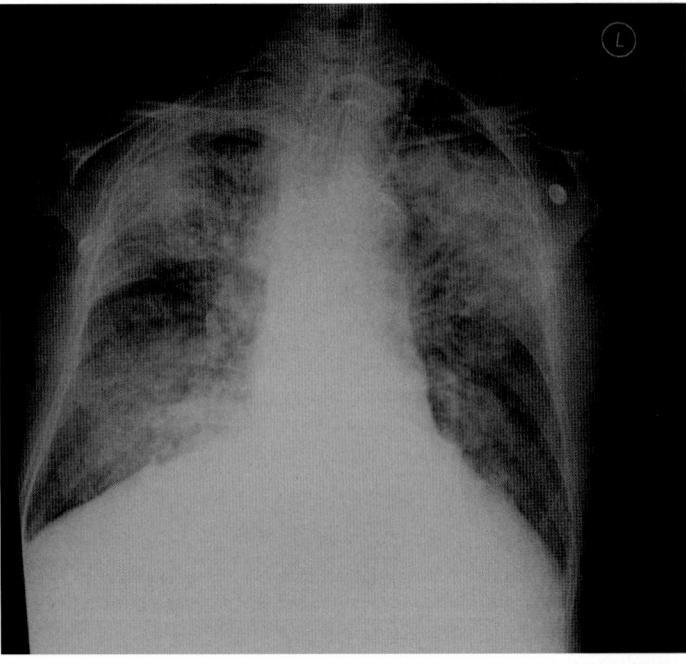

Fig 28.1: PCP. Chest X-ray demonstrates ill-defined opacities in both lung fields.

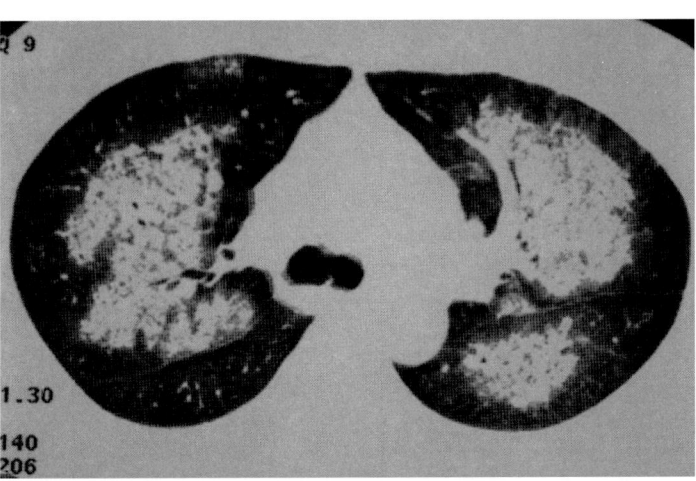

Fig 28.2: PCP. Chest CT demonstrates ill-defined ground-glass densities in both lung fields.

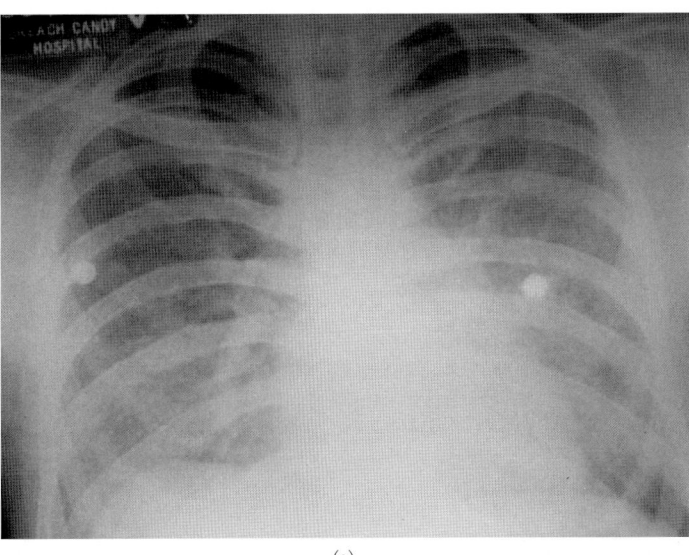

(a)

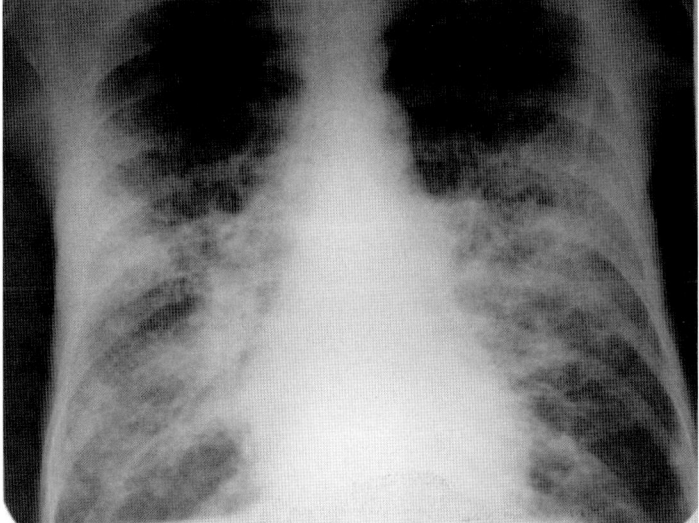

Fig 28.3: PCP. A 43-year-old male patient with a longstanding history of smoking, alcohol abuse and HIV presented with high-grade fever and low oxygen saturation. Chest X-ray demonstrates ill-defined areas of ground-glass densities in both lung fields, essentially in the parahilar location. Bronchoscopic lavage revealed PCP.

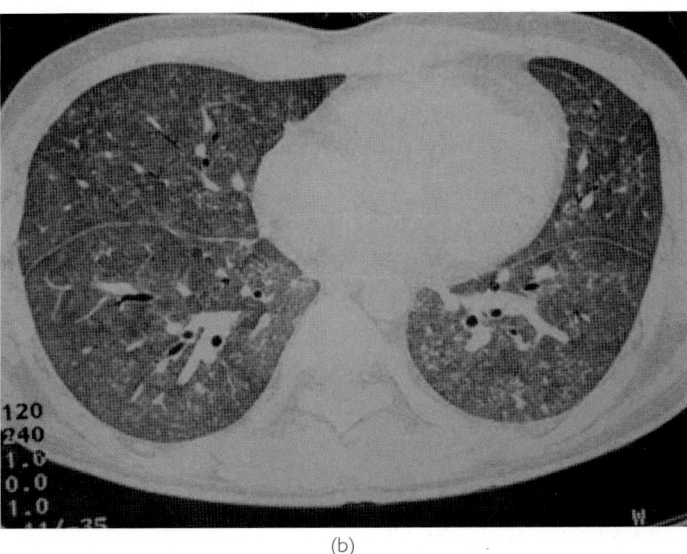

(b)

Fig 28.4 (a) and (b): PCP in a seropositive male with cough, fever and dyspnoea. Chest X-ray (a) reveals diffuse ground-glass densities in both lung fields. HRCT chest (b) confirms diffuse ground-glass densities in both lung fields.

Other diagnostic tests: Increase in lactate dehydrogenase (LDH) and desaturation with exercise are both sensitive but not specific tests.

MICROBIOLOGY

Microbiology is crucial to making a diagnosis. Sputum is often not produced and hence must be induced by nebulization with hypertonic saline. The yield can be improved by performing a BAL. A transbronchial biopsy is seldom performed but increases diagnostic yield further. In our series we had four patients with negative BAL but PCP was proven on transbronchial lung biopsy only. The stains used are Gomori methenamine, Calcofluor white and immunofluorescence staining which we have found sensitive and extremely specific for identifying trophic and cystic forms.

TREATMENT

TMP-SMX (trimethoprim-sulphamethoxazole) in a dose of two double-strength tablets thrice daily (TMP-SMX—160 mg trimethoprim, 800 mg sulphamethoxazole constitutes a double-strength tablet) remains the treatment of choice in PCP. Unfortunately, side-effects are common at the high doses needed and as many as 50% of patients develop major side-effects which demand temporary or permanent discontinuation.

Clindamycin (300 mg TDS/QDS) plus primaquine (15–30 mg OD) is a reasonable alternative and often one that is better tolerated. A large multicentre study by Toma et al. compared clindamycin plus primaquine with TMP-SMX in 87 patients and found it to be better tolerated with similar success rates. Other drugs used include nebulized and intravenous pentamidine (4

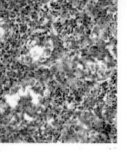

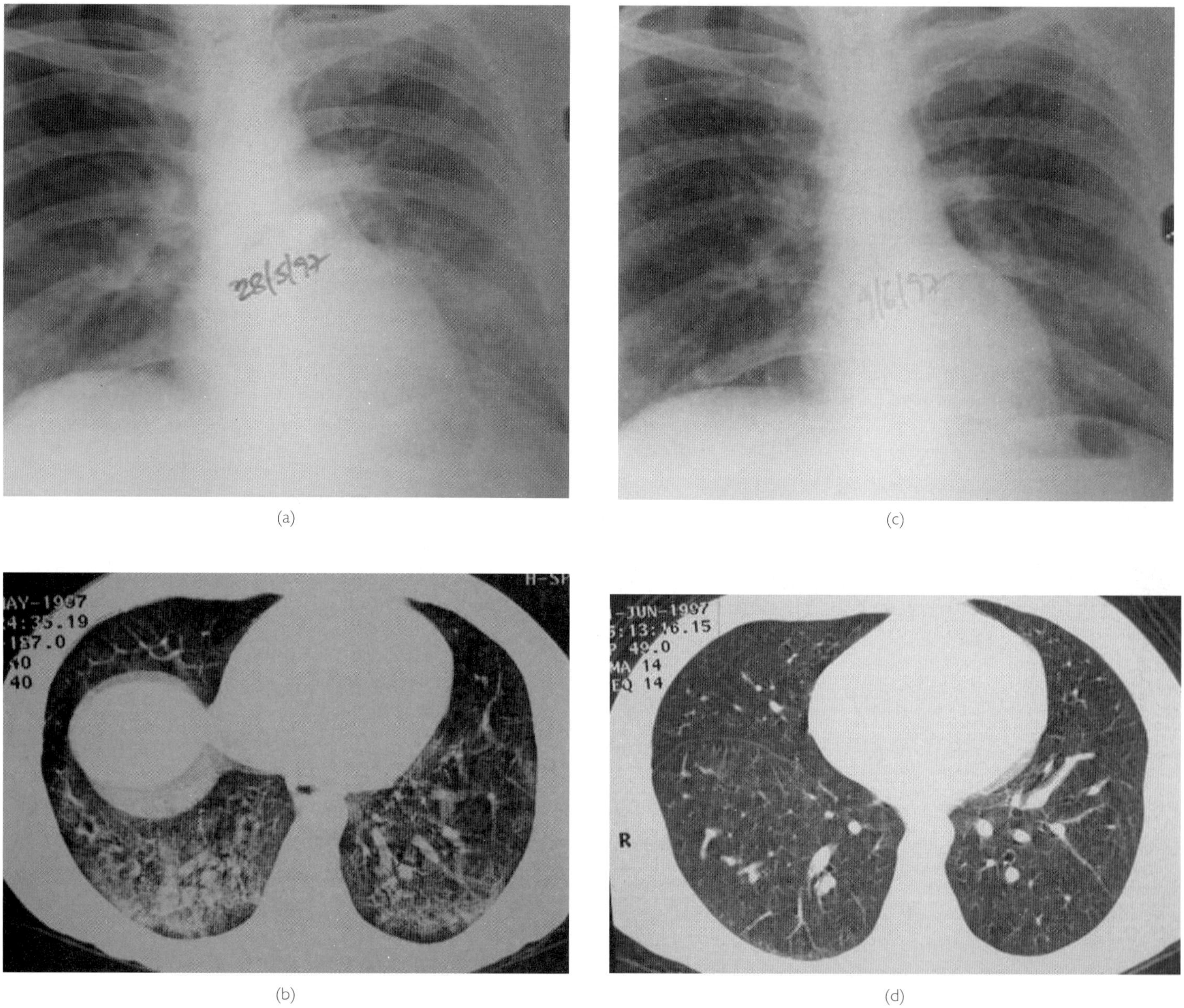

(a)

(c)

(b)

(d)

Fig 28.5 a-d: PCP: Seropositive middle-aged man presented with dyspnoea, cough and fever. Patient was rapidly desaturating. Chest X-ray (a) done on 28/5/97 reveals suspicious ill-defined areas of ground-glass density in both paracardiac regions HRCT (b) reveals ground-glass densities in both lower zones. Sputum revealed PCP. Post-treatment X-ray (c) ten days later on 9/6/1997, reveals total clearing of ground-glass densities, X-ray has returned to normal, HRCT (d) has also returned to normal.

mg per kg IV OD), dapsone (100 mg OD) and atovaquone (750 mg orally thrice daily).

Role of Steroids Data from four clinical studies has shown that steroids are unequivocally useful in moderate to severe PCP. Their use should be reserved for PCP patients who are hypoxic (PaO$_2$ < 70 mmHg) and have been shown in some series to reduce the rate of worsening respiratory failure and death by as much as 50%. They are most effective when given within 72 hours of onset of the disease. They act by blunting the inflammatory response and are used in a dose of oral prednisolone 40 mg bd x five days, 40 mg od x five days, 20 mg od x 11 days.

Antiretroviral (ARV) Therapy The timing of ARV therapy in relation to PCP is controversial. While it was earlier felt best

to complete the TMP-SMX therapy before commencing ARV therapy, evidence from the Adult and Adolescent Spectrum of HIV Disease Project showed concurrent prescription of ARV was associated with improved early survival (OR 0.4).

Outcome There is little doubt that the outcome of PCP has improved. In the Adult and Adolescent Spectrum of HIV Disease Project which looked at 4412 patients with 5222 episodes of PCP, survival at one year improved from 40% in 1992 to 63% in 1998 despite emergence of antibiotic-resistant PCP strains. This improvement in survival, although drugs have stayed the same, is due to widespread use of steroids, better intensive care unit (ICU) care of these patients and earlier introduction of ARVs. Lack of response or inadequate response to specific therapy may be due to one or more of the several factors tabled below.

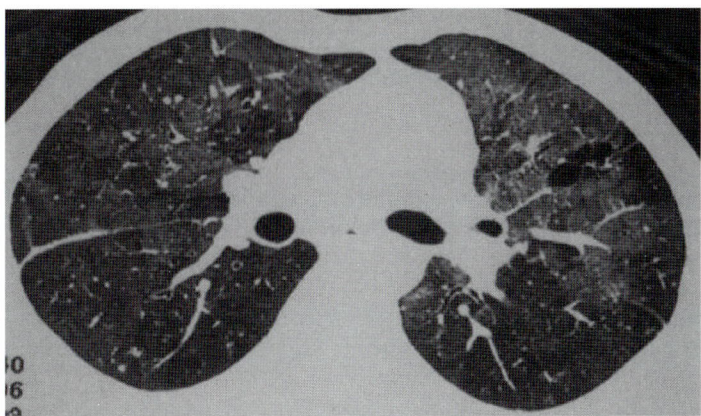

Fig 28.6: PCP. HRCT demonstrates ill-defined ground-glass densities in both lung fields, there are focal areas of sparing in the lung fields. Multiple pneumatoceles, thin-walled air spaces are seen in the left lingula. This combination of ground glass and pneumatoceles is important to differentiate PCP from CMV and other conditions which present with ground-glass densities. The only other condition with ground-glass densities and cysts is lymphocytic interstitial pneumonia (LIP), the cysts in LIP are numerous and diffuse as compared to the few isolated seen in PCP.

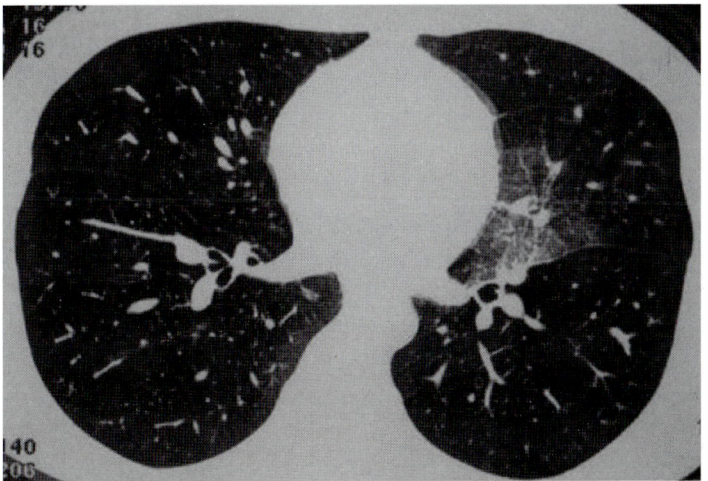

Fig 28.7: PCP. HRCT demonstrates ill-defined ground-glass densities in the left lingula and subtle areas in the right lower lobe paravertebral region. In a seropositive individual these are highly suggestive of PCP.

Table 28.6:
Possible causes of clinical deterioration in HIV patients with PCP infection

1. Severe PCP pneumonia with persistent hypoxia even on ventilator support

2. Iatrogenic

3. Drug induced anaemia/methaemoglobinemia

4. Pneumothorax

5. Associated bacterial/viral (cytomegalovirus) infection

6. Associated infection with Mycobacterium avium intracellulare

7. Very low CD4 count (<50 cells/µL)

8. Pulmonary embolism

9. Inappropriate dosing

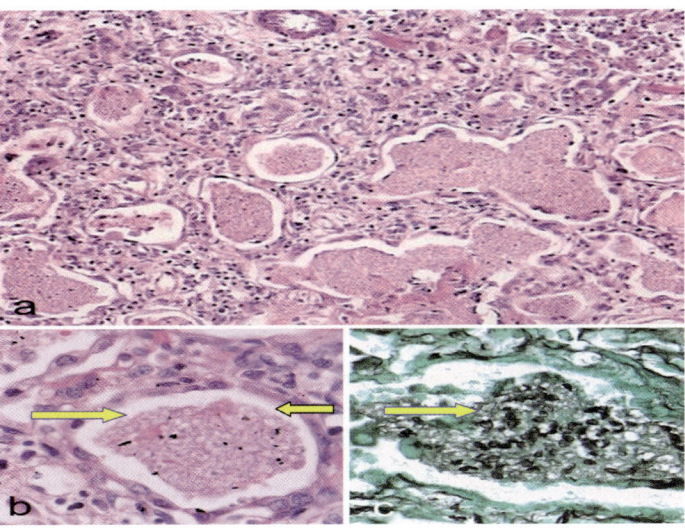

Fig 28.8: PCP. a) & b) Haematoxylin & eosin stain (H&E) 10X, 100X: The alveolar spaces contain typical granular, foamy honeycombed material showing cysts of *Pneumocystis jiroveci*. The alveolar walls are infiltrated with mononuclear cells. c) Methanamine silver stain 100X: Round & oval, black-coloured cysts of *Pneumocystis jiroveci* approximately 4 µm to 5 µm in size seen within the alveolar spaces.

Table 28.7:
Prophylactic Treatment for PCP infection in HIV

Drug	
1. TMP-SMX	1 double strength tablet orally/day
2. Dapsone	100 mg orally/day
3. Pentamidine	Nebulised from-300 mg every 4 weeks
4. Atovaquone	750 mg orally BD
5. Azithromycin	1250 mg orally/weekly

Table 28.8:
Prevention of pulmonary infections in HIV-infected patients

Infection	Drug used
Bacterial Infections	
M. Tuberculosis	Isoniazid (6–12 months)
MAC	Clarithromycin daily
Streptococcus pneumoniae	Immunisation with 23-valent capsular polysaccharide
Fungal infection	Fluconozole

Any patient with HIV and a CD4 count < 200 cell/uL as also any patient with a past history of pneumocystis infection must necessarily be given prophylaxis against PCP. The most effective prophylactic drug is TMP-SMX. Drugs used as the prophylaxis of PCP infection as shown in the table.

Drugs used as prophylaxis against a few other pulmonary infections in HIV patients as shown in the table.

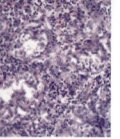

Community-Acquired pneumonia (CAP)

CAP is 10 times more common in HIV-positive patients. CAPs dominate PCP in all African and most Western series. Bacterial infections were the commonest lung infection in the 'Pulmonary Complications of HIV Study'. The incidence of CAP increases with declining CD4 counts. Bacteraemic pneumococal pneumonia is commonly seen and in a study by Gilks *et al.* in the *Lancet*, accounted for 26% of all CAPs in Nairobi. Gram-negative bacilli and *Staphylococcus aureus* increase in importance as immunosuppression increases. Atypical pathogens are relatively uncommon but do occur.

The mortality of CAP in HIV is also approximately four times higher in HIV-positive than negative patients. Relapses are also more frequent and occurred in 22% of Nairobi prostitutes with CAP. TMP-SMX prophylaxis is useful not just in PCP but also in CAP. It was associated with a 67% reduction in the incidence of bacterial pneumonia in patients receiving this drug. Pneumococcal vaccine is recommended but may be ineffective in preventing disease. A study by French *et al.* in the *Lancet* in 2000 showed that the 23 polyvalent vaccine actually increased the risk of developing CAP.

MALIGNANCIES AND IDIOPATHIC NON-INFECTIVE DISORDERS IN HIV INFECTIONS

Malignancies

Kaposi's Sarcoma (KS)

KS is an angioproliferative tumour now known to be associated with infection with human herpes virus 8—HHV 8. HHV 8 has been demonstrated in all forms of KS, the HHV 8 RNA and DNA being present in endothelial cells, mononuclear cells and spindle cells of the lesion. HHV 8 is detectable and shown to replicate in the peripheral blood of patients before symptoms of KS appear. Most patients with AIDS-associated KS have antibodies towards HHV8. HIV is believed to activate this virus which lies dormant in endothelial cells; this is the trigger for angiogenesis which results in the development and proliferation of this vascular tumour. The HHV 8 genome may exert its oncogenic effect in more than one way. The genome contains genes that are homologs to human genes. Among these is a nuclear antigen that binds to P53 and links viral DNA to human DNA during mitosis. The HHV 8 genome also expresses a viral interleukin-8 receptor that induces angiogenesis. Cytokines are required for HHV 8-infected endothelial cells to change to a phenotype that leads to the development and growth of KS. The HIV1TAT protein regulates cytokines which promote the oncogenicity of KS cells. Genetic polymorphism of the Fe-y receptors III A is reported to be associated with an increased risk for developing KS.

KS is more prevalent as the CD4 count declines, but it can occur with comparatively higher CD4 counts as well. In the US, it is 20 times commoner in men who have sex with men. The prevalence has dropped markedly in the West with the introduction of ARV therapy. It is considered rare in India and there are just a few case reports of KS in our country.

CLINICAL FEATURES

KS causes cutaneous, mucocutaneous and visceral lesions, the first two generally preceding visceral lesions by months or years.

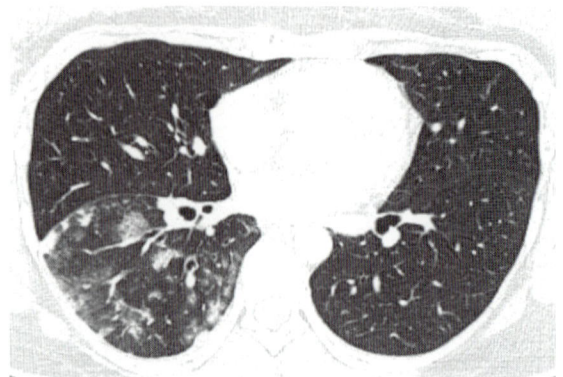

Fig 28.9: Kaposi's sarcoma. HRCT demonstrates ill-defined nodular lesions in the right lower lobe in a subpleural and peribronchovascular location. Transbronchial biopsy revealed a Kaposi's sarcoma.

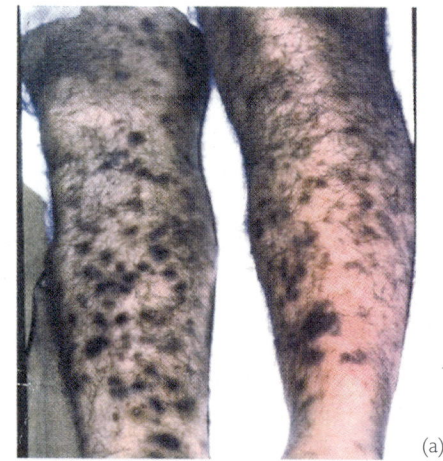

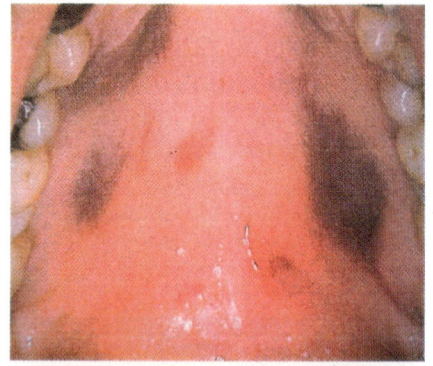

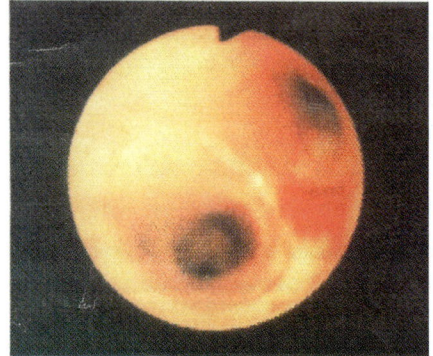

Fig 28.10: Kaposi's sarcoma (a) Involvement of the skin and mucosal lesions of (b) the soft palate and (c) the endobronchial region in a patient with KS.

The lesions appear as red or violet papules or nodules which often fuse to form raised plaques. Any portion of the skin, mucosa or any visceral organ may be involved.

Pulmonary involvement can cause cough, haemoptysis and breathlessness. Though extra-pulmonary involvement is generally evident, 10–15% of KS occurs without skin lesions. CD4 counts are generally < 100/μL. Clinical examination of the respiratory system is usually normal. Typical radiographic features include single or multiple nodules with pleural effusion. HRCT shows peribronchovascular nodules that may be missed on a chest X-ray. Infiltrates and air-space consolidation may also be present. A fibreoptic bronchoscopy classically reveals purplish raised lesions on the mucosa of the airways. Lesions in the larynx and trachea may rarely cause obstruction. KS lesions are highly vascular and as their appearance is distinctive they are best not biopsied.

DIAGNOSIS

Diagnosis is easy when endobronchial lesions are visible through fibreoptic bronchoscopy. It is difficult if endobronchial lesions are absent, more so if there are also no visible skin or mucosal lesions. Pleural effusions may be serous or serosanguinous; they are exudates with a high LDH. In some patients a CT-guided or a thoracoscopic biopsy of a nodule within the lung or a thoracoscopic visualization (and biopsy if thought necessary) of the pleura is needed for a confirmed diagnosis.

TREATMENT

All patients with KS involving the lung require ARV therapy with concomitant chemotherapy. Prophylaxis against pneumocystis infection should be given to all patients. There are two chemotherapeutic regimes in use:

1. Adriamycin (20 mg/m^2), bleomycin (10 mg/m^2) and vincristine (1.4 mg/m^2)—in four to six cycles. Response rates are about 30–50%.
2. Liposomal doxorubicin (40–60 mg/m^2) or doxorubicin (20 mg/m^2) given every two weeks has the same response rate as the first regime with lesser side-effects. The risk of drug to drug interaction with ARV therapy needs to be kept in mind with both regimes.

CLINICAL COURSE

The five-year survival rate of patients with pulmonary KS receiving both ARV therapy and chemotherapy is 50%. Untreated pulmonary KS has a median survival rate of less than six months. Very low CD4 counts < 100 / uL, respiratory distress, hypoxia, all worsen prognosis. Early treatment of HIV disease with ARV therapy is the best prevention for KS and other AIDS-related complications.

Non-Hodgkin's Lymphoma (NHL)

The incidence of NHL in HIV patients has reduced sharply after the introduction of ARV therapy. Even so, it remains an important AIDS-defining illness, particularly in the West. The risk of high-grade lymphoma is increased 600fold and of primary lymphoma within the brain 3500 fold in HIV patients. This marked increase is associated with concomitant infections with Epstein-Barr virus and/or HHV 8 virus. Other risk factors for

NHL are male sex, increased age and a very low CD4 count < 100/ uL. Most NHLs in AIDS are high-grade and belong to either one of the three categories—Burkitt's lymphoma, centroblastic lymphoma and immunoblastic lymphoma. Burkitt's lymphoma can occur with higher CD4 counts compared to other varieties. Also, the incidence of Burkitt's lymphoma has not appreciably changed following ARV therapy.

Pulmonary NHL can occur as a primary within the lung or may occur secondarily as a spread from a primary elsewhere in the body. The development of NHL in HIV patients is probably influenced by co-infection with EBV and by HHV-8 antigenic stimulation and dysregulation of cytokine response.

CLINICAL FEATURES

Secondary involvement of the lung from NHL originating outside the lung always means aggressive advanced Stage IV disease even at presentation. Fever, weight loss and presence of disease in lymph nodes or other organ systems is clinically evident.

Primary lymphoma of the lung may present with systemic features of low-grade fever and a high erythrocyte sedimentation rate (ESR). A Pel-Ebstein type of fever may occur though not as frequently as in Hodgkin's disease. Pulmonary symptoms include cough, breathlessness (when there is increased involvement of the lung) and chest pain. The CD4 counts are generally < 50/uL. Anaemia, leucopenia and thrombocytopenia are frequently present. Imaging studies show single or multiple nodules within the lung parenchyma. Pleural effusion and mediastinal lymphadenopathy may be present.

DIAGNOSIS

A confirmed diagnosis is generally possible through a CT-guided core needle biopsy of a lung nodule. When this is non-confirmatory, a video-assisted thoracoscopic biopsy may be necessary.

TREATMENT

The treatment is as for NHL in general. Two chemotherapeutic regimes are in use

1. Cyclophosphamide, doxorubicin, vincristine and prednisolone (CHOP),
2. Etoposide, prednisolone, vincristine, cyclophosphamide and doxorubicin (EPOCH).

Either one or the other is used in conjunction with ARV therapy.

Primary Effusion Lymphoma (Body Cavity-Associated Lymphoma)

Primary Effusion Lymphoma (PEL) is a variant of NHL which occurs almost exclusively in HIV infections. The pleura, pericardium, and peritoneum may be involved with malignant effusions without identifiable tumour mass in any one of the above. The pleura is more frequently involved. Men are at greater risk, the disease occurring predominantly in men who have sex with men and who are positive for HHV 8. PEL contains HHV 8, EB virus and expresses CD 45.

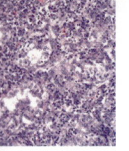

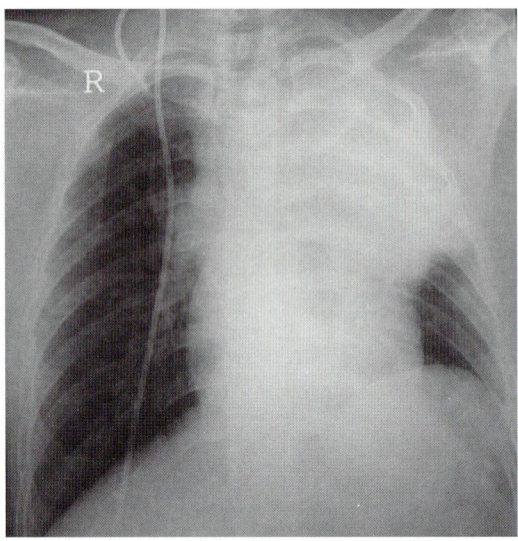

(a)

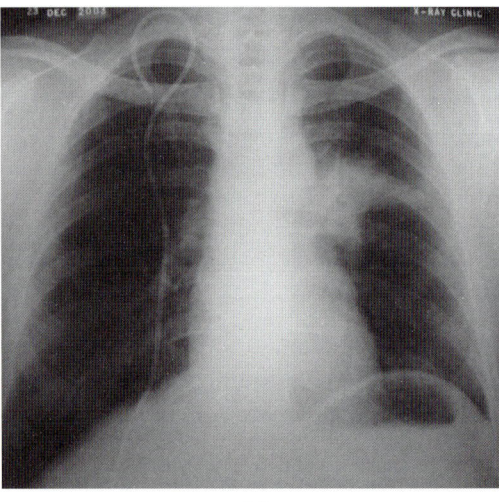

(b)

Fig 28.11: Non-Hodgkin's Lymphoma. Chest X-ray (a) demonstrates a large mass lesion in the left hemithorax superiorly in a seropositive individual. CT-guided biopsy revealed a non-Hodgkin's lymphoma. Post-treatment chest X-ray (b) reveals marked resolution in the mass lesion.

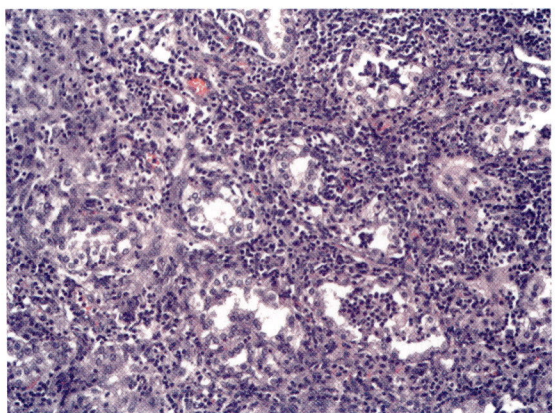

Fig 28.12: NHL. Histopathological specimen reveals a dense interstitial infiltrate of small lymphoid cells. 10X magnification shows primary low-grade B-cell Non-Hodgkin's lymphoma.

CLINICAL FEATURES

Fever, weight loss, and fatigue are presenting features. Pleural effusion causes cough, pleuritic pain and dyspnoea. Imaging shows unilateral or bilateral pleural effusions. CT scans may reveal localized masses of NHL in the lung. PEL remains localized to its site of origin—generally the pleura.

DIAGNOSIS

Diagnosis is based on examination of pleural fluid—its immunohistochemistry and molecular characteristics. Demonstration of HHV 8 is considered essential.

TREATMENT

Treatment is as for NHL and includes chemotherapy with ARV therapy.

Lung Cancer

HIV-positive patients have a two to five old increased risk of developing lung cancer. Though this risk extends to all lung cancers, adenocarcinoma accounts for most cases. Men are at greater risk and as in NHLs, lung cancer in the HIV-positive population tends to present in more aggressive and advanced forms. Unlike NHL or KS, the CD4 counts tend to be well preserved in patients with HIV-associated lung cancer. The risk of lung cancer in HIV-positive patients who smoke is greater than in the normal smoking population. Perhaps smoking added on to HIV infection inflicts greater damage to the lung compared to non-HIV individuals.

CLINICAL FEATURES

Clinical features are the same as lung cancer in general. Patients tend to be younger and the disease is generally more aggressive.

TREATMENT

Treatment for HIV-associated lung cancer is along the same lines as for lung cancer in non-HIV patients.

Multicentric Castleman's Disease

Castleman's disease is a rare lymphoproliferative disorder showing angioproliferation. There are two clinical variants—localized and multicentric. The multicentric form often transforms to NHL.

There is an increased incidence of Castleman's disease in HIV-infected patients. The disease generally occurs in association with KS with a positive HHV 8 infection. Pulmonary involvement in Castleman's disease is exceedingly rare even in the Western world. Neither have we seen one in India and to the best of our knowledge, there is no proven reported case from this country.

Features of the multicentric form of the disease include fever, lymphadenopathy, hepatosplenomegaly and pancytopenia. Pulmonary involvement often causes cough, and breathlessness. Auscultation reveals bilateral basal crackles. CD4 counts vary and need not be very low. There is generally microbiological evidence of HHV 8 infection. Imaging studies show mediastinal adenopathy, interstitial infiltrates and pleural effusion. A lung biopsy is necessary to confirm the diagnosis. Multicentric disease requires chemotherapy with vincristine or etoposide.

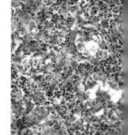

With the use of ARV therapy and chemotherapy, the five-year survival rates reported in the West are close to 50%. NHL is a frequent development.

Idiopathic, Non-infective, Non-malignant Disorders

A large number of these disorders have been described in the literature. These disorders should always be considered when microbiological staining and culture together with molecular techniques fail to reveal an infective organism in HIV patients who have pulmonary infiltrates and clinical features compatible with pulmonary infections. A number of these disorders also occur in non-HIV patients; the clinical features and management in HIV patients is similar to that in non-HIV patients.

Only a few of these miscellaneous disorders are considered here.

Lymphocytic Interstitial Pneumonia (LIP)

LIP is a disease of unknown aetiology occurring in patients with HIV infection and in autoimmune disease. It is commoner in children than in adults and generally occurs with advanced disease associated with severe immunosuppression.

CLINICAL FEATURES
Clinical features are non-specific and include fever, cough and breathlessness. Generalized lymphadenopathy may be present. Clubbing occasionally occurs in children. Radiography of the chest most commonly shows diffuse interstitial infiltrates. Nodular shadows may also be present. Pleural effusion is a frequent occurrence. Chest CT show interstitial infiltrates, diffuse ground-glass shadowing and nodules.

DIAGNOSIS
Diagnosis is one of exclusion. Transbronchial biopsy is necessary for a diagnosis. Biopsy reveals peribronchial, perivascular infiltration of lymphocytes and plasma cells. Septal infiltration is also present and distinguishes LIP from non-specific interstitial pneumonia.

TREATMENT
ARV therapy is believed to cause a regression of this disorder.

HIV-Associated Pulmonary Hypertension

HIV is an important cause of pulmonary hypertension (PH). It is a rare complication, the reported incidence being less than 0.5% which however is significantly greater that the reported incidence of PH in non-HIV patients (0.02%). HIV is assumed to produce vascular changes in the pulmonary arterial tree similar to those observed in primary PH.

The pathogenesis of HIV-associated PH is unclear. HIV is believed to result in increased expression of endothelin 1, a vascular growth factor which may well be responsible for remodelling of the media and adventitia of the pulmonary arterial tree. HIV-related PH can occur at all stages of HIV disease and at any level of the CD4 count.

CLINICAL FEATURES
The main symptom is dyspnoea on exertion. Other symptoms include syncope, fatigue, angina and peripheral oedema. The diagnosis is often made late in the natural history of the disease.

The physical signs are similar to those described under primary PH in the section on 'Pulmonary Vascular Disorders'. Imaging features, echocardiography and electrocardiography (ECG) findings have been described in the same section. Catheter studies are invariably necessary to measure pulmonary artery pressure, pulmonary occlusion pressure and the cardiac output.

DIAGNOSIS
It is imperative to exclude all causes of secondary PH described in the section on 'Pulmonary Vascular Disorders', before making a diagnosis of HIV-related PH. Also, before a young adult is labelled to have primary PH, care must be taken to exclude HIV disease.

TREATMENT
Treatment consists of ARV therapy together with drugs helpful in reducing pulmonary artery pressure. These drugs have been discussed in the section on 'Pulmonary Vascular Disorders' to which the reader is referred. Interaction between sildenafil and protease inhibitors must be borne in mind.

PROGNOSIS
In spite of newer drugs available for treatment, the disease has a downhill course, leading to heart failure within two years.

SUGGESTED READING

Hull MW. Changing global epidemiology of pulmonary manifestations of HIV/AIDS. *Chest.* 1 Dec. 2008; 134(6): 1287–98.

Hussain T. Seroprevalence of HIV infection among tuberculosis patients in Agra, India—a hospital-based study. *Tuberculosis (Edinb).* 1 Jan. 2006; 86(1): 54–9.

Lawn SD. Immune reconstitution disease associated with mycobacterial infections in HIV-infected individuals receiving antiretrovirals. *Lancet Infect Dis.* 1 Jun. 2005; 5(6): 361–73.

Mbulaiteye SM. Epidemiology of AIDS-related malignancies an international perspective. *Hematol Oncol Clin North Am.* 1 Jun. 2003; 17(3): 673–96, v.

Narain JP. Epidemiology of HIV-TB in Asia. *Indian J Med Res.* 1 Oct. 2004; 120(4): 277–89.

Pathni AK. HIV/TB in India: a public health challenge. *J Indian Medical Association.* 1 Mar. 2003; 101(3): 148–9.

Sharma SK. HIV-TB co-infection: epidemiology, diagnosis and management. *Indian J Med Res.* 1 Apr. 2005; 121(4): 550–67.

Slotar D. Pulmonary manifestations of HIV/AIDS in the tropics. *Clin Chest Med.* 1 Jun. 2002; 23(2): 355–67.

Wolff AJ. Pulmonary manifestations of HIV infection in the era of highly active antiretroviral therapy. *Chest.* 1 Dec. 2001; 120(6): 1888–93.

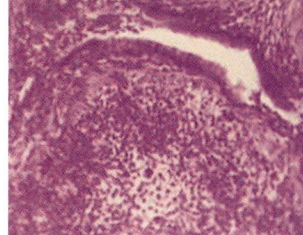

CHAPTER **29** Helminthic Lung Diseases

INTRODUCTION

There are far more people living in the tropical and subtropical areas of the world than in other regions. Besides being exposed to and subject to most diseases and pulmonary infections prevalent in the West and common to the whole world, the billions residing in tropical areas also need to cope with disease and pulmonary infections by and large specific to the tropics.

The battle between 'seed' and 'soil' is most intensely fought in the tropics. This general geographic term refers to regions of the earth lying between the Tropic of Cancer and the Tropic of Capricorn. Some of the most impoverished countries of the globe lie between these equatorial parallels and include India and Sri Lanka, Thailand, Malaysia, Philippines and Indonesia, most South American countries, Central American and Caribbean islands, all of Africa except its southernmost tip and many South Pacific islands. The climate in these 'tropical countries' is characterized by heat and humidity and these climatic conditions coupled with the milieu of poverty and deprivation provide ideal breeding grounds for pathogenic bacteria and parasites and their vectors and intermediate hosts to flourish. Overcrowded, unhygienic living conditions, lack of basic sanitation or access to safe drinking water increase the transmission of these infections. Finally, lack of medical facilities and essential drugs, poorly staffed and funded hospitals and clinics and general lack of infrastructure at all levels of society make practicing medicine in these circumstances a daunting and challenging task. As Maurice King so eloquently pointed out in his monograph, 'The main determinant of the pattern of developing care in tropical countries is poverty rather than a warm climate.'

The impact of respiratory infections in the tropics is considerable. Pulmonary tuberculosis is an example of one disease which though prevalent in most parts of the world continues to exert its most devastating effects on the life and economy of poor third world countries. The same is true for pulmonary infections in HIV-infected patients. Both these conditions have been considered elsewhere in this book.

In some tropical and developing countries childhood mortality may reach 50% in the first five years. At least one-third of these deaths are due to respiratory infections. Exotic diseases are also encountered here; the kind the physician practicing in the West may only vaguely remember from his medical-school days. Why are these obscure conditions relevant to all physicians wherever they may practice? The boundaries of countries are shrinking, international travel is becoming common and affordable, and, as the severe acute respiratory syndrome (SARS) epidemic taught us, respiratory pathogens are oblivious to boundaries not even pausing to acquire a visa!

In the last few decades there have been unparalleled increases in the number of travellers, and populations are now in motion to a degree never before seen in history. Mobile populations include leisure and business travellers, military personnel, long-term expatriates, missionaries etc. Also included are legal and illegal immigrants and refugees from numerous global conflicts and genocides. Members of these populations travel between countries more frequently and rapidly than ever deemed possible. Back in 1995 it was estimated that 1.5 million tourists crossed international borders every day, an annual total of over 500 million. This number is expected to rise to over 1 billion within a decade. As SARS taught us so compellingly, virtually any destination in the world can be reached from any other in only 36 hours of travel. This 36-hour window is well within the incubation period of most infectious diseases, affording ample opportunity for the unrecognized movement of pathogens from place to place and for rapid global spread of microbes. From the microbe's point of view the global village of the 21st century provides global opportunities for disease emergence and transmission.

HELMINTHIC LUNG DISEASES

General Considerations

Parasitic helminths infect billions of people in our world, especially in the tropics, and constitute one of the most important causes of morbidity and mortality. Pulmonary helminthic infections generally manifest with cough, breathlessness and a varying degree of peripheral eosinophilia. An eosinophilic pulmonary infiltrate is often present which may or may not cast a 'shadow' on a radiological examination of the chest. In the West, pulmonary helminthiasis is often missed because of its comparative rarity. On the other hand, in the tropics pulmonary helminthiasis is at times wrongly diagnosed when a radiologically apparent pulmonary infiltrate is associated with peripheral eosinophilia. This is because one fails to take note of the fact that the prevalence of peripheral eosinophilia for several reasons is extremely common in poor tropical countries. A pulmonary infiltrate or shadow may not necessarily be related to either peripheral eosinophilia or proven helminthic infection. It could be due to tuberculosis, other infections or even a non-infective pathology.

In humans, helminths produce a variety of pulmonary diseases, depending chiefly on the nature of the helminthic infection. Also, a pulmonary pathology is observed at a particular phase or stage in the lifecycle of the helminth—a phase or stage which involves a transit or a stay within the lungs for a period

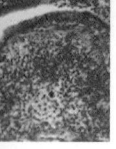

of time. It is important to be aware of the biological behaviour of different helminths in order to arrive at a diagnosis of the pulmonary infections they produce.

Biology and Host-Parasite Relationship

Certain important generalizations need to be kept in mind.

1. Helminths are highly evolved human parasites; they have developed elaborate mechanisms that evade the defences of the host, allowing them to survive in hostile environments.
2. The lifecycle of these helminthic parasites starts with the egg and then goes on to the larval form and the adult worm. Human infection is by ingestion of the egg or the larvae, penetration of the skin by larvae, transmission of larvae by bites of insects or vectors. Man may constitute a definitive host, an intermediate host, an accidental host or the only host, all depending on the kind of parasite considered.
3. Helminths as a rule cannot multiply in the mammalian host. Therefore the higher the worm load to start with, the greater the pathological consequences. There are two important exceptions to this generalization. The helminth *S. stercoralis* can autoinfect an immunocompromised patient, causing a hyperinfection syndrome that is often fatal. An echinococcal infection can disseminate and the parasite can multiply following rupture of a hydatid cyst. The released contents seed other sites causing other multiple lesions.
4. Helminthic parasites which at any stage of their lifecycle migrate through the lungs cause generally both a peripheral eosinophilia and a pulmonary eosinophilic infiltrate. This peripheral and tissue eosinophilia is caused by sensitized T-cell lymphocytes which secrete mediators that induce progenitor cells in the marrow to develop into mature eosinophils. Eosinophilic production and maturation is affected by cytokines, chiefly Interleukin 3 (IL3), Interleukin 5(IL5) and granulocyte/macrophage colony stimulating factor (GM-CSF). The eosinophilic response depends on the integrity of the cellular immune response of the host. When the cellular immune response is poor or well-nigh absent as in severe h*uman immunodeficiency virus* (HIV) infections, the eosinophilic reaction may not occur. Thus, eosinophilia is not observed in strongyloid infections in HIV patients or in other immunocompromised hosts. Cytokines interact with eosinophils through specific receptors on the cell wall of the eosinophil, stimulating both maturity and metabolic activity.
5. Pulmonary manifestations of helminthic disease are due to various factors, again depending on the exact nature of the helminth involved. They could result from the larvae within the lung (as with nematode infection), eggs within the lung (schistosomiasis) or from the actual worm (paragonimiasis). The pathogenesis of pulmonary manifestation may be due to mechanical obstruction, an inflammatory response to the presence of what the lung considers a foreign body, or as a by-product of the host immune response. In fact the pulmonary manifestations of many helminthic infections are due to a combination of Type I, Type III, Type IV immune responses of the host.
6. It is debatable whether humans develop immunity to a helminthic infection. Unquestionably, ascarial infections are

known to recur and filarial infection causing the syndrome of tropical eosinophilia can recur either due to a relapse or re-infection.

PULMONARY MANIFESTATIONS OF NEMATODE INFECTIONS

The pulmonary manifestations of nematode infections typically take the form of pulmonary eosinophilia. *Pulmonary eosinophilia* is characterized by pulmonary infiltration with a predominantly eosinophilic exudate, peripheral eosinophilia and the presence of respiratory symptoms, chiefly cough and breathlessness. The nematode parasite infections presenting with pulmonary eosinophilia are *Ascarial infection, Ankylostomal infection, Filarial infection* and *Strongyloides infection.*

Ascariasis

Ascariasis results from the ingestion of embryonated *A. lumbricoides* eggs which contaminate unwashed vegetables and fruits. The eggs hatch in the gut and the larvae penetrate the gut and reach the lung via the bloodstream. The larvae migrate via the pulmonary capillaries into the alveoli. They then pass up the airways, ascend up the trachea and are swallowed to reach the small intestine where they mature into adult worms.

The presence of larvae in the lungs exerts a hypersensitivity response which is clearly of the Type I kind (Immunoglobulin E (IgE) levels are raised), but probably also involves a Type III reaction. The hypersensitivity response in its entirety is characterized pathologically by an eosinophilic pulmonary infiltrate, peripheral eosinophilia, and the presence of a patchy shadow within the lung on a radiographic examination of the chest. The X-ray chest may however appear normal in a number of patients. The peripheral eosinophilia is not marked and except in rare instances does not exceed a total eosinophil count of 2500/mm³. The clinical symptoms are cough, often paroxysmal, and breathlessness which is often associated with a wheeze, so that a mistaken diagnosis of asthma can be easily made. Fever and general malaise may be present. Very rarely, larvae may be expectorated in the sputum. Once the helminths mature in the gut, eggs of *A. lumbricoides* are detected. Lung functions may show a mild obstructive defect with a fair degree of reversibility.

In the more severe cases the larvae may incite a hypersensitivity pneumonic reaction with a larger shadow occupying part of a lobe. The systemic features are more marked. The larvae are sometimes observed to be fragmented and destroyed, surrounded by a dense cellular exudate chiefly consisting of eosinophils.

The presence of cough, breathlessness, a radiologically observed pulmonary infiltrate or a localized pulmonary shadow (generally in the upper lobe) together with peripheral eosinophilia is often termed Loeffler's syndrome. It denotes a hypersensitivity pulmonary reaction (Type I response) to an antigen and the commonest antigenic stimulus is the larvae of either *Ascariasis lumbricoides* or the larvae of the ankylostomaes. The onset of Loeffler's syndrome caused by intestinal nematodes is generally two to three weeks after infection, around the time the larvae migrate from the pulmonary circulation into the alveoli. Other antigens are also known to cause Loeffler's syndrome. Loeffler's syndrome is self-limiting, the pulmonary

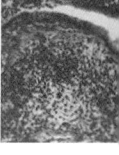

shadow on the chest X-ray generally clearing within three to four weeks. The major mistake frequently made is to consider the pulmonary shadows in Loeffler's syndrome to be due to tuberculosis and to start the patient on six to nine months of anti-tuberculosis therapy. Nothing is lost in waiting for at least four weeks when the possibility of Loeffler's syndrome is suspected. The pulmonary shadows and symptoms disappear by then on their own.

Management is symptomatic. Bronchodilators help and inhaled β_2 agonists give symptomatic relief. No drug acts on the larvae of either Ascarial or ankylostomal infection that cause a hypersensitivity pulmonary response. Albendazole 400 mg once daily or mebendazole 100 mg BD orally daily for three days can eradicate both ascarial and ankylostoma infection once the parasite matures into adult worms in the small intestine. Diethylcarbamazine 100 mg thrice daily for a week has the same curative effect on the adult worm.

Ankylostomal Infection (*Ankylostoma duodenale, Necator americanus*)

The parasite found in the tropics is *Ankylostoma duodenale*. It is the infective larvae of this parasite found in soil which penetrate the skin and through the bloodstream find their way via the pulmonary circulation into the alveoli. Here they excite the same hypersensitivity pulmonary reaction which often presents clinically as Loeffler's syndrome. The pathogenesis, pathology and clinical features are similar to those described under infection with *A. lumbricoides*. Pulmonary manifestations of ankylostomiasis are not as common as in infections with *A. lumbricoides*. The larvae (as in *A. lumbricoides*) then travel up to the airways, up the trachea and are swallowed into the upper gut where they mature into adult hookworms. These worms attach themselves to the duodenal and jejunal mucosa and suck blood causing well-marked iron deficiency anaemia.

Pulmonary Filariasis (Tropical Eosinophilia)

Weingarten in 1943, working at the Breach Candy Hospital in Mumbai, was the first to give the term 'tropical eosinophilia' (TE) to a syndrome characterized by severe spasmodic bronchitis, eosinophilic leucocytosis and disseminated mottling of both lungs. The mystery of this exotic tropical syndrome slowly started to unfold, first with the discovery of the clinical efficacy of diethylcarbamazine, then with the unravelling of its histopathology and natural history and finally with studies in aetiology and immunology. It is now accepted that *'tropical eosinophilia' as seen in India and other tropical countries is merely an unusual variant of human filariasis, caused by Wuchereria bancrofti and Brugia malayi.*

EPIDEMIOLOGY

TE has been reported from filarial endemic regions worldwide. The syndrome is particularly endemic in India, Sri Lanka and Southeast Asia. In India it is most endemic along the western coastal strip around Mumbai, Goa, Kerala, the whole of the eastern coast, and in Bengal, Bihar, Orissa, and areas endemic to filarial infection.

Northwest and Central Africa, Tanganyika, West Indies, the coast of China and the Philippines are other countries endemic

to this syndrome. Travel from endemic to non-endemic areas also results in the syndrome being occasionally recognized in the West.

AETIOLOGY

As mentioned above, the syndrome is a variant of human filarial infection and results from an unusual hypersensitivity reaction to microfilariae liberated by *W. bancrofti* and *Brugia malayi*.

This concept is based on serological, histopathological, therapeutic and immunological studies. The serum of patients with TE shows raised IgE levels and specific anti-filarial antibodies. In its early stages, TE responds to diethylcarbamazine both clinically and with regard to a fall in the specific anti-filarial antibodies. This drug *in vitro* has a destructive effect on both microfilariae and the adult filarial worm. Histopathological studies of the lung, liver and lymph nodes in this syndrome often show degenerating fragmented microfilariae in the midst of an intensive eosinophilic exudate.

The role of animal filarial infection in causing TE has been suggested by several workers. Present evidence suggests that animal filarial infection is rare and has little or no role in the overall problem of TE.

CLINICAL FEATURES

Pulmonary Manifestations Pulmonary manifestations are characterized by paroxysmal cough, breathlessness, wheeze, pulmonary infiltrates on a radiographic examination of the chest and an absolute eosinophil count > 3000–3500/mm³. These symptoms are most marked at night but may also be present in the day. Non-specific features that accompany pulmonary manifestations include low-grade fever, malaise and weight loss. The absolute eosinophil count in hyperacute cases can be as high as 30000–50000/mm³. Laboratory features include filarial-specific IgE and IgG antibodies.

Hyperacute manifestations of TE with focal consolidation resembling pneumonia or bronchopneumonia have been described but are now rarely encountered.

Radiological Examination The radiological findings show reticulonodular shadows chiefly in the mid-zones or bases, prominent hila with heavy vascular markings over the bases, and occasionally, miliary mottling indistinguishable from miliary tuberculosis. In about 20% of patients the X-ray chest may appear normal even though the lung histopathology (on a biopsy) may reveal typical features of TE. The syndrome in the early stages of its natural history invariably responds to diethylcarbamazine. Patients who have not been treated, or have a long history, or who respond inadequately to diethylcarbamazine may progress to chronic respiratory disability due to moderately severe pulmonary fibrosis.

Manifestations Involving Other Systems Other body systems may be involved. Patients may have lymphadenopathy and hepatosplenomegaly due to involvement of the liver and spleen. Occasionally, the presentation is with a low-grade fever, weight loss, abdominal complaints in the form of abdominal discomfort, diarrhoea, the diagnosis being suggested by the very high eosinophil absolute count and the presence of specific anti-filarial antibodies. Even here, a lung biopsy may reveal histopathological features of TE.

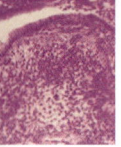

LUNG FUNCTIONS

About 70% of patients show a dominant restrictive pattern; 30% show airways obstruction + restriction. A lowered single breath transfer factor has also been observed in untreated TE. These findings showed marked improvement following a good clinical response to diethylcarbamazine but do not always return to normal. Some patients continue to progress to interstitial pulmonary fibrosis with permanent impairment of lung function. A study of 162 patients over five years by Udwadia revealed an increasing restrictive pattern in patients who had frequent relapses, and in those who responded inadequately to diethylcarbamazine. Patients with a history stretching over five years showed lung functions compatible with moderately severe interstitial pulmonary fibrosis. The degree of fibrosis was not as marked as in fibrosing alveolitis and the PaO_2 did not fall below 65 mm Hg. Pulmonary hypertension and cor pulmonale were not evident.

HISTOPATHOLOGY AND NATURAL HISTORY

This was unravelled for the first time in 1963 when Udwadia and Joshi reported a study of 26 open-lung biopsies in TE. The clinical features of paroxysmal cough, breathlessness, wheeze (resembling spasmodic airways' obstruction), and peripheral eosinophilia are from the very outset characterized by an alveolitis caused by an acute dense eosinophilic exudate. Lung histopathology reveals eosinophilic pneumonia, bronchopneumonia, microabscesses, and granulomas. Lung functions, even at this stage, show a restrictive pattern on which is superimposed a pattern of airways' obstruction. The latter is due to eosinophilic infiltration of the bronchioles, with oedema and disruption of the bronchial mucosa or muscle. Six months to two years after the onset of symptoms, a 'mixed-cell' exudate consisting of eosinophils, mononuclear cells and histiocytes is observed in the lungs. Fibrosis occurs early in the natural history and is slowly progressive. The clinical picture is still readily recognizable because of marked peripheral eosinophilia. Breathlessness on exertion is now the most important symptom. Still later, in patients with a history > two years, the eosinophils in the lung exudate become comparatively sparse, there being an increase in mononuclear cells and histiocytes. Fibrosis is evident and the lung is scarred. Lung functions show a well-marked increasing restrictive pattern. The overall clinical picture is one of moderately severe interstitial pulmonary fibrosis. This results in respiratory disability due to increasing breathlessness on exertion, increasing restriction on lung function tests and is associated with reticulation of the mid-zones and bases of both lungs on a chest X-ray. The pulmonary fibrosis in TE remains patchy and therefore is never as crippling as that observed in cryptogenic fibrosing alveolitis. The incidence and frequency of pulmonary disability in TE is difficult to estimate. Five out of 19 patients with a history of more than two years' duration progressed to a fair degree of pulmonary disability when followed up for five years.

The natural history of TE in endemic zones shows frequent recurrences and relapses. In some patients the peripheral eosinophil count wanes with frequent relapses (the total eosinophil count often being < 2000/mm³), and the predominant symptom is breathlessness on exertion rather than paroxysmal cough and breathlessness. The syndrome if seen at this juncture for the first time is difficult to recognize. It is likely that a

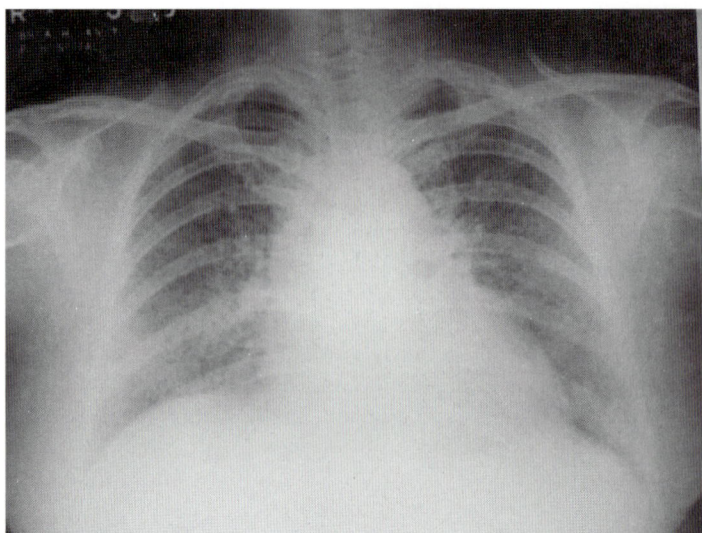

Fig 29.1: Tropical eosinophilia. Chest X-ray demonstrates bilateral reticulonodular opacities indicative of pulmonary eosinophilia.

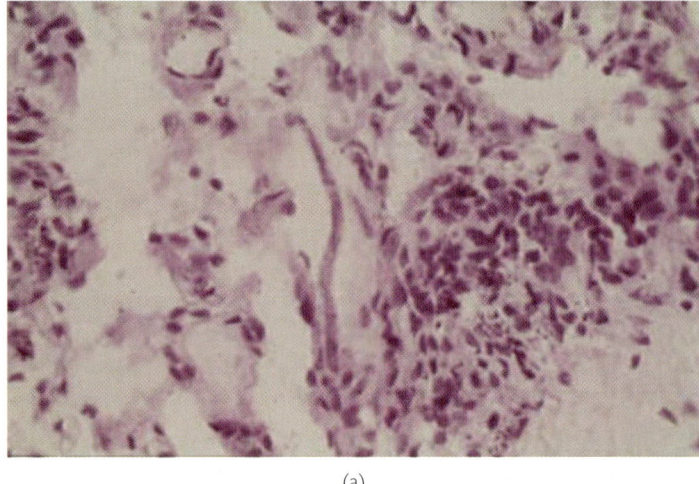

(a)

Fig 29.2a: Tropical eosinophilia showing the presence of a microfilarial parasite within lung parenchyma.

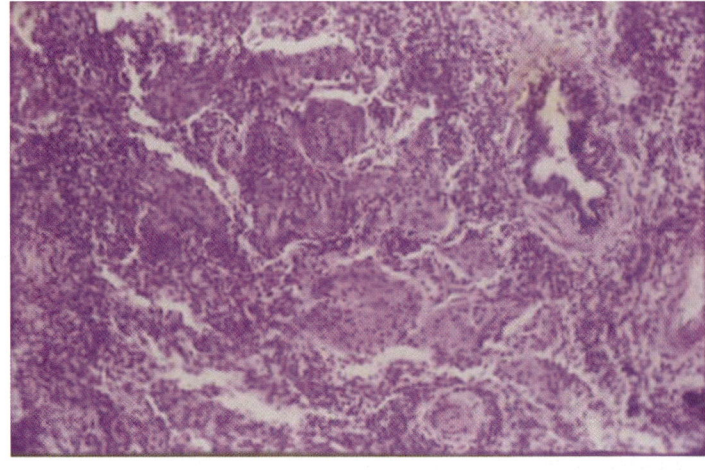

(b)

Fig 29.2b: Tropical eosinophilia. H/P section of eosinophilic pneumonia in a patient with tropical eosinophilia. Note alveoli packed with eosinophils.

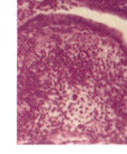

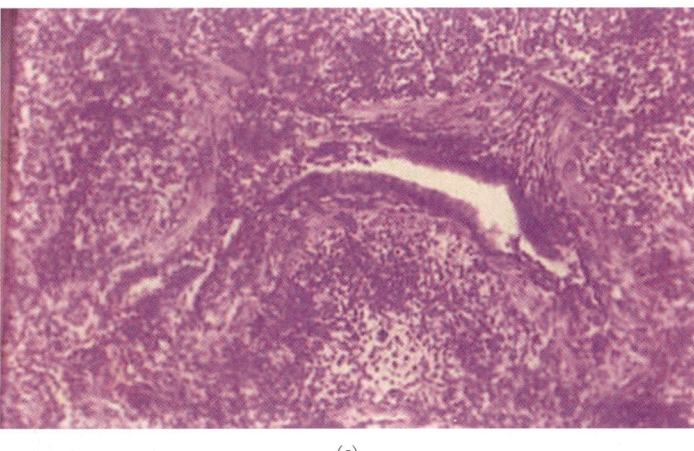

(c)

Fig 29.2c: TE. H/P section showing eosinophilic bronchopneumonia. Note infiltration of the bronchial wall with eosinophils with sloughing bronchial mucosa.

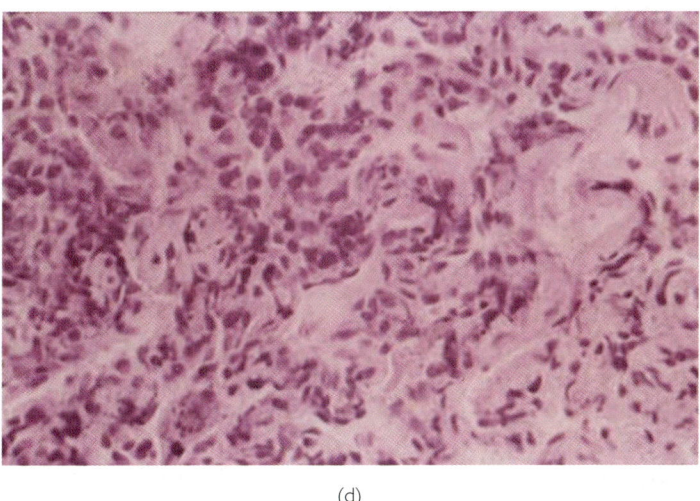

(d)

Fig 29.2d: Tropical eosinophilia. A mixed-cell exudate consisting of eosinophils, mononuclear cells, histiocytes and lymphocytes. This reaction is observed six to nine months after the onset of infection.

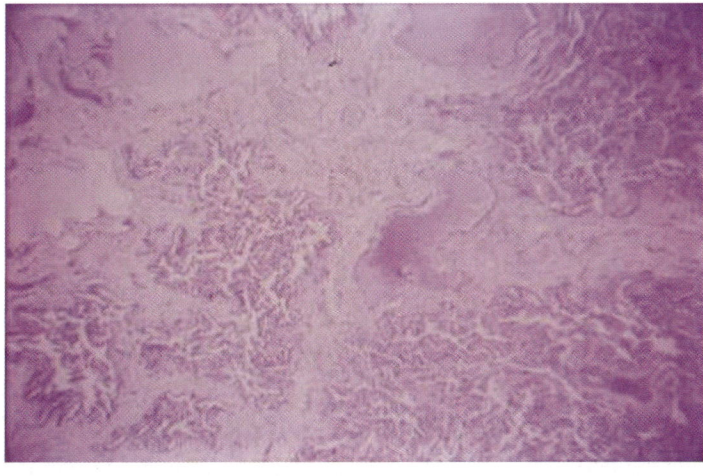

(d)

Fig 29.2e: Tropical eosinophilia. H/P section showing the end-stage of TE. Note well-marked fibrosis, compartmentalizing the lung. The fibrosis is never marked or as diffuse as in interstitial pulmonary fibrosis. Pockets of eosinophilic infiltration are still recognized, but histiocytes predominate.

number of patients in the tropics who masquerade under the guise of 'bronchitis' or 'pulmonary fibrosis', are in fact suffering from the end result of TE.

IMMUNOLOGY

In TE, microfilariae from a mature gravid human filarial parasite (*Wuchereria bancrofti, Brugia malayi*) are periodically released but promptly removed from the circulation and 'trapped' within the lungs. Microfilaremia in the blood is therefore very rarely observed. Within the lungs the microfilariae excite a severe, immunological response characterized by a marked increase in IgE and high levels of filarial-specific IgG, IgM, and IgE in the lower epithelial lining fluid. There appears to be an antibody-dependent mechanism of immune-mediated clearance of microfilariae within the lungs. Type I, Type III and Type IV immunological responses are all involved. The role of the eosinophil is crucial in this response. This cell probably has a dual role—a warrior of distinction that helps destroy the microfilariae, and also a role in the destruction of lung tissue due to release of eosinophilic granule components. Activated eosinophils are capable of releasing major basic proteins, peroxidase and collagenase which injure lung tissue. Eosinophils may also release leukotrienes which induce bronchoconstriction. The role of the mononuclear cell and macrophages in perpetuating inflammation and in increasing fibrosis is an area of fruitful research. The clinical, physiological and histopathological features characteristic of TE are unquestionably related to the immunological host response to microfilariae. If microfilariae succeed in running the gauntlet of the pulmonary circulation, they can excite an immunological response in the lymph glands, liver, spleen and rarely in the muscles and the gastrointestinal tract. Thus, though TE almost always involves the lungs, other organ systems may occasionally also be involved. The reason for the difference between the immunological host response to the same parasite in patients suffering from the usual form of endemic filariasis and in those with TE is an unsolved problem. Racial and genetic factors may play a role, as also the age at which infection occurs and perhaps the frequency of exposure.

The following patterns of human filarial infection can be described:

1. Microfilaremia without any clinical features (asymptomatic)
2. Microfilaremia with the classic features of endemic filariasis—high fever, severe lymphangitis chiefly involving the lower limbs
3. Amicrofilaremia with the clinical features of chronic endemic filariasis
4. Amicrofilaremia with the features of TE

Unfortunately, the term TE is still used by many medical practitioners in the tropics as a 'wastepaper basket' for any patient with cough, breathlessness and a rise in the peripheral eosinophil count. Ideally, the term TE should be abandoned and the overall features described above should be considered either as pulmonary manifestations of filarial infection or pulmonary filariasis. This is however easier said than done, because a) peripheral eosinophilia is so common in the tropics; b) a number of conditions in the tropics (including infestation by other helminths) do also produce eosinophilia, cough and breathlessness; c) The diagnostic confirmation by specific anti-filarial

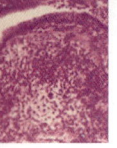

antibodies in pulmonary filariasis is a luxury available in very few laboratories in the tropics. A classification of the causes of pulmonary eosinophilia in the tropics is given later in this chapter.

TREATMENT

Diethylcarbamazine is specific for the treatment of TE. Though a dose of 5 mg/kg/day for 10 days may well be adequate, Udwadia recommends the same dose for a period of four weeks. The drug is remarkably free from major side-effects. A few patients (<5%) even in the earlier part of the natural history respond inadequately and as many as 20% of patients with a longer duration of symptoms extending from two to five years may fail to respond. The lack of response in patients with a long history is understandable as the drug cannot be expected to act on the increasing fibrosis within the lung.

The only five-year follow-up study of a large series of cases showed that the relapse rate in TE following specific therapy was at least 20%. It was impossible to determine in this study how many were true relapses and how many were due to re-infection. In those living in highly endemic zones, we would recommend repeated monthly courses of diethylcarbamazine at three-monthly intervals for a period of one to two years to help reduce the morbidity in TE. The use of corticosteroids in longstanding cases with evidence of pulmonary fibrosis is worth a trial, though their efficacy has not been studied and is therefore uncertain.

Visceral Larva Migrans

Visceral larva migrans is a disease with pulmonary manifestations caused by the larvae of the dog and cat round worms (*Toxocara canis, Toxocara catis*). These round worms infest the dog and cat respectively and the eggs are passed out via the faeces.

These eggs may contaminate food or water and may be ingested by humans. In the intestines the eggs hatch into larvae which penetrate the gut and reach the liver, lungs and other tissues via the systemic circulation. The larvae excite an immunological plus an inflammatory granulomatous reaction, chiefly in the liver and lungs. The larvae after weeks or months may die and become encapsulated and surrounded by an eosinophilic exudate. The lifecycle of these animal parasites is cut short in humans as the animal larvae cannot mature into adult worms in humans.

CLINICAL MANIFESTATIONS

Visceral larva migrans occurs chiefly in children below five years, particularly when there is history of pica in the child. Pulmonary manifestations are characterized by cough, breathlessness, eosinophilic pulmonary infiltrates and well-marked peripheral eosinophilia with an absolute eosinophil count > 3500/mm^3, as in patients with TE. Breathlessness is often associated with wheezing, the clinical picture being indistinguishable from bronchial asthma. Transient pulmonary infiltrates on chest radiography are observed in over 50% of patients. Acute eosinophilic pneumonia and respiratory failure have also been observed. The liver is often enlarged; granulomas may be found on histopathological examination of the liver biopsy material. The central nervous system and other body tissues may be rarely involved. Constitutional symptoms in the form of fever, weight loss, malaise, and muscle pains may be present.

DIAGNOSIS

The clinical features of well-marked pulmonary eosinophilia, hepatic enlargement in a young child with no or poor response to diethylcarbamazine should arouse suspicion of visceral larva migrans. A marked elevation of IgE is generally present. An enzyme-linked immunosorbent assay (ELISA) test using larval antigen has a sensitivity of about 70% and a specificity of 90%.

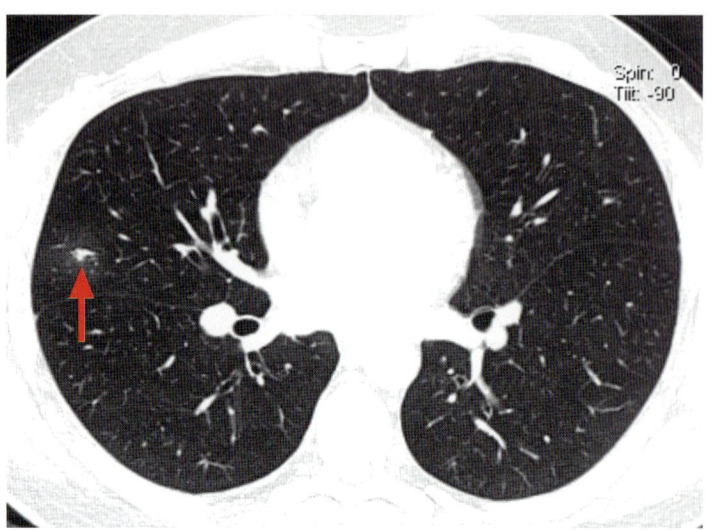

Fig 29.3: Visceral larva migrans. HRCT demonstrates a small linear density with a surrounding halo in the right middle lobe.

MANAGEMENT

There is no specific therapy; anti-helminthic agents are of doubtful use. Diethylcarbamazine, however, should be given a try. The disease is generally self-limiting, though clinical features may last for several months. Corticosteroids suppress and perhaps control the inflammatory response within the body tissues.

Strongyloides stercoralis Infection

Infection with *S. stercoralis* occurs when infective larvae present in the soil penetrate the human skin and travel via the bloodstream into the lungs. The larvae reach the alveoli though the pulmonary capillaries and excite a hypersensitivity lung response that results in the classical clinical features of pulmonary eosinophilia which have already been described. The larvae ascend up the bronchi and the trachea to be swallowed so as to reach the small gut where they mature into adult worms. These adult worms produce rhabditiform larvae which are non-infective and which are passed out in the stools. In the soil these non-infective larvae turn into infective filariform larvae. It is rare for larvae to be found in the sputum and the correct diagnosis must await the presence of larvae of *S. stercoralis* excreted in the stool.

Hyperinfection Syndrome Due to *S. stercoralis* Infection

The most dreaded pulmonary manifestation induced by intestinal nematodes is the hyperinfection syndrome caused by *S. stercoralis*. Invariably, this syndrome occurs only in immunocompromised individuals with a markedly depressed

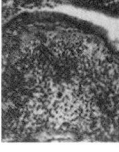

cell-mediated immune response. Very rarely, it has been observed in normal persons. Immunocompromised individuals with depressed cell-mediated immunity include patients with HIV infection, neoplastic diseases such as lymphomas, leukaemia, patients on prolonged corticosteroid therapy for whatsoever reason, and patients who have received organ transplants. In these patients there may well occur a change in the reproductive cycle of the parasite. In immunocompetent individuals, the non-infective rhabditiform larvae have to be passed out into stools and only then can develop into the infective filariform larvae. In immunocompromised patients the change to infective larvae occurs within the host. These numerous infective filariform larvae penetrate the gut, reach the circulation and invade various organ systems, in particular the lungs.

Pulmonary manifestations include severe breathlessness, airways' obstruction with pulmonary opacities on an X-ray chest which may appear as infiltrates, consolidation, cavities or may resemble bronchopneumonia. Tachycardia, tachypnoea and increasing hypoxia are observed. The filariform larvae when they penetrate the gut carry gram-negative gut organisms with them, so that the clinical picture is often combined with that of severe gram-negative sepsis and at times with meningitis due to gram-negative organisms. Interestingly, eosinophilia is absent probably due to poor cell-mediated immunity.

The hyperinfection syndrome caused by *S. stercoralis* is in our experience generally fatal.

MANAGEMENT

Early diagnosis and the stoppage or drastic modification of immunosuppressive therapy (if this is being administered) is imperative. *When an immunosuppressed patient develops pulmonary disease with associated bacteraemia and sepsis, the possibility of strongyloidiasis should be seriously entertained.* Larvae should be carefully searched for in bronchial washings, sputum, duodenal washings and stools. Even reasonable suspicion should warrant the use of specific therapy. Specific therapy consists of albendazole 400 mg orally for seven days. Broad-spectrum antibiotics which cover gram-negative infections should always be used in adequate dosage for 10 to 15 days. More often than

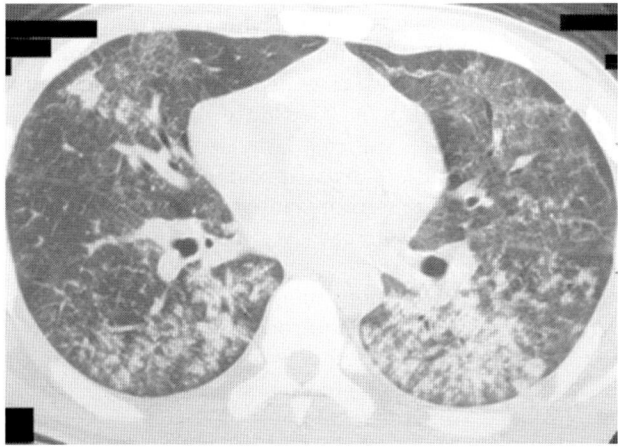

Fig 29.4: Strongyloidiasis in an 18-year-old man with haemoptysis. CT chest clearly delineates the areas of consolidation. BAL revealed larvae of *S. stercoralis*. Reproduced with permission from Martinez S, Restrepo CS, Carrillo JA, et al. Thoracic manifestations of tropical parasitic infections: a pictorial review. *Radiographics*. 2005; 25: 135–55.

not diagnosis is made too late to allow survival. Treatment should be initiated in suspect patients.

PULMONARY MANIFESTATIONS OF TREMATODE INFECTIONS

Schistosomiasis

Schistosomiasis is the second most common cause of mortality among parasite infections after malaria. It affects 150–200 million people causing 500,000 deaths annually. According to the GeoSentinel database that monitors travellers around the world, schistosomiasis is one of the ten leading causes of morbidity among travellers, accounting for 6% of all the cases in sub-Saharan Africa. It is reported that 55–100% of travellers on rafting tours in African rivers become infected. The lungs can be affected in both the acute and chronic stages of the illness.

The disease is caused by three important schistosoma species—*S. hematobium, S. mansoni* and *S. japonica*. The disease is endemic in Egypt, Africa, Saudi Arabia, Brazil, Philippines and the Yangtze valley of China. It remains a rarity in India.

PATHOGENESIS

Infection occurs due to exposure to water-contaminated cercariae excreted by snails. These cercariae can penetrate the skin or the intestinal wall and turn within a few hours into schistosomula which migrate to the lung. Their passage through the lungs often causes an acute hypersensitivity response manifesting clinically as pulmonary eosinophilia. From the lungs they reach the liver where they mature into adult worms. Fecund adult worms then migrate to their final habitat—the vesical plexus around the bladder and uterus (*S. hematobium*) and the mesenteric venous plexus (*S. mansoni* and *S. japonica*). Eggs of *S. hematobium* besides causing a painful cystitis, enter the systemic venous system and are transported to the lung. Eggs of *S. mansoni* and *S. japonica* are first transported to the liver via the portal circulation where they block the portal radicals causing portal hypertension. These eggs reach the lungs through anastomatic channels between the portal and systemic veins only when portal hypertension is well established.

Eggs reaching the lungs block pulmonary arterioles and excite a granulomatous reaction (eosinophils, lymphocytes, macrophages) within the wall of the arterioles. Granulomatous lesions are also formed around eggs situated within the alveoli. Plexifrom lesions consisting of dilated thin-walled vessels are also observed. There is a progressive blockage of the pulmonary circulation as a result of tissue response (endothelial thickening, fibrin deposition, medial wall hypertrophy) to the eggs within the arterioles. The end result is cor pulmonale and congestive heart failure.

CLINICAL FEATURES

During the phase of migration from the skin through the lungs to their final habitat the clinical features are of pulmonary eosinophilia—fever, cough, wheezing, peripheral eosinophilia; the chest radiograph may show areas of mottling. Pulmonary mottling–on a chest X-ray may also be observed due to widespread granuloma formation caused by ova reaching the lungs via the pulmonary vessels.

During the late phase of the infection when schistosomal ova lead to progressive blockage of the pulmonary circulation,

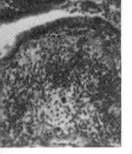

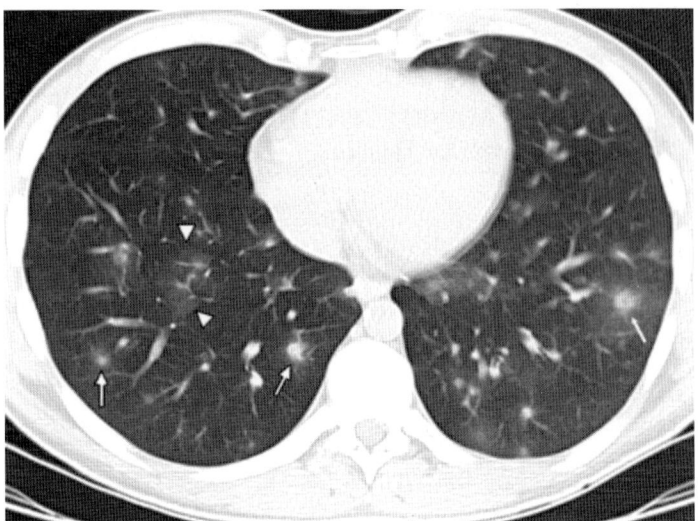

Fig 29.5: CT chest showing early pulmonary schistosomiasis in a 28-year-old man who had travelled to Mali. Initially, the patient had fever and urticaria, after which he experienced dry cough, predominantly at night. Chest CT scan shows multiple nodular lesions with ill-defined borders in the lower lobes. Histological analysis revealed S mansoni. (Courtesy of E. Schwartz, MD, Center for Geographical Medicine and Tropical Diseases, and J. Rozenman, MD, Department of Radiology, Sheba Medical Center, Tel Hashomer, Israel.)

the clinical picture is that of pulmonary hypertension and cor pulmonale. Gross aneurysmal dilatation of the pulmonary artery may be observed at this stage. The pulmonary involvement in the chronic phase almost always occurs in those with hepatosplenomegaly and portal hypertension. The opening of portosystemic collaterals allows passage of massive numbers of eggs from the portal vein directly to the lungs. A granulomatous reaction and fibrosis develop, with an acute necrotizing arteriolitis in the pulmonary vasculature leading to pulmonary hypertension and cor pulmonale. The degree of pulmonary hypertension is usually mild to moderate; but may, on occasion, be severe with some patients progressing to cardiac failure or sudden cardiovascular collapse. Pulmonary hypertension and cor pulmonale develop in 5–25% of patients with portal hypertension. Pulmonary arteriovenous fistulae have also been described in this form of schistosomiasis. The exact incidence of schistosomal pulmonary hypertension and cor pulmonale in endemic areas is unclear, but in a study on hospital populations, between 2–4% of the total cardiac population were diagnosed as having schistosomial cor pulmonale. Finally, a third form of pulmonary schistosomiasis consists of the reappearance of cough, wheeze, eosinophilia and pulmonary infiltrates during the course of treatment with praziquantel. This is a form of Jarisch-Herxheimer reaction and represents an immunological reaction to newly released antigens from dead worms and eggs in the lungs. Treatment of advanced pulmonary hypertension and cor-pulmonale is supportive.

DIAGNOSIS

Stool examination (*S. hematobium*); urine examination (*S. mansoni, S. japonica*) may reveal eggs of the worm. Rectal biopsies may clinch the diagnosis in *S. hematobium* infection. Serology is also of help.

TREATMENT

Praziquantel 40 mg/kg in a single dose is the drug of choice. Pulmonary hypertension and cor pulmonale are however irreversible.

Paragonimiasis

Paragonimiasis is a disease endemic in East Asia, Southeast Asia, Africa, and Latin America (particularly in Peru). Human infection is caused by the lung fluke *Paragonimus westerni* and other paragonimus species endemic in the above mentioned areas. It is believed that 195 million people are at risk and 26.7 million are infected in endemic areas.

PATHOGENESIS

Human infection occurs from eating raw or insufficiently cooked crustacea such as crabs and crayfish which contain the encysted infective parasite (metacercariae). These forms excyst in the duodenum, penetrate the wall of the gut, go through the peritoneal cavity, diaphragm and pleural cavity to enter the lungs, where they mature into adult worms roughly measuring 1.2 × 6 × 5 mm. These trematodes (lung flukes) are hermaphrodites and produce brownish eggs coughed up in the sputum or swallowed and voided in faeces. Outside the human host, the lifecycle goes through a snail intermediate host and then they encyst as metacercariae in freshwater crustacea.

The mature worm tunnels through the lung exciting a granulomatous reaction consisting of eosinophils and neutrophils. The surrounding lung tissue may show consolidation and/or atelectasis. Cystic lesions may enclose the parasite. Secondary infection of these cysts can result in the formation of one or more lung cavities (abscesses) which may communicate with bronchi. The worms as mentioned above lay eggs which again excite a strong hypersensitivity reaction within the lungs. It needs to be mentioned that though the primary site of infection is in the lungs, the worm may also be found in the brain and very rarely in other tissues.

CLINICAL FEATURES

Clinical features depend on the worm load present in a given patient. When the worm load is small, the patient may be asymptomatic, and even the chest X-ray may be normal. When moderate or large, clinical features include fever, breathlessness, chest discomfort, cough with expectoration and haemoptysis. The sputum may be rusty or blood-tinged and may contain eggs. Charcot leyden crystals are frequently present in the sputum.

Chest radiography shows infiltrates, nodular shadows, which may cavitate to resemble one or more abscesses. Fibrosis and areas of atelectasis may be present. Pleural effusion, pneumothorax may also occur, particularly at the time of penetration of the worm into the lung parenchyma. *Computed tomography* (CT) chest often reveals areas of consolidation in one or both the lungs together with associated ground-glass attenuation. The consolidated areas may show cavitation indistinguishable from tuberculosis. Multilocular radiolucencies, cystic or bronchiectatic, usually without fluid levels, giving a so-called soap bubble appearance have been described. Another characteristic radiographic feature described is a ring shadow with a crescent along one border resembling the corona phase

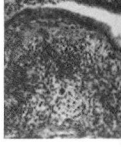

of a solar eclipse. The lesions are predominantly in the bases and peripheries of both lungs. Pleural effusions have been described in 70% of Japanese patients as the Paragonimus worms pass through the pleural cavity on their way to the lungs. Pleural thickening and calcification have also been described. Despite this plethora of pulmonary and pleural manifestations, about 20% of paragonimiasis patients are asymptomatic with the lung lesions being detected at routine health checks.

The main differential diagnosis is from tuberculosis or from a bacterial infection. Diagnosis is based on finding eggs in the sputum, in bronchoalveolar lavage (BAL) fluid or faeces. Serological tests may also help.

TREATMENT
The drug of choice is praziquantel given orally 25 mg/kg thrice daily for two days. Following treatment the stools within a few days stop containing eggs of the parasite and there is improvement both in the symptoms and in the imaging findings. In patients with pleural effusions the fluid must be first drained before administering the drug. Triclabendazole, a new benzimidazole derivative has been recently used in small-scale clinical trials and found to be effective and safe in a single dose of 10 mg/kg.

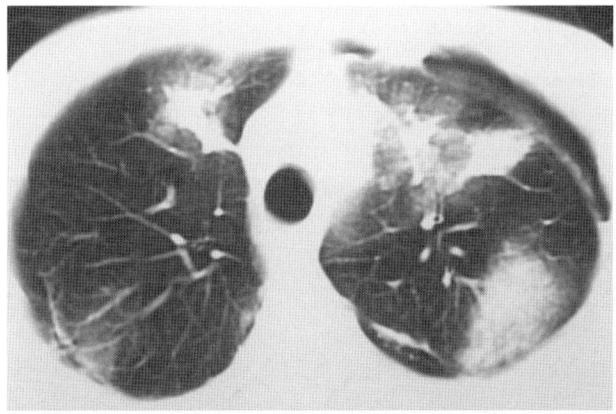

Fig 29.6. Pulmonary paragonimiasis in a 35-year-old man. CT scan demonstrates bilateral ill-defined areas of consolidation and areas of ground-glass attenuation associated with left pneumothorax. Eggs of *P. westermani* were found at bronchoalveolar lavage. Reproduced with permission from Martinez S, Restrepo CS, Carrillo JA, et al. Thoracic manifestations of tropical parasitic infections: a pictorial review. *Radiographics.* 2005; 25: 135–55.

It is seen from the previous descriptions that parasitic nematode and trematode infections often present with pulmonary eosinophilia. Pulmonary eosinophilia can also be due to other causes. The accompanying table lists the causes of pulmonary eosinophilia.

PULMONARY MANIFESTATIONS CAUSED BY CYSTODE INFECTIONS

Hydatidosis (Echinococcosis)

Hydatid disease in humans is chiefly caused by the larvae of the cystode *Echinococcus granulosa*, a worm which is found in the intestines of dogs and wolves. These worms release eggs

Table 29.1: Causes of Pulmonary Eosinophilia
Parasitic diseases
Filaria
Ascaris lumbricoides
Ankylostomal infection
Strongyloidiasis
Toxocara canis and catis
Paragonimiasis
Schistosomiasis
Allergic bronchopulmonary aspergillosis
Hypersensitivity response to
Drugs—penicillin, sulphonamides, trimethoprin-sulphamethaxazole, NSAIDs, carbamazepine, nitrofurantoin, penicillamine
Pollen
Other fungi
Other antigens
Asthamatic pulmonary eosinophilia
Pulmonary vasculitis: Churg-Strauss syndrome
Cryptogenic eosinophilic pneumonia
Hypereosinophilic syndrome

from their gravid segments and the eggs are passed out in the animal's faeces. Humans get infected when they ingest these eggs through contamination of food and water. After ingestion, the eggs on reaching the small intestine hatch larvae which can migrate via the portal vein radicals into the liver where they slowly form hydatid cysts. The larvae could also reach the lungs via haematogenous spread, giving rise to one or more hydatid cysts within the lung. Rarely, haematogenous spread to other organs may also occur. In adults, the liver is the most common site of involvement, followed by the lung. In children the lung is the most common site of hydatid disease.

EPIDEMIOLOGY
Though worldwide in distribution, particularly involving sheep- and cattle-raising areas (where dogs are also present), the disease is frequent in some tropical countries—particularly parts of Africa, South America and Northern India. It is particularly common in the State of Jammu and Kashmir where hydatid of the lung is one pathology which most frequently necessitates thoracic surgery. A study from the Post Graduate Institute of Chandigarh in North India has reported an increasing trend in the sero-prevalence of human hydatid disease between 1999–2003 when compared to the period 1984–98.

PATHOLOGY
The larvae reaching the lung slowly give rise to a space-occupying unilocular cyst which to start with is small but can grow as large as 20cm in diameter. The cyst is most often solitary (in 60–70% of cases), but multiple cysts also occur. They may be unilateral

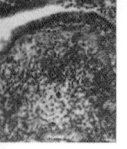
but in 20% of patients, are bilateral. It is uncommon to observe cysts within the liver and the lungs in the same patient. The cyst wall on histology has three layers—

a) The outer pericyst, which is chiefly composed of fibroblasts and fibrous tissue;
b) An acellular middle laminated layer which has a nutrient function;
c) An inner germinal layer which has scoleces and generates daughter cysts. The cyst may lie quiet over years, it may grow to compress neighbouring structures, it may rupture into the lung, bronchus, pleura or rarely into the mediastinum or even the pericardium, causing spread of hydatid disease in these areas.

CLINICAL FEATURES AND COMPLICATIONS

A hydatid cyst in the lung is often asymptomatic being discovered on routine chest radiography. Large cyst or cysts may cause cough, breathlessness and vague chest discomfort. An infected cyst behaves as a lung abscess. Rupture of a cyst invariably produces symptoms. The cyst fluid is immunogenic and following rupture can lead to a hypersensitivity reaction or even anaphylaxis. Bronchospasm, hypotension, tachycardia may occur, and anaphylaxis can be fatal. The cyst may rupture into a bronchus, the contents being coughed up in the sputum. Communication with a bronchus also predisposes to infection of the cyst contents and to purulent expectoration. Rupture may also be associated with consolidation of the neighbouring lung. If the cyst opens into the pleura, pleural effusion results and pleural dissemination follows with hydatid cysts within the pleura and pleural space. Rarely, rupture into the mediastinum leads to hydatids within the mediastinum and rupture into the pericardium to hydatids within the pericardium.

IMAGING FINDINGS

Hydatid cysts appear as round or ovoid cystic, unilocular masses with sharply defined borders which enhance on administration of contrast. The 'meniscus sign' is observed when there is air between the outer pericyst and the middle laminated layer. This occurs when a cyst starts to erode an adjacent bronchus or bronchiole. When a cyst ruptures into a bronchus, an air-fluid level is observed within the cyst; the meniscus sign may or may not be present at the same time. The 'water-lily sign' is typified by the endocyst floating within the cyst.

DIAGNOSIS

The presence of a well-defined cyst, particularly in an endemic area should arouse suspicion and suggest the correct diagnosis. Indirect haemagglutination tests and the Cansoni skin tests are of doubtful use as they lack sensitivity and specificity. ELISA tests are more useful. Multiple lung cysts may need to be differentiated from metastatic lesions. The liquid nature of the contents of the cyst as judged on CT chest should give a correct diagnosis.

MANAGEMENT

The treatment of choice of a large cyst which produces compression or is likely to rupture is surgical resection. This is followed by the use of mebendazole (10–15 mg/kg body weight per day) for eight weeks to take care of any spillage that could have occurred during surgery.

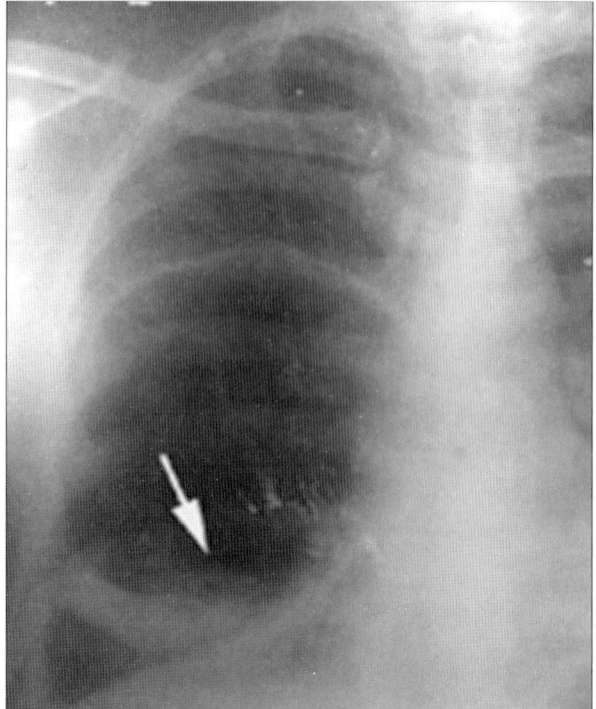

Fig 29.7: Pulmonary Hydatid Cyst.
Chest X-ray demonstrates a large air-filled cavity in the right lower zone with a crumpled membrane in the base of the cyst representing a ruptured pulmonary hydatid.

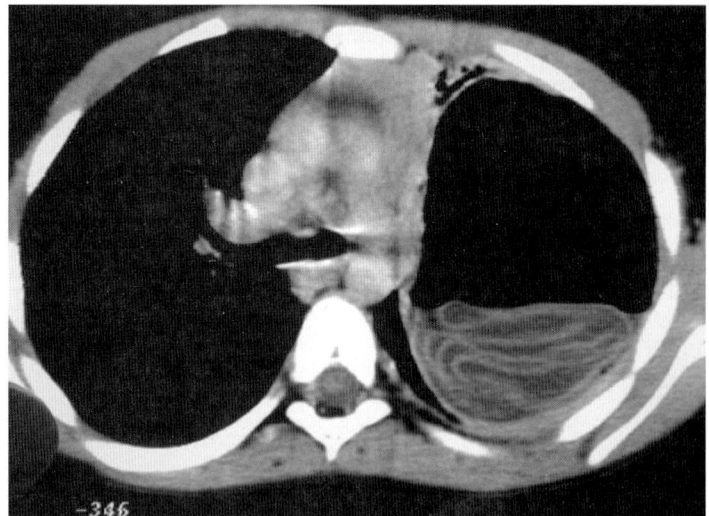

Fig 29.8: Hydatid cyst. CT chest showing the 'water-lily sign', typified by the endocyst floating within the cyst.

When surgery is not indicated or when there are multiple bilateral cysts or when there is dissemination because of rupture of a cyst, one has to rest content with the use of mebendazole in the dose stated above. The course of mebendazole may be repeated several times. Percutaneous aspiration of a cyst followed by an injection of a cysticidal agent such as hypertonic saline or alcohol, with reaspiration has also proved successful. It needs to be done under CT guidance. Mebendazole in the dose recommended should be administered.

SUGGESTED READING

Allen GP Ross, Ph.D. Paul B Bartley, *et al.* Schistosomiasis. *N Engl J Med.* 2002; 346: 1212–20.

Kim TS, Han J. Pleuropulmonary paragonimiasis: CT findings in 31 patients. *AJR Am J Roentgenol.* Sep. 2005; 185(3): 616–21.

Manghani DK, Dastur DK, Udwadia FE. The lung in tropical eosinophilia compared to that in pulmonary hypertension. Fine structural basis of respiratory disability. *Zentralbl. Patholo.* 1992; 138: 108–18.

Martãnez S. Thoracic manifestations of tropical parasitic infections: a pictorial review. *Radiographics.* 1 Jan. 2005; 25(1): 135–55.

Ozvaran MK. Pleural complications of pulmonary hydatid disease. *Respirology.* 1 Mar. 2004; 9(1): 115–19.

Udwadia, FE. Pulmonary Eosinophilia. *J Ass. Phy. India.* 1978; 26(5): 429–37.

Udwadia FE. Tropical Eosinophilia: a review. *Respiratory Medicine.* 1993; 87: 17–21.

Vijayan VK. Tropical pulmonary eosinophilia: pathogenesis, diagnosis and management. *Curr Opin Pulm Med.* 1 Sep. 2007; 13(5): 428–33.

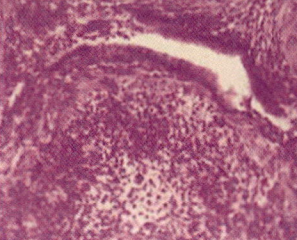

30 Pulmonary Manifestations of Protozoal Infections

PULMONARY MANIFESTATIONS OF MALARIAL INFECTION

Malaria is caused by the Plasmodium species—*P. falciparum, P. vivax, P. ovale* and *P. malariae*. The disease is endemic in sub-Saharan Africa, India, Southeast Asia, the Caribbean, South and Central America. The parasite is transmitted by the female Anopheles mosquito and infects 400–600 million people, causing well over one million deaths annually. Some compute deaths close to two million annually. Deaths are most common among pregnant women and in children under five years living in endemic areas. The majority of deaths are due to *P. falciparum* infection, which can cause a hyperacute fulminant illness that can at times kill the patient within 48 h. Pulmonary manifestations are almost entirely caused by *P. falciparum* infection.

The infecting mosquito injects sporozoites into the host which then travel to the liver and multiply to form schizonts. These schizonts rupture, liberating numerous merozoites into the blood. The merozoites invade the erythrocytes and develop into mature ring forms (which produce symptoms), and ultimately into erythrocytic schizonts. A few merozoites develop into sexual gametocytes. These do not cause symptoms but when ingested by a mosquito feeding on an infected patient, develop within it to sporozoites thus completing the lifecycle.

Pulmonary Manifestations

Malaria continues to ravage large tracts of the tropics and with the rise in world travel is a disorder that must be considered in any traveller with a recent or remote history of tropical travel. Malaria occurs in 300–500 million individuals annually, affecting 40% of the world's population and an estimated 50–70 million Western travellers are exposed to it annually. It continues to result in 1.5–2.7 million deaths annually. Falciparum malaria is a major cause of death in tropical areas.

A mild degree of 'bronchitis' characterized by cough with rhonchi on auscultation is a common feature of all plasmodial infections occurring in 36% of falciparum and 55% of ovale malaria. It is associated with the usual fever with rigors and the disease is mistaken by the unwary as an acute respiratory infection, particularly when the fever is intermittent or continuous as with *P. falciparum* infection.

A recent study of lung functions in uncomplicated symptomatic malaria showed the presence of increased airways' obstruction, impaired ventilation, decreased gas transfer and increased pulmonary phagocytic activity in both *P. vivax* and *P. falciparum* infections.

P. falciparum infections can be associated with far more severe pulmonary complications than those mentioned above. These are briefly described:

1. Even when radiography of the chest seems apparently normal, some patients with *P. falciparum* infection have a low PaO_2, as low as 60–65 mm Hg. This is due to a ventilator perfusion inequality as the PaO_2 and the oxygen saturation rise with oxygen given at 2–4 L/min. Perhaps interstitial oedema and disturbed perfusion to the lungs contribute to this ventilation perfusion inequality.

2. *Acute Lung Injury* The incidence of acute lung injury/*acute respiratory distress syndrome* (ARDS) is higher in those with more severe malaria. Non-cardiogenic pulmonary oedema has been reported in 21% of patients with cerebral malaria and in a third of patients dying of severe malaria. Unlike cerebral malaria which occurs early in the natural history of *P. falciparum* infection, ARDS occurs later, around the same time as renal, hepatic or coagulation failure. Also, unlike cerebral malaria, there may be little or no evidence of significant parasitemia at the time of its occurrence. The reason for its delayed occurrence, at times several days after anti-malarial drugs have been instituted is a mystery. Perhaps the gradual release of cytokines may be responsible for the delayed organ damage. Acute lung injury/ARDS is more common in pregnant women, in children and non-immune adults. In the very severe forms of *P. falciparum*, coexisting cerebral, renal, haematological and coagulation abnormalities may be seen so that these patients are desperately ill with multiorgan failure.

Acute lung injury may vary in severity:

a) In mild lung injury the PaO_2/FIO_2 ratio is between 200 and 300. The increased alveolar arterial gradient in mild acute lung injury observed with *P. falciparum* infection is largely related to a ventilation perfusion inequality rather than to a right to left shunt within the lung. The prognosis is good and recovery occurs provided there is no serious dysfunction involving other systems.

b) Severe acute lung injury (ARDS) as has already been mentioned, is a classic feature of fulminant or hyperacute *P. falciparum* infection. It has however also been recently reported with *P. vivax* and *P. ovale* infection. Increasing tachypnoea, respiratory distress, bilateral crackles, fluffy shadows in both lung fields and severe hypoxia necessitating ventilator support and the use of *positive end-expiratory*

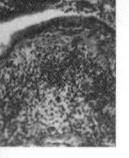

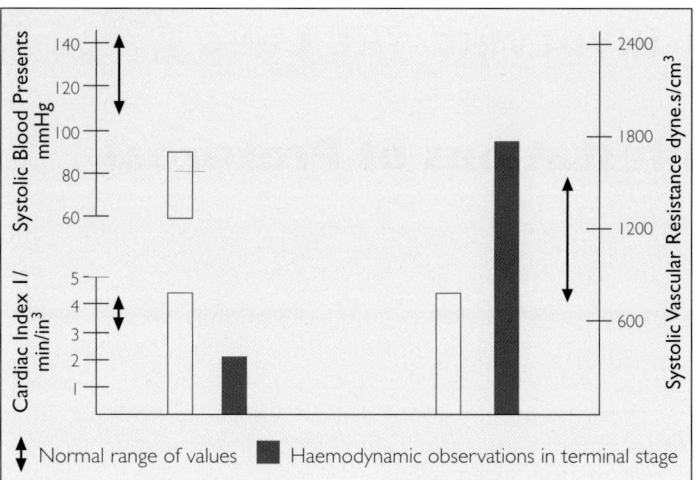

Fig 30.1: Haemodynamic observations in fulminant falciparum infections.

pressure (PEEP) are all present. A right to left shunt within the lungs is a prominent feature of severe ARDS though some degree of ventilation perfusion abnormality correctible by increasing the FIO$_2$ is also invariably observed.

ARDS rarely occurs as an isolated complication of acute *P. falciparum* infection. It is invariably associated with other organ dysfunction, particularly with cerebral malaria.

Haemodynamic studies of patients with hyperacute *P. falciparum* infection with ARDS and other organ dysfunction reveal hypotension, a low central venous pressure, low pulmonary capillary wedge pressure, with a high cardiac index and a low systemic vascular resistance. The findings are similar to those observed in severe bacterial sepsis and septic shock. In patients who ultimately die, there is marked hypotension, a very low cardiac index, with an increase in the systemic vascular resistance and an increase in pulmonary capillary wedge pressure.

c) ARDS at times complicates fulminant *P. falciparum* infection associated with disseminated intravascular coagulopathy (DIC). The latter then forms an important pathogenetic factor of ARDS. The features of DIC dominate the clinical picture in these patients.

The pathophysiology of ARDS is characterized by damage to the alveolar capillary membrane causing non-cardiogenic increased permeability inflammatory oedema. *P. falciparum* infection causes the formation of 'sticky knobs' on the surface of infected red blood cells (RBCs). The 'knobs' consist of host cells with parasitic antigen and help in binding of infected RBCs to endothelial cells of capillaries and venules. Sequestration and sludging of RBCs blocking capillaries and venules ensues, with hypoxic damage to the alveolar capillary membrane. There is also an increased production and liberation of cytokines, in particular tumour necrosis factor alpha (TNFα). TNFα exerts direct cytotoxic effects and also induces the expression in endothelial cells of ICAM-1 and other adhesins which ensure adherence of parasitized RBCs to the alveolar capillary wall.

A recent study on severe falciparum malaria by Krishnan and Karnad *(Ref: Krishnan A, Karnad DR. Severe falciparum malaria: an important cause of multiple organ failure in Indian intensive care unit patients. Crit Care Med. 2003 Sep;31(9):2278–84.)*

from a busy tertiary referral ICU in Mumbai is the largest prospective study to date. Three hundred and one patients with severe falciparum malaria were admitted in the 30-month study period comprising 13% of all ICU admissions in this hospital. ARDS was seen in a relatively higher number (79 patients, 26%) than in any previous study and carried the worst outcome. In this study, ARDS occurred later in the course of the illness (mean 3.1 days, *P* < 0.001) compared with cerebral, renal or coagulation failure.

3. *Pulmonary oedema in P. falciparum* infection can be due to *causes other than ARDS*. Pulmonary oedema can be due to fluid overload, myocardial dysfunction associated with fulminant *P. falciparum* infection, and rarely due to hyperpyrexia. Rectal temperatures which suddenly shoot up to 108° F or 110° F can cause sudden cardiorespiratory failure with fulminant pulmonary oedema. Death can occur within a few minutes to a few hours.

4. *Severe P. falciparum infec*tion, particularly when it occurs in the old, the very young, in pregnant women, or in the malnourished, can cause *marked tachypnoea*. The tachypnoea in the presence of high fever, electrolyte imbalance and poor nutrition leads to respiratory muscle fatigue. Respiratory muscle fatigue results in low tidal volumes, a poor cough reflex with inability to clear airway secretions. Areas of atelectasis develop within the lungs with patchy shadows visible on X-ray of the chest. These patients are prone to sudden respiratory arrest. Elective intubation with ventilator support promptly restores normal gas exchange and the pulmonary shadows disappear quickly, distinguishing this condition from ARDS.

5. *Aspiration pneumonia* is an important complication, particularly in obtunded patients, more so when injudicious attempts are made to feed them orally.

6. *Malarial pneumonia* While consolidation and pneumonitis on a radiograph in a patient with falciparum or vivax malaria usually represent a superadded bacterial pneumonia, Applebaum and Shrager in 1944 described 4% of their patients with a 'malarial pneumonia'. The consolidation was lobular in all except 7% who had lobar consolidation. This complication occurred equally in vivax and falciparum malaria. The existence of malarial pneumonia as an entity remains unproven as no convincing demonstration of parasites in sputum has been made nor has there been conclusive exclusion of other pathogens as causative factors. However, the response of the consolidation to antimalarials alone suggests the possibility of malaria pneumonia existing as a distinct but rare entity.

7. *Pleural effusion* Pleural effusions have frequently been found at autopsy in patients dying of pulmonary oedema and Applebaum described them in 2.5% of his patients with pneumonia. There is only one report of pleural effusion large enough to require drainage.

8. *Secondary bacterial pneumonia* Secondary bacterial gram-negative infections are frequent complications of severe complicated malaria and contribute significantly to morbidity and mortality. As early as 1902 Ross alluded to pneumonia being a common cause of death in patients severely debilitated with malaria, and despite the broad-spectrum of antibiotics available today, this

statement still holds true. Bacterial sepsis and its associated complications must be avidly sought and excluded or aggressively treated to minimize this high mortality rate. Patients with malaria are prone to bacteremia due to ischemic breakdown of the gastrointestinal mucosal barrier and bacterial translocation. In Krishnan's large series of 301 falciparum patients, secondary bacterial sepsis accounted for 39 patients (35 deaths). Sepsis was the commonest cause of death occurring after the seventh day of hospitalization.

9. Patients on ventilator support may develop *nosocomial pneumonia*.
10. *Deep vein thrombosis and pulmonary embolism* are important complications to be watched out for.

There are certain points of importance that perhaps need to be stressed.

1. ARDS as has been stated earlier is invariably associated with multiple organ dysfunction.
2. Once ARDS and organ dysfunction set in, they may continue to evolve even when parasitemia is abolished by specific therapy.
3. In hyperacute cases associated with severe hypotension and cardiovascular collapse, ARDS and the full spectrum of multiple organ failure seen with *P. falciparum* infections may occur without detectable parasitemia. This is because most of the parasites remain sequestered within the capillaries of various organs and there are very few circulating in the peripheral blood. Incomplete treatment at home or in another hospital may also be occasionally responsible for inability to detect parasitemia in the peripheral blood. The moral of the story is that in endemic and hyperendemic areas one is justified in treating a patient whose clinical features are compatible with fulminant *P. falciparum* infection with

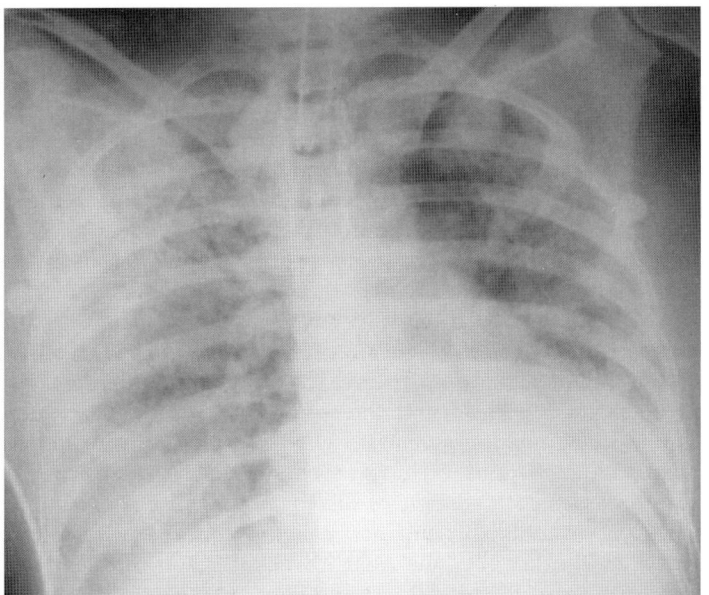

Fig 30.2: *P. falciparum* malaria. X-ray chest showing ARDS in patient with *P. falciparum* malaria. Note bilateral shadows in both lung fields, more in the right than the left.

specific anti-malarial therapy, even if the diagnosis cannot be confirmed.

PULMONARY COMPLICATIONS OF VIVAX MALARIA

The clinical course of vivax malaria is generally benign with lung complications seldom seen. A review of the literature however reveals very rare cases of acute lung injury and pulmonary oedema secondary to vivax malaria. The possibility of mixed infection with falciparum should always be considered in such cases and it is probably prudent to treat such cases as mixed infections even if falciparum cannot be isolated. Other extremely rare pulmonary complications of vivax malaria include one reported case of bronchiolitis obliterans (BOOP) and one case of acute interstitial pneumonia.

PULMONARY TOXICITY OF MALARIA PROPHYLAXIS

Anti-malarial drug toxicity while rare has been reported. With increasing numbers of travellers on malaria prophylaxis during holidays to endemic areas, this must be borne in mind. Sulfadoxine and pyrimethamine hypersensitivity can cause pulmonary eosinophilia, lung infiltrates, allergic alveolitis and non-cardiogenic pulmonary oedema. Methemoglobinaemia is well described after use of primaquine and dapsone.

DIAGNOSIS

Diagnosis depends on demonstration of malarial parasites on blood smears. A thick blood smear examined by an experienced pathologist generally allows a definite diagnosis. A thin smear allows identification of the infecting species. Antigen-detecting assays which identify *P. falciparum*-specific histadine-rich protein are of further help in identifying *P. falciparum* infection.

Finally, the need for vigilance even for physicians and patients from the developed world is exemplified by the case of an elderly resident of Germany who developed a sepsis syndrome and respiratory failure. Falciparum was found in the blood on the sixth day of hospitalization. She had never travelled outside the country but lived close to Frankfurt airport and 'baggage malaria' from imported anopheles mosquitoes in the luggage or airplane was postulated to be responsible for her illness.

PROGNOSIS

Despite these patients being desperately ill with multi-organ failure survival rates are better than those with equivalent organ failure from other causes of sepsis. The overall mortality rate in the experienced ICU in Krishnan's study was relatively low at 24% despite severe organ failure. As expected only 6% of patients with single or no organ failure died whereas mortality rose to 49% in those with multi-organ failure.

TREATMENT

All patients with severe *P. falciparum* infection require critical care. Specific treatment is with intravenous quinine. The IV dose of quinine is 10 mg/kg of quinine base every eight hours for seven days. Artesunate is also being increasingly used. The dose of artesunate is 2.4 mg/kg initially, 1.2 mg/kg 12 h later, then 1.2 mg/kg daily for five days. Whether the use of both is superior to the use of one alone is not proven. The Artemether-Quinine Meta-analysis Study group favoured artesunate as it was found to be more active than quinine in terms of parasite killing, less toxic, and easier to administer. To counter the

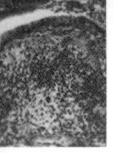
threat of resistance of P. falciparum to monotherapies, and to improve treatment outcome, combinations of anti-malarials are now recommended by WHO for the treatment of falciparum malaria. The following anti-malarial combination therapies (ACTs) are currently recommended:

- artemether + lumefantrine,
- artesunate + amodiaquine,
- artesunate + mefloquine,
- artesunate + sulfadoxine–pyrimethamine.

Note: amodiaquine + sulfadoxine–pyrimethamine may be considered as an interim option where ACTs cannot be made available, provided that efficacy of both is high.

Chloroquine should not be used in India and Southeast Asia for *P. falciparum* infections as in most endemic areas the parasite is resistant to the drug. Widespread resistance to chloroquine has also been reported from Indonesia, Papua New Guinea, parts of Africa, Myanmar and Brazil. Non-severe cases of chloroquine-resistant *P. falciparum* infection can be treated with oral quinine in combination with either doxycycline or clindamycin. The use of ventilator support in ARDS, in severe pulmonary oedema from other causes, and in patients who are tachypnoeic and who show evidence of respiratory muscle fatigue is imperative. Secondary infection whether iatrogenic or otherwise requires appropriate antibiotic therapy. Serious pulmonary complications are associated with dysfunction of other organ systems. All systems require support if the patient is to survive. Persistent hypotension in spite of the use of inotropes and vasopressors is of ominous significance. Renal replacement is invaluable in patients with renal shutdown or in overhydrated patients with poor renal function. Patients with a parasitemia of over 25–30% may require exchange transfusion. In our experience lesser degrees of parasitemia respond to specific treatment with anti-malarials and to expert critical care.

Amoebic Infections

Amoebiasis is caused by the protozoan *Entamoeba histolytica* and is probably the most common cause of mortality among parasitic infections after malaria and schistosomiasis. Amoebiasis is responsible for 50–100,000 deaths annually. The disease is endemic in tropical and subtropical regions, having a high prevalence rate in India, Asia, Africa, South America and Mexico. It spreads by the orofaecal route; contamination of food and water, poor hygiene, poor sanitation and overcrowding help in its dissemination. Globally 10% of the world's population is infected with *E. histolytica* causing significant morbidity and mortality. There are two more points worth noting—

i. Host immunity is negligible in the virginal host. The host antibody response is however useful in preventing subsequent invasive episodes.
ii. Amoebic infection can be fulminant in the very young, in the malnourished, in those on corticosteroids and in the immunosuppressed. We have observed fulminant amoebic infections in some patients with HIV disease.

PATHOGENESIS

Pulmonary manifestations are invariably secondary to an amoebic hepatic abscess. Following the ingestion of cysts, the trophozoites develop in the small gut and are carried with the intestinal contents into the caecum and the large bowel. The trophozoites are motile amoebae which attach themselves anywhere along the mucosa of the large gut (particularly in the recto-sigmoid and caecum). They produce an ulceration of the mucosa because of the proteolytic enzymes secreted by them. Large flask-shaped ulcers are formed which could bleed or perforate. The trophozoites at the base of these ulcers may enter the portal circulation and reach the liver. Here the proteolytic enzymes secreted by the trophozoites produce a lytic necrosis of the liver cells resulting in one or more abscesses. A hepatic abscess is most often in the posterio-superior aspect of the right lobe of the liver. Pulmonary manifestations occur as a direct extension of the hepatic abscess through the diaphragm into the pleural space, or into the lung or into both. A left lobe hepatic abscess may extend through the diaphragm into the pericardium and rarely into the left pleural space. Rarely, trophozoites may enter the systemic circulation via the rectal venous plexus so that there is a haematogenous spread of infection to the lung and very occasionally, to other organ systems, particularly the brain. There are some who believe that haematogenous spread could also occur if the trophozoites of a liver abscess gain access to the hepatic veins or the inferior vena cava. Lymphatic spread of amoebic infection from the liver through the diaphragm into the thorax remains a theoretical possibility.

In our series more than 60% of patients with a large liver abscess had serious pulmonary manifestations. It is uncommon to find overt manifestations of amoebic ulcerative colitis in patients who have pulmonary manifestations of amoebiasis.

CLINICAL FEATURES AND COMPLICATIONS

Pleuropulmonary amoebiasis was first described by Simon in 1890 who reported a patient whose liver abscess ruptured into the lung with *E. histolytica* observed in the sputum. Since then different series from the tropics have reported the incidence of pleuropulmonary involvement to vary from as low as 4% of patients with amoebic liver abscesses to as high as 86%. A consistent observation has been that pleuropulmonary complications occur more commonly in developing countries. Like amoebic liver abscess, pleuropulmonary amoebiasis occurs predominantly in men with a male/female ratio varying from 9:1 to 15:1. Whilst no age is exempt, the age group most likely to develop this complication is young adults in the range of 20–45 years. The onset may be acute, subacute or chronic. Acute onset is heralded by sudden onset of fever with chills, pain over the right hypochondrium, pleuritic right-sided chest pain referred to the shoulder and to the back to the right of the midline. There is leucocytosis with a rise in the erythrocyte sedimentation rate. Clinical examination reveals a right-sided pleural rub, dullness to percussion over the right lower chest below the scapula, with diminished breath sounds, or distant bronchial breath sounds. There is invariably an enlarged palpable tender liver; a gentle tap with the fist over the right lower intercostal spaces often produces exquisite tenderness and pain.

Subacute onset is characterized by low-grade fever, weight loss, a milder degree of leucocytosis, pleuritic chest pain and a variable degree of pleural effusion or the presence of pleuropulmonary complications, the source of which may remain undetected. This is particularly so if the liver is not sufficiently enlarged.

Chronic onset and course are characterized by evening rise of fever, weight loss, pleural effusion which is often wrongly diagnosed as being due to tuberculosis. The presentation could also be that of a chronic lung abscess or pulmonary consolidation, the source of which remains obscure.

COMPLICATIONS

1. Segmental atelectasis of the lower lobe due to upward displacement and fixity of the right dome of the diaphragm are the commonest pulmonary manifestations.
2. A sympathetic pleural effusion is equally frequent. It is sterile on culture.
3. A hepatic abscess may open through the diaphragm into the pleura leading to a pleural exudate and an empyema. A sudden rupture causes sudden severe pleural pain, tachycardia and well-marked dyspnoea. The patients can be gravely ill if the hepatic abscess that has ruptured into the pleural space is large; there is danger of death if there is a simultaneous rupture of the hepatic abscess into the peritoneal cavity. A subacute or slow seepage of the hepatic abscess into the pleural space through the diaphragm leads to subacute or chronic clinical features of a right-sided empyema. Pleural paracentesis often reveals dirty brown pus. Trophozoites of *E. histolytica* may be found in the fluid.
4. The hepatic abscess may go through the diaphragm into the lower lobe of the lung to cause a) *consolidation* of part or whole of the right lobe; b) a lung abscess; the patient coughing up anchovy sauce material in his sputum. The liver and lung abscess may thereby drain and at times heal. Communication between the liver and lung can lead to a *hepatobronchial fistula* or a *biliary bronchial fistula*.
5. Finally, the hepatic abscess may open both into the pleura and lung causing both an empyema and pulmonary complications stated above.
6. A left lobe liver abscess may encroach through the left dome of the diaphragm into the pericardium. Tachycardia of sudden onset with breathlessness is an early sign. It is usually due to a sympathetic pericardial effusion. Actual rupture into the pericardial space of a large left lobe liver abscess is a catastrophe that leads to quick death from cardiac tamponade. A slow leak into the pericardium can however be promptly drained and treated. A simultaneous involvement of the left pleura and rarely of the left lower lobe may also be observed.

It should be noted that pulmonary manifestations generally involve the right lower lobe. Occasionally pulmonary involvement is observed in the middle lobe or at a distance well away from the right dome of the diaphragm. This may well result from a haematogenous spread of trophozoites though the rectal venous plexus into the systemic circulation.

DIAGNOSIS

Pleuropulmonary manifestations involving the right thorax should always arouse suspicion of a possible amoebic infection in patients living in endemic areas. Ultrasound of the liver should enable the

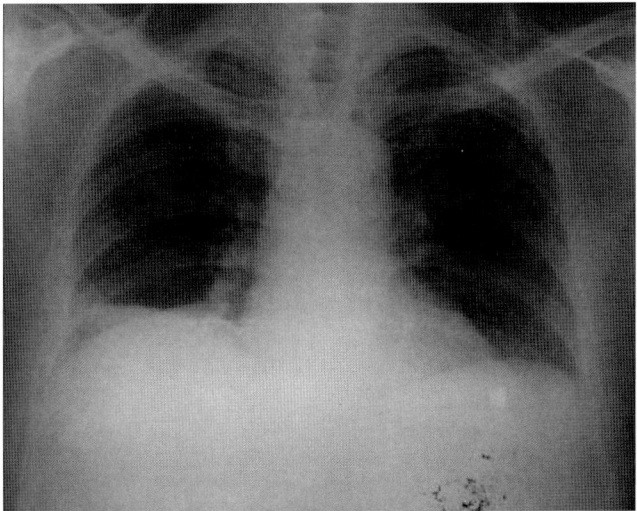

Fig 30.3: Pulmonary complications of amoebiasis. X-ray chest showing an elevated fixed right dome of the diaphragm, segmental atelectasis of the right lower lobe and a right-sided pleural effusion.

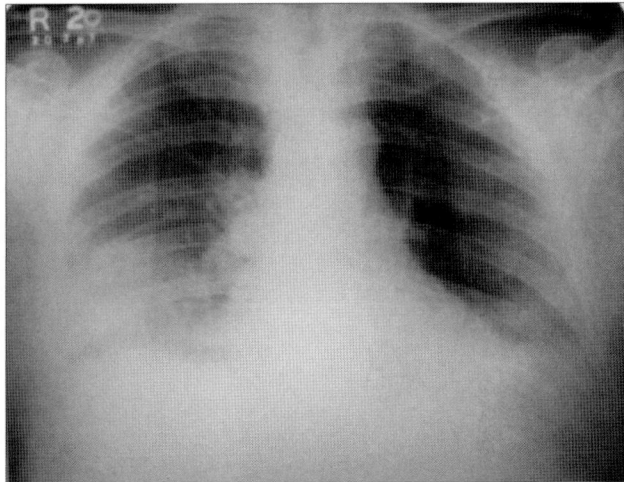

Fig 30.4: X-ray chest showing right lower lobe consolidation in a patient with an amoebic liver abscess.

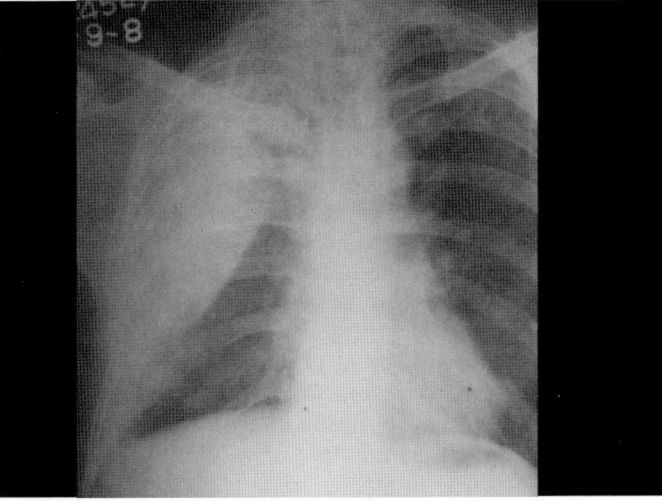

Fig 30.5: Amoebic empyema. X-ray chest showing a right-sided empyema caused by a hepatic abscess opening both into the pleura and lung.

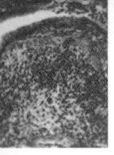

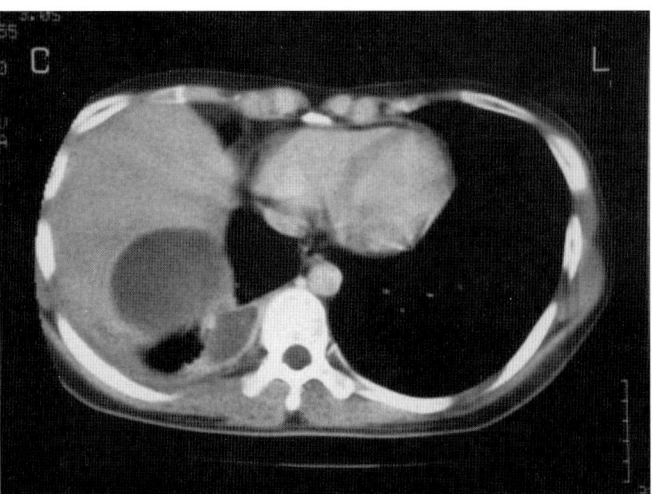

Fig 30.6: Amoebic liver abscess. CT abdomen demonstrates a well-defined hypodense area in the right lobe of the liver, posterior-superior segment. There is extension into the right pleural space; this represents a ruptured amoebic liver abscess.

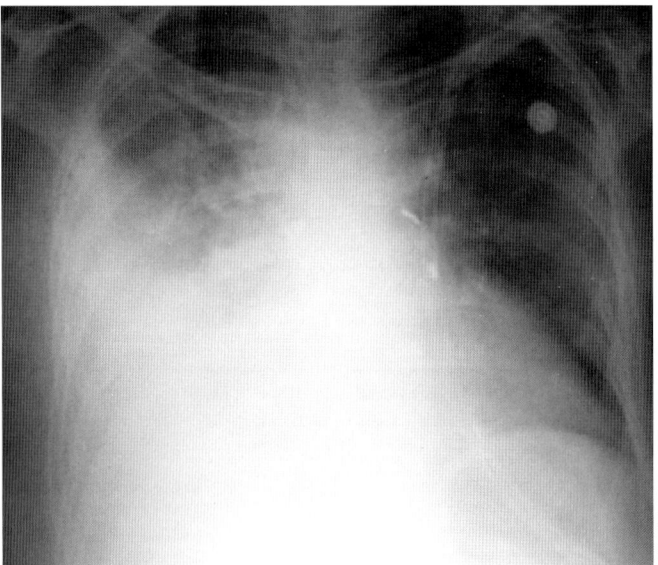

Fig 30.7: Large right-sided pleural effusion of amoebic aetiology. X-ray chest showing right-sided pleural effusion caused by an amoebic liver abscess.

diagnosis of a possible liver abscess as the source of infection. Radiographic features include an elevated right hemidiaphragm which is the commonest radiographic abnormality being found in well over 50% of amoebic liver abscesses. Small sterile right-sided pleural effusions are frequently observed. Basal consolidation is the next most frequent radiographic abnormality; cavitation and abscess formation may occur in the consolidated area. Occasionally, a pulmonary abscess may be seen, distinct from the liver, in any lobe as a result of haematogenous dissemination. Pleural effusions can be small, moderate or massive. If a hepatobronchial fistula forms, an air-containing cavity may be observed under the diaphragm.

CT of the upper abdomen and chest should further clarify the diagnosis. Needle aspiration of a hypoechoic area of the liver draws pus which is reddish brown in colour. Trophozoites

are only rarely found in the liver aspirate or in the aspirate from an amoebic empyema, or in the sputum in patients with a hepatopulmonary or biliopulmonary fistula.

The haemagglutination test for amoebiasis is positive and shows a rising titre over the next few weeks. The test may remain positive for several months. Stools very rarely show trophozoites of amoeba in patients with pleuropulmonary manifestations. The presence of cysts of *E. histolytica* has no meaning as there are many asymptomatic carriers of amoebiasis.

Newer tests that detect DNA of amoebae in pus or pleural fluid are being developed and may prove far more sensitive. A recently developed monoclonal antibody test that can be used in serum or pus samples has been developed.

PROGNOSIS
If promptly treated the prognosis is good, except in fulminant infections, in immunocompromised patients and in children. We have seen one death occur, even though the diagnosis was prompt, treatment adequate and drainage of the pleural space done as per our protocol. Death when it occurs is due to sepsis, and hypotension with associated myocardial dysfunction. Even with expert critical care, multiple organ failure leading to death can occur. Yet some patients recover even when they seem on the verge of death. To quote just one example, an elderly diabetic lady was brought into the ICU with a near cardiac arrest. She was resuscitated and was found to have a liver abscess which had ruptured into the peritoneum, pleura and pericardium. All these spaces were adequately drained as emergency procedures within the ICU and she was given specific anti-amoebic treatment. The huge liver abscess was also drained a few days later with a large drainage tube. She went into multi-organ failure but after a stormy course ultimately survived.

TREATMENT
1. Metronidazole is the specific treatment for all amoebic infections given in a dose of 750 mg thrice daily for 10 to 15 days. In acutely ill patients we prefer to give the drug intravenously. Seizures are an important complication of this therapy.
2. An empyema or a pleural exudate needs to be drained. Thick pus necessitates tube drainage through an intercostal space. CT studies should help correct positioning of the drainage tube.
3. An amoebic liver abscess is the source of pleuropulmonary manifestations. Ordinarily, after a diagnostic tap, the pus within the abscess need not be aspirated. Specific treatment outlined above leads to healing, though imaging studies may reveal a walled-off space in the liver for weeks or even months. If however the abscess is large, 8–10 cm or more, it should be aspirated dry. Even if it fills up again repeated aspirations are only occasionally necessary. Repeated aspirations may however be necessary if an amoebic abscess is complicated by secondary bacterial infection. This is rare, and most often iatrogenic, from improper unsterile aspiration attempts. Very large abscesses which sometimes almost occupy the greater part of the right lobe of the liver may require tube drainage. An important disadvantage of tube drainage is the possibility of introducing secondary bacterial infection.

4. Secondary bacterial infections of pleuropulmonary lesions are rare; if present they require appropriate antibiotic therapy.
5. Amoebic infection within the gut may be asymptomatic. It is important to use diloxanide 500 mg TDS or iodoquinol 650 mg TDS for 20 days to clear the gut of infection.

PULMONARY MANIFESTATIONS OF RARE PROTOZOAL INFECTIONS

Babesiosis

Babesiosis is caused by a tick-borne protozoan parasite *B. babesiosis*. The disease is characterized by a malaria-like illness with fever with chills, leucopenia and thrombocytopenia. The disease is usually mild except in asplenic patients, when it can be severe and even fatal. Pulmonary complications are uncommon but the most frequent manifestation is ARDS. This non-cardiogenic pulmonary oedema is not related to splenic function or the degree of parasitemia. ARDS responds to supportive treatment.

Leishmaniasis

Leishmaniasis is caused by the protozoan termed *Leishmania donovani*. It is endemic in tropical Africa, South America and in eastern India, particularly in the states of Bihar, parts of Bengal and Orissa. The disease is characterized by fever, hepatosplenomegaly, leucopenia, and thrombocytopenia. Bacterial pneumonia may occur as an intercurrent infection. Rarely, the disease causes pulmonary infection in immunocompromised states, e.g. HIV infection. In these patients interstitial pneumonia, ARDS, disseminated intravascular coagulopathy, and hepatic/renal dysfunction may be the presenting features.

SUGGESTED READING

Bora D. Epidemiology of visceral leishmaniasis in India. *Natl Med J India*. Mar.–Apr. 1999; 12(2): 62–8.

Douglas NM. Artemisinin combination therapy for vivax malaria. *Lancet Infect Dis*. 1 Jun. 2010; 10(6): 405–16.

Martãnez S. Thoracic manifestations of tropical parasitic infections:a pictorial review. *Radiographics*. 1 Jan. 2005; 25(1): 135–55.

Shamsuzzaman SM. Thoracic amebiasis. *Clin Chest Med*. 1 Jun. 2002; 23(2): 479–92.

Tan LK. Acute lung injury and other serious complications of Plasmodium vivax malaria. *Lancet Infect Dis*. 1 Jul. 2008; 8(7): 449–54.

Taylor WR. Malaria and the lung. *Clin Chest Med*. 1 Jun. 2002; 23(2): 457–68.

CHAPTER

31   Pulmonary Involvement in Fulminant Systemic Tropical Infections

Pulmonary involvement is observed in severe tropical infections such as *P. falciparum* malaria, salmonellosis, leptospirosis, dengue haemorrhagic fever (DHF), other rare haemorrhagic fevers, melioidosis, plague, and anthrax. *P. falciparum* is one infection which when hyperacute often causes pulmonary complications. These have been already described under protozoal infections.

Typhoid and Other Salmonella Infections

Typhoid fever due to *S. typhi* (*B. typhosus*) is today fortunately detected (at least in metropolitan cities) within the first week and is invariably responsive to ceftriaxone. When diagnosis is delayed pulmonary complications though uncommon may occur.

Respiratory symptoms are common in typhoid infections, being present in about half of all cases at the onset of the disease. Bronchitis causing a dry cough with auscultatory rhonchi is commonly seen. In the tropics, fever lasting a week or more, associated with cough and ausculatory rhonchi is most commonly due to either S. typhi or malaria.

In their classic description of 360 cases of typhoid fever, from 1946, Stuart and Roscoe reported cough in 86% of patients, coryza in 60% and chest pain in 60%. In their series, 8% of typhoid cases were initially diagnosed as 'chest infection'. Pneumonia is the other pulmonary manifestation being reported in 37 of the 154 patients in this series who had a chest radiograph. The pneumonia usually represents a secondary bacterial pneumonia, often due to S. pneumoniae infection, but lobar pneumonia occasionally accompanied by pleural effusion secondary to S. typhi itself or to S. cholerasius, while rare, is well recognized. Empyema is occasionally reported, 18 cases being reported between 1929–80 in world literature, S. typhimurium being the causative organism in the majority of cases. Lung abscess is a rare complication and is mostly caused by S. typhi. Thailand in Southeast Asia is endemic for salmonella infections. Rare pulmonary manifestations reported from Thailand include interstitial pneumonia, necrotizing pneumonia, and large oneumatoceles of the kind seen in staphylococcal pneumonia. We have never witnessed these complications in India. Rare upper airway complications of typhoid that have been described include laryngeal ulceration and glottic oedema.

With increasing international travel to endemic areas, *B. typhosus* and salmonella infections are sporadically seen in the West with the US reporting about 500 cases annually. Non-typhoidal salmonella infection is more common in the US with salmonella typhimurium bacteria being an important pathogen in the HIV-positive and immunosuppressed populations. The course in the immunodeficient patient is different from that in the immunocompetent. The incidence of bacteraemia is high with 75–95% of these patients having positive blood cultures as opposed to 1–4% in the normal host with gastroenteritis. The disease tends not to respond well to antibiotics and often recurs after discontinuation of therapy. Remarkably, *S. typhi* infection is uncommonly reported.

The most dreaded pulmonary complication of *B. typhosus* infection is ARDS, generally observed in the second week of the fever. ARDS presents with the usual features of breathlessness, tachypnoea, auscultatory crackles and radiological features of pulmonary oedema. The patient generally has high fever and there is often evidence of multi-organ dysfunction. Blood cultures for *B. typhosus* are invariably positive in patients with ARDS. The prompt use of ceftriaxone (2 g IV 8-hourly, for 10 days) and appropriate ventilatory support together with support to other organ systems often leads to recovery. Rarely, other salmonella infections (paratyphoid A or B) can also cause ARDS.

TREATMENT
Ceftriaxone 2 g intravenous twice daily and in severe cases thrice daily is the drug of choice in India. Azithromycin 500 mg twice daily orally for 5 days is also generally given in addition. Resistance to the quinolone group of drugs is on the rise and unless sensitivity tests permit their use they should be avoided.

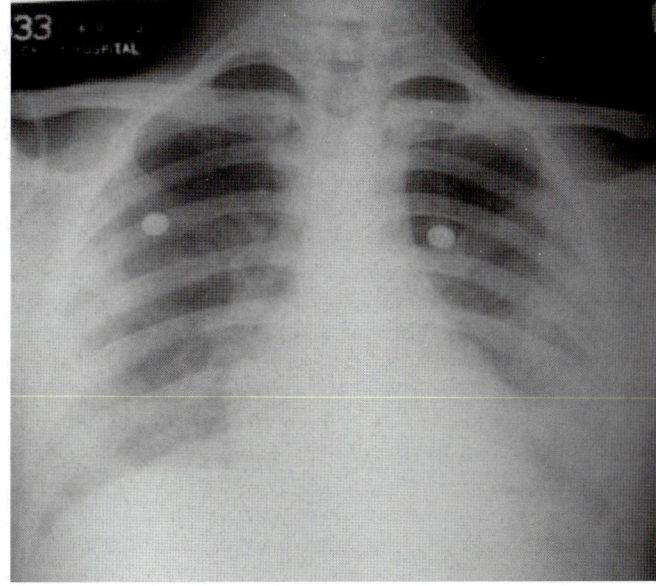

Fig 31.1: ARDS. X-ray chest in a 30-year-old man who had *B. typhosus* infection.

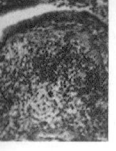

Remarkably, *S. typhi* now is sensitive to chloramphenicol, perhaps because the drug was not used for several years in the treatment of this disease.

Leptospiral Infection

Leptospirosis is a zoonotic disease. Though worldwide in distribution, it is most common in the tropics and in the developing countries of the world. It is a spirochetal disease, caused by spirochetes belonging to the genus Leptospira which comprises a number of serological disease-producing strains. The commonest disease-producing strain in India is Leptospira icterohaemorrhagiae. Human infection occurs from exposure to rat-infected urine containing the organism present in contaminated water or soil. The organism penetrates the skin and thereby gains entry, following which there is bacteraemic spread to various organs of the body, notably the lungs, liver, kidney and the central nervous system.

Leptospirosis is a grave health hazard in tropical and developing countries where rainfall is heavy. It occurs in outbreaks and even larger epidemics during and soon after the monsoon season. In India there are yearly seasonal outbreaks between July and September, particularly where there is heavy flooding from the rains. The disease is endemic in the Indian subcontinent, the whole of Southeast Asia, Andaman Islands, China, Taiwan, South America (particularly in Brazil, Nicaragua) and in Africa. Epidemics in Brazil (1988) and Nicaragua (1995) and periodic yearly epidemics in India have resulted in significant mortality. The disease occurs mainly in farmers exposed to contaminated soil, sewer workers and in city dwellers who have to walk through contaminated water during and following floods caused by heavy rains. People swimming in contaminated swimming pools are also at risk.

PATHOPHYSIOLOGY

The leptospirae invade and proliferate in various organs—chiefly the lungs, kidneys, liver, heart and the central nervous system via the bloodstream.

Lung pathology reveals congestion; an interstitial inflammatory reaction, intra-alveolar haemorrhage or diffuse alveolar damage causing ARDS. Histopathological examination shows changes in the capillary endothelium with swollen endothelial cells with an increase in pinocytotic vesicles. Inflammatory damage to the alveolar capillary membrane is extensive in severe infection and this is responsible for extensive leak of fluid from the capillaries into the interstitial spaces and the alveoli.

CLINICAL FEATURES

Leptospiral infections are characterized by high fever, muscle pain and frequent involvement of the liver (causing hepatitis and jaundice), kidneys (causing an acute nephritic picture with acute renal shutdown) and the central nervous system (causing chiefly a meningitis).

Pulmonary involvement is common and is usually mild, consisting of a non-productive cough or cough with blood-tinged sputum.

Severe lung involvement may take the form of ARDS or severe intra-alveolar haemorrhage. Intra-alveolar haemorrhage resembles ARDS. It may occur (and in fact often does) without serious liver, kidney or CNS involvement. The general presentation is high fever of unknown aetiology suddenly complicated by acute breathlessness, tachypnoea, increasing hypoxia with mottled shadows in both lungs. The shadows may become confluent to resemble pulmonary oedema. A wrong diagnosis of pneumonia, aspiration pneumonia or ARDS is often made. The degree of haemoptysis varies. It may be mild, severe and exsanguinating or may not be evident at all. A BAL study or an endotracheal aspirate if the patient is intubated and put on ventilator support, shows blood-stained fluid with hemosiderin-laden macrophages. The single most important clue to the correct diagnosis of a patient with high fever, sudden onset dyspnoea, hypoxia and bilateral alveolar shadows on an X-ray of the chest is the presence of a marked rise in the creatine phosphokinase (CPK) enzyme in the blood. The rise is generally in the thousands. Serological tests for leptospira and in particular a rising titre of antibodies can only be demonstrated after some days or weeks. There is invariably a slight rise in bilirubin and the liver transaminases. A urine examination may show the presence of albumin and red blood cells.

RADIOGRAPHIC FINDINGS

Radiological findings are non-specific and may be present in the absence of chest symptoms. Common abnormalities include non-segmental pulmonary opacities, occurring peripherally, particularly in the lower lobes. They are believed to represent a haemorrhagic pneumonitis rather than a bacterial pneumonia. Areas of consolidation may also be observed, not necessarily confined to a segment or lobe. Linear opacities extending upwards from the cardiac border are related to areas of atelectasis. These linear opacities may be unilateral or bilateral in distribution.

ARDS when it occurs has the usual bilateral distribution of opacities, at times causing total 'white-out lungs' (see chapter on 'Acute Respiratory Distress Syndrom' (ARDS)). Alveolar haemorrhage is characterized by bilateral extensive alveolar opacities. Smaller areas of alveolar haemorrhage produce more localized shadows that could be mistaken for pneumonia.

DIAGNOSIS

Diagnosis in an endemic area is generally easy. Though lung involvement may occur in isolation, urinary abnormalities, and increase in liver enzymes are generally present. A marked rise in the CPK enzyme is invariably observed. Antibodies to leptospira in the leptospira agglutination test, the ELISA test and the immunofluorescent test may take several weeks to turn positive. A fourfold rise in titre observed between the acute and convalescent sera is diagnostic.

TREATMENT

It is important to make a prompt diagnosis in fulminant cases of intra-alveolar haemorrhage, else death results. Methylprednisolone 0.5 to 1 g IV daily for three days followed by prednisolone orally starting with 60 mg daily and tapered off within two weeks is lifesaving. Clinical and radiological improvement accompanied by rapid relief of hypoxia within a matter of 8 to 12 hours is observed following the very first dose of IV methylprednisolone. Ventilatory support is absolutely necessary till recovery occurs. ARDS requires the usual expert ventilatory support with the use of PEEP. The prognosis is especially grave if other organ systems are involved. Specific antibiotics for leptospiral infection also need to be given. Penicillin G, two

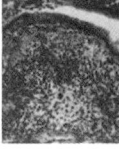

million units 4 to 6-hourly intravenously for 10 days is the drug of choice. In mild to moderate cases oral medication using amoxicillin, erythromycin, doxycycline or ampicillin can be used.

Dengue haemorrhagic fever (DHF)

Dengue haemorrhagic fever (DHF) is a viral infection caused by the transmission of the one of the strains of the dengue virus through the bite of the Aedes aegypti mosquito. The disease has wide distribution in the tropics. It occurs in epidemic form in India, Pakistan, the whole of Southeast Asia, Sri Lanka, Philippines and the Pacific islands. It is also observed in Central and South America and in Africa. The disease in its severe form carries a high mortality.

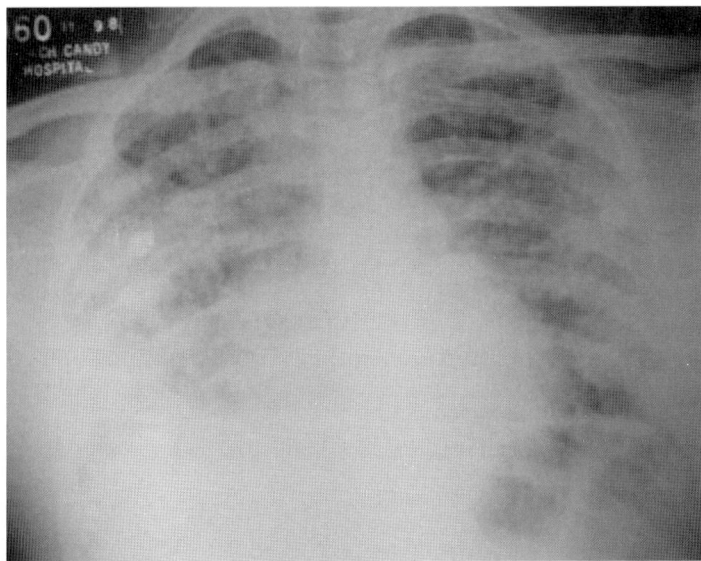

Fig 31.2: Leptospirosis. X-ray chest showing bilateral diffuse alveolar shadows in a patient who had intra-alveolar haemorrhage causing severe hypoxia.

PATHOPHYSIOLOGY

In its severe form, the disease is characterized by a marked increase in capillary permeability leading to leakage of fluid and albumin from the vascular to the extravascular compartment. This leads to a form of severe hypovolaemic shock. The disease is characterized by thrombocytopenia and haemorrhages within the skin and also in internal organs, particularly the gastrointestinal (GI) tract. Capillary leak within the lung is responsible for ARDS.

CLINICAL FEATURES

The usual clinical picture is that of a viral fever with severe aches and pains in the muscles and bones (break-bone fever) which lasts for about a week. Leucopenia and varying degree of thrombocytopenia are invariably present. A skin rash consisting of scatted purpuric spots may or may not be present.

The more severe form of DHF is characterized, to start with, by the above mentioned features and is then followed by the second or toxic phase. This is characterized by a fall in temperature accompanied by features of severe hypovolaemic shock.

Pulmonary manifestations are invariably present in the second or toxic phase, though they may also occur in the initial febrile period. These include non-productive cough, alveolar shadows suggestive of pneumonic consolidation and the rapid evolution of acute lung injury going into ARDS. Tachypnoea disproportionate to the degree of fever invariably points to an impending lung injury even when radiographic examination of the chest shows no significant change.

Pleural effusion occurs in the more severe often fatal cases. They are a manifestation of a generalized capillary leak syndrome and therefore are invariably accompanied by severe shock. The pleural fluid does not contain inflammatory cells, is rich in albumin, the albumin concentration being over 60% of that in blood.

Pulmonary manifestations of DHF include haemorrhage, more often into the pleural space and surprisingly much less frequently into the lung parenchyma. Rarely, bleeding into body spaces may precede purpura, epistaxis, GI bleed or haematuria. Of interest is a young lady of 22 years who presented with fever, leucopenia, thrombocytopenia and who developed tachypnoea and severe abdominal pain five days after the onset of infection. She was strongly positive for the dengue antigen and IgM dengue antibody. Examination and imaging studies revealed bilateral pleural effusion as also fluid within the peritoneal cavity. Examination of the abdomen pointed to an acute abdomen with tenderness, guarding rigidity and ileus. Diagnostic aspiration revealed frank haemorrhage at both these sites. The hemorrhagic fluid accumulated again and again so that she needed drainage tubes in both pleural spaces and in the peritoneal cavity. There was no other bleed at that point in time. The condition was associated with quickly evolving ARDS together with hypovolaemic shock. Recovery ensued following replacement of blood loss, measures to counter shock, ventilator support with PEEP for ARDS and support to other organ systems.

Fulminant DHF is associated with a disseminated intravascular coagulopathy (DIC). Massive bleeding from various sites and into organ systems is observed, including massive pulmonary haemorrhage. Death almost always occurs.

Recovery in DHF is characterized by a return to haemodynamic stability, reduction and stoppage of bleeding and a progressive rise in the leucocyte and platelet count.

DIAGNOSIS

Dengue antigen and the IgM antibody to the dengue virus are positive. The IgM antibody test may however take as long as seven days to turn positive.

TREATMENT

The dengue virus is not susceptible to any antibiotic or antiviral agent. Since leucopenia at times is marked (< 1500/mm^3), secondary infection is possible and known to occur, particularly in the lungs. Appropriate antibiotics are used to counter such infections. Some clinicians use a prophylactic antibiotic cover in patients with severe leucopenia.

Dengue shock is countered by use of IV crystalloids (normal saline, Ringer lactate) and if hypotension is severe, by the use of colloids, in particular IV albumin. Shock with ARDS is indeed a difficult management problem. Restoration of haemodynamic stability is of prime importance, but this can aggravate ARDS. Once shock is overcome, fluid intake should be titrated so as not to exceed the urine output. Ventilator support is

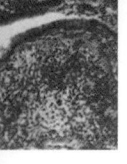

crucial in the management of respiratory problems causing respiratory failure.

Though severe DIC in dengue is almost always fatal, mild derangement in the form of increased activated prothrombin time is countered by the use of intravenous fresh frozen plasma. Severe bleeding with thrombocytopenia < 50,00/mm^3 needs platelet infusions as also packed RBCs to replace blood loss.

Tetanus

Tetanus is an acute often fatal disease caused by the contamination of wounds by C. tetani, a gram-positive motile rod shaped obligate anaerobe. Under anaerobic conditions the vegetative form of the organism produces a powerful neurotoxin which on reaching the nervous systems cause a marked increase in muscle spasm.

The disease is chiefly prevalent in India, Bangladesh, Pakistan, South-east Asia, the African continent, and South America. It is indeed a disease of the poorer countries of the world. Spores of C. tetani are present in soil, particularly fertile soil, in rural areas where human beings and animals live in close proximity often sharing the same shelter.

The description below first briefly considers the prevalence of Tetanus, its pathophysiology, and then discusses the respiratory complications invariably encountered with the disease. Respiratory complications are in fact inherent features of tetanus. They add to its morbidity and mortality and pose problems in management. The management of these respiratory problems involves the basic management of the disease which is therefore finally given brief consideration.

PREVALENCE

In the very early 1990s it was computed that approximately one million cases of tetanus occurred annually in the world, with a global incidence of 18 per 100,000, with a crude fatality rate at all ages being 40–70%. Fifty percent of these patients were neonatal tetanus. The World Bank Development Report states that more than 500,000 reported tetanus fatalities occurred annually in 1993 to 277,000 in 1997. Neonatal tetanus accounted from 20 to 70% of all deaths. For obvious reasons this in an underestimate. The recent WHO report in 2008 shows a significant decline in mortality, the estimated deaths being 163,000 in 2004. The decline is a tribute to the vaccination campaign in mothers and in children. The menace of tetanus with its high fatality remains chiefly in the poorer countries stated above.

PATHOPHYSIOLOGY

Tetanus arises from the contamination of a wound by Cl. tetani. It can arise from the most trivial of wounds as after minor needle injuries, or in more serious wounds as in injuries, in accidents, or in war. Asterile cutting of the umbilical chord, application of various substances by poor ignorant people to the stump of the chord are the common causes of neonatal tetanus. Once the Cl. tetani spores gain entry into a wound, the vegetative form of the organism elaborates a toxin which spreads to adjacent muscles attaching itself to nerve endings in proximity to the wound and in the adjacent muscles. The toxin is internalized and spreads retrogradely along the axons of the peripheral nerves to the anterior horn cells of the related segments of the spinal chord. The toxin also enters the blood stream from where it reaches the nerve endings of all muscles throughout the body, then along the axonal pathways of all peripheral nerves to reach the motor neurone bodies of the whole spinal chord and brain stem. It also reaches the sympathetic chain, the preganglionic sympathetic neurones in the lateral horns and to the parasympathetic centre. After reaching the anterior horn cells the toxin passes retrogradely across the presynaptic cleft to bind to receptor nerve terminals of inhibitor interneurones. It then blocks the release of inhibitor neurotransmitters, chiefly glycine and γ aminobutyric acid (GABA). The motor neurons and the autonomic nerves are now released from all inhibitory control. The unchecked uninhibited motor discharge from motor neurons leads to a marked increase in muscle tone and frequent uncontrolled muscle spasms.

CLINICAL FEATURES

Tetanus can be mild, moderate, or severe. The severity is often graded in ascending order from grade I to grade IV. Grade III and grade IV correspond to severe and very severe tetanus, respectively. Grade III tetanus is associated with marked rigidity, frequent spasms which also involve the muscles of respiration; spasms occur on the slightest touch or other stimuli (light, noise, for example) or even occur spontaneously. Tachycardia, marked tachypnoea (> 40 breaths /min), hypoxemia, dysphagia, and a steady increase in autonomic nervous activity is noted. Grade IV (very severe) tetanus consists of all features of grade III tetanus coupled with violent autonomic disturbances amounting to what have been termed 'autonomic storms'.

Complications in tetanus can involve almost any or every system. Only complications involving the respiratory system will now be considered.

Respiratory Complications

Respiratory complications are extremely common and contribute significantly to morbidity and mortality. They occur frequently and repeatedly, particularly in severe tetanus and are seen more commonly is those treated conservatively than in those managed with tracheostomy and ventilator support.

HYPOXEMIC RESPIRATORY FAILURE

Hypoxemic (Type I) respiratory failure occurs frequently in the natural history of even moderately severe tetanus. It is related to ventilation perfusion abnormalities even in lungs which appear normal on clinical and radiological examination and also to some degree of a right to left shunt.

HYPERCAPNIC RESPIRATORY FAILURE

Patients with severe well-nigh continuous uncontrolled seizures develop hypoventilation with a rise in PaCO$_2$ and a fall in PaO$_2$. Excessive sedation (in the absence of ventilator support) worsens the situation. The hypoxemia can be corrected by oxygen given though nasal prongs or a mask, though the hypercapnia remains unchanged.

Further dangerous life threatening hypoxia often occurs in the presence of other pulmonary complications discussed below. Prolonged or recurrent hypoxia is an important cause of cardiac arrest and death or may produce cerebral damage that can result in coma even when seizures are well controlled.

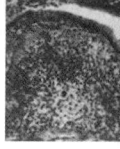

The use of ventilator support prevents respiratory failure and hypoxia due to pulmonary complications.

ATELECTASIS, ASPIRATION PNEUMONIA, PNEUMONIA, BRONCHOPNEUMONIA

These complications are related to the difficulty experienced by patients with tetanus in effectively handling their upper respiratory secretions. The difficulty is related to the following factors:

(a) Marked increase in oral and pharyngeal secretions.
(b) The inability to swallow or spit.
(c) Frequent regurgitation of stomach contents leading to aspiration.
(d) Rigidity and muscle spasms involving the intercostal and all other respiratory muscles prevent the patients from coughing effectively. Tracheobronchial secretions which are often both infected and excessive gather both in large and small airways leading to infected atelectasis.
(e) Muscle spasms and marked rigidity of the respiratory muscles markedly reduce chest wall compliance, restricting ventilation and thereby predisposing to atelectasis.
(f) During the period of prolonged respiratory muscle and laryngeal spasm, there is further accumulation of respiratory secretions within the airways, as well as a fresh reflux of gastric contents. Following prolonged spasms, there often follows a short period of deep breathing resulting in the aspiration of accumulated secretions deep into the lung.

The aspiration is usually patchy, but can be segmental, lobar or, at times, even involve the whole lung. As expected, atelectasis is more frequent in the apical and basal segments of the lower lobes and in the posterior segment of the upper lobe. Diffuse micro-atelectasis is frequently observed in patients with severe tetanus. It is characterized by an increase in the alveolar arterial gradient and in the true venous admixture even though the lungs on clinical and radiological examination appear normal. It should therefore be suspected when the PaO_2 is lower in relation to the FIO_2, in the presence of a satisfactory chest X-ray.

In our experience atelectasis occurring in tetanus is more often than not infected in more than 80% causing aspiration pneumonia, pneumonia, bronchopneumonia. Lung abscess and empyema may also occur. Infecting organisms are usually gram negative bacteria, the most frequent of which are Klebsiella and Pseudomonas aeruginosa. Rarely staphylococci, streptococci, and anaerobes are also found to be responsible for infection in these patients.

LARYNGEAL SPASM

Laryngeal spasm is a common and a dreaded feature of tetanus. If protracted and unrelieved it causes hypoxia, cyanosis, and sudden death. Laryngeal spasms may accompany or follow a bout of generalized spasms, but may occur alone as an isolated feature. It may occasionally occur as the only spasm in a patient graded as mild tetanus. The very first episode of laryngeal spasm may be sudden and severe enough to cause death. Usually laryngeal spasms occur early in the natural history of severe tetanus or at the height of the disease. Occasionally, an unexpected and even fatal laryngeal spasm may occur, when the patient appears well and is on the way to recovery.

APNOEIC ATTACK

Apnoeic spells, even in the absence of laryngeal spasms, can also occur, leading to severe hypoxemia and cyanosis. They may occur with generalized spasms but more importantly may occur by themselves unrelated to episodes of severe spasms. They always signify severe tetanus. If unrecognized and protracted, the resulting severe hypoxia leads to bradycardia, cardiac arrest, and death.

EPISODES OF SEVERE RESPIRATORY DISTRESS

This is a rather unusual respiratory complication observed in both moderate and severe tetanus. It is characterized by episodes of tachypnoea, extreme respiratory distress and is not associated with increasing hypoxemia, nor with hypercapnia, bronchospasm, or increase in secretions within airways. It is also unrelated to atelectasis. The reason for these attacks is obscure. The explanation perhaps lies in the release of inhibitory control over the respiratory centre, or perhaps to the direct action of the tetanus toxin per se on the respiratory centre.

BRONCHOSPASM

Tachypnoea due to bronchospasm is observed in both moderate and severe tetanus. It is partly related to increased secretions in the tracheobronchial tree producing narrowed airways. In severe tetanus, bronchospasm may be a manifestation of increased parasympathetic activity, many of these patients show evidence of increased vagal tone, in particular bradyrhythm induced by tracheal suction.

ACUTE RESPIRATORY DISTRESS SYNDROME

Acute respiratory distress syndrome can be due to two causes. It is often caused by associated gram-negative sepsis. It then occurs later in the natural history of severe tetanus and the clinical and other features of sepsis are evident. It can also occur early in the natural history of tetanus in the absence of sepsis, and then may well be related to the disease itself.

DIAPHRAGMATIC PARALYSIS

Foccata *et al.* reported diaphragmatic paralysis in 37% of 115 patients studied both clinically and radiologically. In 97% of patients the paralysis involved the right dome of the diaphragm. We have however been unable to confirm this finding. Whenever the right dome was raised in our patients it was invariably related to a basal atelectasis.

Complications Related to Ventilator Support

Patients with severe tetanus may need ventilator support for 6 weeks or more. They are critically ill not just with complications involving the respiratory systems, but also complications involving the cardiovascular and often of many other systems. Ventilator support is a challenge to the intensivist and offers him a wealth of experience hardly ever seen with any other disease. Complications include pulmonary infection; significant pulmonary atelectasis (recurrent atelectasis—segmental or sub-segmental is an invariable feature of severe tetanus),

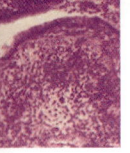

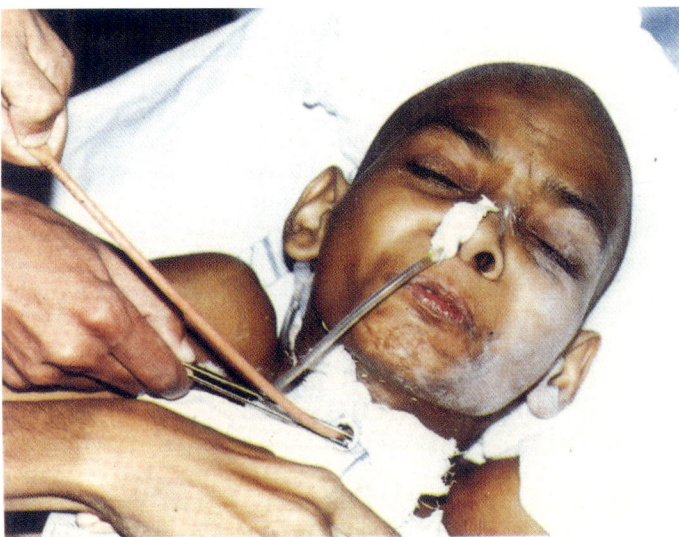

Fig 31.3: Tetanus facies with 'risus sardonicus'.

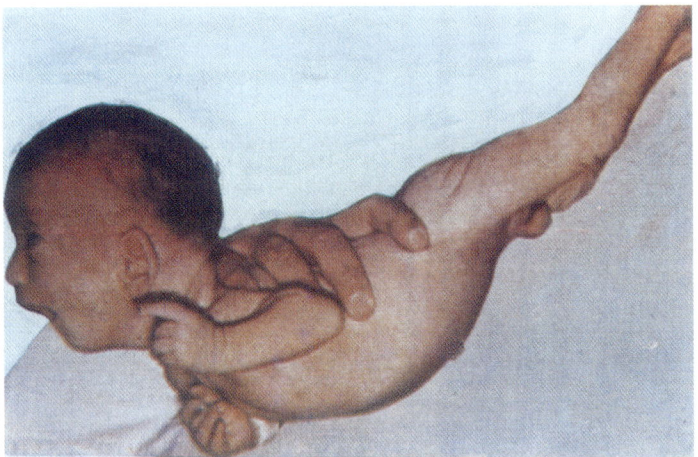

Fig 31.4: Ophisthotonos in neonatal tetanus.

pneumothorax, pneumomediastinum, accidental disconnection of the ventilator in a paralysed patient.

Management

In no disease is the dictum that prevention is better than cure more applicable than in tetanus. Tetanus toxoid vaccination at recommended intervals and the use of tetanus toxoid in pregnant mothers who have not been previously immunized could perhaps help to sharply reduce, if not eliminate, the scourge.

USE OF ANTITOXIN

One thousand units of human tetanus immunoglobulin (if available) is given intravenously. Human tetanus immunoglobulin is free of hypersensitivity reactions. Equine antiserum is unfortunately more easily available in poor countries. A skin test for a hypersensitivity reaction should first be done; fatal anaphylaxis can otherwise occur with use of the equine antiserum.

The details of management of tetanus are beyond the scope of this book. Only management principles are given below.

USE OF SEDATIVES AND MUSCLE RELAXANTS

The use of sedatives and muscle relaxants is the cornerstone of therapy in grade I and grade II tetanus. The objective is to reduce rigidity and control muscle spasms without depressing respiration. Diazepam, a benzodiazepine and a GABA antagonist is the drug of choice in most units. It should be given in a slow IV infusion over 24 hours, the dose titrated to meet the objective stated above. It is best not to exceed a dose of 120 mg to at most 150 mg over 24 hours in adults even if there is marked rigidity. Higher doses will inevitably depress respiration. Lorazepam with a longer duration of action or midazolam with a shorter duration of action can also be used in place of diazepam. Chlorpromazine and phenobarbital are second line drugs that can be used in combination with diazepam.

TRACHEOSTOMY

Tracheostomy is indicated in all patients with grade III and grade IV tetanus. We would also recommend tracheostomy in moderately severe or grade II tetanus as we have seen deaths from sudden uncontrolled laryngeal spasm in these patients.

INDUCED PARALYSIS AND VENTILATOR SUPPORT

All patients with grades III and IV (severe and very severe) tetanus require both a tracheostomy and ventilator support. Our experience (with many patients) has taught us that mortality in severe tetanus can be markedly reduced if the following principles are followed.

1. Ventilator support till such time as spasms cease. Rigidity is markedly reduced and the patients can be successfully weaned. This may take 6 to 8 weeks in some patients. Efficient ventilator support reduces the risk of respiratory complications.
2. The use of neuroparalytic agents to enable effective ventilator support. Pancuranium 2 to 4 mg IV every 30 minutes to 2 hours or vercuranium 0.1 mg/kg is very effective. Alternatively either of these two drugs can be given in a slow titrated IV infusion over 24 hours so that ventilation is well maintained and spasms are well controlled but not necessarily totally abolished.
3. During induced paralysis with ventilator support, our experience with the disease dictates that it is best not to give large doses of IV diazepam. We found that 75 to 100 mg of diazepam is the upper limit of use. Higher doses given over several weeks depress the respiratory and other medullary centres markedly. Sudden death is one of the most important complications of tetanus and resuscitation in these patients is nearly impossible if the medullary centres have been paralysed through large doses of diazepam.
4. Critical Care This is of vital importance. Physiotherapy to the chest given at the time of the maximum effect of the neuroparalytic drug, careful gentle suction to keep the airways open and a constant watch for evidence of atelectasis with prompt efforts to open up an ateletatic segment or lobe are of vital importance. Tracheostomy care needs to be meticulous. Prevention and treatment of iatrogenic infection, particularly involving the respiratory system is equally important. There is no complication in or outside a book on critical care medicine that does not occur in some

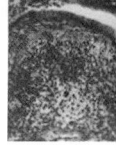

patients with severe tetanus. Looking after and caring for these patients is indeed a great learning experience for the intensivist.

MANAGEMENT OF AUTONOMIC DISTURBANCES

Intravenous beta blockers, heavy sedation, intravenous morphine sulphate, intravenous labetalol, intravenous magnesium sulphate and clonidine have all been tried to control autonomic storms. These drugs do not alter the high mortality. Hypotensive spells are best controlled with a volume load or if needs be by a titrated dose of dopamine to maintain a systolic presure of over 100 mm Hg. Hypertensive spells (BP > 200/100) are controlled by a titrated dose of oral propranolol and if needs be by a calcium channel blocker. IV propranolol should never be used as it can cause sudden death.

Bradyrhythms are treated by a titrated dose of IV atropine; tachyrhythms by a titrated dose of a beta-blocker given orally or by the use of verapamil. Meticulous critical care and ventilator support remain the corner stone of therapy in these very ill patients.

Treatment of complications that arise need expert attention and prompt treatment.

Mortality

The mortality in severe tetanus dropped from 30% to 12 % and the mortality of fulminant tetanus from 100% to 23% in the tetanus ward of a large public teaching hospital using basic equipment for critical care and the management principles outlined above. In a well equipped critical care unit in Mumbai, the mortality of severe tetanus in our unit is as low as 6%. The mortality of severe neonatal tetanus is still between 30% and 70%.

Melioidosis

Melioidosis is an infection caused by the saprophytic bacterium *Burkholderia pseudomallei*. It is endemic in South and Southeast Asia, the incidence being particularly high in northeast Thailand. The country with the highest number of recorded cases is Thailand where the average incidence is 4.4 per 100,000 people. The disease is also endemic in South China, Central and South America and parts of Africa. Human infection probably occurs through contaminated scratches and abrasions or occasionally following aspiration of contaminated fresh water. Agricultural workers and rice farmers in close contact with soil and water are at greater risk. It has been reported in India, particularly from Tamil Nadu and Karnataka. Cases have also been reported from Orissa, West Bengal, Assam, Andhra Pradesh, and Maharashtra.

PULMONARY MANIFESTATIONS

Infection with B. pseudomallei causes acute, disseminated, chronic or localized disease. Though melioidosis is a multisystem disease, the lung is a frequent and most important site of involvement.

In the acute form the lung may be the primary site of involvement or may be part of an acute disseminated disease with multi-organ involvement. Symptoms generally develop within two weeks after exposure. There is sudden onset of fever, breathlessness, cough with productive sputum, pleuritic pain and severe prostration. Haemoptysis may occur. The clinical picture is indistinguishable from a severe community-acquired pneumonia or severe gram-negative sepsis. There is well-marked polymorphonuclear leucocytosis. Radiographic examination of the chest reveals lobar consolidation on one or both sides. The consolidated areas may cavitate to form one or more lung abscesses. Pleural effusion and empyema may be associated features.

Though occasionally the lung may appear as the only organ to be involved, most patients with acute disease have evidence of other organ system involvement. There may be cutaneous abscesses, liver abscess, splenic abscess, abscesses within the brain or bones.

Overwhelming sepsis may supervene ARDS; septic shock, and multi-organ failure are observed in fatal cases.

The subacute form is characterized by low-grade fever, weight loss, cough with expectoration and haemoptysis lasting for weeks or months. These symptoms develop weeks or months after exposure to infection or represent reactivation of latent disease.

Radiographic examination reveals consolidation with cavitation generally involving both upper lobes, the X-ray appearances being indistinguishable from pulmonary tuberculosis or a lung abscess. Pleural effusion and empyema may occur. Even when the lung seems the sole site of involvement, investigations may reveal the presence of one or more abscesses in other organs such as the liver, spleen, bones or the brain. Leucocytosis is generally present.

The chronic form of melioidosis lasts for several months or years with low-grade fever intermingled with apyrexical periods, weight loss, cough, haemoptysis and pleuritic chest pain. Chest radiographs invariably reveal bilateral upper lobes' cavitative disease with fibrosis indistinguishable from tuberculosis. Metastatic spread to other organs may be present or may still occur.

DIAGNOSIS

A clinical diagnosis of melioidosis should always be suspected in upper lobe lesions which resemble tuberculosis when acid-fast bacilli (AFB) smear, culture of sputum or BAL fluid are negative. The diagnosis is confirmed by isolation, identification on culture of B. pseudomallei from the sputum. At times isolation of this organism is easier from the discharge of a metastatic cutaneous lesion or from the aspirate of a metastatic liver abscess.

Blood cultures may be positive in septicaemic patients. It is important for the clinician to specifically inform the microbiologist if he suspects an infection with *B.pseudomallei*. Identification of the organism in sputum samples which have polymicrobial flora is difficult and often missed.

In patients with little or no sputum, indirect haemagglutination tests and complement fixation tests are performed; they have a high diagnostic sensitivity. People living in highly endemic areas such as Thailand have a high incidence of seropositivity for this disease. Therefore in these areas the diagnostic titre needs to be high, preferably 1 in 640 or more, to avoid false positive readings.

TREATMENT

The acute form of the disease or patients with multi-system involvement are best treated with ceftazidime in maximum

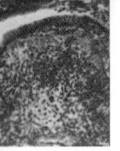
doses of 2 g IV eight-hourly with one other antibiotic. This could be doxycycline (4 mg kg/day) or cotrimoxazole in maximal doses. The antibiotic course should be for two to four weeks. Following this oral antibiotic maintenance thereby is advised for six months to a year. Antibiotic for maintenance therapy could either be doxycycline 4 mg/kg/day or cotrimoxazole (trimethoprin 10 mg/kg/day, sulphamethaxazole 50 mg/kg/day) or amoxicillin clavunate in high doses.

Prolonged courses are necessary because the disease is slow to respond and frequently relapses. Extrapulmonary abscesses may require surgical drainage.

Penicilliosis marneffei

Penicilliosis marneffei is a penicillium that causes disease. Infection with this fungus is rare in India, though a few HIV patients suffering from the infection have been reported from Manipur in North-east India but it has been increasingly reported from Southeast Asia—Thailand, Vietnam, South China and Hong Kong. Though more often seen in immunocompromsied HIV patients, it has also been noted in immunocompetent patients. The organism is found in the soil of the countries stated above.

Human infection through direct skin contact with contamination or through inhalation of infected aerosols.

CLINICAL FEATURES
Pulmonary manifestations include cough with or without dyspnoea. In HIV patients, the clinical manifestations are those of pneumonia, which may be difficult to distinguish from tuberculous infection, cryptococcal infection, cytomegalovirus (CMV), pneumocystis pneumonia (PCP) or even bacterial infection. A prospective BAL study of HIV patients from Chang Mai University Hospital, Thailand revealed that P. marneffei was found in 40% of patients with fungal infections and in 16% of all cases of pneumonia. Radiological examination of the chest usually showed bilateral involvement with areas of consolidation with or without cavitation or non-specific reticulonodular or reticular infiltrates. Besides pulmonary manifestations, infection with this fungal species was associated with fever, anaemia, lymphad-

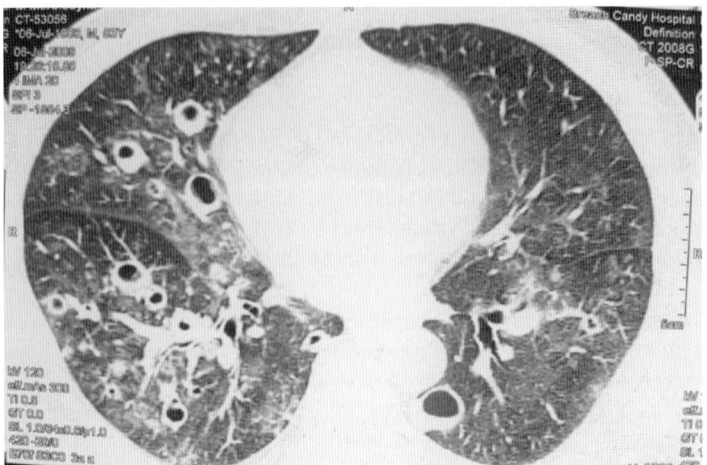

Fig 31.5b: Melloidosis: Lower CT sections reveal well-defined nodular lesions with cavitations as well as air-fluid levels within the lesions. The location of these lesions in the lung bases as well as the well-defined nature of these lesions is not in favour of tuberculosis. Microbiological evaluation of sputum revealed *B. pseudomallei*.

enopathy, hepatosplenomegaly and papular skin eruptions with central umbilication resembling molluscum contagiosum.

DIAGNOSIS
Diagnosis is made by identifying the organism from a gram stain of sputum or BAL fluid. *P. marneffei* appears as a sausage-shaped gram-negative organism with central septation. Yeast forms of this fungus may also be found. Culture of sputum or BAL fluid is highly specific.

TREATMENT
Treatment of choice is Amphotericin B 0.5 mg/kg intravenously given daily for a total dose of approximately 1 g. Itraconazole 400 mg/day given for eight to twelve weeks is also effective. Relapse is frequent in HIV patients; itraconazole 200 mg/day is continued to prevent relapse. Response to treatment is generally observed within two to three weeks.

Plague

Plague is caused by the bacterium *Yersinia pestis*. The disease exists as a bacterial zoonosis with rodents being the chief reservoir. The black rat (Rattus rattus) and the Oriental flea (Xenopsylla cheopis) are the main reservoir and transmitting agent respectively for human plague in India. Plague is endemic in Africa, Vietnam, India, Myanmar, China, Peru and has been reported sporadically from the United States. India has seen several outbreaks since 1994, the worst being an outbreak of pneumonic plague in Surat, Gujarat, which caused 52 deaths and resulted in 876 seropositive cases.

Plague generally presents in the bubonic form—painful large buboes (inflamed lymph glands) develop generally in the inguinal region, occasionally in the axillary region and rarely in the cervical region. Bacteraemic spread may involve the lungs giving rise to pneumonic plague. This is characterized by pneumonia, often involving both lungs. Marked toxicity, severe prostration, hypotension and rapidly evolving cardiorespiratory failure can kill the patient in 24 to 72 hours. Leucocytosis of

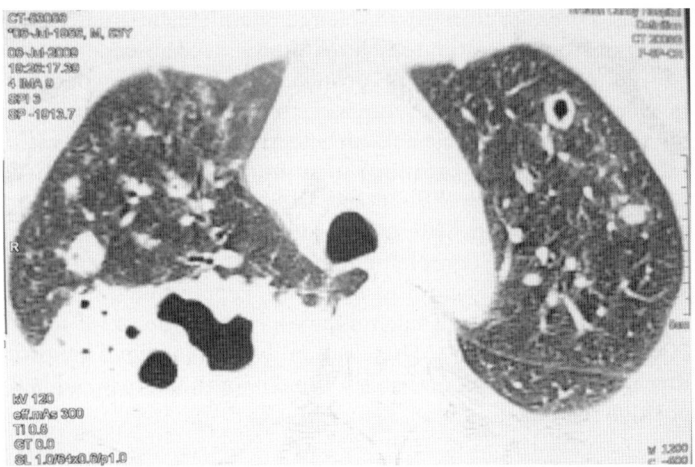

Fig 31.5a: Melloidosis: CT scan of the chest in an individual whose chest X-ray appearances were highly suggestive of pulmonary tuberculosis. The CT confirms the appearance of a large right upper lobe cavitating lesion. Additionally there are multiple nodular lesions with cavitation seen in both upper lobes.

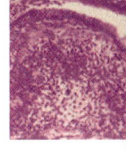

10,000 to 20,000/mm³ is generally present. Thrombocytopenia and DIC can occur.

DIAGNOSIS

This is evident in an established epidemic but may be otherwise difficult. Presence of *Yersinia pestis*, a gram-negative coccobacillus in sputum smear and culture is confirmatory. A passive hemagglutination test or an ELISA test is available in reference laboratories for testing acute and convalescent serum.

TREATMENT

The drug of choice is streptomycin 30 mg/kg given in two divided doses for 10 days. Patients should be nursed in isolation.

Anthrax

This is a disease caused by *B. anthracis* and is commonly seen in domestic and herbivorous animals. Human anthrax is more prevalent when there is direct contact with infected animals. Anthrax spores are hardy and can remain infectious for months or even years. They are transmitted by contact with infectious carcasses, hides, hairs, bone-meal or from contact with soil contaminated by spores. The disease is endemic in India, Pakistan, Iran, Latin America, and Central Africa. In India the disease still remains endemic in Tamil Nadu, Karnataka and Andhra Pradesh. The majority of cases are of cutaneous anthrax. However, human cases of pulmonary anthrax, GI anthrax and septicaemic anthrax have also been reported.

The pulmonary form is best described as inhalation anthrax (also termed wool sorter's disease).

PATHOLOGY

Inhaled anthrax spores are deposited in the alveolar spaces. Macrophages transport these spores to the tracheobronchial and mediastinal lymph glands where they germinate to cause a haemorrhagic mediastinitis with a necrotizing lymphadenitis.

CLINICAL FEATURES

Initial symptoms are those of a flu-like syndrome with fever, cough, malaise and myalgia. The second stage is characterized by severe respiratory distress, cyanosis and profuse sweating.

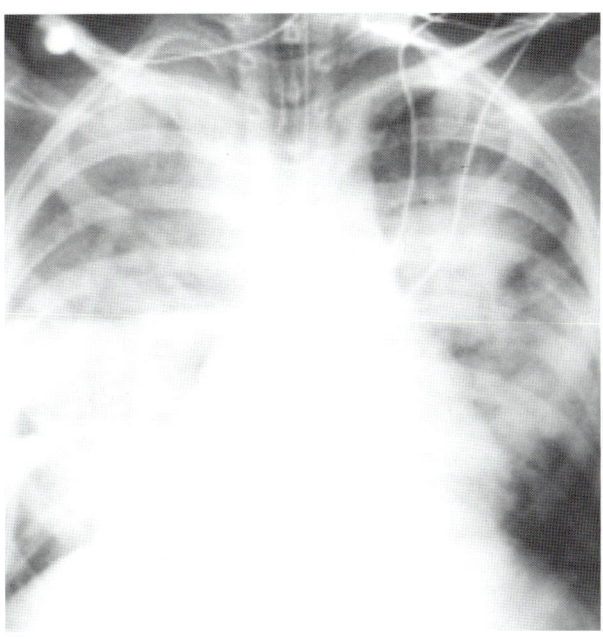

Fig 31.6: Plague. X-ray chest showing diffuse bilateral consolidation involving both lungs.

There is often subcutaneous oedema of the neck; an X-ray of the chest shows symmetrical mediastinal widening with or without a pleural effusion. The mediastinal widening is due to acute mediastinitis and necrotizing lymphadenopathy. Blood culture is often positive for *B. anthracis*. Shock with cardiorespiratory failure occurs within 24 to 48 hours.

PROGNOSIS

The pulmonary form has a dreadful prognosis. Death occurs from increasing hypotension and cardiorespiratory failure.

TREATMENT

Penicillin is the drug of choice, four million units four-hourly administered for two weeks. Intravenous ciprofloxacin (500 mg/day) or IV doxycycline (200 mg/day) may also be used. Intensive support to all organ systems is necessary.

SUGGESTED READING

Cunha BA. Osler on typhoid fever: differentiating typhoid from typhus and malaria. *Infect Dis Clin North Am*. 1 Mar. 2004; 18(1): 111–25.

Halstead SB. Dengue. *Lancet*. 10 Nov. 2007; 370(9599): 1644–52.

Martãnez S. Thoracic manifestations of tropical parasitic infections: a pictorial review. *Radiographics*. 1 Jan. 2005; 25(1): 135–55.

Pande JN, Kabra SK. Dengue hemorrhagic fever and dengue shock syndrome. *Natl Med J India*. 1996; 9: 256–8.

Singhi S, Kissoon N, *et al*. Dengue and dengue hemorrhagic fever: management issues in an intensive care unit. *J Pediatr* (Rio J). May 2007; 83(2 Suppl): S22–35.

Udwadia FE. Tetanus. 1994; Oxford University Press, New Delhi.

Udwadia FE, *et al*. Tetanus and its complications: Intensive care and management experience in 150 Indian patients. *Epidemiology and Infections*; 1987; 99: 675–84.

Udwadia FE, Sunavala JD, Jain M, *et al*. Hemodynamic studies during the management of severe tetanus. *Quart J of Medicine*. 1992; New Series 83, No. 302: 449–60.

Udwadia FE. *Oxford Textbook of Medicine*. 2005; fouth edition, Oxford University Press, New Delhi.

Vijayachari P. Leptospirosis: an emerging global public health problem. *J Biosci*. 1 Nov. 2008; 33(4): 557–69.

White NJ. Melioidosis. *Lancet*. 17 May 2003; 361(9370): 1715–22.

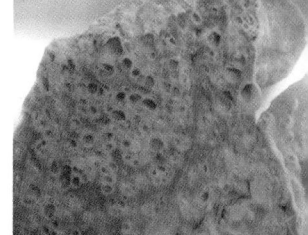

CHAPTER **32** Asthma: Introduction, Epidemiology, Aetiopathogenesis

INTRODUCTION

Asthma is a chronic disease characterized by recurrent attacks of cough, wheeze and breathlessness. It is a public health problem not just for developed countries but across the globe. The World Health Organization (WHO) estimates that 300 million people are afflicted by asthma globally with 250, 000 deaths recorded annually. Asthma is the commonest chronic disease affecting children and, with the related atopic disorders of eczema and atopic rhinitis, constituted a third of all chronic disorders even 30 years ago. Asthma prevalence is increasing across the globe due to increasing exposure to exacerbating factors like airborne indoor or outdoor pollutants and indoor allergens, and decreasing exposure to protective factors like antioxidants, microbial burden and physical exercise. It remains an underdiagnosed and under-treated condition creating substantial burden to patients and their families. Despite all the advances in our understanding and treatment of asthma, it continues to kill, with most asthma deaths occurring in the poorer countries. This chapter will focus on the definition, global and Indian epidemiology, types, aetiopathogenesis, investigations, treatment, and look at special situations like difficult and fatal asthma, asthma in pregnancy, aspirin-induced and exercise-induced asthma.

DEFINITION

Asthma is a chronic inflammatory disorder of the airways in which many cells and cellular elements play a role. The chronic inflammation is associated with bronchial hyperresponsiveness (BHR) that leads to recurrent episodes of wheezing, breathlessness, chest tightness and coughing, especially at night or in the early morning. These episodes are usually associated with widespread but variable airflow obstruction within the lung that is often reversible either spontaneously or with treatment. This definition from GINA (Global Initiative for Asthma) is long but complete, including not just the clinical features but also the key physiological problem (BHR), the inflammation that is the pathological highlight, and the usually but not inevitably reversible nature of the disease.

It encapsulates the huge shift in our understanding of the disease over the last three centuries from the predominantly bronchospastic condition it was postulated to be by Sir John Floyer in his *Treatise of Asthma* in 1698. In fact, it was as early as 1892 that Osler discussed the role of airway inflammation in the pathogenesis of asthma in his *Principles and Practice of Medicine*. Pathological evidence supporting this view appeared as early as 1922. It was only over the last few decades however that our view

of asthma shifted from that of a disease of airway smooth muscle contraction to one characterized by complex interactions between inflammatory mediators and effector cells. Helping us make this paradigm shift have been several key clinical studies, postmortem studies, bronchial biopsy studies and bronchoalveolar lavage (BAL) fluid analysis in asthmatic patients.

EPIDEMIOLOGY OF ASTHMA

Asthma is a complex disease and there are many challenges in studying its epidemiology including the lack of a precise and universal definition and the absence of a single physiological test that is sensitive and specific. Asthma is one of the most common chronic disorders of the developed world. Over the last three decades there has been an increase in the global incidence of asthma and atopy. There is limited data on the epidemiology of asthma from the Asian continent in general, and the Indian subcontinent in particular, though there is a general impression that the prevalence is lower here than in the Western world. Much of our information on the prevalence of asthma in India comes via the ISAAC study (International Study of Asthma and Allergies in Childhood) in which many Asian countries participated. This and similar studies provided important information on the prevalence and burden of asthma in Asia.

Global Epidemiology

The prevalence of asthma varies from country to country depending upon the definition used to diagnose asthma. Currently, asthma is reported in 1.2–6.3% of the adult population in most countries. On the other hand, diagnosed asthma, (i.e. asthma ever diagnosed by a clinician) runs at 12% in the UK, 7.1% in the US and as high as 15% in Australia. The ECRHS (European Community Respiratory Health Survey) studied the geographic variation in asthma and allergies among the adult population of 22 countries across the globe. Both the ECRHS and the ISAAC surveys demonstrated dramatic variations in the prevalence of asthma symptoms from across the globe. Whilst the ECRHS considered representative samples 20–44 years of age from 22 chiefly Western European countries, ISAAC looked at several (eight participating) Asian countries. In the ECRHS study, the highest prevalence of wheeze was found from Ireland (32%) and the lowest from India (4.1%). In the ISAAC study too, the prevalence of asthma in 13–14-year-olds varied widely across countries: from a high of 32.2% in the UK, to a low of 1.6% from India. Thus between them, these

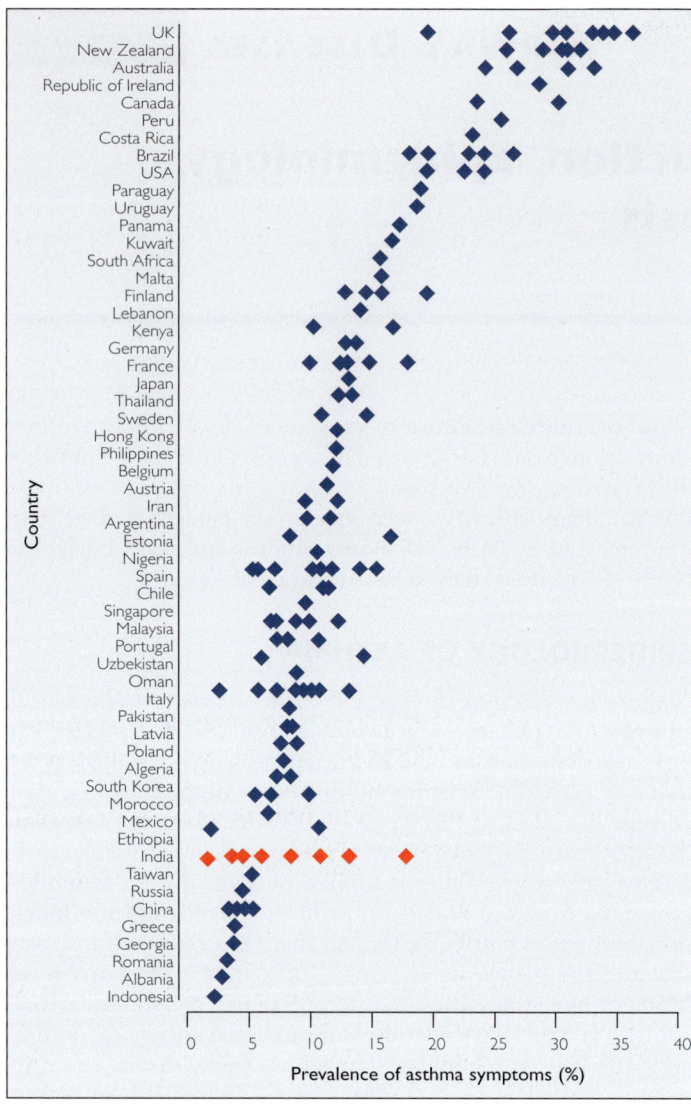

Fig 32.1: 12-month prevalence of self-reported asthma symptoms in differnt countries as reported in ISAAC.

Source: Beasley Richard. Worldwide variation in prevalence of symptoms of asthma, allergic rhinoconjunctivitis and atopic eczema: ISAAC. *The Lancet*. 1998; 351, 9111: 1225–32, 25 April.

two major studies showed that asthma prevalence was clearly higher in the Western world than in the Asian region. The wide variation in asthma prevalence seen in the ISAAC study is shown Figure 32.1. As can be seen India finishes at the lower end of the asthma prevalence league.

Asian Epidemiology

Prior to the 1990s, most of the epidemiological data from Asia was collected in a non-standardized fashion with different types of written questionnaires. This early data showed there was great variation in the prevalence of 'asthma ever' from a low of 1.6% from Guangzhou to a high of 19% from Taiwan. The ISAAC study brought home two important facts. Firstly, that the prevalence of self-reported asthma symptoms in 13–14-year-olds was much lower in Asian countries than in the West. It also demonstrated tremendous variation even among

different countries in the Asian region, with the more affluent Asian countries like Japan and Hong Kong having higher prevalence rates of 10.2 and 10.1% respectively. However, even these higher prevalence rates lagged considerably behind the prevalence rates reported from New Zealand (18.4%) and Australia (17.6%). Even in younger children aged 6–7 years, the Asian rates mirrored those found in the older children.

SECULAR TRENDS IN THE ASIAN REGION

Several studies from the Asian region confirmed the secular trends of increased prevalence of asthma over the years observed in Western countries. The magnitude of increase was particularly striking in, for example, affluent countries like Singapore, where a study by Leung in 1997 showed the prevalence rates of asthma had increased almost threefold from 5.5% in 1967 to 20.7% three decades later.

ETHNIC DIFFERENCES

Another way to assess the possible changing trend of asthma is to assess the same ethnic group living in a different environment. Such studies demonstrate considerable ethnic differences. A study by Leung and Ho in Chinese children aged 12–18 from three locations demonstrated that the prevalence of asthma was highest in the children recruited from Hong Kong. In a similar study on almost 3000 adults from three ethnic groups residing in Singapore, the highest asthma prevalence was found in the Indians (6.6%), whilst the lowest prevalence was found in the Chinese (3%).

Indian Epidemiology

There is very limited information on the prevalence of asthma among adults in India. The first epidemiological study of asthma prevalence from India emerged from Lucknow in 1966. This study was a questionnaire-based study involving a sample size of 5% of the population of Patna. The prevalence of asthma in the adult population between 30–49 years of age was estimated to be 2.78%. More recent knowledge of the epidemiology of Indian asthma comes from a study by Chowgule *et al.*, which was part of the ECRHS survey in Mumbai residents from 1992–95. In this study a one-in-ten random sample of adults aged 20–44 years was selected from electoral rolls. In Phase 1 of this study, 2313 adults were interviewed about symptoms, asthma diagnosis and medications in the preceding 12 months. In Phase 2, family and smoking history, serum Imuunoglobulin E (IgE), skin tests, spirometry and methacholine challenge were performed on a subset of 20% of patients who had completed the Phase 1 questionnaire. Asthma prevalence in Mumbai was found to be higher than in the Patna study, but still relatively low, at 3.5% (physician diagnosis) and 17% using a very broad definition of asthma. The house dust mite was the most common positive skin test (18% prevalence) and the only one of the nine applied that was significantly linked to asthma symptoms and physician-diagnosed asthma. In this study, asthma prevalence was strongly associated with positive house dust mite skin test, family history of asthma and total IgE level. When this study cohort was broken down into four age groups, the youngest group aged 20–24 years had the highest prevalence of doctor-diagnosed asthma. Comparison of these results with the prevalence of asthma symptoms overall in all the 48 participating ECRHS centres reveals that the prevalence of asthma and hay fever in Mumbai was significantly lower than the median for most other centres. The highest prevalence rate of wheeze reported in the questionnaire part of the ISAAC survey was 28% in Melbourne, Australia which was seven times the 4.1% prevalence reported from Mumbai. Thus the ISAAC study established that today, atopic diseases are diseases of privileged countries. The excess in the prevalence of asthma in Western countries is almost totally accounted for by excess in atopic sensitization.

The only other large prevalence study from India comes from a field study conducted at Chandigarh, Delhi, Kanpur, and Bangalore through a two-stage stratified sampling strategy using a previously validated questionnaire. In this large study data from over 70, 000 respondents were analyzed to give asthma prevalence rates of 2.28%, 1.69%, 2.05% and 3.47% from Chandigarh, Delhi, Kanpur and Bangalore respectively with an overall prevalence of 2.38%. Female sex, advancing age, usual residence in urban area, lower socioeconomic status, history of asthma in a first-degree relative and tobacco smoking were all associated with significantly higher odds of having asthma.

More data exists regarding the prevalence of childhood asthma in India. A literature search identified 15 epidemiological studies on the development of asthma in Indian children from 300 potentially relevant articles. Wide differences in samples, primary outcome variables, lack of consistency in age category, rural-urban variation, criteria for positive diagnosis, and study instruments confounded the outcome variables. The mean prevalence was 7.24% (± SD 5.42). The median prevalence was 4.75% [with IQR = 2.65–12.35%]. Overall weighted mean prevalence was found to be 2.74. Childhood asthma among children 13–14 years of age was lower than that in younger children 6–7 years of age. Urban and male predominance with wide inter-regional variation in prevalence was observed. These studies show collectively that the burden of bronchial asthma in Indian children is higher than was previously understood.

IMPACT OF ASTHMA IN INDIA

Even figures of 2–3.5% prevalence applied to a country of over a billion translate into large absolute numbers of Indians with asthma. Thus, based on these studies, at least 25–35 million Indians are asthmatic and the economic burden of this disease in India is thus huge.

India is a vast country of great variation in geographic and climatic conditions, and in socioeconomic and cultural backgrounds. Many large surveys will be needed before a true picture of the prevalence of asthma in this country emerges. Studies from different regions, communities and occupations and from both the rural and urban sectors are needed before a clearer idea of nationwide epidemiology emerges.

TYPES OF ASTHMA

Asthma can be classified into several types:
These include: Childhood asthma, Late-onset asthma, Chronic asthma, Occupational asthma and Difficult asthma. These will all be discussed at appropriate points later.

GENETIC FACTORS

In contrast to single-gene disorders like cystic fibrosis, that exhibit classic Mendelian recessive or dominant inheritance, asthma involves multiple genes and expression is influenced by both complex genetic and environmental factors. The multifactorial nature of asthma has confounded genetic studies and despite intensive efforts, no asthma gene has been identified with any certainty.

Asthma is, however, well known to run in clusters in families. Simply put, the risk that a first-degree family member of a patient with asthma will also develop asthma has been calculated to be two to six times higher than the risk in the general population.

While the search for a specific gene or genes for asthma or atopy remains elusive, the gene that governs airway hyperresponsiveness is located on Chromosome 5q near a major locus that regulates serum IgE levels. Marsh first reported this breakthrough announcement of the link between total serum IgE levels and Chromosome 5q in an article in *Science* in 1994. Studies of asthma genetics from the UK, Japan and the US have also gone on to implicate Chromosome 5q as the region that contains one or more susceptibility genes for asthma. Other candidate regions detected by genome-wide searches include Chromosome 11q (atopy and positive skin tests and total IgE), Chromosome 12q (interferon γ, a mast cell growth factor and the β subunit of nuclear factor-Y), Chromosome 6 (eosinophils), and Chromosome 16 (total serum IgE).

After determining linkage between asthma and a chromosomal region, the next challenge is to screen this region for candidate genes. A candidate gene has to meet four criteria; the gene product must be functionally relevant to asthma, mutations within the gene must alter the function of the gene, asthma must be linked to the chromosomal region harbouring the candidate gene and finally asthma has to show association with different alleles of this candidate gene. A number of candidate genes have been found that meet these criteria. Chromosome 5q itself has been found to contain numerous candidate genes for asthma and atopy including the cluster of cytokine genes (IL-3, IL-4, IL-5, IL-9, and IL-13) as well as the genes coding for the β2-adrenergic receptor, the corticosteroid receptor and the granulocyte-macrophage colony stimulating factor. Other candidate genes include the human leukocyte antigen region at Chromosome 6p, tumour necrosis factor-α (TNF-α), and the cytokine gene cluster at Chromosome 5q31-33.

Thus, approximately a third of the genetic predisposition to asthma has currently been uncovered. To become relevant to clinical asthma, potential asthma susceptibility genes will now need to be tested in cases and controls with different manifestations of disease and disease severity and in representative population samples with different environmental risk factors. Only then will genotype become a predictor of disease that can be understood in the same terms as other epidemiological risk factors.

Pharmacogenetics—The Role of Genetics in the Treatment of Asthma

Additional genes that are associated with the response to asthma treatment have also been isolated. Thus, it is now clear that different asthmatics respond to β_2 agonists in different ways because of differences in the gene encoding the beta-adrenoreceptor. Differences in responses to glucocorticosteroids and leukotrine antagonists are also due to genetic differences in the genes. Thus pharmacogenetics, the genetic variations in individuals that give rise to differing response to drugs, will undoubtedly influence how asthma is managed in the years ahead. A positive association between common arginine-16 variants in the β-adrenergic receptor gene and the responsiveness of asthmatics to β-adrenergic agonists is particularly intriguing. Studies *in vitro* show that the presence of the Gly16 variant increases down-regulation of the β_2-adrenergic receptor following β_2-agonist exposure while conversely the Glu27 variant protected against agonist-induced down-regulation. Intriguingly, studies have shown that the Gly16 variant is more prevalent in asthmatics with nocturnal asthma while homozygous Gly16 individuals are more prone to bronchodilator desensitization. Already, such genetic information has helped push forward the frontiers of therapy. In a study of 16 moderate asthmatics, albuterol responsiveness was correlated with position in 16 genotypes. The authors found that Arg16 homozygotes gave a higher and more rapid forced expiratory volume in one second (FEV1) change compared to Gly16 homozygotes. Similarly, genetic variations may explain the clinical observation that some patients respond well to leukotrine modifiers and some not at all. A series of naturally occurring mutations have been identified within the 5-lipooxygenase gene promoter. In a study of 221 asthmatics, those possessing mutant alleles were relatively resistant to the effects of the leukotrine modifiers.

AETIOPATHOGENESIS

In a susceptible host, a number of factors are consistently recognized as triggers of asthma. Some of the important ones will be discussed here.

Allergens

Part of the reason why the prevalence of asthma is so much higher in the West than in the developing world may have to do with the fact that children in the West spend more time indoors and the indoor environment is changing. A number of allergens have been associated with the indoor environment. The most important of these is undoubtedly the house dust mite. Dust mites are arthropods, which grow throughout the world depending on the climate. They thrive in humid environments and some of the highest levels are found in New Zealand, explaining why asthma prevalence is consistently higher in this country. There are different varieties of house dust mite, with *Dermatophagoides pteronyssinus* being the commonest temperate species while *Blomia tropicalis* is the most important type encountered in the tropics. Many different dust mite allergens have been characterized, the most extensively studied are the Group 1 and 2 allergens Der p1 and Der p 2 which are 25-kD cysteine protease and 14-kD epidydimal proteins respectively. An elegant longitudinal study by Sears confirmed the relevance of the link between allergy to house dust mite and asthma with sensitivity to house dust mite in childhood (by skin test) being associated with persistent symptoms and relapse of asthma in adult life. A positive skin test for house dust mite allergen at age 13 carried a 3.38 odds ratio in univariate analysis for predicting wheeze and asthma by the age of 26. Other indoor allergens of note include dog dander, cat dander and cockroach droppings.

Infections

During infancy a number of viruses have been associated with the inception of the asthma prototype. Respiratory syncytial virus (RSV) and parainfluenza virus produce a pattern of symptoms, including bronchiolitis that parallel many of the features of childhood asthma. RSV causes significant damage to the respiratory tract epithelium, and epithelial necrosis results in decreased effectiveness of the mucociliary elevator, allowing mucus, inflammatory cells and plasma exudate to accumulate within the airway lumen. This combination of epithelial damage and resultant airway obstruction can lead to clinical manifestations of asthma. Several long-term prospective studies have shown that as many as 40% of children hospitalized for documented RSV will continue to wheeze or have asthma in later childhood.

In contrast, there is a growing body of literature to suggest that recurrent infections in childhood, especially parasitic, may protect against the development of asthma. This is the basis of the so-called "Hygiene Hypothesis". This was first proposed by Strachan in 1989 when he demonstrated an inverse relationship between birth order in families and prevalence of hay fever and proposed that infections in early infancy, brought home by older siblings, might prevent sensitization. Conversely, lack of early childhood exposure to infectious agents and parasites increases susceptibility to allergic diseases by modulating immune system development. Clearly, there is biological credibility to this hypothesis in that infection will tend to induce a T-lymphocyte helper 1 (Th1) response, promoting the production of interleukin2 (IL-2) and interferon gamma. These in turn would down-regulate the Th2 response associated with allergy, where a different set of mediators (IL-4, IL-5, IL-10, and IL-13) is generated. This hypothesis has been supported by a number of studies. In Germany, the higher pollution levels in East Germany were associated with an increased frequency of respiratory infections and consequently with less allergy. In Japan, an inverse relationship was found between tuberculin responsiveness and allergy. It is intriguing to postulate that this is one reason behind the relatively low asthma prevalence in India. Almost 50–70% of young Indian adults would be tuberculin skin test-positive and this might help explain the lower asthma prevalence as discussed earlier in the chapter. Similar inverse relationships have been found between allergy and parasitic infections, measles, and hepatitis A infections in childhood. Tuberculosis, measles and parasitic and viral infections are all more common in the tropics providing an explanation for the global differences in the epidemiology of asthma observed in the ISAAC study. As a corollary to the hygiene hypothesis, so-called helminthic therapy using *Trichuris suis* ova and *Necator americanus* larvae has been tried in a number of immunological disorders including Crohn's disease, ulcerative colitis, multiple sclerosis and asthma. *Thus, the essence of the hygiene hypothesis is that modern living is associated with too little microbial stimulation early in life. This lack of stimulation of the immune system leads to deficient down-regulation of immune responses to the ubiquitous allergens that the individual encounters early in life.*

Pollution

It has become fashionable for the media to blame outdoor pollutants as the cause for increasing asthma and related atopic disorders. While various pollutants can incite asthma, there is no evidence to support the assertion that they induce the disease. Indeed, the study by Von Mutius showed clearly that asthma was less prevalent in polluted East German cities than in cleaner West German cities. Whether this difference was due to pollution or to some other aspect of lifestyle or indoor environment has however not yet been established. A study we conducted in Mumbai tried to correlate the levels of SO_2, NO_2, NH_3 and suspended particulate matter (SPM) with asthma hospitalizations over a period of three years in two large private hospitals in different parts of Mumbai. We found no significant correlation between adult asthma hospitalizations and the level of any of these pollutants over the three years under study. Thus as this study demonstrates, no simplistic conclusions can be drawn about the exact role of pollution in asthma; the field is a complex one and further, larger, nationwide studies are needed with a prospective birth cohort design to track individual patient exposure to different pollutants more accurately. Such studies would be incredibly expensive and complex to do but would clarify the intriguing link between asthma and outdoor pollution.

AIR POLLUTION AND ASTHMA EPIDEMICS

The relation of ambient air pollution and epidemics of asthma is exemplified by the asthma epidemics of Barcelona in the 1980s. Doctors were struck by clusters of mid-day emergency room (ER) visits for asthma occurring in hospitals located around the docks. Clever epidemiological detective work implicated the unloading of soya beans in the harbour as the cause; affected patients being more likely to be allergic to soya bean. Pollen counts were discounted as a likely cause because levels were not unusually high at these times. NO_2 and SO_2 levels were highest on the days of the epidemics suggesting a possible synergistic role of air pollution. Soya beans have also been implicated in similar epidemics in New Orleans. Discrete asthma epidemics linked to thunderstorms have also been described in London, Birmingham and Melbourne. Subjects admitted during these epidemics were largely atopic and the levels of air pollution were not exceptional. It is postulated that the dispersal of pollen grains due to aqueous contact after the thunderstorm may release allergens that are small and potent enough to enter the airways and initiate an attack of asthma.

Obesity

Cross-sectional and case-controlled epidemiological studies have shown a modest correlation between obesity and adult asthma prevalence, with relative risk or odds ratios ranging from 1.0 to 3.0. Some studies show that this effect may be especially pronounced in women. One of the largest studies in the field looked at 86,000 women participating in the Nurses' Health Study, and found that over a four-year follow-up, the odds of developing asthma were 2.7 times higher in obese (BMI >30 kg/m^2) than normal weight women. While obesity does not directly cause airway obstruction, it is biologically plausible that it may contribute to airway inflammation. Indeed, obese asthma may be a unique phenotype of asthma, characterized by lack of eosinophilic inflammation, decreased lung volumes, greater symptoms for a given degree of lung function impairment and poor asthma control. Besides, obesity may induce a state of relative glucocorticoid resistance which may lead to obese asthmatics responding sub-optimally to asthma medications. Weight loss has been shown to improve asthma control and the obese asthmatic should be encouraged and helped to lose weight.

Nutrients

Westernization is characterized by profound changes in dietary habits, so it is conceivable that dietary factors may have caused changes in asthma prevalence. The factors implicated include: increased salt intake, increased consumption of vegetable oil (margarine), decreased consumption of antioxidants, and bottle feeding practices. None have been confirmed as yet and none explain sibship size and birth order effect, but they remain intriguing hypotheses.

Exercise

Exercise is a potent stimulus to asthma. Exercise-induced asthma (EIA) is particularly common in children and it is estimated that at least 10–12% of school children have EIA. Exercise-induced asthma is also commonly seen in professional athletes. A survey of athletes for the 1996 Atlanta Olympics found that 16% of athletes had a history or medication use compatible with EIA. The incidence of EIA varies depending on the sport. The highest rates of EIA are found in winter sports, where 35% of ice skaters and as many as 40% of cross-country skiers had EIA. Two different hypotheses have been raised regarding the mechanism of EIA. The hyperosmolarity theory states that water loss occurs from the airway surface liquid of the airways during the hyperventilation of exercise. This water loss leads to the release of mediators that cause bronchoconstriction. The other theory is the airway rewarming theory which states that the hyperventilation of exercise leads to cooling of the airways. After the exercise is complete there is rewarming of the airway because of dilatation of the small bronchiolar vessels that surround the bronchial tree. This influx of warm blood into these vessels leads to congested vessels, fluid exudation in the submucosa and mediator release with consequent bronchospasm. Cross-country skiers have the highest rates of EIA because they exercise over prolonged periods and hyperventilate in cold air. A study of 40 elite cross-country skiers showed that this group of athletes had evidence of a high incidence of airway inflammation and even airway remodelling in bronchial biopsies.

Rhinosinusitis

Several studies dating back to the 1920s have identified rhinosinusitis as a trigger for asthma. A study by Bresciani showed that 100% of severe asthmatics and 88% of patients with mild

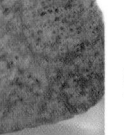
or moderate asthma will have evidence of sinusitis on computed tomography (CT) scan studies. The verdict is still not out on whether this relationship is causal or an epiphenomenon i.e. asthma and sinusitis manifestations of the same disease process. Numerous reports do suggest that medical or surgical treatment of rhinosinusitis does undoubtedly improve coexisting asthma. This suggests that rhinosinusitis may have a role as a trigger of asthma. Proposed mechanisms for a causal relationship between the two conditions include naso-pharyngio-bronchial reflexes which may be vagal nerve-mediated, drip or drainage of inflammatory cells and mediators from the sinus into the lungs, and local upper respiratory inflammation leading to pulmonary inflammation. Thus the clinician must consider the possible presence of rhinosinusitis in every asthmatic.

Gastroesophageal Reflux (GER)

The link between GER and asthma has been known since William Osler first stated that asthma attacks may be due to 'reflex influences from the stomach'. GER symptoms have since been shown to be extremely common in adults and children with asthma, with as many as 65% of consecutive asthmatics in one study having GER symptoms. More importantly, studies have shown asthma symptoms correlate with oesophageal acid events on 24-hour oesophageal pH testing. It is important to realize that GER may be clinically silent in asthmatics. Several studies have found abnormal oesophageal pH tests in large numbers of 'difficult asthmatics', even those without any obvious reflux symptoms. Compared with controls, asthmatics have more frequent reflux episodes and higher oesophageal acid contact times. Studies using oesophageal manometry conclude that approximately 50–80% of adults and children with asthma have GER. GER has also been linked to increased risk of hospitalizations due to asthma in a few studies. There are several reasons why asthmatics could be more prone to GER than the general population. These include increased pressure gradients between the thorax and abdomen, which tend to overcome the lower oesophageal sphincter (LES). Neurogenic reflexes have also been implicated, with autonomic dysregulation and heightened vagal tone releasing more acid in the oesophagus, which in turn triggers airway responses. Heightened bronchial reactivity and micro-aspiration are also postulated mechanisms. Finally, medications like theophylline, albuterol, and oral corticosteroids may all predispose to GER. Studies have shown that GER symptoms increase 170% at night and daytime reflux 24% with theophylline. Nebulized albuterol has been shown to produce a dose-dependent reduction in LES pressure from 17 to 8 mmHg and compromise the amplitude of the oesophageal contractions 5 cm and 10 cm above the LES. Oral corticosteroids when given in a dose of 60 mg per day for seven days have been shown to result in significant increases in oesophageal acid contact time at both the proximal and distal oesophageal pH probes.

If GER is a potential asthma trigger, then aggressive GER therapy should improve asthma symptoms. Field reviewed the combined results of 12 studies looking at the role of anti-reflux therapy in improving asthma symptoms and found that symptoms improved in 69% and medication could be reduced in 62%. Although pulmonary function did not improve, there was objective improvement in evening peak expiratory flow (PEF) rates in 26%. A more recent Cochrane review however failed to demonstrate an improvement in asthma symptoms. Most of the earlier studies used H_2 receptor antagonists and not the more potent proton pump inhibitors currently available today. Hence an important trial from Littner is worth quoting here. This was the only large multicentre, double-blind, placebo-controlled trial in the field and used the highly effective lansoprazole in a dose of 30 mg twice a day or oral placebo and found that treated asthmatics had fewer exacerbations and required significantly fewer oral steroid rescue courses than the controls. Surgical trials have also examined the role of surgery in asthmatics with GER. In a review by Field of 24 trials examining asthma outcomes after anti-reflux therapy, surgery improved GER variables in 90%, asthma symptoms in 79%, and asthma medication use in 80% of subjects. Pulmonary function improvement occurred in 27% of surgically treated patients.

Food Allergy and Additives

Several studies have shown that food allergy and egg allergy in particular in early infancy increases the risk of asthma developing in later life. Food allergy has also been documented as a risk factor for life-threatening asthma. A case control study found that patients with asthma and food allergy had an OR of 8.58 for life-threatening asthma. The foods known to induce this kind of violent asthmatic reaction include egg, milk, peanut, soy, fish, shellfish and tree nuts. It must be clarified that food sensitivities causing asthma are rare. Studies where actual food challenge has been used suggest overall rates are no more than 2–5%. Food additives can also be implicated as triggers of asthma. The Food and Drug Administration (FDA) has listed more than 2500 substances as food additives. Of these only a few are known to be triggers of asthma. The best known of these are the sulphating agents which include additives like sulphur dioxide, sodium sulphite, sodium and potassium bisulphite and metabisulphites. These agents are used as preservatives and antioxidants. About 4% of a random sample of asthmatics will be shown to have sulphite allergy on specific sulphite challenge; however, the risk of reacting to sulphites may be highest in the more severe asthmatics. Tartrazine, a yellow dye is another food additive known to be implicated in asthma. Other colouring agents are also implicated and it is best to advise asthmatics to avoid exposure to all such agents.

Occupational Triggers

Occupational factors have been implicated in almost 20% of asthmatics. Occupational asthma has been discussed in a separate section. (See chapter on 'Common Occupational Lung Diseases'.)

Psychological Stress

Asthma has long been known to have a psychosomatic basis and is considered by some to be the prototype of a psychosomatic disease. Daily diary studies of patients with asthma have shown that life stressors are associated with lower peak expiratory flow rates. That stressful life events increase the risk of onset of asthma comes from a large study of over 10, 000 Finnish university students where stressful life events like death of a family member were shown to promote development of asthma. Rather than stress directly causing the asthma symptoms, it is thought that stress modulates the immune system to increase the magnitude of the airway inflammatory response to allergens. Difficult asthma has also been linked to stress and depression and several studies have shown the link.

Medications as Triggers of Asthma

A number of commonly used drugs have been implicated as triggers of asthma. Aspirin and other non-steroidal anti-inflammatory drugs (NSAIDs) are the most commonly implicated agents. Aspirin-induced asthma will be discussed again later. Other important drugs known to worsen asthma include beta-blockers which are contraindicated in asthma and should never be used as they may trigger severe exacerbations. While selective beta-blockers have been cleared as safe for use in mild asthmatics, we would recommend that it is wise to avoid these drugs completely. A meta-analysis of randomized, blinded, placebo-controlled trials that studied the effects of cardio-selective beta-blockers in patients with mild to moderate asthma showed that even a single dose of such a drug could reduce FEV_1 by 7.5% though this was not accompanied by a concomitant increase in symptoms. Long-term studies are needed to define the safety profile of cardio-selective beta-blockers in asthmatics.

Angiotensin-converting enzyme (ACE) inhibitors are well known to cause cough in as many as 10–20% of patients receiving them. Prior asthma is not a risk factor for developing this side-effect. ACE inhibitors are thus generally safe in asthmatics though there have been stray reports of bronchoconstriction, asthma worsening and bronchial hyperreactivity following the use of these drugs in asthmatics. An analysis of the side-effects to this group of drugs in the New Zealand Adverse Effects Registry showed that cough accounted for 86% of the 596 adverse respiratory events but bronchospasm and dyspnoea occurred in 8% of patients on this drug. Based on this data and case reports it can be concluded that these drugs are safe but the physician must be aware of their potential to occasionally trigger asthma.

PATHOGENESIS OF ASTHMA

Asthma is an inflammatory disorder of the airways, which involves several inflammatory mediators that result in distinct pathophysiological changes. The inflammation, which is a hallmark of asthma, leads to airway hyperresponsiveness and asthma symptoms. The major cells and the mediators involved in the asthma process will be discussed here.

Mediators of Asthma and their Cellular Origin

A complex cascade of mediators is involved in the pathogenesis of asthma. These mediators produce their effects by activating specific cell surface mediators resulting in a complex cascade of signalling events. In this section we will discuss the cells in the bronchial mucosa central to the asthmatic response and the mediators they release.

CELLS

MAST CELLS

Mast cells uniquely populate all vascularized tissue including the upper and lower respiratory tracts. While the role of mast cells in allergic reactions is unequivocal, their precise role in asthma remains controversial. It was believed earlier that mast cells and the mediators they released (histamine, leukotrines, prostaglandins) played a central role in the pathogenesis of asthma. Recent evidence argues against the critical involvement of these cells in bronchial hyperreactivity (BHR) or in the continuing inflammation of asthmatic airways. Mast cell stabilizers like disodium chromoglycate were clinically ineffective and more potent newer mast cell stabilizers have had little or no impact in asthma. Beta agonists which are also potent stabilizers of human mast cells fail to inhibit late asthmatic responses following allergen challenge or to reduce BHR.

MACROPHAGES

Macrophages are present throughout the respiratory tract and may be activated by IgE-dependent mechanisms. They are characterized by their capacity to synthesize large quantities of a broad array of mediators. These include thromboxane, prostaglandins, leukotrine C, platelet activating factor (PAF), chemokines and cytokines, including IL-1, IL-6, tumour necrosis factor (TNF) and granulocyte macrophage colony stimulating factor (GM-CSF) which plays a central role in eosinophil survival and function and regulation of antigen presentation. Macrophages have the capacity to synthesize both pro and anti-inflammatory cytokines depending on the nature of the stimulus. Inhaled corticosteroids alter the balance of these pro and anti-inflammatory cytokines in asthma increasing IL-10 production by the alveolar macrophages.

EOSINOPHILS

Eosinophilic infiltration is a prominent feature of asthmatic airways. It is the eosinophil that is found in large numbers in BAL fluid at the time of a late reaction following allergen inhalation. Eosinophils release a variety of membrane-derived mediators including leukotrine C, PAF, and granulocyte-associated proteins such as eosinophilic cationic protein, which are toxic to the airway epithelium. Activated eosinophils in the airway lumen may thus lead to the epithelial damage that characterizes asthma. Eosinophils also synthesize chemokines such as IL-8, MI-1α (macrophage inflammatory problem) and RANTES (regulated upon activation, normal T-cell expressed and secreted) and MCP-1 (monocyte chemoattractant protein), which are inhibited by glucocorticosteroids.

NEUTROPHILS

The role of the neutrophil in human asthma is unclear. In acute severe asthma, high numbers of neutrophils and increased amounts of neutrophil chemoattractant, IL-8 have been described.

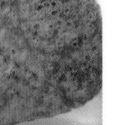

T-LYMPHOCYTES

T-lymphocytes are also prominent cells in asthmatic airways. They release a variety of lymphokines which perpetuate allergic inflammatory responses. Thus, for example, IL-3 is important in differentiating mast cells, IL-4 critical for B-cell activation and IL-5 for maintaining eosinophil survival in tissues.

Inflammatory Mediators

An array of different mediators has been implicated in the pathogenesis of asthma. These account for many of the pathological features of the disease. The important mediators will be discussed in this section.

HISTAMINE

Histamine is released from mast cells and contributes to bronchoconstriction and the inflammatory response.

CHEMOKINES

Chemokines are important in the recruitment of inflammatory cells into the airways and are mainly expressed in airway epithelial cells. Eotaxin is selective for eosinophils whereas thymus and activating regulated chemokines (TARC) and macrophage-derived chemokines (MDC) recruit Th2 cells.

LEUKOTRINES

Leukotrines are potent bronchoconstrictors and proinflammatory mediators mainly derived from mast cells and eosinophils.

CYTOKINES

Cytokines orchestrate and amplify the inflammatory response and determine its severity. Keen cytokines include: IL-1β, TNF-α and GM-CSF. The Th2-derived cytokines include IL-5, IL-4 and IL-13.

NITRIC OXIDE (NO)

Nitric oxide is a potent vasodilator produced from the action of inducible nitric oxide synthase in airway epithelial cells. Exhaled NO is increasingly being used to monitor the effectiveness of asthma treatment as will be discussed in the section on monitoring of asthma.

PROSTAGLANDIN D$_2$

Prostaglandin D$_2$ is a bronchoconstrictor derived predominantly from mast cells. It is involved in Th2 cell recruitment to the airways.

STRUCTURAL CHANGES IN AIRWAYS/AIRWAY REMODELLING

In addition to the inflammatory response, a number of structural changes take place in asthmatic airways over time. These are referred to as airway remodelling. Airway remodelling is defined as an alteration in size, mass or number of tissue structural components that occur during growth or in response to injury or inflammation. These changes represent repair in response to chronic inflammation and may result in irreversible narrowing of the airways. These structural changes are seen in all asthmatics from an early stage. The remodelling theory is important as it offers crucial insights into the permanent biochemical and pathological alterations of asthmatic patients that have been clinically observed for long. It challenges the assumption that asthma is a reversible disease and explains the accelerated decline in FEV$_1$ seen in some asthmatics.

Pathological Features of Lung Remodelling

AIRWAY THICKENING

Reticular basement membrane thickening (RBM) is a characteristic feature of asthma not being found in chronic obstructive pulmonary disease (COPD). Collagen Types I, III, V and fibronectin all contribute to this thickening. The magnitude of deposition has been found to correlate with asthma severity. Thickening of the RBM is an early change being observed in biopsy samples even before the onset of symptoms.

EXTRACELLULAR MATRIX CHANGES

Deposition of proteoglycans and over-expression of GAG hyaluronan have also been noted and it is conceivable that airway geometry and subsequently function and dynamics could be affected by this process.

MYOCYTE CHANGES

Myocyte hypertrophy and hyperplasia have been linked to asthma remodelling. Several studies show the area of the smooth muscle in the airways increases by as much as 50–230% in fatal cases of asthma and by 25–150% in non-fatal cases. Steroid therapy may have a role in reducing the number of submucosal myofibroblasts.

MUCUS GLAND CHANGES

Changes in the subepithelial mucus glands also contribute to airway remodelling. Mucus gland area is increased in subjects with fatal asthma and airway occlusion and plugging secondary to increased mucus production has been a feature noted in several autopsy studies of severe asthma.

CARTILAGE CHANGES

Increase in total cartilage area and structural changes like perichondrial degeneration and fibrosis are changes that have been observed in the remodelled airway.

VASCULAR CHANGES

Changes in airway vasculature are an important component of remodelling. Vascular congestion, dilatation of vessels and even neovascularization are important components of vascular remodelling. Patients who have fatal asthma also have a marked increase in vessel number and diameter. These changes in vessels contribute to airway wall thickening and increased resistance.

CHANGES IN ENERVATION

Recent evidence suggests a loss of nerves containing the potent bronchodilator vasoactive intestinal peptide and an increase in nerves containing the bronchospastic agent substance P.

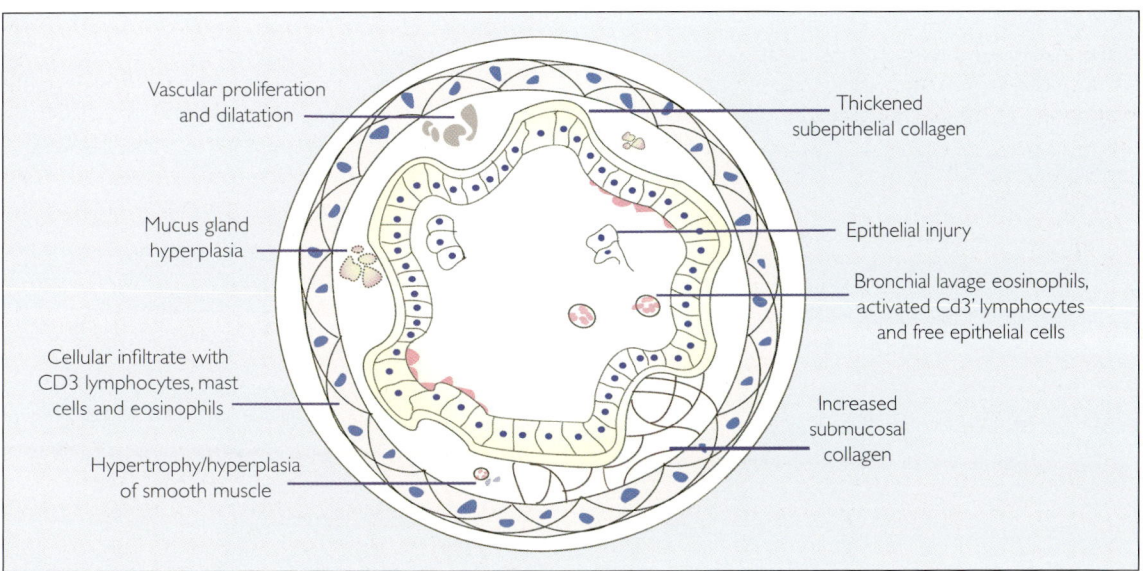

Fig 32.2: The features of airway remodelling in asthma.

SUGGESTED READING

Aggarwal AN, Chaudhry K, Chhabra SK, *et al*. Prevalence and risk factors for bronchial asthma in Indian adults: a multicenter study. *Indian J Chest Dis Allied Sci*. Jan.–Mar. 2006; 48(1): 13–22.

Chowgule RV, Shetye VM, Parmar JR, Bhosale AM, Khandagale MR, Phalnitkar SV, Gupta PC. Prevalence of respiratory symptoms, bronchial hyperreactivity, and asthma in a megacity. *Am J Respir Crit Care Med*. 1998; 158; 547–54.

Gibson PG, Henry HL, Coughlan JL. Gastroesophageal reflux treatment for asthma in adults and children. *Syst Review*. 2003; (2): CDOO1496.

Leung R, Ho P. Asthma, allergy and atopy in three south-east Asian populations. *Thorax*. 1994; 49; 1205–10.

Singh RB. Asthma in India: applying science to reality. *Clin Resp Allergy*. 2004; 34; 686–8.

The International Study of Asthma and Allergies in Childhood (ISAAC) Steering Committee. Worldwide variations in the prevalence of asthma symptoms: the International Study of Asthma and Allergies in Childhood (ISAAC). *Eur Respir J*. 1998; 12: 315–35.

Vishwanathan R, Prasad M, Thakur S, *et al*. Epidemiology of asthma in an urban population; a random morbidity survey. *J Med Assoc. India*. 1966; 46; 480–3.

CHAPTER **33** **Asthma: Clinical Features, Diagnosis**

CLINICAL FEATURES

The classic symptoms of asthma include the triad of cough, dyspnoea and wheeze. These symptoms occur in combination, but on occasion, may occur in isolation. In its classic form, asthma is easy to recognize for both patient and doctor. However, none of these symptoms in isolation or even in combination are specific for asthma, and on occasion the physician may be caught out. Because of the intermittent and non-specific nature of the symptoms, asthma may remain undiagnosed by both the patient and physician.

Cough

Cough may be the sole manifestation of asthma, in which case it is known as cough-variant asthma. Asthmatic cough is often quite distinctive. It is usually dry, intermittent, has diurnal variation often being significantly worse at night and may be triggered by talking, laughing or exercise. When accompanied by wheeze it is easy to diagnose. However, cough is often the sole symptom of asthma and in this setting a high index of suspicion is needed. A history of intermittent seasonal cough or prolonged cough which persists more than a few weeks following a viral URTI (bronchial hyperactivity) is also suggestive of asthma, especially in a young patient with a history of rhinitis or other allergies.

Dyspnoea

Dyspnoea is another cardinal symptom of asthma but may be absent in milder cases. It may be triggered only after exertion in some younger asthmatics with exercise-induced asthma. It can worsen to extreme levels in asthmatics during acute exacerbations of asthma. In chronic asthma, as in chronic obstructive pulmonary disease (COPD), the breathlessness may be constantly present and worsen with even trivial exertion and activities.

Wheeze

Wheeze is the sine qua non of asthma. The old axiom that all that wheezes is not asthma must of course never be forgotten. Other causes of wheeze are tabulated in Table 33.1 and some of these will be discussed in the section on differential diagnosis.

Physical Examination

Because of the intermittent nature of asthma, it must be stressed that physical examination may be completely normal at the time the patient is examined, and in this setting, a history based

Table 33.1:
Clinical conditions associated with Wheeze
1. Asthma
2. COPD
3. Pulmonary oedema
4. Infections such as croup, whooping cough, laryngitis, acute tracheobronchitis
5. Tracheomalacia (laryngeal, tracheal or bronchial)
6. Tracheal and large airway stenosis; tumour obstructing large airway
7. ILD's especially hypersensitivity pneumonitis and sarcoidosis
8. Bronchorreal states: bronchiectasis, cystic fibrosis
9. Foreign body aspiration
10. Vocal cord dysfunction/laryngeal spasm
11. Forced expiration in normal subjects

on the symptoms listed earlier is often sufficient to diagnose asthma. Wheeze is the most prominent abnormal physical finding. Wheezes are continuous adventitious lung sounds that can be heard in several diseases including asthma and COPD. The American Thoracic Society (ATS) defines wheezes as high-pitched continuous sounds with a dominant frequency of 400 Hz or more. The mechanism of wheeze production was first compared to a toy trumpet whose sound is produced by a vibrating reed. The pitch of the wheeze is dependent on the mass and elasticity of the airway walls and on the flow velocity. A more current model of wheeze production is based on the mathematical analysis of the stability of airflow through a collapsible tube. According to this model, the fluttering of the airway walls and fluid together, induced by a critical airflow velocity, produces wheeze. Most wheezes have spectrum peaks with frequencies below 2 kHz, mean frequency between 200–800 Hz and probably occur when airflow in large central airways exceeds a critical velocity. Wheezing can appear monophasic, denoting a single note, or polyphonic. Wheezes are often audible at the patients open mouth or by direct auscultation over the trachea. The clinical value of tracheal auscultation in asthma is well recognized, and the trachea is superior to the lung for detection of wheeze in most asthmatics.

Paradoxically, of all the variables used to measure the severity of asthma, wheeze is the least sensitive. Occasionally, wheeze may be absent even in the face of severe airflow limitation, as occurs during a severe exacerbation. Godfrey found that only 70% of patients with severe airflow obstruction

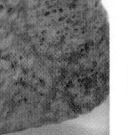

and an $FEV_1 < 1$ L wheeze. The so-called 'silent chest' in an asthmatic portends a severe attack that may well end fatally unless promptly recognized and treated.

CLINICAL FEATURES OF ACUTE SEVERE ASTHMA

Onset

An acute asthma attack is frightening for patient and physician. The onset is often dramatic, for example in the atopic patient who is exposed to high concentrations of a provocating allergen, or in the patient markedly sensitive to aspirin. Such a patient may have a catastrophically sudden attack with extreme chest tightness and inability to breathe. More often though, the acute attack may have been building up over several days or even weeks, before the patient is hospitalized. A study by Bellany revealed that 50% of patients dying of asthma in hospital had been waking up for five nights a week in the week prior to their death, and as many as 35% had been waking up that often in the previous month. Clearly an intensification of treatment at that stage, for example with a short course of steroids, might have prevented the fatal attack.

History

A history of wheeze at night, bad enough to wake the patient from his sleep, must be elicited. Worsening of exertional dyspnoea and increasing requirement of inhaled beta-agonists with diminishing relief after each puff are also pointers to a severe attack.

Examination Findings

The patient with an acute severe attack is distressed and able to speak in short sentences only. He gasps for breath, each breath being an audible struggle, often accompanied by a loud wheeze and sometimes by uncontrollable coughing. He is unable to lie flat and always prefers to adopt the sitting position, often bolt upright and leaning forward as he struggles to breathe. A respiratory rate of >30/min is a bad prognostic sign. On

Table 33.2: Features of a severe attack of asthma
– Inability to complete sentence in one breath
– Obtunded or altered conscious level
– Respiratory rate > 30/min
– Silent chest
– Cyanosis
– Respiratory muscle fatigue; apnoeic spells
– Tachycardia > 110/min
– Systolic paradox > 15 mmHg
– PEF < 30% of predicted or known best
– PaO_2 < 60 mm Hg despite supplemental oxygen at 60% FIO_2
– $PaCO_2$ which is normal or high and rising

auscultation of the chest most patients have loud, widespread, inspiratory and expiratory ronchi but the occasional patient with severe asthma has a silent chest with hardly any audible breath sounds or rhonchi. A silent chest is another grave prognostic sign and denotes obstruction so severe that there is hardly any airflow. Accessory muscles of respiration are in active use as the patient struggles to overcome the airways' obstruction by sternocleidomastoid contraction and intercostal retraction. Cyanosis may be difficult to detect but when present denotes a severe and dangerous attack. Tachycardia is always present and may be worsened by the medication the patient has taken. A tachycardia >110/min denotes a severe attack. The presence of a significant pulsus paradoxus has been shown to reflect lung hyperinflation combined with wide fluctuations in intrathoracic pressure, and when > 15 mmHg reflects a severe attack. The features of a severe attack of asthma are given in Table 33.2.

DIAGNOSIS OF ASTHMA

The diagnosis of asthma is usually based on the presence of characteristic symptoms. However, because the symptoms may be non-specific, and because patients with asthma (especially when the asthma is longstanding) may often have poor recognition of these symptoms, and poor perception of their severity, measurement of lung function abnormalities greatly enhances diagnostic confidence. The following measures of asthma are used in clinical practice.

Peak Expiratory Flow (PEF)

This is a simple, universally available and cheap way to diagnose asthma and assess its severity. Just as blood pressure cannot be measured and treated without recourse to sphygmomanometry, it is unwise to attempt to manage asthma without peak flow recordings. Modern peak flow meters by virtue of their being light and portable are ideally adapted for use by the patient in home settings for objective recording of the day to day variations that are the hallmark of asthma. Careful instructions must be given to the patient in order to maximize the accuracy of PEF recordings. PEF is effort-dependent hence the patient must be urged to put maximal effort into the peak flow manoeuvre. PEF also shows diurnal variation, hence the time the peak flow is measured is crucial and must be recorded. Ideally, patients should be instructed to measure their peak flows in the morning soon after waking when the values will be close to the lowest and at night before retiring when they will be higher. Dips in peak flow are the differences between highest and lowest peak flows occurring on a diurnal basis and are a reflection of how well the asthma has been controlled. One method of describing diurnal PEF variability is by noting the amplitude, i.e. the difference in the maximal and minimal peak flows of the day, expressed as a percentage of the mean daily peak flow value and averaged over one to two weeks. Another method of describing PEF variability, and one that is considered the best index lability in clinical practice, is the minimum morning pre-bronchodilator PEF over one week, expressed as a percentage of the recent best (Min/Max). This measure, which involves only a single daily reading and a simple calculation, correlates better than any other index with airway hyperresponsiveness.

LIMITATIONS OF PEF

Apart from the effort-dependent nature of the test, it must be realized that PEF can underestimate the severity of asthma, especially as airflow limitation and gas trapping worsen. It must also be mentioned that PEF is not interchangeable with other measures of airflow limitation like forced expiratory volume in one second (FEV_1). Another inherent problem with PEF is that the values of PEF obtained with different peak flow meters vary considerably. Finally, the range of predicted values is wide and PEF measurements must be correlated with the patient's previously recorded best (when asymptomatic or optimally treated) to more meaningfully assess the severity of his asthma at that point in time.

UTILITY OF PEF

In a patient whose history is typical of asthma but who is normal when seen by the physician, the suspicion of asthma can most easily be confirmed by giving the patient a peak flow meter to record PEF at home and demonstrate diurnal variations. In nocturnal asthma, a patient is instructed to record his or her PEF when he wakes up with asthma-like symptoms. PEF readings also have a vital role to play in diagnosing occupational asthma and demonstrating environmental triggers in the patient's workplace. Finally, integral to good asthma management is giving each patient with asthma a written plan with instructions on how to escalate asthma medications based on PEF readings at home.

Spirometry

This is the recommended method of measuring airflow limitation. It involves using a spirometer to perform measurements of FEV_1 and forced vital capacity (FVC). Asthma is characterized by a low FEV_1 and a low FEV_1/FVC ratio. After the baseline measurement has been made, reversibility to two puffs of inhaled beta-2 agonist must be documented. An improvement of >12% and >200 ml from the pre-bronchodilator value is diagnostic of asthma. The main advantage of spirometric FEV_1 is that it is easy to perform, requires relatively inexpensive equipment and is reproducible. It must be remembered though that spirometry has many drawbacks as well. It is not as universally available as peak flow meters and is also to some extent effort-dependent. It requires the patient to first take a full inspiration, which some breathless asthmatic patients may be unable to do without coughing. Although most of the flow expired in the first second of the FVC is effort-independent, the initial part of the FVC is effort-dependent and this might slightly affect FEV_1. Hence detailed instructions need to be given by a trained technician and the highest value of three recordings must be recorded. As with other measurements of airway resistance, the FEV_1 is relatively insensitive to obstruction of the peripheral airways. As ethnic differences in spirometric values have been demonstrated, normal values must have been clearly demonstrated for the population studied. Norms for Indians (in Mumbai) have been established by Udwadia *et al.* and it is recommended that these be used in our population as they vary considerably from Caucasian values. Normal ranges are also wider and less reliable in younger patients (<20 years) and in the elderly (age > 70) *(Ref: Udwadia FE et al. The maximal expiratory flow-volume curve in normal subjects in India. Chest. 1986 Jun; 89(6): 852–6).*

Measuring Airway Hyperresponsiveness

Airway responsiveness is a term used to describe the ability of the airways to narrow after exposure to constrictor agents. Often a patient with a history consistent with asthma will have normal spirometry when he or she is examined and in this setting, measures of airway responsiveness to direct airway challenges such as inhaled histamine or methacholine or indirect challenges with inhaled mannitol or exercise challenge may help establish the diagnosis of asthma. These tests of bronchial hyperresponsiveness are sensitive for diagnosis of asthma but not specific as they have been reported to be positive in patients with atopic rhinitis, bronchiectasis, cystic fibrosis and even COPD.

METHODS OF MEASURING AIRWAY RESPONSIVENESS

The original method used was inhalation of an aerosolized pharmacological agent in an aerosol generated by a Wright nebulizer inhaled by tidal breathing for two minutes. Currently, aerosol is generated by a DeVilbiss 646 nebulizer attached to a Rosenthal French dosimeter and inhaled by five inspiratory capacity breaths.

FACTORS AFFECTING THE RESULTS

A number of technical factors affect the response including nebulizer output, particle size and speed, and volume of inhalation. If the patient is on medication that controls bronchial hyperreactivity it will also affect the results and hence beta-agonists and anticholinergic agents must be withdrawn for at least 8 hours and long-acting beta-agonists (LABAs) and anti-histaminics at least 48–72 hours prior to the test. Recent viral infections and ozone may also worsen airway hyperresponsiveness. Therefore in research settings the test should not be performed within six weeks of exposure to these stimuli.

CHOICE OF BRONCHOCONSTRICTOR AGENT

Histamine and methacholine are the two agents used and airway responsiveness to both agents correlates well. Whilst histamine is more easily available, it may result in systemic side-effects like flushing, tachycardia, and headache in high concentration. Another problem with histamine is that tachyphylaxis may be observed following repeated challenges. These side-effects are not noted with methacholine, which is therefore the agent of choice.

MEASUREMENT OF RESPONSE

The response is most commonly measured by assessing the fall in FEV1 or increase in airway resistance following inhalation of the agent at different concentrations.

EXPRESSING THE RESULTS

The usual way of expressing the result is to determine the provocative concentration (PC) of the agent that causes a predetermined drop in FEV1 from the baseline (usually 20%). This is expressed as PC20 FEV_1.

Measuring Allergic Status

Most patients with asthma have a background of atopy. This can be established by checking the patient's Immunoglobulin

E (IgE) levels or performing skin tests to house dust and other allergens. A limitation of these tests is that a positive test does not establish that the disease is allergic in nature or that it is causing asthma, as some individuals have specific IgE antibodies without any symptoms and they may not be causally related.

Non-Invasive Markers of Airway Inflammation

As asthma is currently considered to be an inflammatory disorder of the airways it seems logical to include an assessment of this inflammation in the diagnosis and follow-up of this disease. A number of biomarkers in the blood, urine, sputum, exhaled air and breath condensate have been studied. These are tabulated in Table 33.3 and a short account of exhaled nitric oxide, the most promising biomarker is given here.

Table 33.3: Non-invasive markers of airway inflammation
BLOOD/SERUM:
– Eosinophils
– Eosinophilic cationic protein (ECP)
– Eosinophil peroxidase (EPO)
URINE:
– Leukotriene E4 (LTE4)
– 9α, 11β-PGF2
INDUCED SPUTUM:
– Cell differential
– Soluble mediators (ECP, cysteinyl leukotriene)
EXHALED AIR:
– Nitric oxide
– Carbon monoxide
– Hydrocarbons
BREATH CONDENSATE:
– Hydrogen peroxide
– Leukotriene metabolites
– 8-isoprostane
– Nitrotyrosine

Exhaled Nitric Oxide (eNO)

NO has been the most extensively investigated of all the gases present in exhaled air. Measuring NO has been proposed as a simple, non-invasive method of asthma diagnosis and monitoring. Levels of eNO are elevated in asthmatics and correlate closely with many surrogate markers of disease, including peak flow variability, bronchial hyperresponsiveness and sputum eosinophil count. At a cut-off of 16 parts per billion (ppb), eNO measurement is an accurate way to diagnose asthma in adults. Exhaled NO's high positive predictive value for subsequent exacerbations indicates a direct relationship with asthma pathophysiology. Several recent studies have confirmed the ability

of eNO to predict asthma exacerbations. Exhaled NO levels rise during an acute attack and after allergen exposure in an asthmatic, and then drop after corticosteroid therapy. A study by Jones demonstrated that eNO was associated with a positive predictive value of 80–90% for predicting and diagnosing loss of control. Additionally, serial changes in eNO had better sensitivity than a single measurement. Thus, eNO may have a role in monitoring a patient's response to anti-inflammatory therapy. Traditionally, decisions on an individual's asthmatic treatment have been based on symptoms and lung function. eNO measurements may provide an additional dimension and help tailor and optimize an asthmatic's therapy.

Exhaled NO can be measured easily, quickly, and noninvasively in an office setting and is hence reproducible. The techniques used to measure eNO have become simpler and well-standardized and require about the same amount of time as that taken by spirometry. Thus while eNO measurement has emerged as a promising tool in the diagnosis and management of asthma, a lot remains to be elucidated and many questions remain. The cut-off points for an elevated eNO value remain poorly defined, the variability of eNO measurements in populations and within individuals also needs to be defined. In addition, subsets of asthma patients that may benefit from eNO measurements need to be further investigated.

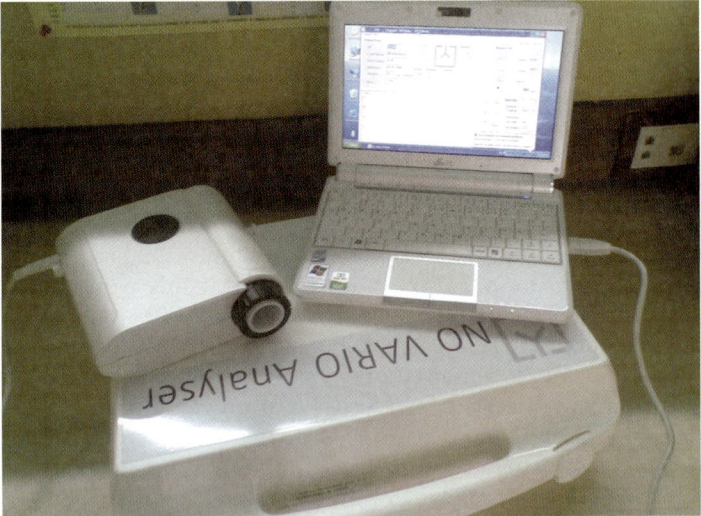

Fig 33.1: Exhaled Nitric Oxide Apparatus.

DIFFERENTIAL DIAGNOSIS

Whilst the typical asthma attack is easy to diagnose there are a number of asthma mimics that must be mentioned here.

COPD

While the distinction of late-onset asthma from COPD is generally straightforward, on occasion, the difference between these conditions may be difficult. Thus, it is easy to distinguish one from another when the asthmatic is a young atopic subject who has never smoked and has intermittent wheeze and variable reversible airflow limitation. But distinguishing asthma from COPD is much more difficult in a patient whose airway obstruction starts at the age of 60, has smoked in the past for a few years, also has a history of atopy when he was younger and presents with chronic cough and fixed airflow limitation.

There are many obvious similarities between these two diseases. Both are chronic diseases characterized by airflow obstruction and both are characterized by inflammatory components. In asthma whilst the inflammation is in response to an inhaled allergen and chiefly involves the eosinophil, in COPD the inflammation is secondary to noxious particles in cigarette smoke and is primarily neutrophilic. Despite the obvious differences between these two diseases, including the natural history, the bronchodilator response and the corticosteroid response, actual distinction between the two may be difficult. In a study by Bellia of 128 confirmed asthmatics, 20% were wrongly misdiagnosed as asthma with diagnostic errors especially common in the elderly. Thus, one out of five elderly asthmatics may receive an incorrect label. The distinction is vital when many therapeutic choices exist. Apart from the wrong diagnosis, it is important to realize that there may be genuine overlap between these two diseases. In the NHAHES survey in the US, 17% of participants reported coexisting asthma and COPD and in the UK a study showed that 19% had more than one obstructive lung diagnosis. The coexistence of these two conditions in the same patient is associated not just with increased disease severity but also increased mortality. Finally, a subset of patients can start off as clearly asthmatic and evolve over the years into COPD. The Tuscon epidemiological study of airway obstructive disease followed up 3000 subjects over two decades and established that adult subjects with active asthma had a 12 times higher risk of acquiring COPD than subjects with no asthma even after adjusting for smoking. In another study from Copenhagen which followed up 228 asthmatics over 26 years, 16% had developed non-reversible airway obstruction with a quarter of patients having reduced transfer factor. The factors at initial enrolment that predicted subsequent development of irreversible airflow limitation included initial lower FEV_1 values, less bronchial hyperreactivity and less reversibility to beta-agonists. Thus, th available literature suggests that around 10–15% of asthmatics will develop fixed airways obstruction. The chances increase if the asthmatic smokes and the asthma is poorly controlled over the initial years. Airway remodelling which has been discussed in an earlier section may help explain why some asthmatics evolve into COPD.

Distinguishing Asthma from COPD

CLINICAL FEATURES
The important clinical differences between these two conditions are outlined in Table 33.4.

Having said this, the clinical distinction is seldom so cut and dry, and symptoms alone cannot reliably distinguish these two conditions.

SPIROMETRY
If the airflow limitation is reversible, this suggests asthma. Having said this, asthmatics may have fixed airflow limitation, especially those with severe or chronic asthma over many years duration and conversely one-third of patients with COPD may show significant (>12%) reversibility after inhaled beta-agonists.

Table 33.4: Clinical differences between Asthma and COPD		
	Asthma	**COPD**
Symptoms	Dyspnoea episodic, cough dry	Dyspnoea persistent and progressive, cough productive
	Wheeze	Breathless on exertion
Onset	Usually childhood	Usually > 45 years
Course	Variable, remissions	Progressive
Smoking	Sometimes	Invariably
Bronchodilator response	Good	Poor
Response to steroids	Good	Poor

Thus both asthma and COPD have a spectrum of reversibility and reversibility alone cannot distinguish the two conditions.

REVERSIBILITY TO STEROIDS
Reversibility to steroids is a defining feature of asthma but here too there are exceptions. Patients with steroid-resistant asthma will, by definition, be refractory to steroids. On the other hand, significant numbers of COPD patients will show a heartening response to inhaled and oral steroids.

DIFFUSION CAPACITY
Diffusion capacity is normal or increased in asthma while it is reduced in patients with COPD. It should be noted that it may also be reduced in smokers without airflow limitation.

AIRWAY HYPERRESPONSIVENESS
Even airway hyperresponsiveness, long considered the hallmark of asthma, may be present in COPD and hence cannot reliably distinguish these conditions. A recent study showed that as many as 60% of patients with COPD had evidence of airway hyperresponsiveness with methacholine.

AIRWAY IMAGING
Airway imaging is not routinely recommended but high-resolution computed tomography (HRCT) scans can accurately distinguish asthma from emphysema.

AIRWAY INFLAMMOMETRY
Airway inflammometry is a research tool but can help distinguish these two conditions as well. Induced sputum in the two conditions shows important differences and exhaled NO is also high in asthma and generally normal in COPD.

Cardiac Asthma

Cardiac asthma is another close mimic of asthma. Distinguishing one condition from the other may on occasions be difficult on clinical grounds alone. Along with a careful history, chest radiography, electrocardiography (ECG) and echocardiography may be useful in distinguishing cardiac asthma from bronchial asthma. Another useful and new test to help distinguish cardiac asthma from bronchial asthma is the BNP assay. This helps detect the presence of heart failure, determine its severity and estimate prognosis. It is a point of care test that is rapid, easy to perform and relatively inexpensive. Results are available in no longer than 15 minutes from most laboratories. The main advantage of the BNP is its negative predictive value, which stands at around 96%. Thus, heart failure can be confidently ruled out when the BNP is normal (around 100 pg/ml). In a recent emergency room survey, doctors admitted to being unsure of the diagnosis of heart failure in 40% of encounters. The BNP was particularly useful in just these settings with a normal BNP ruling out cardiac failure and suggesting the dyspnoea had to be secondary to another cause. The worse the heart failure, the higher the BNP levels and patients admitted with florid congestive cardiac failure (CCF) routinely have levels around 1000 pg/ml. Serial BNP levels correlate with response to therapy and are thus of some prognostic value. Several studies have shown that patients whose BNP levels reduce in response to treatment in hospital have good outcomes whereas those whose hospital stay ends in death or readmission have rising or only minimal decreases in BNP. It must be noted that BNP levels are higher in older patients, women, patients with renal dysfunction and those with sepsis. From a management point of view it is worth pointing out that if there is any doubt if the asthma is bronchial or cardiac it is mandatory to avoid ephedrine and beta-blockers in any form. Other measures like beta-agonists, diuretics and steroids help both conditions.

Vocal Cord Dysfunction

Vocal cord dysfunction is an important mimic of asthma that is discussed here. It occurs predominantly in women aged 20–40 years and seems more common in those in the medical or nursing profession. Many patients have true asthma coexisting as well, which makes the diagnosis even more difficult. During episodes of vocal cord dysfunction, the 'wheeze' is in reality an inspiratory monophasic sound produced at the larynx. The distinction from asthma may be very difficult and some pointers to vocal cord dysfunction are that the sounds resolve with quiet breathing, the patient cannot phonate or cough during the attack, and that there is a normal alveolar arterial gradient during the attack. Other pointers are the absence of hyperinflation on chest radiography and a distinctive inspiratory cut-off on the inspiratory limb of the flow-volume loop. Direct laryngoscopy during an attack is the investigation of choice though this may be difficult to perform. If done, it shows that both vocal cords are in the midline, adducted position during inspiration. On occasion, this finding is only present when provoked after making the patient exercise on a treadmill. Acute attacks can be relieved by breathing an air-helium mixture called heliox. They are all diagnosed late, some even after multiple episodes of ventilator support. As a consequence most develop obesity due to prolonged corticosteroid therapy; iatrogenic Cushing's syndrome is common. These patients have a high incidence of psychiatric problems and hence treatment involves psychiatric help and counselling.

Obstruction to a Large Airway

Intrinsic obstruction produced by a tumour or stenosis or extrinsic obstruction of a large airway (as from a mediastinal mass or an aortic aneurysm) may at first encounter be mistaken for asthma. These patients have a monophonic wheeze (instead of the usual polyphonic wheezes heard on asthma). The flow-volume loop shows a clear flattening of the inspiratory limb of the loop. Other relevant investigations also clarify the diagnosis.

Constrictive bronchiolitis

When idiopathic in origin also presents with cough, breathlessness and wheeze. The HRCT findings (discussed in a separate chapter) should help to differentiate it from asthma.

SUGGESTED READING

Berend N. Mechanisms of airway hyperresponsiveness in asthma. *Respirology.* 1 Sep. 2008; 13(5): 624–31.

Ehrlich RI. Wheeze, asthma diagnosis and medication use: a national adult survey in a developing country. *Thorax.* 1 Nov. 2005; 60(11): 895–901.

Field SK, Gelfand GAJ, McFadden SD. The effect of anti-reflux surgery on asthmatics with gastroesophageal reflux. *Chest.* 1999; 116: 766–74.

Jones SL, Kittelson J, Cowan JO, *et al.* The predictive value of exhaled nitric oxide measurements in assessing changes in asthma control. *Am J Respir Crit Care Med.* 2001; 164: 738–43.

King CS. Clinical asthma syndromes and important asthma mimics. *Respir Care.* 1 May 2008; 53(5): 568–80.

Littner MR, Ballard D, Huang B, *et al.* Twenty four weeks of lansoprazole reduces asthma exacerbations and improves asthma quality of life in subjects with symptoms of acid reflux. *Eur Resir J.* 2002; 20: 428.

Majid H, Kao C. Utility of exhaled nitric oxide in the diagnosis and management of asthma. *Current Opinion in Pulmonary Medicine.* 2010; 16: 1: 42–7.

Pollart SM. Overview of changes to asthma guidelines: diagnosis and screening. *Am Fam Physician.* 1 May 2009; 79(9): 761–7.

Salpeter SR, Ormiston TM, Salpeter EE. Cardioselective beta-blockers in patients with reactive airway disease; a meta analysis. *Ann Intern Med.* 2002; 137: 715–25.

Slaughter MC. Not quite asthma: differential diagnosis of dyspnea, cough, and wheezing. *Allergy Asthma Proc.* 1 May 2007; 28(3): 271–81.

Tilles SA. Differential diagnosis of adult asthma. *Med Clin North Am.* 1 Jan. 2006; 90(1): 61–76.

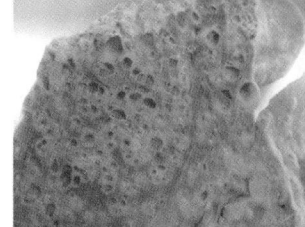

CHAPTER **34** **Asthma: Management**

ASTHMA MANAGEMENT

Global Initiative for Asthma (GINA) guidelines stress the importance of a six-part management plan.

The components are:

1. Educate patients to develop a partnership Education of an asthmatic is an ongoing continual process. It is sobering to note that several studies show that socioeconomic factors like poverty and ignorance are linked to poor asthma control and even asthma deaths. The process of education must include not just the patient but ideally his family as well. Education empowers the asthmatic to understand and manage his disease and helps build up trust and a relationship between the patient and his healthcare provider. Education not only clarifies the nature of the disease and the medications that must be taken but also serves to teach the patient the correct inhaler technique, the importance of monitoring via a home peak flow meter and allays fears and doubts the patient may have regarding the safety and side-effects of the drugs.

2. Assess and monitor asthma severity This is achieved in a number of ways. Symptom reports are the easiest way for the patient to monitor his asthma severity. An asthmatic must be taught that frequent need for reliever medication, nocturnal awakening due to asthma and limitation of activity secondary to worsening asthma are all portends of poor control for which urgent action should be taken. Objective measures of control are based around the peak flow meter at home and every asthmatic must be encouraged to own and monitor his peak flows on an ongoing basis with a written treatment plan geared around changes in peak flow from baseline values. Peak expiratory flow (PEF) monitoring is especially useful in those with poor perception of symptoms. Monitoring in hospital includes spirometry, which is useful for initial assessment, to assess the severity of the airflow limitation and to assess response to therapy.

3. Avoid exposure to risk factors The patient must be urged to avoid exposure to known triggers of asthma including allergens in the environment, food allergens and additives and medications that can worsen asthma whenever possible. This avoidance should extend to even second-hand or passive tobacco smoke, vehicle emissions in polluted areas and irritants in the workplace that may be adding an occupational dimension to the patient's asthma.

It would seem intuitive that establishing a low-allergen environment in the asthmatic patient's home would help in the day to day management of his asthma. Although not

Table 34.1: Allergen avoidance in the home
I. House dust mite reduction measures:
– Cover mattresses, pillows and blankets in impermeable covers
– Plastic covers (feels uncomfortable)
– Water vapor permeable fabrics (mite guard)
– Wash all bedding at 55°C weekly (hot cycle of washing machine) as this is the temperature that kills mites.
– Remove carpets of hoover them frequently
– Acaricides are chemicals that kill mites
– Minimize upholstered furniture, replace with leather
– Keep dust accumulating objects in cupboards
– Replace curtains with blinds
– Hot wash/freeze stuffed toys
– Reduce humidity
II. Per allergen avoidance:
– Get rid of pets
If this is not possible:
– Keep pet out of bedroom
– Have the pet washed twice a week
– Cleaning the upholstered furniture the pet sits on
– HEPA filters in the main living areas and bedroom
III. Avoidance of cockroach allergens:
– Remove waste food
– Seal leaks
– Use of chemicals like diazinon, chlorpyrifos and boric acid

easy to achieve, substantial reductions in allergen load can be achieved, with gratifying improvements in control, by adopting the measures outlined in Table 34.1.

4. Establish medication plans for long-term Asthma Management This stepped care approach to asthma management will be dealt with in detail shortly.

5. Management of acute exacerbations.

6. Provide regular follow-up Continual monitoring is essential to ensure that therapeutic goals are met. At each follow-up an overview of the clinical parameters, a review of home peak flow records and a check of the risk factors and their avoidance, is made.

We will now discuss the following:

I. Asthma medications and the long-term, outpatient-based pharmacological management of asthma.
II. Management of acute exacerbations of asthma in hospital.

ASTHMA MEDICATIONS

Introduction

Medications to treat asthma can be classified into two broad categories: Controllers and Relievers. Controllers are medications designed to be taken long term to control asthma through their anti-inflammatory effects. Relievers are medicines used on an as-needed basis to quickly relieve symptoms, primarily by their bronchodilator properties.

Routes of Administration

Asthma treatment can be administered by a variety of different routes: inhaled, oral or parenteral (subcutaneous, intramuscular, intravenous). What is unique about the therapy of asthma is that it is via the inhaled route that medications are primarily delivered to the patient. One of the biggest changes in asthma management in recent times has been the transition from oral to inhaled therapies as the preferred route of administration. The metered dose inhaler (MDI) was first developed in 1955 by Riker Laboratories. Prior to the advent of the MDI, asthma medication was delivered using a squeeze bulb nebulizer which was fragile and unreliable. The particles this crude device generated were too large for effective lung delivery. Two new technologies converged in the MDI: the chlorofluorocarbon (CFC) propellant and the Meshburg metering valve (originally designed for dispensing perfume). A modern MDI consists of three major components; the canister where the drug formulation resides, the metering valve which ensures a metered quantity of the drug is dispensed with each actuation and the actuator or mouthpiece which allows the patient to operate the device. The propellant used to carry the active drug contained CFCs. These compounds while safe for the patient were proven to be damaging the earth's ozone layer, hence CFC-containing inhalers are being phased out the world over and being replaced by CFC-free inhalers as per the Montreal Protocol signed by more than 160 countries including India. The new inhalers, which will use hydrofluoroalkane (HFA) technology, will replace all CFC-containing inhalers by 2010. Pressurized MDIs are not the only route by which inhaled drugs are delivered to asthmatics.

Other inhaler devices include: breath-actuated inhalers (so called acuhalers and turbohalers), dry powder inhalers (rotacaps and rotahalers), soft mist inhalers and nebulized or wet aerosols. These different inhaler devices differ in their efficiency of drug delivery to the lower respiratory tract and the ease with which the device can be used by the majority of patients. Individual patient preference, convenience, and ease of use determine which inhaler device is the right one for a particular patient. A good physician is duty-bound to spend part of every consultation teaching and rechecking his patient's inhaler technique as large numbers of patients have very poor inhaler techniques despite using their inhalers (with the same poor technique) for years. The steps to be followed whilst using an inhaler are outlined in Table 34.2. Several studies worldwide have identified poor patient inhaler technique as a common and persistent problem. Up to 90% of adult patients have been reported to have inadequate inhaler technique with higher rates of errors in children and the elderly asthmatics. The majority of asthmatics using their inhalers do so too poorly to result in reliable drug delivery. Even healthcare professionals themselves are often not familiar with correct inhaler technique and use. In an oft-quoted study from Iran, of 173 healthcare workers (doctors and nurses) who had their inhaler technique checked, only 7% performed all steps correctly. *(Ref: Nadi E, Zerrati F.*

Table 34.2: Steps in correct MDI technique
1. Take the cap off the inhaler mouthpiece
2. Shake the inhaler
3. Hold the inhaler upright
4. Breathe out
5. Place the inhaler mouthpiece between the lips
6. Activate the inhaler while breathing in deeply and slowly
7. Continue to inhale until the lungs are full
8. Hold the breath for 5–10 seconds
9. Breathe out
10. Gargle immediately after use (while using an inhaled steroid)

Table 34.3: Choice of inhaler device for children with asthma	
Age Group	**Devices Used**
Less than 5 years	– MDI + spacer with face mask – Nebulizer with face mask
5–8 years	– MDI + spacer with mouthpiece – Nebulizer with mouth piece
More than 8 years	– Dry powder inhaler or breath activate inhaler or MDI with spacer and mouthpiece – Nebulizer with mouth piece

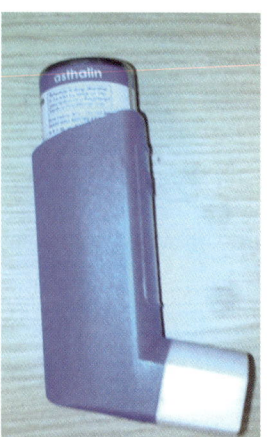

Fig 34.1: Metered dose inhaler.

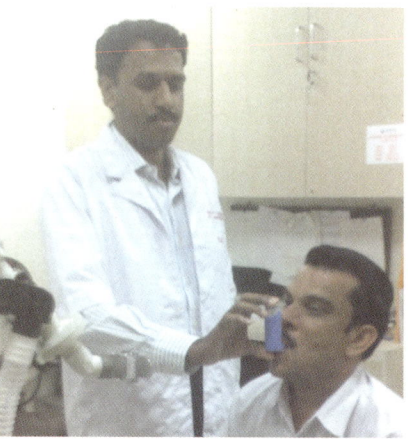

Fig 34.2: PFT technician teaching a patient how to use an MDI.

Evaluation of the metered dose inhaler technique among healthcare providers. Acta Medica Iranica 2005;43: 4: 268–72).

DRUGS USED IN ASTHMA

I. CONTROLLER MEDICATIONS
   – Inhaled corticosteroids
   – Leukotriene modifiers
   – Long-acting inhaled β_2-agonists
   – Theophylline
   – Long-acting oral β_2-agonists
   – Immunotherapy and biological agents

II. RELIEVER MEDICATIONS
   – Rapid-acting inhaled β_2-agonists
   – Systemic glucocorticosteroids
   – Anticholinergics
   – Theophylline
   – Short-acting oral β_2-agonists

Inhaled Corticosteroids (ICS)

Inhaled corticosteroids are currently the most potent anti-inflammatory drugs for the treatment of asthma. They have a number of positive effects in asthma which have been outlined in Table 34.4.

What needs to be clarified to patients and their families is that though these drugs have an amazing impact on asthma as outlined in the Table, they do not cure asthma and within a few months of being discontinued, clinical control deteriorates in a significant proportion of patients.

Table 34.4: Effects of ICS in asthma
1. Controls symptoms
2. Improves quality of life
3. Decreases airway hyperresponsiveness
4. Controls inflammation
5. Reduces frequency and severity of exacerbations
6. Reduces asthma mortality
7. Prevents airway remodelling
8. Possibly alters the natural history of asthma

TYPES OF INHALED STEROIDS

There are several generations of inhaled steroids available in the market. Although they differ in potency and bioavailability, because of relatively flat dose-response relationships in asthma, there is not much clinical difference among the different forms.

The different preparations of ICS available in India and their equipotent daily doses are summarized in Table 34.5.

ICS are remarkably effective in the vast majority of asthmatics at relatively low doses (equivalent of 400 μg of budesonide / day). However, there is a subset of severe asthmatics where much higher doses of ICS will be needed to achieve optimal control. There does seem to be a close relationship between the

Table 34.5: Different ICS preparations available in India		
Drug	Low Daily Dose (μg)	High Daily Dose (μg)
Beclomethasone dipropionate	200-500	> 1000–2000
Budesonide	200–400	> 800–1600
Fluticasone propionate	100–250	> 500–1000
Mometasone furoate	200–400	> 800–1200
Ciclesonide	80–160	> 320–1280

dose of ICS and the prevention of acute severe exacerbations. Higher doses of ICS are often required in smokers as cigarette smoke reduces the responsiveness to ICS.

ADVERSE EFFECTS OF ICS

The commonest side-effects of ICS are oropharyngeal candidiasis, dysphonia and cough from upper airway irritation. These side-effects are reduced if the patient is instructed to gargle after each dose or advised use of a spacer device. Certain inhaled steroids like ciclesonide which are activated in the lungs but not in the pharynx are less likely to induce these local side-effects. When the dose of ICS crosses 400 μg of budesonide or its equivalent, certain systemic side-effects may be noticed. These include: easy bruising, adrenal suppression, decreased bone mineral density, growth suppression in children, cataracts, and glaucoma. Certain ICS like ciclesonide, budesonide and fluticasone at equipotent doses have less systemic side-effects. It is sometimes difficult in disassociating the effects of high-dose ICS from the effect of the frequent courses of oral corticosteroids taken by patients with severe asthma. ICS do not increase the risk of pulmonary infections including tuberculosis. This is a misconception that is common in India where tuberculosis is endemic. It must be stressed that ICS can be safely used in patients with tuberculosis and are not contraindicated even in patients with active tuberculosis.

There has been ongoing debate on the effect of long-term use of ICS on the bone and on growth and these two important side-effects which all asthmatics are concerned about will be put in perspective.

ICS AND OSTEOPOROSIS

There is little doubt that high doses of ICS taken over the years can lead to osteoporosis. In a regression analysis, the lumbar BMD z score decreased by 0.5 SD for each 1-mg increment in the daily dose of inhaled steroid, with most patients (71%) taking inhaled budesonide for more than 10 years. An increased risk of hip fracture in patients taking inhaled corticosteroids (dose-dependent) was also noted in a large cross-sectional study in the United Kingdom, with an OR of 1.19 (after adjusting for use of oral corticosteroids). An almost linear relationship in OR was noted; with the lowest risk at less than 200 μg/day (OR 1.1), to an OR of 1.5 for patients taking 800 to 1600 μg/day, to a further exponential risk for those taking >1600 μg/day (OR of 2). In Canada, a similar case-controlled study found that the risk of hip or upper limb fracture increased significantly, by 12%, for each 1000-μg/day over 1000 μg dose of inhaled corticosteroid.

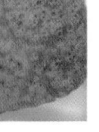

Thus, the risk of osteoporosis with high doses of ICS used over prolonged periods of time is real. Recommendations would include keeping the ICS dose to a minimum by using ICS—long-acting beta-agonists (LABA) combinations, and using calcium and bisphosphonate prophylaxis to prevent osteoporosis in vulnerable patients.

ICS AND GROWTH

There are three phases of normal childhood growth: nutrition-dependent growth of infancy (the fastest growth phase), the growth hormone–dependent linear second phase from infancy to prepuberty, and the pubertal phase, which ends with epiphyseal growth plate maturation.

When used at the recommended dosages of 100 to 200 µg/d of beclomethasone diproprionate and HFA or 200 to 400 µg of beclomethasone diproprionate CFC (with volumetric spacer), no significant differences were found in growth velocities (5.27 vs. 5.71 cm/year). Fluticasone, when used in doses up to 400 µg/d and ciclesonide up to 160 µg/d also did not seem to have significant effects on growth. Long-term studies with budesonide show a transient slowing of growth in the first year of use but no significant effect on final attained adult height. Factors that predisposed to a greater reduction in growth velocity were lower age and lower pre-treatment heights. While most studies document slowing of growth in the early stages of long-term inhaled corticosteroid use, it is reassuring to note that when used in the recommended doses, children on inhaled corticosteroids will attain their anticipated height as adults.

Leukotriene Modifiers

The leukotriene modifiers include montelukast, pranlukast and zafirlukast (which are cysteinyl-leukotriene 1 receptor antagonists) and zileuton which is a 5-lipoxygenase inhibitor). The only preparation available in the Indian market is montelukast. A mounting body of evidence supports the use of these drugs as an alternative treatment in patients with mild persistent asthma. When used alone, they are weak drugs and as controllers are far less effective than even low doses of ICS. Studies attempting to substitute ICS with these drugs have confirmed that this approach risks a worsening in asthma control. Their optimal role is probably as an 'add-on' therapy to ICS, in an attempt to reduce the dose of ICS in patients with moderate to severe asthma. Another role for these drugs is in the asthmatic who remains poorly controlled despite high doses of ICS. In this setting, they may help improve asthma control, though less effectively than the addition of a LABA at this stage.

SIDE-EFFECTS

These are well-tolerated drugs and few if any class-related side-effects have been reported. One of the leukotriene modifiers has been associated with liver toxicity. Monitoring of liver function is recommended when this drug is used. As discussed in the section on vasculitis, earlier fears of an association with Churg-Strauss syndrome have proved unfounded.

Long-acting Beta Agonists (LABAs)

The two drugs in this category are formoterol and salmeterol. Both provide a similar duration of bronchodilatation but formoterol has

a more rapid onset of action than salmeterol, which may make it more suitable for symptom relief as well as symptom protection. These drugs must never be used as monotherapy as they do not influence the inflammation that is the hallmark of poorly controlled asthma. They are most effective when combined with ICS and are the most effective add-on when a medium dose of ICS fails to achieve adequate asthma control. Indeed, in this situation this is a preferred strategy to increasing the dose of ICS. Several studies have shown that this combination of LABA and ICS in medium doses results in better symptom control, improved lung function, decreased nocturnal attacks and reduced exacerbations, than ICS alone. Given the synergy between these two groups of drugs, it is only natural that they be combined in fixed dose inhalers that deliver both drugs in standard doses. Several studies have shown that giving this therapy in combination is as effective as giving each drug separately. Thus, salmeterol and fluticasone are combined into inhalers at different concentrations of fluticasone, and formoterol and budesonide are similarly combined with different concentrations of budesonide varying from 100–400 µg/actuation. This is not only more convenient and cost-effective than giving each drug separately but also ensures that the LABA is always accompanied by ICS, thus increasing safety. The real concerns of LABAs triggering asthma deaths will be discussed separately. The combination of formoterol and budesonide has an additional advantage. It may be possible to use this single inhaler as both reliever and controller as part of the SMART strategy. This strategy advocates the use of a single inhaler (budesonide and formoterol in combination) for maintenance and reliever therapy in the treatment of asthma and has the advantage of being simple (one inhaler instead of two), and prevents LABA monotherapy. The strategy allows anti-inflammatory therapy to increase in line with disease activity when patients have symptoms. Indeed, some studies have shown that this strategy may provide patients with more sustained control than a fourfold increase in ICS alone.

However, the strategy does have the potential of exposing the patient to high doses of LABAs, albeit with concomitant ICS therapy, and vigilance is warranted in the use of this novel and promising solution to better asthma control. The maximum approved dosage per day with this approach (36 µg/day formoterol in adults and 18 µg/day in children below 12 years of age) needs to be emphasized and made clear to the patients when their asthma control strategy includes this single inhaler approach.

LABAS AND THE RISK OF SUDDEN DEATH

An analysis of the controversy:

Inhaled β_2–agonists have been used for almost half a century in the treatment of asthma. Yet their use, especially of the long-acting formulations (LABAs), remains mired in controversy and the verdict on their benefit-to-risk ratio repeatedly questioned. This section attempts to understand the rationale for the debate on their use, and reviews the literature to answer questions raised by both clinicians and patients regarding their use.

THE BENEFITS

LABAs, when used with or without ICS confer beneficial effects to patients with asthma. A Cochrane review that analyzed 85 randomized controlled trials using LABAs found statistically significant improvements in morning PEF rates, asthma symptoms, quality of life, and need for rescue medications when compared to placebo. When used in combination with ICS, there was a significant reduction in asthma exacerbations as well. Guidelines recommend their use in Step 3 or 4 in the management of asthma, i.e. stages associated with a poor level of control despite low-dose ICS.

THE CONTROVERSY

In the 1960s, an epidemic of asthma deaths was noticed in at least six countries, including England and New Zealand. This epidemic coincided with the use of an aerosolized formulation of a high-dose β_2–agonist, isoprenaline, called "Isoprenaline Forte", and was noticed only in countries where this high-dose formulation, containing almost five times the standard dose was used. In the 1970s a second epidemic of asthma-related deaths took place in New Zealand, and this temporally coincided with and was attributed to the use of a new short-acting β_2-agonist fenoterol. The termination of this epidemic also coincided with the withdrawal of the drug from the market.

Salmeterol and Formoterol, the two LABAs in current use were developed by Glaxo-SmithKline (GSK) and Novartis, respectively, in the 1990s. With the apprehension created by the earlier epidemics of asthma mortality associated with β_2–agonists, the Serevent Nationwide Surveillance (SNS) trial was commissioned in the United Kingdom to analyze the safety of salmeterol; 25,189 asthma patients were randomized in a 2:1 ratio to receive either salmeterol 50 μg twice a day or albuterol 200 μg four times a day added to their existing asthma therapy for 16 weeks. The relative risk of death in the salmeterol group was three times that in the albuterol group, although this was not found to be statistically significant.

The largest and the most cited evidence against the use of LABAs comes from the Salmeterol Multicenter Asthma Research Trial (SMART), a study that was conducted as a consequence of the fears raised by the SNS trial. The study was launched in 1996, with the aim of recruiting 60,000 patients. The patients were randomized to receive either salmeterol 42 μg twice a day or placebo in addition to their regular asthma therapy for 28 weeks. In 2003, the study was prematurely terminated because an interim analysis revealed significantly higher rates of secondary outcomes (respiratory-related deaths, asthma-related deaths, combined asthma-related life-threatening experiences) in those receiving salmeterol. Among the 26,355 subjects studied, adverse outcomes were mainly seen in African Americans, and in this cohort, those patients who were not taking ICS prior to randomization were found to be at greatest risk.

Postulated Mechanism of Increased Mortality due to LABAs

Several hypotheses have been postulated to explain increased mortality due to LABAs.

1. Direct cardiotoxicity   Direct cardiotoxicity due to overdosing and concurrent hypoxia. Overdosing with LABAs has been postulated to be a consequence of poorly controlled asthma with worsening symptoms. Tolerance to LABAs resulting from a combination of reduced receptor numbers secondary to receptor internalization and reduced production, along with uncoupling of receptors to downstream signalling pathways following repeated activation is also a possible reason why patients overdose on the drugs. Higher doses of LABAs, coupled with hypoxia have been shown in experimental models to be cardiotoxic, causing fatal cardiac depression and asystole. The reduction of peripheral vascular resistance leading to decreased diastolic blood pressure has also been hypothesized as being a contributory factor to death. Hypokalaemia caused by these drugs can trigger ventricular tachyarrhythmias as well.

2. Genetic factors   Genetic polymorphisms of aminoacid 16 (arginine or glycine) of the β_2 adrenergic receptor play an important role in clinical response to β-agonists. African-Americans more commonly have the Arg/Arg 16 genotype, a genotype that confers an individual with an increased risk of adverse events with the use of LABAs. Prolonged QTc interval, an adverse effect of β_2-agonists, has also been postulated to be seen more frequently in certain races.

3. Masking of inflammation   A likely hypothesis is that the use of these bronchodilators may initially improve symptoms and thus might mask the underlying inflammation, which continues unchecked. It is possibly this worsening inflammation that predisposes these individuals to serious, life-threatening asthma exacerbations.

THE CURRENT EVIDENCE

In a recent meta-analysis that included 215 studies with 106,575 subjects, it was concluded that the odds-ratio (OR) for risk of asthma mortality was 2.7. However, in the subset of patients not prescribed ICS, the OR was 7.3, while in the 63 studies in which subjects were randomized to receive the combination salemeterol/fluticasone or ICS, no mortality was reported among 22,600 patients. Recent Cochrane reviews analyzing the same question have come to a similar conclusion. A meeting convened by the US Food and Drug Administration to review the risks and benefits of inhaled LABAs for asthma concluded that for adults the benefits of combination inhalers outweighed the risks.

Thus, to conclude, the proven benefits of LABAs in the improvement of subjective and objective parameters of asthma control in patients with moderate to severe asthma, and their role in decreasing the need for higher doses of ICS make them valuable drugs in the management of the disease. However, caution needs to be exercised in prescribing them without adequately controlling the inflammation that is the hallmark of the disease. When used along with ICS, they have been found to be safe and effective and can be recommended for use.

Theophylline

Theophylline is traditionally recognized as a bronchodilator, but a growing body of evidence confirms that it also has modest anti-inflammatory properties. While it would not be expected to have any real effect as a first-line controller, it may be beneficial as add-on therapy in patients who are not controlled on ICS alone. Its advantages are that it is a cheap and widely available drug. The main drawback is its toxicity which has been discussed in the section on acute asthma.

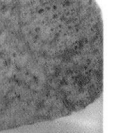

Systemic Glucocorticosteroids

Whilst short bursts of oral steroids lasting for two weeks are often required by many asthmatics, a small fraction of asthmatics may only achieve acceptable control by the addition of a low maintenance dose of oral steroid. If these drugs have to be administered on a long-term basis, attention must be paid to measures that minimize the systemic side-effects.

ANTI-IgE AND OTHER BIOLOGIC THERAPIES

The realization that Immunoglobulin E (IgE) is an important contributor to the pathogenesis of allergic asthma has stimulated the development of anti-IgE therapy in the form of omalizumab. Omalizumab is a humanized monoclonal antibody to IgE that binds free circulating IgE, thus preventing this molecule from binding to receptors on mast cells, basophils and dendritic cells. Blocking the attachment of IgE also downregulates the expression of cell-bound IgE receptors. Omalizumab was the first biological agent approved for the clinical treatment of allergic diseases and has been in clinical use since 2003. As clinical experience with omalizumab grows, it is clear that this is an effective drug in some patients with severe asthma. A recent observational study of 280 patients with severe persistent asthma receiving this drug from 2005–07 reported dramatic reduction in daily symptoms by 76% and nocturnal symptoms by 84%. More important, as in earlier studies with this drug, the main advantage was that exacerbations reduced by 82%, unscheduled health visits by 81% and hospitalizations by 78%. Quality of life also increased after six months of use at an average dose of 450 mg every four weeks. Recent studies also suggest that omalizumab therapy for asthma has the additional benefit of improving allergic rhinitis as well.

The drug has a good safety profile with the frequency of allergic and anaphylactic reactions being no more than 0.41%. Post-marketing analysis data is now available on over 50, 000 patients on this drug and it can safely be concluded that the earlier reports of neoplasms and lymphoma have proved unfounded. The main disadvantages in the Indian context are the high cost and the need for each dose to be given under medical supervision.

Anti-IL5—Mepolizumab

Interleukin-5 (IL-5) is a major cytokine associated with eosinophil recruitment to the airway. Mepolizumab is a monoclonal antibody to IL-5, which decreases peripheral blood eosinophilia when administered to patients with eosinophilic syndromes. Early studies which paved the way for its clinical use showed that mepolizumab resulted in a significant reduction in eosinophils in the blood, airways and bone marrow. Two back-to-back randomized, double-blind, placebo-controlled, parallel-group studies were published in the same issue of the *New England Journal of Medicine* in 2009. The first by Haldar used it in 61 patients with refractory eosinophilic asthma and recurrent severe exacerbations and demonstrated that its use resulted in not just significant reduction in blood and sputum eosinophilia but also significantly fewer exacerbations. The second study from Nair's group in Ontario also repeated these observations and found that the nine patients in the treatment group were able to reduce their prednisolone dose significantly. These two studies show that this phenotype of difficult asthma

with persistent sputum eosinophilia is most likely to respond to this promising new therapy.

Anti-TNF

Tumour necrosis factor alpha (TNFα) is a major TH1 cytokine found in patients with asthma. Monoclonal antibodies to TNF -α such as etanarcept and infliximab have proved to be invaluable in autoimmune conditions like rheumatoid arthritis and ankylosing spondylosis and have recently been assessed in asthma as well. In two small but well-designed studies etanarcept was found to result in significant improvement in forced expiratory volume in one second (FEV_1), forced vital capacity (FVC) and PEF whilst infliximab resulted in a significant decrease in mean diurnal variation of PEF. More recently, golimunab, a human monoclonal antibody against TNF-α was used in 309 patients with severe asthma and although no significant differences were noted in FEV_1 or rate of exacerbations, a post-hoc subgroup analysis indicated that patients with a 12% or greater improvement in FEV_1 at enrolment had fewer exacerbations when treated with this drug.

Anti-IL-4

Pascolimuzab, a humanized anti-IL-4 monoclonal antibody has been through Phase 1 and Phase 2 studies and although it has not demonstrated clinical efficacy further trials are under way.

Anti-CD4

CD4+ cells represent an important source of pro-inflammatory cytokines. Keliximab, a monoclonal antibody to CD4, significantly reduced T-cell proliferation in 22 steroid-dependent asthmatics.

Thus, the biological agents represent an exciting new advance in the management of asthma in certain allergic phenotypes of severe asthma.

Reliever Medications
Rapid-Acting Inhaled β₂-Agonists

These agents are the drugs most used and abused by asthmatics across the globe. By virtue of the quick relief they provide, they are the preferred medication for relief of bronchospasm during exacerbations and are also used for prevention of exercise-induced asthma. The drugs included in this category are: salbutamol, terbutaline, fenoterol, levalbuterol, reproterol and pirbuterol. Formoterol, a LABA with a rapid onset of action is also approved for symptom relief but only when combined with a controller like budesonide as part of the SMART strategy discussed earlier.

It is important to stress that these drugs must only be used on an as-needed basis at the lowest dose and frequency required. Increased requirement and use of these drugs should send a clear signal to the patient and physician that the patient's asthma is sub-optimally controlled and that control needs to be intensified.

The side-effects encountered when these drugs are used in ever-escalating doses include tachycardia, tremors, arrhythmia, and hypokalemia.

Anticholinergics

Anticholinergics include ipratropium bromide and oxitropium bromide. These drugs are less effective relievers in the acute setting than rapidly acting inhaled β_2-agonists but may have some additive effect. They are a viable alternative in the group of asthmatics who cannot tolerate inhaled β_2-agonists because of side-effects.

The major side-effects reported with these agents include dryness of the mouth and a bitter taste.

Theophylline And Oral β_2-Agonists

Short-acting theophylline and oral β_2-agonists (salbutamol and terbutaline tablets and syrups) have some role in relieving asthma symptoms. For millions of Indians who cannot afford or have no access to inhalers, the reality is that these drugs, are often, by default, first-line and sometimes sadly, the sole treatment for their asthma.

ALTERNATIVE AND COMPLEMENTARY MEDICINES IN ASTHMA

Like in any other chronic disease for which there is no cure, there are a profusion of alternative therapies available to the asthmatic. Here we shall only discuss those which have been subjected to the rigors of a clinical trial.

Yoga

Yoga embodies a form of therapy that could conceivably help the asthmatic. It incorporates breathing exercises (pranayama), a cardiovascular component, and relaxation techniques, all of which could be helpful. A recent study from Australia in 2002, was the first to assess the effect of Sahaja yoga, an Indian system of medication based on ancient Yogic principles, in the setting of a controlled clinical trial. In this parallel-group, double-blind, randomized controlled study, subjects were randomly allocated to the Sahaja yoga or control intervention groups. The Sahaja yoga group attended a two-hour yoga session once a week for four months with assessments being undertaken at the conclusion of this period and then again two months later. The study concluded that the patients in the Sahaja yoga group had limited but definite subjective and objective improvement in some measures of their asthma control with improvement in bronchial hyperreactivity of 1.5 doubling doses and some improvement in aspects of the asthma quality of life score. This benefit was not sustained at the two-month follow-up period however. Another older study on the impact of Yoga on asthma showed that it helped lower anxiety and medication use.

Breathing Exercises

The use of breathing exercises in controlling asthma symptoms has been taught and promoted by the American Lung Association in their asthma education series. The type of breathing is 'belly breathing' or diaphragmatic breathing. A more specific form of breathing therapy called the Buteyko breathing technique (BBT), which dates back to 1952, has also been found to be beneficial. Four published clinical trials and two abstracts have evaluated

BBT and although all reported improvements in one or more outcome measures, results have not been consistent and a recent systematic review concluded that no reliable conclusion could be drawn about the benefit of breathing exercises in asthma.

Homeopathy

There have been six trials with a total of around 500 subjects, but a recent Cochrane review indicated that that there is no evidence that homeopathy is of benefit in asthma.

Hypnosis

Because asthma has a strong psychosomatic component it would be expected that any form of relaxation therapy would have a positive impact. In keeping with this, a study in the *British Medical Journal* showed that hypnosis was effective in patients with mild asthma and a strong emotional component. In this study by Ewer, hypnosis resulted in an improvement in symptoms coupled with a reduction in medicine requirement and improved bronchial hyperreactivity.

USING THE AVAILABLE DRUGS CORRECTLY; THE STEPPED CARE APPROACH

This involves assessing the patient's level of control each time he is seen and then stepping up or down the medications to maintain optimal control.

Assessing Control

Control is assessed from daytime symptoms, limitation of activities, nocturnal symptoms, need for reliever/rescue medication and home PEF and office spirometry. Using all of the above, any asthmatic can be classified into three broad categories of control: well-controlled, partly controlled, and uncontrolled, as can be seen from Table 34.6.

Table 34.6: Levels of asthma control			
Characteristic	Well Controlled	Partly controlled	Uncontrolled
Daytime symptoms	Very occasional; not more than once or at the most twice a week and shortlasting	2–4 times/week	More than 4 times a week
Full activity	Unrestricted	Slight limitation	Marked limitation
Nocturnal symptoms	None	May have many nocturnal symptoms	May have many nocturnal symptoms
Need for β_2 agonist inhaler	Not more than twice a week	3–5 times/week	> 4–5 times/week
PEFR	Normal	Normal except during an attack	Reduced, may be markedly so during an attack

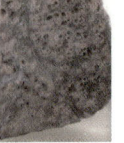

Stepping Up or Down till Control is Achieved

An asthmatic who remains uncontrolled on his or her current regimen should have his treatment stepped up a level till control is achieved. Conversely, if control has been maintained for at least three months, treatment can be stepped down to establish the lowest dose that achieves good control.

The five steps listed in Figure 34.3 provide options of increasing severity as attempts are made to achieve optimal control. In addition, at each step, GINA guidelines permit use of a short-acting beta-agonist as a reliever for quick relief of symptoms. The frequent use of a reliever inhaler is of course one of the components of poor control and is clear indication that control needs to be increased a step.

STEP 1: AS-NEEDED RELIEVER MEDICATION

Treatment with as-needed short-acting beta-agonist inhaler can be recommended only for the patient with mild intermittent asthma who is normal for long periods between episodes. The asthma must be of relatively mild severity and each episode of short duration (no more than a few hours). The patient and even the physician may underestimate the severity and hence if this strategy is to be followed, it is important to document that when the patient is asymptomatic and between episodes, he has normal lung function. In asthmatics intolerant to beta-agonists an alternate though inferior approach is an inhaled anticholinergic or oral theophylline though these have a higher incidence of side-effects and a slower onset of action. An as-

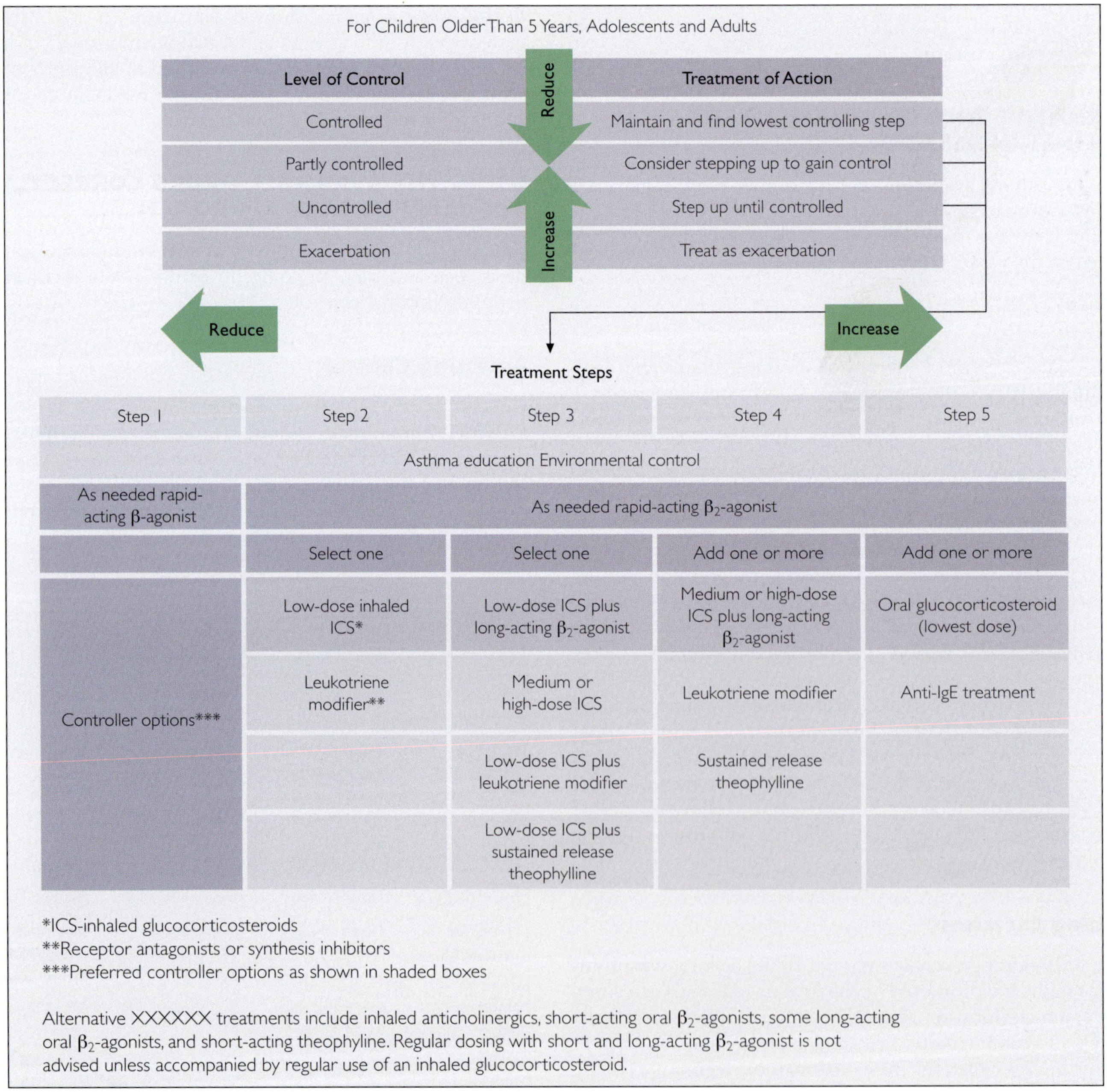

For Children Older Than 5 Years, Adolescents and Adults

Level of Control	Reduce / Increase	Treatment of Action
Controlled		Maintain and find lowest controlling step
Partly controlled		Consider stepping up to gain control
Uncontrolled		Step up until controlled
Exacerbation		Treat as exacerbation

Reduce ←   **Treatment Steps**   → **Increase**

	Step 1	Step 2	Step 3	Step 4	Step 5
		Asthma education Environmental control			
	As needed rapid-acting β-agonist	As needed rapid-acting β₂-agonist			
		Select one	Select one	Add one or more	Add one or more
Controller options***		Low-dose inhaled ICS*	Low-dose ICS plus long-acting β₂-agonist	Medium or high-dose ICS plus long-acting β₂-agonist	Oral glucocorticosteroid (lowest dose)
		Leukotriene modifier**	Medium or high-dose ICS	Leukotriene modifier	Anti-IgE treatment
			Low-dose ICS plus leukotriene modifier	Sustained release theophylline	
			Low-dose ICS plus sustained release theophylline		

*ICS-inhaled glucocorticosteroids
**Receptor antagonists or synthesis inhibitors
***Preferred controller options as shown in shaded boxes

Alternative XXXXXX treatments include inhaled anticholinergics, short-acting oral β₂-agonists, some long-acting oral β₂-agonists, and short-acting theophyline. Regular dosing with short and long-acting β₂-agonist is not advised unless accompanied by regular use of an inhaled glucocorticosteroid.

Fig 34.3: Management Approach Based on Control (reproduced with permission from Global Initative for Asthma, Global Strategy for Asthma Management and Prevention, 2009).

needed beta-agonist is also the standard treatment of exercise-induced asthma.

STEP 2: RELIEVER PLUS SINGLE CONTROLLER

This is the initial treatment for the vast majority of asthmatics with persistent symptoms. The controller of choice is low-dose ICS which is recommended across all age groups as the initial treatment. Alternative but inferior choices are leukotriene modifiers, which are appropriate for patients who are unwilling to use ICS or those asthmatics with severe concomitant atopic rhinitis.

STEP 3: RELIEVER PLUS ONE OR TWO CONTROLLERS

At Step 3, the recommended option is to combine a low dose of ICS with an inhaled long-acting β_2-agonist, either in a single combination inhaler or as two separate inhalers. If the combination inhaler chosen is the formoterol-budesonide combination, then this inhaler may double up for both maintenance and rescue because of formoterol's rapid onset of action. Whether this combination can be used with other combinations of inhaler and reliever requires further study.

Other Step 3 options are to increase to medium doses of ICS or add on a leukotriene mediator or oral theophylline.

STEP 4: RELIEVER PLUS TWO OR MORE CONTROLLERS

GINA guidelines recommend that patients at this step should ideally be referred to a specialist who will re-evaluate the reasons for their poor control thoroughly. The preferred treatment at this step is to combine medium or high-dose ICS with a LABA and in addition add on a leukotriene modifier and/or sustained-release oral theophylline. Unfortunately, in the majority of these difficult asthmatics the change from medium to high doses of ICS provides only little additional benefit but is associated with some systemic side-effects.

STEP 5: RELIEVER PLUS ADDITIONAL CONTROLLER OPTIONS

Options at this stage for the difficult-to-treat asthmatic include low maintenance doses of oral steroids, after careful analysis of their risk-benefit balance, or the addition of biologicals like omalizumab.

Scaling Down Treatment

Just as treatment is scaled up a step to improve control, the GINA guidelines also encourage deescalating a step once control is achieved. Such changes should be made by the doctor in conjunction with the patient, with the latter being made fully aware of the potential consequences, including worsening symptoms and an increased risk of exacerbations. Examples of this kind of 'step down' include:

1. When asthma is controlled with a combination of ICS and LABA, begin by reducing the dose of ICS by approximately 50% whilst continuing the LABA.
2. If control remains, attempt to switch the combination to once daily dosing.
3. An attempt could be made to stop the LABA and continue the low dose of ICS alone as monotherapy.
4. Controller medicine can be stopped altogether if the patient's asthma remains controlled on the lowest dose with no recurrence of symptoms for a year.

HOSPITAL MANAGENENT OF ACUTE SEVERE ASTHMA

Acute severe asthma is a medical emergency. Despite asthma being by definition a reversible disease, deaths from asthma continue to occur during severe attacks. Data from India are not available, but in the UK 2000–4000 people die of asthma every year with death rates on the incline in every age group, being around 4.5% per annum in the 5–34 year group. Fatal and near-fatal asthma will be discussed in a separate section while management of the hospitalized patient with severe asthma will be discussed here.

Oxygen

The majority of patients hospitalized for asthma have hypoxemia of varying degrees of severity at the time of admission. Death when it occurs during an acute asthma attack is almost always a consequence of hypoxemia. Oxygen should therefore be started as promptly as possible. Unlike in chronic obstructive pulmonary disease (COPD), there is little risk of suppression of ventilatory drive, hence oxygen should be given at high flow rates to maintain a $SaO_2 > 95\%$. The oxygen should be well-humidified to minimize bronchial irritation and drying of secretions. Since the main cause of hypoxemia in asthma is V/Q mismatch, inspired oxygen concentrations of 35–50% are usually adequate to reverse the hypoxemia. An oximeter is invaluable in detecting the improvement or deterioration in SaO_2 as the attack evolves, though a baseline arterial blood gas on admission is ideally recommended for every patient hospitalized with severe asthma.

Nebulized Beta-Agonists

Nebulised beta-agonists are the mainstay of treatment of acute severe asthma. They are the agents of first choice to relieve airflow obstruction in acute asthma. They provide more significant bronchodilatation with the most prompt relief, are cost-effective and have fewer side-effects than other agents. The method of delivery has been the topic of much recent discussion. By the time a patient with severe asthma is hospitalized, metered dose inhalers may be less effective because the hyperinflated asthmatic will be too breathless to effectively use his inhaler. These limitations can be overcome by the use of the compressor-driven nebulizer, where drug delivery is less dependent on a coordinated breathing pattern. Also, the more prolonged period of administration permits the delivery of a larger dose. If nebulizer facilities are unavailable, a spacer device may suffice. In a meta-analysis it has been shown that this was at least equivalent to nebulized therapy. The initial dose of salbutamol or terbutaline is 5 mg diluted with 2–3 ml of normal saline. The dosing frequency can be titrated depending on the response. In severely ill patients the nebulization can initially run continuously with the dose being topped up as soon as it is finished. Alternatively, it can be given hourly initially and then repeated every 2–4 hours, monitoring for excessive tachycardia. Theoretically, nebulizers driven by air can worsen hypoxemia if they improve ventilation (by reducing bronchospasm) to a lung unit that is not being perfused. Hence oxygen mains should ideally drive nebulizers, or, if driven by a compressor,

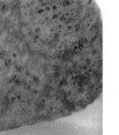

the patient should simultaneously receive supplemental nasal oxygen. If a metered dose inhaler is being used via a spacer, the initial dose is 4–8 puffs of salbutamol, which can be repeated every 15–20 minutes up to three times. In severe disease, the dose can be increased by 1 puff every 30–60 seconds up to 20 puffs as needed. One advantage of the spacer over the nebulizer is that medication given this way can be administered and repeated very quickly (2 minutes versus 10–20 minutes for the wet nebulizer).

Corticosteroids

Corticosteroids have become first-line drugs in the management of asthma, highlighting the recognition of the increased inflammation associated with such attacks. Every asthmatic sick enough to be hospitalized must promptly receive systemic steroid therapy. The use of steroids has been demonstrated in a large Cochrane meta-analysis to favourably affect the outcome of both admitted and discharged patients. What remains in doubt however, even after decades of use, is the optimum dose, route and frequency of administration and the type of preparation used. The onset of action of corticosteroids has been historically felt to be slow and a number of recent studies have looked at high doses of inhaled steroids in the setting of an acute asthma attack. In a study by Rodrigo in patients presenting to the emergency department with acute severe asthma, the addition of high-dose inhaled steroid (flunisolide 1mg every 10 min for 3 hours) to salbutamol led to greater bronchodilatation at 120, 150, and 180 minutes than salbutamol alone. In another important study, Harrison showed that orally administered steroids were equally effective even in severe asthma exacerbations, and provided the patient was not vomiting, were a cheaper and simpler option to intravenous therapy.

We would like to offer the following generalizations based on our personal experience when it comes to steroid therapy in acute severe asthma:

1. Steroids must be administered early, ideally orally by the patient himself, as soon as his PEF drops < 50% of his best level.
2. In hospital they should be administered as soon as the patient is first seen as they take around 6 hours to act. Available data suggests that a clear benefit from corticosteroids is unlikely to be noticed in the first 6 hours of administration and becomes evident only 6–12 hours after the initial dose.
3. In the hospitalized asthmatic who does not have a very severe attack and who is not vomiting, oral prednisolone in a dose of 40–60 mg/day is as effective as intravenously administered steroids.
4. Inhaled steroids may be continued concurrently with systemic steroids though their exact dose and route (spacer versus nebulizer) are unclear. A study by Rowe showed that the addition of inhaled budesonide (800µg bid) to oral prednisolone in patients discharged from the emergency department led to a reduced relapse rate compared to prednisolone alone, with almost 50% reduction in the relapse rate in those on inhaled and oral steroids compared to those on oral steroids alone.
5. In the critically ill asthmatic admitted to the intensive care unit (ICU) we would recommend hydrocortisone in a dose of 200 mg initially, then repeated as 100–200 mg every 6 to 8 hours. Alternatively methyl prednisolone in a dose of 40–80 mg 6 to 8-hourly can be used.
6. There is no evidence that giving much larger doses of steroids significantly speeds up or improves response. The temptation to use heroic doses of steroids must be resisted even when the initial response of the asthmatic seems slow. Indeed, there is a real risk of precipitating an acute steroid myopathy when large doses of steroids are used.
7. Complications following a short-duration, moderate-dose course like the one outlined above appear to be minimal, even when continued over 7–14 days.

Anticholinergics

Ipratropium bromide, the anticholinergic agent most commonly used has a slower onset of action (90–120 min vs 5–15 min) and produces less bronchodilatation than β_2-agonists. A number of large recent studies have examined the additive effect of the two agents, with one from New Zealand showing a greater improvement in FEV_1 (equivalent to 150 ml) in the combination therapy group. Of even greater impact, the combination of anticholinergics and beta-agonists leads to a significant reduction in hospitalization. The initial dose when given by nebulization is 0.5 mg in 2 ml of saline every 15 minutes or even continuously during a severe attack. It may be mixed with the β_2-agonists in the nebulizer chamber. If given via a metered dose inhaler and spacer, the initial dose is 4–8 puffs every 15 minutes, repeated three times.

Intravenous Beta-Agonists

Intravenous beta-agonists are less often required with the realization that beta-agonists administered via the inhaled route, as discussed earlier, offer at least equal and often superior efficacy with greater safety than parenteral therapy with the same agent. It has been argued that in severe asthma with extensive small airway mucus plugging, nebulized medication may not reach the affected airways. Hence the addition of intravenous beta-agonists may be considered when the severe asthmatic remains refractory despite nebulized beta-agonists. Salbutamol is given as an intravenous infusion at 10 µg/min and terbutaline as an infusion at 5 µg/min. When given by this route, beta-agonists have a high rate of adverse effects, especially tachycardia and tremors and must be carefully monitored.

Aminophylline

Intravenous amionophylline is a useful bronchodilator that has been used for many years in the treatment of acute asthma. Although a meta-analysis by Littenberg of 13 adequately designed studies could not find conclusive evidence for supporting its use, we have found it to be an extremely effective agent in the asthmatics who remain refractory to nebulized beta-agonists and steroids. Aminophylline has a very narrow therapeutic margin and its metabolism is affected by multiple factors, making close monitoring of its levels mandatory if it is used. In patients who are not on oral theophylline preparations at the time of admission, a loading dose of 6 mg/kg body weight diluted in 20 ml of 5% dextrose is given slowly over 25–30 minutes. Following this loading dose, an infusion is set up at a rate of 0.6 to 0.9 mg/kg/hour via an infusion pump. The plasma concentration must be monitored and maintained within the therapeutic range of 10–20 µg/ml. Although the bronchodilator effect increases when the serum concentration is maintained at the upper end of the therapeutic range, the toxicity increases too, and we would hesitate to cross a serum level of 10µg/ml. These adverse effects include nausea, vomiting, insomnia, headache, cardiac arrhythmias, convulsions and death. Unquestionably, some of the deaths from asthma in asthma death audits are linked to theophylline toxicity, hence it must be stressed again that the drug must be used with caution, monitoring levels where facilities exist. A number of disease states (liver disease, cardiac failure, pneumonia, and hypoxemia) and drugs (macrolides and most fluoroquinolones) affect theophylline clearance and doses need to be adjusted carefully with even more frequent serum level monitoring in these settings.

Adrenaline

Although adrenaline has been used for acute asthma since 1951, with the current availability of more specific β_2-agonists, it is seldom needed. It remains the drug of choice in certain situations like anaphylaxis with prominent bronchoconstriction. It can also be life-saving in a patient with catastrophic asthma who is given pre-loaded syringes, which they can self-administer, at the start of a sudden attack. The usual dose is 0.5 ml of a 1: 1000 solution given subcutaneously. It may be cautiously repeated if the patient is being monitored in an ICU to a maximum dose of 2 ml.

Magnesium

A number of studies have evaluated the role of intravenous magnesium sulphate but not all have shown a positive effect. A recent meta-analysis has shown beneficial effects in patients who fail to respond to standard therapy and those with more severe asthma ($FEV_1 < 25\%$ at presentation). A study by Sudlow showed that giving 10–20 g over 1 hour to five ventilated asthmatics resulted in significant falls in Ppk from 43 to 32 cm H_2O. There may also be a trend towards female responsiveness, as oestrogen is believed to augment the bronchodilator effect. There is need for further randomized controlled trials to determine the exact role of magnesium in severe asthma.

Unconventional Therapy

In refractory asthma there are scattered reports of the use of inhalational anaesthetics, extra-corporeal oxygenation or bronchial lavage in patients who are on ventilators. The combination of helium and oxygen (heliox) has also been tried and appears to reduce airway pressure.

Mechanical Ventilation in Asthma

INTRODUCTION

Despite all the above measures, a small proportion of patients with acute severe asthma will continue to deteriorate and eventually require mechanical ventilation. Fortunately, only about 10% of asthmatics admitted to hospital will need ICU

Table 34.7: Management of acute asthma
1. Oxygen: high flow to maintain $SaO_2 > 95\%$
2. β_2-agonists: Nebulized initial dose 5 mg salbutamol run continuously in severe attack or every 15 min. MDI: initial dose 4–8 puffs. Can be repeated every 15 min upto 3 times.
3. Anticholinergics: Ipratropium bromide nebulized 0.5 mg every 15 min or continuously if necessary. Can be mixed with β_2 agonists. MDI: initial dose 4–8 puffs every 15 min to be repeated 3 times
4. Corticosteroids: intravenous hydrocortisone 100–200 mg 8 hourly or oral prednisolone 40–60 mg/day
5. Aminophylline: loading dose 6 mg/kg in 20 ml of 5% dextrose IV over 20 minutes, subsequent infusion 0.6–0.9 ml/kg/hr via syringe pump.
6. Adrenaline: 0.6 ml of 1:1000 solution subcutaneously, repeated to a maximum of 2 ml.
7. Magnesium: 2 grams IV
8. Intravenous β_2 agonists: salbutamol 4 µg/kg over 2–5 min and then as an infusion at 0.1–0.2 µg/kg/min.
9. Mechanical ventilation: when indicated.

transfer and no more than 1–2% of them will end up requiring mechanical ventilation.

RATIONALE

When a patient with severe asthma does not respond to all the medical therapy outlined above, the only way to provide adequate oxygenation may be mechanical ventilation. These patients have a propensity to develop severe airflow limitation, making it difficult to exhale all of their inspired gas, resulting in gas trapping which leads to dynamic hyperinflation. This is referred to as intrinsic positive end-expiratory pressure (PEEP) or auto-PEEP. One of the most important principles of mechanical ventilation in this setting is to utilize a strategy aimed at reducing the likelihood of this complication occurring.

NON-INVASIVE VENTILATION (NIV)

Unlike COPD where NIV has a major role, to date, only two small, prospective, randomized studies have evaluated the role of NIV in severe asthma. Both of these studies suggested that in selected asthmatics NIV could be useful as an initial alternative to intubation and ventilation. Further data is needed

Table 34.8: Indications for commencing ventilatory support
– Cardiac or respiratory arrest with apnea or near apnea.
– Deteriorating level of consciousness with inability to protect the airway.
– Increasing respiratory muscle fatigue.
– Cyanosis or worsening hypoxemia ($PaO_2 < 60$ mm Hg despite high flow oxygen)
– Hypercapnia with serial arterial blood gas measurements showing a rising $PaCO_2$.

and without this, the excellent results of NIV in COPD cannot be transposed to acute asthma.

It must be stressed however *that arterial blood gas values alone should never dictate when ventilatory support should commence*. Each patient should be evaluated individually; the trends of serial blood gases viewed in conjunction with the patient's clinical status are far more informative than a single blood gas report in isolation.

INTUBATION

Intubation of the critically ill asthmatic involves considerable risk and hence should be performed deftly and expeditiously by an expert. Many patients have increased bronchospasm and laryngeal spasm during attempted intubation and hence a thorough local anaesthetic spray of the pharynx is important. The patient must be pre-oxygenated and care taken to avoid gastric aspiration. A large-diameter endotracheal tube, ideally > 8 mm should be used to minimize airway resistance and facilitate suction. Sedation before intubation is obtained with a small dose of midazolam and if paralysis is needed, atracurium is preferred.

VENTILATORY STRATEGIES

In an attempt to counter the problem posed by traditional ventilation in asthma, Darioli and Perrret in a landmark paper in 1984 introduced the concept of controlled hypoventilation. Realizing that high peak pressures were to be avoided at any cost they set a limit on the peak inspiratory pressure and achieved this by reducing the tidal volume, respiratory rate, minute ventilation and inspiratory flows. This strategy of deliberate hypoventilation resulted in $PaCO_2$ levels around 60–70 mm Hg that were accepted and tolerated by most patients without complication. Arterial pH was maintained with intravenous bicarbonate if necessary. Adequate oxygenation was maintained by increasing the fraction of inspired oxygen (FiO_2) as necessary. Using this strategy in 34 episodes of mechanical ventilation in 26 asthmatic patients, all survived. Equally important there was no barotrauma in any of their patients. Hypotension, though it occurred in 45% of cases, was usually transient and fluid-responsive.

The fine details of the ventilator settings are not as important as close attention to the basic principles of ventilation in patients with severe asthma: employ low tidal volumes and respiratory rates, prolong expiratory time as much as possible, shorten inspiratory time as much as possible, and monitor for the development of auto-PEEP. Thus, the pressure control mode is used setting the pressure to achieve a tidal volume of 6–8 ml/kg, rate at 11–14 breaths/ minute. An extrinsic PEEP is only used if there is significant auto-PEEP, the set extrinsic PEEP being clearly lower than the auto-PEEP.

DYNAMIC HYPERINFLATION

Dynamic hyperinflation occurs when a machine-preset breath is delivered before the previous expiration is complete so that elastic equilibrium is not reached before the next inspiration starts. This hyperinflation results in the lungs and chest wall operating on a suboptimal portion of their pressure volume curves. Because gas is trapped in the lungs, there is additional pressure at the end of expiration (auto-PEEP or intrinsic PEEP) above the applied PEEP which leads to dynamic hyperinflation. Dynamic hyperinflation may thus be defined as the failure of the lung to

return to its relaxed volume or functional residual capacity at end-exhalation. Dynamic hyperinflation must be assiduously guarded against when ventilating patients with acute severe asthma. It can be clinically assessed by direct auscultation to make sure expiration is complete before the next breath is delivered. It may also be clinically detected by placing a measuring tape across the patient's chest at the level of the nipples and actually noting the increasing chest girth with each breath if dynamic hyperinflation is occurring. The most accurate method to detect and quantify dynamic hyperinflation is by measuring the auto-PEEP generated by the end-expiratory occlusion method, where the expiratory limb of the tubing is clamped off at the end of expiration. This method must be routinely used to assess the severity of dynamic hyperinflation while ventilating any asthmatic.

Excessive dynamic hyperinflation has been linked to development of hypotension and barotraumas, the two dreaded complications of ventilation in asthmatics. Hypotension is frequent and is usually fluid-responsive. It also usually responds to briefly disconnecting the patient from mechanical ventilation. A brief trial of apnoea (30–45 seconds) is usually diagnostic. When hypotension is due to dynamic hyperinflation, a period of apnoea serves to increase venous return and raise the blood pressure. A favourable response to a trial of apnoea should lead to a reduction of the respiratory rate and intravenous fluid administration. If on the other hand a brief trial of apnoea and a fluid challenge fail to promptly improve blood pressure, then a mechanism other than dynamic hyperinflation, such as pneumothorax or myocardial depression is likely.

Barotrauma is the other dreaded complication encountered while ventilating patients with severe asthma. It includes not just pneumothorax, but also interstitial emphysema, pneumo-mediastinum, subcutaneous emphysema, pneumoperitoneum and tension lung cyst. In older series of mechanical ventilation in asthmatics, barotrauma was a frequently observed complication, with pneumothorax occurring in almost a third of all patients. This was undoubtedly the cause of the high mortality reported when ventilating these patients.

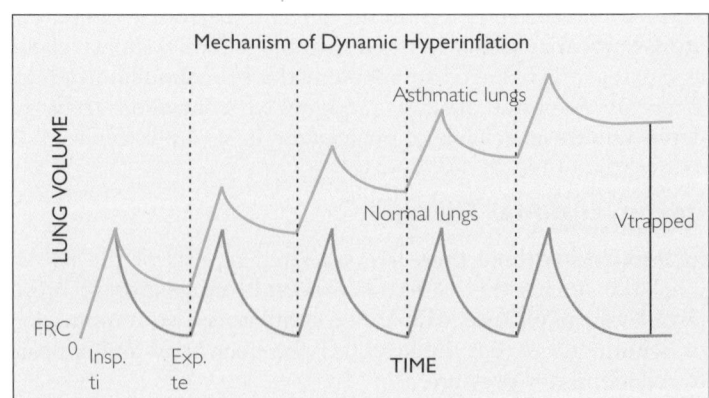

Fig 34.4: Mechanism or dynamic hyperinflation in the setting of severe airflow obstruction. (Adapted from Levy BD, Kitch B, Fanta CH. Medical and ventilatory management of status asthmaticus. *Intensive Care Med.* 1998; 24: 105–117).

WEANING

Most patients with asthma do not require prolonged periods of ventilatory support and once bronchospasm has settled and the asthma attack is felt to have resolved on clinical grounds, weaning may be successfully attempted. Difficult weaning may be secondary to respiratory muscle weakness from hypokalemia, hypophosphatemia, acute steroid myopathy or from prolonged use of neuromuscular blocking agents.

Discharge Planning and Advice

The patient must be discharged when clinically stable. Peak flow monitoring can help predict when the patient may be safely discharged. A study by Udwadia and Harrison showed that patients discharged from hospital when their peak flows are still fluctuating continue to have major and occasionally catastrophic dips in PEF after discharge. In this study, the authors concluded that it was only safe to discharge patients when the diurnal variation in their PEF falls < 20%. Discharging them before this target is reached puts them at risk of further severe attacks of asthma requiring re-hospitalization and even leading to death.

A hospitalization with severe asthma must be looked at as a failure on the part of the treating physician and his self-management plan. The hospitalized asthmatic offers the physician the ideal opportunity to educate the patient about his disease. Healthcare providers should seize this opportunity to review the patient's understanding of the causes of asthma exacerbations and avoidance of its triggers. He should be taught the correct inhaler technique, taught to use a peak flow meter, and given a written treatment plan. In a study of 150 asthmatics discharged from the emergency department with an action plan which included peak flow monitoring, there was a striking reduction in the risk of relapse in the peak flow action plan group (five readmissions in this group versus 55 in those with no plan). A recent systematic review by the Cochrane airway group looked at 23 studies that compared a written self-treatment plan with usual care and showed that a written plan reduced hospitalization, emergency room visits and days off work or school.

But we end this section by quoting the words of Thomas Petty, who said: *'The best treatment of status asthmaticus is to treat it three days before it occurs.'*

HOW IS ASTHMA MANAGED IN INDIA?

In Hospitals

Good guidelines on how to manage asthma exist but are seldom followed. Asthma is a disease that lends itself well to audit, yet there are hardly any audit studies from India. In one such study of acute severe asthma from the Hinduja Hospital, a large private hospital in Mumbai, an audit revealed a number of deficiencies. The authors looked at the hospital records of 80 asthmatics, admitted for an acute exacerbation of asthma over 18 months. A number of deficiencies were identified, chief amongst these being: the respiratory rate was recorded in only 28% of patients, arterial blood gas measurements were made in only 55% and theophylline levels checked in just 22%. Peak flows were recorded in just 2% of patients and pulmonary function test (PFT) measured in just 43%. More worryingly, errors in management were also highlighted with 20% of hospitalized asthmatics not receiving steroids. Attempts are being made, at local hospital level, to close the audit loop by making recommendations based on this audit and then repeating the audit a few years down

the line. It remains to be seen if such studies actually impact on asthma management or remain academic exercises. We would none the less encourage asthma to be audited in similar fashion at other hospitals in the country, with the audit followed by feedback and implementation of action to close the loop.

In the Community

A study called AIRSA (Asthma insights and realities in South Asia), conducted in 2002 contacted 8000 random households in nine Indian cities (including the big metros like Mumbai, Delhi, Kolkata and Chennai) to identify 403 asthmatics. These had a face to face interview for 45 minutes about their asthma control and treatment. The results highlighted major lacunae in the delivery of treatment and care towards asthmatic patients even in some of India's biggest cities. The survey found that the majority of asthmatics were poorly controlled with 60% of those questioned reporting daytime symptoms and 77% experiencing nocturnal symptoms that disrupted sleep at least once a week in the month prior to the interview. Other reflections of the poor asthma control were that 87% reported limitation in sport and 85% had frequent need for reliever medication in the past month; 27% of adult asthmatics and 53% of children with asthma had missed work or school respectively in the past year due to asthma. Indian doctors seemed to be failing in their duties to their patients; only 58% of patients had actually been taught how to use an inhaler and 10% had a written treatment plan. Only 13% of patients surveyed had even heard of a peak flow meter, only 2% owned one of their own and only 28% of patients had ever had a PFT. The most striking deficiency highlighted by the AIRSA survey was that only 2% of respondents used inhaled corticosteroids for their asthma. Thus the current level of asthma control in India falls far short of the GINA-set optimal goals for long-term asthma management.

Factors Contributing to the Problem of Asthma in India

(a) Asthma is felt to be less of a priority   Asthma is not felt to be a priority in this country with its huge burden of tuberculosis and other infectious diseases. However, its impact on the health of large numbers of Indians must not be underestimated. The global burden of disease as measured by disability adjusted life years (DALY) lost is 3.4 for tuberculosis and a not inconsiderable 0.9 for asthma.

(b) Less healthcare spending on asthma   Raj Singh from Chennai has estimated that if the prevalence of asthma is 5% and the average cost of asthma medication is about 30 US$ per month, 30% of the entire expenditure on health in the country would have to be spent on asthma alone. It is felt that about 10% of patients have access to good quality healthcare, which includes inhalers. However, even less, probably no more than 2% actually use inhalers. If the cost of asthma medication were to be reduced, a greater proportion of those afflicted can be expected to benefit. It is little wonder that the average asthmatic in India still relies on outdated drugs like oral beta-agonists instead of inhaled medication. Table 34.9 looks at what asthma drugs cost the average Indian as a percentage of his monthly income.

Table 34.9: What do asthma drugs cost the average Indian? Per capita Indian income = Rs 11,302 Statistical Outline of India, 2000		
Drug	Cost of 1 month tablets/1 MDI	% monthly income
Oral salbutamol	Rs 12	1.3%
Oral theophylline	Rs 21	2.2%
Salbutamol MDI	Rs 80	8.5%
Budesonide MDI	Rs 214	22%
Nebuliser solution	Rs 1080	115%
Nebuliser	Rs 4000	424%
O_2 Concentrator	Rs 60,000	6369%

(c) Attitudes to health and disease also affect perceptions of asthma in India. Asthmatics are treated differently by many competing systems of medicine in India. Thus, Ayurveda, which is followed by large numbers of Indians believes that asthma is caused by an imbalance in one of the three 'humours': Kapha (phlegm), Pitta (bile) and Vata (gas). It is probably these concepts that affect the misconceptions about food many asthmatics in India have. In a survey from Northern India, 88% of parents of children with asthma felt that food was the primary trigger for their children's asthma. A trial we conducted at the Hinduja Hospital of Ayurvedic drugs in 195 asthmatics in 2001, randomized to receive standard versus Ayurvedic treatment was stopped because only 14% of Ayurvedic patients responded compared to 97% of allopathic patients.

(d) Ignorance and superstition The Hyderabad fish 'treatment' of asthma is another classic example of how superstition and ignorance can combine to hinder the correct medical management of asthma. In this ancient custom, spanning over 150 years, the Murrel fish prepared in a holy well with a herbal cocktail, is forced down the throat of hundreds of thousands of asthmatics desperate for a cure. These gullible and desperate asthmatics throng this venue in Hyderabad on the 7 June each year for three consecutive years. The family administering the drug claims this treatment will cure asthma, provided it is accompanied by a special diet over 45 days.

(e) Poorly trained doctors Poorly trained doctors contribute to 'difficult asthma' in India. An audit by Bedi of asthma treated by general practitioners in Punjab, identified an underuse of inhalers and an overuse of ephedrine.

(f) Lack of access It is estimated that only 10% of asthmatics in India have access to optimal care and less than 2% actually use inhaled medication for their asthma.

Thus clearly the way ahead includes greater public spending on asthma, educating doctors and patients and improving access to inhalers to large parts of the population.

SUGGESTED READING

Agertoft L, Pedersen S. Effect of long-term treatment with inhaled budesonide on adult height in children with asthma. *N Engl J Med.* 2000; 343: 1064–69.

FitzGerald JM. Commentary: intravenous magnesium in severe asthma. *Evid Based Med.* 1999; 4: 138.

Global Initiative for Asthma, Global Strategy for Asthma Management and Prevention, 2009. www.ginaasthma.org

Harrison BDWH, Stokes TC, Hart GJ, *et al.* Need for intravenous hydrocortisone in addition to oral prednisolone in patients admitted to hospital with severe asthma without ventilatory failure. *Lancet.* 1986; 8474: 181–4.

Lazarus SC, *et al.* Long-acting beta2-agonist monotherapy vs continued therapy with inhaled corticosteroids in patients with persistent asthma: a randomized controlled trial. *JAMA.* 2001; 285(20): 2583–93.

Manocha R, Marks GB, Kenchington P, *et al.* Sahaja yoga in the management of moderate to severe asthma: A randomised controlled trial. *Thorax.* 2002; 57: 110–15.

Nelson HS, *et al.* The Salmeterol Multicenter Asthma Research Trial: a comparison of usual pharmacotherapy for asthma or usual pharmacotherapy plus salmeterol. *Chest.* 2006; 129(1): 15–26.

Rodrigo G, Rodrigo C. Inhaled flunisolide for acute severe asthma. *Am J Respir Crit Care Med.* 1998; 157: 698–703.

Rodrigo GJ. Comparison of inhaled fluticasone with intravenous hydrocortisone in the treatment of adult acute asthma. *Am J Respir Crit Care Med.* 2005; 171: 1231–6.

Rowe BH, Bota GW, Fabris L, *et al.* Inhaled budesonide in addition to oral corticosteroids to prevent asthma relapse following discharge from the emergency department: a randomized controlled study. *JAMA.* 1999; 281: 2119–26.

Rowe BH, Spooner CH, Ducharme FM, *et al.* The effectiveness of corticosteroids in the treatment of acute exacerbations of asthma: a meta-analysis of their effect on relapse following acute assessment. *The Cochrane Library. 1998*; Issue 4. Oxford: Update software.

Skoner DP, Maspero J, Banerji D. Assessment of the long-term safety of inhaled ciclesonide on growth in children with asthma. *Pediatrics.* 2008; 121: e1–e14.

Stather DR and Stewart TE. Clinical review: mechanical ventilation in severe asthma. *Critical Care.* 2005; 9: 6: 581–7.

Udwadia ZF. Acute severe asthma in *Principles of Critical Care.* 1995. (ed Udwadia FE) Oxford University Press, 265–71.

Udwadia ZF, Harrison BDWH. An attempt to determine the optimal duration of hospital stay following a severe attack of asthma. *Journal of the Royal College of Physicians of London.* 1990; 24: 2: 112–14.

Walters EH, Walters JA, Gibson MD. Inhaled long acting beta agonists for stable chronic asthma. *Cochrane Database Syst Rev.* 2003(4): CD001385.

Walters JA, Wood-Baker R, Walters EH. Long-acting beta2-agonists in asthma: an overview of Cochrane systematic reviews. *Respir Med.* 2005; 99(4): 384–95.

Weatherall M, *et al.* Meta-analysis of the risk of mortality with salmeterol and the effect of concomitant inhaled corticosteroid therapy. *Thorax.* 2010; 65(1): 39–43.

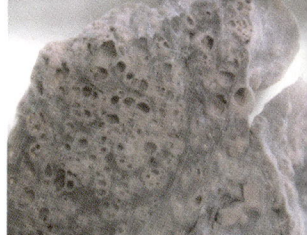

CHAPTER **35** **Asthma: Special Types**

SPECIAL TYPES OF ASTHMA

Difficult Asthma

DEFINITION

Brian Harrison defines difficult asthma as being present in a patient with a confirmed diagnosis of asthma whose symptoms and/or lung function abnormalities remain poorly controlled despite treatment which experience suggests would be effective.

PATHOLOGY

The pathology of severe asthma is distinctive. These patients have persistent airways inflammation and evidence of airway remodelling with structural changes. There is evidence of smooth muscle hypertrophy, thickening of the epithelium and subepithelial fibrosis. Some studies have documented an excess of profibrotic cytokines like TGFβ in the mucosa of the patient with severe and difficult asthma.

How common is it? Fortunately, most asthma is not difficult, but relatively easy to manage. Difficult asthma constitutes only the tip of the asthma iceberg. Of the more than 200 million estimated asthmatics worldwide, only a small fraction can truly be considered difficult. It is however the difficult asthmatic that consumes most in terms of healthcare resources and time.

In Weiss's study showing that the estimated total annual cost of asthma was a staggering US$ 4.5 billion in America in 1992, it was noted that 80% of the costs were attributable to 20% of patients with this problem. Studies from Canada and Australia also revealed that patients with severe and difficult asthma though comprising no more than 10% and 6% of the asthma population accounted for 54% and 40% of the annual cost respectively. Thus the economic burden of asthma is large and derives disproportionately from those with severe disease.

Types of Difficult Asthma

If 'difficult' is defined as 'a task that demands toil or effort, or a problem that is difficult to solve' then a number of types of asthma can be considered to be difficult. Severe asthma is a heterogeneous disease, in which specific severity phenotypes may respond differently to different therapies. The following clinical phenotypes of asthma can be included under 'difficult asthma':

ACUTE SEVERE ASTHMA

Nothing can be more difficult than managing a patient with severe life-threatening asthma in an intensive care unit (ICU).

BRITTLE ASTHMA

Brittle asthma is defined as a form of asthma that causes little or no problem on most days but is associated with frequent

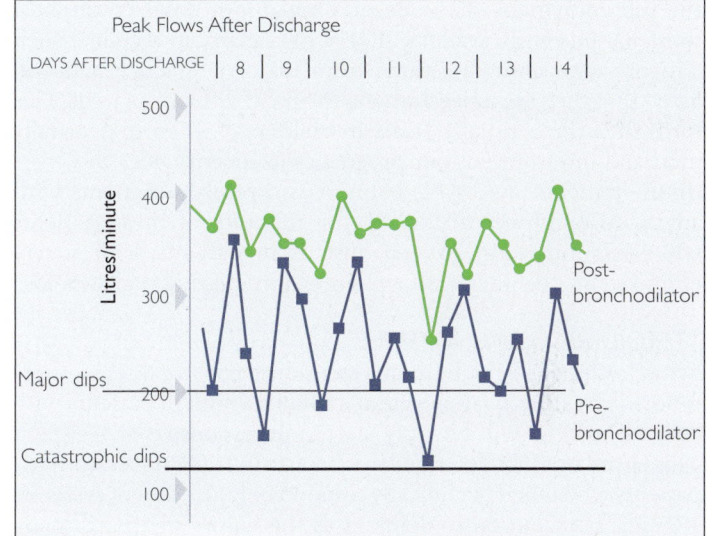

Fig 35.1: PEF in a patient with brittle asthma: These hectic dips in PEF were even more striking when noted that they began just 8 days following discharge from hospital for an acute attack. This lady was readmitted a few days later.

severe attacks requiring unscheduled hospital or physician visits or frequent courses of oral steroids. A common feature in brittle asthma is the apparent difficulty in controlling the variability in airway function as shown in Figure 35.1.

Fortunately, brittle asthma is not common, it has a prevalence of 0.05% of all asthma. A possible genetic component is present in brittle asthma; 50% of patients have lost a first-degree relative from asthma.

Two types of brittle asthma are recognized:

Type 1   Characterized by chaotic peak-flow variability for more than 50% of the time for at least 150 days, despite maximal medical treatment. This type is more likely to occur in females. The majority are atopic, with at least one positive skin-prick test. Pet allergies are common and premenstrual factors may contribute in some women with Type 1 brittle asthma.

Type 2   Characterized by sudden attacks becoming severe within minutes, against a background of apparently good control. This type has no sex predilection. This form of severe asthma is even more rare. Attacks can occur with catastrophic speed and are believed to be Immunoglobulin E (IgE)-mediated.

Both types are difficult to treat and carry a greatly increased risk of death. Multiple hospitalizations and frequent need for mechanical ventilation characterizes both types. Subcutaneous

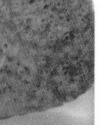

terbutaline, driven by a syringe pump is an intervention that has been found to be of benefit in some patients with brittle asthma. Brittle asthma is really the prototype of difficult asthma and no form of asthma has such a profound impact on the lives, work and psyche of the asthmatic. Psychological disturbance develops in the majority of these patients as shall be discussed later.

CHRONIC ASTHMA

Chronic asthma is another clinical phenotype of difficult asthma. This type of asthma rarely causes severe exacerbations but is 'difficult' by virtue of it causing symptoms that interfere with the full enjoyment of life despite maximum doses of the best therapies currently available. Every physician can recollect such patients with chronic asthma from his own practice and will agree that they are indeed among the most difficult to treat. This form of asthma usually starts in childhood when it is usually mild and intermittent, but progresses in severity over the years till the patients are disabled almost as severely as patients with advanced emphysema. Indeed, the majority of these patients will need long-term oxygen, just as in patients with severe emphysema, together with a maintenance dose of oral steroids.

STEROID-RESISTANT ASTHMA

While asthma is by definition a steroid-responsive disease, there is now increasing awareness that a small fraction of patients with difficult asthma will be truly steroid-unresponsive or resistant. This entity was first described by Shwartz in 1968 in six asthmatic patients who failed to clinically respond to high doses of systemic steroids. He went on to define it as the failure of an asthmatic to improve his forced expiratory volume in one second (FEV1) by 15%, despite an adequate dose of steroid (equivalent of 40 mg prednisolone), with assured compliance, for an adequate duration (two weeks), despite demonstrating > 15% reversibility to an inhaled β_2-agonist. Primary glucocorticosteroid (GCS) resistance is a genetic syndrome, which occurs due to either reduced GCS receptor binding affinity or due to abnormally low numbers of GCS receptors. There is increased activating peptide-1 (AP1) activity in steroid-resistant asthma. AP1 is a transcription factor complex, which is pertinent to asthmatic inflammation. At a cellular level, steroid-resistant asthma is characterized by impaired *in vitro* and *in vivo* responsiveness of monocytes and T-lymphocytes to the suppressive effects of glucocorticosteroids. Secondary GCS resistance is more common and is due to factors like decreased absorption of steroids or increased metabolism due to interaction with other drugs like rifampicin or carbamazapine.

The importance of recognizing an asthmatic to have steroid resistance is considerable. Early identification can lead to institution of alternative therapies. If on the other hand, steroid resistance remains unrecognized, they continue to be treated with high doses of oral steroid with no clinical benefit but considerable cumulative toxicity. These patients often have a good response to long-acting beta-agonists (LABAs) and theophylline and these drugs along with steroid-sparing agents like methotrexate and cyclosporin may be tried.

Approach to the Difficult Asthmatic

A difficult asthmatic requires specialist referral and investigations that encompass the full range of respiratory, imaging, and allergy testing. A multidisciplinary approach is recommended, with close coordination between ear, nose and throat (ENT) colleagues, psychiatrists and counsellors offering psychiatric and psychological assessment, and respiratory physicians deciding on therapy. In the West this is often served by 'difficult asthma clinics' where these patients are carefully assessed. In an interesting study by Heaney from one such difficult asthma clinic at a referral hospital in the UK, of the 80 patients referred with 'therapy-resistant' asthma, 95% were found to have an ENT abnormality, 57% had gastroesophageal reflux disease (GERD), 50% had an ICD-10 (The International Statistical Classification of Diseases and Related Health Problems 10th Revision) psychiatric diagnosis, 30% had an additional diagnosis, which was bronchiectasis in nine patients, chronic obstructive pulmonary disease (COPD) in three and vocal cord dysfunction in three. Indeed, one patient did not have asthma at all despite all the referrals to this clinic having come from chest departments from peripheral hospitals with a chest physician confirming the diagnosis of 'asthma with persisting refractory symptoms'.

Monitoring the Difficult Asthmatic

This is one type of asthma where meticulous monitoring might be rewarded by a reduction in hospitalizations and morbidity. Induced sputum eosinophilia, exhaled nitrogen oxide (NO) levels and other markers of inflammation have all been studied in this group of difficult asthmatics. Exhaled NO has been found to be a reliable, non-invasive and easily measured marker with increasing values serving as a good predictive marker for poor asthma control. Sputum eosinophilia may also be an invaluable marker in further phenotyping severe asthmatics into eosinophilic or neutrophilic categories with the former showing a good response to biological therapies like mepolizumab, an anti interleukin-6 (IL-5) agent, which has been discussed earlier.

Approach to Evaluating the Difficult Asthmatic

We would recommend the following 10-point approach when faced with a difficult asthmatic:

1. Question and re-establish the very diagnosis of asthma: spirometry, flow volume loops, methacholine challenge, and tests of airway conductance and resistance may all be used for this purpose.
2. If there is still any doubt, high-resolution computed tomography (HRCT) and fibreoptic bronchoscopy may be needed.
3. Check for coexisting conditions, cardio-pulmonary diseases like associated bronchiectasis, COPD, Churg-Strauss syndrome or left ventricular dysfunction.
4. Establish if the asthma is 'difficult' because of genuine disease factors: e.g. brittle asthma, steroid resistance etc.
5. If not, is the asthma difficult because of 'doctor'-related factors: being inappropriately treated or undertreated.
6. Are patient-related factors to blame? Is the patient compliant with regard to his therapy? Most often 'difficult' asthma boils down to the patient being noncompliant with his inhaled steroid because he is concerned about potential side-effects. All that is needed in this situation

is to stress the importance and safety of these drugs and spend some time re-educating him. A psychiatric and psychosocial evaluation should be considered in all such patients. Harrison has stressed that underlying depression, denial, personality problems, socioeconomic deprivation, employment problems, marital problems and substance abuse can be found in a significant numbers of these patients and may contribute to the difficulty in controlling their asthma. He has stressed the importance of listening to their problems and concerns and offering sympathy and understanding which may be at least as important as escalating treatment in some of them.

7. Specifically question the contribution of GERD and sinus disease. Both of these have been discussed earlier. Consider 24-hour ambulatory pH monitoring and CT scanning of the sinuses.
8. Check if environmental and occupational factors are worsening the asthma.
9. Are drug-related factors worsening asthma?
10. Finally, are hormonal factors worsening asthma? In significant numbers of women, menstrual factors can contribute to asthma.

Managing the Difficult Asthmatic

The majority of these patients will be on Step 4 treatment, with many requiring in addition oral maintenance doses of steroids. Here too, there are unanswered questions about opting for frequent intermittent high-dose courses each time they exacerbate versus settling for a daily, regular maintenance dose. The risk-benefit comparison of these two strategies in the difficult asthmatic with frequent exacerbations has not been evaluated. What is also unclear is whether there is any clear difference between the different types of oral steroids in terms of long-term side-effects. Another unanswered question is whether the route of administration (oral versus injectable) makes a difference. An interesting recent study by Brinke looked at the role of a single intramuscular dose of triamcinolone in 22 patients with severe asthma who had remained uncontrolled despite > 4 courses of oral steroids in the preceding year. They found that this strategy not only normalized sputum eosinophilia and improved post-bronchodilator FEV1, but also decreased the use of rescue medicine in the following six months. Other studies have looked at high doses of inhaled corticosteroids with fourfold or even much higher than normal doses sometimes re-establishing control. Rodrigo's study showed that repeated and high doses of inhaled fluticasone (3000 μg/hour, administered through an MDI and spacer at 10-minute intervals for three hours) were more effective than intravenous hydrocortisone in acute severe asthma with more rapid onset of action and a greater response.

This is the group of patients where omalizumab and the other biological therapies discussed earlier may have a real role. A variety of non-steroidal agents have also been looked at in this patient group, with agents like methotrexate, troleandomycin, telithromycin, macrolides and cyclosporine all being considered. A Cochrane analysis of two of these agents, methotrexate and cyclosporine A has shown a small benefit, but perhaps certain phenotypes would respond better to one or more of these agents.

A novel and exciting new intervention, bronchial thermoplasty has also recently emerged. This involves controlled thermal energy (at 65°C) being applied via the fibreoptic bronchoscope to the bronchial wall in an attempt to reduce smooth muscle mass. Results of a recent trial by Castro of 288 patients where this procedure was compared to a sham procedure showed it improved asthma-specific quality of life with a reduction in severe exacerbations and healthcare utilization in the post-treatment period. The procedure is done with intravenous sedation in three sessions, about a month apart. The bronchi in the lower lobe of one lung, then the lower lobe of the other lung and finally in both upper lobes together are tackled over the three sessions, each lasting about 30–60 minutes. While fears have been raised about the safety of the procedure in patients with severe asthma, the study by Castro found it well tolerated. Finally, patients with severe asthma increasingly turn to alternative therapies like yoga, acupuncture and behavioural therapy, which prove helpful in the occasional patient.

Fatal and Near-Fatal Asthma (NFA)

Historically, asthma was not considered a fatal disease. Osler declared: 'the asthmatic pants into old age'. Yet, it is now evident that many patients will die of their asthma, some in their youth. No Indian data are available but there are 2000 deaths in a small country like the UK from asthma annually. This works out to almost 1 death from asthma every 4 hours. In the US, deaths from asthma doubled from 0.6 per 100, 000 in 1977 to 1.4 per 100, 000 in 1984. Indeed one of the unanswered paradoxes of asthma is why, despite better understanding of the disease and better drugs, asthma mortality is still on the rise when the mortality of all other non-malignant chronic diseases has declined. Possible explanations for this asthma paradox include increasing incidence of atopy and house dust mite allergen, increasing air pollution, and inappropriate use of inhaled β-2-agonists. None of these on their own are likely to be the real explanation, which is probably that there is a problem in delivering the most crucial disease-modifying agents, inhaled corticosteroids, to the vast majority of asthmatics who need these drugs. A survey by Watson from 24 developing countries in Asia and Africa showed that inhaled steroids were not used by almost 93% of respondents, primarily due to purely economic constraints. As one doctor wrote in his response to Watson's questionnaire: 'The poor die, the rich live, matter of cash, really sad.' Of course it is not only economics that dictate why asthmatics die, for they also die in significant numbers in the developed world. To understand the causes of death here we have to turn to asthma death audits and confidential enquiries. In a review of seven asthma death audits from the UK and one from New Zealand, there were a few messages that came through clearly. Harrison succinctly summarized these under the following three headings:

1. DOCTORS fail to assess the severity of asthma because they fail to make objective measurements (PEF, SaO_2, ABG).
2. PATIENTS fail to appreciate the severity of their asthma and fail to make the measurements they are meant to (PEF). This is because significant numbers of asthmatics under-perceive their asthma and get accustomed to experiencing severe attacks.

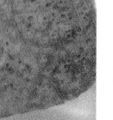

3. As a result of 1 and 2, under-use of the most effective asthma medication, steroids (inhaled and oral) is very common.

Overall, potentially treatable factors occurred in 86% of the patients dying from asthma. An asthma death is always a cause for introspection. Here is a disease, which is by definition meant to be reversible, going on to result in a fatality, that too in a young and productive member of society. What makes it even more poignant is the observation that the vast majority of such deaths could have been prevented.

The factors that come up repeatedly in the asthma audits have been summarized in Table 35.1.

Table 35.1:
Factors contributing to death in asthma death audits
PATIENT RELATED FACTORS:
Most patients dying of asthma have had previous admissions
Most give a long history of asthma
Adverse psychosocial factors found to have been present in significant numbers
Most are poorly compliant with their medications especially ICS
Most tend to over rely and use their reliever inhaler (short-acting β_2 agonists like salbutamol and terbutaline)
Patients become accustomed to a degree of disability
Not all patients with severe obstruction feel unwell
The fatal attack of asthma has often persisted for days or even weeks before admission: 50% were waking up 5 nights a week in the week prior to death and 35% were waking up that often for 1 month prior to the eventually fatal admission
Under use of PEF meters
Delays in reaching hospital
The overwhelming majority of deaths occur at home
DOCTOR RELARED FACTORS:
Doctors underestimate the severity of the attack
Doctors fail to make objective measurements
Underuse of steroids
Underuse of agonists
Overuse of agonists
Injudicious use of sedation
Wrong use of drugs like β blockers and NSAIDs
Failure to monitor theophylline
Uncorrected hypokalemia
Delays instituting mechanical ventilation
Unrecognized complications of mechanical ventilation

Lessons Arising from the Asthma Death Audits

The studies of asthma deaths from New Zealand and the US and the results of the confidential enquiry into asthma deaths

Table 35.2:
Patients at risk of developing fatal or near-fatal asthma (from New Zealand and US death audits and UK confidential enquiries)
Previous life threatening attacks
Severe disease
Hospital admission in the previous year
Unscheduled ER visits in the previous year
Patient non-compliance
Psychosocial problems
Behavioural problems especially denial
Socioeconomic deprivation
3 or more categories of asthmatic drugs prescribed
Requiring frequent courses of oral steroids
Requiring high dose inhaled steroids
Requiring 2 or more canisters of a bronchodilator monthly
Discontinuity of medical care

from East Anglia in the UK, led to the list in Table 35.2 describing the characteristics of a patient at risk of developing a fatal or a near-fatal attack of asthma.

The way ahead lies in Education. Education, not just of patients, but also of doctors and family physicians is of crucial importance. The patient who dies of fatal asthma has been getting up for several nights in the week prior to his eventual death. Recognizing the gravity of this and intervening with a short oral course of steroid might save the lives of such patients. Patients at increased risk of developing fatal or near-fatal asthma can and should be identified. It is this group that needs extra attention and focus even in a busy outpatient department.

These efforts seem to be paying off and there is now light at the end of the tunnel. Despite the increased prevalence of asthma, deaths from asthma over the last two decades seem to be on the decline in many developed countries. This decline has been noticed in all age groups, but particularly in those under the age of 65 years. Special approaches and management strategies in these, the most difficult and challenging of all asthmatics need to be prioritized.

The Pregnant Asthmatic

Asthma is a disease that often complicates pregnancy. Recent studies show that 1–4% of pregnancies may be complicated by asthma. Pregnant women have a higher incidence of adverse maternal and foetal outcomes, and are hence a high-risk group that needs to be carefully monitored and optimally treated.

PHYSIOLOGICAL CHANGES DURING PREGNANCY

Pregnancy results in enhanced production of progesterone, oestradiol and cortisol. Progesterone specifically increases minute ventilation and decreases pulmonary vascular resistance. Changes in lung function noted in pregnancy include reduced functional residual capacity (FRC), reduced residual volume, and reduced total lung capacity. These changes occur even before significant uterine enlargement implying non-direct physiological effects.

FEV_1, and FEV_1/forced vital capacity (FVC) are unaffected by pregnancy hence any change in these parameters can be assumed to be due to respiratory pathology. Minute ventilation can increase by 20–40% and this results in changes in arterial blood gases. The PaO_2 rises to 100–105 mmHg, whilst $PaCO_2$ falls to 32–34 mmHg. The pH is maintained by renal compensation with increased excretion of bicarbonate. Breathlessness is often present in pregnancy, especially in the last trimester and is due to increased work of breathing or increased respiratory drive. Nasal stuffiness is common in pregnancy, due to a combination of nasal hyperemia and oedema and may add to the perceived difficulty in breathing.

EFFECTS OF PREGNANCY ON ASTHMA

Pregnancy can have varying effects on asthma. A third of all asthmatics will worsen, a third actually improve and a third remain unaffected. The same pattern is usually repeated for the pregnant asthmatic in her subsequent pregnancies. Asthma control is often at its worst at the start of the third trimester with the asthma reassuming its pre-pregnancy level about three months post-delivery. Studies show that the severity and duration of asthma attacks are no different in pregnant asthmatics compared to their non-pregnant counterparts, but due to the reluctance of pregnant patients to commence corticosteroids, they have a threefold increased chance of suffering ongoing exacerbations.

EFFECTS OF ASTHMA ON THE MOTHER

Maternal complications associated with uncontrolled asthma include pre-ecclampsia, placenta previa, gestational hypertension, hyperemesis gravidarum, vaginal haemorrhage, toxaemia, induced and complicated labour, increased caesarean sections and prolonged maternal hospital stay. A study showed that asthmatic females have an odds ratio of 1.6 to 2.2 for each of these complications compared to non-asthmatic females.

EFFECTS OF ASTHMA ON THE FOETUS

Oxygenated foetal blood is normally very low in PaO_2 but because of a remarkable compensatory mechanism this is well tolerated (high foetal haemoglobin concentration, leftward shift in oxygen-haemoglobin disassociation curve, a high foetal cardiac output). Critical respiratory disease in the mother such as an asthma exacerbation results in a fall in maternal PaO_2 and a profound decrease in foetal PaO_2 and tissue oxygenation. As the mother gets hypoxemic during a severe asthma exacerbation, maternal compensatory mechanisms will maintain oxygenation to vital maternal organs at the cost of uterine blood flow. Hence foetal distress can occur even in the absence of obvious maternal hypoxia or hypotension. Foetal complications reported during uncontrolled asthma include increased risk of prenatal mortality, intrauterine growth retardation, low birth weight, preterm birth and neonatal hypoxia.

MANAGEMENT OF ASTHMA DURING PREGNANCY

The treatment of asthma in pregnancy is no different from that in a non-pregnant asthmatic. Of course, the benefit from each medication must be shown to outweigh its possible risk. Having said this, we have seen too many pregnant asthmatics treated sub-optimally because of perceived fears of the side-effects of asthma medication on the foetus. It must be stressed to the patient apprehensive about taking her drugs that the greatest risk is from uncontrolled asthma and not the drugs. Inhaled and oral steroids may safely be used depending on the situation and inhaled short- and long-acting β_2-agonists are also safe. Oral beta-agonists are best avoided near term as they may cause hypoglycaemia and palpitation. Epinephrine is also best avoided as it may cause vasoconstriction in the uterus and reduce utero-placental flow. Theophylline may be used, provided its levels are monitored and it is kept at the lower limit of normal. Not enough is known about the leukotriene modifiers to recommend them safely at present.

The Asthmatic with Premenstrual Worsening

A small group of women with asthma may have severe, sometimes catastrophic, worsening in their asthma just prior to their menstrual period. This correlates with falling progesterone levels and increasing oestrogen to progesterone ratios. Progesterone is meant to have anti-inflammatory properties, hence its decrease before menstruation could worsen asthma in some patients. Such patients may also demonstrate some degree of steroid resistance. It is vital to recognize this potential link with menstruation in the young asthmatic who has cyclical exacerbations of her asthma. Hormonal treatment with progesterone, usually in depot preparations through the intramuscular route (Depo-Provera) works best in this setting. Recently, goserelin, a gonadotrophin-releasing (GnRH) analogue has been shown to be effective. On occasion, oopherectomy is the only way to control the catastrophic deterioration in asthma associated with menstruation in some asthmatics.

The Asthmatic Undergoing Anaesthesia

It is imperative to ensure that the asthmatic goes into surgery with his or her asthma optimally controlled. In a recent study examining almost 18,000 day-care surgeries, asthma was present in 5.7% of all patients and these patients had an approximately fivefold increase in the risk of developing postoperative respiratory adverse effects. Intubation and anaesthesia have the potential to induce bronchospasm and worsen pre-existing asthma. Adverse effects included unanticipated admission to ICU, prolonged postoperative stay and unscheduled readmission because of worsening asthma. Poorly controlled and severe asthma, thoracic and upper abdominal surgeries, and general anaesthesia involving tracheal intubation were associated with more perioperative problems in asthmatics. Pulmonary function test (PFT) must be checked prior to the surgery and if found to be poor or if bronchospasm is present preoperatively, it is beat to delay the surgery (if elective) till the asthma is optimally controlled with bronchodilators and even a short course of oral steroids if necessary. Intravenous hydrocortisone should be given to the asthmatic a few hours prior to surgery if preoperative FEV1 is low. Nebulized β_2-agonist should be administered just prior to shifting the patient to the operating theatre and continued in the postoperative period. Close monitoring of the patient by the anaesthetist perioperatively, and the physician postoperatively, is recommended.

Aspirin-Induced Asthma (AIA)

Cases of violent bronchospasm following ingestion of aspirin began to be reported shortly after introduction of aspirin into

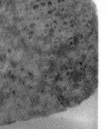

therapy well over a century ago. The association of aspirin sensitivity, asthma and nasal polyposis was first described by Widal in 1922. It was subsequently realized that many other non-steroidal anti-inflammatory drugs (NSAIDs) shared with aspirin the potential to trigger asthma in sensitive patients.

PATHOGENESIS

Allergic Mechanisms Because clinical reactions triggered by aspirin are reminiscent of immediate type hypersensitivity reactions an underlying antigen-antibody mechanism has been suggested. However, skin tests with aspirin are negative and attempts to demonstrate specific antibodies to aspirin have been unsuccessful.

CYCLOOXYGENASE THEORY

This theory proposes that precipitation of asthma attacks by aspirin is not based on antigen-antibody reactions, but stems from the pharmacological action of the drug: namely, specific inhibition in the respiratory tract of the enzyme cyclooxygenase (COX). This enzyme is central to the mechanism of AIA. This would explain why NSAIDs with anti-COX activity invariably precipitate bronchospasm while those that do not affect COX activity do not provoke bronchospasm. It is now known that the COX enzyme exists in at least two isoforms, COX_1 and COX_2 encoded by distinct genes. Aspirin, indomethacin and piroxicam, which can all trigger AIA in small doses, are all more potent COX_1 inhibitors. Specific COX_2 inhibitors (eteroxib) and NSAIDs that are more potent COX_2 than COX_1 inhibitors, like nimesulide and meloxicam are generally well tolerated.

LEUKOTRIENE PATHWAY

Over recent years, the cys-LTs have emerged as major mediators of AIA. In most patients with AIA, basal excretion of cys-LT in the urine is elevated and increases further upon aspirin administration. In addition, following aspirin challenge there is a release of cys-LT into both the nasal cavity and bronchial tree. The terminal enzyme for cys-LT production is LTC4 synthase. In bronchial biopsies from patients with AIA, the expression of this enzyme is fivefold higher than in asthmatics who tolerate aspirin and nineteen-fold higher than in normal subjects.

CLINICAL FEATURES

AIA is a clear-cut syndrome with a distinct clinical picture. Aspirin intolerance is clearly under-diagnosed in the asthmatic population. Based on history alone, it is estimated that 3–5% of adult asthmatics are aspirin-sensitive. This percentage rises to 6–15% if asthmatics are challenged with aspirin. Many asthmatics who test positive after an aspirin provocation test were unaware of aspirin intolerance prior to the test.

The classic triad of AIA is asthma, nasal polyposis and aspirin sensitivity. Rhinitis is the first symptom to develop. It is perennial, difficult to treat, accompanied by sinusitis and may lead to loss of smell in 50% of patients. In the average patient, asthma starts about two years later and intolerance to aspirin and NSAIDs is evident four years later. Apart from triggering nasal discharge and acute severe bronchospasm, aspirin can trigger skin manifestations like urticaria and a scarlet flush in 20% of patients, angioedema in 8% of patients and violent anaphylactoid reactions with shock, hypotension and loss of consciousness in about 5% of patients. Females outnumber males by a ratio of 2.3:1 in most series, with symptoms starting earlier in females than males. Asthma runs a protracted course despite the avoidance of aspirin and cross-reactive drugs.

TREATMENT

Treatment centres around avoidance of aspirin and all NSAIDs as patients with AIA can develop severe and occasionally fatal attacks with not just aspirin but a variety of NSAIDs. The likelihood of an NSAID triggering an asthma attack in these patients correlates with the drug's anticyclooxygenase potency and the dosage. If necessary, patients with AIA can tolerate paracetamol in a dose not exceeding 1000 mg. If an NSAID must be given, a COX_2 inhibitor like rofecoxib is generally felt to be safer.

Several trials have shown that chronic treatment with a leukotriene antagonist may be protective. However, individual AIA cases have been reported who developed bronchospasm after taking NSAID despite being on treatment with montelukast. Inhaled corticosteroids and intranasal fluticasone are also protective. A state of aspirin tolerance can be induced and maintained by aspirin desensitization. Small incremental doses of aspirin are ingested over the course of a few days until 400–650 mg of aspirin is tolerated. Aspirin can then be administered daily, with doses of 80–325 mg used to maintain desensitization. After each dose of aspirin there is a refractory period during which NSAIDs can be taken. This is important in patients with AIA who have chronic arthritis and rheumatic disease in whom these drugs are regularly needed. Nasal inflammatory disease responds best to this strategy, with a study showing that aspirin desensitization delayed re-occurrence of nasal polyp formation by an average of six years in patients who had just completed sinus and polyp surgery.

SUGGESTED READING

Ayres JG, Miles JF, Barnes PJ. Brittle asthma. *Thorax*. 1998; 53: 315–21.

Castro M, Rubin AS, Laviolette M, *et al.* Effectiveness and safety of bronchial thermoplasty in the treatment of severe asthma. *Am J Respir Crit Care Med*. 2010; 181: 116–24.

Demissie K, Breckenridge MB, Rhoads GG. Infant and maternal outcomes in the pregnancies of asthmatic women. *Am J Respir Crit Care Med*. 1998; 158: 1091–5.

Harrison BDW. Difficult asthma. *Thorax*. 2003; 58: 555–6.

Heaney LG, Conway E, Kelly C, *et al.* Predictors of therapy resistant asthma: outcome of a systematic evaluation protocol. *Thorax*. 2003; 58: 7: 561–6.

Schatz M. Asthma during pregnancy: interrelationships and management. *Ann Allergy*. 1992; 68: 123–33.

Watson JP, Lewis RA. Is asthma affordable in developing countries? *Thorax*. 1997; 52: 605–7.

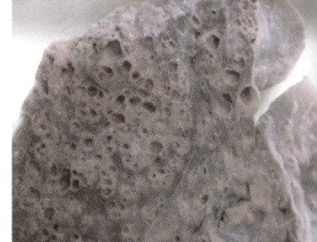

CHAPTER **36**

Chronic Obstructive Pulmonary Disease: Epidemiology, Aetiopathogenesis, Clinical Features, Diagnosis and Imaging

INTRODUCTION

Chronic obstructive pulmonary disease (COPD) is a preventable, treatable, yet progressive inflammatory respiratory disease characterized by airflow limitation which is not fully reversible. COPD is a generic term which holds within it separate disease entities, often producing similar overlapping clinical features.

It is important to elaborate upon key words in the above definition. The disease is considered to be preventable because cigarette smoking (and in India also bidi smoking) is the most important causative risk factor, so that not smoking would sharply reduce its prevalence. Yet COPD does occur in non-smokers and the importance of other risk factors (some of which are to an extent preventable) are being increasingly recognized.

It is important to stress the word 'treatable' with reference to COPD as in the past the disease was considered irreversible and hopeless in its prognosis. This was because patients came for treatment late in the natural history of the disease, at a point in time where treatment was of little or no help. It is now recognized that COPD may be partially reversible and that diagnosis and current treatment at an early stage can and does offer significant relief and benefit to the patient. Yet the disease is not truly curable and in fact is progressive at varying rates in different individuals. The definition given above hinges on the phrase 'airflow limitation which is not completely reversible.' This stresses the underlying disturbance in lung function. The hidden clinical message underlying this phrase is that patients with COPD invariably have breathlessness on exertion and in severe cases breathlessness at rest.

COPD AND ASTHMA

A major difficulty is in distinguishing COPD from bronchial asthma, a disease characterized by airways obstruction which is often completely reversible. Yet patients with longstanding asthma may show lesser and lesser degree of reversibility and some may ultimately end up showing little or no reversibility whatsoever. Asthmatics, with little or no reversibility may be indistinguishable from patients with COPD. Similarly, patients with COPD who show a fair degree of reversibility in their airways obstruction may be difficult to distinguish from asthmatics. There is also a great similarity and overlap in the physiological disturbances underlying chronic asthma and COPD, as also between acute severe asthma and an acute exacerbation of

COPD. Finally, COPD and asthma may coexist; patients with asthma who smoke or are exposed to noxious particles or gases may go on to develop poorly reversible or irreversible airflow limitation. Airflow limitation or airways obstruction (there is a subtle difference between the two terms as is explained later) can therefore be considered as a spectrum; at one end is complete reversibility and at the other end is irreversibility. Patients often fall in between these two ends, there being an overlap at times between asthma and COPD.

ATOPY AND AIRWAY HYPERRESPONSIVENESS

The Dutch Hypothesis

In 1960 Dutch workers hypothesized that COPD patients with severe, nearly fixed airflow limitation and asthmatics shared a common constitutional predisposition of atopy, airway hyperresponsiveness and eosinophilia. This was contrary to Fletcher's findings that failed to show a relationship between the presence of allergy and an accelerated decline in forced expiratory volume in one second (FEV_1) in smokers. Studies in middle-aged smokers have however shown a relationship between airway hyperresponsiveness (as judged by methacholine or histamine test) and an accelerated decline in FEV_1. COPD patients also have an increase in Immunoglobulin E (IgE) and some degree of eosinophilia though this is much less than in asthmatics. There is however, no evidence of atopy (as judged by skin tests) in COPD patients. It is

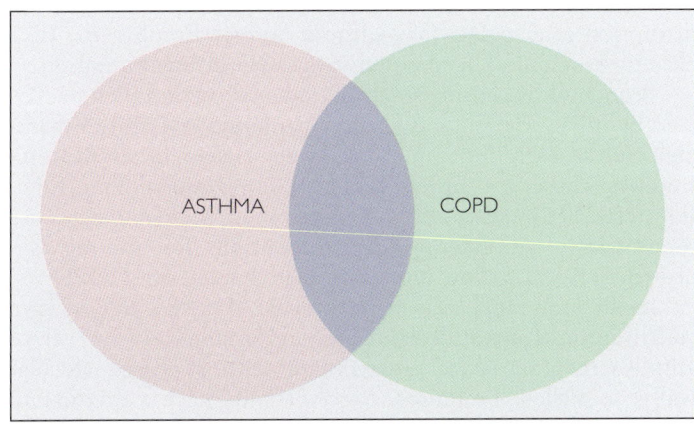

Fig 36.1: Overlap seen in some patients with asthma and COPD.

Table 36.1:
Differences between asthma and COPD

	Asthma	COPD
Aetiology	Sensitizing allergen	Smoking, other noxious particles or gases
Pathology	An inflammatory disease—chiefly eosinophilic infiltrate + CD4 lymphocytes	An inflammatory disease chiefly macrophages, CD8 lymphocytes, neutrophils in the cellular exudate
Disturbances in function	Significant exacerbations of airflow limitation with good or even complete reversibility	Airflow limitation which may worsen during acute exacerbation Not completely reversible—can be poorly reversible or irreversible
Bronchical hyperactivity	Marked (as judged by bronchial provocation tests)	Poor or absent in most patients
Family history	Often present	Not present
Skin allergy	Often present	Not present

debatable whether airway hyperresponsiveness is a cause or an important contributory factor to COPD as the Dutch maintain, or whether airway hyperresponsiveness is the result of COPD, as is believed by others.

It has been mentioned that COPD is a generic name inclusive of other disease entities. These disease entities are chronic bronchitis, small airways obstruction and emphysema. Whereas the defining feature of COPD is airflow limitation, chronic bronchitis is defined in clinical terms; bronchiolitis (causing small airways obstruction) and emphysema are defined in terms of pathological findings.

DEFINITIONS

Chronic bronchitis is clinically (though arbitrarily) defined as chronic cough with sputum on most days for at least three months in each of two consecutive years, when any other cause of chronic cough has been excluded. Chronic bronchitis need not necessarily cause airflow limitation. It can be classified into simple bronchitis characterized by hypersecretion of mucus; mucopurulent bronchitis characterized by recurrent or chronic mucopurulent sputum and obstructive bronchitis where productive cough is associated with airways obstruction.

Emphysema is defined as abnormal permanent enlargement of airspaces distal to terminal bronchioles accompanied by the disruption of alveolar walls without fibrosis. Emphysema (like chronic bronchitis) need not always cause airflow limitation.

Bronchiolitis causing small airways obstruction is characterized by inflammation and fibrosis in airways < 2 mm in diameter. Subtle early inflammatory changes occur in all cigarette smokers; these are undetectable by conventional lung function tests. Yet in susceptible smokers, these subtle changes are progressively amplified, being responsible for the airways obstruction and airflow limitation that characterize COPD.

In an individual case it is difficult to assess the relative contribution of airway disease (large and/or small airways) versus emphysema (air space enlargement with ruptured alveolar walls) to airflow limitation. Most patients have a mixture of both these contributing factors—some more of one and some more of the other. The term COPD was coined in the 1960s to denote airflow limitation from a combination of airway disease and emphysema without assigning the contribution of each of these to the airflow limitation.

The American Thoracic Society and the European Respiratory Society in their statement on the standards for diagnosis and care of patients with COPD have defined the disease as 'a preventable and treatable disease characterized by airflow limitation that is not fully reversible. The airflow limitation is usually progressive and is associated with an abnormal inflammatory response in the lungs to noxious particles or gases, primarily to cigarette smoke. Although COPD affects the lungs it also produces significant systemic consequences' . The Global Initiative for Chronic Obstructive Pulmonary Disease (GOLD) has put forth a similar definition stressing the abnormal inflammatory response of the lung to noxious particles or gases and that extrapulmonary events and co-morbidities may contribute to the severity of the disease in individual patients.

There are two points that need to be stressed before discussion of the epidemiology, pathology, pathophysiology and clinical features of COPD.

1. COPD is not just a disease confined to the lungs; it is in a way a systemic disease with a number of co-morbidities that influence the severity of the illness. These co-morbidities

Table 36.2:
Comorbidities of COPD

Weight loss
Loss of lean muscle mass
Skeletal muscle dysfunction
Osteoporosis
Sleep disorder
Anaemia
Psychosocial problems, in particular anxiety, depression
Association of ischemic heart disease, diabetes, acid peptic disease

are listed below and include weight loss with significant loss of lean muscle as the disease progresses. (Table 36.2).

2. A number of other conditions such as bronchiectasis, bronchiolitis obliterans, cystic fibrosis and sarcoidosis which cause airways obstruction should not be considered under COPD but should be considered in the differential diagnosis. Similarly, burnt out or active tuberculosis with inflammatory damage to the airways, or airway obstruction secondary to or a sequel of any other infective or obstructive pathology is not to be considered under COPD. (Table 36.3).

Yet COPD could well co-exist with many of these other diseases which cause airways obstruction. In many developing countries, including India, several Asian and South American countries, tuberculosis and COPD may both be present in many patients, as risk factors for both these diseases are strongly prevalent. In patients with both these diseases each would be expected to contribute to the degree of pulmonary disability. However, there is little recent information on the result of the interaction between these two common diseases. Earlier works suggest that the degree of airways obstruction in patients treated for tuberculosis increases with age, the number of cigarettes smoked and the extent of initial tuberculous disease.

Table 36.3:
Pathologies other than COPD that can present with chronic airways obstruction and which should be distinguished from COPD
Bronchiectasis
Sarcoidosis
Tuberculosis
Bronchiolitis obliterans
Cystic fibrosis
Other burnt-out infective pathologies
Tropical Eosinophilia
Langerhans' cell histiocytosis (Histiocytosis X)
Lymphangioleiomyomatosis

EPIDEMIOLOGY

COPD is a significant cause of worldwide morbidity and mortality. Both are clearly on the rise. In 1990, COPD was the 12th leading cause of morbidity and the sixth leading cause of death in the world. In 2002, it was the sixth leading cause of morbidity and the fourth leading cause of death. It is projected that by 2020 COPD will be the fifth leading cause of disability and the third leading cause of death worldwide, the first two leading causes being ischemic heart disease and cerebrovascular disease. Its upward climb on the ladder of morbidity and mortality is greater than any of the other chronic diseases.

The prevalence of COPD varies in different countries but is almost certainly more than what is reported. The reasons for this are obvious—for one, in spite of current standard definitions of

the disease, there are different concepts of COPD, particularly in Asian countries; also, spirometric studies to confirm the diagnosis of COPD are often lacking. Diagnosis is often made only when the disease is clinically evident, by which time it is already moderately advanced. Patients with early COPD with few or no symptoms therefore go undetected.

Reports on the prevalence of the disease depend on the method used for survey. In Western countries, prevalence based on the self-reporting of a doctor was as low as < 6% of the population, clearly an underestimation. On the other hand, prevalence based on spirometric studies suggests that 25% of adults aged 40 years or more have airflow limitation.

According to the World Health Report 2002, the global prevalence of the disease is 1013/100, 000, the incidence being 921/100, 000. The prevalence in the Western Pacific region is the highest—1676/100, 000, and is lowest in Africa 179/100,000.

Epidemiological Data in South-East Asia and India

In the developing world compromising South-East Asia, the Asia Pacific region and India, the epidemiological data is scanty, often involving localized areas; also, the data is not easily accessible, as in some South-East Asian countries it is often published in local languages. Nevertheless there is little doubt that the burden of COPD is significantly underestimated in Asian countries. (Figure 36.2).

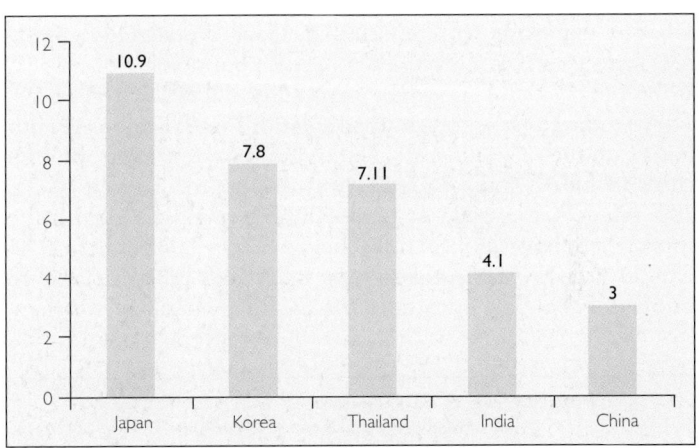

Fig 36.2: Prevalence rate of COPD in South-East Asia.

Source: Adapted from Jindal SK. Emergence of chronic obstructive pulmonary disease as an epidemic in India; *Indian J Med Res*. 2006; 124: 619–630.

Model Estimates of COPD in Asian Countries

Actual scientifically performed studies on the prevalence rate in Asian countries are unavailable. In the absence of such field studies, the Asia Pacific Round Table Group used a statistical model to project the prevalence of COPD in 12 countries in 2000. The rates varied significantly between 11 Asian countries and Australia from a minimum of 3.5% (Hong Kong, Singapore) to a maximum of 6.7% (Vietnam). The overall prevalence in this study was 6.3% which is higher than the rate of 3.9% extrapolated from the WHO study. The estimated rate for China was 65/1000 which was again 2.5 times greater than that estimated by the WHO study. The considerable variation in the prevalence rate of COPD in the Asia Pacific region is due to two factors—most importantly the different smoking habits in these countries and also the proportion of the population living in rural areas.

The high prevalence rates of COPD in many Asian countries projected by the Asia Pacific Round Table Group in turn reflect the increased prevalence of and exposure to risk factors, chiefly cigarette smoking, but also to occupational factors, indoor pollution from biofuels and environmental outdoor pollution. These projected prevalence rates need to be confirmed by actual field studies. Till then these figures can be used by governmental organizations to allocate resources to mitigate the physical and economic burden caused by the disease.

Recent key field studies in Asia include Kim *et al.*, from South Korea in 2005 who reported a prevalence rate as high as 17.2% and of Fukuch *et al.*, from Japan in 2004 who reported a prevalence rate of 10.9%.

PREVALENCE STUDIES IN INDIA

India is a huge country and there is no study that gives a reliable prevalence rate of COPD for the country as a whole. In fact such a study would pose tremendous logistical difficulties and other problems. In the few studies reported from India in the past three decades, the prevalence of COPD was twice as much in men than women with a mean smoking association of 82%. A recent multicentric study on the epidemiology of COPD and its relationship with tobacco smoking and environmental tobacco exposure was reported by S K. Jindal (*Ref:* Jindal SK: Emergence of chronic obstructive pulmonary disease as an epidemic in India. *Indian J Med Res 2006, 12: 619–623*). They studied urban and rural populations in Bangalore (South India) and in Chandigarh, Delhi, Kanpur (all metropolitan cities in North India). COPD was diagnosed in 4.1% of 35, 295 subjects, the male to female ratio being 1.56: 1 and the smoker to non-smoker ratio being 2.65: 1. Prevalence of COPD among bidi smokers was 8.2% and among cigarette smokers 5.9%. The odds ratio for COPD was higher for men,

elderly individuals and in those from the lower socioeconomic strata. They concluded that both cigarette and bidi smoking had a significant association with COPD. In non-smokers, especially women, exposure to indoor air pollution due to the use of biofuels (for heating and cooking) was an important risk factor. More significantly, exposure to environmental tobacco smoke was an established cause of COPD. The risk from environmental tobacco smoke exposure in non-smokers was equally significant in children and adults.

A recent (2005) retrospective study from a chest clinic in Hyderabad showed the prevalence rate of COPD to be 6.85%. The prevalence rate in males was 7.4% and in females 4.64%. A history of 10 pack years of smoking was seen in 87.7% of patients with COPD. Only 12.3% of COPD patients were non-smokers.

COPD Prevalence in the West

It is estimated that approximately 14 million people in the US have COPD. A large national survey (NHANES) carried out between 1988 and 1994 revealed that the prevalence rate of mild COPD (FEV_1/forced vital capacity (FVC) < 70%, FEV_1 > 80% of predicted) was 60% and of moderate COPD (FEV_1/FVC < 70%, FEV1 < 80% of predicted) also 60%. The prevalence rate was higher in men than in women, in whites than in blacks, and increased with age in all groups. Airflow limitation was observed in 14% of smokers, 7% ex-smokers and 3% of non-smokers. Interestingly, a physician's diagnosis of COPD had been made in less than 50% of those who had airflow limitation on spirometry.

In England and Wales, the number of COPD patients is probably well over a million, the prevalence increasing with age and being more in men than in women. A population survey of current smokers between 40–65 years of age revealed that 18% of men and 14% of women had an FEV_1 greater than 2 standard deviation below normal, compared to 7% male and 5% female non-smokers.

The prevalence has increased in women in the UK from 0.8% in 1990 to 1.4% in 1997 though the prevalence in men remained unchanged during this period. These prevalence rates probably reflect an increase in smoking habits in women, a feature also observed in the US and in some countries in Europe.

THE BOLD STUDY

The BOLD (Burden of Obstructive Lung disease) study is an ongoing epidemiological study of COPD. Phase 1 of this study had as its objective the development of a standard methodology to determine the prevalence as also the economic burden of COPD in all countries. The study also includes the determination of the risk factors in COPD, the disability burden and variations in the management of the disease.

Phase 2 of the BOLD study consists of field 'pilot' studies undertaken in China (a developing country) and the US (a developed country). The purpose of these field studies is to validate or modify the standard methodology set out in Phase 1. Once a standard methodology is arrived at, it could be used to provide the prevalence rate within different countries, so as to allow valid comparisons between different countries and between different regions in the world.

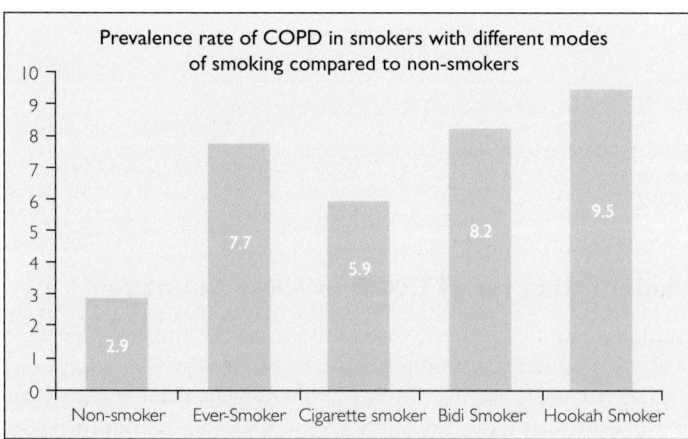

Fig 36.3: Indian scenario: smoking habits.

Source: Adapted from Jindal SK, Agarwal AN, *et al.* A Multicentric Study on Epidemiology of Chronic Obstructive Pulmonary Disease and its relationship with Tobacco Smoking and Environmental Tobacco Smoke Exposure: *Indian J Chest Dis Allied Sci.* 2006; 48: 23–29.

ECONOMIC BURDEN OF COPD

The economic burden of COPD with regard to cost of health-care and the indirect drain on economy due to disability caused by the disease is extremely high in Western countries. For example, in the UK, the NHS bears an estimated cost of £ 819 million with 54% of the costs being caused by hospital admissions and 19% caused by drug treatment. Respiratory disease is the third most common cause of disability, COPD accounting for 56% of these lost days in men and 24% in women. Bronchitis, emphysema, COPD and asthma account for 24.4 million lost working days per year.

Unfortunately, reliable figures for the economic burden in developing countries are unavailable. The World Bank /WHO have introduced a new term called the 'Disability Adjusted Life Years' for determining the economic and social burden of a particular disease, which can then be compared with other diseases. This is a composite of years lost by premature death and the number of years lived with disability, adjusted for the severity of the disability. By this yardstick, respiratory diseases account for over 20% of the global economic cum social burden of all diseases. This is likely to increase in the coming years with COPD projected to be the fifth leading cause of disability and the third leading cause of death by 2020. The dramatic projected rise in the global economic and social burden caused by respiratory diseases in general and COPD in particular, will be chiefly related to the increased morbidity and mortality from tobacco smoking and to an ageing population. Both these factors will operate most of all in the developing world, constituted by India , the Asia Pacific region, the South American continent and perhaps also in Africa. The developing world therefore in the years to come will face a formidable challenge requiring a huge financial outlay on healthcare with regard to COPD and respiratory diseases. The economic burden entailed could well retard overall prosperity and social welfare in these countries.

AETIOLOGY, RISK FACTORS

Cigarette Smoking

The evidence pointing to cigarette smoking as the most important cause of COPD is overwhelming. There are certain features in the relation between cigarette smoking, impaired lung function and COPD that need to be stressed.

1. All cigarette smokers whose respiratory system is exposed to cigarette smoke on a long-term basis show an inflammatory response within the respiratory system. Also, in general, there is a direct relationship between the degree of smoking and impairment of lung function, those smoking more and for a longer duration having a greater impairment of lung function. Yet a great deal of variability exists, in that some heavy cigarette smokers have near normal lung function. Clinically significant COPD can be said to develop in 10–20% of smokers, though currently this figure is felt to be an underestimate. The evolution of COPD in 20% or more of smokers is related to a marked amplification of the inflammatory response to cigarette smoke. The reason for this is debatable and is the subject of research. It needs also be noted that 20% or more of patients with COPD have been lifelong non-smokers, pointing to the role of other aetiological or risk factors in the causation of this disease.

2. Fletcher and colleagues in a prospective eight-year study on working men in London showed that while the average decline in FEV_1 in non-smokers was just 30 ml/year, the average decline in smokers was 60 ml/year. However in the 20% of smokers who developed COPD, the average decline in FEV_1 per year was significantly greater (as high as 100 ml/year) pointing to the increased susceptibility of this group to the effects of cigarette smoke.

   Fletcher and colleagues also showed that stopping smoking led to a normal rate of decline of FEV_1. Recently, the Lung Health Study confirmed the distinct beneficial effect of quitting smoking on the FEV_1, thereby confirming the important role of cigarette smoking in the pathogenesis of COPD.

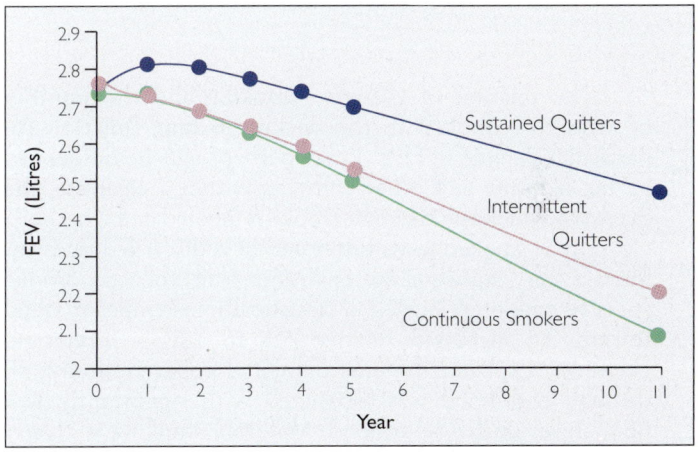

Fig 36.4: Decline in FEV_1 over years in sustained quitters, intermittent quitters and continuous smokers.

Source: Reprinted with permission of the American Thoracic Society. Copyright © Americal Thoracic Society. Nicholas R Anthonisen, John E Connett, Murray Robert (2002). Smoking and Lung Function of Lung Health Study Participants after 11 years. American Journal of Respiratory and Critical Care Medicines. Vol. 166, pp. 675–9. *Official Journal of the American Thoracic Society*, Diane Gern, Publisher.

3. The work of Doll and Petro in the UK provides strong evidence to link smoking with mortality from bronchitis. The death rate for chronic bronchitis in male doctors between 35 and 64 years of age fell between 1953–57 and 1961–65 by 24%, compared to a fall of 4% in other men in the UK of the same age group. These differences in mortality were related to the decrease in smoking habits in doctors between 1961–65.

4. There is evidence that in general the risk of developing COPD increases with the increasing degree of cigarette smoking and increasing exposure to cigarette smoke. Work in India suggests that the same holds true for bidi smoking. The bidi is the Indian equivalent of the cigarette, consisting of a rolled up tobacco leaf stuffed with tobacco powder. Pipe and cigar smokers have higher mortality and morbidity rates than non-smokers, though not as great as cigarette smokers.

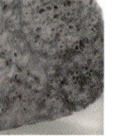

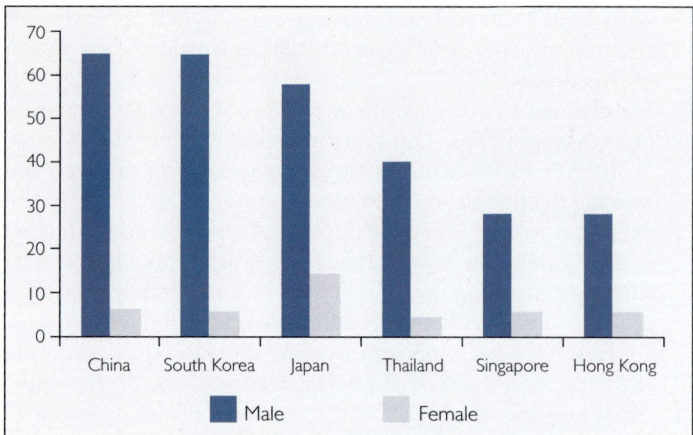

Fig 36.5: Smoking prevalence by country-gender in South-east Asia.

Source: Adapted from COPD prevalence in 12 Asia-Pacific countries and regions: projections based on the COPD prevalence estimation model. Regional COPD Working Group. *Respirology*. 2003 June; 8(2): 192–8.

The relation of cigarette smoking and the number of cigarettes smoked to the decline in lung function (in particular decline in FEV_1) may perhaps also be influenced by tar, nicotine and other contents within a cigarette, the extent to which the cigarette smoke is inhaled and whether a cigarette is smoked to its bitter end or is discarded midway

5. Studies on exposure to environmental tobacco smoke (passive smoking) suggest a statistically insignificant trend towards an increased relative risk to airflow limitation. However, exposure to environmental tobacco smoke all through childhood was associated with significantly low FEV_1 level during adulthood. Maternal smoking is clearly harmful to the foetus, as the newborn child has a low birth weight and presumably reduced lung growth and reduced lung function. To what extent these findings relate to the risk of future development of COPD is difficult to ascertain. Reduced lung function in childhood persisting into adulthood could perhaps accelerate the risk of COPD, particularly in smokers.

Chronic Mucus Hypersecretion

Population studies show that smokers have a greater prevalence of cough and sputum due to hypersecretion of mucus when compared to non-smokers. Petro and co-workers in an eight-year prospective study in London were unable to show a correlation between the degree of mucus secretion and the accelerated decline in FEV_1 or mortality. They however showed that both mortality and morbidity were strongly related to the development of a low FEV_1. However, a more recent study in a general population in Copenhagen (Copenhagen City Lung Study) between 1976–1994 indicated that mucus hypersecretion is associated with an increased risk of hospitalization for COPD and an increased mortality from COPD. This association between mucus hypersecretion and mortality from COPD is even more marked when the airflow limitation increases and FEV_1 decreases. Mucus hypersecretion in patients with an FEV_1 of 40% of predicted value was then associated with four-

fold mortality from COPD compared to a group whose FEV_1 was 80% of predicted.

Bronchopulmonary Infections

COPD patients are prone to recurrent bronchopulmonary infections and one would expect these recurrent infections to accelerate a decline in lung function. However, Fletcher, Petro and colleagues in their prospective eight-year study showed that this was not so. Acute bronchopulmonary infections did cause a temporary decline in lung function which could last for some weeks but which recovered completely. Neither mucus hypersecretion nor bronchopulmonary infections were shown to cause a more rapid decline in FEV_1 after due adjustments were made for age, smoking and the values of FEV_1.

These results have been challenged by the more recent Lung Health Study which showed an association in smokers between lower respiratory tract infection and an accelerated decline in lung function. Other recent population studies in patients with COPD support this finding.

Differences in the degree of airflow obstruction in the population studied by Fletcher and colleagues from that studied by the Lung Health Study and more recent studies probably explain the different findings.

RISK FACTORS FOR COPD IN NON-SMOKERS

For several years research was chiefly concentrated on smoking as the main risk factor for COPD, so that several prevalence studies in COPD were chiefly done on smokers. However, over the past five to seven years many studies have suggested that risk factors other than smoking are also strongly associated with COPD. These factors include indoor and outdoor air pollution, bronchopulmonary infection in childhood, occupational exposure to dust and fumes, history of pulmonary tuberculosis, chronic asthma, intrauterine growth retardation, poor nutrition and poor socioeconomic state. Some of these risk factors are briefly discussed below.

Prevalence of COPD in Non-smokers

The US-based NHANES III study reported the prevalence of COPD in non-smokers to be 6.6% , the diagnosis of COPD being based on a post-bronchodilator spirometric recording of $FEV_1/FVC < 70\%$. This study also suggested that a quarter of COPD patients in the US were 'never-smokers'. A similar proportion of COPD 'never-smokers' was reported from the UK (22.9%) and Spain (23.4%).

Figure 36.6 shows the proportion of non-smoking COPD patients worldwide. The proportion of non-smoking COPD patients is well over 20% and is reportedly as high as 45% in South Africa. In many studies the diagnosis of COPD was based on the FEV_1/FVC ratio being < 70%; in some (including the study from South Africa) it was based on the findings observed on a respiratory symptoms questionnaire. A recent study by Brashier B from the Chest Research Foundation, Pune reported the prevalence of COPD to be 6.7 % and the proportion of COPD patients who never smoked as high as 68.6%. This study was on 12053 subjects over 45 years of age, living in the poorer

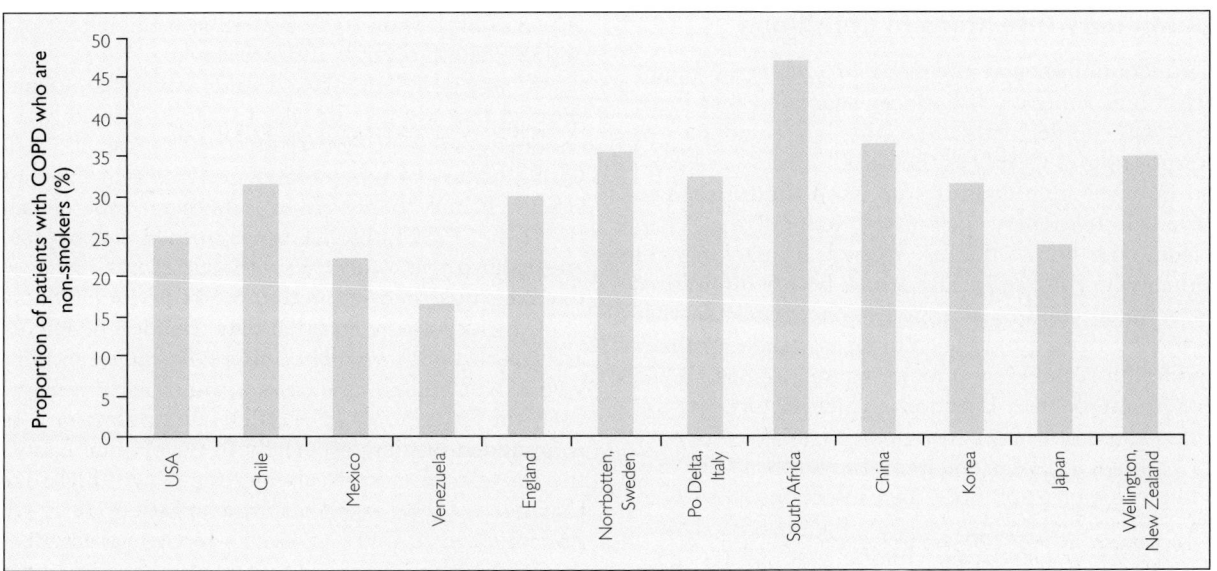

Fig 36.6: Proportion of patients with chronic pulmonary disease (COPD) who are non-smokers worldwide.

Source: Adapted from Salvi Sundeep and Barnes Peter. Chronic obstructive diseases in non-smokers. *Lancet.* 2009; 374: 733–43.

areas of Pune. However, the diagnosis of COPD was based on a respiratory symptoms questionnaire and not on the basis of FEV_1/FVC ratio < 70%.

The overall data strongly suggests that the prevalence and burden of COPD in non-smokers is much higher than what was earlier believed. The risk factors for COPD in non-smokers are considered below.

Indoor Pollution

Indoor pollution is related to the combustion of biomass fuels which are chiefly derived from the use of wood, grass, vegetable matter, animal dung and charcoal. It is not sufficiently realized that worldwide about 50% of all households and 90% of rural households use biomass fuel as their chief source of domestic energy, chiefly for cooking and heating. By this estimate, about 3 billion people in our world are exposed to smoke from incomplete combustion of biomass fuel compared to 1.01 billion who smoke tobacco. More than 80% of households in China, India and Sub-Saharan Africa use this fuel for cooking and 30–75% of homes in South America do likewise. The smoke arising from the burning of biomass fuel is heavily polluted with particulate matter (< 10 um—PM_{10}), nitrogen dioxide, sulphur dioxide, carbon monoxide, formaldehyde, and polycyclic organic compounds, including carcinogens. It therefore appears from the figures stated above that exposure to smoke from these biofuels may be an extremely important global risk factor for COPD. A study suggests that about 50% deaths from COPD in developing countries are due to exposure to smoke from biofuels, of which about 75% are women. Women are at far greater risk for COPD because they use this fuel for cooking and heating purposes. Studies from India, Pakistan, Nepal, and Turkey have amply confirmed this. In North India, where it is bitterly cold in winter, the use of biofuel for heating and cooking in small rooms with little or no ventilation has led to increasingly severe airways

obstruction. Severe COPD with cor pulmonale and right heart failure is observed at a comparatively very young age in these women, in striking contrast to cor pulmonale and right heart failure due to tobacco smoke which generally occurs at a much older age.

Outdoor Air Pollution

The role of outdoor air pollution was recognized following various air pollution episodes, particularly the smog in London in 1952 which led to an excess of deaths from respiratory disease. Though Western countries have cut emission of smoke and sulphur dioxide to an extent, the problem of air pollution in developing countries like India is acute and is likely to increase manifold. The high density of the population in large metropolitan cities (such as Mumbai, Delhi, Kolkata, Bengaluru, Chennai, Hyderabad) together with the ever increasing number of poorly maintained vehicles careening across narrow congested streets, pose a great risk factor to the development of respiratory symptoms and declining lung function. Current studies show an association between high levels of particulate air pollution that exists in several urban centres and respiratory symptoms and hospital admissions in patients with COPD. Air pollution with particulate matter at more than permissible levels (< 100 ug/m³) is the rule rather than the exception in the large cities of India and in many other cities in the world as well. Increased levels of particulate air pollution are associated with deaths from all causes, particularly cardiorespiratory deaths. There is also a clear association between levels of air pollution and exacerbations of COPD. The role of long-term exposure to outdoor air pollution as a risk factor in the development of COPD is perhaps particularly important in the non-smoking group, though evidence to this effect is not conclusive. There is evidence that air pollution can cause mucus hypersecretion but evidence to show that it causes an accelerated decline in FEV_1 is debatable.

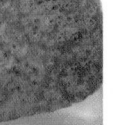

Bronchopulmonary Infections in Childhood

Recurrent bronchopulmonary infections in childhood might adversely affect lung function. It has been suggested that these children grow into adults with unhealthy lungs and have a greater predisposition to COPD as they age.

Children in developing countries are even more prone to recurrent bronchopulmonary infections, particularly when they come from poor homes that use biofuels for cooking and heating. Women who cook and clean in such homes often carry their babies or small children strapped to their back, so that exposure to smoke is as great in the children as in their mothers. Indoor air pollution is therefore a major factor responsible for acute lower respiratory tract infections, which in turn are the most important cause of death in developing countries. Twenty per cent of 12 million deaths in children younger than five years of age are due to lower respiratory tract infections. Nearly all these deaths occur in developing countries, the majority in Asia (42%) and Africa (28%). Here again, children who survive these infections may do so with impaired lung function which might predispose them to COPD in later life.

Occupational Exposure

There is a relationship between occupational exposure to organic and inorganic dusts and to the hypersecretion of mucus leading to symptoms of chronic cough and sputum. A longitudinal follow-up of workers exposed to dust over some years has shown a relation between exposure and a decline in FEV_1.

Occupational exposure probably accounts for at least 10–15% of patients who have chronic respiratory symptoms or show a decline in lung function consistent with COPD. In the big cities of India, workers exposed to dust at construction sites, as also those in flour mills grinding grain and those exposed to dust in numerous dusty occupations, are at special risk of developing chronic respiratory symptoms with persistent airways obstruction. Miners exposed to dust in mines besides being at risk for pneumoconiosis are also at risk for developing cough, sputum and increasing airflow limitation. COPD is a hazard faced by welders due to exposure to welding fumes; workers exposed to cadmium are at risk of developing emphysema.

It needs to be stressed that numerous other factors may interact and perhaps accentuate the effects of occupational exposure. These include smoking and the possible interaction between smoke and dust, as also the effect of air pollution to which many of these poor workers are exposed either at home or in their workplace.

Pulmonary Tuberculosis

There are many who consider that airways obstruction and airflow limitation occurring with active or burnt out pulmonary tuberculosis should not be categorized under COPD. Yet there are many doctors, particularly those working in poor developing countries who question this concept. Pulmonary tuberculosis has been noted to be associated with airflow obstruction during the active phase and also several years after treatment has ended. Airways obstruction is related to the immune response to the mycobacterium that results in airways inflammation and airways fibrosis which is characteristic of COPD. The degree of airways obstruction is correlated with the extent of the disease and the length of time after treatment.

A large population-based study in five Latin American cities showed that the prevalence of COPD (judged by a post-bronchodilator value of $FEV_1/FVC < 70\%$) was 30.7% for patients with a history of tuberculosis and 13.9% in those without this specific history. A history of pulmonary tuberculosis increased the risk of COPD by 4.1 times in men and by 1.7 in women after adjustment for age, sex, ethnicity, smoking habits, exposure to dust, smoke and respiratory morbidity in childhood.

Considering the fact that over 2 billion people in our world are infected with *Mycobacterium tuberculosis* and that there are well over a million new cases of pulmonary tuberculosis every year, the association of COPD with pulmonary tuberculosis is an added burden, especially in developing countries, where the prevalence rate of tuberculosis is very high. The question that needs to be asked and researched upon is whether this phenotype of COPD is similar to that of COPD caused by smoking both with regard to its natural history and response to pharmacotherapy.

Chronic Asthma

It has already been mentioned that in some severe chronic asthmatics, reversibility of airways obstruction is small or even absent, due to remodelling of the airways from thickening and fibrosis of the bronchial walls. The distinction from COPD in these patients may be impossibly difficult. These asthmatic patients have a pattern of inflammation similar to that of COPD, with increased neutrophilis, interleukin-8, proteases, oxidants and a poor response to corticosteroids.

In a retrospective study of more than 300 patients from a rural population in India, it was observed that 75% of patients with poorly controlled asthma, who had received an oral bronchodilator drug alone, had clinical features characteristic of COPD. Therefore inadequate treatment of severe chronic asthma could well be a risk factor for COPD. This risk is even greater in the developing countries of the world where for several reasons severe chronic asthma is poorly treated, thereby perhaps contributing to the overall burden of COPD in these countries.

Socioeconomic Conditions

The risk of COPD is greater in those living in poor socioeconomic conditions. This may be related to exposure to indoor and outdoor pollution, poor housing, diet, exposure to repeated infections and other socioeconomic factors.

Gender

Though historically the incidence of COPD is more in men than in women, recent studies in developed countries suggest a near equal distribution between men and women. In North India, where women are markedly exposed to the combustion products of biofuels, the incidence of COPD in women is significantly higher than in other parts of the country.

Growth and Nutrition

Many studies suggest that the incidence of death from COPD varies inversely with the weight at birth and at the age of one year. It seems that impaired growth of the foetus *in utero* is a risk factor in the future development of respiratory disease including COPD. Similarly, impairment of lung growth during gestation is believed to be a potential factor for the future development of COPD.

Genetic Factors

The only proven genetic factor is the one associated with $\alpha_1$antitrypsin deficiency. Genetic susceptibility is suggested by the increased risk of development of airflow limitation in siblings of patients with COPD. There are other genes reported to be associated with COPD. These include tumour necrosis factor, transforming growth factor beta and microsomal epoxide hydrolase-1. Their association with COPD is inconsistent and their exact role is undetermined. The association of $\alpha_1$antitrypsin deficiency with COPD is described below.

ALPHA-1 ANTITRYPSIN DEFICIENCY

Alpha-1 antitrypsin deficiency is an inherited disease that can affect the lungs and the liver. In the lung it leads to emphysema and COPD starting in young adulthood. The lung disease progresses, causing crippling respiratory disability and premature death from severe respiratory failure in many patients. In the liver, alpha-1 antitrypsin deficiency may result in the benign neonatal hepatitis syndrome. Some with this deficiency develop hepatic fibrosis progressing to cirrhosis of the liver. Hepatocellular carcinoma can be a complication of cirrhosis related to alpha-1 antitrypsin deficiency. Only the pulmonary manifestations of alpha-1 antitrypsin deficiency are dealt with here.

The alpha-1 antitrypsin deficiency molecule is produced in the liver and its main function in the lung is anti-proteolytic, so that it protects the lungs from the proteolytic enzymes which if left unopposed would lead to destruction of lung tissue. The molecule is also believed to regulate immune defence within the lung. A great deal of research has been done on the genetics and the biology of the alpha-1 antitrypsin molecule as also on the pathophysiology of the lung in alpha-1 antitrypsin deficiency. There still remain lacunae on some issues, in particular the reason why only a few patients with this deficiency manifest pulmonary disease.

Genetics

Alpha-1 antitrypsin deficiency is an autosomal recessive disease. The *SERPINA1* gene (formerly known as *PI*), which encodes the alpha-1 antitrypsin protein, is 12.2 kb, located on the long arm of Chromosome 14 (14q31–32.3) and is markedly pleomorphic. The variants are classified depending on their influence on the alpha-1 antitrypsin level in the blood. The M alleles (M1 to M6) are most commonly found; these are considered to be normal 'variants' and are not associated with a fall in alpha-1 antitrypsin levels. Disease occurs as a result of an abnormal mutation of the alpha-1 antitrypsin gene resulting in consequences at several different levels. These include deletion of the gene, degradation of unstable m-RNA transcripts, accumulation of alpha-1 antitrypsin in the endoplasmic reticulum, degradation of the antitrypsin protein before its translocation to the Golgi complex, and finally difficulty in the effective release of alpha-1 antitrypsin.

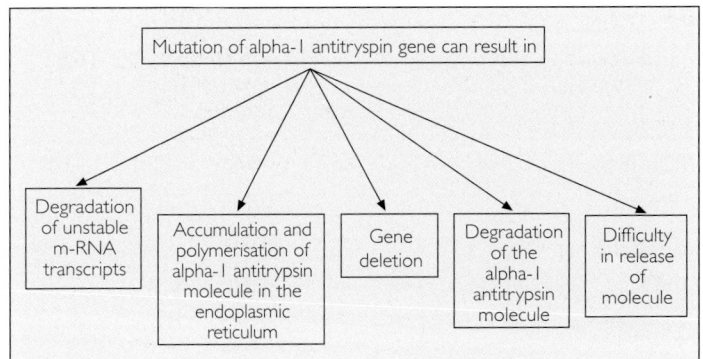

Fig 36.7: Smoking Prevalence by Smoking-Gender in South-east Asia.

The normal serum concentration of alpha-1 antitrypsin is 20–52 µmol/L. It is an acute phase protein whose production is increased during pregnancy, inflammatory diseases and cancer. The released alpha-1 antitrypsin inactivates proteolytic enzymes released in the lungs. Proteolytic enzymes are normally produced in abundance in the lungs as a result of immune responses to airborne pathogens to which the airways and parenchymal lung tissue are constantly exposed. The most important and powerful protease resulting from these immune responses is neutrophil elastase, which is effectively inhibited by alpha-1 antitrypsin in a ratio of 1: 1. There are other important lung protease inhibitors. These include secretory leucoprotease inhibitor (SLPI) and elafin, both of which are present in a much lower concentration when compared to alpha-1 antitrypsin.

Prevalence

INDIA

The prevalence of alpha-1 antitrypsin deficiency in India is underdetermined as there is no significant reliable data on this subject. Perhaps screening of appropriate patients with COPD or bronchitis may unearth more patients than what is apparent today.

NORTH AMERICA, EUROPE

The highest allele frequencies for alpha-1 antitrypsin deficiency are found in the Caucasians of Europe and America. US African Americans have the lowest. Prevalence estimates for typical deficiency genotypes (SZ, ZZ, SS) of the disease in North America and some of the larger European countries are given in Table 36.4.

Among European countries, Spain and Portugal have the highest prevalence estimate for the deficiency genotypes SZ, ZZ, SS.

SOUTH-EAST ASIA

The database for seven countries in South-east Asia is given in Table 36.5. The study consisted of 20 cohorts with a total cohort sample of 4547. The study demonstrated that the PiS and PiZ alleles are found in Malaysia and Thailand, with only the PiS allele found in the Philippines and Singapore, with neither the PiS nor PiZ alleles present in Indonesia, New Guinea or Vietnam. With an estimated total population of 473, 595, 032 for these seven countries, the total population at risk consists of

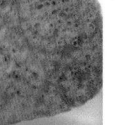

Table 36.4:
Estimated percentage of individuals with alpha-1 antitrypsin genotype SZ, ZZ, SS in the total population of North America and some European countries

Country	SZ	ZZ	SS
France	0.195	0.017	0.578
Germany	0.041	0.010	0.044
Italy	0.075	0.027	0.052
Netherlands	0.044	0.010	0.046
Portugal	0.356	0.019	1.667
Spain	0.360	0.030	1.087
Russia	0.007	0.001	0.009
Sweden	0.113	0.053	0.060
UK	0.065	0.014	0.078
US Caucasian	0.022	0.036	0.052
US African American	0.006	0.002	0.022

Source: Adapted from de Serres FJ, Fernandez-Bustillo E, *et al.* Estimated numbers and prevalence of PI*S and PI*Z alleles of alpha1-antitrypsin deficiency in European countries. *Eur Respir J.* 2006; 27: 77–84.

5, 761, 832 carriers and 93, 062 deficiency allele combinations for PiS and PiZ.

Pathophysiology

It has been shown in all countries that the number of clinically identified patients with lung disease is far less than the anticipated prevalence rate as judged on allele frequencies. However 85% of individuals with the ZZ variants manifest pulmonary disease. The ZZ variants are characterized by the substitution of lysine for glutamic acid at position 342 of the amino acid sequence on the alpha-1 antitrypsin molecule. For this reason, protein synthesis in the endoplasmic cytoplasm of the hepatocytes is delayed, so that 85% of synthesized molecules

polymerize into larger concentrates, only a little of the non-polymerized molecule being released into the blood stream. The anti-proteolytic effect exerted by this small release of the alpha-1 antitrypsin molecule is five times less than what would accrue with normal levels of alpha-1 antitrypsin. Thus the balance between proteolytic activity within the lung and anti-proteolysis is tilted markedly in favour of the former. The released proteases over a few decades destroy the alveolar walls, lung matrix, vessels, giving rise to progressive chronic obstructive lung disease with well-marked emphysema.

The alpha-1 antitrypsin molecule also regulates inflammatory processes in the lung. It exerts an anti-inflammatory effect and perhaps stimulates tissue repair and exerts antibacterial activity.

Current research suggests that polymerized ZZ alpha-1 antitrypsin molecules accumulate not only in hepatocutes but also in peripheral tissue. Bronchoalveolar lavage (BAL) fluid of these patients has revealed the presence of polymerized alpha-1 antitrypsin, suggesting that the anti-proteolytic activity within the lung is further diminished. It has also been contended that the polymerized alpha-1 antitrypsin molecule may exert a pro-inflammatory effect in contrast to the monomer form of the molecule which is believed to have an anti-inflammatory effect.

Clinical Features

PULMONARY MANIFESTATIONS
Cough with expectoration and progressive breathlessness generally occur by the age of 30–40 years. Severe COPD with panacinar emphysema develops over a few decades if the alpha-1 antitrypsin serum concentration is below 35% of the normal mean value (≤ 0.8 g/L or ≤ 11 μmol/L). The course of the disease is punctuated by acute exacerbations with worsening of cough and breathlessness. Acute exacerbations are invariably related to airway or pulmonary infections; the additional release of proteolytic enzymes which remain unopposed adds to increasing destruction of alveolar walls, vessels and lung matrix. The end result is progressive crippling respiratory failure similar to advanced COPD unrelated to alpha-1 antitrypsin deficiency.

Table 36.5:
Estimates of the mean gene frequencies in different countries of Southeast Asia

Country	Cohorts		Mean Gene Frequencies			
	No.	Size	PiM	PiS	PiZ	Total Population
Indonesia	5	724	0.9869	0.0000	0.0000	224,784,210
Malaysia	6	1,886	0.9692	0.0241	0.0013	21,793,293
New Guinea	2	182	0.9973	0.0000	0.0000	20,000
Philippines	1	243	0.9918	0.0021	0.0000	82,841,518
Singapore	1	385	0.9792	0.0065	0.0000	4,151,264
Thailand	4	1,064	0.9591	0.0226	0.0132	61,230,874
Vietnam	1	63	0.9921	0.0000	0.0000	78,773,873
Total	20	4,547	0.9732	0.0159	0.0036	473,595,032

Source: Adapted from Worldwide Racial and Ethnic Distribution of α1-Antitrypsin Deficiency: Summary of an analysis of Published Genetic Epidemiologic Surveys. *Chest.* November 2002; 122: 1818–29.

Physical examination, lung function tests show evidence of airflow limitation with increased lung volumes and reduced CO diffusion capacity. Chest radiography and computed tomography (CT) reveal the classic features of pulmonary emphysema. However, unlike other usual patients with COPD who have predominant emphysematous changes most marked in the upper lobes, patients with ZZ alpha-1 antitrypsin deficiency have emphysematous changes mainly in the lower lobes. As the disease progresses arterial blood gases show hypoxemia and ultimately there is increasing hypoxemic plus hypercapnic respiratory failure.

Ten per cent of patients with ZZ alpha-1 antitrypsin develop bronchial hyperreactivity. Large bullae may be present and pneumothorax remains a potential dangerous complication.

Other Organ Manifestations

Besides hepatitis and cirrhosis of the liver, alpha-1 antitrypsin deficiency is rarely associated with Wegener's granulomatosis, necrotizing panniculitis and aneurysms that may affect the abdominal aorta and/or cerebral vessels.

Diagnosis

Diagnosis depends on measurement of the concentration of alpha-1 antitrypsin in the serum, the normal range being 1.5 to 3.0 g/L or 20–52 µmol/L. It needs to be stressed that the alpha-1 antitrypsin molecule is an acute phase protein and the level is upregulated in inflammatory disease. The C-reactive protein should therefore be measured simultaneously, and if found high, the alpha-1 antitrypsin concentration (even if found to be normal) is unreliable, and needs to be repeated when the C-reactive protein is within normal limits.

If the alpha-1 antitrypsin concentration is below normal, a genotyping is performed. This allows genetic counselling of patients and their families and may help predict the severity and course of the disease.

It is unfortunate that screening of alpha-1 antitrypsin is very rarely practised in hospitals in India. Perhaps screening tests in appropriate patients with COPD would prove that this deficiency is not as rare as is believed.

Treatment

Treatment is similar to that given to any COPD patient. Smoking cessation is imperative, as is exposure to occupational or environmental pollutants. Bacterial infection should be promptly countered with appropriate antibiotics. Lung volume reduction surgery recommended at one time is not generally recommended. Lung transplantation is recommended in severe cases. Replacement therapy with alpha-1 antitrypsin has been used in Europe and America for several years but the evidence for its efficacy is uncertain.

Table 36.6: Features suggestive of alpha-1 antitrypsin deficiency
1. Pulmonary emphysema without risk factors such as smoking, occupational exposure, exposure to dust exposure to combustion products of biofuels, or heavy environmental pollution
2. Pulmonary emphysema at a young age < 45 years
3. Pulmonary emphysema predominately involving the lower lobes
4. Family history of emphysema, or chronic bronchitis or liver cirrhosis in ancestors
5. Chronic active hepatitis or cirrhosis of unknown etiology.

Table 36.7: Aetiology, risk factors in COPD
1. Cigarette smoking, bidi smoking, hookah smoking; cigar, pipe smoking to a lesser extent than cigarette or bidi smoking
2. Indoor and outdoor air pollution
3. Occupational factors
4. Bronchopulmonary infections in childhood
5. Pulmonary tuberculosis
6. Chronic unrelieved severe asthma
7. Genetic factors (α-1 antitrypsin deficiency)
8. Socioeconomic conditions
9. Growth and nutrition (Low birth weight and at age of 1 year; Impairement of lung growth during gestation)

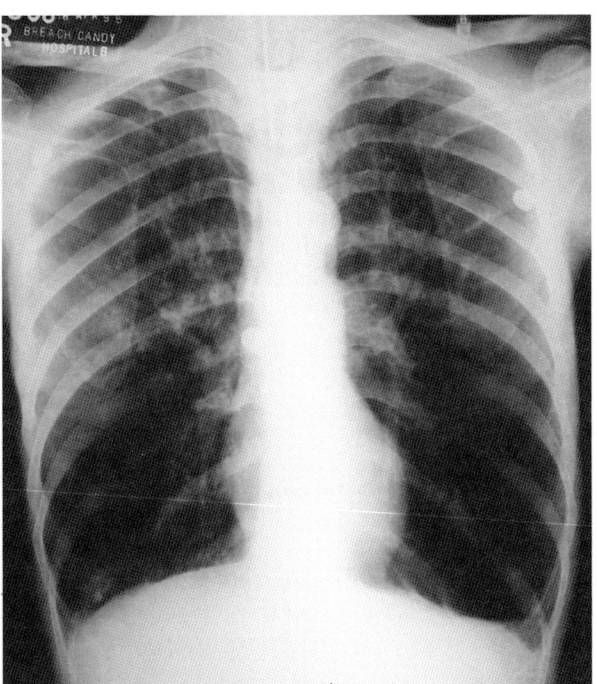

Fig 36.8: Alpha-1 antitrypsin deficiency: Chest X-ray PA view demonstrates large areas of hypertransluscency in the lower zones with a tubular heart and compressed lung in the upper zones.

PATHOLOGY OF COPD

The pathology of COPD can be summarized as an inflammatory response of the lungs to inhalation of noxious particles or gases.

The overall pathological changes within the lungs in COPD can be summarized as follows:

(a) inflammatory changes in the large airways (> 2mm), but more importantly in the small peripheral airways (< 2mm), leading to their obstruction, fibrosis, with ultimate distortion;

(b) loss of support to the airways because of rupture of alveolar attachments to the airways;

(c) loss of elastic recoil of alveoli because of emphysematous changes;

(d) all three of the above occurring in varying degrees in different patients.

Inflammation of the large airways results in chronic bronchitis which has a clinical definition. Inflammation of the peripheral airways leads to bronchiolitis causing obstruction to the small airways. Inflammation leading to enlarged distal airspaces with rupture of alveolar walls leads to emphysema, a pathological entity.

Chronic Bronchitis

The characteristic pathological features of chronic bronchitis are summarized below.

1. Inflammation of the bronchial mucosa and wall There is increased mucous secretion due to inflammatory changes in the central airways—trachea, bronchi, bronchioles > 2 mm in diameter. Mucous is produced by sub-epithelial mucous glands in the large airways and by goblet cells in the airway epithelium. There is an increase in the size and number of the mucous glands and of goblet cells. In healthy subjects goblet cells are chiefly present in the proximal airways and decrease peripherally; in chronic bronchitis goblet cells not only increase in number but extend more peripherally. The increase in number and size of mucous-secreting glands and cells leads to an increased volume of mucous secretion not only in the central airways but also in the peripheral airways, where mucociliary clearance is comparatively inefficient. Inflammation of the bronchial mucosa and submucosa further contributes to excessive mucous secretion. Neutrophilic infiltration is present in the mucosa, submucosa and in mucosal glands; the inflammatory process increases with progress of the disease and during acute exacerbations. Inflammation also involves the bronchial wall. Neutrophils and macrophages are observed in bronchial biopsy specimens together with activated CD8 suppressor cells in contrast to the predominant CD4 cells seen in asthma.

There is in addition metaplasia of the airways epithelium, loss of cilia and disturbed ciliary function resulting in impaired mucociliary clearance. Stagnation of mucous leads not only to obstruction but possible infection. Hypertrophy and hyperplasia of the bronchial muscles with subepithelial fibrosis is also observed.

2) Intraluminal inflammation BAL studies and examination of sputum show evidence of intraluminal inflammation not necessarily associated with airways obstruction. Neutrophils predominate, together with the presence of chemotactic factors which include interleukins and leukotrienes. These inflammatory changes in the central airways induced typically by the noxious influence of cigarette smoke are aggravated during acute exacerbations. The latter are associated with some degree of eosinophilic infiltration of the bronchial mucosa and wall. Neutrophils, macrophages however still predominate in contrast to patients with bronchial asthma where the eosinophil remains the chief inflammatory cell.

Cessation of smoking usually brings symptomatic relief but bronchial biopsy studies indicate that a fair degree of inflammation in the bronchial lumen and wall still persists.

Small Airways Disease

It is believed that silent, often asymptomatic inflammation of the small airways (< 2mm) is one of the earliest changes to occur in patients with COPD. These inflammatory changes may not be detected by routine spirometry and lung function tests. The nature of inflammation is similar to that described in the large airways, being characterized by an exudate of macrophages, lymphocytes, neutrophils, by goblet cell hyperplasia with excessive mucous production, increase in CD8 lymphocytes and an increase in the CD8/CD4 ratio. The small peripheral airways (< 2mm) of the lungs now contribute much more towards airflow resistance. As the inflammatory pathology in the small airways progressively worsens, obstruction increases. There now results a structural remodelling with subepithelial deposition of collagen, increasing fibrosis, scarring and further destruction of the airways.

Resistance to airflow is due to the following factors:

1. Physical obstruction to small airways caused by mucous, cell debris, inflammation, narrowing and distortion.
2. An airflow limitation caused by loss of alveolar attachments to the peripheral airways. These alveoli through their elasticity normally help to hold the peripheral airways open. The loss of this support leads to premature closing of the airways during expiration.

Emphysema

Emphysema is defined as abnormal permanent enlargement of air spaces distal to the terminal bronchioles and is accompanied by destruction of alveolar walls. Emphysema is best understood with reference to the acinar unit, which is that unit of the lung being supplied by a single terminal bronchiole. Emphysema is of three main types:

1. *Centriacinar or centrilobular emphysema*, in which large airspaces formed by ruptured alveoli cluster around the terminal bronchiole.
2. *Panacinar or panlobular emphysema*, in which large airspaces due to ruptured alveolar walls are distributed throughout the acinar unit.
3. *Periacinar or paraseptal emphysema*, where enlarged airspaces are found in the periphery of the acinar unit abutting against a fixed structure such as the pleura or septum or a lung fissure.

Centriacinar or centrilobular emphysema has a greater association with cigarette smoking than panacinar emphy-

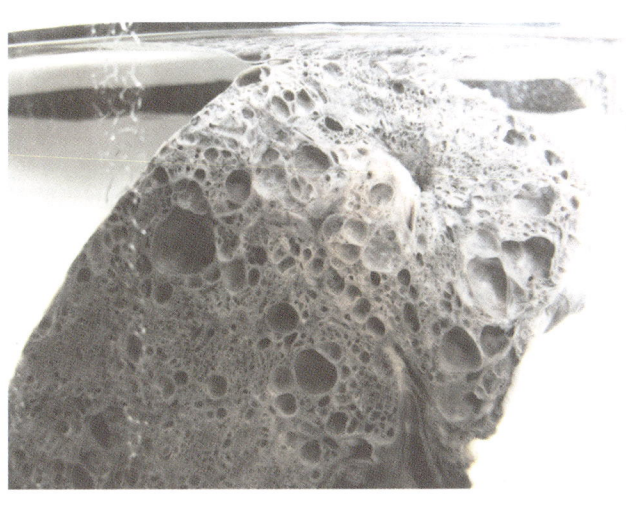

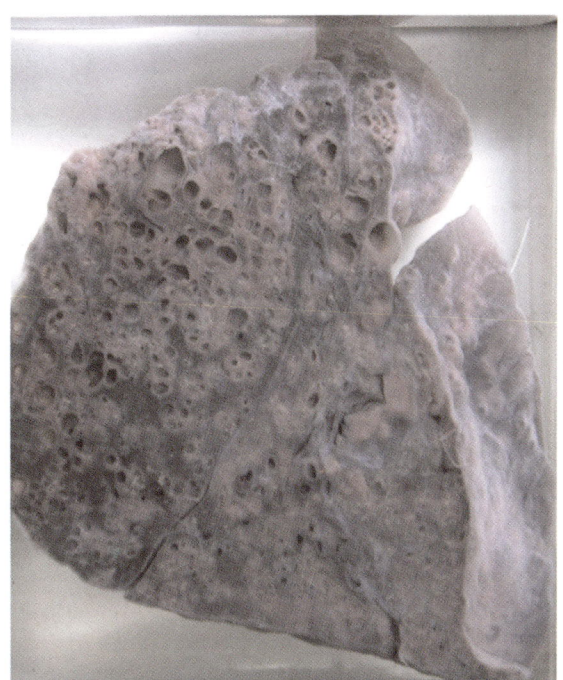

Fig 36.9: Cross-section of lung showing emphysematous changes.

sema, though both types of emphysema can occur with smoking. Patients with centriacinar emphysema have greater inflammation and pathological involvement of the smaller peripheral airways, the distribution of the emphysema being more marked in the upper lobes. Panacinar emphysema is found in patients with alpha-1 antitrypsin deficiency and alpha-1 proteinase inhibitor deficiency. It is most evident in the lower lobes and can also occur in patients who have no genetic abnormality.

Paraseptal emphysema occurs peripherally in the acinar unit and is of significance only when it is sufficiently marked in the subpleural region to cause a pneumothorax.

At times emphysematous areas occur irregularly as a sequel to inflammation resulting in scarring and local deforming of lung tissue unrelated to the acinar unit. This does not come under the present definition of emphysema.

Airspace enlargement in emphysema to start with is only visible microscopically. It can be visible macroscopically only when the airspace enlargement exceeds 1 mm. A bulla is produced by rupture of many adjacent alveolar walls to result in an air space 1 cm or more in diameter. Small bullae may merge with one another to form one or more large bullae which may occupy the greater part of the lobe of a lung. Though the definition of emphysema excludes the presence of fibrosis, some degree of fibrosis is present as a feature of bronchiolitis involving the respiratory bronchioles in smokers.

Vascular Changes

Changes in the vessel walls of the pulmonary arteries occur early in the natural history of COPD. There is thickening of the intima, followed by increase in the smooth muscle of the media with infiltration by inflammatory cells consisting of macrophages and CD8-T-lymphocytes. As the disease

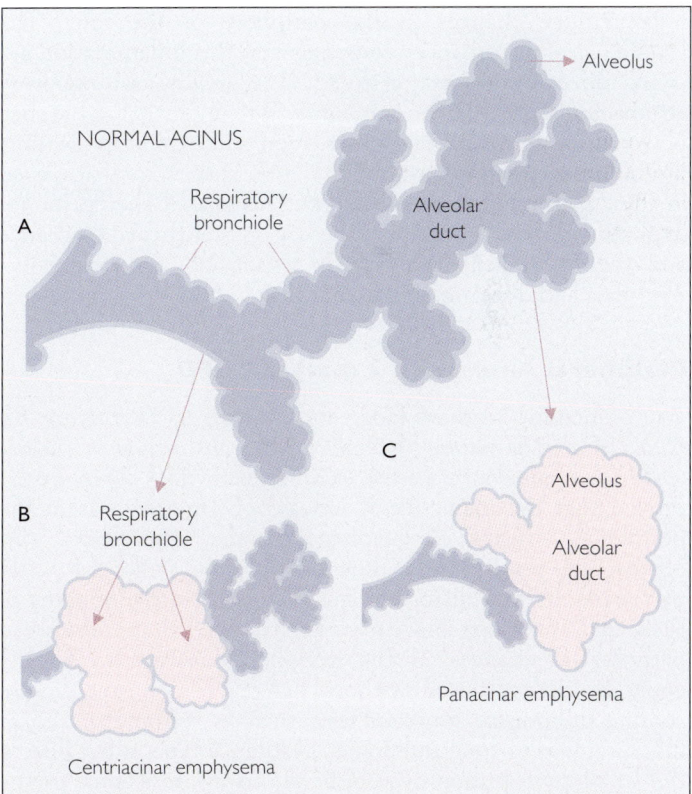

Fig 36.10: Major patterns of emphysema. A. Normal structure within the acinus. B. Centriacinar emphysema with dilation that initially affects the respiratory bronchioles. C. Panacinar emphysema in which large airspaces due to ruptured alveolar walls are distributed throughout the acinar unit.

Source: This figure was published in, Kumar: Robbins and Cotran, *Pathologic Basis of Disease*, professional edition, eighth edition Copyright © 2009 Saunders, An Imprint of Elsevier.

progresses, further thickening of the intima and of the muscle within the media, together with deposition of collagen are noted. Hypoxia and hypercapnia so often observed in advanced COPD produce vasoconstriction. Ruptured alveolar walls lead to reduced cross-section of pulmonary capillaries in the lungs and promote further pulmonary hypertension. Pulmonary hypertension is responsible for right ventricular enlargement and right ventricular dysfunction (cor pulmonale).

PATHOPHYSIOLOGY OF COPD

COPD is a heterogeneous disease in its clinical, physiological and pathological aspects. Its pathophysiology is therefore complex as it is dependent on abnormalities in the central conducting airways (> 2 mm), the peripheral airways (< 2 mm), the lung parenchyma, chest wall mechanics, respiratory and skeletal muscle function and structure. The combination of these abnormalities can culminate in crippling respiratory disability, manifest as progressive breathlessness, and disturbed gas exchange leading to respiratory failure and premature death. The function of the heart and lung are inter-dependent, so that changes in the structure and function of the lungs ultimately result in pulmonary hypertension and right ventricular hypertrophy with or without failure (cor pulmonale).

The starting point of the pathophysiology in COPD is inflammation of the peripheral airways together with destructive inflammatory changes in the periphery of the lung. The physiological disturbances consequent to this inflammation are characterized by obstruction to expiratory air flow and expiratory airflow limitation. There is a subtle but important difference between the terms airways obstruction and expiratory air flow limitation. Expiratory air-flow limitation is the expression used in the current definition of COPD. This is as it should be, for expiratory airflow limitation is the key physiological disturbance and the key mechanism that is responsible for progressive dyspnoea and disability in patients with COPD.

Peripheral Airways (< 2 mm) in COPD

The pioneering work of Hogg and co-workers *(Ref: Hogg JC, Chu f et al: The nature of small-airways obstruction in chronic obstructive pulmonary disease. NEJM 2004; 350: 2645–2653)* proved that the main site of airways obstruction was in the peripheral airways. As explained under 'Pathology', this obstruction results from mucous plugging, inflamed walls, narrowing, fibrosis, distortion and even obliteration of many of these airways. Hogg and co-workers showed that widespread pathological changes in the peripheral airways in COPD could be demonstrated without detectable abnormalities in routine pulmonary function tests such as spirometry and/or measurement of total pulmonary resistance. This is because of the small contribution of peripheral airways resistance to the total resistance at this early stage of the disease. This prompted Mead to term the small airways in the lungs as the 'silent zone'. However, though these peripheral airways lesions were undetected by routine spirometry they can now be detected by special tests for peripheral small airways function. These include measurements of the closing volume (asymptomatic adult smokers have an increase in closing volume compared to non-smokers), volume of isoflow, slope of the Phase III of the single

breath nitrogen washout curve, and frequency dependence of lung compliance (worsening of lung compliance with increased rate of breathing). These are rather esoteric tests performed in special laboratories. Perhaps the only test easily performed and thought to mirror changes in peripheral airways is a reduction in the maximum expiratory flow at lung volume below 50%.

As COPD evolves in its natural history, *in vivo* measurements show a significant increase in total airway resistance, involving both central and peripheral airways. However, central airways resistance is noted to increase by just 50% whereas resistance of the peripheral airways show a fivefold increase.

The inflammation of peripheral airways also involves the periphery of the lung to a varying degree. This inflammation has two effects—a) disruption and loss of alveolar attachments to peripheral airways. It is these attachments which normally hold the peripheral airways open during expiration; b) disruption of alveolar walls (typical of emphysema) resulting in loss of elastic recoil.

Expiratory Air flow Limitation

Air flow limitation implies that expiratory flow cannot increase at a given lung volume by increasing intrathoracic pressure through forcible contraction of respiratory muscles. COPD is characterized by a reduction in the expiratory flow rates, the lower the flow rate at a given lung volume, the more severe the COPD. This reduction is due to two causes—

1. Mechanical obstruction of peripheral airways due to mucus plugging, together with inflammatory changes in the bronchial wall.
2. 'Collapse' of the peripheral airways during expiration because of loss of elastic recoil and loss of alveolar attachments to the airways. Expiratory airflow limitation is therefore far more complex than mere obstruction because it implies dynamic compression of the airways during expiration.

It needs to be pointed out that expiratory air flow limitation occurs in all subjects when the level of maximal flow has been

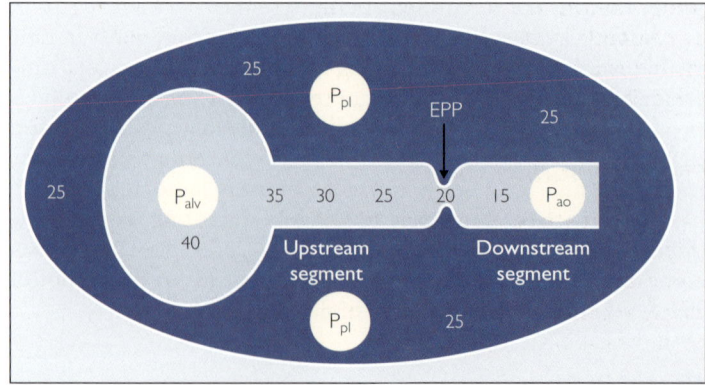

Fig 36.11: Airway collapse resulting in an airflow limitation in a normal individual during forced expiration. Just as an example, pressure within the alveolus is equal to the intrapleural pressure of 25 mm Hg + alveolar recoil pressure (say 15 mm Hg), amounting to 40 mm Hg. Once the pressure within the airway falls below the intrapleural pressure, the airway closes thereby limiting expiratory airflow (See section on Lung Physiology). p_{pl} = intrapleural pressure; P_{alv} = alveolar pressure; EPP = Equal pressure point.

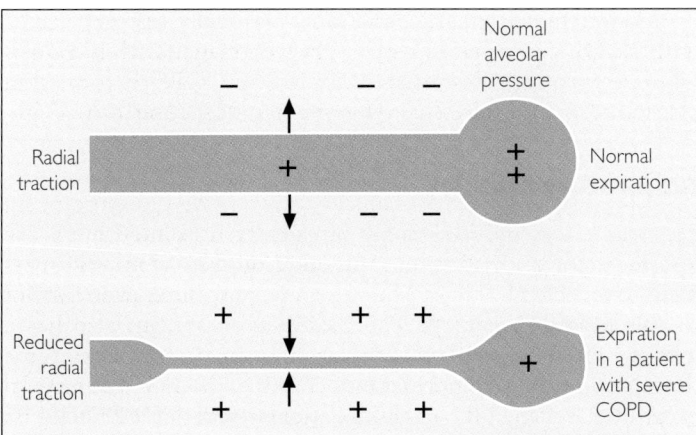

Fig 36.12: Expiration in a normal individual and expiratory airflow limitation in a patient with severe COPD. Alveolar attachments to the airway wall keep the airway open during expiration in a normal individual. In severe COPD there is both a loss of elastic recoil and loss of alveolar attachments to the airway walls. The airways collapse even during normal expiration because of dynamic compression leading to a limitation of the expiratory flow rate.

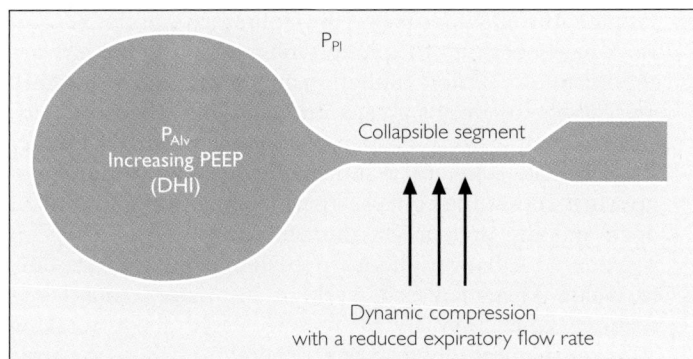

Fig 36.13: Dynamic compression of the airways during expiration resulting in dynamic hyperinflation (DHI).

reached (Figure 36.11). In normal subjects and in patients with mild COPD, airflow limitation occurs as the degree of exercise increases due to increased ventilation. However, in severe COPD expiratory airflow limitation occurs during resting tidal breathing, which is to say that the flow generated during tidal breathing equals the maximum expiratory flow. These patients are unable to increase their tidal volume to meet increased ventilatory demand necessitated by activity, exercise or increased metabolism. The increased ventilatory demand can only be met by an increase in rate. This results in air-trapping, dynamic hyperinflation (as is explained below) necessitating an increase in the work of breathing.

Pulmonary Hyperinflation

Airways obstruction leads to an increase in the 'resistive work' of breathing. The major consequence of expiratory airflow limitation is pulmonary hyperinflation. Pulmonary hyperinflation is characterized by an increase in the functional residual capacity (FRC) above the predicted value. In normal subjects FRC corresponds to the volume at which the inward elastic recoil of the lungs is counterbalanced by the outward elastic recoil of the chest wall. It measures 40% of the total lung capacity.

Static Hyperinflation

In COPD patients the static equilibrium value of the respiratory system is at a higher volume than in normal subjects. This is because of the loss of elastic recoil of the lungs. The outward elastic recoil of the chest raises the resting FRC to the volume of the chest wall.

Dynamic Hyperinflation (DHI)

Dynamic hyperinflation is the mechanism responsible for progressive air-trapping within the alveoli leading to a progressive increase in the intra-alveolar pressure and the FRC. It can occur in severe COPD even when the patient is at rest. In moderately

advanced COPD it can occur when the patient exercises or exerts. Most importantly, it can occur with frightening rapidity during an acute severe exacerbation of COPD. The underlying cause is airways obstruction and expiratory airflow limitation. As explained earlier, a dynamic compression and collapse of the peripheral airways during expiration leads to a reduced rate of lung emptying. In these circumstances an inspiratory effort starts before the prolonged expiration is complete. Air is thus trapped in the alveoli causing a rise in the intra-alveolar pressure. The end-expiratory alveolar pressure continues to rise every time a prolonged expiration is prematurely cut short or interrupted by an inspiration. This progressive rise in end-expiratory alveolar pressure is termed intrinsic PEEP or auto-PEEP; it results in an increase in the FRC and in overinflated lungs.

Dynamic hyperinflation exerts a deleterious effort on the respiratory and circulatory systems—

1. Breathing at higher lung volumes is greatly uncomfortable and causes increasing distress. The work of breathing is significantly increased because of an overinflated chest. An overinflated chest has ribs which are more horizontally placed; also the length tension relationship of the intercostal muscles is far from optimal so that the chest bellows work at a mechanical disadvantage. The low diaphragm and the decreased area of apposition between the diaphragm and the chest wall are further mechanical disadvantages adding to the work of breathing.

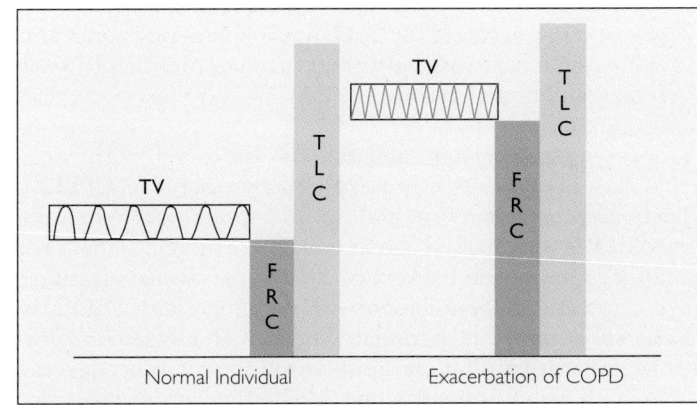

Fig 36.14: Increased FRC with the patient breathing at higher lung volumes in severe COPD.

2. Though it would appear that the expiratory muscles need to work hard because of expiratory obstruction to the airways and expiratory airflow limitation, it is in fact the inspiratory muscles that endure a great workload. This is because with each inspiration the inspiratory muscles need to contract strongly and generate a sufficiently negative intrapleural pressure so that the collapsed peripheral airways are pulled open and the pressure in the central airways and alveoli is rendered subatmospheric, to enable inspiratory air flow to occur. This increased work of inspiratory muscles is required when they are for reasons stated above working at a mechanical disadvantage. Therefore when dynamic hyperinflation is marked (as in an acute exacerbation of COPD), inspiratory muscle fatigue occurs, and may lead to a respiratory arrest.

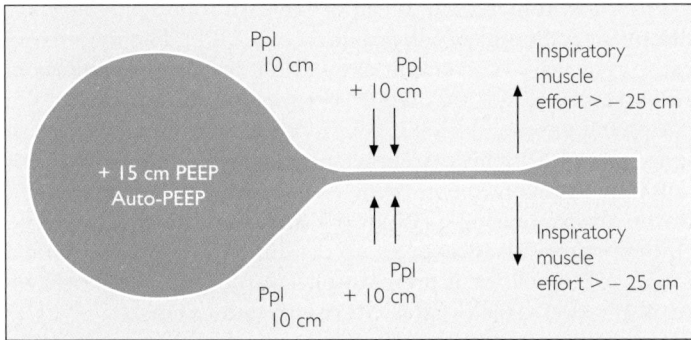

Fig 36.15: An increased inspiratory effort is necessary to open collapsed airways and produce a sufficient negative intrapleural pressure to overcome the positive intra-alveolar pressure so as to allow inspiratory air flow. During expiration the intrapleural pressure of + 10 cm H₂O prematurely closes the airways. Total intraalveolar pressure is 25 cm H₂O. During inspiration the inspiratory muscles must create a negative intrapleural pressure of well over – 25 cm H₂O to allow inspiratory airflow.

3. Increasing dynamic hyperinflation is often associated with hypoxia and hypercapnia because of ventilation-perfusion inequality and alveolar hypoventilation.
4. The markedly hyperinflated lungs associated with severe dynamic hyperinflation squeeze the capillaries in the functioning and perfused alveoli, resulting in an increased pulmonary vascular resistance and precipitating pulmonary hypertension and right heart failure in patients with moderate to severe COPD. Hypoxia and hypercapnia also cause pulmonary vasoconstriction and contribute further to pulmonary hypertension.

Severe dynamic hyperinflation is associated with well-marked rise in the positive end-expiratory pressure (auto-PEEP). This hinders venous return and causes hypotension. When the auto-PEEP is very marked, it exerts an effect similar to that seen in cardiac tamponade (caused by a large pericardial effusion). Severe dynamic hyperinflation with very high auto-PEEP can cause cardiac arrest. Hyperinflated lungs with increase in auto-PEEP can cause barotrauma. Spontaneous pneumothorax is the commonest result of barotrauma. Mediastinal emphysema and interstitial emphysema are two other complications resulting from barotrauma.

Marked hyperdynamic inflation is classically seen in patients with severe exacerbations of COPD, or in patients in a crisis who are incorrectly ventilated. End-stage COPD is also often associated with progressive dynamic hyperinflation.

Respiratory Muscles

The respiratory muscles as has already been pointed out work at a mechanical disadvantage. In addition, loss of muscle mass leads to muscle weakness. Malnutrition contributes even further to this muscle weakness. The flattened diaphragm also has a loss of muscle and fails to generate the usual inspiratory force during inspiration. In normal individuals expiration during tidal breathing is generally passive. Patients with COPD need to use their rib cage muscles and accessory muscles of respiration such as the sternomastoids even during quiet breathing. Global function of respiratory muscles has been shown to be impaired in some studies as judged by measurement of maximum inspiratory mouth pressures. Measurement of transdiaphragmatic pressure during inspiration suggests a reduced inspiratory force exerted by the diaphragm in COPD.

Pulmonary Gas Exchange, Ventilatory Control and Respiratory Failure

The pattern of blood gases in patients with COPD with special reference to Indian subjects is given in the chapter on 'Acute Exacerbation of COPD'. As COPD progresses, there is often hypoxia associated with hypercapnia. Hypoxia is chiefly due to ventilation-perfusion inequalities or mismatch. There may be a slight increase in the shunt but this is of little significance and does not contribute materially to the low PaO_2. Hypercapnia is often observed in advanced COPD and is due to alveolar hypoventilation. There is still a school of thought that believes that the respiratory centre in COPD is insensitive to the rise in $PaCO_2$, compared to normal individuals, so that the ventilatory drive does not increase with increasing $PaCO_2$. All current work, however, suggests that the ventilatory drive in COPD is indeed adequate. In fact Purrel et al., showed that even in very severe end-stage COPD (patients being ventilator-dependent) the ventilatory drive to breathe was not only preserved but was even greater than in stable conditions. Alveolar hypoventilation and CO_2 retention result because the 'load' or the ventilatory demands in these patients cannot be matched by the effort the 'chest bellows' are capable of.

The reason for mismatch between ventilatory demands (the work of breathing) and the effort required to meet these excessive demands are summarized below.

1. Overinflated lungs in COPD can markedly increase the work of breathing.
2. The abnormal configuration of the chest puts the 'thoracic bellows' including the respiratory muscles and the flattened diaphragm, at a mechanical disadvantage. Wasting of the intercostals and weakness of both the intercostals and the diaphragm adds to the inability of the 'effort' to meet the 'load.'
3. There is an excessive load on the mechanically disadvantaged inspiratory muscles of breathing because of premature

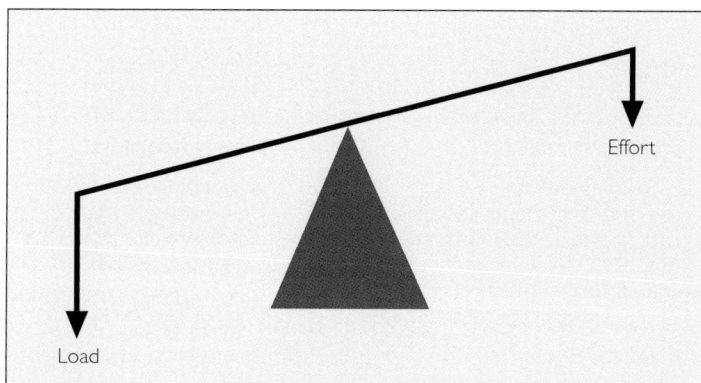

Fig 36.16: The above figure shows how effort does not commensurate with the load.

closure of the peripheral airways during expiration with a resultant increase in intra-alveolar pressure (auto-PEEP).

Yet in clinical practice, one occasionally sees COPD patients who do not seem distressed or who do not make any undue effort while breathing. They seem to be breathing 'lazily'. Perhaps therefore in some patients a poor respiratory drive in relation to increasing $PaCO_2$ may be at least partially responsible for hypercapnia.

As is pointed out in a subsequent section, though in advanced or severe COPD hypoxia and hypercapnia are present either at rest or during an acute exacerbation, about 10–15% of patients with severe COPD manage to keep their blood gases within reasonably normal limits almost right up to the very end of the natural history of the disease.

Cor Pulmonale

Cor pulmonale is defined as right ventricular hypertrophy with or without right heart failure due to disease of the lungs or the pulmonary circulation or due to chronic alveolar hypoventilation from other causes. The commonest cause of cor pulmonale is COPD. As COPD increases in severity it produces pulmonary hypertension which results in right ventricular hypertrophy and failure. Pulmonary hypertension in COPD is due to several factors:

1. Inflammation and narrowing of the walls of pulmonary vessels is an accepted feature of COPD.
2. Rupture of alveolar walls in emphysema reduces the total pulmonary vascular bed and contributes to pulmonary hypertension.
3. Hypoxia and hypercapnia in advanced COPD lead to pulmonary vasoconstriction and pulmonary hypertension. This is so in stable COPD but the marked increase in hypoxia and hypercapnia observed in severe exacerbation of COPD can cause an acute rise in pulmonary artery pressure.
4. Once pulmonary hypertension is well established, the hypertension itself induces further intimal fibrosis and medial wall hypertrophy.
5. Finally, thromboembolic complications are common in COPD and when present add to pulmonary hypertension.

Right ventricular hypertrophy with right heart failure is the end result. Some degree of tricuspid incompetence is also often present. Oedema and later, ascites are due to increased systemic venous pressure and hormonal changes leading to salt and water retention.

SYSTEMIC EFFECTS OF COPD

COPD is not just a disease confined to the lungs. It has important systemic effects which influence morbidity and mortality. These systemic effects are marked in patients with severe COPD. They include weight loss, skeletal muscle wasting and dysfunction of the muscles of respiration, including the diaphragm. Weight loss is associated with a poor prognosis. Loss of muscle mass has been shown to be related to systemic inflammation caused by inflammatory mediators, such as tumour necrosis factor, interleukins such as IL-6 and free oxygen radicals leading to oxidative stress. Other systemic effects of COPD include anaemia, osteoporosis, nutritional deficiencies, psychological problems, in particular depression and perhaps a higher risk of cardiovascular disease.

PATHOGENESIS

There are three important factors contributing to the pathogenesis of COPD—

1. An amplification of the inflammatory response within the peripheral airways and lung parenchyma.
2. Increased oxidative stress within the lungs
3. An imbalance between proteases and antiproteases

Nature of the Amplified Inflammatory Response

The specific pattern of inflammatory response in COPD involves macrophages, neutrophils, T-lymphocytes, B-lymphocytes, and eosinophils. These cells release pro-inflammatory mediators which amplify inflammation and produce both structural and functional damage within the airways and lung parenchyma. Secretion of chemotactic factors attracts macrophages, lymphocytes and neutrophils to the site of inflammation within the respiratory tract.

Inflammatory Cells in COPD

MACROPHAGES
These are derived from mononuclear cells within the blood but differentiate into macrophages within lung tissue. Macrophages are present in the lumen of the small airways, within the wall and in the lung parenchyma. They produce inflammatory mediators and proteases which amplify the inflammatory response to the irritant effect of cigarette smoke, or other noxious particles or gases.

NEUTROPHILS
They are chiefly present in the lumen of the airways and show a marked increase within the lumen during periods of acute exacerbations. An increase in number is also related to COPD severity. Neutrophils may also be present in the walls and in lung tissue but to a much lesser extent.

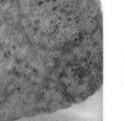

T-LYMPHOCYTES

There is a marked increase in CD8 lymphocytes, a lesser increase in CD4 lymphocytes, so that there is an increase in the CD8–CD4 ratio. The CD 8+ cells together with the TH_1 cells secrete γ interferon and express the chemokine receptor CX R3. CD8 cells are capable of damaging and destroying alveolar cells through a direct cytotoxic effect.

B-LYMPHOCYTES

There is an increase of B-lymphocytes in lymphoid follicles and in the peripheral airways, perhaps resulting from chronic bacterial colonization and infection within the airways.

EOSINOPHILS

Eosinophils are never as prominent as in bronchial asthma. They are increased within the sputum and within the airways during exacerbations.

EPITHELIAL CELLS

Epithelial cells within the airways may also be activated by the irritant effect of cigarette smoke or other noxious particles or gases to produce inflammatory mediators.

Inflammatory Mediators

These can be classified into three classes:

1. *Chemotactic factors*
2. *Pro-inflammatory cytokines*
3. *Growth factors*

Chemotactic factors include a) lipid mediators such as leukotrienes B4 (LTB4) which are chemotactic to neutrophils and T-lymphocytes; b) chemokines like interleukin—8 (IL-8), which attract neutrophils and monocytes to the site of inflammation.

Pro-inflammatory cytokines include tumour necrosis factor (TNF-α), interleukins (IL-8 and IL-6). The interleukins increase inflammatory response and are believed to perhaps contribute to the systemic effects of COPD.

Growth factors include transforming growth factor which helps fibroblasts lay down fibrous tissue. The latter distorts peripheral airways contributing to airways obstruction.

THE ROLE OF OXIDATIVE STRESS

Oxidative stress plays an important role in amplifying inflammation in COPD. Oxidants are produced by cigarette smoke and other irritant particulate matter; these oxidants are released into the area of inflammation by neutrophils and macrophages. The proof of increased oxidative stress lies in the increase in biomarkers (hydrogen peroxide and B-isoprostane) of oxidative stress in the breath, sputum and systemic circulation of COPD patients. A possible reduction in endogenous anti-oxidants in COPD may well worsen the effects of oxidative stress.

The adverse effects of oxidative stress in the lungs include increased inflammation, increased mucus secretion, inactivation of antiproteases, and oedema due to exudation of plasma from capillaries. The mechanism by which oxidative stress is translated into the adverse effects stated above is explained thus. Nitric oxide is generated by inducible nitric oxide syn-

Table 36.8: Inflammatory cells and inflammatory mediators in the pathogenesis of COPD	
Inflammatory cells	**Inflammatory Mediators**

1. Neutrophilis
  a. Present in lumen of airways
  b. Increase mucous secretion
  c. Release proteinases
  d. Increase in number with increasing severity of disease
	1. Chemotactic factors
	  a. Lipid mediators e.g. leukotrienes (LT) B4 which attract neutrophilis, T lymphocytes
	  b. Chemokines like IL-8

2. Macrophages a. Present in lumen and wall of airways, in lung tissue and in BAL fluid	2. Proinflammatory cytokines e.g. IL-8 which amplify the inflammatory process in the lung responsible for systemic effects

3. T lymphocytes
  a. Increase in CD8 cells and CD8/CD4 ratio
  b. CD8 and Th1 cells secrete interferon γ and express CXCR3
  c. CD8 cells cytotoxic to alveolar cells
	3. Growth factors e.g. trans forming growth factor (TGF4) which may be responsible for fibrosis

4. B lymphocytes-present in peripheral airways and lymphoid follicles as a response to infection and chronic bacterial colonization	
5. Eosinophils-increased in sputum and airways during exacerbation of COPD	
6. Epithelial cells may be activated to produce inflammatory mediators.	

thase expressed in the peripheral airways and lung parenchyma of COPD patients. The interaction between superoxide anions and nitric oxide leads to the formation of peroxyl nitrite which mediates many of the adverse effects of oxidative stress on the lungs. It is further believed that oxidative stress may lead to an increased expression of inflammatory genes and a marked decrease in the anti-inflammatory action of corticosteroids due to a reduction in the histone deacetylase activity in the lung of COPD patients.

PROTEASE–ANTIPROTEASE IMBALANCE

There is evidence that COPD is characterized by an imbalance between proteases which break down connective tissue and antiproteases which protect against this. Protease-mediated destruction of elastin present within connective tissue is an irreversible, established feature of emphysema. Proteases are derived from both inflammatory and epithelial cells. The three important groups of increased proteases in COPD are the serine proteases (represented by neutrophil elastase and proteinase 3), the cysteine proteinases (cathepsins B, K, L, S), and the matrix metalloproteinases (MMP-8, MMP-9, MMP-12).

The antiproteases that counter the serine proteases are $alpha_1$ antitrypsin, $alpha_1$ chymotrypsin, and secretory leukoprotease inhibitor. The antiproteases that counter the cathepsins are cystatins, and those countering the MMPs are the tissue

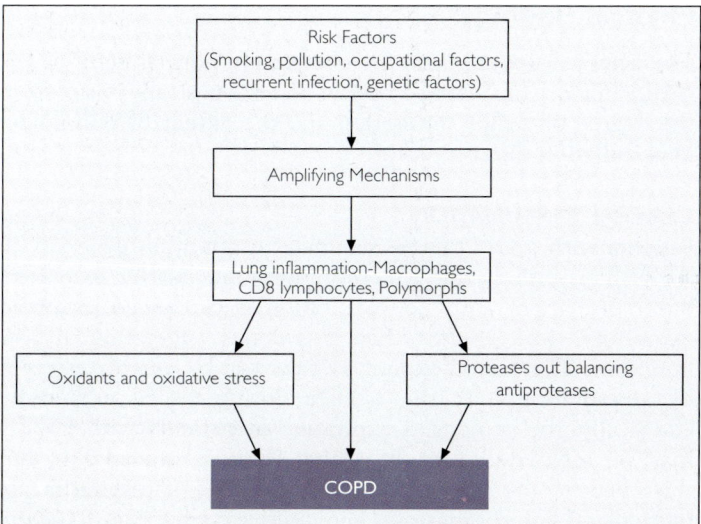

Fig 36.17: Pathogenesis of COPD.

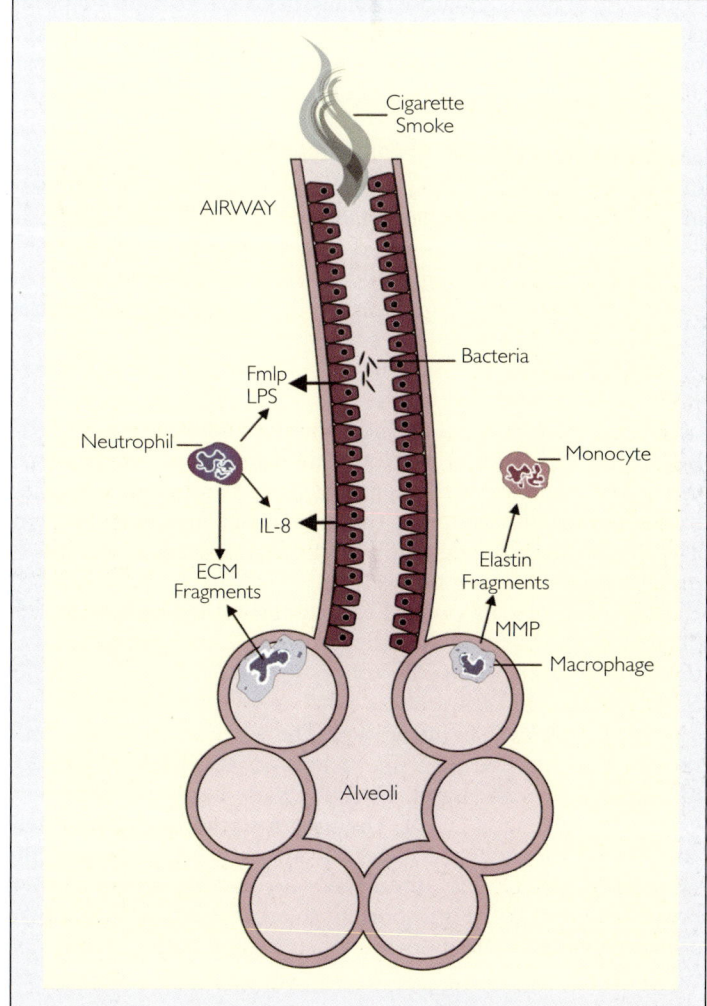

Fig 36.18: Mechanism of inflammatory cells accumulation in the lung in COPD—Neutrophils are recruited to the airways in response to bacterial products such as lipopolysaccharide (LPS) and IL-8 (from latent viral infections). Inflammatory cell recruitment within the alveolar space is related to activated constitutive marcrophages releasing proteineases that produce extracellular matrix fragments (ECM) that are chemotactic for neutrophils and macrophages.

inhibitors of MMP (TMMP 1–4). The proteases outbalance the antiproteases leading to a poorly checked destruction of connective tissue within lung parenchyma, and rupture of the alveolar walls with resultant emphysema.

CLINICAL FEATURES

A history of risk exposure is important. Smoking cigarettes, bidis, hookahs, cigars, and pipes is the first and greatest risk. The patient often gives an incorrect assessment of the number of cigarettes or bidis smoked. Smoking history corroborated by a close relative or friend is therefore essential. In most non-smokers a history of indoor and outdoor urban pollution should be sought as also history of occupational exposure, particularly to dust. Indoor exposure to biofuels might have occurred several years before actual symptoms develop.

Symptoms

The two main symptoms of COPD are breathlessness on exertion and cough with expectoration, sometimes accompanied by a wheeze. Breathlessness initially is only on exertion like climbing stairs, walking uphill or walking fast on the level. It gradually worsens so that in the end-stage of the disease the patient is breathless at rest, often sitting up the whole day and night, every breath a struggle. The symptom of breathlessness on exertion in COPD signifies at least moderate airways obstruction and airflow limitation. Yet the perception of the uncomfortable sensation associated with breathlessness and the increased workload of breathing vary in different individuals, so that a COPD patient with well-marked airflow limitation may clinically be less dyspnoeic than one with lesser

Category	Degree of Dyspnoea	Effect
0	None	Not troubled by shortness of breath except with strenuous exercise
1	Slight	Troubled by shortness of breath when hurrying on the level or walking up a slight hill
2	Moderate	Walks slower than people of the same age on the level because of shortness of breath
3	Moderately severe	Has to stop because of shortness of breath when walking at own pace on the level
4	Severe	Stops for breath after about 100 yd or after a few minutes on the level
5	Very severe	Too breathless to leave the house or breathless when dressing or undressing

Table 36.9: Modified MRC dyspnoea scale

Based on information to classify the severity of dyspnoea according to the categories proposed by the Medical Research Council (MRC)

Source: Mahler DA, Wells CK. 1988. Evaluation of clinical methods for rating dyspnoea. *Chest*. 93: 580–86.

disease. However, once the FEV_1 is less than 35–40% of its predicted value, patients with COPD are breathless even on minimal exertion. In well-established disease, breathlessness is often worsened in the winter months, or following increased air pollution or an increased exposure to dust. The degree of breathlessness can be assessed using the Medical Research Council Dyspnoea Scale or the Borg Scale.

The O_2 cost diagram is more sensitive to the change in breathlessness with progression of the disease than the MRC scale. The patient marks on a 10-cm line, the point beyond which he or she feels breathless. The distance between 'zero' and the marked point enables a score to be obtained.

Cough may be dry or productive, being associated with mucoid sputum. A careful history in smokers generally reveals the presence of cough even before breathlessness appears, the patients ignoring this as a smoker's cough, till such time as breathlessness on exertion ensues either in the natural course of the disease, or is triggered by pulmonary infection. Cough may be severe enough to cause fracture of the ribs, particularly in advanced disease or in osteoporotic patients.

Chest discomfort is often complained of, particularly during periods of exacerbation of breathlessness. This discomfort or tightness may resemble ischemic cardiac pain; it is probably related to the increased workload of breathing borne by intercostal muscles working at a mechanical disadvantage.

Pleuritic chest pain should always suggest the possibility of pneumonia, pulmonary infarction or pneumothorax. Haemoptysis may occur with a complicating acute pulmonary infection but should always prompt the search for bronchogenic carcinoma, particularly in smokers. Weight loss with muscle wasting is a frequent feature of advanced COPD, due to poor nutrition and/or increased metabolism. Patients with severe disease are unable to sleep because of breathlessness and cough. Psychiatric disturbances, in particular depression are frequently observed.

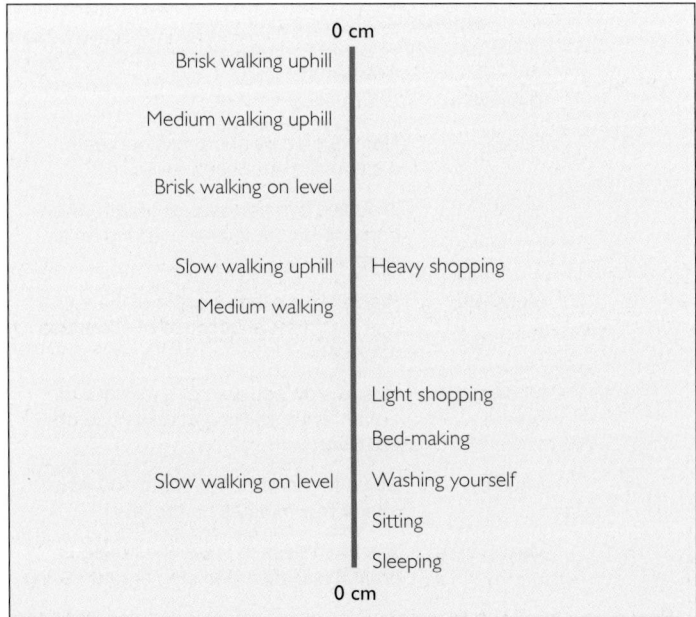

Fig 36.19: Oxygen-cost diagram.

Physical Findings

The physical findings may be completely normal early in the natural history of COPD. Physical findings basically ensue from the degree of airflow limitation and the extent of pulmonary hyperinflation that is present.

GENERAL EXAMINATION

Patients with COPD come for medical attention generally in the fifth or sixth decade. The respiratory rate is often increased, but more importantly the expiration is prolonged, a forced expiratory time greater than 5 seconds suggesting airflow limitation. The forced expiratory time can be roughly assessed by auscultation over the trachea during forced expiration. Classically, the prolonged expiration in patients with COPD may be associated with breathing through pursed lips, but this need not be so. The accessory muscles of respiration, in particular the sternomastoids, show active contraction. In severe COPD the nails, lips and tongue may be cyanosed. Clubbing of the nails is absent and when present should suggest underlying bronchiectasis or a bronchogenic carcinoma. The patient may be drowsy or even comatose because of CO_2 retention. Flapping tremors of the hands or of the whole upper limbs (asterxis) may be observed for the same reason. Rarely, CO_2 retention can lead to papilloedema and seizures.

EXAMINATION OF THE RESPIRATORY SYSTEM

In advanced COPD the chest is barrel-shaped with an increase in the anteroposterior chest diameter. This is due to kyphosis, an elevated sternum, elevated and horizontally placed ribs, a prominent sternal angle and a wide subcostal angle. The elevation of the sternum reduces the space (normally three finger breadths) between the suprasternal notch and the cricoid cartilage. These peculiarities in the shape of the chest are due to overinflated lungs. Besides the use of the accessory muscles of breathing there is often an indrawing of the intercostal spaces and of the suprasternal notch during inspiration. This is due to the marked increase in the negative intraplueral pressure caused by the strong contraction of the intercostals during inspiration. The flat position of the diaphragm often tugs the lower costal margin inwards during inspiration.

Palpation reveals poor chest expansion. Percussion reveals decreased cardiac and hepatic dullness. In advanced COPD the cardiac dullness may be totally lost. Auscultation typically reveals prolonged expiration with a wheeze more marked during expiration than inspiration. The wheezes are polyphonic though this may be difficult to appreciate. Crackles are also often heard over the bases, chiefly in early inspiration. In many cases with advanced COPD the breath sounds are diminished. An auscultatory wheeze is not always heard. In fact, patients with advanced COPD often have no audible wheeze when breathing normally. It is important to ask the patient to perform a forced expiratory manoeuvre when a 'tight' wheeze may just be audible.

CARDIOVASCULAR SYSTEM

The heart and lung are closely linked and increasing COPD produces changes in the circulatory system.

Carbon dioxide retention produces a hyperdynamic circulation with tachycardia, a high pulse pressure and a large volume pulse. Pulsus paradoxus though considered an important physical finding, is not often clinically detectable. The marked swings in intrapleural pressure during inspiration (markedly negative intrapleural pressure) and expiration (positive intrapleural pressure) are responsible for the paradoxical pulse. The jugular venous pressure is clinically difficult to gauge because of marked swings during inspiration (the veins collapse sharply) and expiration (the veins fill, mimicking a rise in pressure). The apex is not generally palpable. The heart sounds are often faint but once cor pulmonale occurs, a right ventricular gallop (third heart sound) is often heard close to the lower left sternal border. A systolic murmur of tricuspid incompetence (increasing in inspiration) may be present and the pulmonary second sound at the base may be accentuated. The presence of marked pulmonary hypertension leads to a dilated pulmonary artery with pulmonary incompetence, manifested by a blowing diastolic murmur (Graham Steele murmur) best heard in the second, third left intercostal spaces close to the left sternal border. These are the classical findings of cor pulmonale. But there are a number of patients with COPD and cor pulmonale where few or none of these auscultatory findings are elicited. Their absence does not exclude cor pulmonale.

When right heart failure occurs, the liver is enlarged and tender. The liver however may be felt well below the costal margin due to the low diaphragm in COPD patients even without heart failure. Pitting oedema of the feet is a crucially important physical finding. In the absence of any other obvious cause that explains this finding, it invariably means right heart failure due to cor pulmonale.

It needs to be noted that before the term COPD came into being, patients with this disease were classified into two separate phenotypes—the blue bloater and the pink puffer. The 'blue bloater' was puffy in the face, was often cyanosed, was not unduly 'tachypnoeic, breathing in a lazy and in a not too disturbed fashion. He was both hypoxic and had carbon dioxide retention, and was prone to developing pulmonary hypertension, cor pulmonale and right heart failure with well-marked oedema due to fluid retention. The blue bloater was considered to be chiefly bronchitic with regard to his pathology. We know today that the pathology here is not just in the large airways but is maximum in the small airways leading to increase in airways resistance.

The 'pink puffer' on the other hand was tachypnoeic, could be seen breathing hard using all his accessory muscles. He however kept his arterial blood gases within normal limits almost up to the very end of the natural history of the disease. He was considered to have more of emphysema as the predominant underlying pathology.

It soon came to be realized that such watertight compartments were unsatisfactory, because most patients had varying components of inflammation of the small airways leading to obstruction + airflow limitation *and* emphysema with airflow limitation. In fact this is the reason why the common generic term COPD was given to the disease.

ASSESSMENT OF LUNG FUNCTION

The assessment of lung function is of vital importance for the following reasons—

1. The diagnosis of early COPD may be missed on a clinical examination. COPD even today remains grossly under-diagnosed for this very reason.
2. An objective diagnosis of COPD needs basic spirometric tests.
3. The degree or severity of COPD can be assessed and followed up objectively through spirometric studies.

SPIROMETRY

In the very early stages, as for example in asymptomatic smokers, the subtle increase in resistance in the peripheral airways can only be made out by special tests (e.g. measurement of closing volume, frequency dependence of compliance) which may be abnormal. These tests are difficult to perform, have a high coefficient of variability and are not advised in routine clinical practice. However, by the time a patient starts to complain of breathlessness, spirometric changes obtained through routine spirometry become evident. The American Thoracic Society (ATS), the European Respiratory Society (ERS) and the Global Initiative for Obstructive Lung Disease (GOLD) have defined COPD to be present in spirometric terms when $FEV_1/FVC < 70\%$. This ratio used in spirometric definition holds true irrespective of age, sex and ethnicity. The FEV_1 as a percentage of the predicted value is used to assess the degree or severity of COPD. FEV_1 values within $\pm 20\%$ of the predicted range are considered to be within normal limits.

The spirometric classification of the degree of COPD severity is given in Table 36.10.

There is indeed an interesting direct relationship between the degree of COPD as judged by the degree of fall in the predicted values of FEV_1 and the degree of inflammatory changes in the small airways as observed in pathological studies.

It is important to note that the speed of inspiration and the presence and duration of the end inspiratory pause before the forced expiration can influence both the FVC and FEV_1 values. If the forced expiratory manoeuvre is preceded by a slow inspiration and a long (4–5 sec) inspiratory pause, the forced expiratory flows (FVC, FEV_1) are lower than when the

Table 36.10: Spirometric classification of the degree of COPD severity		
I	Mild COPD	$FEV_1/FVC < 70$; $FEV_1 \geq 80\%$ of predicted
II	Moderate COPD	$FEV_1/FVC < 70$; $FEV \geq 50\%$ and $< 80\%$ of predicted
III	Severe COPD	$FEV_1/FVC < 70$; $FEV_1 \geq 30\%$ and $< 50\%$ of predicted
IV	Very severe COPD	$FEV_1/FVC < 70$; $FEV_1 < 30\%$ of predicted

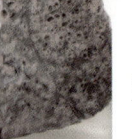

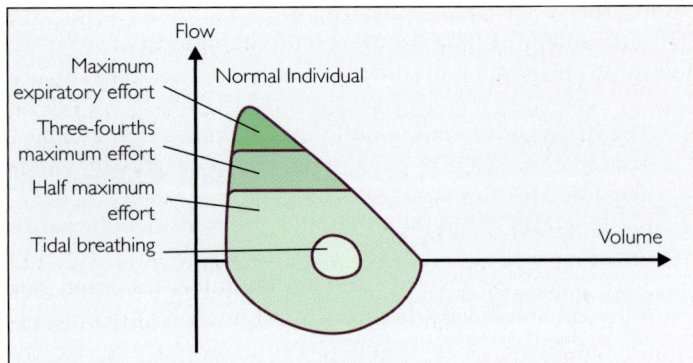

Fig 36.20: Flow-volume loop of a normal individual.

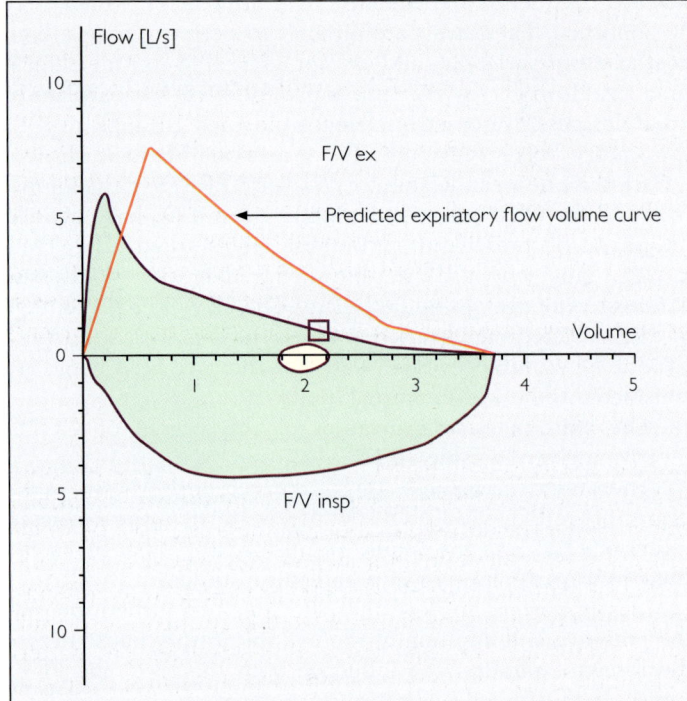

Fig 36.21: Flow-volume loop showing mild COPD.

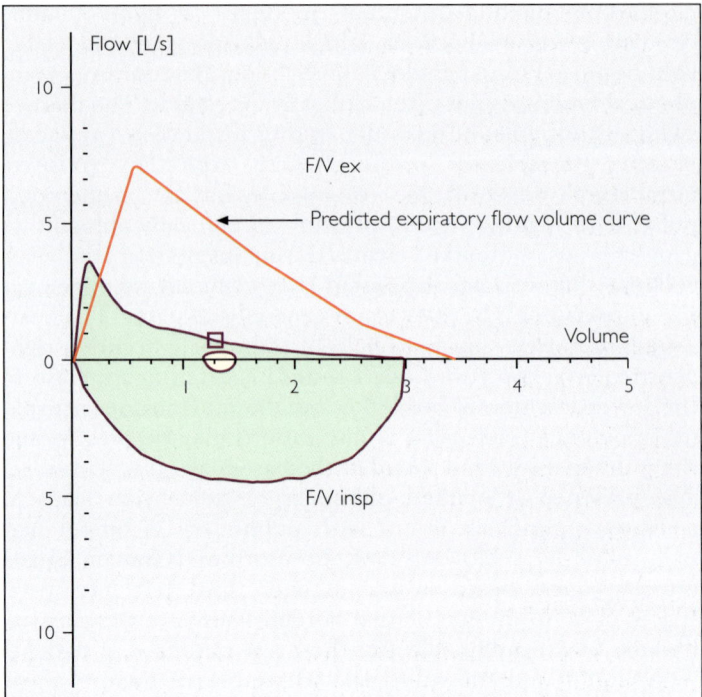

Fig 36.22: Flow-volume loop showing moderate COPD.

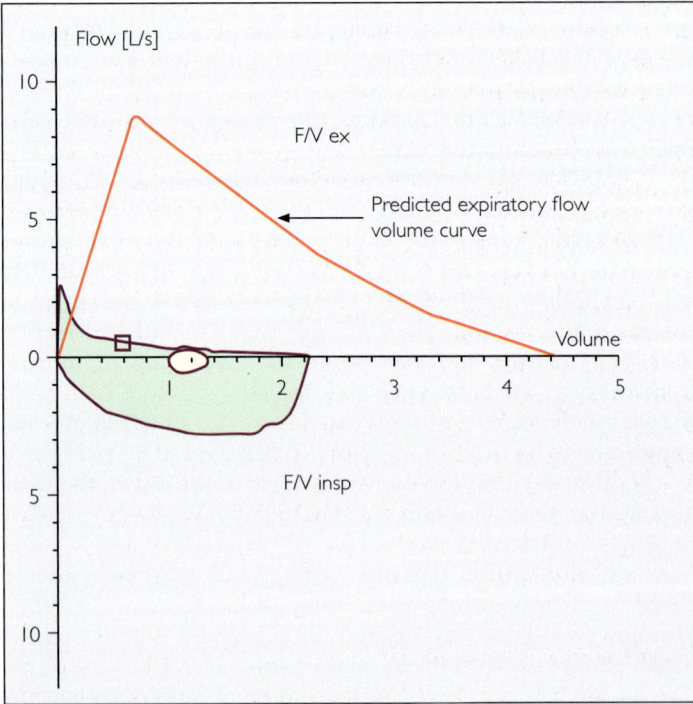

Fig 36.23: Flow-volume loop showing severe COPD.

Note: Increasing upward concavity of expiratory curve with increasing severity of COPD.

forced expiratory manoeuvre is preceded by a fast inspiration and without an inspiratory pause. The necessity to standardize procedures during spirometry is clearly evident. To obtain maximal flows the inspiration should be at maximum speed, followed by a forced expiration without any inspiratory pause.

Testing Reversibility of Airways Obstruction and Airflow Limitation

1. *Use of an Aerosolized Bronchodilator* It is important to test for the degree of reversibility to distinguish COPD from asthma. Asthma generally shows good or even complete reversibility, while COPD shows incomplete, poor or no reversibility. There are some who advocate repeating the forced expiratory manoeuvre after four to five puffs of a β_2-agonist through a metered dose inhaler; others would prefer to nebulize the patient with salbutamol and then repeat the

forced expiratory manoeuvre. In some patients the addition of an anticholinergic drug to a β_2-agonist produces a further increase in FEV_1. Reversibility should be tested at the time of diagnosis. It need not be tested at subsequent follow-ups. A change in FEV_1 > 200 ml is considered to be more than random variation, and only then should a change in FEV_1 be taken as significant. In addition to this absolute change in FEV_1, an increase in the FEV_1 by 12% or more is considered significant according to the ERS, ATS and GOLD guidelines. The British Society Guidelines suggest an absolute increase in FEV_1 by 200 ml and an increase of 15% over the baseline value to be significant. Roughly 30% of patients with COPD show significant reversibility.

2. *Reversibility to Corticosteroids* Use of corticosteroids to test reversibility in COPD has not been included in the recent guidelines on the assessment and management of the disease. The corticosteroid test does however reveal significant reversibility in some patients with COPD who show no reversibility on using aerosolized or nebulised bronchodilators. Prednisolone in a dose of 30 mg is given for two weeks and standard spirometry is repeated to note the change in FEV_1 as also the degree of change present.

Lung Volumes

The RV, FRC, TLC and ratio of RV/TLC are all increased due to air trapping and hyperinflation of lungs. Using helium techniques to measure static lung volumes might give false low values as the inspired helium may not have sufficient time to equilibrate within the air spaces. Lung volumes measured through body plethysmography are more accurate. This technique measures trapped air in large air spaces, air in poorly ventilated alveoli and gives higher lung volume readings compared to the helium technique.

Flow-volume loops Flow-volume loops show that the expiratory flow rates at different lung volumes are reduced because of airflow limitation; they also show the degree of airflow limitation in COPD patients.

Measurement of lung volumes can prove to be of immense use in some patients with severe COPD due to marked airways obstruction and airflow limitation. In these patients the FVC on routine spirometry may be markedly reduced, so that the FEV_1 almost approximates the FVC and the FEV_1/FVC is greater than 70%. A mistaken spirometric interpretation of severe restrictive disease can be made if the lung volumes are not measured. If the lung volumes were to be measured in these patients the RV is found to be markedly increased often with some degree of increase in TLC. The low FVC in these patients is due to a marked increase in the RV. It is of crucial importance to measure lung volumes in these patients to avoid a wrong diagnosis.

Inspiratory Capacity (IC)

Greater stress is being placed in noting the Inspiratory Capacity (a neglected spirometric variable) in COPD. Recent studies have shown the following—

1. The IC reflects the FRC so that any change in the FRC is accompanied by an opposite change in IC provided the TLC is by and large constant. Millie Emily and Casanova *et al.*, found that a reduced IC correlated both with dyspnoea and exercise capacity in COPD. The lower the IC the greater the dyspnoea and the poorer the exercise capacity in COPD.

2. The IC is a good predictor of maximal tidal volume during exercise and so of maximal exercise ventilation.
3. There appears to be a significant inverse correlation between $PaCO_2$ and IC in COPD patients who have significant expiratory airflow limitation.
4. The IC is simple to measure and can reflect changes in hyperinflation (either following use of a bronchodilator or an increase in ventilation).
5. The IC could help evaluate the status and progress of COPD. A progressive reduction in IC would indicate reduction in exercise capacity and therefore a progression of the disease. Measurement of IC could perhaps also help assess the efficacy of therapy in COPD. Measurements of FEV_1 and IC should be analyzed to provide better information on lung function in COPD.

CO Transfer

The carbon monoxide transfer factor (TLCO) in advanced COPD is invariably reduced because of a reduction in 'ventilated' lung volumes and an inequality in the ventilation-perfusion ratio. However, the diffusion capacity of CO normalized to ventilated alveolar volume (TLCO/VA/ KCO) may remain normal, except in the presence of emphysema when it is reduced. A reduced TLCO/VA, KCO excludes bronchial asthma.

The changes in static pressure volume curves of the lungs in COPD in the presence of emphysema consist of an increase in static compliance and a reduction in static transpulmonary pressure at any specific lung volume.

Arterial Blood Gases

Arterial blood gas studies are essential to determine the presence and degree of hypoxemia and hypercapnia in patients with COPD. A lowered PaO_2 and an increased $PaCO_2$ generally occur when the FEV_1 falls below 50% of predicted values. But there are many exceptions to this generalization and some patients continue to ventilate well and keep their CO_2 within limits even when the FEV_1 is less than one litre. The pattern of blood gases in Indian subjects and their change during an

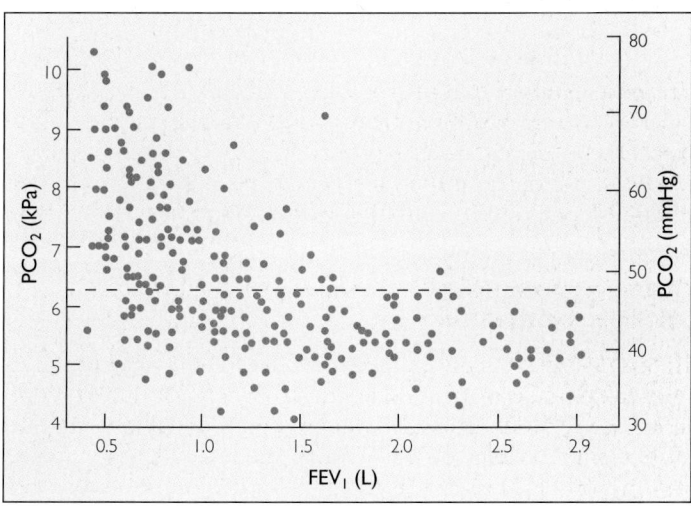

Fig 36.24: Relationship between FEV_1 and PCO_2 in COPD. Reproduced with permission from *Respiratory Medicine*, second edition, volume 2, ed. Brewis RAL, Corrin B, Geddes DM, Gibson GJ. 1995. WB Saunders Company Ltd. © Elsevier.

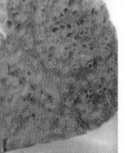

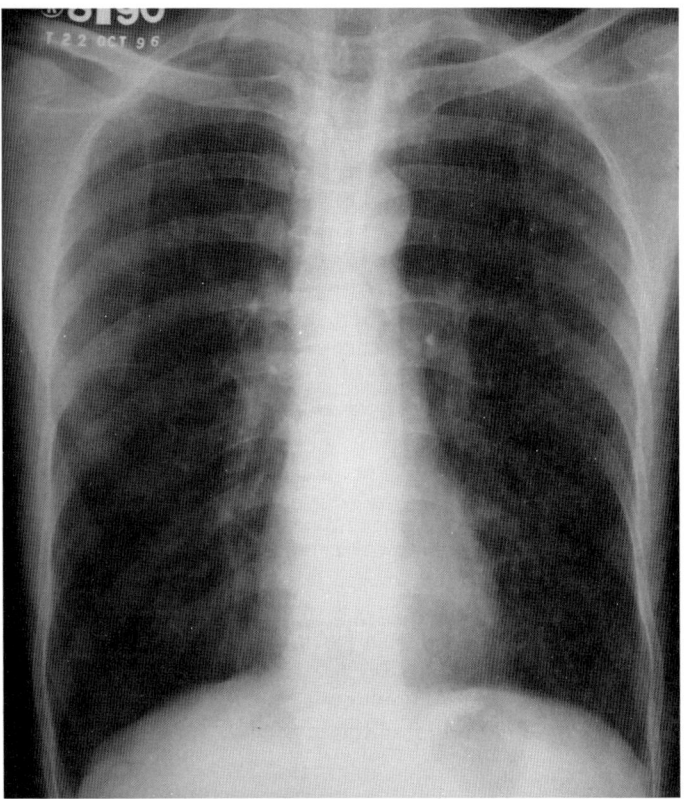

Fig 36.25: COPD—PA view demonstrates a tubular heart, flattened domes of diaphragms, hyperinflated lungs and visibility of the tenth rib. All are classical features of COPD.

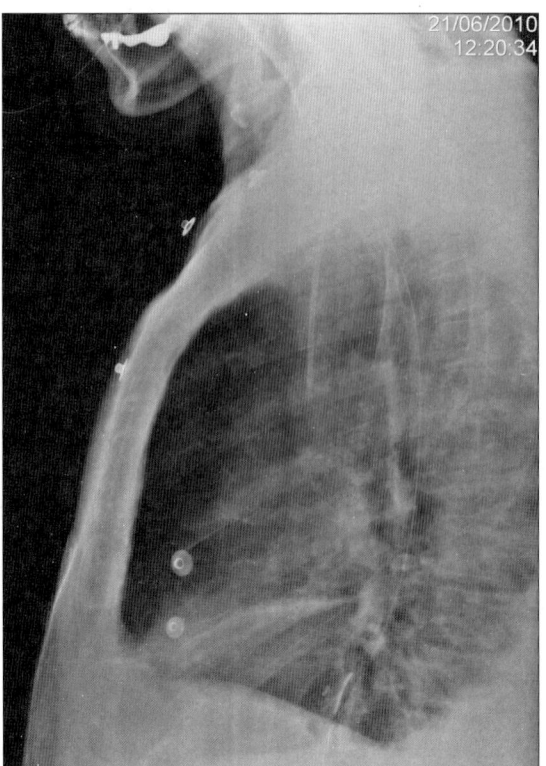

Fig 36.27: COPD—Lateral view of chest demonstrates a markedly widened retrosternal air space.

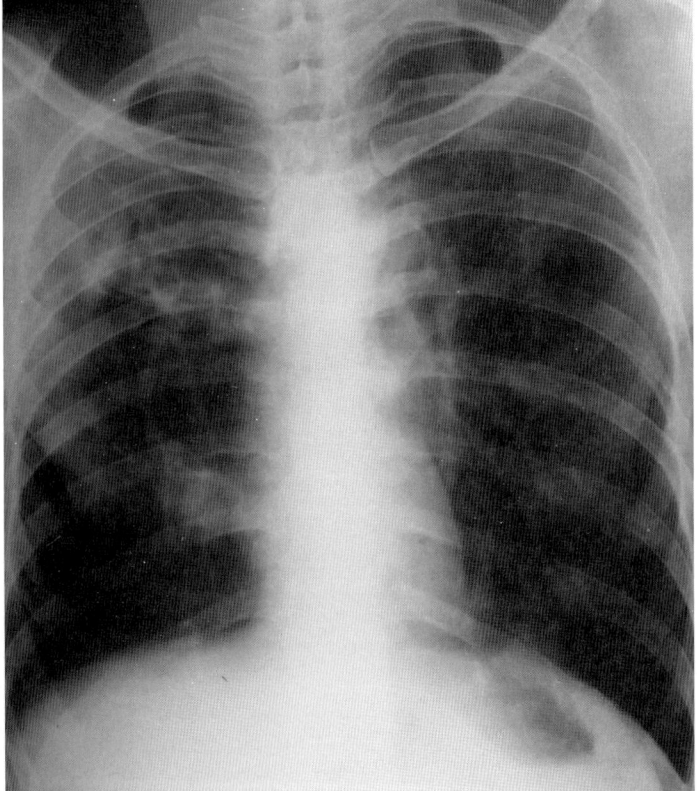

Fig 36.26: Emphysema: Chest X-ray PA view demonstrates extensive luscent areas in both lower zones representing areas of emphysema. Note compressed lung in upper and mid-zones.

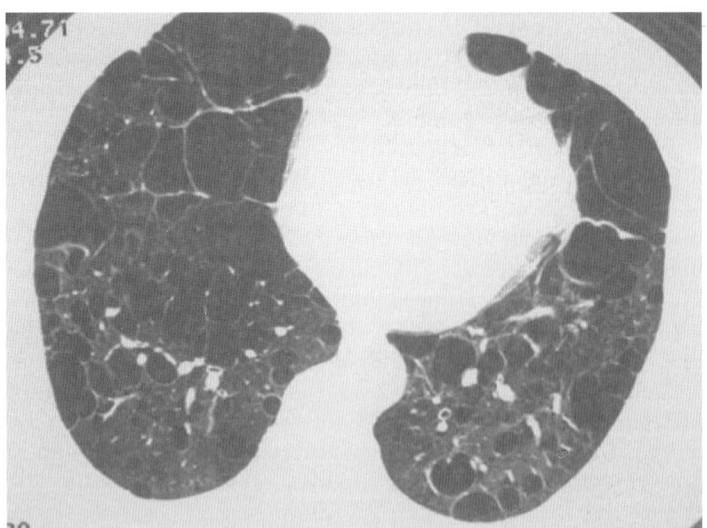

Fig 36.28: Emphysema. Extensive thin-walled bullae in both lung fields.

acute crisis associated with an exacerbation of COPD are considered later.

Exercise and COPD Patients with COPD have higher oxygen consumption for a given workload compared to normal individuals due to increase in the work of breathing. These patients also have an increase in dead space; minute ventilation therefore needs to be increased if the $PaCO_2$ is to be kept within normal range. As COPD worsens, expiratory air flow limitation occurs even during normal tidal breathing. (Figure

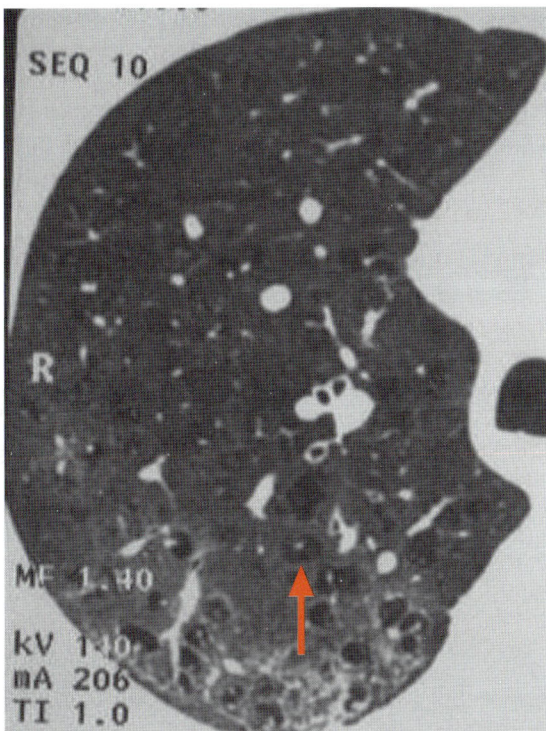

Fig 36.29: Centrilobular emphysema-HRCT demonstrates thin-walled well-defined luscencies in the posterior aspect of the right lung. These air spaces demonstrate a vessel in the central portion of the air space representing a centrilobular vessel. This is a classical sign of centrilobular emphysema.

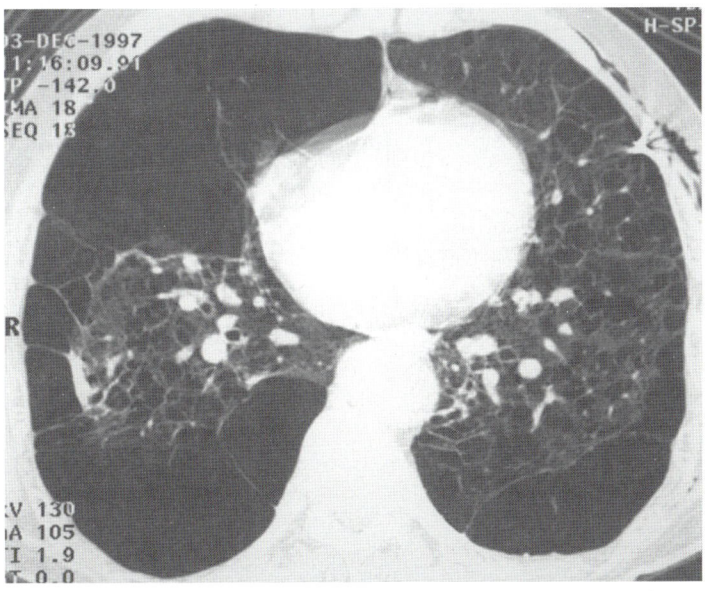

Fig 36.30: Emphysema. HRCT demonstrates extensive emphysema in the form of centrilobular emphysema and paraseptal emphysema, compressing lung parenchyma.

36.23) Such patients cannot meet the increased ventilatory demand by increasing their tidal volume. They can only do so by increasing the respiratory frequency or increasing inspiratory flow thereby causing an upward shift in the end-expiratory volume so that expiratory flow rate can increase. Each of these

manoeuvres will lead to increased inflation of the lungs and a further increase in the workload of respiratory muscles which are already working at a mechanical disadvantage. Increasing dyspnoea would limit their exercise. Exercise is at times also limited by leg muscle fatigue pointing to skeletal muscle dysfunction in COPD.

Exercise increases cardiac output and the increased perfusion of poorly ventilated alveoli lowers V/Q ratios causing hypoxemia and in some instances hypercapnia.

Exercise Test

Exercise testing is quite unnecessary for the diagnosis of COPD. Exercise testing may however offer valuable information on the behaviour of the heart-lung combination during the stress of an increased workload. There are three types of tests—

1. *Progressive Symptom Limited Exercise Test* The patient is exercised on a treadmill or cycle with a progressively increasing workload. The patient stops when symptoms prevent further continuation of exercise. A maximum test is defined as one where the heart rate reaches 80% of predicted and the ventilation 90% of predicted. Blood pressure and ECG recordings done simultaneously help assess cardiovascular factors that may contribute to limitation of exercise capacity
2. *Self-Paced Exercise Test* The commonly used test is the six-minute walk test which is useful only in moderately severe COPD when the FEV_1 is < 1.5L. These patients would be expected to have an exercise tolerance of less than 600 meters in six minutes. We would recommend measuring the O_2 saturation at the end of the six-minute walk. The heart rate, blood pressure and auscultating the heart for a third heart sound in particular may help detect cardiovascular abnormalities. The six-minute walk test has a coefficient of variation of about 8%.
3. *The Shuttle Walking Test* In this test, the patient performs a paced walk between two points 10 meters apart (the shuttle). The pace of the walk is increased at regular intervals until the patient stops the walk because of breathlessness. The number of completed shuttles is noted.
4. *Steady State Exercise Test* The patient is exercised at a sustainable state of maximal activity for three to six minutes. Blood gases, V_D/V_T are measured during this test. This test is not necessary for clinical assessment.

Sleep Studies

Nocturnal hypoxemia is often observed in patients with moderate to severe COPD. The association of obstructive sleep apnoea with COPD is fairly frequent and these patients can suffer dangerous hypoxic spells during sleep. Sleep studies are indicated in these patients.

Other Investigations

1. 2D Doppler Echocardiography is often used in suspected or definite cor pulmonale. The tricuspid gradient is used to measure right ventricular systolic pressure and to estimate the pressure gradient across the tricuspid regurgitant jet recorded by the Doppler ultrasound. Right ventricular

dimensions, systolic and diastolic function can also be assessed along with the degree of pulmonary hypertension.

2. A complete blood count with a determination of the PCV will detect the presence of polycythemia. Polycythemia is always secondary to fairly longstanding hypoxia with a PaO_2 generally < 55 mm Hg. Polycythemia should be suspected when PCV is > 47% in women and > 52% in men, the Hb is > 16 g/dl in women and > 18 g/dl in men. It is important to recognize polycythemia as it contributes to cerebrovascular accidents, cardiovascular episodes and features of peripheral vascular disease.

3. Alpha$_1$ antitrypsin deficiency should be looked out for in all patients < 45 years of age with an early onset of emphysema and in all patients with a family history of premature emphysema.

SUGGESTED READING

Chan-Yeung M, Ait-Khaled N, *et al*. The burden and impact of COPD in Asia and Africa. *Int J Tuberc Lung Dis*. 8(1): 2–14.

Global Initiative for Chronic Obstructive Lung Disease. Global Strategy for the Diagnosis, Management, and Prevention of Chronic Obstructive Pulmonary Disease. Global Initiative for Chronic Obstructive Lung Disease. 2006.

Hogg JC, Chu F, Utokaparch S, Woods R, Elliott WM, Buzatu L, Cherniack RM, Rogers RM, Sciurba FC, Coxson HO, *et al*. The nature of small-airway obstruction in chronic obstructive pulmonary disease. *N Engl J Med*. 2004; 350: 2645–53.

Lopez AD, Shibuya K, Rao C, Mathers CD, Hansell AL, Held LS, Schmid V, Buist S. Chronic obstructive pulmonary disease: current burden and future projections. *Eur Respir J*. 2006; 27: 397–412.

Mannino DM. COPD: epidemiology, prevalence, morbidity and mortality, and disease heterogeneity. *Chest*. 1 May 2002; 121(5 Suppl): 121S–126S.

Salvi Sundeep S, Barnes Peter. Chronic Obstructive pulmonary disease in non-smokers. *Lancet*. 2009; 374: 733–43.

Surinder K. Emergence of chronic obstructive pulmonary disease as an epidemic in India. *Indian J Med Res*. Dec. 2006: 619–30.

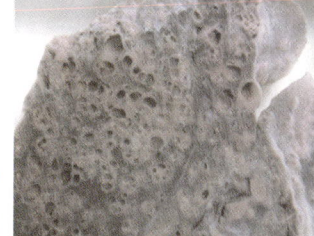
CHAPTER **37**

Acute Exacerbation of Chronic Obstructive Pulmonary Disease

Acute exacerbations of chronic obstructive pulmonary disease (COPD) are in-built features in the natural history of the disease, punctuating its course from time to time. They significantly increase both morbidity and mortality, the in-hospital mortality of COPD exacerbations being as high as 10%. In the UK, COPD exacerbations are the most common cause of medical hospital admissions, amounting to 15.9% of the hospital admissions at a huge cost to the national exchequer. In large metropolitan cities in India, COPD exacerbations are an important and frequent cause of admission to critical care units. Approximately 1 in 15 patients reporting to the Emergency department in a busy Mumbai hospital comes with worsening of symptoms of COPD.

Acute exacerbations are more frequent and often more severe in patients with increasing severity of COPD. The annual frequency of exacerbations in different patients having the same severity of COPD varies for unknown reasons. Predisposition to acute exacerbations may well be related to increasing severity of the disease, greater inflammation of the small airways, greater exposure to and perhaps greater susceptibility to infection and to the presence of lower airways bacterial colonization.

DEFINITION

An acute exacerbation of COPD is an acute worsening of symptoms associated with worsening lung functions that could in some patients precipitate acute respiratory failure or the acute worsening of chronic respiratory failure. Respiratory failure (acute or acute on chronic) is often the culminating feature of an acute severe exacerbation of COPD. It is important to stress this fact as it entails an awareness for diagnosing this event and necessitates expert critical care in management.

The guidelines of the Global Initiative for Chronic Obstructive Lung Disease (GOLD) define an exacerbation as 'an event in the natural course of the disease characterized by a change in the patient's dyspnoea, cough and/or sputum that is beyond day to day normal variations, is acute in onset and may warrant a change in medication in a patient with underlying COPD'.

PATHOPHYSIOLOGY

The pathophysiology has been detailed in an earlier section. Acute exacerbations are associated with increased inflammation within the peripheral airways and the lungs. Clinically, this is manifest by worsening dyspnoea and sputum production. Pathological features include an even more intense inflammatory exudate and oedema of the mucosa of the peripheral airways, an increase in tone of the bronchial muscle and increased mucous production. The acute increase in obstruction to the airways and the further increase in airflow limitation, if sufficiently severe, produce dynamic hyperinflation. As has been already explained in an earlier section, dynamic hyperinflation in acute severe exacerbations can occur with frightening rapidity, the patient becoming increasingly uncomfortable and dyspnoeic, because he has to breathe at progressively high lung volumes. The work of breathing is substantially increased, well beyond what it was prior to the exacerbation, and there is further impairment of respiratory muscle function. The 'effort' expended by the chest bellows and the respiratory muscles is not commensurate with the extra 'load' of breathing. This results in alveolar hypoventilation and hypercapnic respiratory failure. Hypoxia is also worsened in severe exacerbations because of increasing ventilation-perfusion inequality.

Not all acute exacerbations are severe, the degree of exacerbation being probably dependent on the degree of small airways inflammation present in the stable state.

Moderate and severe COPD (Grade III, Grade IV) is associated with a greater degree of inflammation of the small airways, when compared to Grade I and Grade II COPD. This may well be the reason why acute exacerbations are generally more severe in patients with Grade III, Grade IV COPD.

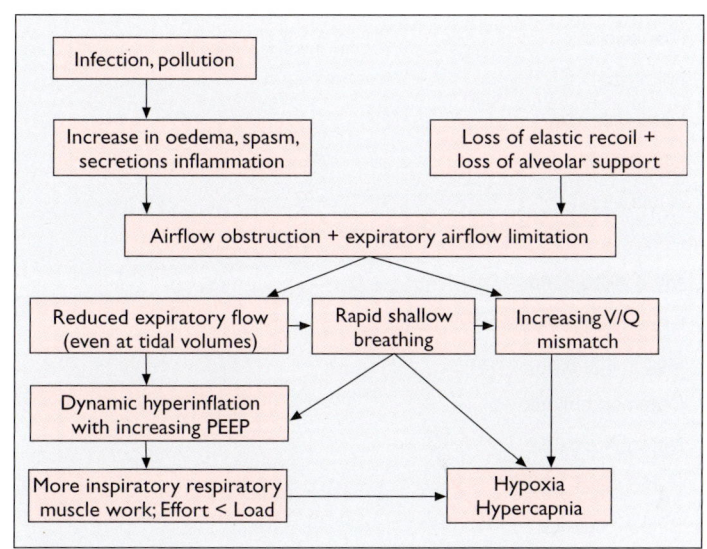

Fig 37.1: Pathophysiology of ARF in exacerbation of COPD.

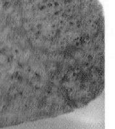
ETIOLOGY

The commonest cause of an acute exacerbation in COPD is infection. The common bacteria causing infective exacerbations are *Streptococcus pneumoniae, H. influenzae*; in older patients, *Klebsiella pneumoniae* and *P. aeruginosa* are often the infecting agents. There is growing incidence of *Moraxella catarrhalis* as a causative infective agent, both in the West and the developing world. Molecular biology using polymerase chain reaction (PCR) techniques has provided evidence for an increasing role of viruses in the aetiology of acute exacerbations. The commonest responsible virus is the rhinovirus. Other viruses include the respiratory syncitial virus, coronavirus, influenza virus and the adenovirus. The role of atypical organisms, in particular mycoplasma and chlamydia is unclear.

Acute exacerbations have also been noted to occur following an acute increase in indoor pollution, exposure to increased outdoor pollution, and due to sudden increase in exposure to an occupational risk factor. One reason for increased incidence of exacerbations during winter is excessive outdoor pollution which blankets large cities in India at almost ground level. Exposure to pollution from exhausts of cars in traffic jams can lead to acute exacerbations, and is another reason for the emergency visits to hospitals. A sudden and marked spurt in the number of cigarettes smoked has been known to cause an acute exacerbation of COPD.

Table 37.1: Common organisms and pollutants responsible for acute exacerbation of COPD
Bacteria
Streptococcus pneumoniae
Haemophilus influenzae
Moraxella catarrhalis
Pseudomonas aeruginosa
Viruses
Rhinovirus
Influenza
Parainfluenza
Coronavirus
Adenovirus
RSV
Atypical bacteria
Chlamydia pneumoniae
Mycoplasma pneumoniae
Common pollutants
Nitrogen dioxide
Particulates
Sulphur dioxide
Ozone

CLINICAL FEATURES

An acute exacerbation of COPD is characterized by a clear worsening of respiratory symptoms, well beyond what the patient is used to experiencing. These symptoms chiefly include increased dyspnoea, increased cough with an increase in sputum volume, purulent sputum and an increase in wheeze.

Physical findings include all the features observed with airways obstruction and airflow limitation described earlier. Tachycardia, tachypnoea, excessive use of accessory muscles of respiration, in-drawing of intercostal spaces during inspiration with paradoxical breathing are all seen in severe exacerbations. Expiration is clearly prolonged and there is an audible wheeze. Rapidly increasing dynamic hyperinflation will cause an actual measurable increase in the circumference of the chest, increasing tachycardia, hypotension, marked distress and difficulty in breathing, the breath sounds ultimately being reduced to short gasps. Auscultation in the presence of rapidly progressive dynamic hyperinflation may reveal faint or absent breath sounds, the expiratory wheeze often being inaudible. Periods of apnoea may interrupt the breathing which is often irregular. Central cyanosis may be evident because of increasing hypoxia. Hypercapnia may progressively worsen, leading often, though not always to flapping tremors and confusion. Rhythm disturbances may occur in the form of multiple atrial or ventricular extrasystoles, supraventricular tachycardia, chaotic atrial tachycardia, atrial fibrillation and even ventricular tachycardia.

Severe acute exacerbations can precipitate right heart failure, particularly in patients with Grade III and Grade IV COPD. This is related to pulmonary vasoconstriction and pulmonary hypertension caused by acute hypoxia and hypercapnia in an individual who often has a baseline increase in pulmonary vascular resistance due to inflammatory changes in the small airways, periphery of the lungs and the pulmonary vessels. The most important and early sign of right heart failure in COPD patients is oedema of the feet for which there is no other obvious cause. The oedema can worsen and can be so marked as to be generalized. In severe exacerbations in Grade III and Grade IV COPD, electrocardiography (ECG) shows a P pulmonale often associated with clockwise rotation. There may be evidence of right ventricular enlargement and/or a right bundle branch block pattern. These ECG findings are acute, for they generally regress after recovery and often return to a stable state. Echocardiography may corroborate right ventricular systolic dysfunction, some degree of functional tricuspid incompetence and pulmonary hypertension.

Acute exacerbations of COPD are not necessarily severe; some are indeed mild, easily manageable at home. Apart from a worsening of symptoms more than what is usual for the patient, physical signs are limited to those caused by a modest increase in airways obstruction and airflow limitation.

The duration of acute exacerbations varies. Milder exacerbations often treated at home may be relieved within four to seven days with adequate treatment, though full recovery with return to baseline symptoms may take as long as three to four weeks in some of these patients. Recurrence rate varies in different individuals for unclear reasons. In a cohort of patients with moderate to severe COPD followed up after acute exacerbation, 22% suffered a recurrence within 50 days

Table 37.2:
Clinical features of acute severe exacerbation of COPD

Increase in dyspnoea, cough, sputum

All the clinical features of severe airflow limitation

Features of hypoxia and hypercapnia

Featurs of right heart failure may be present

Table 37.3:
Causes of hypoxemia

V/Q mismatch causing an increased alveolar arterial O_2 gradient

Alveolar hypoventilation

Small shunts amounting to 4–10% of the cardiac output

Low P_vO_2 (observed in some patients with cor pulmonale and severe heart failure)

Table 37.4:
Causes of hypercapnia

1. Alveolar hypoventilation increased load and the inability of the respiratory muscle (inspiratory in the main) to meet this load. Inspiratory work of breathing is doubled in acute respiratory failure (ARF); increase in auto orintrinsic PEEP accounts for more than half of this increase in the work of breathing

2. V/Q mismatch

3. Change in the pattern of breathing-smaller tidal volume with an increase in respiratory rate. This may be an adaptive mechanism to avoid increasing ventilation and respiratory muscle activation to the point where muscle fatigue ensues.

Source: Orozco Levi. *European Respiratory Journal.* 2003, 22: 410–578.

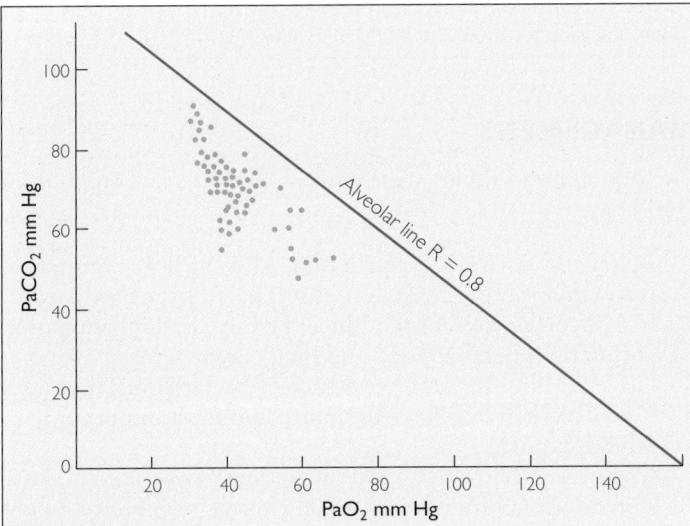

Fig 37.2: ABG in 64 patients with Grade III to Grade IV COPD who developed an acute exacerbation of COPD. Note severity of hypoxemia and hypercapnia present in most patients with Grade III–IV COPD in an acute severe exacerbation.

Source: *Diagnosis and Management of Acute Respiratory Failure*, 1979. Oxford University Press, Oxford, Delhi, Bombay.

of the first (index) exacerbation. Perhaps an initial exacerbation may well increase susceptibility to a subsequent one.

INVESTIGATIONS

Investigations are done with three objectives in mind—

1. To determine the severity of the exacerbation
2. If infection is the cause, to determine if possible the infective agent responsible for the exacerbation
3. To exclude other complications which can cause an acute respiratory crisis in COPD; a crisis that may be clinically indistinguishable from that caused by exacerbation of COPD.

Investigations include a routine complete blood count (CBC), erythrocyte sedimentation rate (ESR), and C-reactive protein. The latter is believed to be an important marker for the presence and degree of the underlying inflammation in the peripheral airways. X-ray chest and ECG are always done routinely. O_2 saturation, arterial blood gases, and pH are vital tests. The O_2 saturation will serve as a guide to the degree of hypoxia, but it is often impossible to diagnose the presence and degree of CO_2 retention without actually determining the $PaCO_2$. In severe exacerbations causing acute respiratory failure or acute on chronic respiratory failure, arterial pH is of vital importance. An arterial pH < 7.25 is perhaps the most important single factor associated with high mortality.

In severe exacerbations, it is important to determine the baseline function of organ systems. Serum creatinine, blood-urea-nitrogen (BUN) levels and serum electrolytes need to be done. Sputum microscopy and culture may help (though not necessarily so) in arriving at the organism responsible for an acute infective exacerbation. It is of particular help if *P. aeruginosa* or *Klebsiella pneumoniae* is grown on culture, as this will dictate the correct choice of antibiotics.

Spirometry is not useful in severe exacerbations as the patient is too ill to allow reliable results. Also, baseline spirometric readings of a patient admitted in an emergency are not generally available.

PROBLEMS IN DIAGNOSIS

Problems in diagnosis are not infrequent in patients who on clinical examination appear to have an acute exacerbation of COPD. The major difficulty encountered is to distinguish left ventricular dysfunction and failure in a patient with COPD from an acute severe exacerbation of COPD. This difficulty is compounded when acute left ventricular failure is the sole manifestation of ischemic heart disease, without a preceding history of anginal pain and without clear evidence of ischemia on the ECG. Both COPD and ischemic heart disease often manifest in similar age groups. Interestingly, patients with COPD who develop acute left ventricular failure often present with tachypnoea and marked wheezing rather than the usual crackles of pulmonary oedema. An X-ray chest may be unhelpful and in fact misleading, because occasionally predominantly unilateral pulmonary oedema may be seen in COPD patients who develop acute left ventricular failure. The unilateral pulmonary oedema is often misdiagnosed as pneumonia. Investigations are often non-contributory. We have found echocardiography notoriously unreliable and even misleading in the diagnosis of diastolic dysfunction in acute left ventricular failure.

A case history illustrates this well. Mr S, a heavy cigarette smoker with Grade III to Grade IV COPD was admitted with classic features of an acute exacerbation of COPD due to an acute pulmonary infection. He went into acute respiratory failure with severe hypoxia, hypercapnia and respiratory cum metabolic acidosis. Medical management including non-invasive ventilator support failed to help. He was intubated and put on mechanical ventilator support. He could not be weaned off support for over 10 days. Every night there was a crisis characterized by sudden tachypnoea so that he would clash with the machine. There was marked bronchospasm during tachypnoeic spells, no change in the X-ray chest, with the central venous pressure (CVP) remaining within the normal range. A tracheostomy was done and ventilator support continued. One night he had an exceptionally severe bout of tachypnoea with marked wheezing and increased desaturation, requiring a significant step-up in the fraction of inspired oxygen (FIO_2). On this occasion the tracheal aspirate was frothy and copious, pointing to pulmonary oedema. Left ventricular failure due to ischemic heart disease was diagnosed. A coronary angiography showed a tight stenosis in the proximal left anterior descending artery. An angioplasty with stenting was performed. The patient could be weaned off the ventilator support within the next two days. It is now five years since the episode. He is on continuous oxygen therapy and has a reasonable quality of life.

Pulmonary embolism complicating COPD can also mimic an acute exacerbation. Here again when pulmonary embolism occurs in a patient with COPD, breathlessness is invariably associated with severe wheezing. A negative D-dimmer test is a strong point against pulmonary embolism. When in doubt, a pulmonary angiography should be done.

Acute pneumonia, lobar atelectasis due to mucus plugging, are other pulmonary pathologies that can precipitate severe acute respiratory failure. The clinical diagnosis may be missed as an acute exacerbation of COPD causing acute respiratory failure.

Even a shallow pneumothorax in a patient with moderate to severe COPD can induce acute respiratory failure. This is because an overinflated lung (as occurs in COPD) does not easily collapse even with a good-sized pneumothorax. The pressure within the pneumothorax may be high but it appears quite shallow on the X-ray. This is one reason why any patient with a diagnosis of acute exacerbation of COPD admitted to the hospital, or reporting to the emergency department, should always have an X-ray chest done. It is almost impossible to clinically detect a shallow pneumothorax in a patient with COPD. The only reliable sign is diminished breath sounds over the area of the pneumothorax, but unequal breath sounds over both lungs are not uncommon in COPD, even without pneumothorax.

It is obvious that each of the three complicating conditions listed above can worsen lung function in patients with COPD. This is because each of these conditions will cause tachypnoea. Tachypnoea in moderate to severe COPD if often characterized by an expiration which is incomplete, being interrupted by the next inspiration. This will lead to progressive air-trapping, hyperinflated lungs with all the consequent deleterious effects on the work of breathing.

Acute severe asthma may in the absence of a good history be difficult to distinguish from an acute severe exacerbation of COPD when the patient is seen for the first time in an emergency. In fact some severe asthmatics have very poor reversibility in airways obstruction and airflow limitation, exactly resembling patients with COPD. Fortunately, the management remains exactly the same.

A number of other complications occurring outside the respiratory system may produce an acute respiratory crisis with respiratory failure in patients with well-marked Grade III and IV COPD. For example, narcotic drugs, anaesthetics, sedatives, tranquilizers even in small doses can depress the ventilatory drive sufficiently to lead to increasing hypercapnic respiratory failure and a mistaken diagnosis of acute exacerbation of COPD. Trauma causing rib fractures or fractures of the femur, acute systemic infections and sputum retention from any cause are other complications that cause an acute respiratory crisis in COPD patients.

It is therefore a cardinal principle in medicine that if a patient with well-marked COPD develops acute respiratory failure or acute on already existing chronic respiratory failure, a careful search for all possible causes must be made. An acute exacerbation of COPD is an important and common cause for the above scenario, but it certainly is not the only cause.

Table 37.5: Problems in diagnosis
Association of LV dysfunction and failure in patients with COPD
Complication of pulmonary embolism in a patient with COPD
Complication of a pneumothorax in a patient with COPD
Pneumonia, atelectasis, presenting with acute respiratory failure (ARF) in COPD
Acute severe asthma
Non-respiratory causes triggering ARF in COPD

MANAGEMENT

The principles in the management of an acute exacerbation of COPD are:

1. Relief of airways obstruction and airflow limitation through a more intensive use of inhaled bronchodilators
2. Use of corticosteroids to reduce the increased inflammation within peripheral airways and lung parenchyma
3. Use of antibiotics in the presence of bacterial infection
4. Use of oxygen to relieve dyspnoea and most importantly to relieve hypoxia
5. Use of ventilatory support in patients who are in acute respiratory failure or in acute on chronic respiratory failure in spite of conservative treatment mentioned above.

We consider the role of the physiotherapist invaluable in patients who have a great deal of sputum but are unable to expectorate it.

Treatment is tailored to the degree of severity of the acute exacerbation. Mild exacerbations may just need intensified

Table 37.6:
Conditions other than acute exacerbation of COPD which are known to precipitate an acute respiratory crisis in COPD patients

Respiratory Conditions

Pneumonia

Pulmonary atelectasis

Pneumothorax

Pleural effusion

Pulmonary thromboembolism

Sputum retention from any cause

Non-respiratory Conditions

Acute left ventricular failure

Use of respiratory depressants, drugs, tranquilizers

Post-operative

Trauma (fracture ribs, fracture femur)

Systemic infections

Severe blood loss

Note: Severe systemic infections increase metabolism thereby increasing ventilatory demands. There is an increase in the 'load' on respiratory muscles leading at times to respiratory failure.

Prolonged immobility (as after trauma) can lead to basal atelectasis, sputum retention and worsening lung function.

Blood loss with hypovolemic shock leads to low pulmonary artery pressure with increased V/Q abnormalities, leading to increasing hypoxia.

bronchodilator therapy. If the sputum is purulent, antibiotics need to be given after collecting sputum for culture/sensitivity but without waiting for the results. If the exacerbation seems more than mild, corticosteroids need to be administered. Controlled oxygen is given for the relief of both hypoxia and dyspnoea. It is the first important therapeutic measure in hypoxic patients, and should be started promptly in a patient admitted with acute respiratory failure. Persistence or increasing respiratory failure in spite of conservative management necessitates the use of ventilator support. Non-invasive ventilator support is preferable, but invasive ventilator support should not be delayed if indications so exist.

Inhaled Bronchodilator Therapy

Mild exacerbations of COPD are often controlled merely by increasing the frequency of inhaled bronchodilators. Both short-acting β_2-agonists and an anticholinergic-ipratropium bromide can be used, preferably through a spacer device, though there is no evidence that the use of both is more effective than the use of either one or the other. Severe exacerbations necessitate the administration of levosalbutamol (1.25 mg 8-hourly) and an anticholinergic agent like ipratropium (500 mcg 8-hourly) through a nebuliser, even though again there is no evidence that this is superior to the use of a metered dose inhaler with a spacer device. Patients in our part of the world who come in with an acute severe exacerbation may have never used a metered dose inhaler and find it impossible to do so effectively at this juncture. Women in particular find it difficult to use the

metered dose inhaler even when the COPD is stable. Patients with severe exacerbations are extremely dyspnoeic, have a poor inspiratory effort and very small tidal volumes. Very little of the drug reaches the airways in spite of using a volume spacer with the metered dose inhaler. The relief in dyspnoea due to reduced airways obstruction following a switchover from a metered dose inhaler with a spacer device to the nebulised administration of the drugs, is at times too obvious to be disbelieved.

The frequency of nebulisation of salbutamol is generally four times a day, perhaps repeated once in the middle of the night if necessary.

Theophylline

Oral theophylline should be given or continued (if the patient is already on the drug) for its bronchodilator effect in the milder forms of acute exacerbation of COPD. In the more severe forms of acute exacerbation, intravenous aminophylline 0.25g to at the most 0.75g intravenously over 24 hours through an infusion pump may be given, particularly when there is marked bronchospasm. Great care must be taken particularly in patients who have received oral theophylline during the stable phase of COPD. Theophylline levels in the blood should be carefully monitored and should not exceed 15 mg/dl.

Use of Corticosteroids

Systemic corticosteroids are indicated in all except the very mild exacerbations that respond well to inhaled bronchodilator therapy alone. A number of randomized trials indicate that the use of steroids relieves airways obstruction producing a rapid improvement in forced expiratory volume in one second (FEV_1). Other outcome effects such as hospitalization, length of hospital stay, and oxygenation are variable. Their effect on mortality has not been determined. Corticosteroids act through their anti-inflammatory effect. The generally accepted dose is 40 mg prednisolone orally for 10 to 14 days. Critically ill patients, or those in whom absorption of the drug is suspect because of vomiting should be given methyl prednisolone 40 mg 8-hourly intravenously till improvement occurs, following which oral prednisolone is used. Nebulised budesonide also acts through its direct anti-inflammatory effect on the airways. It is however difficult to ascertain to what extent the drug reaches the peripheral airways, where inflammation is most marked. In severe exacerbations, budesonide should not substitute the use of systemic corticosteroids.

Antibiotics

Antibiotics should be used whenever the sputum is purulent—coloured yellow or green. These patients should be given antibiotics promptly without awaiting culture sensitivity reports. The choice of antibiotics depends on the organism generally prevailing in patients with acute exacerbation of COPD in a particular locale. The antibiotics used should cover the common organisms generally responsible for acute exacerbations—*Streptococcus pneumoniae*, *H. influenza* and *Moraxella catarrhalis*. In elderly individuals, gram-negative infections are not uncommon, particularly those due to *P. aeruginosa* and

Klebsiella. An appropriate cover for gram-negative infections is then necessary. Viral infections (the rhinovirus in particular) are being increasingly recognized as a cause of acute exacerbations of COPD. Antibiotics are of no use when this is so.

The question often arises—does one use empiric antibiotic therapy in patients with severe acute exacerbation, particularly in those with acute respiratory failure, when there is no evidence of bacterial infection? Rightly or wrongly, we do so, as some patients who have infection may have no sputum and the danger of not treating a possible infection in such critically ill patients, particularly when they are old and feeble is great. When such patients need intubation and ventilatory support, suction through the endotracheal tube has often revealed dirty yellow or green tracheobronchial secretions. Interestingly, a meta-analysis of six sufficiently well-designed randomized trials by Sant and colleagues confirmed a statistically significant benefit that favoured the use of antibiotics. Duration of antibiotic therapy is generally not more than four to seven days.

Controlled Oxygen Therapy

Oxygen through nasal prongs or a Venturi mask is used to relieve dyspnoea, but most importantly to relieve hypoxia. Patients with Grade III, IV COPD who develop a severe acute exacerbation are invariably hypoxic and often hypercapnic. The PaO_2 very often is < 55 to 60 mm Hg. These patients always need oxygen and are at risk of death from worsening hypoxia. It should be a cardinal rule to administer oxygen immediately, and as the very first measure in any acutely ill patient with COPD. Oxygen should be administered in a controlled manner and should be carefully supervised. Uncontrolled oxygen therapy can be lethal in these patients. Intensive care is crucial for survival. The objective is to increase PaO_2 to a safe level of 60 mm Hg or ensure an oxygen saturation of 90%, without the arterial pH falling below 7.25. Controlled oxygen therapy can be given through a Venturi mask which allows an FIO_2 of 24%; this can be increased through Venturi masks that allow an FIO_2 of 26% or even 28–30%, or more, if dangerous hypoxia is unrelieved. Oxygen given through nasal prongs at a flow rate of 1–2 L/min is a cheap, convenient and effective alternative, as this generally equates to an FIO_2 of 24–27%.

The response to controlled oxygen therapy (starting with an inspired oxygen content of 24%, (and increasing to 26% or even 28–30% if dangerous hypoxia is unrelieved), falls into the following three patterns:

(a) Relief of hypoxemia, with a fall in the $PaCO_2$ and an overall clinical improvement.
(b) Relief of hypoxemia, but an initial increase in the $PaCO_2$ with a further fall in arterial pH to not less than 7.25. The $PaCO_2$ then steadies at a higher level, or returns to pre-treatment levels. After a couple of days, the $PaCO_2$ generally falls below pre-treatment levels. The initial rise in $PaCO_2$ with a fall in arterial pH, is usually observed during the first night after starting oxygen therapy, and is associated with increasing drowsiness, dullness, confusion and apathy. Thereafter, there is a gradual fall in the $PaCO_2$ to pre-treatment or even lower levels and a return of pH towards normal, occurring *pari pasu* with clinical improvement.

(c) Relief of hypoxemia, but a rapid, progressive, marked increase in the $PaCO_2$ with an increasing respiratory acidosis (pH < 7.25). This response is to be expected if oxygen is administered in an uncontrolled manner, using high oxygen concentrations. It can however also occur with carefully controlled and supervised oxygen therapy (O_2 concentration between 24–28%). The severe respiratory acidosis and the marked rise in the $PaCO_2$ can prove lethal in these patients.

Unfortunately, it is generally the severely hypoxic patient with a fairly high $PaCO_2$ to start with, who is more prone to developing a progressively increasing, dangerously high $PaCO_2$ with a dangerously low arterial pH (< 7.2).

It is important to understand why uncontrolled oxygen therapy (and in some patients even controlled oxygen therapy) can lead to a sharp rise in $PaCO_2$. It used to be believed that the essential drive to breathe in these patients was due to the prevailing hypoxia, because the respiratory centre was considered to be relatively insensitive (compared to normal subjects) to the rise in $PaCO_2$. Giving a high FiO_2 (uncontrolled oxygen) would remove the hypoxic stimulus to breathe, so that the patient would have a further rise in $PaCO_2$. This is not true; the ventilatory drive in these patients is even more than normal. Uncontrolled O_2 therapy produces vasodilatation in the pulmonary capillaries due to relief of hypoxia. This leads to a further V/Q mismatch with low ventilation-perfusion ratio. It is the increasing alveolar hypoventilation due to the above cause that leads to a sharp rise in $PaCO_2$.

Table 37.7: Blood gas patterns observed in acute exacerbation of COPD
Hypoxia + hypercapnia during crisis
• hypercapnia persists after recovery from acute exacerbation
Hypoxia + hypercapnia during crisis; normocapnia after recovery
Hypoxia but no hypercapnia during crisis

Patients who on conservative management (outlined earlier), and on controlled oxygen therapy show poor relief in hypoxia or show a progressive rise in the $PaCO_2$ with a fall in the arterial pH < 7.25, require mechanical ventilator support. Ventilator support could be of two types—non-invasive and invasive. It should be noted that many patients with severe Grade IV COPD have a persistent hypercapnia between 50–60 mm Hg even in a stable state. It is unwise to attempt to reduce very high $PaCO_2$ seen during an acute exacerbation to normal levels. These patients tolerate a $PaCO_2$ between 50–60 mm Hg fairly well.

Non-invasive Mechanical Ventilation

Non-invasive positive pressure ventilation (NIPPV) has been proven to be useful in several studies of acute respiratory failure caused by an acute exacerbation of COPD. Studies show that the use of NIPPV is associated with a lesser risk of nosocomial infections, less antibiotic use, and a lower mortality when compared to patients who are equally ill but did not receive NIPPV.

NIPPV has the ability to increase alveolar ventilation, rest muscles of respiration, reduce work of breathing and prevent respiratory muscle fatigue. Potential benefits include an increase in tidal volume, a fall in respiratory rate, improved oxygenation, a fall in $PaCO_2$ and greater patient comfort. When these benefits occur, they do so within a few hours of initiating NIPPV. Perhaps the most important advantage of NIPPV in an acute crisis of COPD is that it obviates the need for endotracheal intubation and invasive mechanical ventilation, which is far more inconvenient to the patient, and has more risks—particularly the risk of nosocomial infection.

Having said this, it is our considered opinion that many patients admitted to intensive care units (ICUs) in this country for an acute exacerbation of COPD are offered NIPPV when ventilatory support is not required—i.e. these patients would have recovered on conservative measures outlined above. Also, many such patients are offered NIPPV when they in fact needed prompt intubation and invasive ventilator support.

The indications in our unit for initiating NIPPV in an acute crisis of COPD are:

(i) Respiratory rate > 30/minute
(ii) Respiratory distress due to moderate or severe dyspnoea
(iii) pH ≤ 7.30 and/or a $PaCO_2$ > 60 mm Hg, provided these values fail to improve or worsen after a trial of 6 to 8 hours (or even earlier) of conservative measures.

Non-invasive mechanical ventilation should not be used as the mode of ventilatory support if the patient is obtunded, breathes poorly or irregularly, is unable to protect the airway, has copious respiratory secretions, and has a risk of aspirating gastric contents. We also prefer to intubate and ventilate those whose PaO_2 < 45 mm Hg and who are admitted with a pH < 7.20. Patients who show an acute rise of $PaCO_2$ of > 70 mm Hg are often obtunded, and in our opinion, are more effectively managed by endotracheal intubation and invasive ventilator support. Endotracheal intubation and ventilation should obviously be also resorted to when NIPPV fails to prove of benefit within 6 to 10 hours of its initiation, or even earlier, if the patient worsens on this mode of support.

IMPLEMENTATION OF NIPPV

NIPPV can be offered through either a light-fitting face mask or a nasal mask. Each has its own advantages. We prefer the face mask in patients with severe respiratory failure. A wide variety of ventilatory modes can be used in NIPPV. We prefer the BiPAP mode because it allows for good gas exchange and effectively reduces both the work of breathing and patient distress. Pressure support ventilation (PSV) is perhaps an equally useful mode and is generally better tolerated than the assist-control mode. In a BiPAP mode, to start with, the inspiratory pressure (IP) is kept at 8 to 10 cm above the end-expiratory pressure (EP), so that if the EP is 5 to 7 cm H_2O, the IP is 12 to 15 cm H_2O. The pressure can then be adjusted to allow for effective alveolar ventilation and good gas exchange.

If the PSV mode is used for NIPPV, the inspiratory pressure support to start with is kept on 15 to 20 cm H_2O. A small

PEEP of 4 to 5 cm H_2O may be of help in patients who have a large auto-PEEP, as it helps reduce inspiratory effort to generate inspiratory airflow in these patients.

Weaning from NIPPV is accomplished by progressively decreasing the level of inspiratory pressure support if the PSV mode is used, or by allowing the patient to be intermittently off NIPPV for increasing lengths of time.

Intubation and Mechanical Ventilation

Patients who show a sharp progressive rise in the $PaCO_2$ with a pH < 7.2 on controlled oxygen therapy, or those whose dangerous hypoxia stands unrelieved on conservative therapy or NIPPV, are best intubated and put on mechanical ventilator support. Selection of cases for this mode of treatment is difficult. It would be disastrous for a patient and his family if after starting mechanical ventilation, it becomes impossible to wean the patient off ventilator support. In our opinion, the best indication whether to opt for invasive ventilator support or not, is the activity and state of health of the patient under basal conditions. If the patient's activity was hopelessly poor under basal conditions to start with, (i.e. he was more or less confined to his bed due to poor respiratory reserve), it is unwise to opt for invasive ventilator support, and the family should be advised accordingly. If he was reasonably active prior to the crisis that brought him to the ICU, he should be offered ventilator support.

Endotracheal intubation in patients showing poor response to antibiotics, bronchodilators, physiotherapy and controlled oxygen therapy, offers two advantages. It allows proper access for suctioning of respiratory secretions, and it allows mechanical ventilator support.

Mechanical ventilation is difficult in patients with chronic airways obstruction. We prefer and recommend the assist/control mode in patients with severe acute respiratory failure, so that total support and appropriate choice of ventilator settings

Table 37.8:
Indications and contraindications for NIPPV
Indications for NPPV
Respiratory rate > 30/minute
Respiratory distress due to moderate or severe dyspnoea
pH ≤ 7.30 and or a $PaCO_2$ > 60 mm Hg, provided these values fail to improve or worsen after a trial of 6 to 12 hours of conservative treatment
Contraindications to NPPV
Obtunded patient
Breathes very poorly, irregularly
Unable to protect the airway
Copious respiratory secretions
Risk of gastric aspiration
Hypotension; CVS instability
pH ≤ 7.20 with an acute rise of $PaCO_2$ > 70 mm Hg

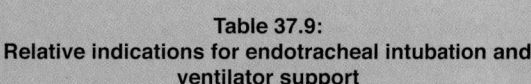

Table 37.9:
Relative indications for endotracheal intubation and ventilator support

Indications for NPPV

1. Respiratory rate > 40/min
2. Respiratory muscle fatigue
3. Mental obtundation
4. A silent chest—respiratory arrest
5. Hypotension
6. Falling pH < 7.25
7. PaO_2 < 50 mm Hg
8. Rising $PaCO_2$ > 70 mm Hg

Table 37.10:	
Principles of mechanical ventilation in patients with COPD with acute respiratory crisis	

Ventilator Settings	Objectives
• Low tidal volumes of 350 ml (6–7 ml/kg) MV < 5–6l/min	• Prevents overinflation
	• Prevents dynamic hyperinflation and progressive increase in auto-PEEP
• Rate: 12–14/min	• Decrease peak inflation pressure
	• Reduces risk of barotraumas
• Flow rate 40–60 l/min	
• I:E ratio of 1:3	• Allows good distribution of inspired gas, allows time for expiration
• FIO_2 of 50–70%	• Allows quick correction of hypoxia
• Sedate or use pancuronium	• Allows machine to take over, and prevents clashing with the machine

Note: (i) Lower $PaCO_2$ very gradually over 24 hours or even longer to 50 mm Hg—a PaO_2 of 60 mmHg suffices.
(ii) If weaning is difficult, use pressure support ventilatioin.

can be provided. Sedation and rarely, neuromuscular paralysis may be necessary for effective respiratory support. As recovery proceeds, or in patients who are not very ill, PSV may be used. The principles for successful ventilation are outlined in Table 37.10.

(a) *Small tidal volumes* of 300–400 ml are used with minute ventilation not exceeding 5–6 l/min. Lung protection measures require that peak pressures are not unduly high and that the plateau pressure does not exceed 30 cm H_2O. The FIO_2 is increased to 50 or 60% so that dangerous hypoxia is quickly corrected. It is unnecessary to aim for an oxygen saturation > 90%. The low tidal volumes prevent dynamic hyperinflation, thereby preventing a further increase in auto-PEEP which is invariably present in these patients (see section on pathophysiology). Low tidal volumes also lead to lower peak inflation pressures. This is a great advantage, as high peak pressures if transmitted to the intrapleural space, cause a sharp reduction in the venous return and the cardiac output, and can produce

sudden severe hypotension. In fact, hypotension should be carefully looked out for, particularly after starting ventilation. A fall in the arterial pressure should prompt one to further reduce the inflation pressure by further reducing the tidal volume. The blood pressure should also be raised by volume expansion or by using inotropic support. Once the patient is on mechanical ventilation with the hypoxia corrected by a high FIO_2, an increase in $PaCO_2$ need not be feared. Under these circumstances, death usually does not occur due to a high $PaCO_2$.

Sensitivity The optimal triggering threshold is difficult in an acute COPD crisis in the presence of dynamic hyperinflation (i.e. auto-PEEP). This is because the patient has to generate a negative pressure at least equal to the level of auto-PEEP before interfacing with the preset sensitivity on the ventilator. If the auto-PEEP is high, the required inspiratory effort (before reaching trigger sensitivity) to initiate airflow is significant and this can lead to patient-ventilator dyssynchrony. Yet if the trigger sensitivity is kept very low, the ventilator could be triggered very frequently and inappropriately. If the auto-PEEP is significantly raised, extrinsic PEEP is applied at a level well below the level of the auto-PEEP. This helps to reduce the effort needed to initiate inspiratory flow.

(b) *Ventilator requirements* are so adjusted so as to bring down the raised $PaCO_2$ level very slowly over 24–48 hours. It is generally unnecessary to reduce the $PaCO_2$ to < 50 mm Hg unless the basal $PaCO_2$ levels were normal. A sudden drop in the $PaCO_2$ is dangerous as it causes a sudden shift from respiratory acidaemia to metabolic alkalosis and alkalaemia. This can precipitate dangerous arrhythmias and cause sudden death.

(c) The flow rates used in such patients are usually between 40–60 l/min, and the inspiration: expiration ratio is initially set at 1:3.

(d) Patients should not be allowed to clash with the machine; they can be safely given pancuronium, or sedated once they are put on ventilator support.

(e) Mechanical ventilator support is generally necessary for a period of three to seven days. The maximum period over which we have used ventilator support, and then finally succeeded in weaning the patient, has been six weeks. An elective tracheostomy is preferred if ventilator support needs to be extended for more than seven days, or if the patient has thick copious secretions which cannot be easily suctioned through the endotracheal tube.

(f) Weaning is generally carried out by the traditional methods. We have used intermittent mandatory ventilation, and PSV, but have never been totally convinced of their absolute necessity. The patient is taken off ventilator support when he can maintain an adequate gas exchange on his own. This generally happens when infection has been controlled, airways obstruction has decreased, and V/Q abnormalities have been significantly rectified.

(g) Older patients with ischemic heart disease often need careful cardiovascular support. The presence of associated left ventricular failure with pulmonary oedema, together with generalized water retention is not uncommon in these patients. It is indeed remarkable how good ventilator support with improvement in blood gases initiates a

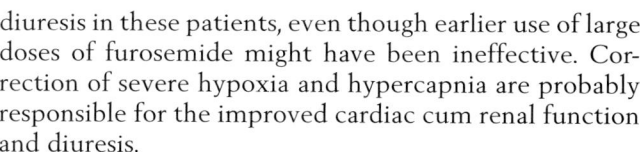

diuresis in these patients, even though earlier use of large doses of furosemide might have been ineffective. Correction of severe hypoxia and hypercapnia are probably responsible for the improved cardiac cum renal function and diuresis.

(h) Expert nursing, humidification of inspired oxygen and persistence with the regime outlined earlier, are all essentials of good respiratory care in these patients.

Our mortality in patients with acute respiratory failure in COPD who require invasive ventilator support is about 20%.

Treatment of Complications during Acute Respiratory Failure in Exacerbation of COPD

A number of complications may arise in critically ill patients with acute respiratory failure resulting from an acute exacerbation of COPD. These are listed in Table 37.11.

These should be promptly diagnosed and treated. The most dangerous complications outside the respiratory system are cardiac arrhythmias and hemodynamic instability.

Cardiac Arrhythmias

Cardiac arrhythmias are frequently observed in these patients. Supraventricular tachycardia, multifocal atrial tachycardia and atrial fibrillation are common; AV dissociation and multiple ventricular extrasystolies may also occur. The mortality rate is significantly higher in patients having arrhythmias.

Hemodynamic Instability

Patients with COPD often suffer from pulmonary hypertension. An acute exacerbation of COPD worsens pulmonary hypertension due to hypoxic vasoconstriction, dynamic hyperinflation, or the presence of auto-PEEP during mechanical ventilation. A sharp increase in pulmonary artery pressure leads to severe right ventricular dysfunction, right-sided heart failure, with a fall in both systolic and mean arterial blood pressure. An intravenous fluid challenge expands the intravascular pulmonary bed and improves right ventricular pump function. It should be the initial step in the management of hypotension and hemodynamic instability in an acute crisis of COPD. If the hemodynamic state fails to improve, we prefer to use inotropic support with dobutamine. Ventilator adjustments to reduce dynamic hyperinflation and auto-PEEP are also necessary.

Table 37.11:
Complications during acute respiratory failure in COPD
Pulmonary infection
Fluid, electrolyte and acid-base disturbances
Respiratory acidosis with hypokalaemic metabolic alkalosis
Severe water logging can occur due to salt and water retention
Cardiac arrhythmias
Right sided heart failure
Hypotension if there is marked auto-PEEP
Pneumothorax
Complications due to mechanical ventilation
Gastrointestinal bleeds
Pulmonary thromboembolism
Mental depression

Table 37.12:
Management of acute respiratory crisis in patients with COPD
1. Improve ventilation, correct ventilation-perfusion mismatch, relieve severe hypoxia and correct low pH
Controlled oxygen therapy (24–30% oxygen)
Treat infection with antibiotics
Relieve airways obstruction—nebulize salbutamol 4 hourly, ipratropium bromide 8 hourly
Use corticosteroids
Theophylline
Physiotherapy to help drain copious secretions and prevent sputum retention
Ventilator support when so indicated
Cardiovascular support when necessary
2. Treat complications encountered during acute respiratory failure
Correct fluid and electrolyte disturbances
Management of cardiac complications eg. arrhythmias, hypotension, right-sided heart failure and pulmonary thromboembolism
Treat GI bleeds
Drain even a shallow pneumothorax

SUGGESTED READING

Brochard L. Non-invasive ventilation for acute exacerbations of COPD: a new standard of care. *Thorax*. Oct. 2000; 55 (10): 817–8.

Elliott M. Noninvasive ventilation in acute exacerbations of COPD. *European Respiratory Review*. EW, 2005; 14: 39–42.

Niewoehner DE. Interventions to prevent chronic obstructive pulmonary disease exacerbations. *Am J Med*. 20 Dec. 2004; 117 Suppl 12A: 41S–48S.

Puhan MA, Scharplatz M *et al*. Respiratory rehabilitation after acute exacerbation of COPD may reduce risk for readmission and mortality—a systematic review. *Respir Res*. Jun. 2005; 6: 54.

Rizkallah Jacques, Paul Man S, *et al*. Prevalence of Pulmonary Embolism in Acute Exacerbations of COPD: A Systematic Review and Metaanalysis. *Chest March*. 2009; 135: 786–93.

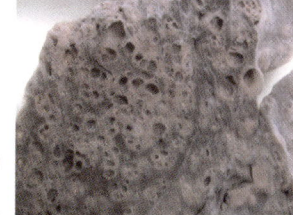
CHAPTER **38**

Chronic Obstructive Pulmonary Disease: Management

By definition, chronic obstructive pulmonary disease (COPD) is incurable yet treatable. Current-day treatment affords significant symptomatic relief, and in particular helps to reduce dyspnoea, increases effort tolerance and improves the quality of life.

Patient compliance with regard to medications prescribed, as also with regard to a disciplined lifestyle and the cessation of smoking (in smokers) is essential for a successful outcome.

Objectives of Management are—

1. *Prevent progression* The only way to achieve this objective is to abolish as far as possible all risk factors. Cessation of smoking in smokers is the key to prevent COPD as also to prevent progression of established COPD in smokers.

2. *Relieve symptoms* The main symptoms are breathlessness, poor exercise tolerance, cough often with mucoid or mucopurulent sputum. Symptomatic relief is provided by the appropriate use of aerosolized bronchodilators, the use of inhaled corticosteroids, and the use of pulmonary rehabilitation.

3. *Prevent and treat exacerbations* Exacerbations are inbuilt in the natural history of COPD. Their prevention and treatment is of paramount importance and have been considered in a separate chapter.

4. *Prolong life* The use of oxygen in patients who are hypoxic has been clearly shown to prolong life. Oxygen also relieves dyspnoea and improves exercise tolerance thereby improving the quality of life.

5. *Diagnose and treat any complications* (besides acute exacerbations) that can precipitate acute respiratory failure or can result in acute on chronic respiratory failure in patients with severe COPD. This has been dealt with in the chapter on acute exacerbation of COPD.

6. *Improve general nutritional state* This requires an appropriate diet and graduated exercise under a pulmonary rehabilitation programme.

7. *Search for and treat co-morbidities* like ischemic heart disease, diabetes, liver cell dysfunction, renal dysfunction, any one of which may have an indirect deleterious bearing on COPD.

8a. *Symptomatic management of severe hypercapnia* in COPD patients with chronic hypercapnic respiratory failure.

8b. *Treatment of right heart failure* arising from cor pulmonale in end-stage COPD with appropriate medications.

9. *Surgical measures* in a select subset of COPD patients.

PREVENT PROGRESSION

Smoking, occupational factors, indoor pollution due to combustion of biofuels and outdoor environmental pollution are the main risk factors. These should be mitigated or abolished. Smoking and indoor pollution can and should be completely abolished. Occupational factors may often be impossible to remove in their entirety but they can and should be appropriately mitigated. Outdoor pollution is impossible for individuals to control, but when feasible, a change of workplace or residence from a very heavily polluted area to an area with little or no pollution may help.

Cessation of smoking is crucial to prevent further progression of COPD and to preserve both lung function and exercise tolerance. Smokers who are susceptible to the adverse effects of cigarette smoke have a sharper decline in lung function, in particular the forced expiratory volume in one second (FEV_1) compared to non-smokers. The Lung Health Study revealed that cessation of smoking in these patients reduces the rate of decline of FEV_1 to that of non-smokers. Cessation of smoking does not cure COPD

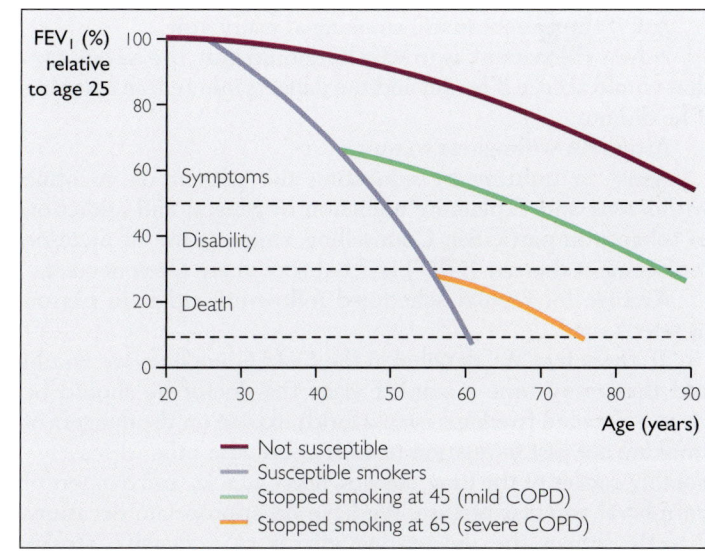

Fig 38.1: Decline in lung function in cigarette smokers and the effects of smoking cessation. Lung function declines more rapidly in smokers who are susceptible to the adverse effects of cigarettes compared with nonsmokers. Discontinuing smoking in both a 45-years-old with more severe disease reduces the accelerated decline in lung function and delays progression of symptoms. COPD, Chronic obstructive pulmonary disease. *(Modified from Fletcher C, Petro R: The natural history of chronic airflow obstruction. BMJ 1977; 1: 1645–1648.)*

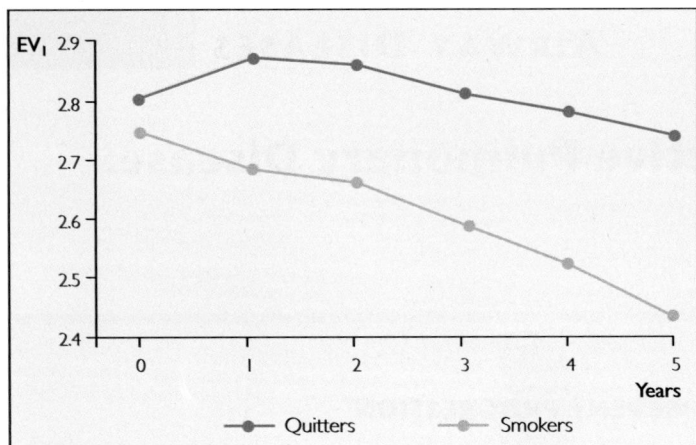

Fig 38.2: Effect of smoking cessation on lung function. The forced expired volume in 1 sec (FEV₁) improved in the year after smoking cessation. *(From Anthonisen et al. Effects of smoking intervention and the use of an inhaled anticholinergic bronchodilator on the rate of decline of FEV₁. The Lung Health Study. JAMA 1994; 272: 1497–1505).*

or reverse the inflammatory damages already present in the small airways and in the lung periphery. Pulmonary function may however show some improvement and not uncommonly the patient feels more comfortable in breathing.

Smoking Cessation Programme

It is important to ascertain the exact habits of patients (both from the patient and for greater accuracy from close relatives or associates), and to assess how motivated they are to quit. An approach to smoking cessation consists of the five 'As' detailed in the Gold guidelines.

Ask if the patient is still smoking at every visit.

Advise the patient as to why he should quit, the advantages that would accrue if he did and the dangers inherent in smoking if he did not.

Assess his willingness to quit.

Assist in quitting by educating the patient on nicotine withdrawal and explaining addiction in general and addiction to tobacco in particular. Counselling, support, use of nicotine replacement therapy (NRT) and bupropion are often needed.

Arrange for regular scheduled follow-up; either in person or telephone.

To these five 'As' detailed in the Gold Guidelines we would add that every time a smoker visits the doctor he should be given a detailed (perhaps even a lurid) exposé on the dangers of smoking not just in relation to COPD but also other diseases—notably cancer of the lung, strokes, heart attacks, and dangers of peripheral vascular disease. We have on appropriate occasions directly shown the devastating effects of a massive stroke, cancer of the lung, gangrene of a foot, to help a smoker realize the danger of smoking so that he is further motivated to quit the habit.

It must be admitted that the pressure of work in very busy outpatient departments of large hospitals in metropolitan cities of India and other developing countries leaves little time for a detailed discussion with a smoker on the dangers of smoking. Merely asking him to quit at every visit rarely helps. In fact,

in our experience nothing helps (and this includes the use of nicotine replacement patches and bupropion) unless the patient is sufficiently motivated to stop. The aim of the treating doctor is to first arouse this motivation and reinforce it with every visit.

The Lung Heart Study showed that patients who were likely to achieve and maintain smoking cessation were married, were accompanied by a relative, friend at counselling sessions, and/or had made previous long-term attempts to quit. Those who were likely to fail had made several short-term attempts to quit, had extra-stressful lives and were still using nicotine patches as replacement therapy one year after quitting. Perhaps the main difference underlying those who quit from those who do not is the different degree of motivation in these two groups, as also external influences together with personality factors influencing the motivation.

Nicotine Replacement Therapy (NRT) and the Use of Bupropion

In the West, NRT is reported to result in twice the quit rate compared to placebo. NRT is available as a chewing gum or a skin patch. In the West it is also available as a nasal spray and an inhaler. The combination of counselling, the use of NRT and of bupropion is reported to result in the highest rate for smoking cessation. Bupropion is given in a dose of 150 mg BD for six to eight weeks. Headache is a frequent side-effect, seizures have been occasionally reported, so that it is best avoided in epileptics. Side-effects of nicotine are not uncommon with NRT, particularly in patients smoking less than 10 cigarettes per day. In patients with ischemic heart disease (angina, recent myocardial infarction), acid peptic disease, and in pregnant or breast-feeding women, NRT is avoided or used with great caution.

Varenicline is a new drug used as an alternative to NRT; it acts as a partial agonist to nicotine acetylcholine receptors and is given in a dose of 1 mg 12-hourly for 12 weeks. Randomized trials have shown a better rate of smoking cessation with varenicline than with either placebo or bupropion. Nausea was the main adverse effect observed. Higher suicide rates have been reported in patients on varenicline.

PHARMACOTHERAPY

Use of Bronchodilators

Bronchodilators provide symptomatic relief and improve exercise tolerance and capacity. They do so by reducing air-trapping and lung hyperinflation, increasing inspiratory capacity and increasing flow rates during expiration. The FEV₁ may show a significant increase (over 15%), but symptomatic relief may be present even when the FEV₁ is unchanged.

Recommendations on the use of bronchodilators as given in the GOLD guidelines are dependent on the severity of the disease. In mild COPD (GOLD Grade I) short-acting bronchodilators are used for symptomatic relief. The choice of short-acting bronchodilators includes inhaled β₂-agonists, inhaled anticholinergic drugs or both.

Patients with increasingly severe COPD (Grade II-IV) have persistent symptoms and require in addition a long-acting inhaled bronchodilator (a long-acting β₂-agonist or anticholinergic). Further therapy (third-line therapy) in this group (in addition to inhaled long-acting β₂-agonist + anticholinergic) includes the use of an inhaled corticosteroid and/or oral theophylline. The choice of pharmacological therapy in this group depends on the frequency of acute exacerbations, the presence of any untoward side-effects with any one of the drugs used and the patient's preference.

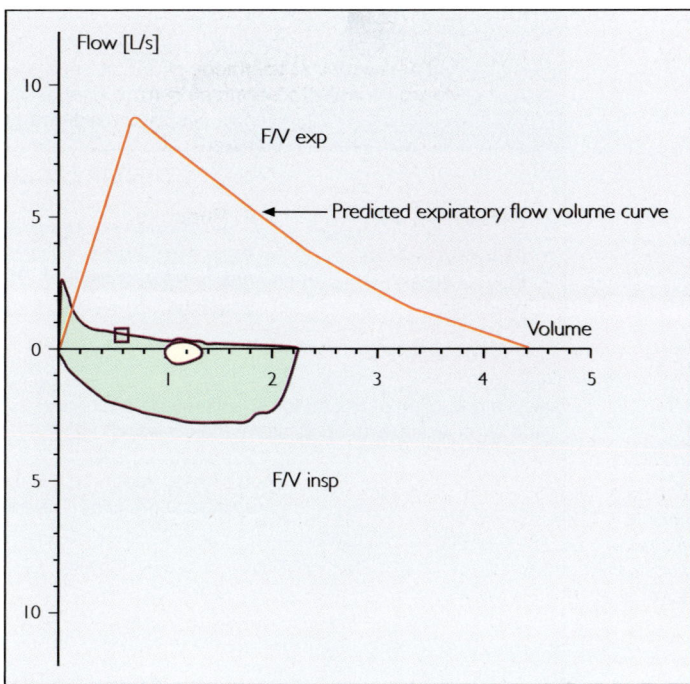

Fig 38.5: Flow-volume loop showing severe COPD.

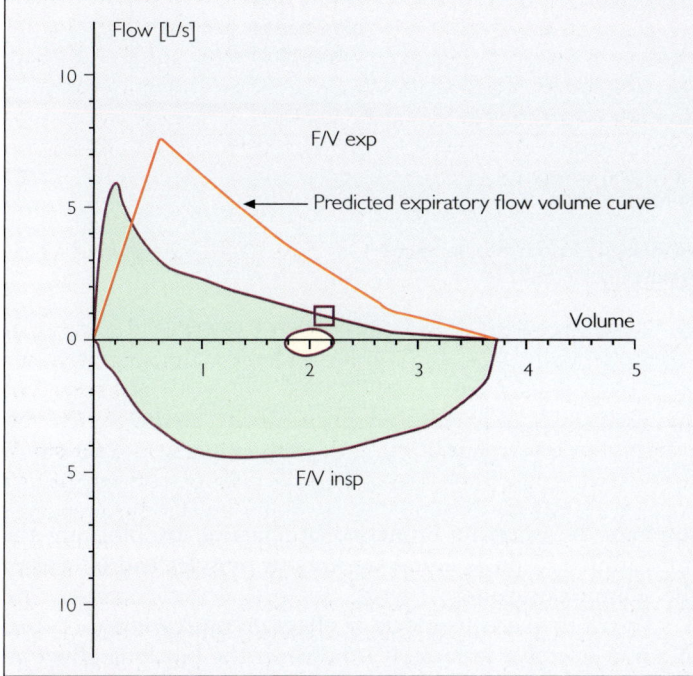

Fig 38.3: Flow-volume loop showing mild COPD.

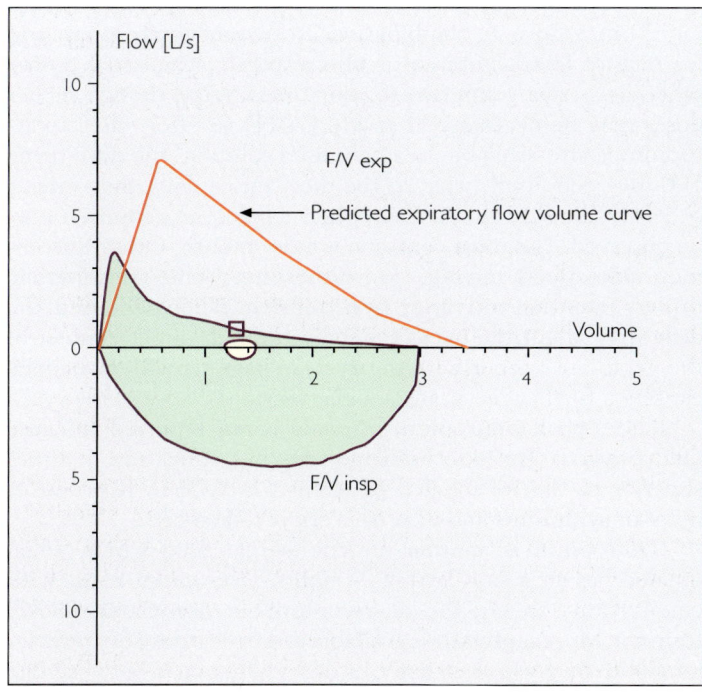

Fig 38.4: Flow-volume loop showing moderate COPD.

β₂-agonist Bronchodilators

SHORT-ACTING β₂-SPECIFIC AGONISTS (SABAs)

SABAs bin2d to and stimulate the β₂ receptors thereby causing smooth muscle relaxation within bronchi and bronchioles. The mechanism of action is through activation of adenyl cyclase thereby increasing the concentration of intracellular cyclic adenosine monophosphate. SABAs have a rapid onset of action which reaches a peak in 5 to 15 minutes, the effect lasting for four to six hours. Salbutamol (Albuterol) is the SABA available for inhalation in most countries of the world. In India it is available as a metered dose inhaler (MDI), 100 µg/dose, and as a solution for nebulisation (2.5 ml = 2.5 mg). It is used in a dose of one to two puffs thrice or at most four times a day; in mild COPD it is used as and when necessary for symptomatic relief. Salbutamol can also be nebulised, with the nebulised solution containing 2.5 mg of the drug. Salbutamol is also available as a long-acting oral preparation in the form of a tablet or syrup.

Side-effects of inhaled SABA include tachycardia, palpitation, hypertension, electrocardiography (ECG) changes that may occasionally resemble those of subendocardial infarction, and chest discomfort. These effects are due to the binding and stimulation of the β₂ receptors of the heart. Tremor of the hands, nervousness, anxiety, gastrointestinal discomfort, gastrooesophageal reflux may also be observed due to systemic absorption of the drug. Hypokalemia is another feature of SABA therapy and is an important effect to be borne in mind, particularly in critically ill patients.

The major disadvantage of SABA is that frequent use leads to a downgrade of the β₂ receptors resulting in tachyphylaxis. They should therefore not be used more than four or at most six times a day. If tachyphylaxis is suspected the drug should be stopped for some days following which it often regains its efficacy.

Table 38.1:
Therapeutic recommendations at each stage of COPD as defined by the GOLD Guidelines
(Reproduced with permission from Global initiative for COPD: Global strategy for the diagnosis, management and prevention of COPD, 2006)

THERAPY AT EACH STAGE OF COPD*			
I: Mild	**II: Moderate**	**III: Severe**	**IV: Very severe**
• $FEV_1/FVC < 0.70$ • $FEV_1 \geq 80\%$ predicted	• $FEV_1/FVC < 0.70$ • $50\% \leq FEV_1 < 80\%$ predicted	• $FEV_1/FVC < 0.70$ • $30\% \leq FEV_1 < 50\%$ predicted	• $FEV_1/FVC < 0.70$ • $FEV_1 < 30\%$ predicted or $FEV_1 < 50\%$ predicted plus chronic respiratory failure
Active reduction of risk factor(s); influenza vaccination ⟶			
Add short-acting bronchodilator (when needed) ⟶			
	Add regular treatment with one or more long-acting bronchodilators (when needed): Add rehabilitation		
		Add inhaled glucocorticosteroids if repeated exacerbations	
			Add long-term oxygen if chronic respiratory failure. Consider surgical treatments

Note: *Postbronchodilator FEV_1 is recommended for the diagnosis and assessment of severity of COPD.

Levalbuterol tartarate is the R-enantiomer of albuterol. The reason for its development is to reduce the adverse effects believed to be related to the S-enantiomer which is present in the racemic mixture. However, clinical studies show that Levalbuterol like other β_2 agonists can produce cardiovascular side-effects. Levalbuterol is available as an MDI of 45 µg/dose and as a solution for nebulisation.

Long-Acting β_2 Agonists (LABAs)

Salmeterol and formoterol are the LABAs available. They, like SABAs, produce bronchodilator effects by direct stimulation of the β_2 receptors. Salmeterol binds preferentially to the lipophilic sites of the β_2 receptors, takes 30 to 60 minutes to reach its maximum bronchodilator effect which lasts for 12 hours. Formoterol binds equally to hydrophilic and lipophilic sites of the β_2 receptors. It has a rapid onset of action in about 5–15 minutes lasting for 12 hours. Salmeterol is available as 50 ug/dose DPI preparation inhaled twice daily. The regular twice daily use of LABA gives symptom relief to stable COPD patients which may or may not always be reflected in improved lung function.

It should be noted that the regular use of LABA has been implicated in acute exacerbations of severe asthma and in increased asthma deaths. It is possible that tachyphylaxis due to the prolonged regular use of LABA might be responsible for possible adverse effects. Admittedly these adverse effects have as yet not been reported in patients with COPD.

Anticholinergic Bronchodilators

The commonly used anticholinergic bronchodilator is ipratropium bromide, a quaternary ammonium derivative of atropine sulphate. It exerts its bronchodilator action by blocking the muscarinic receptors in airway smooth muscles and in cells of the submucous glands.

The drug exerts its blocking effect on muscarinic receptors in a non-selective fashion. It is however the blocking effect on the M_3 receptors in bronchial smooth muscle that is responsible for reduction in bronchomotor tone. There is however no change in mucus secretions following the use of anticholinergic bronchodilators. Ipratropium is available as an MDI containing 20 mcg/dose. A combination 20 mcg of ipratropium and 50 mcg of levosalbutamol is also available. The usual dosing schedule is two puffs two to four times a day, though higher doses may be necessary in severe COPD to offer relief. Ipratropium is also available as a nebulised solution, the dose being 500 mcg nebulised twice, at the most thrice daily. Side-effects of anticholinergic drugs even when inhaled or nebulised may be observed. The most common is a dry mouth. Other uncommon side-effects include skin rashes, headache, constipation, urinary retention and rarely, hypertension. When nebulised, the drug may affect the eyes (generally through direct contact of the nebulised vapour with the eyes) in patients with glaucoma, causing a further rise in intraocular tension.

The use of ipratropium bromide is not reported to cause tachyphylaxis. Its bronchodilator effect is equal and at times superior to that of inhaled β_2-agonists in COPD. It produces relief of symptoms and improves effort tolerance.

Tiotropium is another anticholinergic drug which when inhaled has an action lasting 24 hours. Tiotropium binds with equal avidity to M_1, M_2 M_3 receptors but dissociates quickly from the M_1 receptors. It is available as a 9 mcg/dose dry powder inhaler to be given once daily. Its onset of action is between one to three hours and lasts for 24 hours. Clinical studies suggest that tiotropium is more effective than the scheduled doses

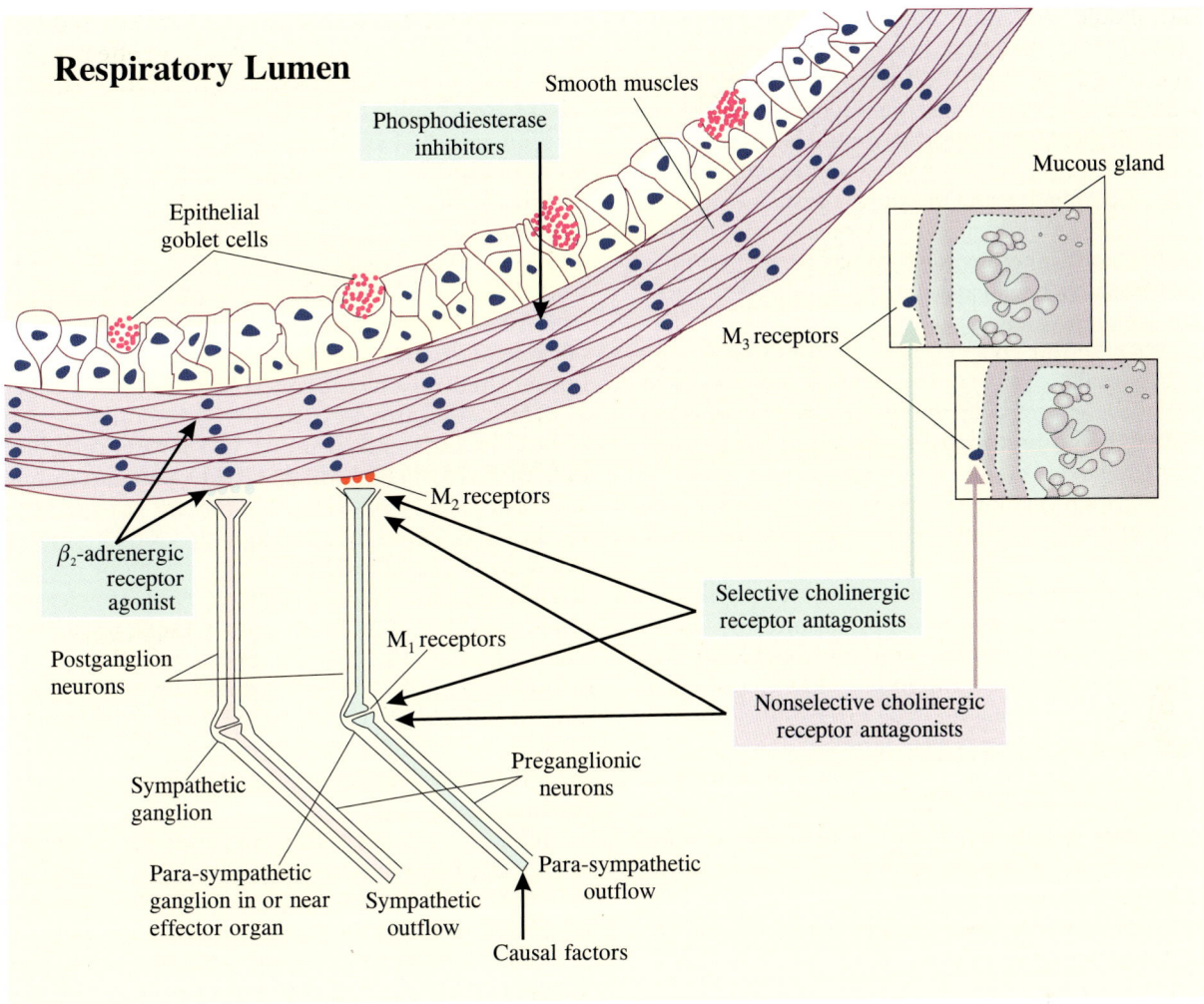

Fig 38.6: Sites of action of β₂ agonists and anti-cholinergic bronchodilators.

of ipratropium bromide in improving lung function, relieving symptoms and decreasing the incidence of acute exacerbations. Clinical studies also suggest that tiotropium has a better bronchodilator effect and causes a greater improvement when compared to salmeterol in COPD. The use of tiotropium is not reported to be associated with tachyphylaxis.

USE OF β₂-AGONIST COMBINED WITH ANTICHOLINERGIC BRONCHODILATOR

The combination of an inhaled β₂-agonist (either SABA or LABA) and an inhaled anticholinergic drug is superior to either one or the other in causing bronchodilatation and symptom relief. In patients who remain significantly symptomatic with the use of either one or the other of these bronchodilators, a combination of β₂-agonist plus an anticholinergic drug should be used, either on a regular or on an intermittent basis.

THEOPHYLLINE

Theophylline was the main drug used as a bronchodilator before the advent of inhaled β₂-agonists. It then fell into relative disuse in the West but has now regained its rightful place in the management of COPD. Theophylline is a modest bronchodilator when given orally, but it has additional

properties that are being increasingly acknowledged. The drug stimulates the central respiratory drive, is believed to improve diaphragmatic function, reduces diaphragmatic and respiratory muscle fatigue, is a diuretic and in addition has anti-inflammatory effects. A recent review shows that it improves forced vital capacity (FVC), FEV$_1$, O$_2$ consumption, PaO$_2$, and PaCO$_2$ in COPD patients. It is cheap, easily available and is therefore particularly useful to the poor and underprivileged of developing countries such as India, where for several reasons patients in this category are either averse to the use of an inhaled bronchodilator and/or do not manage to use the MDIs in the correct manner.

The mechanisms of action of theophylline are not completely understood. The bronchodilator effect is probably mediated through the inhibition of the two isoenzymes phosphodiesterase III and phosphodiesterase IV. Its non-bronchodilator prophylactic action is probably due to the antagonism of adenosine receptors unrelated to inhibition of phosphodiesterase. The drug is metabolized by the cytochrome P450 oxidases. Though the drug unquestionably has side-effects, the oral preparation in a dose of 400 mg to at the most 600 mg/day in our experience is well tolerated in Indian subjects. Theophylline levels in the blood should not exceed

20 mg/dl and should preferably range close to 15 mg/dl. Side-effects like nausea, vomiting, loss of appetite can occur even when the drug level is in the therapeutic range. Many medications like macrolides and most quinolones interfere with theophylline metabolism. The physician should be aware of the important ones that do so. Besides nausea and vomiting, side-effects include abdominal pain, diarrhoea, gastrooesophagel reflux, anxiety, tremors, nervousness, insomnia and muscle cramps. The two most dangerous toxic effects are arrhythmias, in particular ventricular tachycardia and generalized seizures. Unfortunately, though these dangerous complications are apt to occur when serum concentration of the drug is over 20 mg/dl, and generally over 30 mg/dl, this is not always so. Besides, either of these two dangerous toxic effects may occur suddenly without being preceded by any other minor side-effects mentioned above. Perhaps future studies may prove or disprove the contention that lower serum concentration of the drug may be equally effective in COPD without the danger of adverse side-effects.

The GOLD guidelines advocate the use of theophylline in COPD patients who remain symptomatic despite the use of LABA. Theophylline offers greater symptom relief, improves effort tolerance and increases expiratory flow rates when combined with LABA. Stopping the drug reverses this trend. *In developing countries, theophylline is often introduced as a baseline drug, starting in patients with mild COPD and continuing all through to patients with severe COPD.*

Second-generation inhibitors of phosphodiesterase IV are under study. Cilomilast, piclamilast, rofumilast are some of the newer formulations that have a bronchodilator effect and anti-inflammatory properties with fewer gastrointestinal side-effects.

Use of Corticosteroids

It is generally accepted that the long-term use of oral corticosteroids is not indicated and should be strictly avoided in stable COPD patients as their use produces no benefit and results in significant side-effects. It is equally accepted, as is discussed in the previous chapter, that the short-term use of systemic or oral corticosteroids for 10 to 14 days helps recovery in acute exacerbations of COPD.

THE ROLE OF INHALED CORTICOSTEROIDS IN STABLE COPD
The role of inhaled corticosteroids (ICS) has been studied in several large studies of patients with COPD including the Copenhagen study, ISOLDE study, EUROSCOP and the Lung Health Study. Between them these studies have included almost 5000 patients with COPD and some generalizations are possible.

Inhaled corticosteroids **do not** slow the inexorable decline in lung function that is a feature of COPD. A recent meta-analysis of 12 trials showed that the change in FEV_1 was an insignificant 51 ml (mean) at three years.

Inhaled steroids **do** have a very important effect on reducing the frequency of exacerbations of COPD. Annual rate of exacerbation in COPD patients getting ICS is 0.99 events/year vs. 1.32 events in those on placebo. ICS also provide symptom relief and improve effort tolerance in patients subject to acute exacerbations. Thus patients on ICS are significantly less likely to be re-hospitalized. This may translate into reduced mortality and better quality of life. This protective effect of ICS may take some time to be established. In the ISOLDE study, the effect was apparent only after three years.

This effect of ICS on reducing exacerbations may be the main reason behind the improvement in quality of life reported in patients on ICS. It is also certainly the cause of the reduction in mortality observed in patients on ICS. David Sin and colleagues pooled data from seven randomized controlled studies of at least 12 months duration to obtain a database of over 5000 patients. They showed ICS reduced all-cause mortality by 27%, the effects being more pronounced in women, former smokers and patients with moderate or severe COPD.

Thus, currently, for patients with COPD, it may no longer be relevant to ask whether ICS have a role, but the question that remains, is which COPD patients should be given ICS? The answer based on our present knowledge is that ICS should be reserved for symptomatic COPD patients, probably in GOLD Class III and IV (FEV_1 < 50% of predicted value), who have repeated exacerbations. They are clearly NOT recommended for all patients with COPD, not only because of the additional cost, but also because COPD patients (unlike asthmatics) tend to be elderly, and are more prone to all the adverse effects of ICS. Another word of caution against the routine use of ICS in COPD came from a recent study showing an increased incidence of pneumonia in patients of COPD on inhaled steroids.

Inhaled corticosteroids come in various formulations. Those chiefly used are fluticasone, budesonide, beclamethasone, triamcinolone. The most frequent side-effects are the development of thrush in the oropharynx and hoarseness of voice. The possibility of osteoporosis and occurrence of cataracts due to systemic absorption of the steroid need to be considered in older subjects.

Inhaled corticosteroids are not to be used as monotherapy. They are used in combination with LABA. Clinical trials suggest greater improvement in symptoms and in lung function with use of both these agents when compared to either drug used alone. The commonest combination used (and approved by FDA) is fluticasone proprionate 250 ug and salmeterol 50 ug inhalation powder. One to two puffs twice daily is the regular maintenance dose advocated in patients with COPD associated with bronchitis.

Mucolytic Agents and Antioxidants

Cough with mucoid or mucopurulent expectoration is an important symptom in COPD. There is no proven effective mucolytic agent available today for COPD patients. DNAse is effective in reducing acute exacerbations of acute infective bronchitis in cystic fibrosis but is ineffective in COPD patients. A recent large randomized controlled trial of orally administered acetylcysteine was shown to be ineffective in retarding or arresting deterioration of lung function or preventing exacerbations in COPD.

Steam when inhaled is perhaps the best mucolytic agent and when practised every morning often enables the patient to expectorate sputum; it serves as a bronchial toilet and often results in symptomatic relief.

PULMONARY REHABILITATION

Pulmonary rehabilitation has been defined by a National Heart, Lung and Blood Institute workshop as:

A multidimensional continuum of services directed to persons with respiratory disease and their families usually by an interdisciplinary team of specialists with a goal of achieving and maintaining the individual's maximum level of independence and functioning in the community. *(Ref: Fishman A.P. Pulmonary rehabilitation research NIH workshop summary. Am J Respiratory Care, 994: 149; 825–833.)*

Pulmonary rehabilitation is unfortunately a neglected aspect of therapy even in large centres in India and other developing countries. This is due partly to a lack of appreciation and awareness of its role in producing symptomatic relief in COPD patients and partly because of lack of expertise in implementing and organizing a truly beneficial programme.

It is an accepted fact that a carefully implemented rehabilitation programme can provide added benefits over and above the benefits due to medication. The most important benefits observed in COPD patients are a relief or reduction of dyspnoea and an improved exercise capacity. Studies have also shown a reduction in hospital stay and decrease in health costs. There is a decrease in mental depression so frequently seen in patients with severe COPD, an increased independence in performing daily chores and activities, resulting in an overall improved quality of life. It needs to be stressed that pulmonary rehabilitation programmes even in the best centres do not improve lung function, airflow limitation or the basic inflammatory pathology that leads to inevitable progression of the disease. This should be explained both to the patient and to those primarily responsible for the patient's healthcare.

PATIENT SELECTION

Candidates selected for pulmonary rehabilitation often have the following features:

1. Well-marked dyspnoea and poor exercise tolerance or capacity. These patients fall in Grade III-IV severity of COPD. Lung functions are not always an appropriate guide; respiratory symptoms do not always correlate with the degree of reduction in FEV_1. However, patients with an FEV_1 of < 35% would almost certainly benefit with a rehabilitation programme.
2. Patients who have frequent hospitalizations or frequent visits to the emergency department.
3. Patients in need of psychosocial help and adjustment.

Should patients who insist on smoking be admitted to a rehabilitation programme? It is indeed doubtful if any substantial benefit is likely to occur, particularly in heavy smokers. Their commitment to the programme is always suspect. Yet a rehabilitation programme if regularly attended, may be an ideal ground for motivating such patients to stop smoking, and giving them social and emotional support to help them to do so.

It is important to ensure a thorough examination and investigation of a patient before selection for a rehabilitation programme, so as to exclude co-morbidities such as significant ischemic heart disease, hypertension, or arthritis that may preclude exercise.

Table 38.2:
Patient selection for pulmonary rehabilitation

Thorough assessment to exclude significant ischemic heart disease, valvular heart disease, arrhythmias, arthritides is done. Following this, selection of patients with

1. Well-marked dyspnoea and poor exercise tolerance—Grade III/IV severity of COPD
2. Dyspnoea and reduced effort tolerance in patients with Grade II COPD
3. Patients who have frequent hospitalizations or frequent visits to the emergency department
4. Patients in need of psychosocial help and adjustment

Note: Respiratory symptoms (dyspnoea, poor exercise tolerance) do not always correlate with degree of reduction in FEV_1.

Though this section deals with pulmonary rehabilitation in COPD, the rehab programme is also applicable to other respiratory diseases like bronchial asthma and interstitial lung disease.

Finally, rehabilitation is a multidisciplinary approach carried out by a team headed by a coordinator. It should include a physician, an experienced exercise trainer, nurses, physiotherapists, respiratory therapists, psychiatrists and dieticians. The team should provide a coordinated plan of rehabilitation, a plan which most importantly is individualized for each patient's disability and needs, and also a plan which is set to achieve realistic goals and does not promise impossible results. Only then is patient participation good and effective.

Features of Rehabilitation

Realistic patient-centred long-term and short-term goals should be set and aimed at after a thorough overall assessment. Many centres prefer to put the patient through an exercise test to unearth significant ischemic heart disease or development of arrhythmias.

1. Exercise Training   Exercise training, starting at a low level with a slow increase (if that is possible) improves exercise capacity and reduces dyspnoea. The only type of exercise to the lower extremities is in the form of walking or cycling. Training programmes to gradually increase exercise capacity follow the same regime as in healthy individuals. An exercise trainer and physiotherapist supervised by a physician help to provide this graded exercise.
2. Breathing Exercises   Breathing exercises help in reducing dyspnoea—the uncomfortable feeling associated with breathing. Pursed lip breathing, diaphragmatic breathing, controlled rhythmic breathing improve tidal volume, reduce air-trapping and hyperinflation and thereby reduce the work of breathing. Yogic breathing exercises are truly beneficial, provided they do not involve holding the breath or using forced expiratory manoeuvres. Coordinating breathing with special activities, learning not to hold the breath, breathing rhythmically and ensuring a full expiration during any activity help to reduce dyspnoea. Training to use

proper body mechanics to conserve energy and to reduce energy requirements is particularly useful in those with poor respiratory reserve. When necessary, oxygen inhalation during training sessions helps the patient increase his workload during exercise sessions, adding to the benefits of rehabilitation.

PSYCHOLOGICAL COUNSELLING

COPD particularly when marked often causes psychological stress in the form of anxiety and depression. Psychiatric help and counselling can prove of significant benefit.

EDUCATION

Education is centred on:

(a) A healthy, disciplined, and if needs be a suitably modified lifestyle.
(b) A behavioural approach requires education on the technique and timing of medications which are carefully incorporated into the patient's daily activities.
(c) Individual and group instructions are important features of this programme.

NUTRITIONAL GUIDANCE

COPD patients lose muscle mass and body weight. In fact a loss of body weight (< 90% ideal) is a marker for increased mortality in this disease. Nutritional guidance to improve muscle mass is of help in these patients. On the other hand, patients who are overweight clearly benefit with nutritional guidance that allows them to lose weight. In those patients where body weight is not a problem, a balanced diet with enough calories to meet caloric expenditure during exercise is provided.

The optimal duration of a rehabilitation programme has not been established. Most programmes have two to three sessions a week, for a 6 to 12-week period. Patients with severe symptoms benefit with longer programmes. Ideally, an exercise rehabilitation programme should be inbuilt in the daily life of every COPD patient.

OXYGEN THERAPY (ALSO SEE CHAPTER ON 'OXYGEN THERAPY')

Oxygen therapy improves survival in patients with COPD who have significant hypoxia or hypercapnia. Studies in 1980 clearly proved the survival benefits of long-term oxygen therapy. Studies also showed that survival was greater in those who received oxygen all through the day and night compared to those who only received nocturnal oxygen. The inclusion criteria generally accepted by health workers and health insurers for ambulatory continuous oxygen therapy are, stable obstructive pulmonary disease on optimal medical therapy who have a $PaO_2 < 55$ mm Hg or a $PaCO_2$ of 56–59 mm Hg together with a PCV > 55% (erythrocytosis) and right heart dysfunction—P pulmonale, peripheral oedema.

The objective of oxygen therapy is to increase the PaO_2 to > 60 mm Hg (O_2 saturation of 90%). A pulse oximeter is useful to ensure that oxygen flow is adequate to permit saturation

Table 38.3: Features of pulmonary rehabilitation
1. Realistic patient-centered long-term and short-term goals and objectives
2. Exercise training
Graduated exercise under close supervision. Walking or cycling as exercises for the lower limbs. Use of oxygen when necessary during exercise training
3. Breathing exercises and training
Pursed lip breathing with slow complete expiration followed by a slow inspiration Diaphragmatic breathing, rhythmic breathing during activity, allowing for full expiration. Yogic breathing exercises. Proper use of body mechanics to conserve energy and reduce energy requirements in conjunction with rhythmic breathing
4. Psychological counseling to counter in particular anxiety, depression
5. Education

(a) A healthy, disciplined and if needs be a suitably modifed life style
    (b) Education on the technique and timing of medications
    (c) Individual and group instructions
    (d) Reinforce motivation to quit smoking in smokers

6. Nutritional guidance
7. Outcome evaluation
8. Exercise as an inbuilt programme in daily life even after rehabilitation programme is complete (6–12 weeks)

Table 38.4: Indications for continuous oxygen therapy in patients with COPD		
Stable obstructive pulmonary disease on optimal medical therapy + $PaO_2 < 55$ mm Hg with O_2 saturation < 90%	or	$PaCO_2 > 55$ mm Hg together with a PCV > 55%; Right heart dysfunction— P pulmonale, peripheral oedema.

> 90% at all times—during rest and activity. Oxygen flow at night may need to be increased to allow a saturation of 90%. Besides clearly improving survival, oxygen relieves dyspnoea at rest and during activity, reduces pulmonary hypertension, improves cognition and significantly improves the quality of life.

Some patients with COPD may not meet the requirements for use of oxygen at rest in the day. They may however desaturate well below 90% during activity or exercise, or may show significant desaturation during sleep at night, even in the proven absence of obstructive sleep apnoea. These patients require to be given oxygen during exercise as also during sleep to enable the oxygen saturation to be >90%. Nocturnal hypoxemia is particularly dangerous as it can induce dangerous arrhythmia, pulmonary hypertension, poor cognition during the day associated with hypersomnolence. Oxygen is often used intermittently to relieve breathlessness after exertion or activity even in the absence of hypoxemia or right heart failure. Though of no proven benefit, there should be no objection to its use if the patient feels quicker relief.

Finally, are the criteria laid down for continuous oxygen therapy in COPD too stringent? There are practising physicians who feel that this is indeed so. Many would advocate therapy for 16 hours or more out of 24 hours if the PaO_2 is < 60 mm Hg (O_2 saturation < 90%) and the $PaCO_2$ > 50 mm Hg even in the absence of erythrocytosis or right ventricular dysfunction.

In patients who have significant hypercapnia, oxygen administration should be controlled, as uncontrolled therapy using high oxygen flow rates may relieve hypoxia but worsen hypercapnia, rendering the patients increasingly drowsy or even comatose. Controlled oxygen is best delivered by a ventimask, or through nasal prongs at a flow rate of 1–2 L/min.

Sources of oxygen include concentrators which obtain oxygen through concentration of air, compressed gaseous oxygen, or liquid oxygen. Compressed gas cylinders need to be replaced when the oxygen within is used up. Liquid oxygen is costly and is quite unsuitable for developing countries. For ambulation, lighter versions of the compressed oxygen systems are available.

Oxygen is ordinarily administered as a continuous flow of gas. Oxygen however reaches the lungs only during inhalation, oxygen delivered during expiration being wasted. Demand delivery devices are available which trigger the flow of oxygen (giving a pulsed dose of oxygen) only when a patient inhales or inspires, thereby reducing oxygen wastage. Demand delivery systems are being increasingly incorporated in portable oxygen systems. These allow oxygen to last for longer periods of time when patients use these portable systems for ambulation or activity outside their homes. The flow rate needs to be adjusted with the demand-delivery systems, (also called pulse-dose), as oxygenation using the demand delivery system is not always equivalent to continuous oxygen flow delivery.

The role of oxygen in COPD should be carefully explained to COPD patients who require it. This educational aspect can be reinforced during the pulmonary rehabilitation programme.

The five-year survival rate of COPD patients who require continuous oxygen therapy is poor, with a life expectancy of 50% at the end of five years.

Control of Hypercapnia

The end-stage of advanced COPD is often characterized by mounting hypercapnia, with its added feature of drowsiness, which could progress to a comatose state. Hypercapnia often worsens during the night so that the patient is difficult to arouse in the mornings. The excessive drowsy state leads to a poor cough reflex, sputum retention, which in turn causes pulmonary infection with an exacerbation of COPD. Non-invasive ventilatory support at night using a BiPAP machine often helps to prevent an undue rise of $PaCO_2$. This leads to greater alertness in the morning and a better quality of life. If needs be, a BiPAP machine may need to be used during some hours in the day as well, again to prevent an undue rise in $PaCO_2$.

Treatment of Right Heart Failure due to Cor Pulmonale

Symptomatic treatment consists of salt restriction, restriction of fluid intake and the use of loop diuretics such as frusemide.

Digoxin may be used, but is of doubtful benefit. Aldactone 50–100 mg/day may help in salt and water excretion, but care must be taken to avoid hyperkalemia. Relief of hypoxia and hypercapnia is important, as this reduces to an extent the vasoconstrictive aspect of pulmonary hypertension and thereby helps right ventricular function. Measures to reduce hyperinflation of the lungs also help to reduce pulmonary hypertension. It is of practical importance to note that markedly hypercapnic patients who are severely waterlogged because of right heart failure due to cor pulmonale often do not respond to even large doses of diuretics. The response is however often dramatic (with regard to sharp reduction of generalized oedema) when these patients are ventilated so that $PaCO_2$ is brought down to reasonable levels (45–55mm Hg).

Treatment of arrhythmias, recognition and treatment of complicating pulmonary infections and of pulmonary thromboembolism are important aspects of management.

Table 38.5: Treatment of right heart failure in COPD
1. Continuous oxygen
2. Salt and water restriction
3. Loop diuretics
4. Aldactone (check for hyperkalemia)
5. Ventilatory support in patients with marked hypercapnia who are severely waterlogged-diuresis often ensues
6. Digoxin (doubtful value)
7. Measures to reduce hyperinflation of lungs
8. Treatment of complicating arrhythmias
9. Prophylaxis and treatment of pulmonary thromboembolism

LUNG VOLUME REDUCTION SURGERY

Lung volume reduction surgery (LVRS) is useful in a subset of patients with emphysema who have localized bullae, chiefly in the upper lobes. The bullae serve no purpose; in fact they contribute to an increased dead space and thus to alveolar hypoventitlation. The National Emphysema Treatment Trial (NETT) has shown that when lung volume reduction was undertaken in a select subset of patients with emphysema there was an overall survival advantage when compared to medical therapy with a five-year risk ratio of death of 0.86 ($p = 0.02$). Survival, exercise capacity improved in the subset of patients with upper lobe predominant disease and low exercise capacity. Patients with upper lobe predominant disease with good exercise capacity had further improvement in exercise capacity together with an improvement in quality of life, but not in survival. The NETT also identified a high-risk group characterized by FEV_1 < 20% of predicted, and either a homogenous distribution of emphysema or a CO-diffusing capacity (DLCO) <20% of predicted. These patients had a significant operative mortality and surgery was not recommended.

The NETT study was the largest randomized controlled trial (RCT) with 1218 patients. This study showed a 6.6%

Table 38.6:
Indication and contraindications for lung volume reduction surgery

Indications:

1. Severe emphysema confined to upper lobes and low exercise capacity inspite of optimal medical treatment

2. Low exercise capacity with no upper lobe disease

3. Upper lobe disease and fair to good exercise capacity

Contraindications:

1. $FEV_1 < 20\%$ of predicted, and either a homogenous distribution of emphysema or a CO diffusing capacity (DLCO) < 20% predicted

2. High exercise capacity with no upper lobe disease

lower absolute mortality rate in the bilateral LVRS group compared to the medical arm. The inclusion criteria for LVRS in this study included:

- High-resolution computed tomography (HRCT) evidence of bilateral emphysema, upper lobe predominance
- $FEV_1 <= 45\%$, TLC $>= 100\%$, RV $>= 150$, 6MWD $>= 140$ m
- $PaO_2 >= 45$ mm Hg, $PaCO_2 <= 60$ mm Hg
- Non-smoking $>= 4$ months, BMI $<= 31.1$ kg/m^2
- Prednisolone $<= 20$ mg/ day

Note: 6MWD-6-minute walk distance

LUNG TRANSPLANTATION

COPD is the most common indication for lung transplantation. Transplantation can be done for single or both lungs depending on the severity of the disease and the patient's age. Indications for lung transplantation are—

1. Advanced COPD patients who are severely symptomatic in spite of optimal medical therapy;
2. One or more of the following:
   $FEV_1 < 25\%$ of the predicted value
   $PaCO_2 > 55$ mm Hg; pulmonary hypertension; right heart failure
3. A life expectancy < 2 years;
4. Age < 55 years for heart lung transplant; < 60 years for a bilateral lung transplant; <65 years for a single lung transplant.

Lung transplantation is contraindicated if there is a history of malignancy within the past two years, persistence of substance addiction within six months of surgery, presence of Hepatitis B, C or HIV infection and dysfunction of any other organ system.

The survival rate after transplantation varies in different centres but averages as follows:

90% at the end of one year
65–90% at the end of two years
41–50% at the end of five years.

A successful lung transplant leads to an improved quality of life and significant improvement in both lung function and exercise capacity. Patients remain on immunosuppressive drugs and are thus prone to infection. Rejection is another complication that can occur soon after transplantation or may occur months or years later. Unfortunately, there are no centres performing lung transplants in India.

MORTALITY

COPD is the only important chronic disease where the death rate continues to increase steadily. As already mentioned, it has been projected to be the third leading cause of death by 2020. In 2002, the WHO estimated the global mortality from COPD as 44.2/100, 000. Mortality was highest in the Western Pacific region (79.8/100, 000) and lowest in Africa (18.1/100, 000). In all regions, mortality was higher in men than in women except in the West Pacific region.

COPD accounted for 140, 000 deaths in the United States; the mortality increased with age and for patients > 45 years. The current trend shows a slight decrease in mortality in men, and a slight increase in mortality in women. In the United Kingdom in 2003, there were 26, 000 deaths from COPD which represents 4.9% of all deaths. Mortality rates were higher in urban compared to rural areas.

Mortality figures from South East Asian countries are similar or even higher than in the West. It is believed that just as there is an underestimation of prevalence figures of COPD, there is an equal underestimation of mortality figures. This is because COPD is often given as a contributory cause of death rather than a primary cause. Also, terms such as chronic bronchitis and emphysema are often given as the cause of death instead of COPD; this lowers the reported mortality rates for COPD. The epidemiological data gathered from mortality rates given in national statistics of developing countries may therefore be unreliable. Even so, the mortality rates are forbiddingly high.

In China, death from chronic respiratory disease ranks as the first cause of death. In 1994 the mortality rate for the

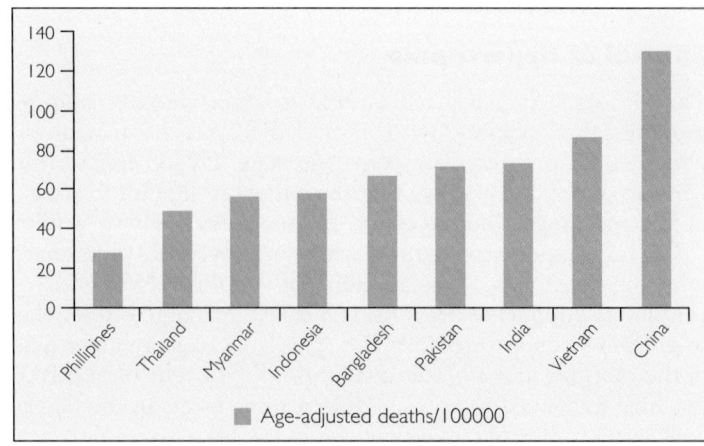

Fig 38.7: Age-adjusted deaths/100000 due to COPD in South-east Asia.

Source: Adapted from Lopez AD, Mathers CD, Ezzati M, Jamison DT, Murray CJ. *Global burden of disease and risk factors*. 2006. Washington: The World Bank.

whole population was 161.57/100,000 in the rural areas and 94.4/100,000 in urban areas. In Thailand, the mortality rate ranged from 500 to 4400/100,000 in men aged 51 and older and 600 to 3400/100,000 in women. In Singapore between 1991–98, COPD deaths were reported to be 16.3/100,000 in individuals > 55 years, being four times higher than in women. In Hong Kong, the death rate from COPD in 1997 was 31.1/100,000 of the population and in Japan COPD mortality in 1999 was 10.4/100,000.

SUGGESTED READING

Almagro P. Recent improvement in long-term survival after a COPD hospitalisation. *Thorax*. 1 Apr. 2010; 65(4): 298–302.

Barnes PJ. Emerging pharmacotherapies for COPD. *Chest*. 1 Dec. 2008; 134(6): 1278–86.

Burge PS, Calverley P. Inhaled steroids in obstructive lung disease in Europe, the ISOLDE trial: protocol, and progress (abstract). *Am J Respir Crit Care Med*. 1994; 149: A312 .

Grimes GC. Medications for COPD: a review of effectiveness. *Am Fam Physician*. 15 Oct. 2007; 76(8): 1141–8.

Global Initiative for Chronic Obstructive Lung Disease. Global Strategy for the Diagnosis, Management, and Prevention of Chronic Obstructive Pulmonary Disease. Global Initiative for Chronic Obstructive Lung Disease; 2006.

Pauwels RA, Lofdahl CG, Pride NB, Postma DS, Laitinen LA, Ohlsson SV. European Respiratory Society study on chronic obstructive pulmonary disease (EUROSCOP): hypothesis and design. *Eur Respir J*. 1992; 5: 1254–61

Reardon J. Pulmonary rehabilitation for COPD. *Respir Med*. 1 Dec. 2005; 99 Suppl B: S19–27.

Vestbo J, Lange P, Sorensen T, Gronlund C, Viskum K. The Copenhagen City Lung Study—a clinical trial of inhaled corticosteroids in COPD: design and progress (abstract). *Am J Respir Crit Care Med*. 1995; 151: A466.

Vestbo J; TORCH Study Group. The TORCH (towards a revolution in COPD health) survival study protocol. *Eur Respir J*. Aug. 2004; 24(2): 206–10.

Welsh EJ, Cates CJ, Poole P. Combination inhaled steroid and long-acting beta2-agonist versus tiotropium for chronic obstructive pulmonary disease. *Cochrane Database Syst Rev*. May 2010; 12(5): CD007891.

Cystic fibrosis is a fatal or life-limiting autosomal recessive genetic disease. In its epidemiology it has an ethnic distribution, being most common in the Caucasian race with a frequency of 1 in 3, 300 live births. It is less common in the black population, the incidence being 1 in 17, 000. The incidence in African-Americans is believed to be in 1 in 15, 000 and in Asian-Americans 1 in 31, 000. The disease is believed to be comparatively rare in India and South East Asia. This may or may not be factual. Its apparent rarity at least in India may well be related to a lack of awareness of the problem, so that diagnostic tests for the disease, particularly in adolescents and young adults presenting solely with respiratory features, are not performed. The Indian scenario with regard to cystic fibrosis is briefly discussed later in the chapter.

Cystic fibrosis involves many organ systems giving rise to a variety of clinical features. Involvement of the respiratory system is however generally most pronounced so that the clinical presentation of cystic fibrosis is often dominated by progressive respiratory disease.

The underlying abnormality in cystic fibrosis is defective chloride transport in sweat glands and respiratory epithelium and other epithelial cells. An increase in sweat sodium and chloride in cystic fibrosis provides an early available diagnostic marker for the disease. The genetic defect responsible for the disease was discovered as late as 1989. The cause of cystic fibrosis was then proven to be due to a mutated gene encoding a defective chloride channel in epithelial cells. This has unquestionably improved our understanding of cystic fibrosis and given us at least some insight into the different manifestations involving different organ systems encountered in this disease.

GENETICS

Cystic fibrosis is caused by a mutation on a gene on Chromosome 7 which encodes a protein responsible for ion transport across epithelial cells. This protein is named the cystic fibrosis transmembrane regulator or (CFTR). Numerous genetic mutations have been described with regard to this gene; most of these mutations are rare. The CFTR mutations are grouped into five classes.

Class I	CFTR is not synthesized
Class II	CFTR is inadequately processed
Class III	CFTR is unregulated
Class IV	CFTR shows abnormal conductance
Class V	CFTR is partially defective in its production or processing

Over 60% of patients with cystic fibrosis in the West have a Class II mutation caused by deletion of phenylalamine in Portion 508 (F508) of CFTR. F508 Δ CFTR is incorrectly folded and trapped in the endoplasm and is then proteolytically degraded, thereby losing its function. The little CFTR that escapes this degradation reaches the membrane of the epithelial cells and shows functional activity.

It has been shown that patients who carry two severe mutations causing a loss of function of CFTR (Class I, II, III) have the typical features of cystic fibrosis characterized by pancreatic insufficiency, elevated sweat chloride and early age of diagnosis. On the other hand patients who have just one mild mutation with partial function of CFTR do not have pancreatic insufficiency, have sweat chloride values close to upper limits of normal and are diagnosed at a later age. Class IV and V mutations have been shown to be linked with pancreatic insufficiency. Attempts to correlate specific mutations with lung disease have shown significant variations with regard to severity of lung involvement. Because of this wide variation, it has been suggested that environmental factors and/or genes other than the one related to CFTR may perhaps play a role in the evaluation, progression and severity of the disease.

PATHOPHYSIOLOGY

The pathophysiology of cystic fibrosis is best understood by contrasting the normal ionic transport within the airways mucosa with that of the deranged ionic transport in cystic fibrosis.

In normal subjects, airway epithelial cells secrete chloride and absorb sodium chloride. This is regulated through 'channels' by the CFTR. The balance between 'secretion' and 'absorption' determines water transport and allows an adequate layer of airway surface liquid which supports the thin mucous layer present over epithelial cells. This mucous layer is constantly escalated upwards and out of the airways through regulated ciliary movement.

In patients with cystic fibrosis, absence or dysfunction of the CFTR leads to reduced chloride secretion and increased absorption of sodium chloride. This is detrimental for water transport so that the airway surface liquid which supports the mucous layer present over epithelial cells is lacking. In the absence of the airway surface liquid, respiratory cilia are dysfunctional and there is a breakdown of mucocilary transport. Mucous which becomes increasingly viscous accumulates and plugs the smaller airways. This is the basic and primary pathological event in cystic fibrosis.

Sequentially, there is now trapping of inhaled bacteria in the poorly moving viscous mucous. These microorganisms

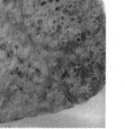

produce an ongoing inflammation in the small airways. Airways inflammation, obstruction, distortion, with progressive lung damage leads ultimately to hypoxic or hypoxic cum hypercapnic respiratory failure.

INFECTING ORGANISMS IN CYSTIC FIBROSIS

There is generally a small spectrum of infecting organisms that perpetuate inflammation in cystic fibrosis. The commonest isolate is *Ps. aeruginosa*, followed by *S. aureus* and *H. influenzae*. Initially these organisms form non-mucoid colonies. However, the mucous in cystic fibrosis lacks oxygen, leading to anaerobic growth of bacteria and a switch of the above organisms from the non-mucoid form to the mucoid form. The mucoid forms produce a fine biofilm which hinders the action of antibiotics on these bacteria and also enables them to resist killing by the immunological responses of the host.

As the disease progresses and worsens, other multi-resistant bacteria may come on the scene. These are *Stenotrophomonas maltophilia*, *Alcaligenes xylosoxidans*, and the *Burkholderia cepacia* complex. These organisms are isolated in 10% of patients with cystic fibrosis. Occasionally, non-tuberculous mycobacteria (*M. avium intracellulare*) are isolated. It is a matter of dispute whether these organisms are colonizers or are responsible for infection, inflammation and progress of the disease. Perhaps they may be playing a dual role. The *B. cepacia* complex is recognized to be an unusual but dangerous organism. This organism, normally present in soil and water, causes chronic infection only in cystic fibrosis and chronic granulomatous disease. It is a multi-resistant organism with poor or no response to antibiotic therapy and worsens the progress in patients with cystic fibrosis. There is evidence that in patients with cystic fibrosis, the *B. cepacia* complex can cause cross-infection by spreading from one patient to the other. What is more, 10–15% of patients with cystic fibrosis who are infected by the *B. cepacia* complex develop the 'cepacia syndrome' characterized by a necrotizing pneumonia, marked leucocytosis, bacteraemia and an almost 100% mortality.

There are a few important features in relation to inflammation of the airways in cystic fibrosis. Firstly and importantly, inflammation of the airways starts very early in the first months of life in a patient with typical cystic fibrosis. It antedates symptoms of respiratory disease by a long period of time stretching from months to years. Secondly, the inflammatory process is neutrophilic and sustained. There is an exaggerated inflammatory response to both bacterial and viral pathogens. Whether the absence or defect of the cystic fibrosis membrane regulator plays a direct role in inducing this inflammatory response or whether it only plays an indirect role by causing mucous plugging is a matter of dispute. Unquestionably, it is persistent exaggerated sustained inflammation within the airways which determines the downhill course of cystic fibrosis.

CLINICAL FEATURES

Cystic fibrosis has a wide spectrum of symptoms which involve the respiratory system, gastrointestinal system and in adults the reproductive system.

The classic triad in cystic fibrosis consists of cough with sputum, steatorrhea and failure to thrive. Pulmonary symptoms may not be present at birth but may occur later in childhood, adolescence or even later. At times clinical features of the disease may only involve the lungs, evidence of steatorrhea due to pancreatic insufficiency not being clinically manifest in 10–15% of patients. As the child matures into an adult, infertility due to azoospermia caused by obstructed or absent vas deferens is almost always present.

Cystic fibrosis is generally not evident at birth except in 10–15% of patients who present with meconium ileus. Meconium ileus is actually a manifestation of pancreatic insufficiency though it is not associated with more severe manifestations of pancreatic disease. The respiratory and non-respiratory features of cystic fibrosis are tabled separately.

This section chiefly deals with the respiratory manifestations of cystic fibrosis. The chief symptom of respiratory involvement is cough, which to start with occurs during exacerbations, but later becomes chronic and is associated with productive sputum. The sputum is mucoid but during periods of infection it becomes purulent and coloured yellow or green. Persistent untreated infection results in persistent cough with purulent expectoration. Minor haemoptysis may occur during exacerbations. As the disease progresses there is increasing breathlessness on exertion. Pansinusitis is often present.

Some patients have hyperactive airways and so have wheezing, paroxysmal bouts of cough and a fair degree of reversibility of airways obstruction. They are often diagnosed and treated as 'asthma'; the underlying disease remaining undetected.

As the disease progresses there is worsening dyspnoea, bouts of fever due to recurrent or persistent infection. Bronchiectasis chiefly involving the upper lobes is observed. Weight loss or failure to increase weight (in childhood and adolescence) is invariably present. The nails are often clubbed.

The end-result is hypoxemic respiratory failure and still later hypoxemic plus hypercapnic respiratory failure. This generally occurs when the FEV_1 is < 30% of predicted value. Cor pulmonale occurs late in the illness.

Patients with cystic fibrosis invariably have a sinusitis involving almost all paranasal sinuses. The sinusitis may be clinically manifest or may be silent being diagnosed on imaging studies.

IMAGING

Although the disease is present at birth, radiographic abnormalities may not become apparent for years. The earliest findings are recurrent pneumonia, mucoid impaction, bronchiectasis and focal atelectasis. The involvement is predominantly in the upper lobes. With time there is advancement in the disease process with progressive worsening of radiographic abnormalities. The hila may be enlarged due to adenopathy or pulmonary hypertension.

COMPUTED TOMOGRAPHY (CT) PICTURE
The findings vary with duration and severity of disease. The predominant findings are of bronchiectasis with or without mucoid impaction mainly in the upper lobes. Due to chronic inflammatory changes, there is bronchial wall thickening with peribronchiolar inflammation. There may be mosaic perfusion due to bronchial wall thickening involving the smaller airways. Focal areas of consolidation and atelectasis are often seen. Pulmonary hypertension develops late in the course of the

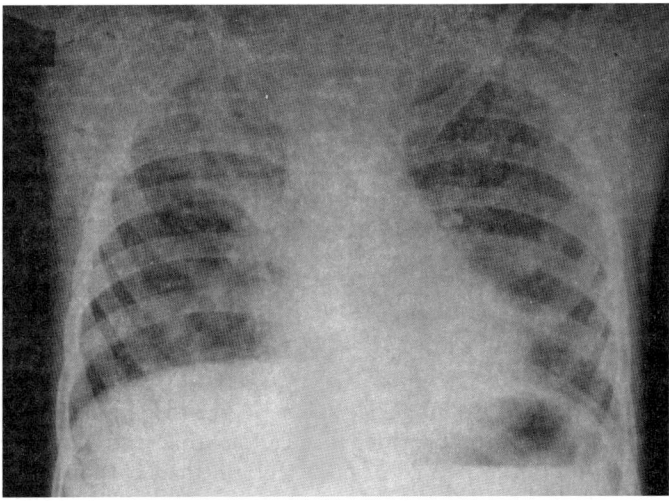

(a)

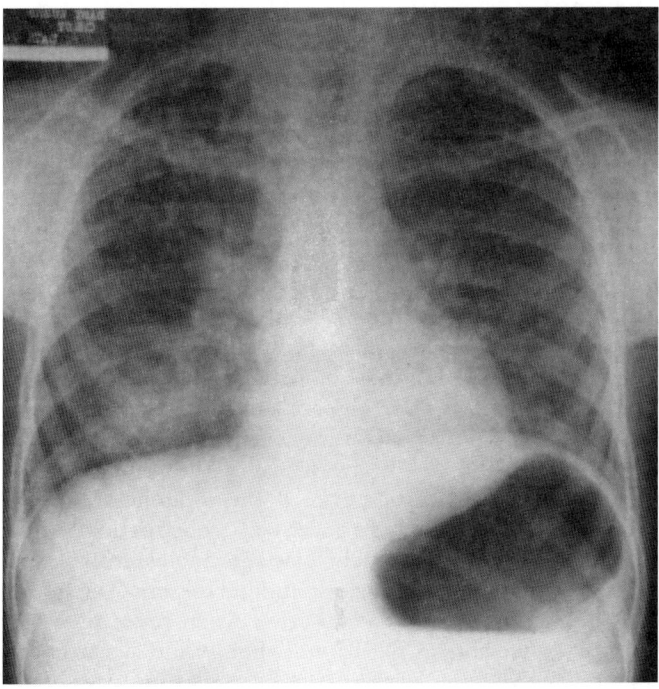

(b)

Fig 39.1: Cystic Fibrosis (a) Chest X-ray demonstrates an ill-defined area of consolidation in a three-year-old boy, (b) two years later he presented with right lower zone consolidation. Serial chest x-rays done later revealed extensive bilateral opacities as a result of bronchiectasis and mucoid impaction. Note, the peripheral lungs demonstrate hyperinflation. This is an example of a young boy initially presenting with repeated consolidations and then progressing to extensive bronchiectasis.

disease. There may also be hypertrophy of the bronchial arteries contributing to episodes of haemoptysis.

DIAGNOSTIC TESTS

1. *The sweat sodium chloride test* A suspicion of cystic fibrosis should prompt the measurement of sweat sodium and chloride. Abnormal ion transport in this disease is reflected

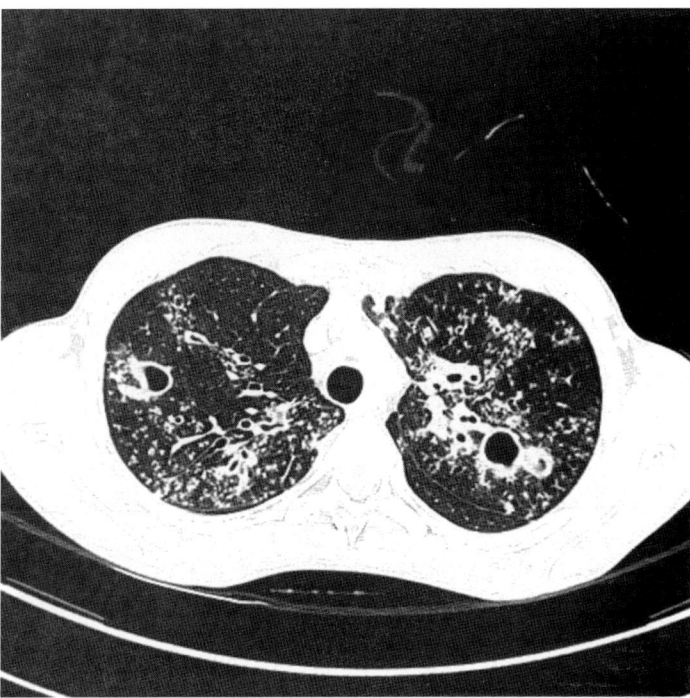

Fig 39.2: Cystic Fibrosis—High-resolution CT demonstrates extensive cylindrical and cystic bronchiectasis in the upper zones bilaterally. Note multiple small nodules as a result of peribronchial inflammation of small airways.

Table 39.1: Respiratory features of cystic fibrosis
1. Chronic productive cough with increasing periods of purulent expectoration
2. Colonization and infection with S. aureus, Ps. aeruginosa
3. Airways obstruction with progressive reduction in FEV_1
4. Radiological abnormalities with bronchiectasis involving chiefly the upper lobes
5. Clubbing
6. Pansinusitis
7. Hypoxemia or hypoxemic + hypercapnic respiratory failure

Table 39.2: Non-respiratory features of cystic fibrosis
1. Gastrointestinal disease
Meconium ileus, distal intestinal obstruction syndrome
Steatorrhoea due to pancreatic insufficiency
Pancreatitis
Failure to thrive, hypoalbuminemia
Deficiency of fat-soluble vitamins
Biliary cirrhosis
2. Infertility due to azoospermia caused by obstruction to the vas deferns

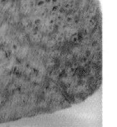
in the high sodium and chloride levels in sweat. Chloride content of sweat > 60 mmol/L on repeated testing is diagnostic of the disease. Sweat chloride content between 30–60 mmol/L is a borderline result which may be observed in patients with cystic fibrosis.

2. *Genotyping of the most common CFTR mutations.*

3. *Assessing CFTR function by measurement of the nasal potential difference.* This tests needs to be done only if the sweat test and the CFTR genotyping are not diagnostic. The transport of sodium and chloride across the nasal mucosa produces an electrical potential difference. Changes in potential difference as a result of stimulation or inhibition of ion channels by nasal perfusion can be measured. The normal nasal mucosa gives a different response when compared to cystic fibrous mucosa. This test is difficult, highly technical and requires special expertise.

4. *Most patients with cystic fibrosis have pancreatic insufficiency.* This can be tested by fat estimation of stools over 48 to 72 hours, to prove the presence of steatorrhoea and by decreased concentration of chymotrypsin or pancreatic-specific elastase in faeces.

5. *Imaging studies (X-ray, CT) of the chest and of paranasal sinuses.*

6. *Sputum cultures* typically show the presence of *S. aureus* or *Ps. aeruginosa* or *H. influenzae*, particularly during infection exacerbation.

Table 39.3: Diagnostic tests for cystic fibrosis
1. The sweat sodium chloride test; sweat chloride > 60 mmol/L
2. Genotyping of the most common CFTR mutations
3. Assessing CFTR function by measurement of the nasal potential difference
4. Fat estimation of stools over 48 to 72 hours, determining concentration of chymotrypsin or pancreatic specific elastase in faeces
5. Imaging studies (X-ray, CT) of the paranasal sinuses and of the chest
6. Sputum culture
7. Seminal fluid test for azoospermia

Western studies suggest that in 5–10% of patients the diagnosis of cystic fibrosis is not made until adulthood. These patients do not have the classic features of cystic fibrosis and may present with involvement of just one system—sterility due to azoospermia from obstructed vas deferens, recurrent acute pancreatitis or chronic airways disease with bronchiectasis. Pancreatic insufficiency is not present in these patients and the sweat chloride test is not clearly diagnostic. Mutations of the CFTR gene test through commercial genetic screening panels in these adults are also not those classically associated with cystic fibrosis. Perhaps, mutations of the CFTR gene in adult patients are mild and therefore escape the genetic screening panels conventionally used for this disease. The nasal potential difference may prove of diagnostic use in these patients, only the test is highly technical requiring special expertise.

The presence of obstructive azoospermia should always prompt genetic testing for cystic fibrosis. However, a diagnosis of cystic fibrosis should only be made in these adults if proper diagnostic criteria are met—sweat chloride > 60 mmol/L, two CFTR causing mutations, nasal potential difference observed with cystic fibrosis.

Western studies claim that despite sophisticated diagnostic tests a definite diagnosis of cystic fibrosis cannot be made in a number of adults who have clinical features suggestive of the disease including typical cystic fibrosis bronchiectasis.

Indian Scenario

Though the precise incidence of cystic fibrosis among Indians is unknown, current evidence suggests that the disease is more common in people of Indian origin than is thought. Of the 3500 new cases registered in the Paediatric Chest Clinic from 1995–2002 at the All India Institute of Medical Science, Kobra and his colleagues diagnosed cystic fibrosis in 120 (3.5%) children. The diagnosis was based on a sweat chloride > 60 mEq/L and a positive genetic test for DF 508 mutation.

Respiratory features included repeated attacks or persistent pneumonia in almost all patients, airways obstruction with hyperinflated lungs in 83%, crepitations on auscultation in 92% and wheezing in 25%. Organisms cultured from sputum in order of frequency were *Ps. aeruginosa*, *S. aureus*, Klebsiella spp.

Failure to thrive, malabsorption and malnutrition were prominent clinical features outside the respiratory system. DF 508 mutation was positive in 45 chromosomes out of 240 tested, the frequency of this Delta F mutation was 19%—less than that observed in Caucasian patients. Remarkably, cystic fibrosis was advanced in most patients at the time of diagnosis.

Almost certainly, the disease in India and perhaps in Southeast Asia is not as uncommon as is believed. The apparent rarity is due to the lack of awareness of the problem and the lack of diagnostic facilities even if the awareness is present. The disease, presenting with airways obstruction, chronic respiratory systems or bronchiectasis in adolescents or young adults is missed for the above-mentioned reasons. The question also arises whether in India and other Asian countries a forme fruste of cystic fibrosis exists, with borderline sweat chloride tests and with lesser degree of CFTR mutation, or mutations not considered typical for the disease. A greater in-depth study of patients presenting with chronic airways obstruction, recurrent respiratory infections or bronchiectasis of the type and distribution seen in cystic fibrosis or of patients with obstructive azoospermia may perhaps prove rewarding.

Natural History of Lung Disease in Cystic Fibrosis

Pathological abnormalities in the small airways precede clinical symptoms. These abnormalities take the form of mucous plugging with dilatation distal to the obstructed small airways. Chronic productive cough is associated with a steady decline in lung function. Acute exacerbations are triggered by infection and as the disease progresses a well-nigh permanent colonization with *S. aureus* and *Ps. aeruginosa* is observed. Exacerbations cause a worsening of symptoms, a decline of FEV_1 and if unrecognized and untreated may cause a permanent further decline in lung function. A greater awareness of this fact has led to more vigorous treatment of pulmonary manifestations of this disease. Evaluation of clinical features, periodic FEV_1 measurements and imaging studies are important in assessing the outcome of these patients. Some patients progress to hypoxemic cum hypercapnic respiratory failure with cor pulmonale in spite of assiduous care.

MANAGEMENT OF PULMONARY FEATURES OF CYSTIC FIBROSIS

There is no cure for cystic fibrosis. Treatment is symptomatic. Principles of treatment are—

1. Early initiation of treatment
2. Combating the cycle of mucus retention, infection and inflammation
3. Recognition and treatment of acute exacerbations

Ensuring Patency of Airways

1. Physiotherapy is of critical importance. Percussion, vibration, positive expiratory pressure and postural drainage all come of use. Physical activity and exercise should be encouraged under supervision.
2. Reduction of airways secretions N-acetyl cysteine has been used as a mucolytic agent though most workers in this field believe that it has little effect because secretions in cystic fibrosis have very little mucus and more pus.

   Recombinant human DNase administered by inhalation reduces sputum viscosity, improves lung function and reduces the number of exacerbations in mild and moderately severe disease. Nebulised hypertonic saline is believed to have the same effect as DNase.

Treatment of Airway Infection

Treatment of airways infection is of crucial importance. The organisms most frequently responsible for infection are *S. aureus*, *H. influenzae* and most of all, particularly in advanced disease, *Ps. aeruginosa*. The following points are noteworthy—

1. Acute exacerbations of the disease are related to infection and need immediate antibiotic treatment.
2. Threshold for administering antibiotics should be low; else each exacerbation can cause further permanent damage.
3. Anti-staphylococcal antibiotics should be given for three to four weeks. There is insufficient evidence to use anti-staphylococcal antibiotics as prophylaxis. In fact prophylactic therapy may perhaps promote the emergence of *Ps. aeruginosa*.
4. *Ps. aeruginosa* is the prominent colonizer and infective agent in cystic fibrosis in adult patients. Patients generally become chronically infected with mucoid strains of this organism and this has a significant negative impact on the disease.
5. It is impossible to eradicate chronic infection caused by *Ps. aeruginosa*, but early antibiotic therapy against this organism is an important advance in management. Inhaled antibiotic therapy with tobramycin together with oral therapy with ciprofloxacin has been used successfully to reduce the incidence of chronic *Ps. aeruginosa* infection.

6. Inhaled antibiotic therapy with tobramycin or colistin or one alternating with the other is the treatment of choice for maintenance therapy in patients infected with *Ps. aeruginosa*. In addition to inhaled antibiotics, Azithromycin 500 mg once or twice daily is reported to reduce exacerbations of *Ps. aeruginosa* infection in this disease. The reason for this is unclear. It may be related to the anti-inflammatory effect of the macrolide or the drug may have an effect on the organisms growing in biofilms, even though the drug has no efficacy against *Ps. aeruginosa* when tested in routine cultures.
7. Acute exacerbations of severe infection are treated with an intravenous combination of piperacillin + tazobactum with an aminoglycoside. Less severe exacerbations are treated with oral ciprofloxicin. Some centres treat chronically infected patients with intravenous antibiotics for two to three weeks every three months on a continuous basis. There is insufficient evidence to advocate use of this protocol.
8. Occasionally, patients with cystic fibrosis are infected by other gram-negative organisms. These include *Burkholderia cepacia* complex, and *Stenotrophomonas maltophila*. Their relation to progression of disease in patients with cystic fibrosis is undetermined. Patients chronically infected with *B. cepacia* respond to doxycycline or trimethoprim-sulphamethaxazole during minor exacerbations. More severe exacerbations may require intravenous meropenem, inhaled tobramycin in 'combination' with ceftazidime or chloramphenicol. Prolonged antibiotic therapy extending for several weeks may be necessary before clinical response occurs. The occurrence of the cepacia syndrome in 10–15% of patients of cystic fibrosis infected by the *B. cepacia* complex has already been commented upon.

   S. maltophilia is best treated with trimethoprim-sulphamethaxazole combined with ticarcillin clavulanate or levofloxacin.

Treatment of Inflammation

Cystic fibrosis is characterized by an intense neutrophilic inflammation of the airways. Prednisolone in a dose of 1 mg/kg given on alternate days was found to reduce decline in lung function in patients infected with *Ps. aeruginosa*. However, serious side-effects which included hyperglycaemia, growth retardation in children and cataract were observed. Treatment with prednisolone should therefore only be reserved for patients who have hyper-reactive airways. Hyper-reactive airways are observed in about 25–30% of patients with cystic fibrosis.

Inhaled corticosteroids are widely used but have not been shown to improve lung function in cystic fibrosis.

Gene Replacement Therapy

Cystic fibrosis is caused by gene mutation leading to deficient or absent CFTR. Therefore gene replacement therapy if successful would be both appropriate and specific. Gene therapy trials have targeted the respiratory system using adenovirus and cationic lipids as vectors. A transient effect on CFTR expression and function has been observed in human trials but there is no long-lasting effect. Gene therapy therefore cannot be recommended as a specific treatment for cystic fibrosis as yet.

Lung Transplantation

Lung transplantation is the only treatment available for end-stage cystic fibrosis. A patient should be ill enough so that there is a survival benefit if given a lung transplant, yet he or she should not die while on the waiting list. An $FEV_1 < 30\%$ of predicted value in a patient receiving maximum medical treatment for the disease is accepted as an indicator for a double-lung or heart-lung transplant. The above value of FEV_1 is associated with a median survival rate of two years. Generally, survival is better for adults than for children. Survival is particularly poor in patients infected with *B. cepacia* so that some centres consider the presence of this infection as a contraindication to surgery. Current data from the International Society for Heart and Lung Transplantation (ISHLT data) has shown a one-year survival rate of 80%, five-year survival rate of 55% and 10-year survival rate of 35% after lung transplantation.

Table 39.4: Drugs in cystic fibrosis		
Pathogen	**Antibiotic used**	**Dosage**
1. S. aureus		
MSSA	Amoxicillin/clavulanate	625 mg BD orally 1.2 g 8 hourly iv
MRSA	Linezolid	600 mg BD
2. H. influenzae	Cefuroxime	500 mg BD orally
	Ceftriaxone	1–2 g 12 hourly iv
3. Ps.aeruginosa	Ciprofloxacin	500 mg BD orally
	Piperacillin/tazobactum	45 g 8 hourly iv
	Nebulised tobramycin	300 mg BD
	Nebulised colistin	150 mg BD

TREATMENT OF RESPIRATORY COMPLICATIONS IN CYSTIC FIBROSIS

Pneumothorax

Pneumothorax is a complication in patients with more severe disease and is related to rupture of an emphysematous area in the lung. A chest tube drain is invariably necessary. The lung may not expand readily because of the underlying fibrosis.

Pneumothorax may be recurrent and pleurodesis may be necessary with talc or tetracycline. If pneumothorax with air leak still persists, a video-assisted thoracoscopic surgical procedure needs to be done to close the leak.

Haemoptysis

Haemoptysis is usually a symptom of infection but can also occur from the dilated bronchial circulation in bronchiectatic areas of the lung. Use of antibiotics to counter infection and of Vitamin K is advisable. Massive haemoptysis which is life-threatening is best treated with bronchial embolization once the site of bleeding is localized through angiographic studies. It is important to secure the airway in a patient with severe haemoptysis.

Allergic Bronchopulmonary Aspergillosis

Aspergillus is frequently present in sputum cultures of patients with cystic fibrosis without being responsible for any symptoms. However, some patients with cystic fibrosis have hyper-reactive airways; an exacerbation of this hyper-reactivity is at times related to allergic bronchopulmonary aspergillosis. The diagnosis may be difficult as cough, wheezing, bronchiectasis, presence of aspergillus in the sputum are common in patients with cystic fibrosis. The presence of fleeting pulmonary shadows, markedly elevated immunoglobulin E (IgE) specific to aspergillus, positive skin test and precipitins against aspergillus support the diagnosis of allergic bronchopulmonary aspergillosis.

Corticosteroids in a dose of 30 to 40 mg daily tapered over two weeks improve both symptoms and the FEV_1. Itraconazole can be used as adjunctive therapy, though its efficacy has not been proven in cystic fibrosis.

Bronchiectasis

Bronchiectasis is not a complication but a feature of progressive cystic fibrosis.

Treatment of Other Features of Cystic Fibrosis

Cystic fibrosis in its full form causes pancreatic insufficiency, malabsorption, with malnutrition and infertility due to obstructive azoospermia. These need attention and treatment for overall success in the management of the disease.

SUGGESTED READING

Dovey M. Oral corticosteroid therapy in cystic fibrosis patients hospitalized for pulmonary exacerbation: a pilot study. *Chest.* 1 Oct. 2007; 132(4): 1212–8.

Gregg AR. Genetic screening for cystic fibrosis. *Obstet Gynecol Clin North Am.* 1 Jun. 2002; 29(2): 329–40.

Michel SH. Nutrition management of pediatric patients who have cystic fibrosis. *Pediatr Clin North Am.* 1 Oct. 2009; 56(5): 1123–41.

Robinson TE. Imaging of the chest in cystic fibrosis. *Clin Chest Med.* 1 Jun. 2007; 28(2): 405–21.

Sueblinvong V. Novel therapies for the treatment of cystic fibrosis: new developments in gene and stem cell therapy. *Clin Chest Med.* 1 Jun. 2007; 28(2): 361–79.

Wilmott RW. Cystic fibrosis. *J Pediatr.* Sep. 2005; 147(3).

CHAPTER **40**   **Allergic Bronchopulmonary Aspergillosis**

Aspergillus species are fungi whose spores are ubiquitous in our environment, being present in house dust, in dust at construction sites and most of all in decaying organic matter such as hay and compost. There are close to 250 species of aspergillus but only a few cause human disease. *Aspergillus fumigatus* is the commonest cause of pulmonary aspergillosis but a few other species (*Aspergillus flavus, Aspergillus niger, Aspergillus clavatus, Aspergillus nidulans, Aspergillus terreus*) can also cause disease of the lungs and the paranasal sinuses. The nature of pulmonary disease caused by Aspergillus infection is determined by the host-immune response and the virulence of the fungus. Three forms of pulmonary aspergillosis have been described—

1. Invasive aspergillosis including necrotising pulmonary aspergillosis.
2. Saprophytic aspergillosis causing aspergillomas—fungal aspergillus balls typically occurring in preformed lung cavities and in bronchiectatic spaces.
3. Allergic aspergillosis which includes allergic bronchopulmonary aspergillosis (ABPA), allergic aspergillus sinusitis, and extrinsic allergic alveolitis.

Invasive aspergillosis and aspergilloma have been dealt with in the chapters on 'Non-Bacterial Pneumonia' and 'Pneumonia in the Non-HIV Immunocompromised Patient'. Extrinsic allergic alveolitis due to aspergillus is dealt with in the section on 'Interstitial Lung Diseases and Other Diffuse Lung Diseases'. This chapter deals with ABPA and allergic aspergillus sinusitis.

ALLERGIC BRONCHOPULMONARY ASPERGILLOSIS (ABPA)

This disease was first described by Hanson and colleagues from the Brompton Hospital, London in 1952. It is characterized by a hypersensitivity host response to intermittent or continuous colonization of the bronchi by hyphae of *Aspergillus fumigatus*. This hypersensitivity response leads to eosinophilic infiltration of the periphery of the lung (eosinophilic pneumonia), plugging of bronchi with mucus plugs often containing hyphae of the fungus and an inflammation of the bronchial walls which in time to come can lead to bronchiectasis. In the vast majority of cases, ABPA is associated with bronchial asthma; the incidence of ABPA is higher in patients with cystic fibrosis, in pre-existing idiopathic bronchiectasis and in individuals with atopic disorders.

Epidemiology

There are a number of asthmatics who show an immediate type cutaneous hypersensitivity to the *Aspergillus fumigatus* antigen

but just a few of these develop ABPA. The reason for this is not known. The prevalence of ABPA in an asthmatic population is probably between 1–2%; it is as high as 7–14% in corticosteroid-dependent asthma. Cystic fibrosis is an uncommon disease in India, but in the West, ABPA complicates 8–10% of patients with cystic fibrosis. Very occasionally, ABPA is diagnosed in non-asthmatics. This is either due to the fact that these patients have a mild asthma of which they are unaware or even if they do not have asthma they are atopic individuals.

Pathogenesis

Aspergillus spores are 2–3 mm in diameter and when inhaled are principally deposited in the proximal large bronchi where humidity and temperature (37°C) provide optimal growth conditions for *Aspergillus fumigatus*. The fungal spores within the bronchi turn into hyphae and colonize the bronchial wall. Epithelial damage within the bronchi with impaired ciliary function observed in both bronchial asthma and in cystic fibrosis probably encourage colonization and therefore predispose to ABPA. The fungal hyphae are believed to further impair ciliary function thereby helping even more in colonization. This effect is mediated by gliotoxin, produced by Aspergillus as also perhaps by other toxins. Adhesion of *A. fumigatus* to the bronchial wall may be also important for colonization and the development of ABPA in susceptible individuals. Adhesion of *A. fumigatus* to extracellular matrix has been observed, in particular to fibronectin and other subepithelial components exposed after tissue damage within the bronchial wall.

Though fungal metabolites may enhance inflammation they are not central to the pathogenesis of ABPA. The pathogenesis is almost completely based on the immunological response of the host to the antigen-colonizing fungus within the airways of the patient. The immunological response is a Type I response, a Type III response and a Type IV T-cell-mediated response.

ABPA is almost always associated with a markedly elevated level of both non-specific and Aspergillus-specific Immunoglobulin E (IgE). A Type I reaction is proposed with degranulation of mast cells and release of histamine, leukotrienes and other cytokines.

There is not just an increase in IgE levels, but also a polyclonal antibody response to the Aspergillus antigen, resulting in high levels of both total and specific IgG and IgA as well. The local high concentration of antigen and specific antibody leads to local immune-complex deposition—a Type III immune response results, causing an inflammatory exudate that damages the bronchial wall.

A Type IV immune response is also believed to underlie the pathogenesis of ABPA. The aspergillus antigen is processed

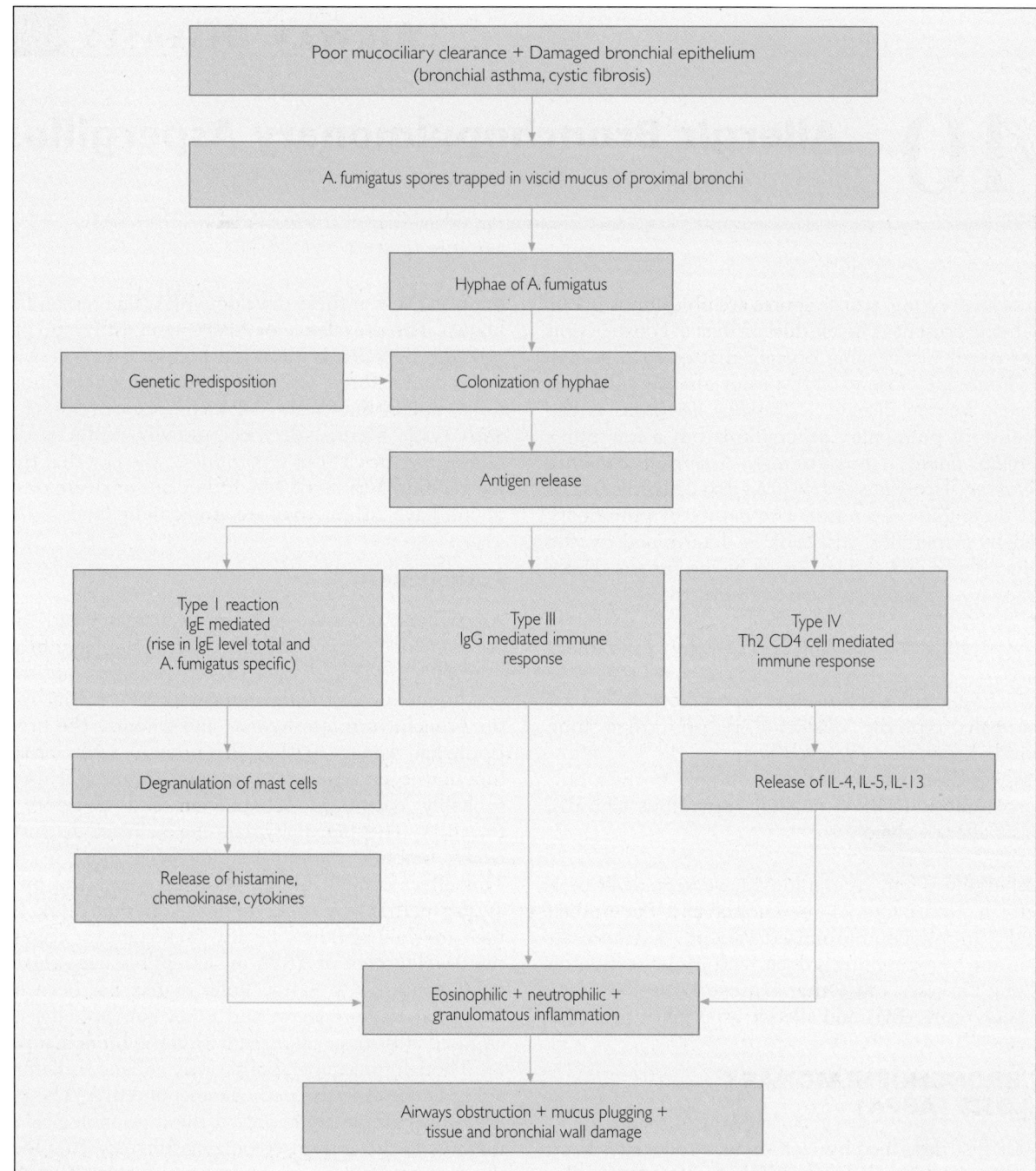

Fig 40.1: Pathogenesis of ABPA.

and presented to T-cells with activation of TH2 CD4—T-cell response. The TH2 cytokines lead to submucosal inflammation featuring both the abundant prevalence of eosinophils together with granuloma formation.

The question that arises is why do only some individuals with asthma develop ABPA while the majority do not. One reason may be genetic predisposition in those asthmatics who develop ABPA. T-cell antigen responsiveness has been observed only with specific HLA-DR subtypes. Six HLA-DR subtypes have been identified accounting for most cases of ABPA. The pathogenesis of ABPA is illustrated in Fig 40.1.

Pathology

Three features are of note—

1. Eosinophilic infiltration of the lung parenchyma which is responsible for fleeting radiological shadows. The eosinophilic infiltration is compatible with an eosinophilic pneumonia.

2. Occlusion of bronchi, by mucus plugs containing Charcot Leyden crystal (eosinophilic degradation products), Curschmann's spirals and fungal hyphae. Mucus plugging can

lead to atelectasis of a lung segment, a lobe or rarely, the whole lung.

3. The bronchial walls show infiltration with eosinophils, granuloma formation, leading to thickening of the walls, fibrosis and bronchiectasis, typically proximal, and chiefly involving the upper lobes.

Clinical Features

ABPA occurs chiefly in patients with asthma. It is more frequent in adults with pre-existing asthma but also occurs in asthmatic children and has been reported in infants as well. It is an important complication of cystic fibrosis, a disease which fortunately is uncommon in our part of the world. Rarely, it may occur in non-asthmatic but atopic individuals. ABPA has the following presentations—

1. The classic presentation is that of an exacerbation of asthma with fever, malaise, cough with expectoration of brownish or brownish black viscid pellets of sputum containing hyphae of aspergillus. Imaging findings are compatible with ABPA.
2. Acute exacerbation of bronchial asthma or an acute severe asthma. A diagnostic search for ABPA is at times rewarding in this setting.
3. Asymptomatic presentation Asthmatic symptoms are no worse and may even appear better to the patient, the diagnosis of ABPA being suggested by findings on an incidental radiological examination of the chest.
4. Repeated episodes of ABPA in an asthmatic patient may lead to proximal bronchiectasis. The symptoms and signs of bronchiectasis may predominate over those of asthma, and the clinical features of repeated episodes of bacterial bronchopulmonary infection may be difficult to distinguish from episodes of allergic bronchopulmonary aspergillosis.

In the hope of aiding diagnosis and management, ABPA has been classified into five stages. Stage I—acute; Stage II—remission; Stage III—exacerbation; Stage IV—corticosteroid-dependent asthma; Stage V—fibrotic end-stage chiefly involving the upper lobes.

Individuals with features consistent with ABPA but with no radiological evidence of bronchiectasis are termed seropositive ABPA (ABPA-S). Those with radiological evidence of bronchiectasis are termed ABPA-B. It is difficult to ascertain whether ABPA-B is the natural sequel or the end result of ABPA-S followed over a varying period of time, or whether the ABPA-S and ABPA-B are two different clinical patterns of the disease.

Diagnosis

Diagnosis of ABPA is often made on clinical grounds. It however needs to be confirmed by radiological and serological findings. Diagnostic criteria laid down in the US are generally accepted. These include major and minor criteria. The presence of six of the eight major criteria or the first five of the major and one of the minor is considered to be diagnostic of the disease.

Table 40.1:
Diagnostic criteria for allergic bronchopulmonary aspergillosis
Major Criteria (ARTEPICS)
A = Asthma
R = Radiographic fleeting opacities
T = Skin test positive for aspergillus type I response
E = Eosinophilia
P = Precipitin antibodies—IgG in serum
I = IgE in serum elevated > 1000 ng/ml
C = Central bronchiectasis
S = Serum Aspergillus fumigatus specific IgG and IgE
Minor Criteria
Presence of Aspergillus in sputum
Expectoration of brownish black mucus plugs
Delayed skin reaction to Aspergillus antigen (Type III)
The presence of six of the eight major criteria make the diagnosis almsot certain   *The disease is further classified as ABPA-S or ABPA-CB on the absence or presence of central bronchiectasis respectively.*

It needs to be remembered that while most of these criteria may be present during the acute phase (Stage I) or during an exacerbation (Stage III) they may not all be evident during remission (Stage II) or in the burnt out fibrotic stage (Stage V). Perhaps less stringent diagnostic criteria may therefore be clinically more practical. These include a positive serology in the form of a positive Aspergillus skin test with positive precipitins and/or evidence of Aspergillus in the sputum together with a definite history of fleeting pulmonary shadows on an X-ray chest. The major difficulty arises in distinguishing uncomplicated asthma from ABPA with a normal chest radiographic appearance at the time of examination. Table 40.1 gives the diagnostic criteria for ABPA.

SKIN PRICK TEST
The skin prick test using standardized extracts of *A. fumigatus* antigen is positive in all patients with ABPA. A positive test detects specific IgE and is characterized by a positive wheal and flare of 3 mm or more (when compared to the negative control) within 15 minutes. The skin prick test is extremely sensitive but is not specific for ABPA as 25% of patients with uncomplicated asthma also have a positive test.

SERUM IgE AND IgG LEVELS
There is a marked rise in total IgE level—far more than in uncomplicated asthma. The rise is due chiefly to a non-specific increase in IgE. IgE specific to *A. fumigatus* is also raised and the absence of rise in this specific IgE makes the diagnosis of ABPA unlikely. The total IgE is generally > 1000 IU/ml though during remission lesser values may be obtained. In the latter group of patients, a follow-up during exacerbation is often

associated with a rise of IgE > 1100 IU/ml. There is also a rise in specific IgG in ABPA. It needs to be stressed that although *A. fumigatus*-specific IgE and IgG are generally higher in ABPA than in uncomplicated asthma there is a considerable overlap between these two groups.

SERUM PRECIPITIN ANTIBODIES

IgG precipitin antibody to *A. fumigatus* is found to be positive in 70% of patients with ABPA. It is less sensitive compared to the Aspergillus prick test, but is more specific. Even so, the precipitin test is also positive in a very small proportion of healthy individuals, in 10–12% of asthmatics and in 27% of patients with farmer's lung.

PRESENCE OF A. FUMIGATUS IN SPUTUM

The detection of hyphae of *A. fumigatus* in patients with asthma (on smear and/ or culture) is confirmatory of ABPA as it clearly points to a colonization of the bronchial wall with the fungus. Unfortunately, hyphae are not always found in the sputum of patients with ABPA. They are more likely to be seen on culture during exacerbations. Even then, sputum containing hyphae of *A. fumigatus* is produced intermittently in patients with ABPA so that a negative sputum examination does not exclude the diagnosis.

Radiographic Changes

Abnormalities in the chest X-ray may be transient or permanent.

TRANSIENT CHANGES

These are of two kinds—

1. Transient pulmonary infiltrates of eosinophilic pneumonia. These are typically not segmental in distribution, fleeting in character, changing positions spontaneously and invariably accompanied by well-marked peripheral eosinophilia. At times the infiltrates are perihilar and when large simulate a tumour mass or marked hilar adenopathy.
2. Areas of atelectasis due to mucus plugging of bronchi. These areas of atelectasis may be segmental, lobar or rarely, whole lung atelectasis. The atelectatic area opens up on coughing up a mucus plug or after bronchoscopic removal of the mucus plug. Persisting occlusion of one or more bronchi is likely to lead to bronchopulmonary damage—bronchiectasis + fibrosis.

PERMANENT CHANGES

These include the following—

1. Parallel line (tram-line) shadows extending from the hilum outwards represent dilated bronchi with thickened walls. In cross-section, dilated bronchi may appear as ring shadows or as cysts of proximal saccular bronchiectasis. Presence of associated fibrosis may cause volume contraction, chiefly of the upper lobes.
2. When large dilated bronchi are filled with mucus they cast a shadow similar to a gloved finger or gloved fingers (if there is more than one bronchus so impacted) appearance. Mucus

may be expectorated from these bronchi but there remains a permanent distortion and thickening of the bronchial walls.

It is important to realize that changes on a radiological examination of the chest in some patients of ABPA may be inconspicuous, even in the presence of well-marked bronchiectasis that is brought out only on a computed tomography (CT) of the chest. Again, upper lobe changes with fibrosis and bronchiectasis can also occur in asthmatics who develop tuberculosis or sarcoidosis, or in patients who have cystic fibrosis not complicated by ABPA.

CT Findings

High-resolution CT (HRCT) of the chest is imperative for the diagnosis of ABPA.

1. HRCT is vastly more sensitive than the chest X-ray in detecting bronchiectasis. Bronchiectasis chiefly involves the upper lobes and is classically central in character. In our experience exclusively, central bronchiectasis seldom occurs in any pathology other than in ABPA, though admittedly there is some disagreement with others on this statement. In advanced cases the bronchiectasis can be more widespread.
2. Pulmonary infiltrates (transient) are observed on a CT chest when none appear on an X-ray chest. Areas of eosinophilic consolidation may at times resemble tumour masses, particularly when situated in the parahilar region.
3. Areas of distal atelectasis and mucus plugging of bronchi may be observed on an HRCT of the chest but may not be evident on an X-ray chest. Mucus impaction may manifest in cross-section as centrilobular nodules.

The distinction between skin test-positive uncomplicated asthma and ABPA may be difficult on clinical grounds. HR CT studies may help. It is suggested that dilated bronchi in more than three lobes, the presence of mucus impaction and centrilobular nodules favour the diagnosis of ABPA.

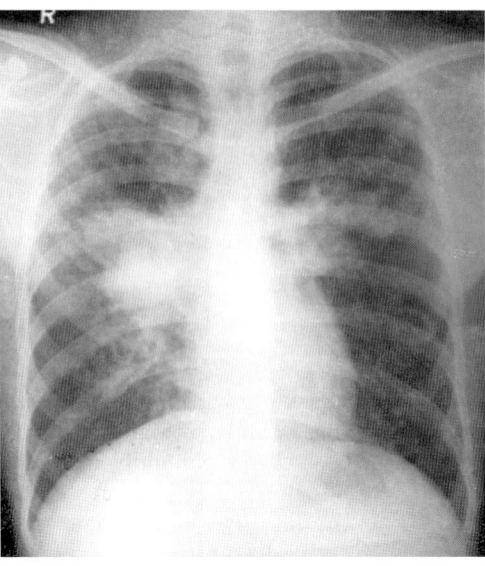

Fig 40.2: ABPA; Chest X-ray demonstrating well-defined tubular densities in the hilar and parahilar regions, finger in glove appearance, typical of central bronchiectasis with mucoid impaction in ABPA.

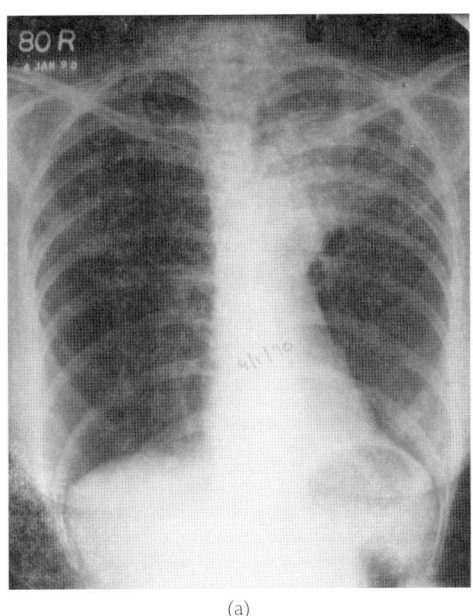

(a)

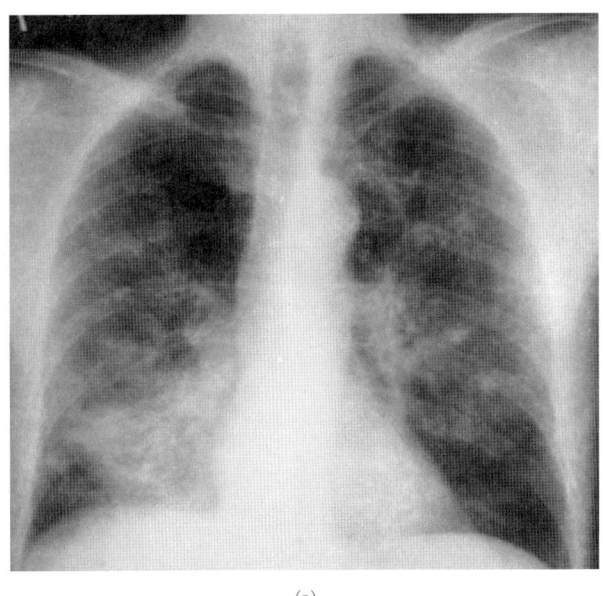

(a)

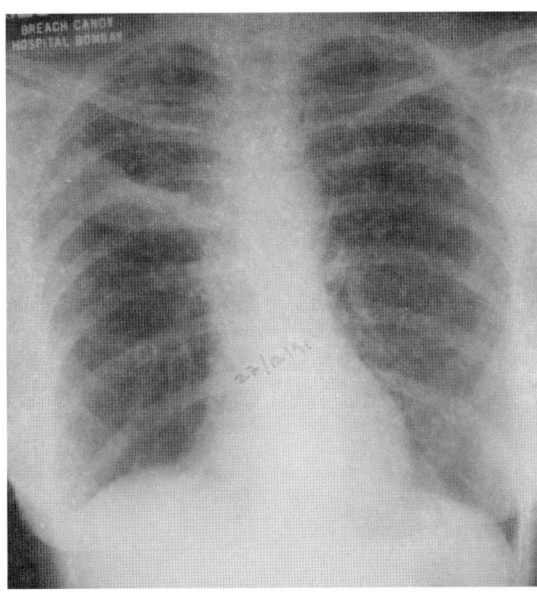

(b)

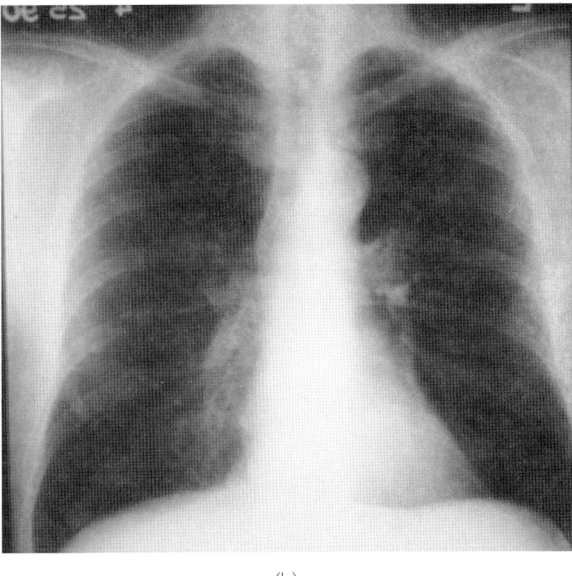

(b)

Fig 40.3: ABPA: (a) Elderly asthmatic lady presented with left upper lobe collapse as evidenced by an ill-defined opacity in the left upper zone (b) One and half years later she presented with right upper lobe partial collapse. Fleeting collapse consolidations are typical of ABPA.

Fig 40.4: ABPA: (a) Chest X-ray reveals ill-defined areas of consolidation in the right lower lobe as well as patchy areas of consolidation in the left lung. Serum IgE levels were very high. Patient was treated for ABPA (b) Chest X-ray subsequently demonstrated complete resolution.

Management

Treatment consists of—a) management of acute exacerbation, b) prevention of recurrent exacerbations, c) control of underlying disease—asthma or cystic fibrosis.

Pulmonary Function Tests

Lung function tests show airways obstruction, worse during exacerbation with improvement during remission. The occurrence of fibrosis and bronchiectasis may lead to a superadded restrictive defect. It has been suggested that worsening airways obstruction in chronic asthma, particularly when there is little or no reversibility should warrant a search for complicating ABPA.

Management of Acute Exacerbations

Acute exacerbations of ABPA are controlled with systemic, or oral administration of corticosteroids in a dose of 0.5 mg/kg/day. This needs to be combined with intensive

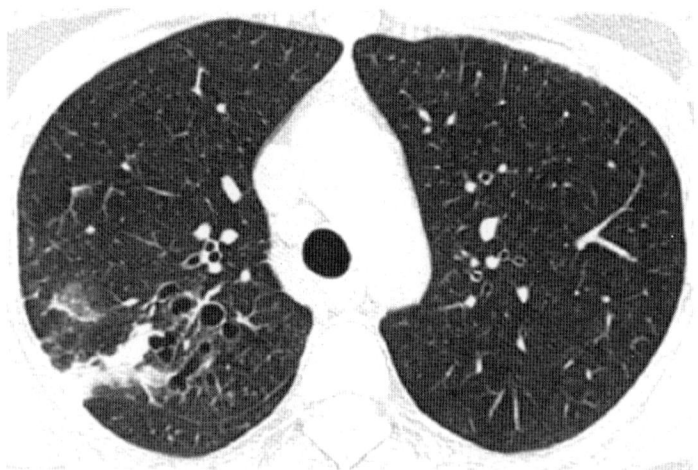

Fig 40.5: ABPA. CT chest reveals tubular branching consolidation in the right middle lobe with dilated bronchi in the right middle lobe and left lingula. The tubular branching structures represent dilated bronchi with mucoid impaction.

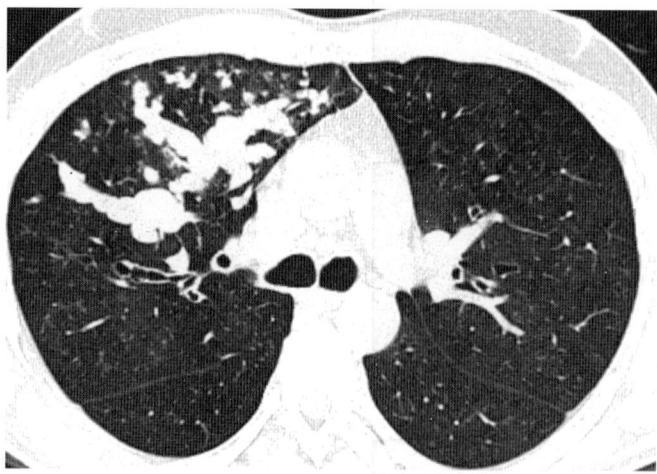

Fig 40.6: ABPA: HRCT chest demonstrates dilated bronchi in the right upper lobe with tubular consolidation along the periphery. Dilated central bronchi with mucoid impaction is typical of ABPA.

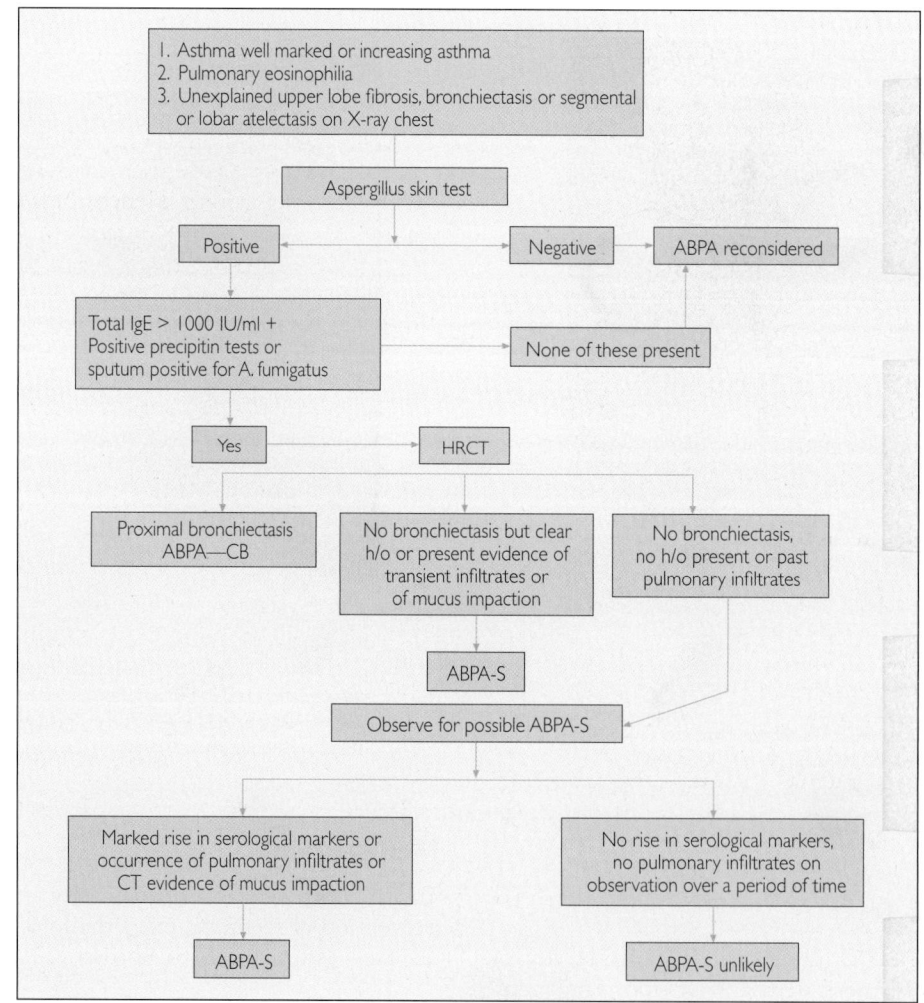

Fig 40.7: Approach to diagnosis of ABPA.

bronchodilator therapy plus physiotherapy. In patients with severe bronchospasm, nebulised salbutamol/ipratropium—three to four times daily is more effective than the use of aerosolized inhaled bronchodilators. Budesonide is also often used though whether it adds to the effect produced by systemic corticosteroids is doubtful. Systemic corticosteroids (together with bronchodilator therapy and physiotherapy) produce prompt relief. Pulmonary infiltrates clear, areas of atelectasis open up. If however after a week of the intensive therapy stated above, evidence of bronchial obstruction with major atelectasis persists, bronchoscopic removal of impacted mucus must be done, else persistent bronchopulmonary damage is likely to occur. Bronchoscopy may need to be repeated in some patients to ensure effective opening up of mucus-plugged bronchi.

The duration of the use of oral steroids in the treatment of an acute exacerbation of ABPA is best tailored to the patient's response. The dose of 0.5 mg/kg/day is continued till there is good clinical response, radiological clearing of shadows and a significant fall in the IgE levels.

The dose is then slowly tapered off and stopped after a further period of one to two months. There are in fact no evidence-based studies to offer more precise guidelines.

Itraconazole is recommended as an anti-fungal agent even during acute exacerbations of ABPA to reduce the antigen load and thereby reduce both antigenic stimulation and the inflammatory response. Results on its use are conflicting; the drug may perhaps reduce the frequency of exacerbations.

Prevention of Recurrent Exacerbation

The use of systemic corticosteroids in the treatment of acute exacerbation of ABPA is clearly defined. However, the prophylactic use of oral corticosteroids to prevent recurrence and thereby prevent or reduce bronchopulmonary damage and the associated decline in lung functions remains debatable.

The argument for using long-term corticosteroid therapy is that many episodes of radiological relapse may not be associated with symptoms. Treatment given only during symptomatic episodes would miss out the asymptomatic episodes, so that further bronchopulmonary damage would pass unnoticed. There is evidence that a sharp rise in IgE levels is followed by an exacerbation of ABPA. Monitoring of IgE levels and obtaining a chest X-ray when there is a sharp rise in the IgE levels may detect such an asymptomatic exacerbation allowing appropriate steroid treatment during these episodes. It needs to be kept in mind that probably only a minority of patients with ABPA are at risk of progressive pulmonary damage. Also, reports of the benefits of long-term corticosteroid use are based chiefly on retrospective uncontrolled studies while the side-effects of long-term steroids can often be crippling. The possible danger of invasive aspergillosis on using long-term steroid therapy should also not be discounted.

The recommendation we follow is to use systemic steroid therapy only during exacerbations according to a regime already outlined above. If IgE levels can be monitored, a sudden rise in IgE should necessitate a radiological examination of the chest, more so if there are worsening asthmatic symptoms. It there is strong suspicion of a recurrence of ABPA, a short

course of corticosteroids on the lines stated above can be given. Admittedly, a follow-up of IgE levels in asthmatics living in developing countries is an impossibly difficult task.

Long-term maintenance corticosteroid therapy should perhaps be considered only in those who have very frequent exacerbation of ABPA and in those who show progressive bronchopulmonary damage.

Various inhaled and oral anti-fungal agents have been tried with a view to prevent or reduce exacerbations of ABPA with variable results. A randomized double-blind trial of itraconazole in corticosteroid-dependent ABPA showed a small but significant benefit in terms of IgE concentration, radiological resolution, lung function and symptoms' score after 16 weeks, with further benefit during a following open-label period (*Ref: Stevens, DA, Schwartz, HJ, Lee, JY, et al. A randomized trial of itraconazole in allergic bronchopulmonary aspergillosis. N Engl J Med 2000; 342, 756–762*). Long-term controlled studies are awaited. Though itraconazole is fairly well tolerated, liver toxicity can occur; liver functions need to be monitored if the drug is used. The use of other anti-fungal agents effective against Aspergillus like voriconazole perhaps merit study.

Control of Underlying Disease

Underlying asthma needs to be optimally controlled. Mucus plugging with the formation of bronchial casts is far more likely to occur in narrow airways than when the airways have a normal or near normal calibre. Hence the need to control asthmatic symptoms and improve expiratory airflow rates as far as is possible. This necessitates the use of inhaled corticosteroids and β_2-agonists, preferably a combination of salmetrol and fluticasone. In some patients adequate control of asthma necessitates the use of a maintenance dose of oral corticosteroids.

Similarly, good control over cystic fibrosis is important when ABPA complicates this disease. It is indeed difficult to diagnose ABPA in patients with cystic fibrosis. Symptoms of ABPA and symptoms caused by an infective exacerbation of cystic fibrosis bronchiectasis are similar. CT findings of ABPA may also be present in cystic fibrosis. Aspergillus skin test and the precipitin test are positive in some patients with cystic fibrosis. However, pulmonary infiltrates do not usually occur with infective exacerbations of cystic fibrosis bronchiectasis. If these infiltrates do occur and if they clear with steroids they lend support to the diagnosis of ABPA.

The complication of ABPA in a patient with cystic fibrosis may present difficulties for a possible future lung transplant. Even colonization of the airways with Aspergillus without ABPA may present difficulties. If sputum cultures are positive for Aspergillus in the pre-transplant period, the patient is treated with oral itraconazole and nebulised amphotericin. This is continued for a month after transplant surgery.

ALLERGIC ASPERGILLUS SINUSITIS

Allergic Aspergillus sinusitis has the same histological features as ABPA. Clinically, patients present with a sinusitis not responding to antibiotic therapy. X-ray of the paranasal sinus shows opaque sinuses and CT of the sinuses shows soft tissue densities filling the sinuses without any bone destruction. Nasal polyps are often present. The Aspergillus skin test is positive; the precipitin test is also positive in the majority of patients. Treatment with oral steroids is very effective and obviates the need for surgical intervention.

SUGGESTED READING

Agarwal R. Allergic bronchopulmonary aspergillosis. *Chest*. 1 Mar. 2009; 135(3): 805–26.

Bedi RS. Allergic bronchopulmonary aspergillosis: Indian perspective. *Indian J Chest Dis Allied Sci*. 1 Apr. 2009; 51(2): 73–4.

Rosenberg M, Patterson R, Mintzer R, Cooper BJ, Roberts M, Harris KE. Clinical and immunologic criteria for the diagnosis of allergic bronchopulmonary aspergillosis. *Ann Intern Med*. 1977; 86: 405–14.

Shah A. Allergic bronchopulmonary aspergillosis: a review of a disease with a worldwide distribution. *J Asthma*. 1 Jun. 2002; 39(4): 273–89.

Stevens, DA, Schwartz, HJ, Lee, JY, *et al*. A randomized trial of itraconazole in allergic bronchopulmonary aspergillosis. *N Engl J Med*. 2000; 342, 756–62.

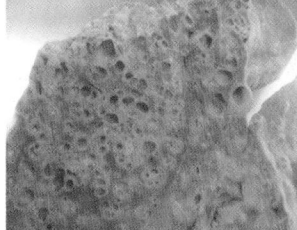

CHAPTER **41** **Bronchiolitis**

GENERAL CONSIDERATIONS

Bronchiolitis is an inflammatory narrowing and obstruction of the small (< 2 mm in size) conducting airways. The inflammation is the result of an 'insult' or 'damage' to the bronchiolar epithelium due to an infective, non-infective or undetermined cause. Inflammatory cells and granulation tissue may be present in the lumen, within the bronchiolar walls as also peribronchially. The sequel to this inflammation is often a narrowing, a distortion and in some cases a total obliteration of the involved small conducting airways. In most instances involvement of the small airways is chiefly proximal to the respiratory bronchioles. Among notable exceptions are patients with diffuse panbronchiolitis and the entity termed respiratory bronchiolitis in smokers, where the brunt of the inflammatory pathology is borne by the respiratory bronchioles and the adjacent alveoli. Involvement of the respiratory bronchioles together with an alveolar infiltrate is also noted in bronchiolitis obliterans with organising pneumonia (BOOP), also termed cryptogenic organising pneumonia (COP).

SEMANTICS

The semantics in relation to bronchiolar disorders is confusing as different descriptive terms are either synonymous or perhaps overlap, or represent different stages of the same disease. For example, terms which are synonymous and in use are constrictive bronchiolitis, obstructive bronchiolitis, obliterative bronchiolitis and bronchiolitis obliterans. Again the term bronchiolitis obliterans has been applied to two different histological patterns of bronchiolar fibrosis as also to different clinical syndromes ranging from progressive airways obstruction (constrictive or obliterative bronchiolitis), to a predominant infiltrative process involving the alveoli and producing a restrictive lesion (BOOP) or cryptogenic organising pneumonia (COP).

Bronchiolar abnormalities may also exist as a feature of parenchymal lung involvement as in bronchopneumonia, or as an associated feature of involvement of the more proximal airways as in bronchiectasis. Secondary bronchiolar involvement is also observed in interstitial lung disease, such as sarcoidosis, extrinsic allergic alveolitis, and Langerhans' cell histiocytosis. Finally, inflammation involving the small airways in chronic obstructive pulmonary disease (COPD) is the major factor responsible for airflow limitation in this disease.

Table 41.1 gives an overall perspective of disorders or diseases involving the bronchioles. *The subsequent discussion centres solely on primary bronchiolitis.*

Table 41.1: Bronchiolar wall disorders
I. Primary bronchiolitis—disorder or disease confined anatomically to the bronchiolar wall
II. Secondary bronchiolitis in which interstitial lung disease is associated with significant bronchiolar involvement
1. Cryptogenic organising pneumonia
2. Extrinsic allergic alveolitis
3. Respiratory bronchiolitis with interstitial lung disease
4. Other interstitial lung diseases e.g. sarcoidosis, Langerhans' cell histiocytosis

PRIMARY BRONCHIOLITIS

Primary bronchiolitis constitutes a group of bronchiolar wall disorders in which the pathology is anatomically limited to the bronchioles. This is in striking contrast to secondary bronchiolitis, where bronchiolar wall abnormalities are secondarily associated features of different interstitial lung diseases or are prominent components of obstructive airways' diseases such as COPD and asthma.

Primary bronchiolitis can be further classified into **1. Constrictive bronchiolitis** (also termed obstructive bronchiolitis or bronchiolitis obliterans) and **2. Other forms of primary bronchiolitis.** These include diffuse panbronchiolitis, mineral dust bronchiolitis, respiratory bronchiolitis, follicular bronchiolitis, and other rare forms of primary bronchiolitis.

CONSTRICTIVE BRONCHIOLITIS (OBSTRUCTIVE BRONCHIOLITIS, BRONCHIOLITIS OBLITERANS)

Constrictive bronchiolitis is characterized histologically by constriction followed by obliteration of the small airways. This histological end-result can occur in different clinical settings with different aetiological factors. When no obvious cause is evident the disease is termed cryptogenic constrictive bronchiolitis or cryptogenic bronchiolitis obliterans. Known aetiological factors are connective tissue disorders (rheumatoid disease, systemic lupus erythematosus in particular), acute viral infections, inhalational injury, as a complication in recipients of heart-lung and bone marrow transplants and as a toxic effect of certain drugs. Rarely, obliterative bronchiolitis is observed in association with inflammatory bowel disease, neuroendocrine cell hyperplasia, multiple carcinoid tumours and paraneoplastic pemphigus.

Table 41.2: Etiology of constrictive bronchiolitis
1. Cryptogenic
2. Connective tissue disorders (perhaps the most common cause in clinical practice)
Rheumatoid arthritis, SLE, polymyositis, systemic sclerosis
3. Acute viral infection
Respiratory syncitial virus, adenovirus, influenza, parainfluenza virus, other viruses
4. Inhalational injury
Toxic gases (e.g. oxides of nitrogen, ammonia, SO_2, chlorine, phosgene etc)
5. Allograft recipients
Heart lung transplants, lung transplant, bone marrow transplant
6. Drugs
Gold, penicillamine, busulfan, cocaine
7. Associated with other diseases
Inflammatory bowel disease, neuroendocrine cell hyperplasia, carcinoid tumors, paraneoplastic pemphigus

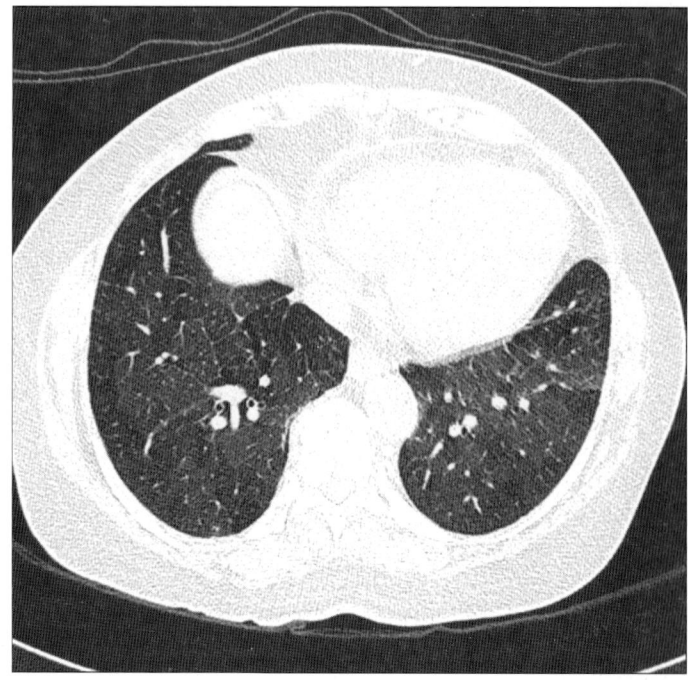

(a)

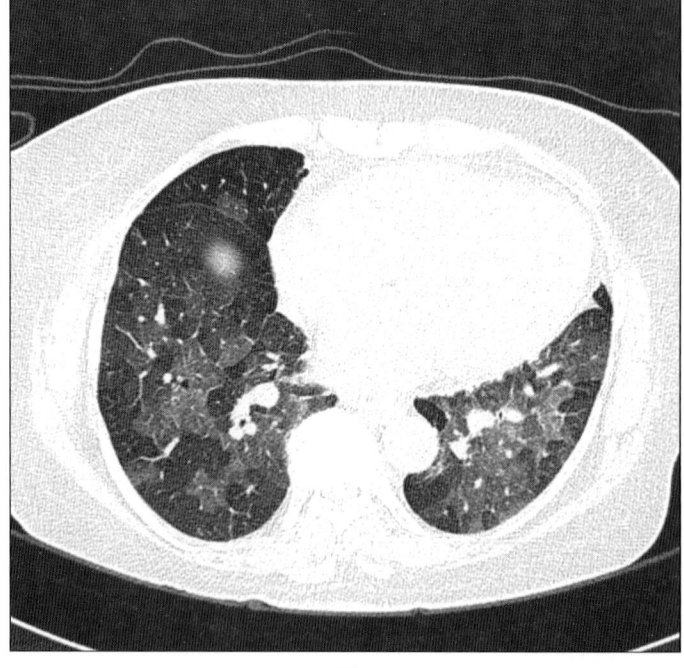

(b)

Fig 41.1: Bronchiolitis obliterans: Inspiratory HRCT (a) demonstrates subtle areas of decreased lung attenuation in the lung periphery bilaterally. Expiratory CT (b) demonstrates marked air-trapping in the subtle areas seen on the inspiratory CT scan.

Histopathology

Histopathology of constrictive bronchiolitis is characterized by a distinctive pattern of peribronchiolar fibrosis which first constricts bronchioles and then obliterates their lumen. This histological feature is common to all aetiological factors. The fibrotic process surrounds the bronchioles, strangling the small airways through external compression and constriction. Even in advanced severe cases, the disease is patchy in its distribution and can therefore be missed if the appropriate areas of the lung have not been sampled. Transbronchial biopsy often does not allow a correct diagnosis which can only be made by a video-assisted thoracoscopic biopsy.

ACUTE INFECTIVE BRONCHIOLITIS

Acute infective bronchiolitis is seen mostly in infants and children as a feature of acute viral infection. In fact it is the commonest respiratory disease in infancy occurring in epidemic form in the winter months. It is also observed in India and other developing countries, but its prevalence remains undetermined because of the general difficulty in performing reliable virological studies. The respiratory syncitial virus is the commonest cause of acute bronchiolitis in infants and children. Other viruses such as the adenovirus, influenza and parainfluenza virus can also do so. Acute bronchiolitis has also been reported following mycoplasmal and chlamydial infection.

Acute bronchiolitis in adults is uncommon though it can occasionally be caused by the viruses stated above. Symptoms in adults are generally not severe when compared to infants and children, perhaps because the small airways in adults contribute less to total pulmonary resistance. Acute bronchiolitis may also be seen in adults following aspiration, (particularly of gastric acid as in Mendelson's syndrome), inhalational injuries and bone marrow transplant and Steven Johnson's syndrome.

Pathology

The mucus membrane of the bronchioles in acute infective bronchiolitis is acutely inflamed, with oedema and necrosis of the epithelial cells. In viral bronchiolitis (in particular respiratory syncitial viral infection), the respiratory epithelial cells produce

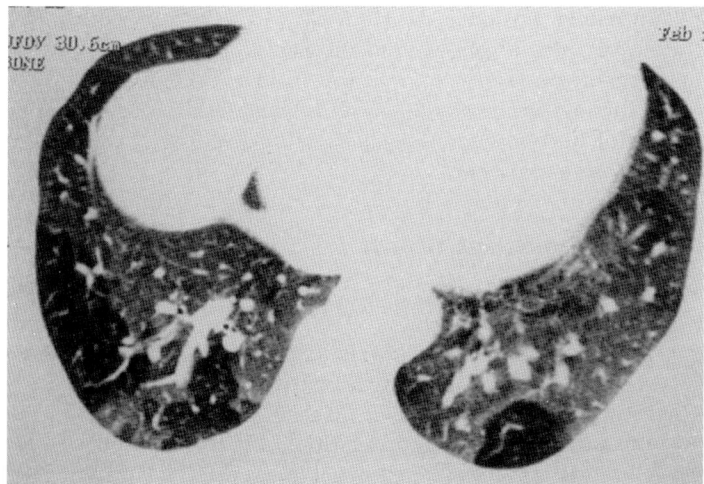

Fig 41.2: Bronchiolitis obliterans: Focal areas of air-trapping on an expiratory HRCT. Note small-sized vessels in luscent areas.

several chemokines such as macrophage inflammatory protein 1α, several pro-inflammatory interleukins and RANTES (regulated upon activation, normal T-cell expressed and secreted). These cytokines recruit and activate eosinophils, lymphocytes, macrophages, neutrophils and natural killer cells at the site of inflammation. Inflammatory oedema of the bronchiolar wall, increased mucus secretion and hyper-reactivity of the small airways form the end-result.

Clinical Features

Clinical features are characterized by tachypnoea, tachycardia and breathlessness with prolonged expiration. Wheeze may be audible at a distance and there may in some infants and children be severe respiratory distress with indrawing of the intercostal spaces during inspiration, flaring of the alae nasi and use of accessory muscles of respiration. Rhonchi, together with crackles are the usual auscultatory signs. Radiography of the chest typically reveals hyperinflated lungs. High-resolution computed tomography (HRCT) of the chest in acute infective bronchiolitis reveals ill-defined centrilobular nodules. These nodules relate to inflamed bronchioles impacted with secretions, coupled with peribronchial inflammation. The inflamed bronchioles cause linear branching lines on imaging study. Focal areas of consolidation may be present.

Treatment

In most instances the disease is mild. Treatment is then supportive. When severe and in the presence of respiratory distress the patient needs to be hospitalized and given supplemental oxygen. Bronchodilators, corticosteroids and antiviral agents need to be used. The overall mortality is generally not more than 1%.

In a few patients, acute infective bronchiolitis may result over a period of time in progressive constrictive bronchiolitis. This is observed in particular with adenovirus infection as also after measles and influenza A infection. Occasionally, Macleod's syndrome may evolve as a sequel of acute infective bronchiolitis.

OTHER CAUSES OF CONSTRICTIVE BRONCHIOLITIS

Inhalational Injury

Constrictive bronchiolitis is a frequent complication of inhalation of toxic gases—In the Bhopal gas tragedy, nercotizing bronchiolitis following inhalation of methyl isocynate gas (MIC) led to a crippling obliterative bronchiolitis in a number of patients. Other toxic gases that cause inhalational injury (characterized by constrictive bronchiolitis) include NO_2, chlorine, ammonia and SO_2. Constrictive bronchiolitis presenting as increasing airways' obstruction may be observed several weeks after the initial insult.

Transplant Recipients

Patients with allogenic bone marrow transplant, heart-lung transplant or lung transplant may develop constrictive bronchiolitis as a chronic rejection phenomenon. Constrictive bronchiolitis is a major cause of death in lung transplant patients. It occurs in over 50% of lung transplant patients over five years. Confirmation of the diagnosis of this complication is often not possible, as transbronchial biopsy in constrictive bronchiolitis generally yields negative results. Diagnosis is based on the clinical and objective evidence of airways obstruction; a fall in FEV_1 below 20% of its previous stable value being considered significant.

Connective Tissue Disorders

Rheumatoid disease is the commonest connective tissue disorder causing constrictive bronchiolitis. The course of the disease varies. In some patients it is rapidly progressive, in others the progress is slow. Constrictive bronchiolitis generally occurs in patients with longstanding disease. It is possible that sub-clinical forms of obliterative bronchiolitis may be present in a larger number of patients than what is suspected. Penicillamine and gold (both uncommonly used today) used as therapy for rheumatoid disease have been known to cause obliterative bronchiolitis.

Association with Other Diseases

The association of constrictive bronchiolitis with inflammatory bowel disease, neuroendocrine cell hyperplasia, carcinoid tumourlets and paraneoplastic pemphigus is rare and though reported, has not been witnessed by us as yet.

Finally, when no aetiological factor can be implicated one is left with the diagnosis of **cryptogenic constrictive bronchiolitis** or **cryptogenic bronchiolitis obliterans**. It is a rare disease occurring mostly in women. In some patients there is a history of a mild flu-like infection in the recent past, but a confirmed aetiological diagnosis generally cannot be substantiated.

PATHOGENESIS

As mentioned earlier different aetiological factors causing constrictive bronchiolitis ultimately lead to the same histopatholgical end-result. The pathogenetic mechanisms may however vary. For example, inhalational injury has a direct chemical toxic effect on mucosal cells and also on the bronchiolar wall structure. Viral infections cause an inflammatory reaction, cytokine production, leading to eventual fibrosis. In constrictive bronchiolitis following lung transplants, the pathogenesis is based on alloreactivity to HLA antigens, airways inflammation, viral infections and airway ischemia. Constrictive bronchiolitis occurring in patients with pemphigus, a paraneoplastic syndrome is characterized by deposition of IgE on epithelial cells and acantholytic changes. Multiple pathogenetic mechanisms, some of which are known and some not yet evident may ultimately lead to the same end-result.

CLINICAL FEATURES

Patients with constrictive bronchiolitis present with progressive breathlessness and cough. There may be few or no physical signs; few crackles may be heard over the bases. If lung function tests are not done, the diagnosis may well be missed in early cases. Lung functions show airways obstruction with air trapping. There is well-marked reduction in the mid and late expiratory flow rates. Residual volume and total lung capacity are both increased. Diffusing capacity is reduced. Aerosolized bronchodilators cause no improvement in the airways obstruction.

CHEST RADIOGRAPHY

In the early part of the natural history, the chest X-ray may be passed off as normal. As the disease progresses there is hyperinflation with peripheral attenuation of vascular markings. Serial radiographs of the chest show increasing lung volumes. Thickening of the bronchial walls may occasionally be observed.

HRCT of the chest shows a mosaic pattern due to areas of decreased attenuation and vascularity. Images during expiration show evidence of air-trapping. Thickened bronchiolar walls with distal bronchiectasis may occur. The mosaic appearance is due to decreased perfusion in areas of bronchiolar obstruction and redistribution of blood to normal areas. Mosaic appearance of the lung described above though a classic feature of constrictive bronchiolitis, is also observed in pulmonary vascular disease, and airway disease. HRCT imaging with contrast enhancement of pulmonary vasculature helps in the differential diagnosis.

NATURAL HISTORY

In most patients the disease is progressive and ultimately leads to respiratory failure and death.

TREATMENT

Bronchodilators are generally ineffective and response to corticosteroids, both oral and inhaled is poor.

Management of post-transplant obliterative bronchiolitis consists of increasing the dose of immunosuppressants in the hope of slowing or countering the rejection phenomenon. The use of statins has been reported to reduce the risk of rejection in the lung transplant patients.

OTHER FORMS OF PRIMARY BRONCHIOLITIS

Bronchiolitis due to Mineral Dust Exposure

Inhalation of mineral dusts generally results in pneumoconiosis (a restrictive lung pathology). However, mineral dust can sometimes be deposited in the bronchioles, particularly in respiratory bronchioles and in alveolar ducts, inciting a chronic inflammatory response with fibrosis at the site of deposition, thereby causing a well-marked airways' obstruction. A number of inorganic dusts can result in this form of bronchiolitis. These dusts include iron, talc, mica, aluminium, silica and coal. The degree of fibrosis depends generally on the local dust burden the patient experiences.

Respiratory Bronchiolitis

Respiratory bronchiolitis is a specific disease of the small airways related to smoking. The distinguishing features of this smoking-related disease is the presence of pigmented macrophages within the lumen of respiratory bronchioles and adjacent alveoli. The disease is invariably asymptomatic except when it is associated with interstitial lung disease—respiratory bronchiolitis-associated interstitial lung disease. It may then cause cough and breathlessness.

Radiographic examination of the chest is normal in respiratory bronchiolitis. An HRCT of the chest shows centrilobular nodules. No treatment is required other than cessation of smoking.

Follicular Bronchiolitis

Follicular bronchiolitis is characterized by the presence of hyperplastic lymphoid follicles with reactive germinal centres along bronchiolar walls. It is a frequent accompaniment of bronchiectasis involving the large airways. However, it also occurs as a feature of primary lymphoid hyperplasia. In these patients peribronchial lymphoid hyperplasia and infiltration may extend into the adjacent interstitium so that there is an overlap with lymphoid interstitial pneumonia.

Follicular bronchiolitis may be idiopathic in origin or is secondary; occurring with rheumatoid arthritis, immunodeficiency states including AIDS and in poorly defined hypersensitivity reaction

CLINICAL FEATURES

Breathlessness on exertion is the usual symptom. Physical signs may be absent or may reveal scattered crackles over both lungs.

Radiography of the chest may appear normal or may reveal bilateral small nodular or reticulonodular infiltrates. Mediastinal adenopathy may be present. HRCT of the chest may reveal centrilobular nodules—1 to 10 mm in size, together with peribronchial nodules and ground-glass opacities. The nodules and ground-glass opacities are diffuse and bilateral in distribution. Bronchial walls may show thickening.

TREATMENT

Treatment is directed to the underlying cause. If no cause is evident corticosteroids and immunomodulation have been tried with varying success. Recently, erythromycin has been reported to be of use.

RARER FORM OF BRONCHIOLITIS

Three rarer forms of primary bronchiolitis have been reported.

The first is aspiration bronchiolitis due to repeated aspiration of foreign particles causing chronic inflammatory bronchiolitis. Most patients are elderly or bedridden.

OCCUPATIONAL AND ENVIRONMENTAL LUNG DISEASES

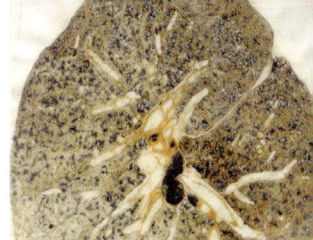

CHAPTER 67   # Environmental Pollution*

DEFINITION

Pollution is the introduction of contaminants into an environment that causes instability, disorder, harm or discomfort to the ecosystem i.e. physical systems or living organisms.

FORMS OF POLLUTION

The major forms of pollution are listed below along with the particular pollutants relevant to each of them:

- Air pollution, the release of chemicals and particulates into the atmosphere. Common gaseous air pollutants include carbon monoxide, sulphur dioxide, chlorofluorocarbons (CFCs) and nitrogen oxides produced by industry and motor vehicles. Photochemical ozone and smog are created as nitrogen oxides and hydrocarbons react to sunlight. Particulate matter or fine dust is characterized by their micrometre size PM_{10} to $PM_{2.5}$.

  In addition, there is the danger of atmospheric pollution caused by mines (coal, metals and other substances), factories (manufacturing or processing asbestos, cotton and numerous chemicals) and finally by dust, particularly in the hot Gangetic northern plains of India and in desert areas as in Rajasthan. Atmospheric pollution from factories, chemical plants, and mines pose not just a danger to workers but to people living environmentally close to these areas.
- Water pollution, by the release of waste products and contaminants on to the surface which run off into river drainage systems, leaching into the groundwater, liquid spills, waste water discharges, eutrophication and littering.
- Soil contamination occurs when chemicals are released by spill or underground leakage. Among the most significant soil contaminants are hydrocarbons, heavy metals, herbicides, pesticides and chlorinated hydrocarbons.
- Littering
- Radioactive contamination, resulting from 20th century activities in atomic physics, such as nuclear power generation and nuclear weapons research, manufacture and deployment.
- Noise pollution, which encompasses roadway noise, aircraft noise, industrial noise as well as high-intensity sonar.

*Thanks are due to Dr HV Ravimohan, Specialist OH, Southern Region, Bangalore, Hindustan Unilever Limited for background research on the topic of this chapter.

I also thank Dr PK Sishodiya, Director, Institute of Miner's Health, Nagpur for according permission to use the chest radiographs dealing with silicosis and progressive massive fibrosis as well as Dr GK Kulkarni, CMO Siemens, India for providing a set of slides based on the ILO International Classification of Pneumoconiosis.

- Light pollution, includes light trespass, over-illumination and astronomical interference.
- Visual pollution, which can refer to the presence of overhead power lines, motorway billboards, scarred landforms (as from strip mining), open storage of trash or municipal solid waste.
- Thermal pollution is a temperature change in natural water bodies caused by human influence, such as use of water as coolant in a power plant.

The major stress in this chapter will be on atmospheric pollution.

Table 67.1: Index of air pollution (Air Quality Index)		
Air Quality Index (AQI) Values	**Levels of Health Concern**	**Colours**
0 to 50	Good	Green
51 to 100	Moderate	Yellow
101 to 150	Unhealthy for Sensitive Groups	Orange
151 to 200	Unhealthy	Red
201 to 300	Very Unhealthy	Purple
301 to 350	Hazardous	Maroon

The US EPA calculates the air quality index (AQI) on the basis of five pollutants, viz. ozone, suspended particulate matter, carbon monoxide, sulphur dioxide and nitrogen dioxide. An AQI value of 100 generally corresponds to the national air quality standard for the pollutant.

ADVERSE EFFECTS OF POLLUTION

Health Effects

Adverse air quality can kill many organisms including humans. Ozone pollution can cause respiratory disease, cardiovascular disease, throat inflammation, chest pain, and congestion. The World Health Organization estimates that about two million people die prematurely every year as a result of air pollution, while many more suffer from breathing ailments, heart disease, lung infections and even cancer. Fine particles or microscopic dust from coal or wood fires and unfiltered diesel engines are rated as one of the most lethal forms or air pollution caused by industry, transport, household heating, cooking and ageing coal or oil-fired power stations.

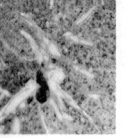

In India, air pollution is believed to cause 527,700 fatalities a year. Studies have estimated that the number of people killed annually in the US could be over 50,000.

Environmental Effects

Pollution has been found to be widespread in the environment. Though increased concentration of SO_2, oxides of nitrogen, particulate matter, ozone, and smog have a direct effect on the respiratory system, it is of interest to note how they also contribute to pollution of the ecosystem in other ways. The need to control air pollutants is therefore of great importance.

The overall pollution of the ecosystem resulting from the increased concentration of atmospheric pollutants is summarized below.

- Sulphur dioxide and nitrogen oxides can cause acid rain which lowers the pH value of soil.
- Nitrogen oxides are removed from the air by rain and fertilize land which can change the species composition of ecosystems.
- Soil can become infertile and unsuitable for plants. This will affect other organisms in the food web.
- Smog and haze can reduce the amount of sunlight received by plants to carry out photosynthesis and leads to the production of tropospheric ozone which damages plants.

- Invasive species can out-compete native species and reduce biodiversity. Invasive plants can contribute debris and biomolecules (allelopathy) that can alter soil and chemical compositions of an environment, often reducing the competitiveness of native species.
- Carbon dioxide (CO_2) emissions cause ocean acidification, the ongoing decrease in the pH of the earth's oceans as CO_2 becomes dissolved.
- The emission of greenhouse gases leads to global warming which affects ecosystems in many ways.

The Environmental Protection Index (EPI) gauges different countries on 25 parameters which fall into 10 categories that include environmental health, air quality, water resource management, biodiversity and habitat, forestry, fisheries, agriculture, and climate change.

Environmental Pollution in India

India ranks 123rd in pollution control according to the 2010 Environmental Performance Index (EPL), reflecting the strain that rapid economic growth imposes on the environment.

The World health Organization (WHO) air quality guidelines recommend the following standards:

			Concentration in Ambient air		
S. No.	**Pollutant**	**Time Weighted Average**	**Industrial, Rural and other Area**	**Ecologically sensitive area (Notified by govt of India)**	**Methods of measurement**
1	Sulphur Dioxide $\mu g/m^3$	Annual* 24 hours**	50 80	20 80	Improved West and Gaeke Ultraviolent Fluorescence
2	Nitrogens Dioxide $\mu g/m^3$	Annual* 24 hours**	40 80	30 80	Modified Jacob & Hahheiser (Na-Arsenite) Chemiluminiscence
3	Particulate matter (Size less than 10 μm) $\mu g/m^3$	Annual* 24 hours**	60 100	60 100	Gravimetric TOEM Beta attenuation
4	Particulate matter (Size less than 2.5 μm) $\mu g/m^3$	8 hr* 1 hr*	40 60	40 60	Gravimetric TOEM Beta attenuation
5	Ozone $\mu g/m^3$	8 hr* 1 hr*	100 180	199 180	UV Photometric Chemiluminiscence Chemical Method
6	Lead $\mu g/m^3$	Annual* 24 hrs**	0.5 1.0	0.5 1.0	AAS/ICP Method after sampling on EPM 2000 Or equivalent filter paper. ED-XRF Using Teflon filters
7	Carbon Monoxide $\mu g/m^3$	8 hr* 1 hr*	02 04	02 04	Non dispersive infrared (NDIR) SPectroscopy

Table 67.2:
Revised National Ambient Air Quality Standards (NAAQA—2009)

SCHEDULE VII. RULE 3(3B) NATIONAL AMBIENT AIR QUALITY STANDARDS 16TH NOV 2009
Ministry of Environment and Forests

(contd...)

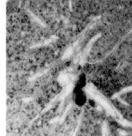

Table 67.2 (contd...)

SCHEDULE VII. RULE 3(3B) NATIONAL AMBIENT AIR QUALITY STANDARDS 16TH NOV 2009 Ministry of Environment and Forests					
S. No.	Pollutant	Time Weighted Average	Concentration in Ambient air		
			Industrial, Rural and other Area	Ecologically sensitive area (Notified by govt of India)	Methods of measurement
8	Ammonia $\mu g/m^3$	Annual* 24 hrs**	100 400	100 400	Chemiluminiscence Indophenol blue method
9	Benzene $\mu g/m^3$	Annual*	05	05	Gas chromatography based continuous analyzer. Adsorption and description followed by GC analysis
10	Benzo (a) pyrene particulate phase only $\mu g/m^3$	Annual*	01	01	Solvent extraction followed by HPLC/GC Analysis
11	Arsenic (SO2) $\mu g/m^3$	Annual*	06	06	AAS/ICP method after sampling on EPM 2000 or equivalent or filter paper
12	Nickel $\mu g/m^3$	Annual*	20	20	AAS/ICP method after sampling on EPM 2000 or equivalent or filter paper

Note: *Annual arithmetic mean of minimum 104 measurements in a year at a particular site taken twice a week 24 hourly at uniform intervals.
** 24 hourly or 8 hourly or 0.01 hourly monitored values as applicable shall be compiled with 98% of the time in a year, 2% of the time they may exceed the limits but not on two consecutive days of monitoring. Note that whenever the monitoring results on two consecutive days of monitoring exceed the limit for the respective category, it shall be considered adequate reason to institute regular or continuous monitoring and further investigation.

Table 67.3: The WHO Air Quality Guidelines	
$PM_{2.5}$	10 $\mu g/m^3$ annual means 25 $\mu g/m^3$ 24-hour mean
PM_{10}	20 $\mu g/m^3$ annual mean 50 $\mu g/m^3$ 24-hour mean
O_3	100 $\mu g/m^3$ 8-hour mean
NO_2	40 $\mu g/m^3$ annual mean 200 $\mu g/m^3$ 1-hour mean
SO_2	20 $\mu g/m^3$ 24-hour mean 500 $\mu g/m^3$ 10-minute mean

Source: WHO Air quality guidelines for particulate matter, ozone, nitrogen dioxide and sulfur dioxide—Global update 2005—Summary of risk assessment.

CAUSES OF ENVIRONMENTAL POLLUTION IN INDIA

Vehicular Growth in India

Air pollution and the resultant impacts in India could be broadly attributed to the emissions from vehicular, industrial and domestic activities. Air quality has been, therefore, an issue of concern in the backdrop of various developmental activities. Due to uncontrolled urbanization in India, environmental degradation has been occurring very rapidly and causing shortages of housing, worsening of water quality, excessive air pollution, noise, dust and heat, and the problems of disposal of solid wastes and hazardous wastes. The situation in cities like Mumbai, Kolkata, Chennai, Delhi and Bangalore, is becoming worse year by year.

Following the trends of urbanization and population growth in Indian cities, people buying more vehicles for personal use have perpetuated an increase in vehicles that contribute to vehicular emissions containing pollutants such as sulphur dioxide, nitrogen oxides, carbon monoxide, lead, ozone, benzene, and hydrocarbons.

Air-borne emissions emitted from various industries are a cause of major concern. These emissions are of two forms, viz. solid particles (SPM) and gaseous emissions (SO_2, NO_2, CO_2, etc.). Heavy polluting industries were identified which are included under the 17 categories of highly polluting industries for the purpose of monitoring and regulating pollution from them.

The Ministry of Environment and Forests has developed standards for regulating emissions for various industries including thermal power stations, iron and steel plants, cement plants, fertilizer plants, oil refineries, pulp and paper, petrochemicals, sugar, distilleries and tanneries.

Impressive growth in manufacturing (7.4% average over the past 10 years) is a reflection of growth trends in the fields of electronics and information technology, textiles, pharmaceuticals, basic chemicals etc. These industries, belong to the 'red category' of major polluting processes designated by the Central Pollution Control Board (CPCB), and have significant environmental consequences in terms of air emissions. The economic boom has also led to an increase in investments and activities in the construction, mining, and iron and steel sectors. This in turn, is causing a significant increase in brick-making units, sponge iron plants and steel re-rolling mills that involve highly polluting processes.

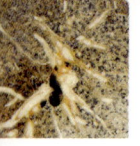

Domestic Sector—Indoor Air Pollution

A considerable amount of air pollution results from burning of fossil fuels. According to National Family Health Survey-3, more than 60% of Indian households depend on traditional sources of energy like fuel-wood, dung and crop residue for meeting their cooking and heating needs. Burning of traditional fuels introduces large quantities of CO_2 in the atmosphere when the combustion is complete, but if there is an incomplete combustion followed by oxidation, then CO is produced, in addition to hydrocarbons.

Burning of wheat and rice straw and other agricultural residue has also contributed to loss of soil fertility, apart from causing air pollution.

Ambient Air Quality Trends in India

Annual average concentration of SO_2 levels are within the prescribed National Ambient Air Quality Standards (NAAQS). During the last few years, a decreasing trend has been observed in nitrogen dioxide (NO_2) levels due to various measures taken for vehicular pollution control such as stricter vehicular emission norms. Vehicles are one of the major sources of NO_2 in the country. Annual average concentra-

tions of Respirable Suspended Particulate Matter (RSPM) and Suspended Particulate Matter (SPM) exceeded the NAAQS in most of the cities.

Environmental Impact

India is a fast-growing economy and has many future developmental targets, several of which are directly or indirectly linked to energy and therefore could lead to increased greenhouse gas emissions. Though the contribution of India to the cumulative global CO_2 emissions is only 5%, impacts could be severe at the local level.

Acid rain is the direct consequence of air pollution caused by gaseous emissions (CO, SO_2, NO) from industrial sources, burning of fuels (thermal plants, chimneys of brick-kilns or sugar mills.) and vehicular emissions. The most important effects of acid rain are damage to freshwater aquatic life, vegetation and damage to buildings and material. In India, the main threat of an acid rain disaster springs from our heavy dependence on coal as a major source of energy. Even though Indian coal is relatively low in sulphur content, what threatens to cause acid rain in India is the concentrated quantity of consumption, which is expected to reach very high levels in some parts of the country by 2020.

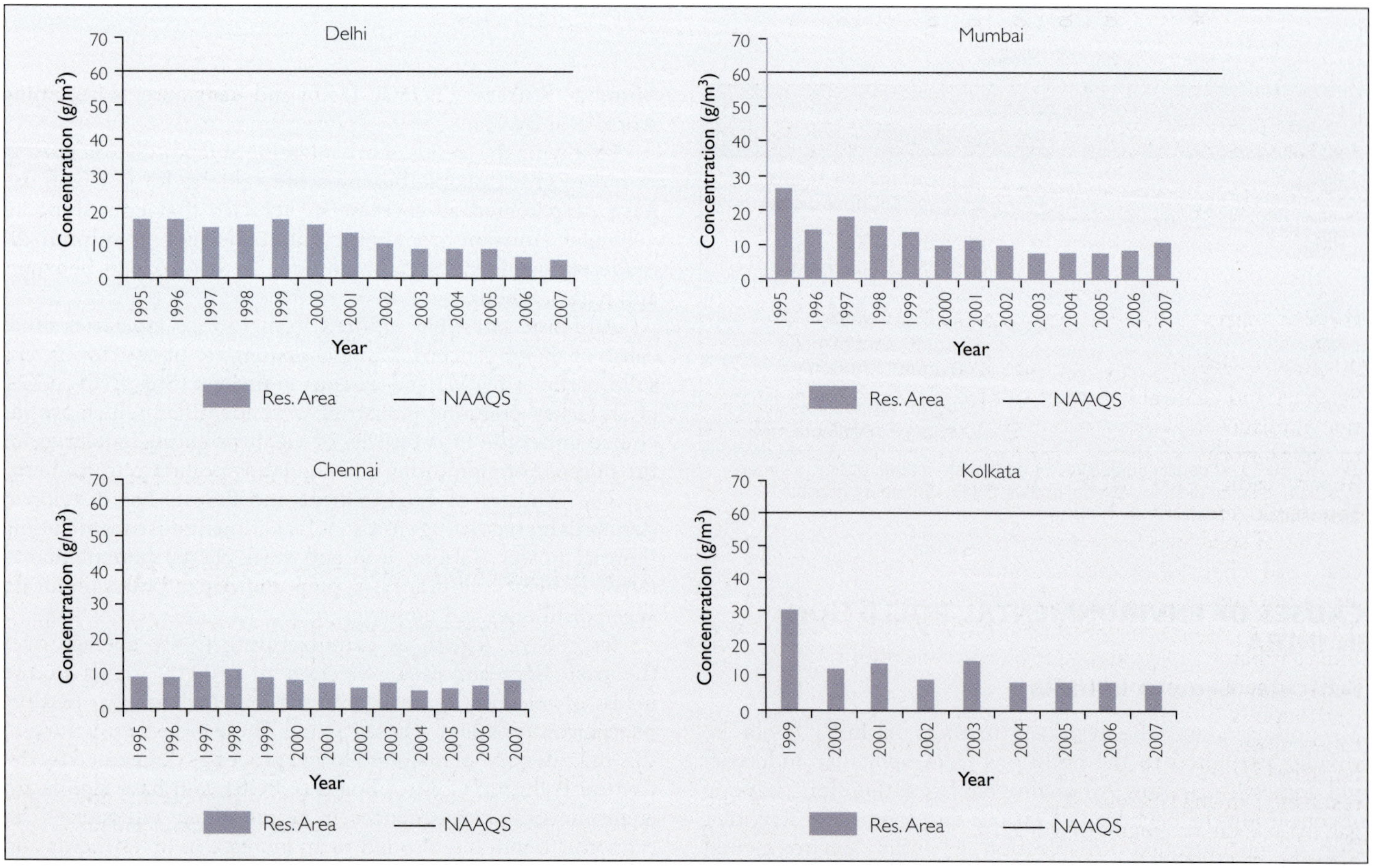

Fig 67.1: Trends in annual average concentration of SO_2 in residential areas of Delhi, Mumbai, Chennai, and Kolkata.

Source: Central Pollution Control Board, 2008.

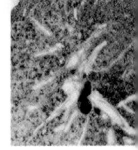

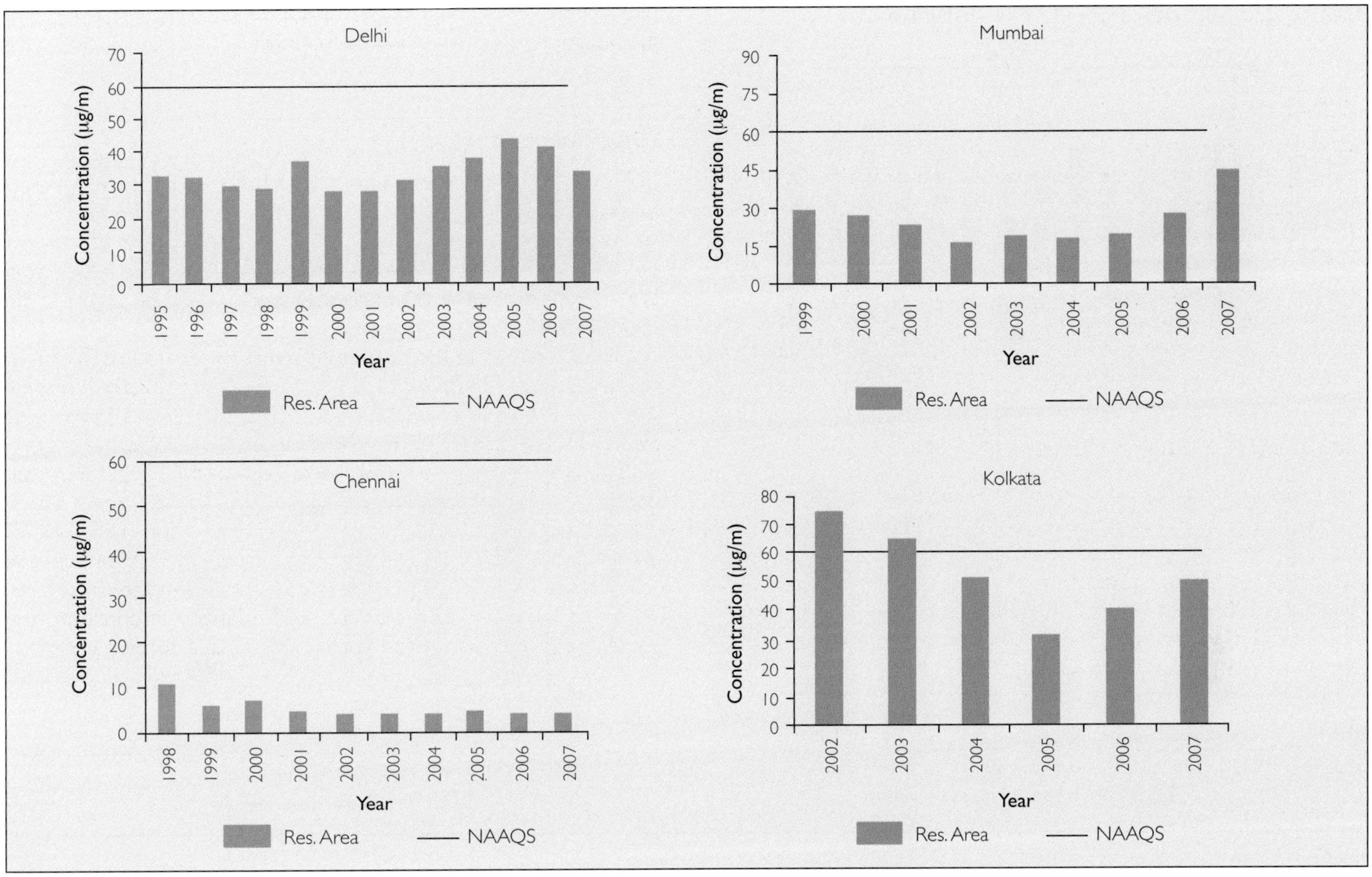

Fig 67.2: Trends in annual average concentration of NO$_2$ in residential areas of Delhi, Mumbai, Chennai, and Kolkata.

Note: Data for 2007 for Chennai, Kolkata and Mumbai is the average of data available as on date.
Source: Central Pollution Control Board, 2008.

Health Impact of Environmental Pollution

A study conducted by the All India Institute of Medical Sciences and Central Pollution Control Board in Delhi showed that exposure to higher levels of particulate matter contributed to respiratory morbidity. [Source: State of Environment Report India 2009 MOEF—Ministry of Environment and Forests Government of India]

Use of solid fuel (wood, animal dung, crop residue/grasses, coal, and charcoal) exposes people to high levels of toxic air pollutants, which result in serious health consequences. National Family Health Survey-3 (NFHS) found that 71% of India's urban households and 91% of rural households use solid fuels for cooking purposes.

There is a great deal of variation in the prevalence of tuberculosis (TB) according to the type of cooking fuel the household uses. It ranges from a low of 217 per 100,000 residents, (among households using electricity, liquid petroleum gas, natural gas, or biogas), to a high of 924 per 100,000 (among households using straw, shrubs, or grass for cooking). High TB prevalence is also seen amongst households using agricultural crop residue (703/100,000) or other fuels not specified.

Studies have found that besides TB, acute respiratory infections, chronic obstructive pulmonary disease, asthma, lung cancer, ischemic heart disease and blindness can also be attributed to indoor air pollution.

Climate change may alter the distribution and quality of India's natural resources and adversely affect the livelihoods of its people. With an economy closely linked to its natural resource base and climatically sensitive sectors such as agriculture, water and forestry, India may face a major threat because of the projected change in climate.

THE POLLUTION CONTROL APPROACH

Pollution control is a term used in environmental management. It means the control of emissions and effluents into air, water or soil. Without pollution control, the waste products from consumption, heating, agriculture, mining, manufacturing, transportation and other human activities, whether they accumulate or disperse, will degrade the environment. In the hierarchy of controls, pollution prevention and waste minimization are more desirable than pollution control.

Comprehensive Waste Management

Under the pollution control perspective, waste is regarded as an undesirable by-product of the production process which is to

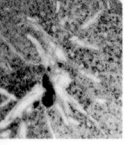

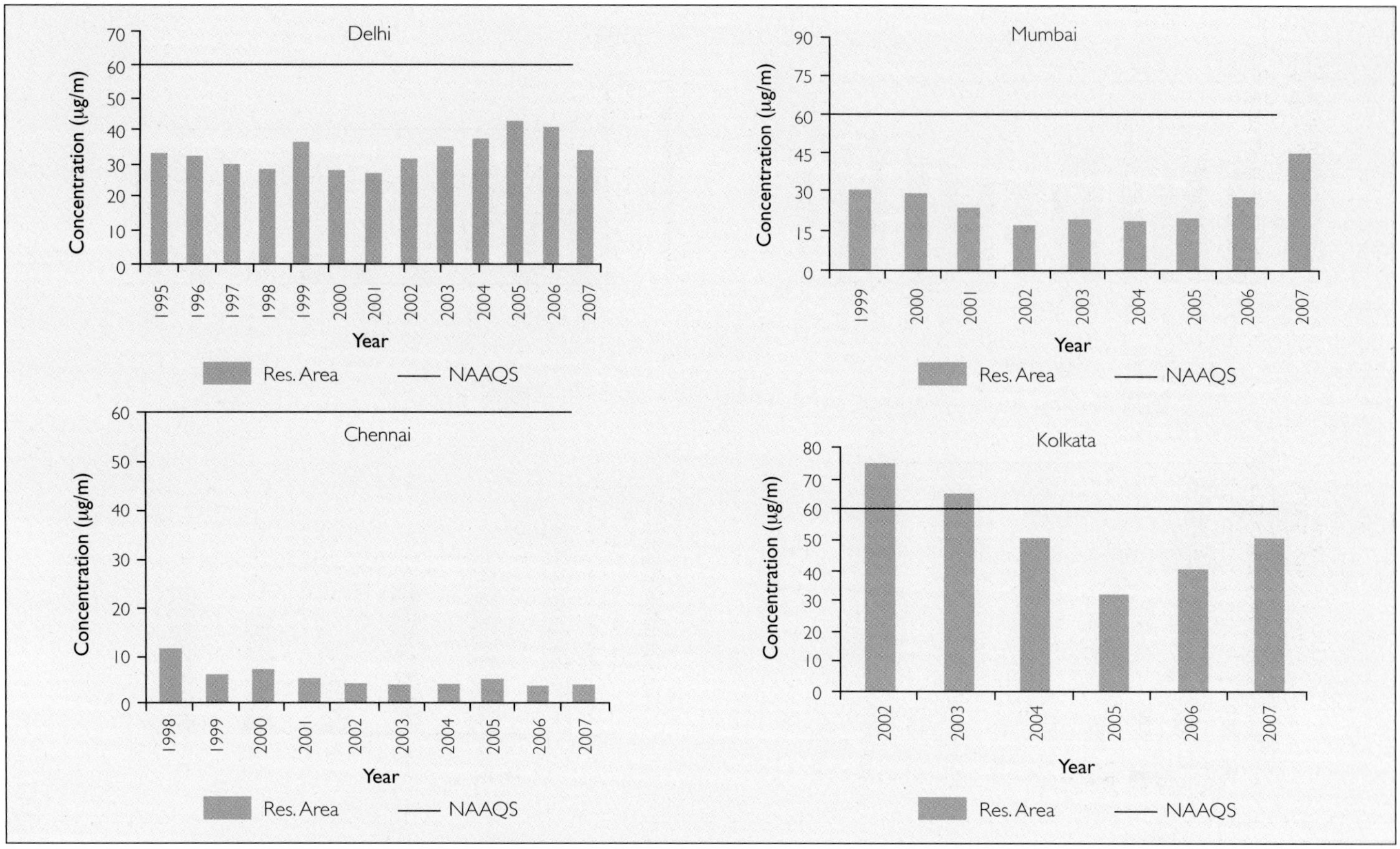

Fig 67.3: Trends in annual average concentration of SPM in residential areas of Delhi, Mumbai, Chennai, and Kolkata.

Note: Data for 2007 for Chennai, Kolkata and Mumbai is the average of data available as on date.
Source: Central Pollution Control Board, 2008.

be contained so as to ensure that soil, water and air resources are not contaminated beyond levels deemed to be acceptable.

While the pollution control approach has achieved considerable success in producing short-term improvements for local pollution problems, it has been less effective in addressing cumulative problems that are increasingly recognized on regional (e.g. acid rain) or global (e.g. ozone depletion) levels.

The aim of a health-oriented environmental pollution control programme is to promote a better quality of life by reducing pollution to the lowest level possible. Environmental pollution control programmes and policies, whose implications and priorities vary from country to country, cover all aspects of pollution (air, water, land and so on) and involve coordination among areas such as industrial development, city planning, water resources development and transportation policies.

As environmental pollution control technologies have become more sophisticated and more expensive, there has been a growing interest in ways to incorporate prevention in the design of industrial processes with the objective of eliminating harmful environmental effects while promoting the competitiveness of industries. Among the benefits of pollution prevention approaches, clean technologies and reduction in the use of products or processes that lead to toxic pollutant effects would reduce worker exposure to health risks.

POLLUTION PREVENTION APPROACH

The pollution prevention approach focuses directly on the use of processes, practices, materials and energy that avoid or minimize the creation of pollutants and wastes at source, and not on 'add-on' abatement measures. The corporate commitment plays a critical role in the decision to pursue pollution prevention.

As per the reports from the Ministry of Environment and Forests, spreading awareness and empowering people to take decisions at the local level, is an effective way of dealing with the environmental problems of India. Their decisions will enable initiatives that will benefit them as well as the local environment. It has been seen that solutions always emerge whenever governments involve people, using a participatory approach to solve problems.

Community-based natural resource management initiatives, coupled with policy reforms, can prove to be an effective mechanism for improving access to, and productivity of, natural resources. The success of joint forest management and irrigation user groups in India provides enough evidence that social capital and participatory processes are as crucial to environmental protection as financial resources and development programmes.

In the last few years, several measures relating to environmental issues have been introduced. They have targeted a

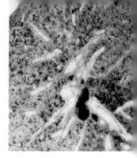

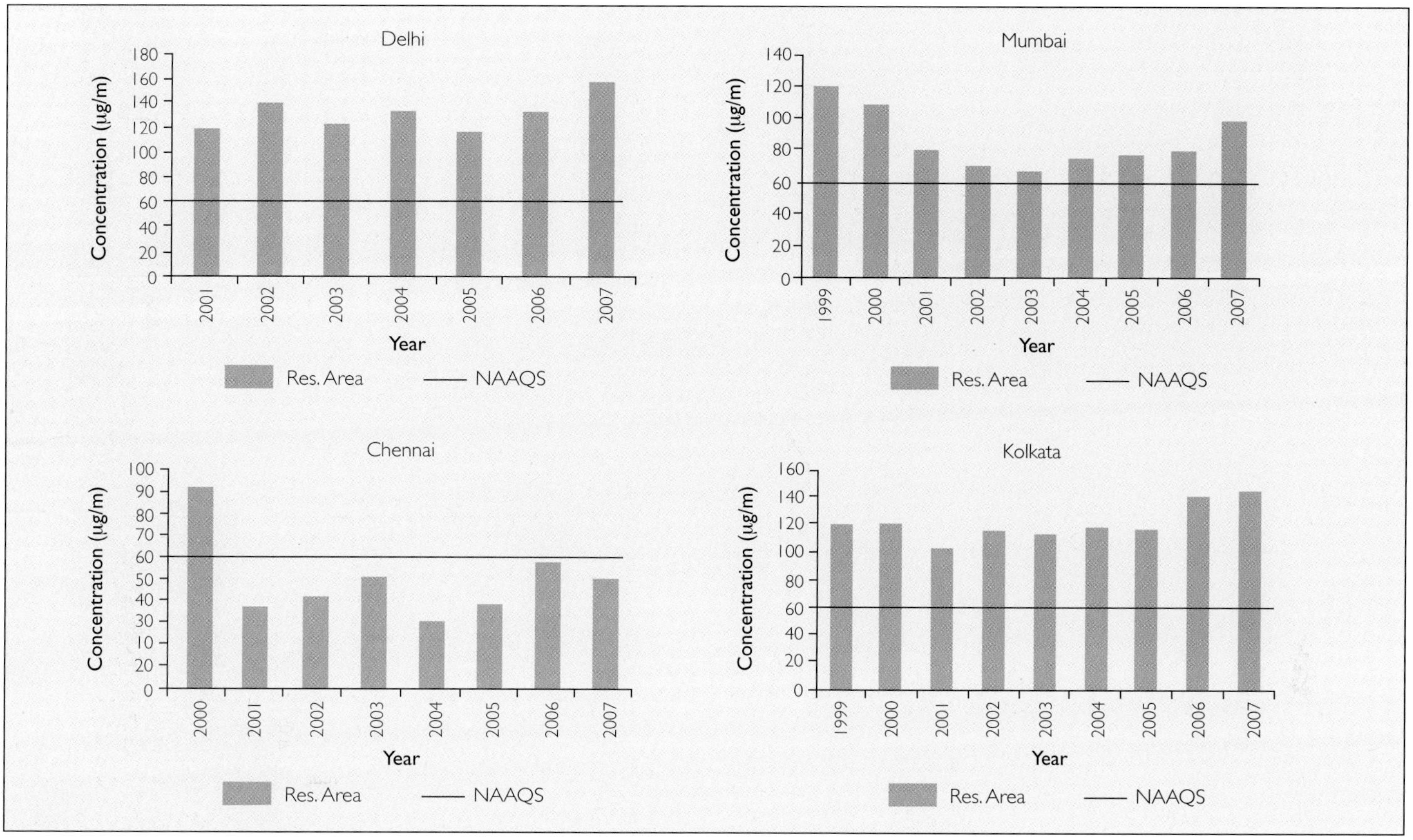

Fig 67.4: Trends in annual average concentration of RSPM in residential areas of Delhi, Mumbai, Chennai, and Kolkata.

Note: Data for 2007 for Chennai, Kolkata and Mumbai is the average of data available as on date.
Source: Central Pollution Control Board, 2008.

significant increase in the capacity of renewable energy installations, improving the air quality in major cities (the world's largest fleet of vehicles fuelled by compressed natural gas has been introduced in New Delhi) and enhancing afforestation.

Other similar measures have been implemented by committing additional resources and realigning new investments, thus steering economic development onto a climate-friendly path.

SUGGESTED READING

Asthmatic symptoms among pupils in relation to winter indoor and outdoor air pollution in schools in Taiyuan, China. *Environ Health Perspect*. Jan. 2008; 116(1): 90–7.

Badrinath KVS, Kiran Chand TR, Krishna Prasad V. Agriculture Crop Residue Burning in the Indo-Gangetic Plains: A study using IRS-P6 AWiFS satellite data. *Current Science*. 2006; 91(8): 1085–89.

Brunekreef B, Beelen R, Hoek G, *et al*. Effects of long-term exposure to traffic-related air pollution on respiratory and cardiovascular mortality in the Netherlands: the NLCS-AIR study. *Res Rep Health Eff Inst*. Mar. 2009; (139): 5–71; discussion 73–89.

Committee of the Environmental and Occupational Health Assembly of the American Thoracic Society, Health effects of outdoor air pollution. *Am J Respir Crit Care Med*. Jan. 1996; 153(1): 3–50.

Curtis L, Rea W, *et al*. Adverse health effects of outdoor air pollutants. *Environ Int*. Aug. 2006; 32(6): 815–30. *Epub*. 30 May 2006.

Khatri SB, Holguin FC, Ryan PB, Mannino D, Erzurum SC, Teague WG. Association of ambient ozone exposure with airway inflammation and allergy in adults with asthma. *J Asthma*. Oct. 2009; 46(8): 777–85.

Ministry of Environment and Forests Government of India. 2009 http://www.moef.gov.in, http://envfor.nic.in.

Taylor-Clark TE, Undem BJ. Ozone activates airway nerves via the selective stimulation of TRPA1 ion channels. *J Physiol*. 1 Feb. 2010; 588 (Pt 3): 423–33. *Epub*. 14 Dec. 2009.

WHO Air quality guidelines for particulate matter, ozone, nitrogen dioxide and sulfur dioxide—Global update 2005—Summary of risk assessment.

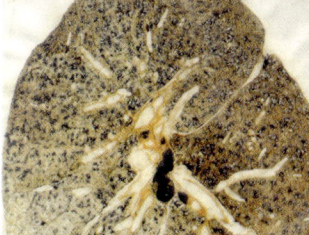

OCCUPATIONAL AND ENVIRONMENTAL LUNG DISEASES

CHAPTER **68** **Inhalational Lung Injury**

Environmental pollution caused by smoke and the release of chemical gases, fumes and other noxious substances into the atmosphere can cause marked irritation and injury to the respiratory tract or could result in asphyxiation. Rarely, irritation and injury to the respiratory tract can occur several years after exposure, as with asbestos, an occupational hazard that not only involves asbestos factory workers, but also affects those living in the vicinity from environmental and atmospheric pollution with the asbestos fibre. Another example of a delayed prolonged effect on the respiratory and other systems related to atmospheric pollution is the Bhopal disaster following the leak of methyl isocyanate gas (MIC) from an industrial plant manufacturing a pesticide in early December 1984.

EPIDEMIOLOGY

Inhalation of smoke causing either death from asphyxiation or severe irritation of the respiratory tract constitutes the commonest inhalational injury to humans. Smoke arises from fire and though domestic, industrial and other fires occur all over the world, they are most common in poor developing countries and affect far more people in these countries than in the Western countries of the world. This is because of inherent far greater fire-risks in dilapidated crowded houses and housing colonies and the comparatively poorer infrastructure which renders fire-fighting difficult and doubly dangerous. Hundreds of thousands in India and other poor developing countries of the world risk inhalation of smoke from domestic and other fires (as in unsafe cinema houses, bars, dance halls, etc).

The number of individuals exposed to dangerous pollutants in the world, particularly in India and other economically growing countries of the world such as China, Southeast Asian countries, South America and the African continent must perhaps run into several million. Why is this so? In India, the gross domestic product (GDP) per capita has increased from $1000 in 1984 to over $ 3000 in 2007 and it continues at a growth rate close to 8% per year. Rapid industrial development has contributed to this growth but it has been at the cost of great environmental degradation and a marked increase in public health risks. Chemical factories spout pollutants into the city atmosphere posing known and unknown hazards to people in the vicinity. Disaster, possibly very nearly akin to the Bhopal disaster, according to many environmentalists, waits just round the corner!

RISK FACTORS

Inhalation of smoke emanating from domestic fires to huge conflagrations as in wars, terrorist attacks, or fires in huge factories housing incendiary material are important examples. Inhalation of chemical fumes occurs particularly in poorly ventilated factories or when they escape the confines of a factory and pollute the atmosphere. Sources of occupational exposure to major chemicals causing injury to the respiratory tract are given below.

Factors that influence the toxic effects of chemicals include the inherent chemical toxicity of the substance, its particle size and concentration, its solubility and the duration of exposure. Water-soluble chemicals afflict the upper airways because they dissolve on reaching these sites. The less water-soluble chemical fumes reach the peripheral airways and exert maximum injury at these sites. The sources of inhalation exposure with regard to a few important noxious chemicals and gases are given below. The first six are examples of irritants and the last three of asphyxiants.

Table 68.1: Exposure to industrial toxic gases	
Gas	**Important Sources**
Chlorine	Textile, paper, sewage treatment, swimming pools, chemical factories producing chlorine
Sulphur dioxide	Atmospheric pollution, chemical manufacture, smelting, power plants
Oxides of nitrogen	Air pollution, welding, agriculture, chemical and dye manufacture
Ammonia	Plastics, agriculture, manufacture of explosives
Hydrogen chloride	Manufacture of acid, fertilizer, textiles, dyes, rubber industry
Hydrofluoric acid	Insecticides, fertilizers, metal working, pharmaceuticals
Carbon monoxide	Smoke inhalation, smelters, miners, home fires
Hydrogen cyanide	Metallurgy, electroplating, plastics, polymethane manufactures
Smoke	Fires (as explained in the text) incomplete combustion of waste produces sought to be destroyed by fire

DIAGNOSIS

Inhalational injury produces either inflammation of the respiratory tract or asphyxia. Inflammation of the respiratory tract may involve the upper respiratory passage—the nose, sinuses, pharynx, larynx, trachea and the large bronchi. Inhalation injury may skip or mildly involve the upper respiratory passage and exert

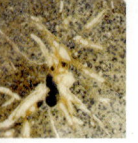

a major effect on the lower respiratory tract—the bronchioles, terminal bronchioles, respiratory bronchioles and the alveoli. Inflamed nasal passages, cough, hoarseness of voice, stridor may be present; rhonchi are often heard on auscultation.

Involvement of the lower air passages and alveoli leads to breathlessness, wheezing and crackles over the lungs on auscultation. Some chemical fumes such as ammonia, chlorine and the dreadful MIC gas in the Bhopal tragedy produce a chemical burn. This can lead to severe diffuse alveolar damage resulting in non-cardiogenic pulmonary oedema (ARDS) and severe bronchial and bronchiolar damage that over a period of time leads to bronchiolitis obliterans or severe progressive fibrosing bronchiolitis. Death can occur within a few hours or few days or the patient may be left with crippling sequelae characterized by well-marked pulmonary fibrosis with restrictive lung disease, or progressive bronchiolitis obliterans causing obstructive lung disease or a combination of both restrictive and obstructive lung disease. The extent of the injury and disease can be gauged clinically, by radiographic examination of the chest and by lung function tests. Routine spirometry, lung volumes, carbon monoxide (CO) diffusion tests will determine the presence of airways obstruction, involvement of small airways in the obstructive pathology, as also the presence of restrictive lung disease. The lung functions will also enable the clinician to determine whether the patient has a combination of airways obstruction and restriction. High-resolution computed tomography (HRCT) of the chest (if facilities are available) will reveal more than a radiography of the chest—the nature of alveolar shadows, the presence of pulmonary oedema as also the presence

of air-trapping because of obstructed bronchi. The flow-volume loop will pick up large airways' obstruction that may occasionally be the chief cause of breathlessness. Severe parenchymal injury to the lung in the form of diffuse alveolar damage, or ARDS will result in increasing hypoxemia necessitating not only the inhalation of oxygen but also ventilator support.

The presence of headache, dizziness, vomiting, and chest pain but with few physical findings in the chest suggests a systemic poisoning with something like cyanide or hydrogen sulphide. Cyanosis or a cherry pink colour of the mucosa with a normal PaO_2 and normal O_2 saturation suggests cyanide poisoning. Hypoxemia (low O_2 saturation) with a normal PaO_2 points to CO poisoning. Both cyanide and CO poisoning are associated with a low pH and an increase in blood lactic acid.

Diagnosis of the nature of the compound inhaled is usually obvious as this is easily determined depending on how and where the poisonous gas originated, in relation to the manufacture of a particular chemical or product. At times this is difficult and may need to await the results of a careful investigation and analysis.

Some disasters may be associated with inhalation of toxic gases which injure the respiratory tract as also of asphyxiants such as smoke.

Individuals with persistent symptoms need a careful follow-up involving clinical examination, pulmonary function tests and imaging studies. Sequelae of some of the toxic irritant gases include pulmonary fibrosis which may be progressive, bronchiolitis obliterans causing obstructive lung disease or a combination of both. Severe sequelae can lead to persistent hypoxemia, varying degree of breathlessness and poor effort tolerance.

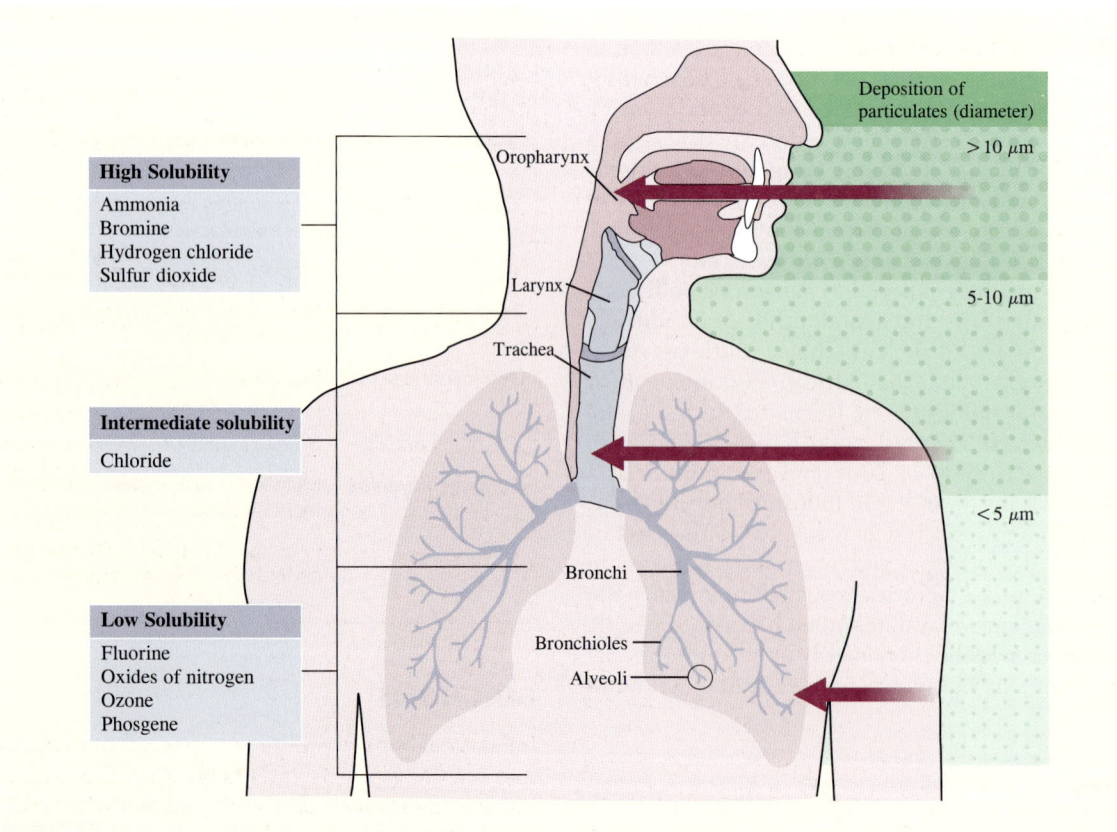

Fig 68.1: Distribution of various gases and particulate matter in the respiratory tract.

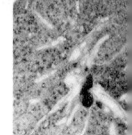

THE BHOPAL TRAGEDY—INHALATION OF METHYL ISOCYNATE

The Bhopal tragedy was and is one of the worst industrial accidents in history. On 2 December 1984 at 11 pm while most of the residents of Bhopal were asleep, there was a small leak of methyl isocyanate (MIC) gas and increasing pressure in the storage tank. Negligent events were direct contributing factors to the start of the disaster—a) a safety device to neutralize toxic discharge from the MIC systems had been turned off; b) a faulty valve allowed one ton of water to mix with 40 tons of MIC; c) a refrigerating unit used to cool the MIC storage tank had been drained off its coolant for use in another part of the plant; d) the gas flare safety system was out of order.

The pressure and heat from the marked exothermic reaction in the storage tank of MIC continued to build. At 1 am on 3 December, a loud reverberation arose as the safety valve gave way and the MIC gas escaped into the early morning air, and within a few hours the streets of Bhopal were littered with corpses of men, women, children and animals (cows, dogs) and birds. Three thousand eight hundred people died almost immediately (mostly in the slum colony adjacent to the Union Carbide factory). Estimates of the number of people killed in the first few days after the escape of MIC gas are as high as 10,000 with 15,000 to 20,000 premature deaths occurring in the subsequent two decades. More than 500,000 people were exposed to the gas and several epidemiological studies showed a marked increase in both morbidity and mortality in this exposed population. This is unquestionably an underestimate, as many exposed people left Bhopal soon after the tragedy, never to return and were lost to follow-up.

Immediate Respiratory Effects of MIC

Acute fulminant toxic chemical inflammation of the lower respiratory tract summarizes the immediate respiratory effects of MIC. These consisted of diffuse alveolar damage with non-cardiogenic pulmonary oedema (ARDS), pneumonitis and pneumothorax (observed in some patients). The chemical burn involved the bronchial mucosa, in particular the smaller bronchioles and the terminal and respiratory bronchioles causing an acute inflammatory bronchiolitis.

In patients with marked exposure, acute respiratory distress, severe hypoxemia and death occurred within a matter of hours. Those with lesser exposure developed ARDS, pneumonitis, bronchiolitis, increasing difficulty in breathing, and increasing hypoxemia within 24 to 72 hours. Some with ARDS who managed to be taken to the sparse (poorly equipped) critical care units in the city survived with ventilator support together with support to other systems.

Late effects on the respiratory system consisted of increasing pulmonary fibrosis and airways' obstruction due to obliterative bronchiolitis. Some developed more of the former, others more of the latter; many had a combination of both obstructive and restrictive lung disease as judged by imaging studies and by lung function tests.

The question that was asked soon after the tragedy was whether MIC gas was the sole toxic agent involved in the disaster. To start with, the immediate crisis was compounded by the ignorance of people and doctors as to what gas was involved and what were its immediate and long-term effects. At every turn, the Union Carbide Company which owned and ran the plant withheld scientific data from the doctors, authorities and people at large. When MIC is exposed to 200°C heat it forms degraded MIC that contains the very deadly hydrogen cyanide (HCN). There was evidence that the storage tank temperature did reach 200°C or more. The corpses that littered the vicinity had a cherry red colour of blood and of viscera at autopsy; many victims responded to the administration of sodium thiosulphate, an antidote to cyanide poisoning but not effective against MIC toxicity. Almost certainly cyanide poisoning was responsible for some of the very quick deaths occurring after escape of the overheated MIC gas.

MCI toxicity had far-reaching effects on other organ systems of the body which are briefly tabled below. These include the induction of genetic chromosomal abnormalities, the effects of which may haunt the descendants of this tragedy for generations to come.

Table 68.2: Early effects on the respiratory system (0–6 months) after exposure to MIC
Respiratory distress
Diffuse alveolar damage, ARDS
Pneumonitis, acute bronchiolitis
Pneumonia
Hypoxemia which may be severe enough to cause death
Secondary pulmonary or bronchopulmonary infection

Table 68.3: Early effects on the organ systems other than the respiratory system (0–6 months) after exposure to MIC	
Gastrointestinal system	Abdominal pain, anorexia, persistent diarrhoea
Ocular	Chemosis, redness, photophobia, corneal ulcers
Psychological	Neurosis, anxiety states
Neurobehavioural	Impaired audio and visual memory, impaired vigilance and impaired response time, impaired reasoning and spatial ability, impaired psychomotor co-ordination
Genetic	Increased chromosomal abnormalities

Source: Broughton Edward. The Bhopal Disaster and its aftermath: A review. *Environmental health*. 2005. 4: 6.

The reasons for briefly describing the genesis of the Bhopal disaster are:

1. The inseparable links between the medical, human, social, moral and ethical aspects of this disaster. It is indeed incredible that the norms followed for workers and public safety by large international manufacturing companies in their own Western countries are set aside in poor developing

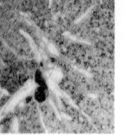
Table 68.4: Late effects on the respiratory system (6 months) after exposure to MIC	
1. Obstructive airways disease due to obliterative bronchiolitis	
Lung function tests	Airways obstruction
Imaging studies	Hyperinflated lungs on X-ray
	Air-trapping in many areas of the lung on CT chest causing a mosaic appearance of the lung fields
2. Restrictive airways disease due to pulmonary fibrosis	
Lung function tests	Restrictive pattern
Imaging studies	Pulmonary fibrosis
3. Combined airways obstruction + airways restriction	
Lung function tests	Combination of obstruction and restriction
Imaging studies	Features of air trapping, bronchial fibrosis, pulmonary fibrosis
4. Chronic hypoxemic respiratory failure or hypoxemic + hypercapnic respiratory failure in those severely afflicted	

Table 68.5: Late effects on the organ systems other than respiratory system after exposure to MIC	
Ocular	Persistent watering of eyes, corneal opacities
Reproductive	Increased pregnancy loss, increased infant mortality, decreased foetal weight
Genetic	Increased chromosomal abnormalities
Neurobehavioural	Impaired associate learning, motor speed, precision

Source: Broughton Edward. The Bhopal Disaster and its aftermath: A review. *Environmental health*. 2005, 4: 6.

countries. Such double standards betray a total lack of ethical, moral and social responsibility. In a settlement mediated by the Indian Supreme Court, the Union Carbide Company agreed to pay $470 million to the Indian government to be distributed to the claimants affected by this disorder as the final settlement. Edward Broughton believes that the liability of the same company in the United States would have exceeded $10 billion if a similar disaster had occured in that country.

2. Despite more stringent laws passed in India since the Bhopal disaster, many small-scale industries and large manufacturing establishments continue to produce toxic chemicals within city limits or just outside large heavily populated cities not only in India but in most poor developing countries of the world and in China. The world (and in particular the poorer countries of the world) has not yet learnt a lesson from the Bhopal disaster.

3. The Bhopal tragedy emphasizes the dire need for improving public health infrastructure and planning for disaster management in India and other poor countries of the developing world.

4. Economic growth and industrial development should not be at the cost of environmental degradation and public health risks, if a repetition of this great tragedy is to be averted.

OTHER CHEMICAL IRRITANTS

The effects of some important chemical irritants on the respiratory systems are now briefly described.

Chlorine

Chlorine is a soluble gas liberating chloride and oxygen free radicals when in contact with water. At low levels of exposure it causes irritation of the conjuctiva and the mucosa of the upper respiratory passage. Higher exposure leads to pulmonary oedema within 6 to 24 hours. Chemical inflammation of the airways leads to airflow obstruction. Breathlessness, wheezing and crackles are heard over the lungs. Imaging may reveal pulmonary oedema or evidence of air-trapping. Clinical evidence of serious respiratory tract involvement (including the development of pulmonary oedema) may occur six to eight hours after exposure to the gas so that observation of the patient for a length of time is imperative.

Treatment is supportive; oxygen, nebulized salbutamol and ipratropium bromide for airways obstruction are of help. Intravenous corticosteroids are of use in patients with severe chemical injury to the airways. In some severe cases pulmonary oedema may necessitate ventilator support.

Sulphur Dioxide

Fossil fuel combustion leads to the formation of sulphur dioxide and sulphuric acid. Various industrial processes such as smelting, chemical manufacture, paper manufacture, metal refining lead to possible exposure to this noxious agent. Exposure to sulphur dioxide or fumes of sulphuric acid leads to burning of the eyes, conjunctivitis, corneal ulcers, cough, chest pain, chest tightness and breathlessness due to pharyngeal inflammation and chemical inflammation of the airways. Greater exposure leads to pulmonary oedema. The chemical inflammation of the airways can lead to bronchiolitis obliterans. This leads to permanent airways obstruction and is particularly observed in smelter workers following overexposure to this agent.

Oxides of Nitrogen (NO, NO_2, N_2O_4)

Oxides of nitrogen can produce fatal respiratory injury to workers who come in contact with high concentration of this gas. Occupations at risk include welders using acetylene torches, exposure to fumes in the manufacture of dye, nitric acid and lacquers.

The most dangerous and important exposure to oxides of nitrogen occurs in silo-fillers disease. This occurs when corn is stored in silos so that it ferments. Fermented corn releases oxides of nitrogen which are strongly irritant to the respiratory system. In contact with water within the lung, oxides of nitrogen form nitric and nitrous acid. The dissociation of oxides into nitrates, nitrites and free radicals is strongly irritant to the mucosa of the airways and the lung parenchyma. Exposures greater than 150

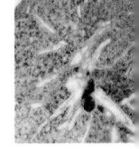

ppm are generally fatal leading to death from pneumonia and pulmonary oedema. A lesser degree of exposure leads to cough, breathlessness, tightness in the chest due to bronchiolitis and pneumonitis. An even lesser degree of exposure may just lead to irritation of the eyes, conjunctivitis and pharyngitis.

Symptoms after significant exposure may be delayed and relapses may occur after three to six weeks with symptoms of cough, breathlessness and tightness of the chest. Chronic bronchitis has been reported to occur in some patients.

Treatment is supportive, aerosolized bronchodilators and the use of corticosteroids for airways obstruction resulting from bronchiolitis may help.

Ammonia

Ammonia though a noxious gas is generally transported as a liquid. Fumes of ammonia in contact with water in the respiratory mucosa form a strong alkali, ammonium hydroxide. Acute irritation of the mucosa is followed by a chemical inflammation, sloughing of the mucosa of the larynx, trachea, bronchi and the smaller airways. Laryngeal oedema causes stridor. Bronchial inflammation can lead to bronchiolitis and later to bronchiolitis obliterans. Parenchymal inflammation can lead to a chemical pneumonitis and ARDS. Treatment is with bronchodilators, and oxygen therapy. Intubation may be necessary to protect the airways form impending laryngeal obstruction due to progressive laryngeal oedema.

Hydrogen Chloride

Hydrogen chloride (HCl) is a strong acid and when it comes in contact with the respiratory mucosa, it induces a severe inflammation of the airways. HCl exposure is encountered in the manufacture of textile, rubber, dye, and fertilizers. High levels of exposure cause airways' obstruction due to mucosal oedema, pneumonitis and pulmonary oedema.

Hydrofluoric Acid

Hydrofluoric acid like other strong acids or alkalis is highly corrosive, even more corrosive than sulphuric acid or ammonia. Hydrofluoric acid is water-soluble, releases H^+ ions and has a strongly corrosive effect on the airways and lung parenchyma. There is rapid damage to the airways, parenchymal lung damage leading to pneumonia, bronchopneumonia, ARDS and death. ARDS may occur after a lapse of some hours after exposure.

CHEMICAL ASPHYXIANTS

Carbon monoxide, hydrogen cyanide, and hydrogen sulphide are examples of chemical asphyxiants which interfere with delivery and/or utilization of oxygen resulting in asphyxiation at the tissue level.

Carbon Monoxide Poisoning

Carbon monoxide is a colourless, odourless, tasteless gas produced by incomplete combustion of carbon and other organic materials. Inhalation of CO is an important cause of accidental and suicidal deaths all over the world. Common sources of CO are car exhausts, and smoke from all types of fire. In the developing world, combustion of coal, wood and other biofuels is an important source of CO and an important cause of CO poisoning. Inhalation of methylene chloride (seen in paint strippers) can also lead to CO poisoning.

MECHANISM OF TOXICITY

Haemoglobin has 240 times greater affinity for CO than for oxygen. CO therefore avidly combines with haemoglobin to form carboxyhaemoglobin, thereby reducing the oxygen-carrying capacity of blood. Also, the oxygen dissociation curve shifts to the left and modifies oxygen binding sites. As a result, the affinity for remaining haem groups for oxygen is increased. The leftward shift and distortion of the oxygen dissociation curve results in a far greater tissue hypoxia than what would result from a reduced oxygen-carrying capacity of blood.

CO may also inhibit cellular respiration due to reversible binding to cellular cytochrome oxidase.

CLINICAL FEATURES

Acute exposure leading to a carboxyhaemoglobin concentration of 10% generally does not cause symptoms. Ten to thirty per cent may produce headache, dyspnoea and at times confusion. Symptoms are more prominent in the elderly; patients with cardiorespiratory disease are at greater risk. High concentrations of carboxyhaemoglobin in the blood as after acute, prolonged or severe exposure to CO cause increasing confusion, agitation, seizures and coma. Hyperventilation, Cheyne Stokes breathing, pulmonary oedema and respiratory failure may occur. There is marked metabolic acidosis.

Neurological examination, besides revealing an altered mental state or an altered state of consciousness, is often characterized by hypertonia, hyperreflexia and bilateral extensor plantar responses. The condition is often mistaken for a brainstem infarct. Rarely, focal signs in the form of monoplegia or hemiplegia may be present.

Cardiovascular features include myocardial ischemia, and infarction, particularly in older patients with cardiovascular disease. Arrhythmias which include atrial fibrillation, ventricular asystole and various degrees of heart block can occur. ST depression and prolonged QT interval may be seen on the electrocardiograph (ECG).

Severe hypoxemia may result in a hearing loss due to ischemia to the cochlea. Acute renal failure is a known complication of severe CO poisoning, related to hypoxemic damage to renal tubule cells. Carboxyhaemoglobin greater than 60% leads to coma, seizures and death from cardiorespiratory arrest. The important features of CO poisoning are listed in Table 68.6.

DIAGNOSIS

The possibility of CO poisoning should always be kept in mind depending on the history and the situation in which the patient is discovered. The possibility of CO poisoning due to a gas leak and accidental poisoning from incomplete combustion of biofuel is often missed. Spectroscopic examination of blood for CO-Hb confirms the diagnosis. The presence of hypoxemia with low O_2 saturation in the presence of a normal PaO_2 also suggests the correct diagnosis.

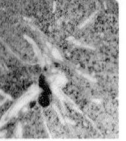

Table 68.6: Features of acute CO poisoning
• Headache, agitation, confusion, seizures
• Drowsiness, coma
• Cheyne stokes breathing
• Pulmonary oedema, respiratory failure
• Metabolic acidosis
• Arterial hypoxemia with a normal P_aO_2
• Spasticity, hyperreflexia, extensor plantar
• Myocardial ischemia, infarction
• Arrhythmia, atrial fibrillation, heart block, ST-T changes, prolonged QT on ECG
• Hearing loss
• Acute renal failure

Table 68.7: Delayed effects of CO poisoning
Neuropsychiatric complications
1. Changes in higher functions—intellectual deterioration, impairment of memory, aggressiveness, abnormal behaviour
2. Cerebral, cerebellar, midbrain damage
3. Parkinsonism
4. Hearing loss following ischemia to the cochlea

DELAYED EFFECTS

Following recovery from the effects of acute exposure to CO, delayed neuropsychiatric problems may develop insidiously over a matter of weeks. These include features of cerebral, cerebellar and mid-brain damage. Cerebellar signs and spasticity are most often seen.

Impairment of higher functions may occur in the form of impairment of memory, intellectual deterioration, aggressive and abnormal behaviour. Parkinsonism is a known sequel to CO poisoning.

TREATMENT

Treatment consists of removal of the patient from the site of exposure and inhalation of 100% oxygen with a tight-fitting mask. Comatose patients, severely hypoxemic with poor respiration should be intubated and given mechanical ventilator support with 100% oxygen. Oxygen at high concentration should be continued till the carboxyhaemoglobin is below 10%.

Hyperbaric oxygen if available may be used, leading to a quicker replacement of carboxyhaemoglobin with oxyhaemoglobin. Controlled studies have not shown a clear benefit with hyperbaric oxygen compared to endotracheal intubation and ventilator support with a fraction of inspired oxygen (FIO_2) of 100% oxygen.

Supportive treatment is important. Convulsions should be countered by intravenous diazepam. Intravenous corticosteroids and mannitol may be used for cerebral oedema.

Hydrogen Cyanide

Fumes of hydrogen cyanide are released following combustion or pyrolysis of plastic and polyurethane. Individuals engaged in this occupation and exposed to the fumes are at grave risk of HCN poisoning. The fumes are absorbed through the skin and respiratory tract. Cyanide binds to the cytochrome oxidase, paralyses the tricarboxylic acid cycle so that the utilization of oxygen by tissue cells and cellular respiration cease.

CLINICAL FEATURES

Minor exposures (50 ppm) cause headache, tachycardia, tachypnoea and tightness in the chest.

Major exposures (> 100 ppm) cause dyspnoea, tightness in the chest, confusion, seizures, pulmonary oedema, ataxia, apnoea, coma and death. Cardiac arrest, respiratory arrest and death can occur within minutes

DIAGNOSIS

Diagnosis rests on a history of relevant occupational or environmental exposure. The skin and blood may have a cherry pink colour and a smell of almonds may be recognized by those with a good sense of smell.

The arterial blood gases show a metabolic acidosis, a normal PaO_2, a normal O_2 saturation and an increase in the blood lactate level.

TREATMENT

The patient should be removed from the site of exposure and given oxygen with a tight-fitting mask. If transported to the hospital alive, endotracheal intubation and ventilator support with an FIO_2 of 100% is recommended. Support to the cardiovascular and all other systems is of crucial importance.

Specific antidotes include cobalt salts (dicobalt acetate), sodium thiosulphate and sodium nitrite and hydroxocobalamin. Cobalt salts form inert salts with cyanide and constitute the treatment of choice. They are unavailable in most units.

Thiosulphate detoxifies by conversion of cyanide to thiocyanate; 12.5 g (25 ml of a 50% solution) is given intravenously over 15 minutes.

Sodium nitrite converts a portion of the haemoglobin to the methaemoglobin which binds cyanide. It is administered intravenously, 300 mg (10 ml of a 3% solution) over three minutes. Inhalation of amyl nitrite may be of some use.

Hydroxocobalamin—1 mole of hydroxocobalamin inactivates one mole of cyanide but on a weight for weight basis,–50 times more hydroxocobalamin is needed than cyanide. Concentrated hydroxocobalamin is unavailable in India and perhaps in most countries of the world. If available it is given in a dose of 5 g intravenously over 30 minutes. The dose may be repeated in severe poisoning.

Hydrogen Sulphide

Hydrogen sulphide is a colourless gas that smells of rotten eggs. The gas is found in mines and sewers so that workers in mining and with sewage may be exposed to it. It is also liberated from decomposing fish (a hazard to fishermen with decomposing fish in the hold of their boats) and from manure systems.

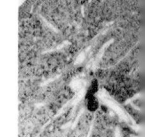

MECHANISM OF ACTION

It acts by inhibition of cytochrome oxidase within the cells thereby stopping cellular respiration, a mode of action similar to cyanide.

CLINICAL FEATURES

Headache, drowsiness, sore throat, and blurred vision with coloured halos around the light occur with lesser degree of exposure. Exposure to higher concentration leads to confusion, seizures, cyanosis, coma and death.

TREATMENT

The patient should be removed from the site of exposure (the rescuer must have appropriate breathing apparatus) and be given 100% oxygen through a tight-fitting mask. Intravenous sodium nitrite (as given in cyanide poisoning) is of help though its mechanism of action is not well understood.

SUGGESTED READING

Broughton Edward. The Bhopal Disaster and its aftermath: A review. *Environmental Health* 2005, 4: 6.

Miller K. Acute inhalation injury. *Emerg Med Clin North Am*. 1 May 2003; 21(2): 533–57.

Niven AS. Inhalational exposure to nerve agents. *Respir Care Clin N Am*. 1 Mar. 2004; 10(1): 59–74.

Parrish JS. Toxic inhalational injury: gas, vapor and vesicant exposure. *Respir Care Clin N Am*. 1 Mar. 2004; 10(1): 43–58.

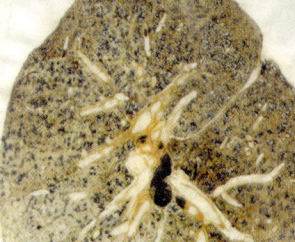

OCCUPATIONAL AND ENVIRONMENTAL LUNG DISEASES

CHAPTER 69 — Clinical Disorders at High Altitude

PHYSIOLOGICAL CHANGES AT HIGH ALTITUDE

Ascent to higher altitude causes hypoxemia. The barometric pressure (P_B) at sea level is 760 mm Hg and the pressure of inspired oxygen (P_IO_2) is 150 mm Hg. With normal alveolar ventilation (V_A) the $PaCO_2$ = 40 mm Hg. Assuming that R = 1, the alveolar oxygen pressure (P_AO_2) is 110 mm Hg. This figure is evident from the equation

$$P_AO_2 = P_IO_2 - PaCO_2 / R$$

The P_IO_2 at sea level being equal to (P_B – 47 mm Hg) × 0.21 = 150 mm Hg; where 21% being the concentration of oxygen in air breathed at sea level; 47 mm Hg being water vapour pressure.

Assuming a normal alveolar-arterial gradient of 10 to 15 mm Hg in a healthy individual the partial pressure of oxygen in the arterial blood (PaO_2) would be P_AO_2 – 10 mm Hg = 100 mm Hg.

As one ascends the barometric pressure of air breathed decreases. The higher the altitude the lower the barometric pressure, the lower the P_IO_2, resulting in a proportionate decrease in the P_AO_2 and PaO_2. Table 69.1 gives an approximate effect of reduced P_IO_2 on PaO_2 at varying altitudes.

Table 69.1:
Appoximate effect of reduced P_IO_2 at different altitudes

Altitude (metres)	P_B mm Hg	P_AO_2 mm Hg	PaO_2 mm Hg
Sea level	760	150	100
1620	620	120	70
3500	500	95	55
8848 (Mount Everest)	253	43	26

A PaO_2 of 26 mm Hg would be close to the lowest limit compatible with life, without breathing an increased concentration of oxygen. Yet there have been some amazing successful attempts at reaching the summit of Mount Everest without the use of supplemental oxygen.

ACUTE RESPONSE TO HYPOXIA

Hypoxia among several other effects increases the ventilatory rate, through stimulation of the peripheral chemoreceptors in the carotid and aortic bodies. The carotid body is composed of highly specialized aerobic tissue cells which depend on mitochondrial oxidative phosphorylation for the production of adenosine triphosphate (ATP). The production of ATP is linked to oxygen consumption. Deprivation of oxygen as in hypoxemic states leads to the inability of mitochondria to produce ATP. Inhibition of mitochondrial function has been shown to stimulate afferent activity of the carotid body. Afferent nerve impulses travel via the carotid sinus nerve to reach the respiratory centre in the brain; efferent discharge from the centre leads to an increase in the respiratory rate.

There are two views with regard to the oxygen sensor responsible for the immediate and rapid response to hypoxia. One view holds that the oxygen sensor is mitochondrial cytochrome oxidase which through oxidative phosphorylation transmits information to the rest of the cell. The other view holds that glomus cells within the carotid body have sensitive potassium channels, whose conductance is lowered with decreasing oxygen pressure. Perhaps both mitochondrial cytochrome oxidase and potassium ion channels act as sensors and are responsible for the sensitivity to change in oxygen pressure.

In the 1960s, Lahire and Milledge working at high altitudes in the Himalayas and Servinghaus and co-workers working in the South American high mountains with natives living at these altitudes noted that these subjects showed a diminished or blunted ventilatory response to an acute reduction in the inspired PO_2. It was uncertain whether this was related to genetic factors or whether this was an acquired trait related to exposure to chronic hypoxia. The conclusion was that the adaptive response to acute hypoxia was more due to environmental than genetic factors.

CHANGES IN THE PULMONARY CIRCULATION

The pulmonary circulation is a low-pressure, high-flow, high-volume circulation which easily accommodates the whole cardiac output that passes through it, not only at rest but also at exercise. This is because of the very low vascular resistance of the pulmonary vessels compared to the high vascular resistance observed in the systemic circulation. Hypoxia observed at high altitude alters the haemodynamics of the pulmonary circulation. It causes vasoconstriction of the pulmonary vessels resulting in both systolic and diastolic pulmonary hypertension. The higher the altitude the more severe the pulmonary vasoconstriction, and the higher the pulmonary hypertension. This has been observed in several studies. Though the pulmonary vasculature is supplied by both sympathetic (vasoconstrictor) and parasympathetic (vasodilator) fibres, vascular tone is chiefly governed by the PO_2 and PCO_2 in the alveoli. A fall in the alveolar PO_2 leads to pulmonary vasoconstriction and a shunting of blood away from alveoli with a low P_AO_2 to those which have a normal P_AO_2. A rise in alveolar PCO_2 (P_ACO_2) also causes well-marked vasoconstriction of the pulmonary vessels and pulmonary

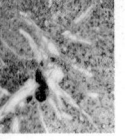

hypertension, in strong contrast to dilatation of the systemic vessels when the $PaCO_2$ is raised.

Exercise at high altitude (as for example in climbers negotiating a steep slope) further increases pulmonary arterial pressure and pulmonary hypertension. The pulmonary hypertension caused by acute hypoxia lasting for just a few hours, regresses with a return to normal pulmonary artery pressures once acute hypoxia is relieved. If hypoxia continues for several weeks as in mountaineers on a mountaineering expedition, pulmonary artery pressure does not decline quickly after return to lower altitudes or to sea level. It takes days, perhaps weeks before pulmonary vasoconstriction and muscularization of the pulmonary vessel walls regress and the pulmonary artery pressure returns to normal. Prolonged hypoxia (as in an expedition to the Himalayas) leads not only to pulmonary hypertension but right ventricular hypertrophy. The latter also regresses over time on a return to sea level.

EFFECTS OF LIVING AT HIGH ALTITUDE

People living at a high altitude (9000 to 12000 feet above sea level) have an increase in pulmonary artery pressure so that there is an appreciable increase in the gradient between the pulmonary artery diastolic pressure and the left atrial pressure (as judged by the capillary wedge pressure or the pulmonary artery occlusion pressure through a Swan-Ganz Catheter). This may not be always evident at rest but is promptly brought on at exercise. Chronic hypoxia in patients living at high altitude leads to increased levels of erythropoetin which causes well-marked polycythemia. Chronic hypoxia also stimulates ventilation, thereby causing hypocapnia and a rise in arterial pH. There is also an increase in 2–3 diphosphoglyerate. The increased affinity of haemoglobin (Hb) for oxygen caused by respiratory alkalosis is balanced to an extent by the decreased affinity of Hb for oxygen caused by an increase in 2–3 diphosphoglycerate. As mentioned earlier, studies have shown that over time the increased ventilatory response to hypoxia is often blunted in people living at high altitudes.

CLINICAL DISORDERS OF HIGH ALTITUDE

Clinical disorders of high altitude include acute mountain sickness (AMS), high-altitude pulmonary oedema, high-altitude cerebral oedema and chronic mountain sickness. While these are generally observed at a height of 10,000 feet or greater, they may occasionally be observed at altitudes of just 8,000 feet. All these entities are of crucial importance to India for several reasons. There are a number of tourist resorts, places of tourist interest and religious temples on sites at altitudes more than 8,000 feet. These include Gulmarg, Khilanmarg, the Kolhoi glacier in Kashmir, religious sites as the Amarnath Caves (Kashmir) and Mount Kailash along Lake Mansarovar, which is at an altitude of 14,900 feet. Gangotri, another important pilgrim town on the Greater Himalayan range is at an altitude of 12,313 feet. Leh, the capital of Ladakh stands at an attitude of 11,483 feet. Tanglang La, probably the highest motorable pass travelled by lay people, tourists and soldiers which connects Leh to Manali in Northeast India is as high as 17,469 feet.

Jawans of the Indian army live on and guard the Siachen glacier which is at an altitude of 18,875 ft. The recently fought Kargil war in which Pakistani soldiers were ferreted out successfully by Indian jawans was fought at high altitudes.

Finally, the largest numbers of climbing expeditions in the whole world are directed to reaching the formidable heights of Himalayans peaks. These include for example, Mt. Everest, Mounts K2, Annapurna, Nanga Parbat and several others.

Mountaineers also climb Alpine peaks and many of the high peaks in the Andes in South America, Kilimanjaro in Africa, as also mountain peaks in North America, Australia, and other high mountains.

ACUTE MOUNTAIN SICKNESS

Acute mountain sickness (AMS) affects healthy individuals who ascend too rapidly to high altitudes. The incidence depends on the rate of ascent and the altitude reached, the quicker the ascent and higher the altitude the greater the likelihood of AMS. The incidence of AMS has unquestionably increased with the sharp rise in tourist traffic and quicker modes of travel to high-altitude resorts and for other reasons already stated above. Among trekkers trekking to the Mt. Everest base camp the incidence was 43% at 4300 meters and was noted to be higher in those who had flown to an airstrip at 2800 meters compared to those who had trekked all the way up to the base camp.

Clinical Features

Symptoms begin within 2 hours to a few days after reaching high altitude. The first and invariable symptom is headache. There is an inability to sleep, sleep being disturbed by nightmares. Nausea, vomiting and malaise are often observed. In mountaineers, a reduced or poor climbing ability is noted. This mild or benign form of AMS resolves in three to five days and then generally does not recur unless the individual goes on to an even higher height. In some individuals AMS takes on a very serious form and progresses to high-altitude pulmonary oedema and/or high-altitude cerebral oedema. Unless promptly treated these conditions are generally fatal.

Pathogenesis

The pathogenesis of AMS is related to two factors. The trigger factor is unquestionably hypoxia due to high altitude. Yet AMS may occur after a few days of reaching a high altitude, and hypoxia should be maximum on immediately reaching a particular altitude. The reason for the delay in symptoms is therefore not easily explained. The second factor is cerebral oedema. Symptoms in AMS are similar to those observed with increased intracranial pressure, notably the occurrence of headache and vomiting. Also, evidence of increased intracranial pressure has been observed in patients with high-altitude cerebral oedema. The current concept is that even in the usual AMS, subclinical pulmonary oedema and a mild degree of cerebral oedema are responsible for the presenting symptoms of the disease. There is also perhaps an increased capillary permeability in patients with AMS as periorbital oedema, puffiness of the face and dependent oedema may be observed.

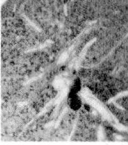

Prevention

Ascent should be gradual. It is advised that over 10,000 feet, ascent should not exceed 1000 feet per day with a rest period of preferably two to three days. Some manifest AMS on further ascent even after the precautions; others can climb higher with lesser periods of acclimatization. If symptoms of AMS occur ascent should stop. If symptoms persist or become more severe, rapid descent to a lower altitude is advisable.

Acetazolamide and dexamethasone are the two established drugs for prevention. Acetazolamide (250 mg) for several days after arrival may reduce headache, improve sleep and reduce or abolish other symptoms. The drug may also be started as a preventive measure for AMS two to three days before arrival at a high altitude. Dexamethasone 4 mg, six to eight-hourly, is also of use, particularly in patients allergic to sulpha drugs. Acetazolamide and dexamethasone may well have an additive effect. Drug therapy should continue till acclimatization occurs after two to four days.

Treatment

Mild AMS is treated symptomatically, headache being relieved by paracetamol or by the use of non-steroidal anti-inflammatory drugs such as ibuprofen. Acetazolamide and dexamethasone are the drugs to use if symptoms are bothersome or for rapidly evolving symptoms. If high-altitude pulmonary oedema or high-altitude cerebral oedema occur, urgent management as described below should be instituted, else death results.

HIGH-ALTITUDE PULMONARY OEDEMA

In most individuals AMS is a nuisance which resolves on its own in a few days. In a small minority of individuals ascending to high altitude, a potentially lethal complication is high-altitude pulmonary and/or high-altitude cerebral oedema. The frequency depends on the rate of ascent, the altitude reached and the rest periods at lower level altitudes to allow for acclimatization. It is less likely to occur in those already living at higher altitudes compared to 'lowlanders'. Individuals who have experienced high-altitude pulmonary oedema are at greater risk of developing high-altitude problems on a repeat ascent. Individuals who are acclimatized to high altitudes (for example, soldiers stationed at an altitude of 17,500 feet) lose their acclimatization when they descend to sea level. They remain at risk for high-altitude pulmonary oedema or high-altitude cerebral oedema if they are once again posted at that altitude. The crucial point to remember is that athletic fitness or prowess in no way influences or affords protection from high-altitude pulmonary oedema. Men and women at all ages may succumb though younger individuals seem more at risk than others.

Clinical Features

Symptoms typically occur in young individuals who have ascended to a high altitude quickly (without a period of acclimatization) and who exert unduly or are very active on arrival. Symptoms of AMS may precede high-altitude pulmonary oedema but not necessarily so. Initial symptoms are breathlessness and cough. The cough is initially dry, then productive, the patient expectorating frothy sputum often tinged with blood. Breathlessness increases rapidly and the patient shows evidence of central cyanosis. Tachycardia, tachypnoea and later, hypotension occur. Auscultation reveals crackles starting at the bases and then involving the whole of both lungs. The jugular venous pressure is elevated. Palpation reveals right ventricular heave, while auscultation reveals an accentuated pulmonary component of the second heart sound. Dependent oedema may be present. The whole scenario may evolve with frightening rapidity, often within a matter of a few hours. Death occurs from gross pulmonary oedema, severe hypoxemia, the patient often lapsing into coma towards the end.

Pathogenesis

It is now accepted that high-altitude pulmonary oedema is not due to left ventricular failure, the pulmonary artery occlusion pressure being always reported as normal.

The accepted pathogenesis is that high-altitude pulmonary oedema is caused by severe, quickly evolving hypoxic pulmonary vasoconstriction causing severe pulmonary hypertension. The hypoxic pulmonary vasoconstrictive response is uneven within the lungs. In areas where the vasoconstrictive response is very severe, the alveoli (in these areas) are protected from pulmonary oedema. In areas where the pulmonary vasoconstriction though present is less marked, the increased blood flow is associated with pulmonary oedema. Oedema in these areas may be due to several causes—increased intra-capillary pressure, flow-related damage to capillary walls, sheer stress damaging capillary walls. Increased permeability of capillary endothelium due to kinins or cytokine release may also play a role.

Prevention

The prophylactic use of nifedipine 20 mg twice daily prior to ascent and then 20 mg thrice daily has been shown to reduce the incidence of high-altitude pulmonary oedema. The mean pulmonary artery pressure is reduced. Surprisingly, nifidepine is of no use in the prophylaxis of AMS.

Inhaled β_2 agonists are also believed to reduce the risk of high-altitude pulmonary oedema.

Treatment

The following are the principles of management:

1. Recognition of the problem in its incipient stage. A dry cough and breathlessness portend disaster if the significance of these symptoms is not promptly realized.
2. Immediate descent to a lower altitude.
3. While arrangements for the above are made, supplemental oxygen should be administered at a high flow rate through a mask with a reservoir bag, so as to allow an $FIO_2 > 90\%$.
4. Nifedipine 10 mg sublingually is tried. If there is no undue hypotension the dose is repeated every 15 minutes.
5. The use of intravenous frusemide in a titrated dose, to increase urine output and help reduce pulmonary oedema may be of some help.

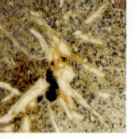

6. The role of sildenafil (which lowers pulmonary artery pressure) both for prophylaxis and treatment awaits evaluation.

7. Some well-equipped mountaineering expeditions include a portable hyperbaric chamber. If available, it should be used while awaiting arrangements for quick descent.

HIGH-ALTITUDE CEREBRAL OEDEMA

High-altitude cerebral oedema (HACE) in its early stage is characterized by persistent headache, nausea, vomiting and is indistinguishable from AMS. The occurrence of blurred vision and ataxia is a warning of a potentially lethal, quickly-evolving cerebral oedema. Truncal ataxia (ataxia on sitting is often a prominent symptom. Confusion, hallucinations, and obtundation progressing to an unconscious state occur. Plantars are often extensor and the fundus on examination reveals papilloedema. There may be associated features of high-altitude pulmonary oedema. If not promptly recognized and treated death preceded by coma is inevitable.

Treatment

Swift descent to a low altitude or to sea level is (as in high-altitude pulmonary oedema) of crucial importance.

Supplemental oxygen should be given as explained under high-altitude pulmonary oedema.

Dexamethosone 4 to 8 mg, four to six-hourly intravenously or intramuscularly is given in the hope of reducing cerebral oedema.

Mannitol IV 150 to 300 ml given as a quick infusion (if available) may also help.

Frusemide 40 to 80 mg intravenously may be of marginal benefit. Portable hyperbaric chamber if available should be used while awaiting arrangement for descent.

CHRONIC MOUNTAIN SICKNESS

Chronic mountain sickness (CMS) affects residents at a high altitude. It was first described by Carlos Monge who reported polycythemia in those living at high altitude in the Andes (Monge's disease).

CMS is commoner in males and occurs generally in middle and later life. Its main features are severe polycythemia with Hb concentration > 20 g/dl and with hematocrits as high as 80%. The cause is chronic hypoxia operating over a long period of many years.

Patients generally have neuropsychiatric symptoms, consisting of headache, dizziness, inability to concentrate, fatigue and poor effort tolerance. Symptoms characteristically disappear on descent to sea level but reappear on a return to high altitude.

In severe CMS, the lips and mucosa appear cyanosed (because of the marked increase in reduced Hb), the conjuctiva shows marked congestion and the fingers are clubbed. Florid signs are particularly observed in Andes Indians who have the highest prevalence rate of CMS.

Milder forms of CMS (in those residing at not very high altitudes) may have few or even no symptoms, the problem being suspected in residents at high altitude who are discovered to have polycythemia. Patients with mild disease bear a close resemblance to patients with chronic obstructive pulmonary disease with hypoxemia and secondary polycythemia.

Treatment

The clinical features improve if those severely afflicted were to shift residence to sea level. But for many residing at high altitudes this is not practical. These patients should have repeated phlebotomies to lower the hematocrit if possible to < 50% and the Hb < 16 g/dl. This provides relief from many of the neuropsychiatric symptoms observed in severe cases. Supplemental oxygen is also of help.

The long-term use of respiratory stimulants such as medroxyprogesterone has been advocated as an alternative to phlebotomy. Acetazolamide is not as effective as in AMS, but may be used to increase O_2 saturation during sleep and perhaps reduce the haematocrit. The role of sildenafil and of newer drugs used for the reduction of pulmonary hypertension is yet to be evaluated.

SUGGESTED READING

Basnyat B, Murdoch DR. High-altitude illness. *Lancet.* 7 Jun. 2003; 361(9373):1967–74.

Luks AM. Travel to high altitude with pre-existing lung disease. *Eur Respir J.* 1 Apr. 2007; 29(4): 770–92.

Sartori C, Allemann, *et al.* Salmeterol for the prevention of high-altitude pulmonary edema. *N Engl J Med.* 2002; 346: 1631–6.

Singh I, Roy SB. High altitude pulmonary edema: Clinical, hemodynamic, and pathologic studies. In: *Biomedical Problems of High Terrestrial Elevations*, Hegnauer A (ed.), Federal Scientific Technical Information Service, Springfield, Va 1962. p.108.

Voelkel, N. High-altitude pulmonary edema. *N Engl J Med.* 2002; 346: 1606–7.

CHAPTER **70** | # Adverse Drug Reactions on the Lung

Almost all drugs which are therapeutically effective can produce adverse effects, some more than others. One is reminded of Osler's saying: 'If all drugs in the pharmacopoeia were thrown into the sea, it would be bad for the fish and good for man.' The pharmacopoeia has increased by geometric progression since Osler's time. More so today than in earlier years, the saying is a reminder to all physicians to use drugs only when indicated (easier said than done) with due circumspection and with a keen awareness of their adverse effects.

A large number of drugs produce adverse effects on the lungs and it is impossible to detail each of them in this chapter. Adverse reactions may involve the airways, the lung parenchyma, the pleura, the pulmonary circulation and the mediastinum. Drugs can also cause a systemic adverse reaction, the reaction within the lung being just a part of this reaction. An example is drug-induced systemic lupus erythematosus (SLE) or drug-induced vasculitis which also involves the lung.

This chapter will go on to state the importance of recognizing an adverse drug-induced reaction on the lung and the difficulties in diagnosis; it then briefly gives the mechanisms involved in these adverse reactions. The patterns of clinical presentation of adverse reactions are then described, followed finally by adverse reactions caused by certain important frequently used individual drugs.

IMPORTANCE OF RECOGNIZING AN ADVERSE DRUG REACTION ON THE LUNG

Recognition is important for several reasons—

1. It prevents further unnecessary diagnostic tests and further unnecessary use of extra drugs. Stopping the drug and observing the reversal or persistence of suspected adverse reactions would be the right approach.
2. Recognizing the incriminating drug and stopping it would prevent further damage to the lung.
3. Some adverse lung reactions to drugs are treatable; this can only happen if they are correctly recognized.

DIFFICULTIES IN DIAGNOSIS

Diagnosis of drug-induced lung disease even if one were keenly aware of this entity can be difficult for the following reasons:

1. Drug-induced lung toxicity may mimic clinical features of pulmonary involvement from the underlying disease.
2. An important drug-induced lung toxicity is pneumonitis. An immunocompromised patient may develop pneumonitis

due to an infective agent. There are no distinguishing features clinically or radiologically between these two forms of pneumonitis. The importance of excluding an infective aetiology before considering drug-induced lung toxicity cannot be overstressed. Unfortunately, this may not always be possible.

3. Ill individuals are often given a number of drugs each of which may have potential adverse effects on the lung. To determine causality in relation to a specific drug may be impossibly difficult.
4. A wrong diagnosis of drug-induced lung toxicity can have an adverse effect on the patient's recovery just because an effective and important drug is withdrawn when it should have been continued.

Table 70.1: Diagnosis of drug induced pulmonary toxicity
1. Awareness of possible pulmonary toxicity in related to drug use
2. Pattern or nature of lung toxicity and whether it is associated with the drug in use
3. Compatible clinical, lung function and imaging features
4. Exclusion of other pathologies in particular infective aetiologies. BAL study necessary in most cases
5. Measurable effect of drug withdrawal

MECHANISM OF DRUG-RELATED LUNG TOXICITY

Underlying mechanisms are as follows:

1. Adverse effect on the airways causing smooth muscle contraction, bronchospasm, dyspnoea.
2. Increase in endothelial permeability resulting in pulmonary oedema.
3. Drug induced inflammation through a drug metabolite or drug + haptene; the inflammation could involve the lung parenchyma, the airways, or the pleura.
4. Increased fibrinogenesis which can lead to pulmonary fibrosis, bronchiolitis obliterans, pulmonary hypertension, veno-occlusive disease, the pathology and clinical features depending on the site of fibrogenesis with resulting fibrosis.
5. Severe bleeding within the lungs or pleural space caused either by anticoagulants or in rare instances by a drug-induced capillaritis.

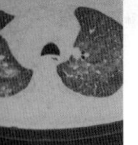

Table 70.2:
Nature and site of drug induced lung toxicity

I. Parenchymal Injury

    Hypersensitivity pneumonitis

    Eosinophilic pneumonia

    Diffuse alveolar injury

    Granulomatous inflammation

    Organising pneumonia

    Diffuse alveolar haemorrhage

    Pulmonary fibrosis

II. Airway Injury

    Acute bronchospasm

    Upper airways obstruction

    Obliterative bronchiolitis

    Cough

III. Pleural Injury

    Pleural effusion

IV. Injury to the pulmonary circulation

    Pulmonary hypertension

    Obstruction to the pulmonary circulation through various causes

V. Drug induced SLE

VI. Neuromuscular disorders

DRUG-INDUCED ADVERSE EFFECTS ON THE LUNG

ADVERSE EFFECTS ON THE LUNG PARENCHYMA

Hypersensitivity Pneumonitis

Hypersensitivity pneumonitis can be caused by a number of drugs, the important ones being nitrofurantoin, methotrexate, sirolimus, gold.

Hypersensitivity pneumonitis can occur acutely as is seen with methotrexate or gold toxicity or it could be subacute as with adverse effects related to nitrofurantoin and sirolimus.

Systemic features include fever, malaise, and arthralgias. Respiratory symptoms which accompany or follow systemic features are dry cough with breathlessness. Pneumonitis is often bilateral though one lung may be more involved than the other. Severe forms of hypersensitivity pneumonitis as in methotrexate toxicity can lead to acute respiratory failure.

Radiography of the chest shows multiple shadows, the mid-zones and bases being more involved. High-resolution computed tomography (HRCT) of the chest reveals multiple streaky linear interstitial shadows, intralobular shadows with ground-glass opacities.

The more acute cases often show areas of alveolar consolidation with air bronchograms; the alveolar shadows may be focal, diffuse or rarely, lobar in distribution.

The clinical and imaging findings are in no way specific for lung-induced toxicity. Similar findings occur with diverse lung infections. It is vital to exclude an infective aetiology, particularly in patients who are immunosuppressed because of their background disease or because of immunosuppressant therapy or because of both. Bronchoalveolar lavage (BAL) study to detect a possible infectious aetiology in addition to the clinical and imaging findings is almost always necessary in patients who have no sputum.

Histopathological confirmation through a transbronchial or thoracoscopic biopsy is usually not necessary. Biopsy studies when done show interstitial inflammation with a mononuclear infiltrate, the pathology resembling that of non-specific interstitial pneumonia.

Treatment consists of withdrawal of the drug. Corticosteroids are unquestionably effective and should be used in the presence of breathlessness, hypoxia and diffuse lung involvement. Most physicians would use corticosteroids on any patient who is symptomatic from interstitial pneumonia. Complete recovery ensues after drug withdrawal. The drug in question should never be exhibited again as drug toxicity towards the lung can be even more violent. This is particularly so with reference to methotrexate.

Diffuse Alveolar Damage

Diffuse alveolar damage (DAD) is a dangerous form of drug toxicity involving the lungs. It occurs acutely or subacutely and is a complication following the use of antineoplastic drugs in multidrug chemotherapeutic regimes. The condition is often termed as the 'chemotherapy lung'. Drugs incriminated in causing this adverse reaction are bleomycin, mitomycin C, busulphan, cyclophosphamide, chlorambucil, and melphalan. Many other antimitotic drugs are believed to have the potential to cause DAD. These include antimetabolites like azathioprine, methotrexate, 6-metacaptopurine. Others in the category are the newer nitrosoureas like etoposide and the taxanes tyrosine kinase inhibitors such as gefitinib and imatinib and the granulocyte monocyte colony-stimulating factors (so often used to counter severe leucopenia following the use of antimitotic drugs).

DAD is characterized by dyspnoea, cough, and diffuse infiltrates which on radiographic examination of the chest cause a diffuse haze, and on CT scan diffuse bilateral ground-glass opacities. In its most severe form DAD manifests as acute respiratory distress syndrome (ARDS) with respiratory distress, increasing hypoxemia and total white-out lungs. Patients with solid tumours and a high tumour load are at risk after chemotherapy (particularly the first chemotherapy). They may develop the tumour lysis syndrome where lysis of tumour cells can result in DAD and even multiorgan failure.

The differential diagnosis of drug-induced DAD is from fluid overload, left ventricular failure, transfusion-related lung injury, alveolar haemorrhage and infections. Infections could be bacterial, viral, fungal or parasitic; opportunistic infections are especially important in patients with mitotic disease who are on antimitotic drugs.

Biopsy is generally not possible as these patients are very ill. Histopathology determined from autopsy studies shows varying degree of cellular inflammatory exudate, diffuse alveolar damage, alveolar oedema and hyaline membrane formation.

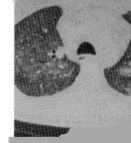

Treatment is supportive. Ventilator support is often necessary. Corticosteroids may be used but the response is unpredictable. The offending chemotherapeutic agent should never be used again.

Eosinophilic Pneumonia

Eosinophilic pneumonia is a classic and generally easily recognizable complication of drug therapy. The drugs known to cause eosinophilic pneumonia are minocycline, sulpha drugs, non-steroidal anti-inflammatory drugs (NSAIDs), anti-epileptics (like carbamezapine, phenytoin), antidepressants and a few others. Eosinophilic pneumonia is characterized by fever, cough, breathlessness, eosinophilic pulmonary infiltrates and peripheral eosinophilia. A BAL study is useful as the BAL fluid contains an excess of eosinophils.

The condition may be mild or even asymptomatic, being discovered on radiographic examination as a peripheral shadow which disappears after drug withdrawal, in two to four weeks. On the other hand, the condition may be severe with diffuse pulmonary infiltrates causing dyspnoea and respiratory failure. Eosinophilic pneumonia may be accompanied by an eosinophilic pleural effusion. The more serious forms of eosinophilic pneumonia are sometimes observed following use of minocycline and occasionally following use of nitrofurantoin.

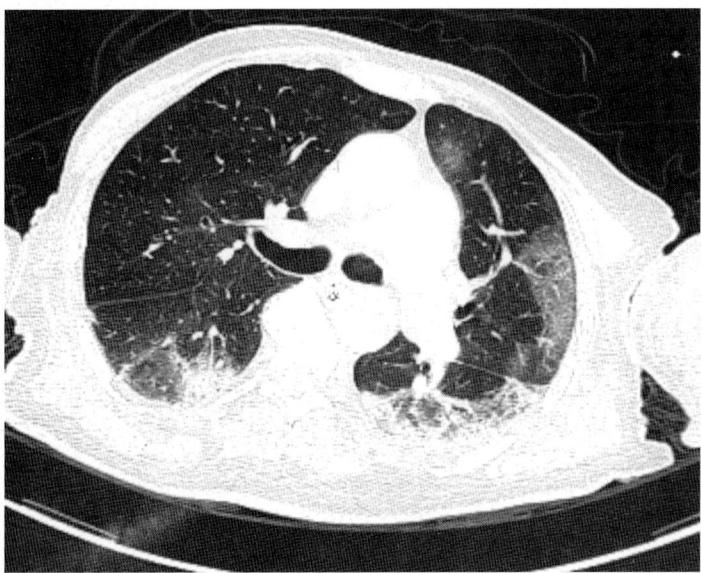

Fig 70.1: Eosinophilic pneumonia following a sulpha drug. CT chest shows ill-defined areas of ground-glass densities in the left upper lobe anteriorly in a subpleural location as well as bilateral, subpleural areas of air space opacification posteriorly. The patient had well-marked eosinophilia. The shadows disappeared after stopping the drug.

A few patients (generally on minocycline or anticonvulsants), in addition to eosinophilic pneumonia, develop a severe cutaneous drug rash together with systemic symptoms probably related to the eosinophilic involvement of other organ systems. This is the DRESS syndrome—drug rash with eosinophilia and systemic symptoms. The syndrome should be promptly recognized; the offending drug should be stopped and treatment

with corticosteroids instituted. The outcome of drug-induced eosinophilic pneumonia is good if promptly recognized and the offending drug is withdrawn. Corticosteroids hasten resolution and should always be used in symptomatic patients with diffuse pulmonary infiltrates.

Granulomatous Infiltrative Lung Disease

This is a rare pulmonary reaction observed with a few drugs, notably interferon α, β, etanercept, methotrexate and sirolimus. The granulomatous inflammation manifests as micronodular or linear pulmonary infiltrates which may be associated with hilar and mediastinal adenopathy. The picture bears a resemblance to sarcoidosis. The SACE level may be elevated. Transbronchial biopsy shows a granulomatous lesion suggesting the diagnosis.

Organizing Pneumonia

Organizing pneumonia (OP), also called bronchiolitis obliterans with OP is an uncommon reaction to drugs. It has been reported after treatment with amiodarone, nitrofurantoin, statins and interferon α, β. The disease manifests as single or multiple opacities within the lung. The opacities may be migratory. Clinical, radiological, histopathological features are the same as in idiopathic OP. OP responds well to drug withdrawal and corticosteroid therapy.

Diffuse Alveolar Haemorrhage

Diffuse alveolar haemorrhage (DAH) is characterized by bleeding into the alveoli. This causes dyspnoea and when severe results in hypoxemic respiratory failure. Haemoptysis, at times exsanguinating, is often present, but not always so. A sharp drop in haemoglobin is observed. BAL studies show blood-stained fluid with hemosiderin-laden macrophages. DAH is seen following

1. Use of anticoagulants, abciximab, fibrinolytic agents, clopidogrel, sirolimus
2. In drug-induced severe thrombocytopenia e.g. following use of abciximab
3. A capillaritis occurring in isolation or as part of a drug-induced micropolyangiitis as following use of penicillamine, hydrazaline.

TREATMENT

Besides drug withdrawal severe DAH requires respiratory support. Pulsed doses of intravenous methyl prednisolone 0.5 G IV daily for three days are helpful when bleeding is related to capillaritis. Bleeding related to coagulation defects needs appropriate replacement of clotting factors, and that related to thrombocytopenia needs infusion of platelet concentrates.

Pulmonary Fibrosis

Pulmonary fibrosis is most often seen as a delayed reaction to antimitotic drugs. The drugs proven to cause pulmonary fibrosis are bleomycin (the most frequent cause), as also busulphan, chlorambucil, cyclophosphamide, nitrosoureas BCNU and

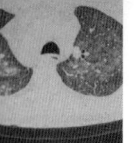

CCNU. Besides drugs used in oncology, the one other major drug known to result in pulmonary fibrosis is amiodarone.

Drug-induced pulmonary fibrosis can develop acutely with rapidly evolving fibrosis within the lung, or soon after drug therapy, or develop insidiously so as to manifest several months or even years after drug therapy.

Clinical features include progressive breathlessness, cough and dry velcro crackles at bases. Severe fibrosis as with bleomycin toxicity or in a few patients with amiodarone toxicity can cause crippling breathlessness and hypoxic respiratory failure.

Chest radiography shows basal interstitial shadows. HRCT shows a reticulo-nodular pattern, subpleural fibrosis with honeycombing at the bases. Fibrosis induced by cyclophosphamide has a predilection for the apices with retraction of the chest wall over the upper lobes. Drug withdrawal is imperative. A varying degree of improvement with corticosteroids is observed if the problem is detected early. Advanced pulmonary fibrosis (the condition being undetected or detected late), shows no response to steroid therapy. Lung transplant is an option to be considered in these patients.

Pulmonary Oedema

Pulmonary oedema as a manifestation of drug toxicity is due to drug-induced increased capillary permeability. Drugs incriminated include antimitotic drugs docetaxel, andgemcitabine; pulmonary oedema occurs during or soon after use of these antimitotic agents. Pulmonary oedema has also been observed after the use of hydrochlorothiazide salicylates, interleukin-2, high doses of intravenous beta agonists or following blood transfusion or transfusion of blood products (transfusion-related acute lung injury, TRALI). Drugs used for ovarian stimulation for purpose of in-vitro fertilization can lead to dangerous pulmonary oedema due to a pronounced capillary leak (ovarian hyperstimulation syndrome).

Clinical manifestations are cough, breathlessness and in severe cases hypoxemic respiratory failure. Imaging appearances are those of diffuse bilateral shadowing as is seen with any form of pulmonary oedema.

Treatment consists of drug withdrawal, use of oxygen and in severe cases, ventilator support.

ADVERSE EFFECT ON AIRWAYS

Acute bronchospasm

The three most common drugs causing acute bronchospasm are aspirin, nonsteroidal anti-inflammatory drugs (NSAIDs) and beta blockers. Although acute bronchospasm with severe breathlessness can occur without warning in an individual who is not asthmatic, more often than not it occurs in those who have asthma or chronic obstructive pulmonary disease. These drugs should therefore be avoided in asthmatics. The triad of nasal polyposis, with nasal allergy, asthma often difficult to control, and intolerance to aspirin or NSAID is an established entity. Bronchospasm after inadvertent use of aspirin or NSAID in asthmatics may occur within minutes or after a few hours. If may be severe enough to cause death from asphyxia.

Beta blocker-induced bronchospasm in asthmatics may also cause severe airways obstruction which may be resistant to β_2 agonists because of the prevailing β blockade.

Upper Airways Obstruction

Angiotensin-converting enzyme (ACE) inhibitors are known to occasionally cause angio-oedema with upper airways obstruction. This may occur at any time in the course of therapy. Angio-oedema results in swelling of the tongue and back of the throat with an obstructed upper airway.

Anaphylaxis from any drug to which a patient is severely allergic can cause upper airways obstruction together with severe bronchospasm and even seizures.

Treatment consists of promptly securing the airways, use of adrenaline, anti-histaminics, corticosteroids and the use of resuscitative measures and supportive care.

Bronchiolitis Obliterans

Bronchiolitis obliterans is reported to be a rare complication following the use of penicillamine in rheumatoid arthritis. It causes progressive dyspnoea and cough. Physical examination may be normal or there may be scattered auscultatory high-pitched squeaks or crackles. Chest radiography shows hyperinflated lungs. HRCT shows clear evidence of air trapping with a mosaic appearance. The pathology consists of narrowing of the smaller bronchioles through lymphocytic infiltration of the walls and fibrosis. Drug withdrawal should be prompt; use of corticosteroids may help.

Cough

ACE inhibitors produce a troublesome dry cough in about 30% of patients using the drugs. Angiostensin II receptor antagonists can also cause cough but less frequently than the ACE inhibitors. Cough usually occurs within a month of therapy, but can occur much later as well. The pathogenesis is not clear. It is not generally associated with airways obstruction. Stopping the drug abolishes cough. It takes two to three weeks for symptoms to abate completely.

ADVERSE EFFECTS ON THE PLEURA

Drugs causing an eosinophilic pneumonia described earlier can also cause an eosinophilic pleural effusion.

A pleural exudate may accompany the pulmonary toxicity of amiodarone, methotrexate and nitrofurantoin.

Ergot compounds and methlysergide may cause well-marked bilateral pleural thickening and fibrosis leading to fibrothorax, which may evolve gradually over months or years. Increasing dyspnoea is the presenting clinical feature. Pleural pain may be accompanied by a pleural rub. Imaging studies (best visualized on CT) show extensive pleural thickening with underlying areas of rounded atelectasis. Lung function studies show a restrictive pattern.

ADVERSE EFFECTS ON THE PULMONARY CIRCULATION

Diffuse alveolar haemorrhage has been dealt with earlier. Pulmonary hypertension was the dreadful effect observed following the use of the anorectic drug, aminorex. It took several years before this dangerous toxic effect was realized. Newer anorectic drugs fenfluramine, dexfenfluramine also cause pulmonary hypertension.

Pulmonary veno-occlusive disease is a rare condition characterized by obliteration of pulmonary venules. It causes pulmonary oedema and later, pulmonary hypertension. Progressive dyspnoea and pulmonary congestion in the absence of cardiomegaly are the main features. The disease has been reported following use of a number of cytotoxic drugs, following radiation, or following marrow transplant.

Acrylate glue used to obliterate intracranial arteriovenous fistulas in the brain or elsewhere may spill into the systemic circulation and then go on to plug several pulmonary vessels, causing chest pain and dyspnoea.

In the same manner, cement injected to stabilize a vertebral body involved in an osteoporotic fracture or fracture from metastasis or multiple myeloma, can result in pulmonary embolism.

Use of silicon injection for breast enlargement or for changing body shape can also cause vascular damage to the pulmonary circulation and result rarely in alveolar haemorrhage.

THE DRUG-INDUCED SYSTEMIC LUPUS ERYTHEMATOSUS SYNDROME

The systemic lupus erythematosus (SLE) syndrome is known to occur after the use of some drugs, the most common being isoniazid, hydralazine, procainamide and diphenylhydantoin. Interferon and TNF α antibody have also been reported to do so. The incidence of pleuropulmonary symptoms is high with drug-induced SLE, whereas renal and neurological involvement is rare. Antibodies to histones are believed to be present in drug-induced SLE. Withdrawal of the offending drug leads to a disappearance of SLE.

NEUROMUSCULAR ADVERSE EFFECTS

Aminoglycosides, muscle relaxants, neuroleptics, corticosteroids, opiates, either inhibit the neural drive or induce a neuromuscular blockade, or cause peripheral neuropathy or a myopathy. Hypoventilation with hypercapnic respiratory failure may follow.

SPECIFIC DRUGS

The drugs briefly discussed below are rather arbitrarily chosen. They however are in frequent use and therefore their adverse effects need to be always kept in mind.

Nitrofurantoin

This drug is very frequently used for treatment of urinary tract infection and as prophylaxis against urinary tract infection in certain circumstances. Even though adverse effects on the lung are rare (< 1%), they should be recognized as and when they occur.

Two forms of lung toxicity occur. The first is an acute hypersensitivity pneumonitis, the clinical and radiological features of which have been already described. Pleural effusion may accompany the pneumonitis. Systemic symptoms in the form of fever, chest pain, arthralgia and occasionally a macular rash may be present in association with cough and dyspnoea. Peripheral eosinophilia is present in most cases.

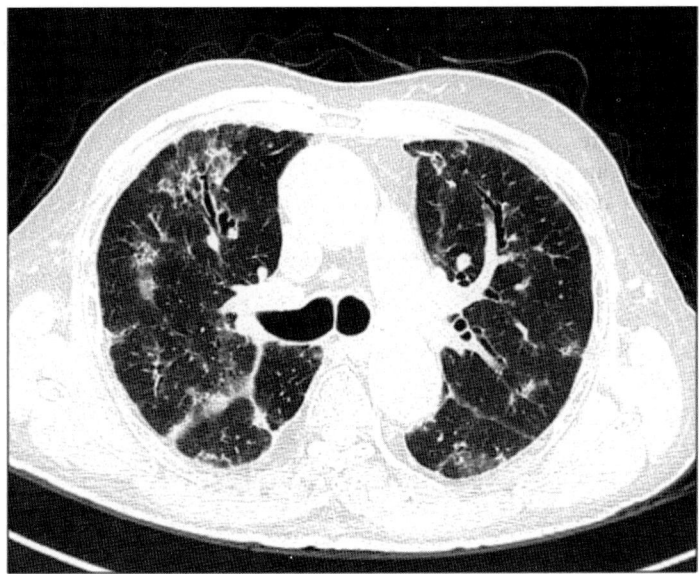

Fig 70.2: Nitrofurantoin toxicity. CT chest shows ill-defined peribronchial areas of air-space opacification with ground-glass densities and mild prominence of the bronchi bilaterally.

The second form is one which is often missed. It can occur after months while on therapy and is characterized by cough and breathlessness on exertion. Systemic features and peripheral eosinophilia are generally absent. Chest radiography shows interstitial infiltrates; occasionally, patchy opacities in peribronchovascular distribution are observed. Anti-nuclear antibodies may be present in the chronic form.

The prognosis is good for hypersensitivity pneumonitis if the drug is withdrawn. The chronic form of pneumonitis may persist in a number of patients even after drug withdrawal. Corticosteroids may help but their effect is not predictable.

Aspirin (Salicylates)

Severe aspirin-bronchospasm has already been described. Another adverse effect often missed is the occurrence of non-cardiogenic pulmonary oedema. This only occurs when salicylate levels are very high, generally > 40 mg/dL, as in individuals who have taken an overdose of aspirin with a suicidal intent or in older individuals who have dosed themselves for long and perhaps indiscriminately on salicylates for effective pain control. The clinical features are confusion, tachypnoea, auscultatory crackles more marked over the bases, together with metabolic acidosis and respiratory alkalosis. Chest radiography shows the presence of pulmonary oedema. A lack of awareness will lead to a missed diagnosis or a late diagnosis. The combination of metabolic acidosis + respiratory alkalosis should always arouse suspicion of salicylate intoxication. Treatment consists of forced alkaline diuresis and supportive care. Pulmonary oedema recedes once salicylate levels decline.

Amiodarone

Amiodarone is perhaps the most frequently used anti-arrhythmic drug today. Its adverse effects involve the eye, the liver, the thyroid gland, the skin and most important of all, the

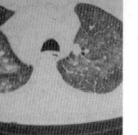

lung. Pulmonary toxicity occurs in 5–15% of patients and is the major reason for drug withdrawal. Several forms of amiodarone lung toxicity are observed. The commonest adverse reaction in the lung is an interstitial pneumonia starting and progressing slowly after weeks or months of drug therapy. The higher the maintenance dose the greater the risk. Maintenance doses of 400 mg/day or more carry greater risk. The clinical features are cough, breathlessness, auscultatory crackles over lower lobes, restrictive lung function and basal interstitial lesions on imaging studies.

The second form of amiodarone toxicity is an acute reversible pneumonia in which one or more pneumonic patches in the lung are associated with fever, cough, chest pain, breathlessness, leucocytosis and a raised erythrocyte sedimentation rate (ESR).

The third is the hyperacute life-threatening form producing the clinical and imaging features of acute respiratory distress syndrome (ARDS). This form generally occurs after cardiac surgery when high doses of IV amiodarone are given to counter arrhythmias during and after surgery. It also occurs when high IV doses of the drug are given over several days in patients with cardiac disorders (most often acute myocardial infarction) to counter dangerous recurrent arrhythmias. We have seen this toxicity develop within four to seven days of drug administration. The lung injury is perhaps aggravated in patients on ventilator support, particularly patients on large tidal volume and high FIO_2. The ARDS picture may resolve, or it may go on to a crippling irreversible pulmonary fibrosis, causing death. Occasionally, progressive pulmonary fibrosis occurs as an adverse reaction without the patient having experienced the acute drug toxicity just described. Amiodarone has also been reported to cause the clinical and radiological features of organizing pneumonia.

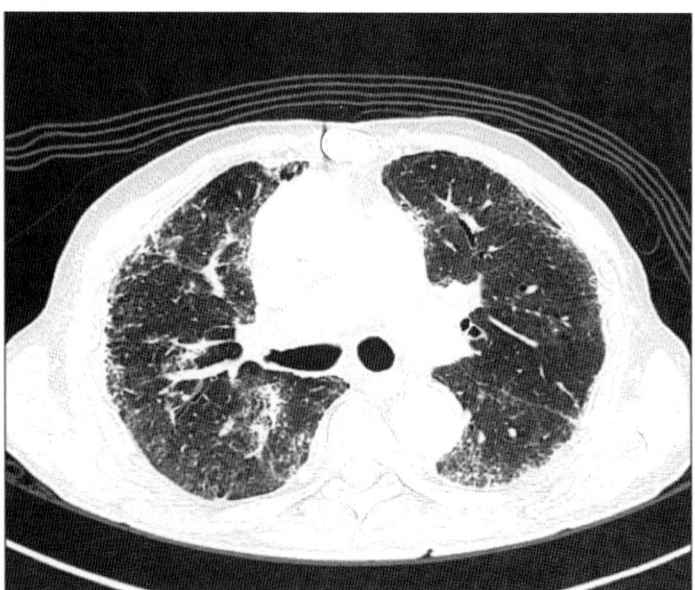

Fig 70.3: Amiodaraone toxicity. CT chest reveals ill-defined subpleural, reticular and peribronchovascular interstitial opacities with associated ground-glass densities. This patient was on amiodarone for several months and came with the history of increasing breathlessness. Pulmonary functions revealed a restrictive ventilatory pattern.

The usual slowly progressive chronic interstitial pneumonia caused by amiodarone is manifested on chest radiography by asymmetrical interstitial infiltrates, most marked over lung bases. In acute pneumonia there are both interstitial and alveolar shadows. The hyperacute form is characterized by bilateral fluffy shadows which progress to the usual radiological appearance of white-out lungs seen in ARDS. When amiodarone produces the adverse effects of organizing pneumonia, radiological appearances take the form of infiltrates, nodules or alveolar opacities that may be migratory in nature.

Gallium scans are positive in pulmonary toxicity following amiodarone and as mentioned earlier, lung function tests show restriction with a reduced CO diffusion.

DIAGNOSIS

The usual forms of pulmonary toxicity are generally recognizable provided the clinician is aware of their occurrence. The difficulty arises in recognizing the acute toxicity characterized by bilateral interstitial and alveolar opacities ultimately indistinguishable from ARDS. The difficulty is compounded in the presence of a critical illness following cardiac surgery or because of a primary cardiac problem. The differential diagnosis is between pulmonary oedema due to left ventricular failure, pulmonary infection and amiodarone toxicity. If good diuresis after frusemide produces no changes in the clinical and radiological picture, left ventricular failure is unlikely. Clinical examination and echocardiographic studies also help in the diagnosis of left ventricular dysfunction. It is indeed difficult to exclude nosocomial infection in these patients. Also, a patient may grow organisms from the endotracheal aspirate and yet have acute amiodarone toxicity. Presence of evolving fibrosis always points to amiodarone toxicity.

Once amiodarone toxicity is strongly suspected the drug should be withdrawn. This is particularly important if the acute or hyperacute forms of pulmonary toxicity are considered likely. Mere stoppage of the drug is not sufficient for resolution of the toxic effects on the lung, because the half-life of the drug is as long as 60 days. Corticosteroids 40 to 60 mg/day are given till resolution is observed and then slowly tapered over three to four months, else pulmonary toxicity may return because of the long half-life of the drug.

Mortality is high in the hyperacute form or in patients with ARDS who progress to crippling pulmonary fibrosis. Overall mortality is believed to be around 10%.

Two less commonly used drugs considered below are gold and d-penicillamine; both used in the treatment of rheumatoid disease. D-penicillamine is also used in the treatment of Wilson's disease.

Oral and Parenteral Gold

Both oral and parenteral gold can cause pulmonary toxicity. The most common manifestation is acute hypersensitivity pneumonitis, but occasionally organizing pneumonia is also observed. Pulmonary toxicity generally occurs within six months of therapy. Clinical features include cough, breathlessness and a skin rash; peripheral eosinophilia may also be present. Chest radiography shows bilateral diffuse reticular infiltrates. Drug withdrawal together with the use of corticosteroids is effective.

Fortunately, gold is rarely used today so that pulmonary toxicity following gold hardly to occurs.

D-Penicillamine

This drug, like gold, is very rarely used today. It serves as an illustration of possible pulmonary toxicity encountered in clinical practice. Lung toxicity attributed to d-penicillamine takes two forms.

1. Obliterative bronchiolitis which has been briefly described earlier and which is reported to occur only in patients with rheumatoid arthritis
2. Pulmonary renal syndrome which resembles Goodpasture's syndrome, only anti-glomerular basement membrane antibodies are absent. Patients developing pulmonary renal syndrome have acute respiratory distress, diffuse intraalveolar haemorrhage and haemoptysis. Treatment is with corticosteroids the use of immunosuppressants like cyclophosphamide or azathioprione and the use of plasmapheresis.

Infliximab and Etanercept

These are monoclonal human antibodies directed against tumour necrosis factor alpha (TNFα). Excessive production of the latter is responsible for inflammatory reactions central to the evolution of a number of diseases such as rheumatoid arthritis, ulcerative colitis and Crohn's disease. Both infliximab and etanercept are capable of producing long-lasting remissions in severe forms of the above diseases. These drugs however increase the risk of reactivation of infections caused by intracellular organisms, mainly tuberculosis and in special endemic areas fungal infections such as histoplasmosis.

Tuberculosis when it occurs does so within weeks or months of starting the drug, suggesting reactivation of the disease rather than fresh infection. Both pulmonary and extra-pulmonary tuberculosis may occur and may be difficult to treat.

Great circumspection is therefore required before using these drugs, particularly in developing countries such as India where the prevalence of tuberculosis is very high. A history of tuberculosis in the recent past, a positive Mantoux test or a positive 'Gold test' need to be considered in patient evaluation before starting therapy. Chemoprophylaxis with isoniazid or isoniazid and rifampicin also needs to be considered provided the regime does not seriously affect liver cell function.

There have been reports of non-necrotizing granulomatous lung disease, pulmonary fibrosis and ARDS in patients with rheumatoid arthritis who have been started on anti-TNF antibody therapy. These have been reported within a few weeks or months of therapy. A conclusive association between these disorders and the anti-TNF antibody therapy has not been established.

Antimitotic Cytotoxic Drugs

There has been a profusion of new and newer antimitotic cytotoxic drugs used as chemotherapy against cancer, solid tumours, lymphomas and haematological malignancies. It is well-nigh impossible to keep track of their adverse effects including toxic effects on the lungs. Their use and the recognition of side-effects on various organ systems including the lungs belong chiefly to the field of oncology. We will rest content by briefly describing the adverse effects on the lungs of a few commonly used antimitotic cytotoxic drugs.

Bleomycin

Bleomycin is used in chemotherapeutic regimes for a number of malignancies, particularly haematological malignancies. The drug is known to cause pulmonary fibrosis, the incidence of this toxicity being 5%. The incidence is 15% if sub-clinical toxicity as judged by lung function tests and HRCT is also taken into account. Though lung fibrosis is the chief toxic effect, acute hypersensitivity pneumonitis may also be occasionally observed.

There are certain important risk factors governing the occurrence and severity of pulmonary fibrosis. These are age > 70 years, rapid infusion instead of slow infusion of the drug, total dose of the drug received, the use of supplemental oxygen and multi-drug regimens. Although toxicity can occur with low doses, chances of toxicity increase with increasing dosage. Clinical features of pulmonary fibrosis include cough and increasing breathlessness. Auscultation reveals basal crackles. Severe fibrosis leads to hypoxemic respiratory failure. Chest radiography reveals diffuse interstitial infiltrates with small lung volumes. CT chest reveals subpleural fibrosis, interstitial thickening with fibrosis extending upwards to involve the greater part of the lungs. Alveolar shadows occur if the drug produces a hypersensitivity pneumonitis. CT changes may be seen even when the chest radiography is normal. Lung functions show a restrictive lesion with impaired CO transfer.

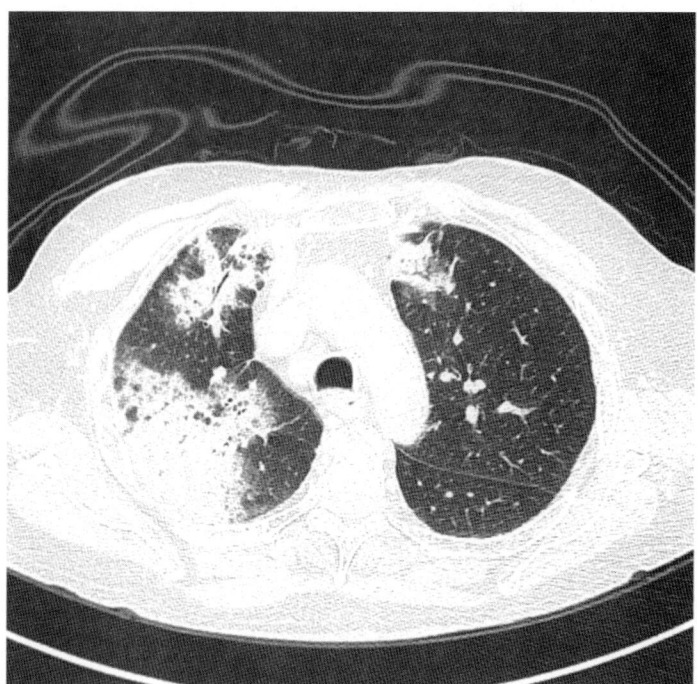

Fig 70.4: Bleomycin toxicity. CT chest reveals ill-defined areas of subpleural and peribronchovascular air-space opacification with air-bronchograms representing an organizing pneumonia. Bleomycin can also give rise to well-marked bilateral interstitial pulmonary fibrosis.

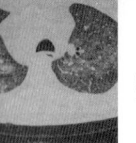

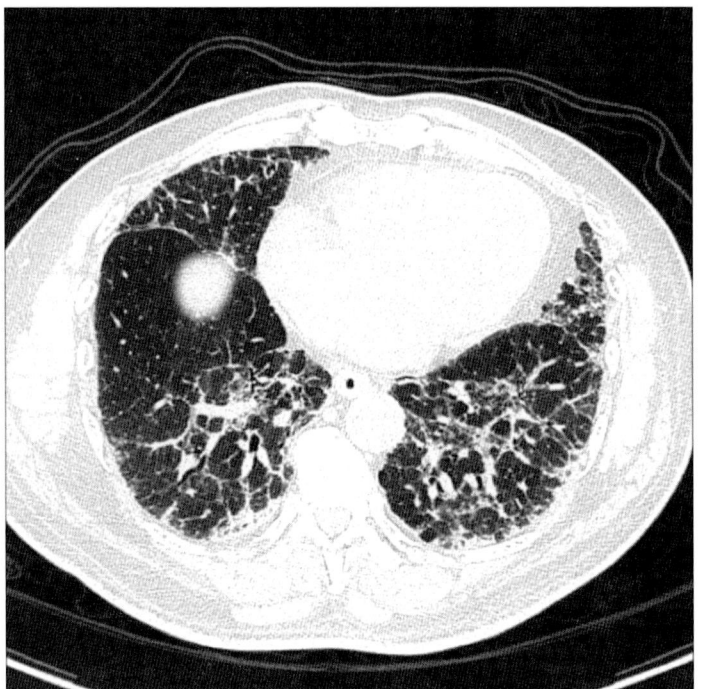

Fig 70.5: Bleomycin toxicity. HRCT chest demonstrates thickening of the peribronchovascular and subpleural interstitium as a result of interstitial fibrosis induced by bleomycin.

The mortality with bleomycin toxicity is around 10%. Patients who have received a large total dose have a higher mortality, severe fibrosis being associated with a mortality as high as 50%.

Treatment involves discontinuation of the drug, use of corticosteroids and avoiding supplemental oxygen. Chest radiation therapy should not be given as a treatment for malignant disease of the breast or lung. Even with improvement in the lung condition, respiratory symptoms may persist to a lesser extent together with some degree of impaired lung function.

Cyclophosphamide

Cyclophosphamide is widely used to treat a variety of malignancies and autoimmune disorders. Pulmonary adverse effects are interstitial pneumonia and pulmonary fibrosis. The latter may be progressive, particularly when higher doses are used. Some patients with cyclophosphamide toxicity develop upper lobe fibrosis, pleural thickening with indrawing of the upper chest. The histopathology is characterized by interstitial oedema, interstitial cellular infiltrates, alveolar damage and fibrosis. The prognosis is generally poor; corticosteroids may offer some relief.

Methotrexate

Methotrexate besides being used in the treatment of lymphomas, leukaemias and other malignancies, is frequently used in the treatment of inflammatory disorders, particularly rheumatoid arthritis.

The most dangerous complication is a hypersensitivity pneumonia termed the 'methotrexate lung'. Risk factors include

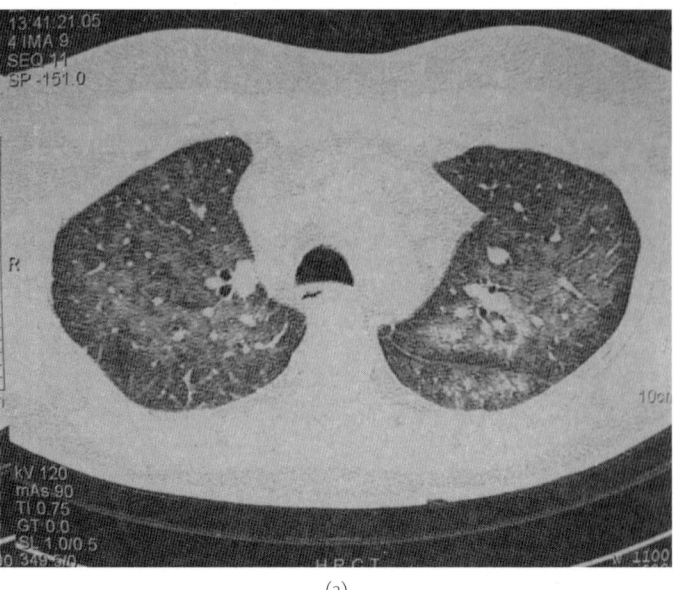

(a)

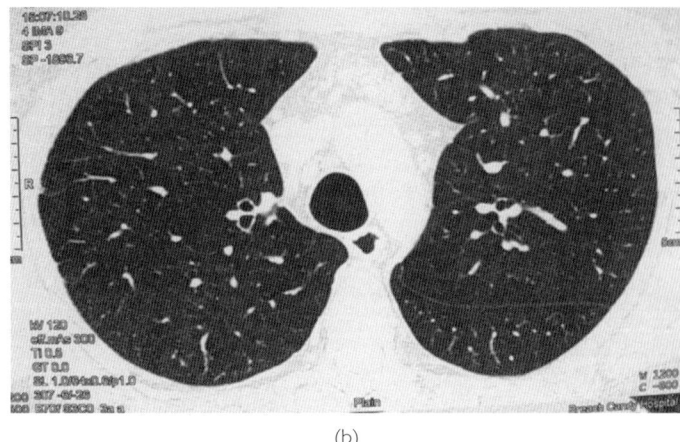

(b)

Fig 70.6: Methotrexate toxicity. (a) CT chest reveals diffuse ill-defined areas of ground-glass densities in both lung fields (b) CT chest following resolution of ground-glass densities after withdrawal of methotrexate.

its use in combination chemotherapy, some combinations being reported to be associated with a high incidence of methotrexate toxicity. 'Methotrexate lung' is a subacute illness developing over a few weeks and is characterized by fever, malaise, dry cough and breathlessness. Auscultatory basal crackles are often heard. The chest radiograph shows diffuse bilateral reticulonodular alveolar shadows. Peripheral eosinophilia may be present. Occasionally, there is progressive interstitial fibrosis. Overall mortality is approximately 10%.

Transbronchial lung biopsy reveals extensive infiltration with lymphocytes and loosely formed granulomas. BAL studies show the presence of T-helper cells and occasionally T-suppressor cells.

The drug should be promptly omitted. Re-introduction of the drug after recovery can cause a fatal relapse of hypersensitivity pneumonitis. The response to corticosteroids is good. There is a suggestion that methotrexate toxicity is immunologically mediated rather than due to a direct toxic effect on the lung.

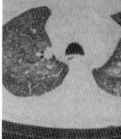

Mitomycin

Mitomycin is one other drug like bleomycin which causes severe interstitial pneumonia and fibrosis, the incidence of pulmonary toxicity being approximately 4%.

When mitomycin is used with vinca alkaloids it can cause acute pneumonitis with diffuse alveolar damage. Clinically, this is characterized by episodes of severe respiratory distress several hours after this combination therapy is administered. In some cases intubation and ventilator support is required. Radiography of the chest shows extensive bilateral infiltrates. Following the use of corticosteroids and supportive care, improvement generally occurs over some weeks. However, a number of these patients (close to 50%) are left with pulmonary fibrosis similar to that observed with use of mitomycin alone.

A rare mitomycin toxicity is mitomycin-induced microangiopathic haemolytic anaemia with intra-alveolar haemorrhage. The condition is characterized by dyspnoea, hypoxia and diffuse pulmonary infiltrates. Treatment is with corticosteroids and plasmapheresis. Fortunately, the drug is now less frequently used in lung cancer.

Taxanes

Taxanes are newer anti-neoplastic drugs used for different cancers, notably cancers of the lung, breast, ovary and cancers of the head and neck. Pulmonary toxicity takes the form of bronchospasm and dyspnoea. Urticaria, skin rash and hypotension may also be observed. Prior use of corticosteroids and H_2 blockers has reduced the incidence of these reactions.

Rarely, acute pneumonia has been observed as a dangerous toxic effect. Treatment consists of omission of the drug and the use of corticosteroids. Prognosis in general is good.

CONCLUSION

The diagnosis of pulmonary toxicity related to drugs is difficult because a number of diseases produce pulmonary manifestations similar to the pulmonary toxic effects of drugs used to treat these diseases. The simultaneous association of pulmonary infection, progression of a mitotic lesion are compounding factors which make the diagnosis of pulmonary drug toxicity difficult. Unfortunately, radiographic findings are non-specific and histopathologic studies are not always helpful. Invasive biopsy procedures carry a grave risk in very ill people. Nevertheless all possible investigations, in particular a BAL study, need to be done to ensure that an infective aetiology is not missed, more so as many of the drugs detailed in the chapter are often used in immunocompromised patients.

The key diagnostic factor is awareness of pulmonary toxicity related to a number of drugs and a keen suspicion of their possible occurrence under certain circumstances.

Periodic lung function tests done on patients exposed to drugs with a potential for pulmonary toxicity may help early detection. A restrictive lesion with a fall in CO diffusion may well be a pointer to interstitial lung disease caused by drugs. Toxicity caused by bleomycin, mitomycin, amiodarone is believed to be increased with the use of supplemental oxygen. Supplemental oxygen should be avoided with these drugs unless absolutely necessary.

SUGGESTED READING

Camus P. Drug induced and iatrogenic infiltrative lung disease. *Clin Chest Med*. 1 Sep. 2004; 25(3): 479–519.

Costabel U. Bronchoalveolar lavage in drug-induced lung disease. *Clin Chest Med*. 1 March 2004; 25(1): 25–35.

Epler GR. Drug-induced bronchiolitis obliterans organizing pneumonia. *Clin Chest Med*. 1 Mar. 2004; 25(1): 89–94.

Lee-Chiong T Jr. Drug-induced pulmonary edema and acute respiratory distress syndrome. *Clin Chest Med*. 1 Mar. 2004; 25(1): 95–104.

Limper AH. Chemotherapy-induced lung disease. *Clin Chest Med*. 1 Mar. 2004; 25(1): 53–64.

Schwarz MI. Drug-induced diffuse alveolar hemorrhage syndromes and vasculitis. *Clin Chest Med*. 1 Mar. 2004; 25(1): 133–40.

Vahid B. Pulmonary complications of novel antineoplastic agents for solid tumors. *Chest*. 1 Feb. 2008; 133(2): 528–38.

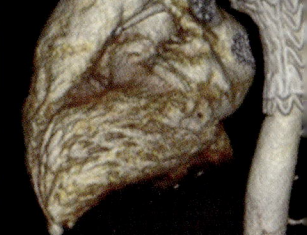

TRAUMA AND CHEST WALL DISORDERS

CHAPTER **71** ## Trauma to the Chest

Trauma to the chest when severe can lead to significant morbidity and mortality. In civilian life chest trauma is largely due to accidents–chiefly road or rail, through violence, as in assault, riots and terrorist attacks are clearly on the rise all over the world. In most severe accidents there is polytrauma when more than one organ system is involved. The morbidity and mortality worsen when trauma to the chest is associated with trauma to other systems. The mortality also worsens with age, especially after the sixth decade, particularly in the presence of co-morbid disease involving the respiratory or cardiac systems.

PREVALENCE

The World Health Organization (WHO) report (Global Status Report on Road Safety) states that over 1.2 million people die in road accidents every year and 20–25 million suffer non-fatal injuries. India's record with regard to road vehicular accidents is dismal. Road fatalities increased between 2003 and 2008 from 84,000 in 2003 to 1.18 lakhs in 2008; 4.69 lakh people were injured in road accidents, nearly four times the total death toll. This is almost certainly an underestimation, many non-fatal accidents or even fatal accidents go unrecorded. Andhra Pradesh has the highest death rates due to road accidents (12%), followed by Maharashtra and Uttar Pradesh (11% each). In most fatal accidents chest wall trauma was the main or contributory cause of death. The WHO states that India has topped the global list of deaths in road accidents, leaving behind the world's most populous country, China. This is particularly disturbing considering the comparatively low density of overall vehicular traffic in the country compared to many other countries in the world. India's vehicular population is just 5% of the world's, and yet as has already been stated, the country has the highest incidence of road accidents, with over a lakh fatalities and five or even perhaps 10 times that number injured or admitted to hospital. The increased incidence of accidents with injury to one or more organ systems in all developing countries (including India) is because of rapid urbanization and industrialization and the need for mechanized transport. Even in rural India, the impact of injuries and deaths caused by accidents is increasingly evident because of mechanization of agriculture and the increased use of vehicular transport.

In road traffic accidents, chest trauma is responsible for death in 30% of cases. Isolated chest trauma in good trauma centres in the Western world has a mortality close to 10%; the mortality is over 20% when two or more organ systems suffer injury.

Care for trauma is ideally organized at two sites. The first and extremely important is the site of the accident and the next is the intensive care unit of ideally a trauma centre or failing that an intensive care unit of any reasonably well-equipped hospital.

Analysis shows that prompt attention to serious chest trauma after an accident significantly improves mortality. The first one to six hours are crucial and prompt attention at the site of accident is vital. Though this is possible in the developed countries of the West, it is well nigh impossible in India and many other developing countries. Even in large cities like Mumbai and Delhi it may take hours before accident victims find their way to a good hospital because of the traffic jams that are routine on all busy city roads. Helicopter service to send emergency medical teams to the site of the accident or to transport the victim to a well-equipped medical centre is almost non-existent in the poorer countries of the world.

APPROACH TO CHEST TRAUMA

Initial Assessment

A quick but careful examination of the patient is necessary to assess the extent and severity of injuries. As with any emergency, immediate attention is focused on the airway, the breathing and the circulation. Is the airway patent? If not, it should be rendered so. An unconscious patient generally requires an oropharyngeal airway; secretions, blood, should be aspirated form the oropharynx, and in emergency situations endotracheal intubation may be necessary. The possibility of trauma to the cervical spine must always be kept in mind; so that flexion of the cervical spine is avoided during intubation. If the airway is patent, is the breathing satisfactory? If not, respiration needs to be supported—mouth-to-mouth respiration, or when possible bag-mask respiration, and in an intensive care unit endotracheal intubation with ventilator support. Equally important is to determine with urgency whether the circulation is adequate. Most accident victims are hypovolemic. It is important to secure a venous line and start an intravenous infusion with normal saline or Ringer lactate, at the same time sending blood to the laboratory for all appropriate tests.

The heart and lungs combine to supply oxygen to the organs and tissues of the body. Serious injury to either results in hypoxemia. The most important question to determine in chest trauma is the presence and the degree of hypoxemia. This may indeed be difficult. Central cyanosis may be clinically difficult to determine even in the presence of severe hypoxemia, particularly so in a patient who is pale following blood loss, or in the presence of severe peripheral vasoconstriction due to shock.

Life-threatening hypoxemia in chest trauma can be due to either one or more of several causes—blocked airway, tension pneumothorax, hemothorax, lung contusions, fractures of the sternum and/or multiple ribs causing a flail chest, myocardial injury or hemopericardium. Each of these causes must be

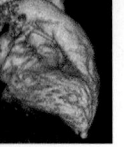

carefully looked out for and excluded. A tension pneumothorax can kill within a short time. Initially, there is marked tachypnoea, tachycardia and hypotension. If not dealt with quickly it leads to gasping breathing and cardiac arrest with an electromechanical dissociation. The most important physical sign is poor or absent breath sound over the affected lung coupled with displacement of the mediastinum to the opposite side. The percussion note over the chest is hyper-resonant. A hemothorax is suspected from signs of blood loss coupled with a stony dull note over the affected side of the chest. Lung contusions should be suspected when there is tachypnoea and evidence of hypoxemia in spite of a patent airway and absence of pneumothorax or hemothorax. A flail chest is immediately evident as there is a sucking in of the flail segment on inspiration and a puffing outwards of the flail segment on expiration. The patient is dyspnoeic and in severe cases increasingly hypoxemic. Finally, hypoxemia may be related to injury to the myocardium, or to the hemopericardium causing a cardiac tamponade. A large contusion involving the myocardium is akin to an infarct and can lead to a low cardiac output and shock. Cardiac tamponade due to hemopericardium should always be suspected in a crush injury to the chest. Tachycardia, shock due to a low cardiac output, dyspnoea, increased jugular venous pressure in the presence of shock and the presence of pulsus paradoxus should suggest a correct diagnosis.

It goes without saying that while the clinical assessment described above is being made, a vein should be secured, and an intravenous infusion of a crystalloid started. Blood is sent for grouping, matching and for appropriate investigations. Arterial pH and blood gases should be determined and an X-ray chest urgently done. If the patient is conscious and is capable of standing, an X-ray in the standing position is desirable; if not, a portable chest X-ray in the ICU is done as quickly as possible. All vital signs including oxygen saturation and electrocardiography (ECG) are continuously monitored. Table 71.1 gives the causes, important clinical manifestations and X-ray chest appearance of life-threatening conditions causing hypoxemia in chest trauma.

Emergency Management

Immediate attention is given to the airway, to supporting ventilation and maintaining adequate circulation.

Tension Pneumothorax

Tension pneumothorax jeopardizes ventilation and circulation. It should be actively looked out for and if present should be promptly relieved by the emergency insertion of a large-bore cannula needle, leaving the cannula *in situ* till an intercostal tube connected to an underwater seal has been introduced. An X-ray of the chest should confirm the presence of tension pneumothorax but in critical situations the pneumothorax needs to be drained as an emergency procedure without awaiting an X-ray of the chest.

Hemothorax

Clinical examination supported by an X-ray chest should confirm the presence of a hemothorax. A small hemothorax can be treated by chest aspiration, but more often than not, catheter drainage through a large-bore silicon catheter inserted through the sixth intercostal space in the mid-axillary line is necessary. Depending on the degree of injury, large quantities amounting to more than a litre of blood may be drained from the pleural space. Prompt blood replacement is necessary. Usually, the blood loss lessens with time, then ceases, and the patient continues to improve. If blood loss continues unabated, an emergency thoracotomy may be mandatory to control bleeding under vision.

Myocardial Injury or Contusion

Contusion involving the myocardium behaves like a myocardial infarct. The ECG may show non-specific ST-T changes or show the typical features of an ST-elevated myocardial infarct. The cardiac enzymes are elevated. Myocardial contusion should be treated if necessary with adequate inotropic or vasopressor support, together with all the other care one takes in a patient with a myocardial infarct.

Lung Contusion

Lung contusions are common in chest trauma. Severe lung contusions in both lungs are most often seen after blast injuries and penetrating injuries caused by shotgun or high-velocity missile wounds. Blunt injury to the chest may also cause contusion of the underlying lung and this may occur without fractures of either the sternum or ribs.

Severe lung contusions are often associated with other major injuries involving multiple body systems. The mortality with severe lung contusions is indeed very high as they result in marked ventilation-perfusion disturbances and severe hypoxemic respiratory failure.

Mild contusion may only be detected on an X-ray chest; however, what appears to be mild in a very early X-ray may turn out to be much larger in subsequent radiographs of the chest. Patients with severe lung contusion (particularly involving both lungs) present with tachypnoea and progressive hypoxemia. Radiographs of the chest show fluffy shadows, which may become confluent with time. Though mild contusion may be managed using a high-flow oxygen mask, severe contusion requires intubation and ventilator support, the fractional inspired oxygen (FIO_2) being adjusted so as to keep the O_2 saturation > 90%. At times it is impossible to keep a PaO_2 of even 40 mm Hg on an FIO_2 of 100%. The contused lung is easily prone to fluid overload which makes management of patients who are in shock doubly difficult. The potency of airways must be ensured and infection rigorously combated. Both inotropic and vasopressor support may be necessary. An ECG may show ST-T changes of a non-specific nature or show the typical features of ST-elevated myocardial infarction if there is associated myocardial contusion.

Cardiac Tamponade

Cardiac tamponade can kill quickly if not promptly recognized. Clinically, a low output state in the presence of a raised central venous pressure should point to a tamponade. In fact chest trauma is one condition where significant tamponade may exist with a central venous pressure which is normal, or in the upper limit of normal. The normal or even low central

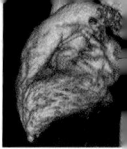

Table 71.1: Immediate complications of chest trauma	
Complications	Clinical Features
Obstruction to trachea or main bronchus	Stridor, tachypnoea, indrawing of intercostal spaces, hypoxemia (if obstruction unrelieved and severe)
Tension Pneumothorax	Severe increasing dyspnoea, absent breath sounds over affected lung, displaced mediastinum, hyper-resonant note over the lung, cardiovascular collapse, typical X-ray chest
Hemothorax	Shock due to blood loss; stony dull note over affected chest. Chest X-ray shows fluid which on aspiration is blood
Cardiac tamponade	Tachycardia, hypotension with other features of low output state. JVP raised, or even normal in presence of hypovolemia or shock; enlarged cardiac silhouette on X-ray of the chest. Echocardiography reveals pericardial fluid
Lung Constusion	Tachypnoea, hypoxemia, hemoptysis, chest X-ray shows airspace consolidates of varying size
Flail Chest	Unstable flail segment showing paradoxical motion, progressive dyspnoea, hypoxemia

venous pressure in the presence of tamponade is because of hypovolemia caused by associated blood loss, or because of shock due to trauma to other organ systems. A normal-sized cardiac silhouette on a chest X-ray does not exclude cardiac tamponade. An echocardiogram can be of immense diagnostic value. Careful aspiration of blood from the pericardial space is necessary. If bleeding recurs or continues, a surgical procedure entailing the insertion of a drain into the pericardial space through a pericardial window becomes necessary.

Flail Chest

A severe flail chest causing dyspnoea with life-threatening hypoxemia is dealt with promptly by intubation and positive pressure ventilator support. This complication is dealt with at greater length later in the chapter (Table 71.1).

Replacement of Blood and Maintenance of Fluid Electrolyte Balance

Serious chest trauma is often accompanied by trauma to other organ systems, by blood loss, fluid loss and disturbance in electrolyte balance. These factors should be recognized and corrected pari-pasu with treatment of the life-threatening complications described above.

Polytrauma requires the attention and help of appropriate specialists. A protocol for priority of treatment should be agreed upon. Serious abdominal trauma may warrant an urgent laparotomy, an intracranial injury may require urgent craniotomy as a priority. If surgery for polytrauma is necessary, it is best to undertake as many procedures as possible in one anaesthetic cum operative session, with due regard to patient safety. In the presence of critical chest injury, fractures of long bones can be stabilized temporarily by skin traction; operative reduction, fixation can be done when the patient has a stable circulation and respiration.

Besides the immediate life-threatening emergencies mentioned above, it is important to bear in mind other lurking threats and complications associated with chest trauma. These include in the main, closed aortic rupture (Figure 71.1), ruptured or torn trachea or bronchus, rupture oesophagus and rupture diaphragm. These may not be immediately evident and may make their presence felt later. Some of these complications necessitate a thoracotomy, the timing of which should be decided upon by the treating team of physicians and surgeons.

OTHER PULMONARY COMPLICATIONS

Lobar or Segmental Atelectasis

Lobar or segmental atelectasis is perhaps the most frequent complication occurring within 48 hours of chest trauma. It results from the inability of the patient to take deep breaths and inability to cough and keep the airways clear of secretions. Relief of pain and good physiotherapy generally suffices to open up the atelectatic lobe of the lung. If lobar atelectasis persists, bronchoscopic aspiration is warranted. Repeated bronchoscopy to aspirate secretions is undesirable and may do more harm than good.

Pneumothorax

Tension pneumothorax may be overlooked in the presence of more life-threatening emergencies. This is particularly so when attention is focused on an associated serious head injury causing unconsciousness which precludes any complaint of pain or breathlessness. Bilateral simple pneumothoraces can produce serious cardiorespiratory embarrassment. They should be evident on an X-ray of the chest and should be treated by chest tube drains connected to underwater seals.

Flail Chest

Double fractures of three or more contiguous ribs or a combination of fracture of the sternum and ribs causes a flail segment in the thoracic cage. As mentioned earlier, during inspiration the flail

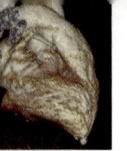

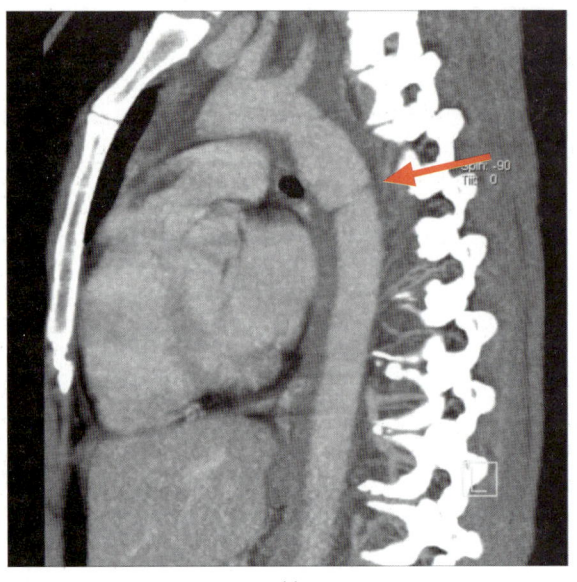

(a)

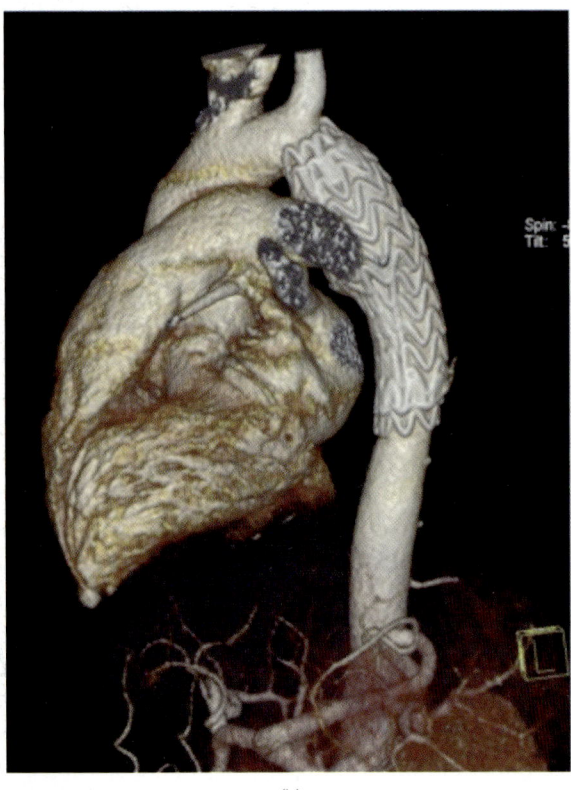

(b)

Fig 71.1: Aortic Transection (a) An 18-year-old girl riding pillion on a motorcycle was thrown off following a head-on collision. CT angiography revealed an aortic transection as evidenced by focal intimal tear in the descending aorta at the level of the aortic isthmus, a typical site for blunt aortic injury (b) An aortic stent was placed across the isthmus intimal tear. This is a post-stent CT angiogram demonstrating the stent in situ.

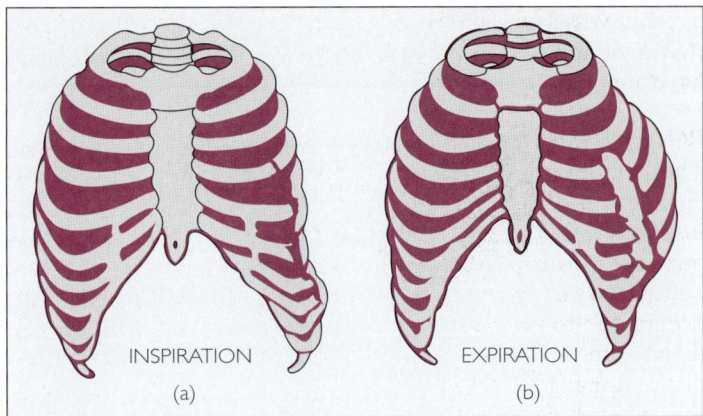

Fig 71.2: Diagram showing a flail segment (a) sucked in during inspiration and (b) pushed out on expiration.

trauma to the chest following automobile accidents or following other forms of crush injury. The next most important cause is fractures of the sternum and/or ribs caused by over-aggressive cardiopulmonary resuscitation. Rarely, multiple pathological fractures of contiguous ribs may also cause a flail chest.

DIAGNOSIS

The diagnosis of flail chest is obvious from the nature of the paradoxical movement of the flail segment during spontaneous breathing. Chest radiography reveals multiple fractures of the ribs. A computed tomography (CT) scan provides more information with regard to associated injuries to the lung, pleura and other mediastinal structures. In fact pulmonary contusion, pneumothorax and hemothorax occur in over 50% of patients with flail chest. Trauma serious enough to cause a flail chest is often associated with traumatic fracture of long bones, intra-abdominal injuries and rupture of the aortic arch

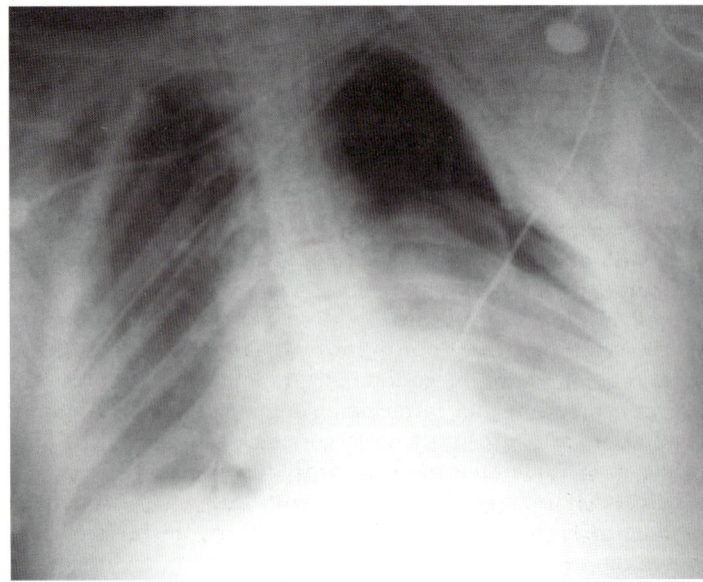

Fig 71.3: Flail Chest: Chest X-ray portable AP view. Chest X-ray demonstrates multiple rib fractures involving the left upper ribs, which appear to have 'caved in'. There is evidence of a large pnuemothorax on the left side with extensive subcutaneous emphysema. Also note fractures of right upper ribs posteriorly.

segment is sucked inwards rather than expanding outwards with the rest of the thoracic cage, while during expiration it is pushed outwards when the rest of the chest moves inwards. (Figures 71.2, 71.3) The most common cause of a flail chest is

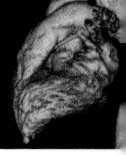

or other vessels within the mediastinum. Patients with multiple traumatic injuries and lung contusions complicating flail chest have a mortality > 50%.

PATHOPHYSIOLOGY

The paradoxical movement of the flail segment is related to changes in intrapleural pressure during breathing. During inspiration the negative intrapleural pressure inflates the lungs but exerts a deflationary effect on the rib cage. In spite of this deflationary effect, normal rib cage expansion during inspiration occurs due to outward forces exerted by the insertions of the diaphragm as it descends during inspiration, due to the action of the upper intercostal muscles on the upper rib cage and to the outward recoil of the thoracic cage at high inspiratory lung volumes. Following contiguous double fractures of three or more ribs, the flail segment is uncoupled from the rest of the thoracic cage, so that the deflationary effect of increased intrapleural negative pressure during inspiration is no longer countered by factors that promote chest wall expansion. Therefore, the increase in the negative intrapleural pressure during inspiration sucks the uncoupled flail segment inwards. During expiration the intrapleural pressure becomes more positive and the flail segment moves outwards. This paradoxical movement of the flail segment is worsened if there is obstruction to the airways which increases the negativity of the intrapleural pressure during inspiration, or in the presence of lung contusions which cause a decrease in lung compliance.

Most flail segments are laterally placed due to rib fractures of the lateral chest wall. Fractures separating the sternum from the ribs produce anteriorly placed flail segments; posterior flail chest segments occur with fractures of the posterior portion of the ribs. Posterior flail chest segments are associated with comparatively less paradoxical movement because of the splinting effect of the back muscles.

The danger of a flail chest is that it sets into motion events that can lead to respiratory failure. This can be due to several causes—

1. Reduction in vital capacity and functional residual capacity by as much as 50% occurring as a result of the paradoxical movement of the flail segment.
2. Severe chest pain, which can lead to hypoventilation. Inability to cough and clear secretions from the airways because of pain leads to regional atelectasis over the flail segment and generalized microatelectasis due to poor inspiration and low tidal volumes. Hypoxemia results from ventilation-perfusion imbalance, and a vicious cycle of increasing hypoventilation and increasing hypoxemia is set into motion.
3. The atelectatic areas within the lung increase the elastic load on the respiratory muscles.
4. A further increase in the work of breathing is due to shortening of the muscles of inspiration because of the flail segment. These muscles therefore work at a mechanical disadvantage and are more prone to respiratory muscle fatigue. The oxygen cost of breathing is increased.

Thus a combination of hypoventilation, hypoxemia due to ventilation-perfusion imbalance, respiratory muscle inefficiency, and respiratory muscle fatigue is responsible for progressive hypoxemic + hypercapnic respiratory failure.

TREATMENT

Control of pain is critical as it prevents both hypoventilation and atelectasis, which is central to the development of respiratory failure. Pain control allows the patient to cough, clear secretions and allows efficient physiotherapy. Narcotics need to be titrated with great care so as to prevent hypoventilation and excessive drowsiness. Intercostal nerve blocks can provide good analgesia. Epidural anaesthesia can also be used in selected patients for pain relief.

Supplemental oxygen to keep oxygen saturation > 90%, physiotherapy that allows an efficient bronchial toilet, and careful fluid replacement are all necessary. In patients where paradoxical movements of the flail segment are not marked and when the flail segment is not large, the above conservative management may successfully prevent or counter respiratory failure and promote recovery.

Mechanical Ventilation Mechanical ventilation is necessary— a) when the flail segment is large with a marked paradoxical movement of the segment; b) when respiratory failure is present or imminent in spite of the conservative therapy outlined above.

Non-invasive ventilation should be tried if the patient is breathing spontaneously; relief of pain through regional anaesthesia or through other means is necessary. Non-invasive ventilation (CPAP) when appropriately used can effectively stabilize the flail segment and abolish its paradoxical movements during the respiratory cycle.

Positive pressure ventilatory support following endotracheal intubation or tracheostomy is advised when there are multiple large flail segments, when non-invasive ventilatory support fails, when there is well-marked hypoxemic + hypercapnic respiratory failure, or when there is associated shock, intracranial injury or associated intra-abdominal injury. Ventilatory support needs to be given till such time as the flail segment or segments are sufficiently stable to allow weaning.

Chest Wall Stabilization The chest wall can be stabilized in selected patients by a number of surgical procedures such as external fixation of the chest wall with wires, staples or steel plates. Surgical fixation improves respiratory mechanics and reduces the duration of mechanical ventilatory support. Selection of patients for surgical fixation depends on the experience of the unit concerned. Large flail segments, multiple segments, and patients whose flail segments fail to stabilize on mechanical ventilator support are potential candidates for surgery.

Patients undergoing thoracotomy for intra-thoracic injuries are often candidates for surgical stabilization of the flail segment at the time of thoracotomy.

Mediastinal and Subcutaneous Emphysema

Mediastinal emphysema may be associated with a pneumothorax following blunt or penetrating injury to the chest. Severe mediastinal emphysema is often associated with a tear in the trachea or a rupture of a bronchus or the oesophagus. Positive pressure ventilator support worsens mediastinal emphysema. The diagnosis is evident on a radiological examination of the chest.

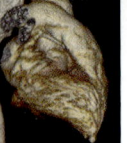

Table 71.2: Management of flail chest
1. Relief of pain—drugs, regional anaesthesia, epidural anesthesia
2. Oxygen
3. Physiotherapy
4. Ventilator support for respiratory failure
a. Non-invasive suppot (CPAP)
b. Invasive ventilator support when indicated
5. Surgical fixation of flail chest

Table 71.3: Indicators for invasive ventilatory support after endotracheal intubation or tracheostomy in flail chest
1. Failure of non-invasive ventilation support
2. Multiple or large flail segments
3. Well-marked hypoxemic + hypercapnic respiratory failure
4. Associated shock, intracranial injury, intra-abdominal injury

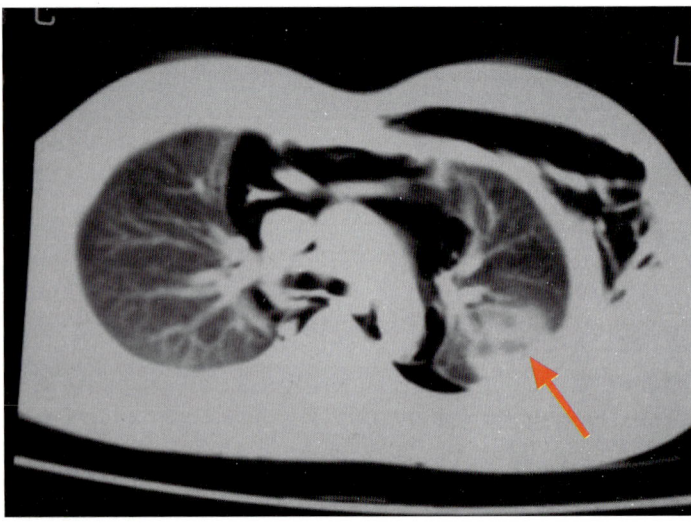

Fig 71.4: Chest Trauma. CT chest lung window demonstrates extensive subcutaneous emphysema on left side. Extensive mediastinal emphysema as evidenced by air in the mediastinum outlining the mediastinal vasculature. An ill-defined area of altered attenuation is seen in the left upper lobe representing a pulmonary contusion.

Extension of air from the mediastinum occurs first into the neck and then to the face. A crepitus is felt on palpation of the face and neck. The subcutaneous emphysema when marked leads to a swollen 'crepitus-filled face', the air then travelling subcutaneously to involve the chest, upper limbs and even the abdomen.

Treatment consists of dealing with the root cause of mediastinal emphysema and appropriate drainage of the pleural space in the presence of a pneumothorax, which is usually an association of mediastinal emphysema.

Rupture of the Trachea or Bronchus or Oesophagus or any combination of these structures

These need appropriate surgical intervention and are all associated with marked increase in mortality and morbidity.

Rupture of the Diaphragm

Traumatic closed severe rupture of the diaphragm leads to the herniation of abdominal contents into the chest and requires surgical repair as soon as the diagnosis is made.

Traumatic Rupture of the Thoracic Duct

Traumatic chylothorax is rare, but should nevertheless be anticipated in severe crush injuries of the chest and in falls from a height which may involve hyperextension of the spine. Chylothorax becomes evident some days after the injury, manifesting as a large-sized pleural effusion which on aspiration is milky because of the presence of chyle.

Conservative treatment generally results in effectively reducing the flow of chyle into the pleural space. Chest tube drainage may be necessary. The reader is referred to the section on 'Diseases of the Pleura'.

Adult Respiratory Distress Syndrome

ARDS is indeed an important complication of chest trauma, particularly in the presence of lung contusion. It is characterized by increasing tachypnoeas, tachycardia, increasing hypoxemia, crackles over both lungs accompanied by fluffy shadows on a radiological examination of the chest. The patient is increasingly hypoxemic, the hypoxemia being uncorrected by high-flow oxygen therapy. Endotracheal intubation and ventilator support is vital. The subject is dealt with at length in a separate section.

IMPORTANT THERAPEUTIC MEASURES IN CHEST TRAUMA

These have been mentioned earlier but need to be doubly stressed. They include:

Relief of Pain

Relief of pain has already been touched upon. It is of vital importance as it enables the patient to cough, take deep breaths and permits efficient, effective physiotherapy. Usual analgesics generally fail to relieve pain and narcotics may relieve pain but depress respiration. An epidural block using 5 to 8 ml of 0.5% bupivicaine or an intravenous Fentanyl drip or both together, may provide significant relief.

Bronchoscopy, Endotracheal Intubation, Tracheostomy

Fibreoptic bronchoscopic aspiration of thick secretions helps to keep the airways patent. Repeated bronchoscopic aspiration however tends to cause or increase infection. When the airways

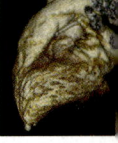

are prejudiced, endotracheal intubation or tracheostomy becomes necessary. Suction of secretions then becomes easy; the patient can receive humidified oxygen and if needs be sedated and ventilated.

Physiotherapy

Expert physiotherapy to the chest often makes the difference between life and death. Effective physiotherapy is not possible without effective pain relief.

Thoracotomy

Thoracotomy may be considered necessary as an emergency measure or electively done at the appropriate time. Indications for thoracotomy are listed in Table 71.4.

Table 71.4: Indications for thoracotomy
1. Rupture of trachea or main bronchus
2. Uncontrolled hemothorax
3. Severe cardiac tamponade due to a massive haemopericardium
4. Closed rupture of the aorta (stenting the aorta if thought appropriate may suffice)
5. Ruptured oesophagus
6. Ruptured diaphragm with herniation of abdominal contents into the chest
7. Thoraco-abdominal injury: e.g. injury involving the liver, spleen or other abdominal viscera; pleura and peritoneal taps reveal blood

SUGGESTED READING

Meredith JW. Thoracic trauma: when and how to intervene. *Surg Clin North Am*. 1 Feb. 2007; 87(1): 95–118, vii.

Miller LA. Chest wall, lung, and pleural space trauma. *Radiol Clin North Am*. 1 Mar. 2006; 44(2): 213–24, viii.

Ullman EA. Pulmonary trauma emergency department evaluation and management. *Emerg Med Clin North Am*. 1 May 2003; 21(2): 291–313.

CHAPTER **72** **Chest Wall Disorders**

SCOLIOSIS AND KYPHOSCOLIOSIS

General Considerations

Curvature of the spine is the commonest deformity that results in a chest wall deformity. Scoliosis is characterized by a lateral curvature of the spine. Kyphosis is a backward curvature of the spine in the anteroposterior plane and lordosis, a forward curvature in the anteroposterior plane. Most patients with scoliosis have a crowding of the ribs on the side of the convexity, so that the condition is often mistakenly labelled as kyphoscoliosis. However, at times scoliosis and kyphosis coexist, leading to a true *kyphoscoliotic spinal deformity*.

Prevalence

Scoliosis with more than a 35° angle affects 1 in 1000 of the population in the United States, an angle greater than 70° having a prevalence of 0.1 per 1000. Females are more often affected with more severe scoliotic deformities compared to males.

An epidemiological study to determine the prevalence of scoliosis in school children in lower Assam revealed an incidence of 0.2% with a female to male ratio of 2.2:1. The idiopathic variety was the commonest form of scoliosis which occurred mainly in the thoracic spine. The highest number of cases was observed between the ages of 11 and 13 years and in over 70% of cases, the patients or their parents were unaware of the deformity. (*Ref: KC Saikia, A Duggal et al. Scoliosis: An epidemiological study of school children in lower Assam. Indian J Orthop 2002; 36:243–5.*)

Etiology

1. Idiopathic   In more than 80% of patients, the cause of scoliosis is unknown, the scoliosis being therefore considered as idiopathic. A proposed classification of idiopathic scoliosis is based on the age of onset of the lateral curvature of the spine—infantile (from birth to 3 years), juvenile (3–11 years) and adolescent (11 years and older). The angle of lateral curvature may vary from less than 30° to over 70°. Females are more often afflicted with significant scoliotic deformity compared to males and the defect is often observed to increase with age. Congenital scoliosis is generally related to developmental defects of the spine such as partial or fused vertebrae or hemi-vertebrae; or genetic syndromes such as the Klippel-Feil syndrome and spondylocostal dystonia.
2. Genetic   The genetic basis of idiopathic scoliosis is uncertain. Perhaps, there is a genetic predisposition which is responsible for a different growth pattern in the spine. A possible genetic factor (among perhaps other multifactorial causes) is suggested by an increase in the incidence of scoliosis not only among first-degree relatives, but also to a lesser extent in second and third-degree relatives as well.
3. Congenital Scoliosis   Congenital scoliosis is observed in association with congenital heart disease and congenital renal tract disease.
4. An Association with Neuromuscular Disease   Scoliosis is invariably associated with poliomyelitis which has affected the spinal muscles unequally. It is commonly observed in muscular dystrophy (particularly of the Duchenne variety), in myopathies, syringomyelia and Friedreich's ataxia.
5. An Association with Other Syndromes   There are a number of syndromes or diseases known to be associated with scoliosis. The important ones include neurofibromatosis, Marfan's syndrome, osteogenesis imperfecta, Klippel-Feil syndrome, Ehlers-Danlos syndome and the rare various forms of mucopolysacharidosis.
6. Disease or Trauma   An important cause of both kyphosis and kyphoscoliosis in India and other developing countries is tuberculosis of the spine (Pott's spine) which results in the formation of a kyphotic 'gibbus', and at times also causes scoliosis. Trauma to the spine or surgery on the spine for whatever reason can also lead to a scoliotic deformity. Thoracoplasty for pulmonary tuberculosis was a frequently performed surgical procedure several decades ago. It often led to well-marked scoliotic deformity of the spine.
7. Tumours or Granulomatous Disease   These are indeed rare causes of a lateral curvature to the spine; they include tumours such as large osteomas, chordomas and very rarely eosinophilic granuloma of the spine.

The causes of scoliosis are listed in Table 72.1.

Table 72.1: Causes of scoliosis
1. Idiopathic
2. Congenital
3. Genetic
4. An association with neuromuscular disease Muscular dystrophy (particularly of the Duchenne variety), myopathies, syringomyelia and Friedreich's ataxia, poliomyelitis (among several others)
5. An association with other syndromes Neurofibromatosis, Marfan's syndrome, osteogenesis imperfecta, Klippel-Feil syndrome. Ehlers-Danlos syndrome and the rare various forms of mucopolysaccharidosis.
6. Disease or trauma Pott's spine, surgery on the spine, thoracoplasty
7. Tumors or granulomatous disease Osteomas, chordomas and eosinophilic granuloma of the spine.

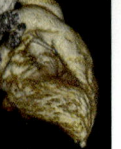

KYPHOSIS

Kyphosis is invariably acquired and is often age-related, so that it is an accompaniment in many individuals past 60 years. Marked kyphosis sometimes results from osteoporotic fractures of the thoracic vertebrae, either related to age, use of corticosteroids or other causes. Tuberculosis involving multiple contiguous vertebrae can lead to a pronounced 'gibbus' resulting in a serious kyphotic deformity.

Pathophysiology

Marked chest wall deformity (whether scoliotic or kyphotic or kyphoscoliotic) always adversely affects cardiorespiratory function. A thoracic curve > 70° imposes serious limits to ventilatory function. The effects of a severe scoliotic deformity are generally more marked than that of a pure kyphotic deformity. The ventilatory defect is of a restrictive nature. The vital capacity, the total lung capacity, inspiratory capacity and expiratory reserve volume are all reduced. In a pure scoliotic deformity, the residual volume though reduced is relatively better preserved. The forced expiratory volume in one second/forced vital capacity (FEV_1/FVC) is generally also preserved but occasionally there is a degree of obstruction to the airways in adults with severe idiopathic scoliotic deformity. The obstructive element when present is due to the association of hyper-reactive airways, smoking, occupation, environmental pollution or other factors. Factors which influence the degree of restrictive ventilatory defects are the number of vertebrae involved in the curve, involvement of the upper and mid-thoracic vertebrae rather than the lower dorsal vertebrae, severity of the kyphosis and Cobb angle.

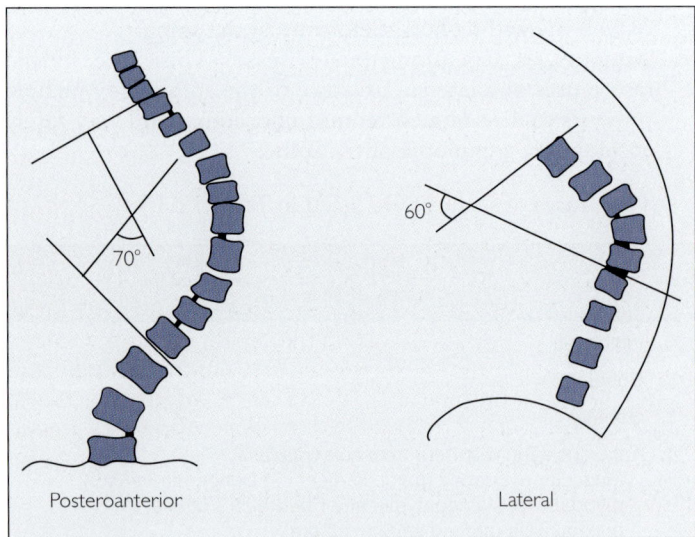

70°

60°

Posteroanterior   Lateral

Fig 72.1: Posteroanterior radiograph depicting the lines constructed to measure the Cobb angle of scoliosis and the lines drawn on the lateral radiograph to measure the Cobb angle of kyphosis (Based on data Rochester DF, Findlay LJ. The lungs and neuromuscular and chest wall disorder in Murray and Nadel (eds). *Textbook of Respiratory Medicine.* WB Saunders, 1988).

Lung Compliance

Though there is no direct pathology within the lungs, the decrease in lung expansion because of the chest deformity and the ensuing hypoventilation produce a fall in compliance. As hypoventilation becomes more marked and as chest wall compliance decreases with increasing scoliotic or kyphotic deformity, cough becomes increasingly ineffective and areas of microatelectasis and segmental atelectasis ensue, causing a further fall in lung compliance. Atelectasis due to hypoventilation is even more frequent in scoliotic patients whose deformity is due to neuromuscular disease. Recurrent chest infections involving the airways (causing bronchospasm and increased respiratory secretions) introduce an element of airways obstruction, while involvement of the parenchyma (as in pneumonia) further reduces lung compliance setting off a vicious cycle terminating in increasing respiratory failure or causing acute or chronic respiratory failure.

Carbon monoxide diffusion or the transfer factor is reduced, yet the Krogh constant (KCO) (i.e. diffusion lung capacity for carbon monoxide (DLCO)/accessible alveolar volume) is increased. This is because the thoracic deformity and the ensuing stiffness of the chest wall squeezes more air out of the affected lung than blood, so that accessible alveolar volume is reduced.

Table 72.2: Pulmonary function tests in severe idiopathic thoracic scoliosis	
Forced vital capacity (FVC)	Reduced
Forced expiratory volume in first second (FEV_1)	Reduced
FEV_1/FVC ratio	Generally normal, occasionally reduced
Total lung capacity	Reduced
Expiratory reserve volume	Reduced
Maximal inspiratory capacity	Reduced
DLCO	Reduced
KCO (DLCO/accessible alveolar volume)	Increased
Chest wall compliance	Reduced
Respiratory muscle strength	Reduced

Chest Wall Compliance

Chest wall compliance is reduced and the greater the deformity, the greater the fall in the chest wall compliance and greater the increase in the work of breathing.

As a consequence of the chest wall deformity, the respiratory muscles are shortened and work at a significant mechanical disadvantage. The effort required of the inspiratory muscles to meet the 'load' (i.e. ventilatory demands) is ultimately inadequate so that hypercapnic respiratory failure ensues. There are some who believe that impaired central ventilatory drive contributes to hypoventilation, the centre being less responsive to an increase in $PaCO_2$ because of chronic CO_2 retention. It is

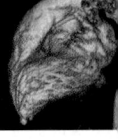

however more likely that in most patients the ventilatory load is far too much for the 'effort' the mechanically disadvantaged respiratory muscles are capable of. This is the prime reason for ventilatory failure in patients with chest wall deformities. In fact ventilatory drive is often increased in patients with scoliosis who develop hypoxemic + hypercapnic respiratory failure.

The ventilatory drive may however be primarily affected in brainstem disorders, amyotrophic lateral sclerosis or the ventilatory drive even if more than normal may fail to be translated into effective inspiratory muscle contraction in patients with neuromuscular disorders.

End Result

The end result as mentioned above is hypoxemic cum hypercapnic respiratory failure. Features of ventilatory failure in patients with well-marked scoliotic deformity generally first appear during sleep when loss of intercostal muscle tone further reduces the 'effort' vis-à-vis the ventilatory 'load'. Ventilatory failure finally supervenes both during the day and night.

Pulmonary artery pressure increases with progressive hypoxemia and hypercapnia, with the final development of chronic cor pulmonale and right heart failure. Nocturnal dips in O_2 saturation during sleep are associated with a further rise in pulmonary artery pressure. Whether these dips with their associated rise in pulmonary artery pressure influence a gradual overall permanent increase in pulmonary artery pressure is undetermined. Death results either from progressive respiratory failure, chronic right-sided heart failure or from a complicating pulmonary infection. Chronic cor pulmonale is the commonest cause of death.

Clinical Features

It is vital to ascertain that there is no other cause of a scoliotic, kyphoscoliotic or kyphotic deformity before dubbing it as idiopathic. Search should in particular include the clinical possibility of Marfan's syndrome, the presence of café au lait spots to suggest neurofibromatosis and a careful radiological study for the presence of hemivertebrae, a Klippel-Feil syndrome suggesting the presence of congenital scoliosis.

A full neurological examination is important. A careful cardiovascular examination in early onset scoliosis may reveal the presence of congenital heart disease which may be associated with congenital scoliosis.

Patients should be viewed in the standing position and also when bending forward to obtain an indication of the lateral deformity of the scoliotic, kyphotic or kyphoscoliotic spine.

Patients with symptoms related to chest wall abnormalities complain of progressive breathlessness on exertion, cough often with expectoration. With progression of the deformity, there is hypoventilation with features of hypoxemia and hypercapnia. A worsening of nocturnal hypoventilation during sleep, most marked during rapid eye movement (REM) sleep, causing a further rise in $PaCO_2$ is often responsible for nocturnal confusion, poor quality of sleep and early morning headache.

Right heart enlargement may be difficult to determine clinically but is evident on echocardiographic studies. Right-sided heart failure and progressive chronic hypercapnic respiratory failure constitute the end stage of the disease.

Most patients with chest wall deformities do not have cardiorespiratory problems. It is however important to determine which patients are likely to do so. Patients who have a vital capacity of < 50% of predicted value at the time of presentation are more likely to progress to pulmonary and later cardiac decompensation compared to those with a higher vital capacity. It has also been shown that of the patients with cardiorespiratory symptoms related to scoliosis, 90% had an early onset scoliosis (before the age of five years). Finally, a fall in vital capacity > 15% on assuming the supine position indicates weakness of the diaphragm.

High-risk patients require a careful follow-up. This should include—

1. Clinical assessment—degree of breathlessness, chest expansion, symptoms of nocturnal hypoventilation, careful examination of the chest and cardiovascular system. Oedema of the feet unless otherwise explained, is generally due to right heart failure.
2. Lung function tests, in particular FVC and FEV_1 using an office spirometer, and peak flow measurements through a peak flow meter.
3. Arterial blood gas analysis at periodic intervals.
4. Radiography of the chest and spine as and when deemed necessary.
5. Periodic electrocardiography (ECG) and echocardiography for evidence of right ventricular hypertrophy and right ventricular systolic and diastolic dysfunction.

Management

CONSERVATIVE MANAGEMENT

Conservative management consists in the use of specially fitted braces which help to create a normal thoracic kyphosis, extend the spine and derotate the scoliosis. The design and fit of the brace is individualized and is best left to the discretion of the orthopaedic team. Conservative treatment is only possible if the spinal curvature is not marked and not progressive. The earlier the onset of scoliotic deformity, the greater the propensity for the deformity to progress.

Smoking should be strongly prohibited. Influenzal and pneumococal vaccines are indicated, particularly in patients with limited ventilation. Exercise under supervision should be encouraged and these patients may perhaps benefit from a pulmonary rehabilitation programme. Patients with Marfan's syndrome and associated scoliosis should avoid undue exercise and keep their blood pressure under close control, preferably with beta adrenergic blocking drugs, as the risk of aortic dissection is significantly high in these patients.

SURGERY

Surgery is indicated in marked deformity and to prevent progression. Thoracic scoliosis > 50 degrees is generally unacceptable; lesser degree of scoliosis may be associated occasionally with a greater degree of rotation of the ribs so as to result in an ugly deformity.

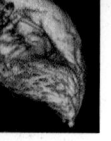

The current surgical approach provides rod instrumentation to stabilize the curve, and spinal fusion to prevent growth. The details of surgical procedure are beyond the scope of this chapter. Nevertheless fitness for surgery has to be decided by the physician. Preoperative investigations include lung functions, ECG, chest radiography, echocardiography, arterial blood gas analysis and the presence or absence of nocturnal hypoventilation. If nocturnal hypoventilation is present, a period of non-invasive ventilatory support before surgery is believed to help. Surgery unquestionably should be performed by experienced orthopaedic surgeons in units which can provide excellent cardiorespiratory support.

Severe scoliosis accompanying Duchenne muscular dystrophy often presents special surgical problems. Surgery should be attempted only if FVC is not too compromised, preferably not < 30% of predicted value. These patients generally need non-invasive ventilator support during the postoperative period, and excellent physiotherapy coupled with cough-assist devices.

MANAGEMENT OF VENTILATORY FAILURE

There is evidence to show that ventilatory failure caused by abnormalities of the chest wall or neuromuscular disease involving the muscles of respiration is successfully treated by the use of non-invasive ventilatory support (NIV). Five-year survivals in patients who receive NIV are as high as 80–100% in post-polio patients and in those with kyphoscoliotic deformity caused by TB spine. If NIV support is offered before the onset of pulmonary hypertension, patients have a normal or near normal life span and can often continue at work. In a retrospective study on patients with kyphoscoliosis receiving either long-term oxygen therapy (LOT) or NIV, those on NIV had a better survival rate at the end of one year and a greater improvement in $PaCO_2$ and PaO_2. A more recent Swedish study also showed that patients on NIV had a survival rate three times greater than those on LOT. Oxygen should be added to the NIV if the latter by itself does not increase O_2 saturation to > 90% even when there is control over the $PaCO_2$. NIV support reduces discomfort and the feeling of breathlessness.

Pregnancy in scoliotic patients can be fraught with danger if the vital capacity is < 1.25L or less than 50% of predicted value. This is observed chiefly in patients with early onset scoliosis starting at adolescence. Pregnancy is contraindicated in the presence of pulmonary hypertension and hypoxemia. If a ventilatory problem arises in pregnancy, labour or in the post-partum period, NIV should be used.

SUGGESTED READING

Crawford AH. Scoliosis associated with neurofibromatosis. *Orthop Clin North Am.* 1 Oct. 2007; 38(4): 553–62, vii.

Demetracopoulos CA. Spinal deformities in Marfan syndrome. *Orthop Clin North Am.* 1 Oct. 2007; 38(4): 563–72, vii.

Gonzalez C. Kyphoscoliotic ventilatory insufficiency: effects of long-term intermittent positive-pressure ventilation. *Chest.* 1 Sep. 2003; 124(3): 857–62.

Gupta MC. Degenerative scoliosis. Options for surgical management. *Orthop Clin North Am.* 1 Apr. 2003; 34(2): 269–79.

Hedequist DJ. Surgical treatment of congenital scoliosis. *Orthop Clin North Am.* 1 Oct. 2007; 38(4): 497–509, vi.

Saikia KC, A Duggal, *et al.* Scoliosis: An Epidemiological study of school children in lower Assam. *Indian J Orthop.* 2002; (36): 243–5.

CHAPTER

73

Central Nervous System and Neuromuscular Disorders Involving the Respiratory System

A large number of central nervous system (CNS) and neuromuscular disorders are capable of involving respiratory muscles, causing hypoventilation, respiratory failure or even respiratory muscle paralysis. A discussion of each of the very many would amount to writing a neurological textbook. Therefore a brief description of important representative examples is given below together with a rather lengthy table so as to give an overall perspective of the problem. CNS and neuromuscular disorders involving respiratory muscles may be acute or chronic, though occasionally chronic disorders may have an acute presentation.

CNS DISORDERS

ACUTE DISORDERS

The two major examples that need serious consideration are Stroke and Head or Spinal Cord injury.

Stroke

Brainstem strokes can disturb the pattern of breathing. Lesions of the dorsolateral medulla damage the respiratory centre and can produce apnoea that is soon fatal. If the dorsolateral position of the medulla is spared automatic or reflex breathing is preserved. Lateral medullary infarct arising from an occlusion of one of the distal vertebral branches is characterized by normal breathing or hypoventilation during waking hours and severe hypoventilation or even apnoea during sleep—Ondine's curse. Rarely, Ondine's curse may occur as an isolated abnormality'—a form of central sleep apnoea.

Strokes affecting the cerebral hemisphere affect the voluntary pathway of respiration and also reduce movements of the contralateral diaphragm. Massive cerebral infarcts or cerebral haemorrhage is associated with marked cerebral oedema that seriously jeopardizes respiration. Temporal herniation with pressure on the brainstem or a lateral shift or torsion of the brainstem can lead to hypoventilation apnoea and death within a matter of minutes. Massive strokes can also cause pulmonary oedema. Whenever respiration is jeopardized or the airway is obstructed as a result of secretions or because of palatal or pharyngeal paralysis, the patient needs prompt intubation and ventilator support. Intubation with induced hyperventilation through a positive pressure machine is often implemented to lower the PaCO$_2$ between 20–25 mm Hg to help reduce cerebral oedema in patients with massive strokes. Its effectiveness is generally limited to 24 to 48 hours.

Head and/or Spinal Cord Injury

Acute injury to the brain or spinal cord when severe can be associated with a total or near total loss of respiratory muscle function requiring prompt intubation and ventilator support. Other complications include—

1. Ventilation-perfusion inequalities leading to progressive hypoxemia. Hypoventilation and partially obstructed airways are responsible for this event.
2. Neurogenic pulmonary oedema which is believed to result from an excessive β adrenergic discharge, systemic hypertension, pulmonary vasoconstriction and increased capillary permeability. This is indeed a form of acute respiratory distress syndrome (ARDS) and again needs intubation with ventilator support. Incidentally subarachnoid haemorrhage can also cause neurogenic pulmonary oedema. Occasionally, pulmonary oedema is a presenting feature of subarachnoid haemorrhage, which can be missed if a careful CNS examination has not been done.

Spinal Cord Injury

Cervical cord injury causes quadriplegia. The latter also results from anterior spinal artery thrombosis or hematomyelia involving the cervical cord. In a transection, during the period of spinal shock the function of the intercostal muscles and the abdominal muscles is completely lost. Diaphragmatic paralysis results if the lesion is at C3 to C5 level. Diaphragmatic function is preserved if the lesion is below the above level. In these patients there is a paradoxical movement of the chest on inspiration, the upper chest being drawn in because of paralysis of the intercostal muscles. When the diaphragm is paralysed there is a paradoxical movement of the abdomen and the patient is severely hypoxemic in the supine posture. Though ventilatory function improves after the initial period of spinal shock, high cervical cord injuries necessitate urgent intubation and ventilatory support.

CHRONIC CNS DISORDERS

Multiple Sclerosis

Multiple sclerosis is a demyelinating disease, very common in the West. It is not as uncommon as it was believed to be in India, being particularly observed in the Zoroastrian community of the country. Demyelinating plaques can occur anywhere within the

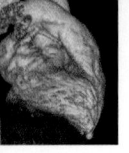

CNS and/or spinal cord, symptoms and signs depending on the situation and size of these plaques. Rarely, plaques within the medulla may be so situated as to impair either reflex automatic breathing or voluntary breathing. More often, medullary involvement in multiple sclerosis leads to lower cranial nerve palsies with danger of aspiration pneumonia. A demyelinating plaque in the region of C3, C4, C5 can cause diaphragmatic weakness or paralysis and multiple plaques within the thoracic segment of the spinal cord can result in a fair degree of respiratory muscle weakness. Acute respiratory failure may be precipitated if pulmonary infections complicate an exacerbation of the disease.

Parkinson's Disease

Parkinson's disease, common all over the world, has many respiratory complications. Aspiration of upper respiratory secretions or food or liquids is frequently observed in advanced disease due to difficulty in swallowing. This results in repeated episodes of aspiration pneumonia. Stiffness of the intercostal and other respiratory muscles together with abnormal control of breathing leads to dyspnoea, tachypnoea, reduced tidal volume and reduced lung volumes. Patients with Parkinsonism also have an instability of the large airways so that flow volume is saw-toothed both in the inspiratory and expiratory limbs. It is very important to bear in mind that the therapy with L-dopa can precipitate respiratory dysfunction in Parkinsonian patients, sometimes within an hour of administrating a dose. Patients may develop tachypnoea and dyspnoea due to respiratory dyskinesia characterized by choreiform movements, and rigidity due to akinesia of the respiratory muscles.

Multiple System Atrophy or Shy-Drager Syndrome

Multiple system atrophy or Shy-Drager Syndrome is characterized by Parkinsonism coupled with autonomic nervous system disturbances—chiefly urinary retention and marked postural hypotension. Abnormalities in breathing patterns are also observed. These include abnormal control of breathing, irregular respiratory rate, Cheyne-stokes breathing, central hypoventilation and rarely, apneustic breathing. The most dangerous complication that can cause death is bilateral abductor paralysis which manifests as stridor, and obstructive sleep apnoea.

DISEASES INVOLVING THE BRAIN AND/OR ANTERIOR HORN CELLS

Rabies

Rabies, a fatal disease, still remains a grave problem in poor developing countries though a few cases continue to be reported in North America and very rarely in Western Europe as well. It is for all practical purposes a universally fatal disease caused by the rabies virus which gains entry through the bite of a rabid animal or through their lick over abraded skin. The incubation period varies form several weeks to several months, at times as long as a year. The reader is referred to a text in Medicine or Neurology for a detailed description of the disease. However, in 20% of cases, the inflammation the virus induces is initially confined to the spinal cord, where it produces a clinical picture indistinguishable from the Guillain Barré syndrome. There is progressive, quickly evolving ascending paralysis with involvement of the respiratory muscles leading to respiratory arrest. If life is prolonged through ventilator and other supports, an encephalopathy with coma results.

Immediate treatment of the wound caused by bites or licks over abraded skin and post-exposure prophylaxis is vital in subjects likely to be exposed to the virus. This consists of the prompt use of the rabies vaccine and of human rabies immunoglobulins.

Poliomyelitis

Poliomyelitis though extinct in many parts of the world is still reported from poor developing countries. Respiratory complications of the paralytic form of poliomyelitis are observed with extensive involvement of the anterior horn cells in spinal poliomyelitis or when there is involvement of the medulla. Respiratory involvement takes the form of respiratory paralysis. This may occasionally occur with frightening suddenness and rapidity. Rarely, it occurs as the first manifestation of the disease when limb power is normal and limb reflexes are still present. Extensive paralysis in these patients is then manifested over the next 24 to 48 hours. The gravity of the situation can be missed to start with, a ghastly mistake of dubbing the difficulty of breathing as 'functional' being occasionally made.

CHRONIC DISORDERS

Amyotrophic Lateral Sclerosis

This progressive degenerative disorder is characterized by anterior horn cell involvement of the spinal cord and/or the motor nuclei of the cranial nerves together with lateral (pyramidal) tract involvement.

Respiratory involvement takes various forms. In many patients respiratory muscle strength is preserved even though the limbs are extensively paralyzed, the patient being wheel-chair-bound or even bedridden. Motor neurone involvement is characterized by muscle weakness and fasciculations. Involvement of the motor nuclei in the brainstem is typically characterized by paralysis of muscles supplied by the 9th, 10th 11th nerves with fasciculations in the tongue. Long tract involvement is characterized by spasticity and extensive plantar responses. Aspiration pneumonia is a frequent accompaniment of medullary involvement. Paresis or paralysis of the abdominal muscles leads to weakness of expiratory muscles. Involvement of anterior horn cells of C3, C4, C5 leads to diaphragmatic paralysis. These patients become hypoxemic when supine and need to be propped up in bed.

Very rarely, acutely involving respiratory paralysis may be the first manifestation of motor neurone disease due to involvement of the motor neurons of C3, C4, and C5. Again, a diagnosis of functional difficulty in breathing is mistakenly made. Fluoroscopy however reveals paresis or paralysis of the diaphragm. Basic lung function tests reveal reduced forced vital capacity (FVC) and a careful neurological examination will generally unearth a degree of muscle weakness, perhaps with evidence of muscle fasciculation. An electromyography (EMG) study will confirm the diagnosis.

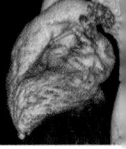

Post-Poliomyelitis Muscular Atrophy

About 20% of patients with previous poliomyelitis develop further muscle weakness as late as 20 to 40 years after the attack of poliomyelitis. This is due to denervation of regenerated motor units over a long period of time. This loss of muscle strength is gradual and if it involves respiratory muscles, it can cause respiratory failure. When kyphoscoliosis is an associated feature of poliomyelitis, further respiratory dysfunction due to hypoventilation results as has been described earlier.

Spinal Muscular Atrophy

These are rare disorders only occasionally encountered by respiratory physicians. Spinal muscular atrophy (SMA) is of three types. Type I and Type II are also termed Werdnig-Hoffman Disease. In Type I, SMA begins before six months of age and causes respiratory paralysis by the age of two years. Type II begins before the age of two years, is slower in evolution and leads to respiratory failure in late childhood. The association of scoliosis or kyphoscoliosis worsens hypoventilation and respiratory failure. Type III also called **Kugelberg-Welander disease** begins before the age of two years and causes late respiratory failure due to respiratory muscle weakness and associated kyphoscoliosis. All forms of SMA cause more pronounced weakness in the lower limbs, most marked in the proximal muscles. The disease is an autosomal recessive one and arises from an anomaly on Chromosome 5.

DISORDERS OF NERVE ROOTS AND/OR PERIPHERAL NERVES

ACUTE DISORDERS

Guillain Barré Syndrome

The Guillain Barré syndrome is characterized by extensive demyelinating polyradiculoneuropathy. Generally no proven aetiology can be found though the disease has been reported due to the Epstein Barr virus, cytomegalovirus, other viruses, and mycoplasmal infection. The condition has also rarely, other verses, been reported to precede or be associated with Hodgkin's disease, non-Hodgkin's lymphoma and other malignancies.

Muscle weakness commences in the lower limbs and ascends upwards with varying rapidity in many patients so as to involve the respiratory muscles. Proximal muscle weakness in limbs is often more marked than the distal. Deep reflexes are lost starting with the lower limbs and then involving the upper limbs. Rarely, a descending variant of the disease may be observed. Sensory loss is minimal, generally affecting the distal lower limbs. Maximal muscle weakness takes place between two days to two weeks in a majority of patients. Motor cranial nerves may also be involved. A third nerve palsy associated with cerebellar signs is another variant of this syndrome (Miller-Fisher variant). Autonomic dysfunction is observed in severe cases and is characterized by episodes of hypertension, hypotension and rarely arrhythmias. Cerebrospinal fluid examination shows a significant rise in proteins with perhaps a slight increase in lymphocytes.

Respiratory failure is chiefly due to respiratory muscle weakness. Aspiration causing atelectasis or aspiration pneumonia contributes to respiratory failure.

Mechanical ventilator support is necessary when there is respiratory muscle paresis. The tempo of the disease should be evaluated so that elective intubation with ventilator support can be offered without awaiting an emergency of well-nigh rapidly evolving apnoea that could be disastrous.

Specific therapy consists of plasma exchange preferably followed by intravenous immunoglobulins. Most patients recover completely but 15% are left with residual weakness and less than 2–5% develop relapsing episodes of demyelianation.

Critical Care Polyneuropathy and Myopathy

Critical care polyneuropathy and/or myopathy is assuming increasing importance in patients under intensive care for several days or weeks. It is characterized by a subacute reversible axonal neuropathy giving rise to weakness of the lower limbs or all four limbs. Respiratory muscle paresis or paralysis is observed in severe cases and is an important cause for difficulty in weaning patients off ventilator support. Deep reflexes are generally absent. EMG points generally to an axonal neuropathy. Muscle biopsy shows changes of denervation and/or myopathic changes. Cerebrospinal fluid (CSF) examination is normal. Complete recovery may take weeks and necessitates physiotherapy and prolonged rehabilitation.

Phrenic Nerve Injury

Damage or compression of the nerves induces bilateral diaphragmatic paralysis. The commonest cause of the injury is following open-heart surgery; other causes include massive intrathoracic surgery, mediastinal tumours and severe mediastinal infection.

Bilateral diaphragmatic paralysis following open-heart surgery or intrathoracic surgery is characterized by inability of the patient to be weaned off ventilator support. The patient becomes extremely tachypnoeic and hypoxemic without ventilator support in the supine posture and improves when he sits upright. Recovery invariably occurs over time; we have seen complete recovery of diaphragmatic paralysis following open-heart surgery after as long as six months of ventilator support.

Rarer Neuritic Pathologies

Diphtheria due to Corynebacterium diphtheriae causes an inflammatory membrane involving the tonsils, pharynx. Occasionally, the larynx is also involved causing life-threatening airways obstruction. Diphtheria toxin may occasionally affect the heart causing cardiomyopathy or arrhythmias and/or affect the peripheral nerves causing a peripheral neuropathy. A demyelinating polyneuropathy may develop four to eight weeks after the initial infection, at times involving the respiratory muscles and causing respiratory failure. Neurological features, particularly those causing respiratory paralysis are indeed rare even in developing countries. They may take 12 to 36 weeks to resolve.

Herpes Zoster is generally due to the reactivation of the varicella zoster infection. It causes a unilateral vesicular eruption involving one or two sensory nerve roots. The motor neurone

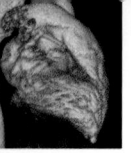

of the root or roots affected may occasionally also be involved resulting in flaccid paralysis. Involvement of the motor neurone of either C3, C4 or C5 may result in hemidiaphragmatic paralysis. This may result in dyspnoea but does not cause respiratory failure. Occasionally, the eruption caused by herpes zoster is sparse and can be missed. Unexplained hemidiaphragmatic paralysis may at times be related to herpes zoster infection.

Metabolic Causes

Two important metabolic causes that cause respiratory muscle weakness and respiratory failure and that always need to be remembered include electrolyte disturbances in the form of hyperkalemia, hypokalemia, and hypomagnesemia. Hyperkalemia has many causes, the most important being acute or chronic renal failure. These patients can have acute hyperkalemia with acute respiratory paralysis and profound cardiac disturbances. Drugs such as angiotensin-converting enzyme (ACE) inhibitors, aldactone, contribute to the sharp rise in serum potassium.

The second rare but important metabolic cause of acute respiratory paralysis is acute intermittent porphyria which causes an axonal neuropathy, at times severe enough to involve the respiratory muscles and cause acute respiratory failure.

Toxic Causes

Rare toxic causes of acute neuropathy causing acute respiratory failure are toxins transmitted by fish—cigatoxin produced by algae and transmitted by fish, saxotoxin transmitted by shell fish and tetradotoxin produced by puffer fish. Thallium toxicity besides causing various organ system disorders can cause an axonal neuropathy that can result in respiratory failure.

DISORDERS INVOLVING THE NEUROMUSCULAR JUNCTION

ACUTE DISORDERS

Organophosphorus Poisoning

Organophosphorus poisoning is the commonest cause of suicidal poisoning in India. Poisoning follows ingestion of organophosphorus insecticides. It can also occur from inhalation or absorption of the poison by the mucous membrane. Organophosphorus compounds are anti-cholinergic, and initially cause a severe cholinergic crisis with marked papillary constriction and involvement of major body systems. Severe hypotension and pulmonary oedema together with bradyrhythms are observed. There is widespread skeletal muscle weakness due to dysfunction at the post-synaptic neuromuscular level. The patient might appear to recover following full support to all systems and the use of pralidoxime, but after two to four days often manifests with cranial and proximal muscle weakness and respiratory failure. Specific therapy includes intravenous atropine, titrated to enable the pupil to return to and keep its normal size and the intravenous use of pralidoxime. Ventilator support as also inotropic and vasopressor support is mandatory in all severe cases. Over-atropinisation should be guarded against, as it causes serious problems.

Snake Bite

The cobra and the krait are common snakes in India, Africa, Southeast Asian and other developing countries. A bite from either of these snakes results in an injection of a neurotoxin which induces paralysis by preventing release of acetylcholine at the neuromuscular junction. Symptoms start within 1 to 12 hours of the bite. There is to start with ptosis, blurred vision, dysphagia and a rapidly progressive descending paralysis which also involves the respiratory muscles causing acute respiratory failure. The patient invariably remains conscious to the very end.

Specific therapy consists of prompt use of polyvalent antivenom serum (4–6 vials as initial dose), prompt ventilatory support to counter respiratory paralysis and support to organ systems as and when necessary. If death does not occur the paralysis regresses over two to seven days. A bite from a King Cobra can kill within less than 15 minutes to half an hour if the venom happens by chance to be directly injected into a vein.

Tick paralysis also follows a bite from a tick which secretes a neurotoxin that blocks the release of acetylcholine. An ascending paralysis is observed after a latent period of three to five days. Respiratory muscle involvement leads to respiratory muscle paralysis and acute respiratory failure. Removal of the tick rapidly reverses the paralysis. Ventilator support is necessary till recovery ensues.

Botulism

Botulism is indeed a rare disorder in India. It is caused by the release of an exotoxin produced by Clostridium botulinum, a Gram-positive spore-bearing anacrobe frequently and widely present in soil. The disease is chiefly caused by the consumption of improperly cooked food containing the exotoxin and spores. Canned food is particularly suspect when followed by symptoms described below. Rarely, botulism occurs from contamination of a wound by spores of the organism or by the exotoxin or from contaminated drugs given intravenously or intramuscularly. It has been reported to occur following colonization of the gastrointestinal (GI) tract by Clostridium botulinum in the first six months of life. The exotoxin after hematogenous distribution, enters the neurons, binds irreversibly to calcium channels and blocks release of acetylcholine at neuromuscular junctions and at postganglionic parasympathetic nerve terminals.

After an incubation period of a few hours to a few days in food-borne disease, and up to about two weeks in wound botulism, symptoms become manifest. There is usually but not necessarily nausea and vomiting to start with, followed by blurred vision and a rapidly progressive descending paralysis. Respiratory muscle involvement leads to acute respiratory failure.

Botulism should always enter into the differential diagnosis of a Guillain Barré syndrome (GBS) particularly when there is a descending paralysis instead of the generally expected ascending paralysis observed in the GBS. Blurred vision is another important differential feature; ptosis is frequent in botulism but occurs only in one of the variants of GBS. Extensive paresis or even paralysis of the GI tract and the bladder results from blockage of acetylcholine release at the postganglionic parasympathetic nerve terminals.

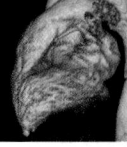

Diagnosis is by isolating the organism from contaminated food or from gastric aspirates in food-borne poisoning and from the wound and the serum in wound botulism.

Specific therapy consists of the use of specific antitoxin, which is unavailable in most countries outside America and Western Europe; penicillin in high doses and ventilatory support are necessary till the effect of the poison wears off.

CHRONIC DISORDERS

Myasthenia Gravis

Myasthenia gravis is the commonest chronic neuromuscular disorder met with in clinical practice. It is due to antibodies against acetylcholine receptors, so that though acetylcholine is secreted at the neuromuscular junction it cannot exert its effect.

The classic feature is increased fatiguability and weakness following use of the affected muscles. The disease may be confined to causing a ptosis, or diplopia, with features of a third nerve palsy being often noticed towards the evening or following a long stretch of reading. It could also be associated or solely confined to muscles innervated by the lower cranial nerves, or by involvement of skeletal muscles causing proximal muscle weakness, or the disease may be generalized and then presents with involvement of not only muscles supplied by the cranial nerves but also with skeletal muscle weakness. Occasionally, the only symptom is fatiguability and at the time of examination muscle power may be passed off as normal. Notably, in all forms of presentation, including severe paralysis of limb muscles, the deep reflexes are preserved, and there is no sensory loss.

Involvement of respiratory muscles with respiratory failure occurs under the following circumstances:

1. A slow progression of the disease involving skeletal muscles and/or muscles innervated by the cranial nerves, ultimately involving the respiratory muscles (intercostals and diaphragm).
2. An acute myasthenic crisis can result in acute respiratory failure. A myasthenic crisis is characterized by worsening of symptoms generally related to a triggering factor. Triggering factors include intercurrent infections, surgery, stress, non-compliance in taking the anticholinesterase drug pyridostigmine, or the use of certain drugs, in particular aminoglycosides which potentiate the disturbance in nerve conduction defect at the neuromuscular junction.
3. At times, the disease presents as an emergency or in the ICU with rapidly evolving acute respiratory failure due to respiratory muscle paralysis in a patient who may have no preceding symptoms suggestive of myasthenia. Myasthenia gravis should always enter into the diagnosis of acute respiratory failure when no obvious cause is found.

Diagnosis rests on a clinical examination, presence of antibodies to acetylcholine receptors and characteristic EMG findings pointing to increased fatiguability of muscles on nerve stimulation. It is noted that in about 5% of patients the antibodies to acetylcholine receptors may not be present.

In an acute crisis occurring in an untreated patient, pyridostigmine 2 to 5 mg intravenously results in a prompt improvement of muscle weakness. An X-ray and computed tomography (CT) of the chest should always be done to determine the presence or otherwise of an enlarged thymus or a thymoma.

TREATMENT

Treatment consists of the use of anti-cholinesterases like pyridostigmine 60 mg thrice daily, prednisolone, starting with a low dose and increasing over a few weeks to 30 to 40 mg daily. Intravenous immunoglobulin and plasma exchange are also of help.

In an acute myasthenic crisis causing respiratory failure particularly after surgery, ventilator support becomes mandatory. It is best to omit pyridostigmine and to reintroduce it when the respiratory muscles have been rested and weaning is about to start.

In patients with chronic well-marked myasthenia which produces paresis of respiratory muscles (not needing ventilator support) standard therapy consists of the use of pyridostigmine orally, corticosteroids increased gradually over weeks to a dose of 100 mg on alternate days with azathioprine in a dose of 2 mg/kg body weight. The steroid is reduced by 5 mg every three weeks so that ultimately if possible the patient is maintained on azathioprine and pyridostigmine alone.

In spite of therapy some patients worsen over years and ultimately fail to respond to all therapy. Death is invariably due to respiratory failure, often worsened by intercurrent infection in the lungs or elsewhere.

DISORDERS OF THE MUSCLES

ACUTE DISORDERS

An important cause of rapidly evolving generalized muscle weakness is the use of high-dose corticosteroids, more so if these patients have in addition received neuromuscular blocking agents during ventilator support. This combination when continued for a length of time can be lethal particularly in elderly patients. When the administration of steroids is considered imperative, it is wise to avoid neuromuscular blocking agents or limit their use as these combinations can lead to grave problems in weaning because of paresis of respiratory muscles. In the medical ICU this is most commonly observed in patients treated for acute severe asthma who have been given corticosteroids in large doses and have required both sedation and neuromuscular agents for effective ventilator support.

CHRONIC DISORDERS

Inflammatory Myopathies

The commonest disorders encountered in clinical practise giving rise to respiratory muscle weakness and hypoventilation, are polymyositis, dermatomyositis and inclusion body myositis. All these inflammatory myopathies are characterized by skeletal muscle weakness, more marked in the proximal muscles. Diagnosis is made by clinical examination, antibodies to JO_1 antigen, EMG studies, rise in creatine phosphokinase (CPK) levels and by muscle biopsy. The reader is referred to the section on 'Pulmonary Manifestations of Systemic Diseases'. The shrinking lung syndrome observed in systemic lupus erythematosus is due to atrophy with fibrosis of the diaphragmatic muscle.

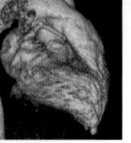
Chronic Inherited Mypopathies

These include Duchenne's muscular dystrophy, the fascioscapu-lohumeral myopathy and myotonic dystrophies. The reader is referred to a neurological text for a description of each of these neurological disorders

Respiratory failure is seen most frequently in Duchenne's muscular dystrophy, most patients with this disease being wheelchair-dependent in their early teens. Tidal volume as also lung volumes in these patients start to diminish by the age of 12. Though there is hypoventilation they may remain fairly stable for a decade or so. Initially there is nocturnal hypoxemia, followed by hypoxemia and hypercapnia during both day and at night during sleep. Scoliosis adds to the problems both in lung functions and chest wall mechanics. Death generally results from an acute respiratory crisis triggered by a chest infection. Non-invasive ventilator support should be considered early in the course of respiratory failure.

Respiratory failure in myotonia dystrophica occurs in advanced disease and is due to respiratory muscle weakness. Rarely, episodes of dyspnoea are related to myotonia of the respiratory muscles which can be alleviated by anti-myotonic treatment. Obstructive sleep apnoea may add to the respiratory problem. These patients are extremely sensitive to anaesthetic drugs and may require temporary postoperative ventilator support after a surgical procedure.

Congenital Myopathies

These are of several types and are characterized by typical abnormalities on muscle biopsy. The commonest form develops in infancy and childhood causing generalized muscle weakness and respiratory failure. The other less common forms of congenital myopathies are generally not associated with respiratory failure.

Metabolic Myopathies

Metabolic myopathies are indeed rare but again should always be considered in the differential diagnosis of any patient with respiratory failure of obscure aetiology.

Acid maltase deficiency (Pompe's disease) occurring in adults may present with respiratory failure, which is frequent and generally caused by dysfunction of the diaphragm.

Mitochondrial myopathies form a very rare group of systemic diseases due to various anomalies of DNA. We have never seen one but the following mitochondrial anomalies have been reported to be associated with respiratory failure, which is occasionally triggered by anaesthetic agents or respiratory depressants to which these patients are extremely sensitive. These mitcochondrial myopathies are Kearns-Sayre syndrome, mitochondrial DNA depletion syndrome and the syndrome which goes by the abbreviation MELAS—Mitochondrial myopathy, encephalopathy, lactic acid acidosis and stroke-like syndromes.

PATHOPHYSIOLOGY

Neuromuscular disorders ultimately lead to poor respiratory muscle function, hypoventilation and respiratory failure. In some disorders this is acute, in others, slowly evolving and chronic.

It needs to be kept in mind that even chronic neuromuscular disorders may occasionally present with acute respiratory failure as the initial event. It also needs to be mentioned that to start with there is no underlying lung pathology, but as hypoventilation and with it respiratory failure worsens, the risk of aspiration pneumonia increases. Once this transpires a vicious cycle occurs leading to worsening respiratory failure unless appropriate measures are promptly taken.

The figure below illustrates the various points at which neuromuscular disorders may ultimately affect respiratory muscle function.

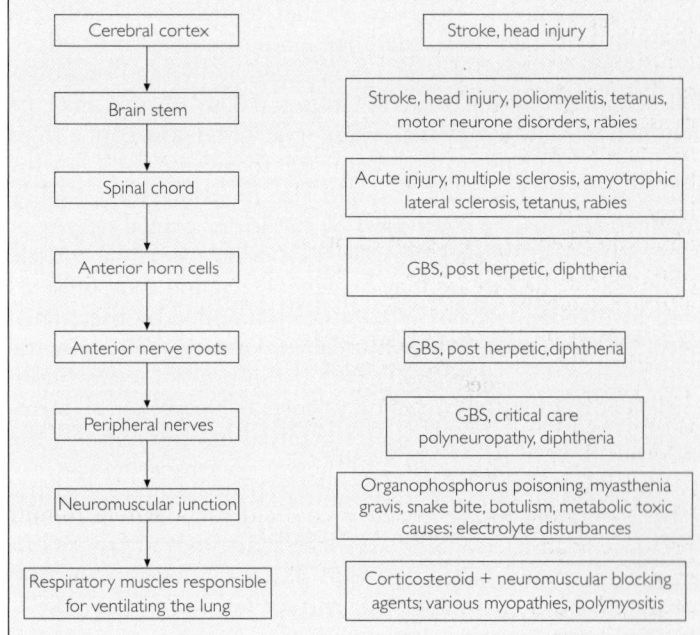

Fig 73.1: The vertical column to the left illustrates the chain of nervous impulses that ultimately reach the respiratory muscles enabling them to ventilate the lung. The column to the right gives a few examples of disorders that act at various sites disturbing, slowing or stopping this chain of nervous impulses.

DIAGNOSIS

The diagnosis of respiratory failure is easy in a patient with a previously known chronic neuromuscular disorder. However, it must be kept in mind that a smouldering chronic neuromuscular disorder may occasionally present with quickly evolving respiratory muscle paralysis and acute respiratory failure. Even if there is no past history of known neuromuscular disease, a careful history and physical examination is imperative. A history of fatiguability on exertion, difficulty in getting up from a low chair or stool without the use of the upper limbs or a difficulty in swallowing are important clues. A history of ingestion of possible contaminated food (botulism) or of poisonous shellfish (contaminated oysters, squid and rarer fish), or of exposure to ticks should be sought. In the villages of India and in other poor tropical countries the possibility of snakebite should also be kept in mind. A history of dyspnoea on exertion is obviously not specific for respiratory muscle involvement in neuromuscular disease. Dyspnoea at rest is however a crucial

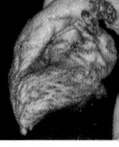

clue if the lungs during examination are found to be clinically normal. Dyspnoea at rest in a patient with neuromuscular disease is an indicator of acute respiratory failure or impending respiratory failure. Paralysis of both leaflets of the diaphragm causes orthopnoea; the patient is unable to lie down supine, though for some inexplicable reason some of these patients are able to lie down on their side.

Paresis of respiratory muscles due to neuromuscular disease often leads initially to hypoventilation and hypercapnic respiratory failure at night, followed later by hypoxemic hypercapnic respiratory failure, both in the day and night.

PHYSICAL EXAMINATION

A meticulous examination of the central and peripheral nervous system should be done. Examination should particularly search for muscle weakness, whether more proximal or distal, presence of fasciculations, evidence for lateral column involvement, presence of atrophy or wasting, presence or absence of deep reflexes. Wasting of the biceps in the presence of an exaggerated biceps tendon reflex is classically associated with amyotrophic lateral sclerosis, though compressive cord lesions at the C5 level could do likewise. Evidence of ptosis which becomes apparent only when the patient is made to fix his or her gaze upwards for a time is excellent evidence of underlying myasthenia. Poor gag reflex, poor movement of the palatal fold suggest involvement of either the lower cranial nerves, or is seen in polymyositis. The latter is at times clinically unmasked only if the patient is observed to get up from a low stool, as this proves difficult without the use of the upper limbs.

Examination of the chest should be meticulously performed. The respiratory rate should be counted for a whole minute; presence or absence of the use of accessory muscles of respiration should be noted. The degree of chest expansion should be observed both on inspection and palpation. Diaphragmatic paralysis besides being characterized by the inability to lie flat is characterized by dyspnoea, tachypnoea and paradoxical respiration wherein the diaphragm is sucked inwards during inspiration and pushed out during expiration. Paresis of diaphragmatic leaflets is suggested by the absence of the outward movement of the diaphragm during inspiration. *A serial count of numbers at as fast a speed as possible after making the patient take a maximum inspiratory breath is an excellent bedside test to determine the presence and progress of respiratory muscle paresis or paralysis.* This of course holds true only if there is no underlying parenchymal lung disease, cardiac disease or any other disease responsible for the difficulty in breathing.

In the differential diagnosis of neuromuscular disease causing acute respiratory failure often associated with paralysis of the skeletal muscles, one should consider GBS, acute myasthenic crisis, paralytic poliomyelitis, acute corticosteroid myopathy, critical illness polyneruopathy and myopathy, acutely evolving polymyositis, acute hypokalemic or hyperkalemic paralysis, botulism, cobra or krait snakebite, and acute intermittent porphyria. Poisoning with various known and perhaps lesser known toxins can also present in the same manner. A GBS may also rarely occur in association with concurrent malignancy (particularly a small cell lung cancer) and preceding or accompanying malignant lymphoproliferative disease.

The important chronic neuromuscular disorders which may occasionally present with an acutely evolving respiratory paralysis causing acute respiratory failure are myasthenia gravis, polymyositis or dermatomyositis and rarely, amyotrophic lateral sclerosis.

Acute diaphragmatic paralysis due to phrenic nerve involvement can cause isolated acute respiratory failure. This is observed after open-heart surgery and after major surgery on the thorax or mediastinal structures. Each of these conditions should be carefully excluded in patients presenting with acute respiratory paralysis causing acute respiratory failure.

IMAGING

Elevation of the dome of the diaphragm can occur with diaphragmatic paralysis, but can also result from basal atelectasis. In diaphragmatic paralysis the sniff test reveals a paradoxical movement of the diaphragm, the diaphragmatic leaflets moving upwards during an inspiratory sniff instead of the usual brisk downward movement. A subpulmonic pleural effusion can give the appearance of a raised diaphragm. Imaging studies in particular an HRCT of the chest gives the correct diagnosis.

ARTERIAL BLOOD GAS STUDIES

The distinguishing feature of hypoventilation causing respiratory failure is hypoxemic hypercapnic respiratory failure. To start with, respiratory failure occurs in sleep. Nocturnal hypercapnia manifests with sleepiness during the day, confusion at night and early morning headaches.

Lung Function Tests and Tests to Assess Inspiratory and Expiratory Muscle Strength

CHANGES IN LUNG STUDIES

Lung volumes Respiratory muscle weakness leads to a fall in vital capacity (VC), forced vital capacity (FVC), end-expiratory lung volume, the functional residual capacity (FRC) and the total lung capacity (TLC). The residual volume (RV) may be normal or even slightly increased. In the absence of lung or skeletal disease, a reduced VC should point to respiratory muscle weakness. The VC test is not a very sensitive test as respiratory muscle strength needs to be reduced substantially (by over 50%) to cause a significant fall in the VC. The RV/TLC ratio is increased but this is not due to obstructive airways disease. The pressure volume curve in patients with respiratory muscle weakness is shifted to the right, so that a large increase in inspiratory pressure near TLC or a large increase in expiratory pressure close to RV produces comparatively small changes in lung volume.

LUNG COMPLIANCE AND CHEST WALL MECHANICS

In acute respiratory muscle weakness, the fall in lung volumes is associated with normal lung compliance. In chronic or longstanding respiratory failure the following changes in lung compliance and chest wall mechanics occur:

a. Reduced lung compliance
b. Reduced chest wall compliance
c. Lung elastic recoil is higher than normal at any given lung volume

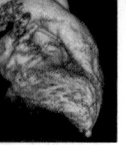

d. Lung elastic recoil pressure in higher than normal at TLC which itself is significantly reduced.

The reduction of lung compliance is due to stiffening of the lung elastin tissue due to prolonged hypoventilation together with microatelectasis so often seen in poorly expanded lungs, as also the occurrence of segmental atelectasis related to shallow breathing and ineffective cough. The fall in chest wall compliance is believed to be related to the stiffening of the costosternal and costovertebral joints due to prolonged poor excursions of the chest wall. The low compliance of the lung and chest wall, in addition to lessened movement of the chest during the respiratory cycle because of respiratory muscle weakness is responsible for the low TLC.

THE FLOW-VOLUME LOOP
The flow-volume loop shows the following abnormalities:

a. A reduction in the peak expiratory flow
b. Delay in reaching the peak expiratory flow
c. A sharp drop in expiratory flow rate towards end of expiration
d. The forced inspiratory flow in one second is less than the forced expiratory flow in one second (FEV_1) because of weakness of the inspiratory muscles.

DIFFUSION CAPACITY FOR CARBON MONOXIDE (DLCO)
The DLCO is reduced, but as mentioned earlier the transfer coefficient KCO or DLCO/VA is typically increased. In patients with neuromuscular diseases, a sniff test below 30% of normal is generally associated with hypercapnic respiratory failure. If the maximum transdiaphragmatic pressure generated during a sniff test is < 30 cm H_2O there is again a strong likelihood of hypercapnic respiratory failure.

SERIAL NUMBER COUNTING TEST AFTER TAKING A DEEP INSPIRATION
This is an extremely useful test for inspiratory muscle strength particularly in acutely evolving respiratory weakness. The patient is asked to take as deep an inspiratory breath and is asked to number serially 1, 2, 3, as fast as possible. Most normal individuals can easily count up to 30 and much more in a single breath. Inability to go beyond 20 and in particular a falling number count when tested at intervals is a good guide to inspiratory muscle weakness.

TESTS FOR EXPIRATORY MUSCLES (SEE CHAPTER ON 'MECHANICS OF VENTILATION')
The P_{EMAX} is an index of expiratory muscle strength though values below normal are difficult to interpret.

COUGH TEST
It is best to gauge the strength of a patient's cough clinically at the bedside. The patient is requested to cough as loudly as possible after a deep inspiration. With a little practice one can judge whether the cough is weak or normal. Serial observations in patients with acutely evolving respiratory muscles weakness are of great help.

REDUCED MUSCLE STRENGTH AND FUNCTION
Reduced lung volumes may occur in lung pathologies other than in patients with pure respiratory muscle weakness, so that direct measurement of muscle strength may be necessary. Strength of inspiratory and expiratory muscles should be evaluated as the decline in respiratory muscle strength need not be necessarily the same. Inspiratory muscle weakness leads to dyspnoea and hypoxemic cum hypercapnic respiratory failure. Expiratory muscle weakness is responsible for a poor ineffective cough that predisposes to aspiration, microatelectasis and segmental atelectasis.

TESTS FOR INSPIRATORY MUSCLES
The easiest test for inspiratory muscle strength is to determine the P_{IMAX}. A P_{IMAX} less than 50% of predicated is often associated with CO_2 retention. There are however fallacies that may enter in performing the test in patients with respiratory muscle weakness (e.g. air leak around the mouth piece) and difficulties in interpretation as some normal patients may also have a low P_{IMAX}.

Sniff Nasal Inspiratory Pressure Test and the Sniff Diaphragmatic Pressure Test have been described in the chapter 'Respiratory Muscle Function Testing'.

MANAGEMENT
1. Treatment of the cause. This is possible in just a few of the neuromuscular disorders causing respiratory paresis and respiratory failure. In most patients with neuromuscular disorders there is no specific treatment and no adequate measure that can prevent respiratory failure in the natural history of the disease (see chapter on 'Acute Respiratory Failure in Adults').
2. Mechanical ventilation. Mechanical ventilation is indicated in chronic hypoxemic hypercapnic respiratory failure or in an acute crisis related to pulmonary infection, retention of secretions within the lungs, or following an abrupt increase in metabolism as with fever or infection from any cause. Patients in acute crisis are dyspnoeic, tachypnoeic and develop acute CO_2 retention. Endotracheal intubation with ventilator support helps in handling the crisis successfully. Endotracheal intubation and ventilator support is also indicated in respiratory paralysis or near-paralysis following head injury and spinal cord injury. Weaning or transfer to non-invasive ventilatory support may be possible in a number of patients.

Patients with GBS with quickly evolving increasing respiratory muscle involvement should in our opinion be intubated and placed on elective ventilator support. *It is better to anticipate rather than await disaster.* Tracheostomy should not be unnecessarily delayed as many patients with GBS require ventilator support for weeks or even months. The longest period of ventilator support in GBS we have successfully managed was over nine months. Almost always weaning is possible even after long periods of ventilator support.

Acute myasthenic crisis also often needs intubation with ventilator support, which generally is necessary for a few days to at the most a few weeks.

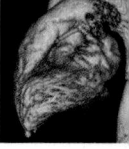

Patients with chronic neuromuscular disease who develop over a period of observation slowly progressive chronic respiratory failure are managed comfortably on non-invasive ventilator support. Non-invasive ventilator support to start with may be necessary only at night. As respiratory failure worsens, support becomes necessary both during day and night. It is best not to delay non-invasive ventilator support once there is persistent hypercapnia.

In amyotrophic lateral sclerosis, non-invasive ventilator support should be introduced once hypercapnia occurs. When the brainstem is involved so that the patient is unable to swallow and cannot handle upper airways secretions, tracheostomy becomes necessary. Invasive ventilator support prolongs life but the quality of life is indeed poor and the situation should be carefully explained to the patient as he has the right to make the choice—to ventilate invasively or not.

Irrecoverable Diaphragmatic Paralysis

Cervical cord lesions at C5, C6 level, or severe irrecoverable bilateral phrenic nerve damage as after open-heart or thoracic surgery, or patients with central alveolar hypoventilation, are indications for diaphragmatic pacing. The phrenic nerves are stimulated by intra-thoracic implanted electrodes, the receiver being activated by radio-frequency waves generated by an external power source. The method is costly, requires special expertise; we have no experience in this field.

PHYSIOTHERAPY

Physiotherapy is vital for survival both in acute respiratory failure and in chronic respiratory failure due to neuromuscular cause. The airways should be kept free of secretions through careful suction and gentle percussion and vibration to the chest. Frequent change of posture is essential. Cough must be encouraged. This may be impossible with severe respiratory muscle paralysis. Manual assistance to cough is given through squeezing of the chest and by a gentle yet sudden upper abdominal thrust timed with opening of the glottis. Mechanical insufflation followed by desufflation may help. It is done by first using a positive pressure insufflation followed by an abrupt negative pressure which causes desufflation. Cough-assist devices are fairly popular abroad. In our opinion, the best method and the least inconvenient method to the patient who fails to cough and clear secretions in spite of expert physiotherapy is to perform a tracheostomy through which secretions can be sucked and the airways kept open.

SUGGESTED READING

De Jonghe B. Critical illness neuromuscular syndromes. *Crit Care Clin.* 1 Oct. 2006; 22(4): 805–18; abstract xi.

Hemachudha T. Human rabies: a disease of complex neuropathogenetic mechanisms and diagnostic challenges. *Lancet Neurol.* 1 Jun. 2002; 1(2): 101–9.

Horowitz BZ. Botulinum toxin. *Crit Care Clin.* 1 Oct. 2005; 21(4): 825–39, viii.

Maramattom BV. Acute neuromuscular weakness in the intensive care unit. *Crit Care Med.* 1 Nov. 2006; 34(11): 2835–41.

Postpolio syndrome and anesthesia. *Anesthesiology.* 1 Sep. 2005; 103(3): 638–44.

Simonds AK. Recent advances in respiratory care for neuromuscular disease. *Chest.* 1 Dec. 2006; 130(6): 1879–86.

van Doorn PA. Clinical features, pathogenesis, and treatment of Guillain-Barre syndrome. *Lancet Neurol.* 1 Oct. 2008; 7(10): 939–50.

Yazici Y. Clinical presentation of the idiopathic inflammatory myopathies. *Rheum Dis Clin North Am.* 1 Nov. 2002; 28(4): 823–32.

CHAPTER **74** ## Sleep Related Breathing Disorders

INTRODUCTION

We spend a third of our lives asleep but it is now clear that sleep is not always the tranquil resting state it is imagined to be. We now know, the lives of millions are disturbed and disrupted by the consequences of sleep-disordered breathing.

Sleep disorders involve any difficulties related to sleeping, including difficulty falling or staying asleep, falling asleep at inappropriate times, excessive total sleep time, or abnormal behaviours associated with sleep.

TYPES OF SLEEP DISORDERS

The International Classification of Sleep Disorders (ICSD), published in 2004 lists 85 sleep disorders, each presented in detail and with a specific diagnostic test. These have been classified as follows into the following eight major categories:

1. The insomnias
2. The sleep-related breathing disorders
3. The hypersomnias not due to a breathing disorder
4. The circadian rhythm sleep disorders
5. The parasomnias
6. The sleep-related movement disorders
7. Isolated symptoms, apparently normal variants and unresolved issues
8. Other sleep disorders

This chapter will focus on obstructive sleep apnoea (OSA) and central sleep apnoea (CSA) as these are the two major sleep-related breathing disorders.

OBSTRUCTIVE SLEEP APNOEA

History

What is so remarkable about OSA is that it should have been so obvious and common yet escaped recognition by the medical community till it was first described by Gastaut in a neurology journal in 1965. Yet, Charles Dickens, an astute observer of the human condition, must be given the credit for first describing this disorder, well over a century before its first medical report. Dickens was only 21 at the time, yet he went on in 1836, to describe in his first book, *The Pickwick Papers*, a textbook description of a person with OSA. In Joe the fat boy, we see an uncannily accurate description of OSA almost 130 years before the world of medicine had acknowledged its existence. The snoring and the irresistible urge to fall asleep, the two cardinal symptoms of OSA are summed up when he has a character say:

'Asleep! He's always asleep. Goes on errands fast asleep, and snores as he waits at table.'

Definition

OSA is defined as repetitive episodes of upper airway obstruction occurring during sleep, usually associated with a reduction in SaO_2, with features of snoring and daytime sleepiness. The apnoea-hypopnoea index is the most commonly used criterion to quantify the severity of OSA. According to the American Association of Sleep Medicine, OSA exists when the patient has five or more obstructed breathing events (apnoeas or hypopnoeas) per hour of sleep with an appropriate clinical presentation.

Epidemiology

OSA is a difficult disease to study, as the standard diagnostic test, polysomnography, is expensive and cumbersome. Until the American Academy of Sleep Medicine Task Force published recent guidelines in 1989, there was no clear consensus regarding diagnostic classification. Thus worldwide there have been only a few good-quality epidemiological studies.

Global Epidemiology

Initial studies in the eighties and early nineties involved short case series or prevalence studies in selected cohorts rather than in the general population. These early studies sought to determine the 'lower limit' of prevalence by conducting polysomnography in small subsets comprising only people with self-reported OSA symptoms selected from sample surveys and then assuming that all cases of OSA had been identified. Although such studies were undermined by the low sensitivity of screening questions, even these lower limits of prevalence established the importance of studying OSA further. Stradling analyzed these early epidemiological studies in a review and noted that the prevalence of OSA varied from 1–4% in adult males. Since then, studies on much larger population-based samples have shown an even higher prevalence. The landmark epidemiological study that brought OSA to the attention of physicians and the lay public was the Wisconsin Sleep Cohort Study in 1993 by Terry Young and colleagues. These authors showed that based on a sample of 625 adults, 9% of women and 24% of men had Sleep Disordered Breathing (SDB) with an average of at least five or more apnoeas and hypopnoeas per hour of sleep. OSA, defined as SDB plus the cardinal symptom of excess daytime sleepiness (EDS) occurred in 2% of women and 4% of men. This study put OSA on the world map by demonstrating that it was a

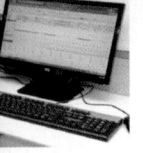

widely prevalent disorder. When one factored in the major cardiovascular impact of this potentially disabling condition, it became clear that undiagnosed OSA represented a potential public health hazard that had to be addressed. Since Young's study there have been several other studies of prevalence from across the developing world but direct comparison is difficult due to considerable variations in methodology. Different studies have, for example, studied different patient populations, used different diagnostic tools, and often used different definitions of OSA. These differences in methodology must be borne in mind when making comparisons. Many prevalence studies have had one or more methodological weaknesses including selection biases, varying definitions of OSA, failure to distinguish types of apnoeas, failure to control for confounding variables, and small sample sizes. These inherent weaknesses in the available studies have made direct comparisons difficult.

Asian Epidemiology

It had initially been perceived that OSA might not be common in the Asian populations due to the fact that obesity, the major risk factor for OSA, is less prevalent than in Western communities. However, this is not the case. Several studies comparing OSA in Asians and Caucasians have shown that Asian subjects have greater severity of illness, as indicated by higher respiratory disturbance indices compared to Caucasian patients matched for age sex and body mass index (BMI).

A study by Ng looked at the prevalence of OSA in the three major ethnic populations in Singapore; Chinese, Malays and Indians. This study established that Indians living in Singapore had the highest prevalence rates (4.5%), significantly higher than the prevalence in Malays (3.7%) and Chinese (1.6%). This was the first study to suggest that Indians, as a race, had a predisposition to OSA. An important study by Hilloowalla hinted that Indian craniofacial anatomy might be the factor predisposing this race to OSA. He compared 75 skulls of Indian origin to 98 Tuscan skulls and noted important cephalometric differences. This pointed to a possible osteogenic aetiology of OSA in Indians.

Indian Epidemiology

OSA is a disease that is strongly affected by racial factors and it seems vital to establish the prevalence in a country of 1.2 billion Indians. India also has amongst the largest populations with ischemic heart disease, diabetes and hypertension and the potential impact of untreated OSA on these sub-populations of Indians is clearly a cause for concern.

There is almost no data on the epidemiology of OSA from India. Possible reasons for this include lack of awareness and formal training in sleep medicine and the cost and lack of availability of polysomnography (PSG). Although the first sleep laboratory in the country was established only in 1991, there has been a rapid and exponential increase in the number of private and public sleep laboratories since then. The labs are mainly concentrated in the big metros and the numbers are still very limited for a country of one billion. An occasional study has looked at the prevalence of OSA in patients referred to and assessed at sleep clinics but an accurate idea of the prevalence of OSA in the general population was until recently lacking. A recent population-based study by Udwadia published in 2004 will be discussed in more detail here, as it was the first epidemiological attempt to study the prevalence of OSA in India.

The authors chose 700 consecutive healthy Indian male residents of Mumbai, aged 35 to 65 years coming as outpatients to the Hinduja Hospital for a routine health check-up between December 1999 and December 2000. None of these patients were coming to the hospital because of suspected sleep problems. Most were undergoing health checks as part of company policy or for insurance reasons.

A two-stage sampling scheme was designed to optimize the study's precision. In the first stage subjects were given a specially designed comprehensive 32-part questionnaire adapted to local conditions and translated into local languages where needed. It sought detailed information on the cohorts sleep habits, snoring, daytime sleepiness, nocturnal choking and associated medical conditions. Physical examination was done thereafter with measurements of BMI, neck girth and blood pressure. All questionnaires were collected and analyzed by a doctor on the same day. Based on the responses, subjects were classified into habitual snorers and non-snorers. All (100%) snorers and 25% of non-snorers were contacted and offered a sleep study if they consented. The type of sleep study chosen was a limited, home-based, semi-supervised sleep study performed on a Compumedics P series 10-channel system. This was considered a more practical and economical approach than a full electroencephalogram (EEG)-based polysomnography in the hospital. The home-based Compumedics system had been validated in several home-based studies and gave polygraphic recordings of nasal and oral airflow, electrocardiographic (ECG), thoracic and abdominal effort, tracheal sounds, limb movement, body position and oxyhaemoglobin level by pulse oximetry.

The results of the study were as follows: 700 questionnaires were given out and 658 were completed and returned giving an initial response rate of 94%. All 171 snorers and 122 non-snorers (25% contacted) were asked if they would undergo sleep testing at home. A total of 254 subjects agreed (151 of the snorers and 103 non-snorers) giving a good participation rate of 87%. Habitual snoring was seen in 26% of the study population, nocturnal choking/witnessed apnoeas in 5% and daytime hypersomnolence in 22% of the study population. The mean age of the sample was 47.84 years, and the mean BMI was 24.56. The mean Epworth score of snorers was 8.39 and that of non-snorers was 6.05.

The prevalence of SDB was 19.5% and that of Obstructive sleep apnoea-hypopnoea syndrome (OSAHS) was 7.5% in healthy urban Indian males between 35–65 years of age. These prevalence rates are among the highest reported from epidemiological studies across the globe and are higher than in most Western and Asian studies. In this study, BMI, neck girth, and a history of diabetes mellitus were significantly associated with SDB, and a history of snoring, EDS, nocturnal choking, recurrent awakening from sleep, unrefreshing sleep and daytime fatigue were all associated with OSA.

REASONS FOR THE HIGHER PREVALENCE FOUND IN INDIANS

The exact causes of this unexpectedly high prevalence are unclear. It must first be pointed out that this data cannot be extended to the country as a whole as only urban Indian men

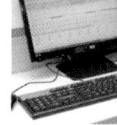

in Mumbai were studied. The study population represents men that are better educated and employed, have higher incomes and are of better socioeconomic class than rural Indians. Also, urban Indian males are significantly more obese (BMI of 24) than their rural counterparts (BMI of 20). Obesity is a major risk factor for OSA in white populations. In this study, a higher BMI was a risk factor for SDB and OSA in Indian subjects as well. However, it is worth stating that 46% of our subjects with SDB had a BMI of less than 30, the Western cut-off for obesity whereas 27% of subjects with SDB had a BMI less than 27, which is the cut-off point for obesity in Asians. These observations suggest that a significant number of patients, though not obese by Western or Asian standards, still had SDB and OSA. This leads the authors to postulate that other craniofacial risk factors for SDB, such as oropharyngeal narrowing, retrognathia or micrognathia, and pharyngeal collapsibility, might assume greater pathogenic significance in Indian subjects and may be responsible for our higher prevalence rates.

In agreement with other Western studies, this study found neck girth to be an important predictor of OSA and found that the risk of SDB is 5.34 times higher for subjects with a neck girth of 17 inches or more.

Other subsequent Indian epidemiological studies: The only other epidemiological studies from India reported lower prevalence rates. The first by Sharma in 2006, reported a prevalence rate of 13.7% for SDB and 3.6% for OSA in a community-based prevalence study in a semi-urban community in Delhi. The second, from Reddy in 2009 again from an urban Delhi population reported the prevalence of SDB to be 9.3% and that of OSA to be 2.8% (4% in males and 1.5% in females).

CONCLUSIONS

Thus there is a divergence in the prevalence rates reported from India with higher prevalence rates in the study from Mumbai in western India, and lower rates from the two Delhi-based studies from northern India. These differences could be real differences as it is possible that different regions and populations in a country as diverse as India could have different prevalence rates. The other explanation could be methodological. The Mumbai study was performed only in men belonging to a higher socioeconomic status with a home-based system, which could have introduced an element of selection bias. The Delhi studies were in both sexes in a community-based setting and had fully supervised PSG performed in a sleep laboratory. Irrespective of which rates are more accurate, these studies have established that OSA is indeed at least as prevalent and possibly even more prevalent in India compared to the West. The high prevalence rates found in these studies might have major public health implications in a developing country with limited health resources. Indian men in this age group have among the highest rates of ischemic heart disease and hypertension worldwide. When compared to whites, blacks, Hispanics and other Asians, coronary artery disease rates among Indians worldwide are two to four times higher at all ages. India also has the largest population of individuals with diabetes (approximately 25 million) and the potential impact of untreated OSA on this population might be considerable. Further studies in populations from different races, in different communities (urban and rural) from all regions of this vast country are urgently needed before a clearer picture of OSA in India emerges. Finally,

Indian cranial anthropometric studies are needed to determine if our facial structure uniquely predisposes Indians to a higher prevalence of OSA.

Clinical Features

The cardinal symptoms of OSA are disruptive snoring, EDS, nocturnal choking and witnessed apnoeas.

SNORING

Snoring is a cardinal symptom of OSA. It is defined as an inspiratory vibration of the soft tissue of the oropharynx. It denotes partial obstruction of the upper airway. Not all snorers have OSA of course; it is estimated that at least 60% of men over the age of 40 snore. The snoring of OSA is distinctive in its quality. It is often disruptively loud, loud enough to drive the spouse out of the bedroom and sometimes out of the house. In one study in the US, almost 50% of all patients slept in separate bedrooms from their partner. Its intensity is often noted to be > 50 db when measured by PSG. An astute partner will describe the snoring as intermittent, more in the supine than the lateral position, of a waxing and waning quality, and sometimes interrupted by long periods of ominous silence when it is felt the patient seems to have stopped breathing altogether. While snoring on its own has a low diagnostic accuracy for OSA, the pattern of snoring just described is very predictive of a positive sleep study. Most snorers are unaware that they snore and there is poor agreement between snorers and their bed-partners when it comes to this symptom. Women are less likely to admit to snoring and patients from poorer socioeconomic backgrounds are also less likely to complain of it or be questioned regarding their snoring habits. In any case, snoring is the most common complaint precipitating referral to a sleep laboratory. A patient and sometimes his spouse may not be forthcoming with a history of snoring hence asking each patient if they snore should be part of each and every medical history. OSA is one of the least diagnosed diseases and we must train ourselves and our medical students that it would be negligent not to enquire about snoring and sleepiness from every patient we encounter. This is even more important with the realization that snoring alone (i.e. even non-apnoeic snoring) may be an independent risk factor for hypertension, cardiovascular disease and cerebrovascular disease.

EXCESSIVE DAYTIME SLEEPINESS (EDS)

EDS is the second major symptom of OSA. Like snoring, it is a non-specific symptom and occurs in a host of other conditions enumerated in Table 74.1. In OSA it is often but not always present. In patients with severe OSA it is an overwhelming urge to sleep in situations that the patient himself acknowledges are inappropriate. Thus we have had patients who routinely fall asleep whilst driving, those who fall asleep whilst addressing a meeting, in the midst of signing a cheque and even, on one occasion, whilst climbing a ladder.

NOCTURNAL CHOKING

Nocturnal choking is another important but non-specific symptom of OSA. It occurs in a few other conditions as outlined in Table 74.2. However, it is a frightening symptom and will often alert the patient and his spouse into consulting a doctor.

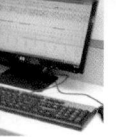

Table 74.1:
Causes of excessive daytime sleepiness
1. Sleep deprivation
2. OSA
3. Narcolepsy
4. Idiopathic hypersomnolescence
5. Nocturnal myoclonus
6. PLMD (Periodic limb movement disorder)
7. Psychological (20% depressed patients)
8. Drugs and alcohol
9. Hypothyroidism
10. Post-viral fatigue syndrome

Table 74.2:
Causes of nocturnal choking
1. Pulmonary edema (paroxysmal nocturnal dyspnoea)
2. Nocturnal asthma
3. OSA
4. GERD causing laryngeal spasm

WITNESSED APNOEA

Witnessed apnoea is the most specific symptom of OSA. Apnoeic episodes may be reported by as many as 75% of bed partners. Episodes of loud snoring often terminate in an apnoea. A characteristic pattern observed in OSA is that of loud snoring or brief gasps that alternate with episodes of silence that typically last 20–30 seconds. An apnoea is defined as complete cessation of breathing for a period of at least 10 seconds. Many apnoeas are longer, some stretching to almost 60 seconds or beyond. An apnoea terminates in an arousal and these cycles of apnoea and subsequent arousal fragment the patient's sleep resulting in sleep that is of very poor quality.

OTHER SYMPTOMS

A host of other symptoms and signs are reported in OSA. These include:

- Restless, non-refreshing sleep
- Diaphoresis usually in the neck and chest area
- Nocturia, with one study reporting a third of all patients with OSA getting up four to seven times at night to urinate
- Morning headaches, a study from a headache clinic found OSA to be the commonest cause of morning headaches. None of these patients had been previously investigated for OSA.
- Gastro-oesophageal reflux is common in patients with OSA and is believed to be due to the raised intra-abdominal pressure observed in patients with OSA related to increased breathing efforts during periods of apnoea.

CLINICAL PRESENTATIONS OF OSA

The following are some of the clinical presentations we have encountered where OSA must be clinically suspected:

- Unexplained respiratory failure (pulmonologist)
- Unexplained pulmonary hypertension or cor pulmonale (pulmonologist)
- Unexplained polycythemia (haematologist)
- Confusional state (neurologist)
- Nocturnal seizure (neurologist)
- Nocturnal arrhythmia (cardiologist)
- Post-anaesthetic respiratory failure (anaesthetist)
- Post-extubation problems (anaesthetist)
- Nocturia, enuresis (urologist)
- Impotence in a male (andrologist)

Thus, as can be seen, OSA can present to a wide range of specialists.

Diagnosing OSA

HISTORY

The cardinal symptoms mentioned earlier must be inquired about in the history. Clinical pointers or risk factors that increase the index of suspicion are obesity, male sex and age > 65 years. A positive family history also increases the risk of OSA two to fourfold. First-degree relatives of OSA patients have a 21–84% chance of having OSA themselves compared to 10% of the controls. This genetic predisposition is likely to be expressed through craniofacial anatomy, though obesity is also often genetic, and both these factors can explain why OSA often runs in families.

Physical Examination

BMI

BMI must always be measured. This is often used to define and quantify obesity and in one study, a BMI of >25 kg/m² had a sensitivity of 93% and specificity of 74% for OSA. Having said this, these Western figures may not translate to Indian populations. In Udwadia's study, 46% of subjects with OSA had a BMI less than 30, the Western cut-off for obesity, whereas 27% had a BMI less than 27, which is the cut-off for obesity in Asians. Thus the important lesson emerging from these observations is that while obesity makes it more likely that the Indian patient has OSA, the absence of obesity does not rule it out.

NECK GIRTH

Neck girth must always be measured. The importance of a larger neck girth in producing upper airway incompetence during sleep has been documented in patients with sleep apnoea in a number of studies and the mechanism is presumably external compression of the pharynx by adipose tissue. In agreement with these Western observations, the study by Udwadia found that the risk of SDB is 5.34 times higher for subjects with a neck girth of 17 inches.

UPPER AIRWAY EXAMINATION

Upper airway examination should be part of the evaluation of any OSA suspect. This should include a look at the nose for any gross septal deviation, polyps or growths. Dentition must be checked especially the presence of retrognathia and dental overjet. The oropharynx should be examined for the presence of tonsillar hypertrophy, uvula size, length, and height. Oedema

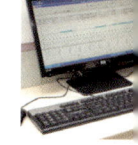

or erythema of the uvula indicates repetitive vibration trauma from snoring. Macroglossia must also be checked for, as it is another cause of partial airway occlusion. It is rare to get an actual structural abnormality but patients with OSA have what can best be described as a 'crowded' oropharynx. Finally, micrognathia and retrognathia can predispose to OSA and must always be checked for.

Clinical scales have been used for standardizing oropharyngeal clinical evaluation, the most frequently used scale being the Mallampati scale. Whether one uses a scale or not, routine visual examination of the upper airway and facial structure will allow the trained observer to suspect OSA in certain patients.

NOCTURNAL OXIMETRY

Nocturnal oximetry has often been used as a 'poor-man's sleep study'. It may be an adequate screening test in a patient with a high pre-test clinical suspicion of OSA. It will, however, miss OSA in significant numbers (almost a third) of patients; a study by Douglas showed that it diagnosed only 66% of all patients with OSA. Many of the patients missed by oximetry had moderately severe OSA and benefited from treatment.

POLYSOMNOGRAPHY

Symptoms and signs alone are not reliable enough to make a definite diagnosis of OSA. A study showed them to have a combined sensitivity of around 60% and specificity of around 70% when diagnosing OSA. Routine tests like radiography, pulmonary function test (PFT) and arterial blood gas analysis add little to this. Hence the only way to confirm a clinical suspicion of OSA is by performing PSG. The nocturnal, laboratory-based PSG is the gold standard for the diagnosis of OSA. It also quantifies the severity of OSA and can grade it into mild moderate or severe. A PSG involves recordings of airflow, ventilatory effort (chest and abdominal movements), oxygen saturation, body position, electrocardiography, electromyography, and electroencephalography (EEG). All these are measured dynamically, through the night. In the standard laboratory-based PSG, a technician is present throughout the night to monitor the patient for the entire study. There are a number of variations however. In patients with obvious OSA diagnosed in the early part of the night, a 'split-night' study can be performed with the continuous positive airway pressure (CPAP) titration being performed in the second half of the night. In some centres, a more limited study is performed without the EEG leads, as these are not crucial when it comes to diagnosing OSA. Sometimes, for reasons of manpower or financial constraints, a partially supervised study is done where the technician sets the patient up for the night and then leaves once the patient falls asleep, returning in the morning to disconnect him from the machine. Finally, with the pressure on beds in many hospitals, home sleep studies are being increasingly performed. Many patients often prefer this as they feel they would sleep more naturally in their own homes than in the artificial confines of a hospital. Modern, lightweight PSG machines are very portable and this has facilitated testing at home. Proponents of home sleep studies thus point out the increased accessibility, reduced cost, enhanced patient convenience and better sleep in a familiar environment. Critics point out that equipment problems cannot be sorted out leading to the occasional technical study failure, and that non-OSA disorders cannot be diagnosed. Irrespective of how

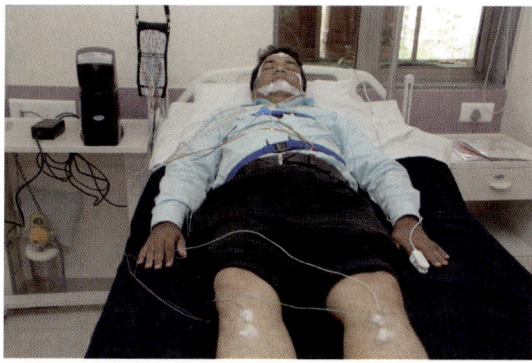

Fig 74.1: PSG being performed at a hospital.

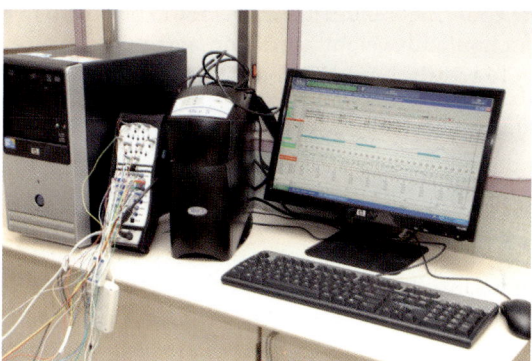

Fig 74.2: PSG monitoring equipment.

or where the test is performed it must be stressed that a doctor trained in sleep medicine must carefully interpret it.

IMPACT OF OSA

Cardiovascular

The association between OSA and cardiovascular morbidity has been evident since the first patients with OSA were investigated in the laboratory. Normal sleep induces reduction in blood pressure, heart rate, stroke volume, cardiac output, peripheral resistance and sympathetic activity. OSA causes cyclical surges in all these variables due to exaggerated negative intrathoracic pressure, hypoxia and recurrent arousals. Coincident with apnoea termination is a surge in blood pressure well over 40 mm Hg, coupled with a rise in heart rate which is probably consequent upon the arousal-related increase in sympathetic tone. It is believed that in patients with OSA, the initial step is absence of the normal nocturnal dipping, then nocturnal hypertension sets in, and sustained hypertension finally follows this.

HYPERTENSION

Fifty to ninety-six percent of OSA patients have hypertension, and conversely, about 40% of hypertensive patients have occult OSA. If a population of patients with refractory hypertension is considered, this figure is even higher. Ample evidence has emerged, not just from animal studies but also from several well-designed longitudinal epidemiological studies, of the link between these two conditions. The landmark Wisconsin Sleep Cohort Study by Peppard, prospectively studied 709

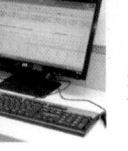

participants for the development of hypertension. The authors found a linear dose-response relation between the severity of OSA and the odds of developing hypertension four years later, with an apnoea-hypopnoea index (AHI) of 5–15 conferring a 2.03 times odds ratio for the development of hypertension. More interestingly, even at a minor AHI of 1–4.9/h, a level that would not even be labelled OSA, the odds ratio already increased from 1 to 1.6 with further rise being exponential. A similar relationship between OSA and the risk of hypertension is seen in other studies. There is also evidence that successfully treating OSA with CPAP reduces blood pressure in patients with hypertension. Thus, the lessons to the physician, based on the cumulative research in the field, is to suspect OSA in every patient with hypertension, screen for it if there are other risk factors (obesity, snoring, thick neck) and treat with CPAP once it is confirmed. Indeed, CPAP should be added to exercise, salt reduction and weight reduction as a non-pharmacological measure to reduce hypertension.

CORONARY ARTERY DISEASE

Several studies report a high prevalence of OSA in patients with coronary artery disease (CAD). While this connection may be indirect, because of shared co-morbidities like obesity and hypertension, there is some evidence that there may be a direct link as well. OSA itself may promote atherogenesis. The evidence for this is based on the increased C-reactive protein (CRP) and endothelin levels seen in patients with OSA. Studies have shown that patients with OSA have a greater prevalence of increased carotid wall thickness and calcified carotid artery atheromas. A study by Hung from Australia of 101 consecutive men with myocardial infarction (MI) who consented to a sleep study three weeks after their infarction showed that an AHI>5.3 was a more powerful predictor of MI (RR 23.3), than the more traditional risk factors like hypertension (RR 7.8), or smoking (RR 11.1). In patients with established CAD, severe OSA may trigger acute nocturnal cardiac ischemia. A study by Franklin documented the presence of OSA in 9 of 10 patients with severe disabling nocturnal angina despite optimal drug therapy. Treatment with CPAP therapy abolished the nocturnal angina.

CARDIAC ARRHYTHMIAS

Sleep apnoea is associated with an increased incidence of brady and tachy arrhythmias, the majority of these arrhythmias recorded in patients with severe OSA and hypoxia, mainly in rapid eye movement (REM) sleep. Heart blocks with Stoke Adams syndrome have also been recorded in patients with severe OSA. CPAP therapy has been shown to be curative in a sample of patients primarily referred for pacemaker implantation for bradyarrhythmias in sleep, most of whom were subsequently diagnosed to have OSA. Atrial fibrillation (AF) is also seen more frequently in patients with OSA, with a study from the Mayo Clinic showing that 49% of patients with AF referred for cardioversion had OSA (OR 3.42), a rate significantly higher than in general cardiology clinic controls matched for age, sex, weight and diabetes.

CONGESTIVE CARDIAC FAILURE

SDB is common in congestive cardiac failure (CCF). Several studies have looked at the prevalence of OSA in patients with systolic heart failure and found that as many as 50–60% of CCF patients have some form of SDB. This is most commonly central sleep apnoea (Cheyne Stokes breathing), but OSA and mixed obstructive and central apnoeas are also frequently seen. A single study looked at the incidence of SDB in isolated diastolic failure and reported that 50% of these patients had OSA as well. At the Hinduja Hospital we prospectively studied 70 patients hospitalized for CCF. Sleep studies were performed on them prior to discharge and we found OSA to be present in 59% and CSA in 20% of these patients. The significance of the impact of SDB in CCF is considerable. Sleep disordered breathing adds to the considerable fatigue that patients with CCF routinely face. It can also be considered a marker of severe CCF and sets up a worsening cycle of heart failure, predisposing these patients to arrhythmias and death. Indeed, Cheyne Stokes respiration (CSR) is recognized to be an independent risk factor for mortality in CCF. CSR in CCF is associated with worse left ventricular ejection fraction (LVEF), higher pulmonary wedge pressures, more arrhythmias and significantly higher mortality and worse survival than in matched patients with CCF and normal nocturnal breathing. When it comes to treatment, there is good news. CPAP at a pressure of 5–12 cm H_2O can have a positive impact. Another non-invasive device used to treat CSA in patients with CCF is adaptive pressure support servo ventilation. This device provides varying amounts of ventilatory support during different phases of periodic breathing. In small studies, treating OSA or CSA with CPAP has been shown to substantially improve not just symptoms like dyspnoea and fatigue but also substantially improve LVEF. Hence the results of the much-anticipated 11-centre CANPAP (Canadian CPAP study for patients with CSA and heart failure) study which showed that CPAP over two years in these patients ultimately failed to improve survival were disappointing and unexpected. Several criticisms have been made about the design of this trial including the fact that patients treated with CPAP did not receive a titration study but received CPAP at 5–10 cm H_2O. Another possible explanation is that this study was underpowered to conclude with certainty that CPAP is ineffective in this patient population. A post hoc subgroup analysis of this data revealed that patients on CPAP did have significant improvements in performances in the six-minute walk test and LVEF, hence the last word on treatment with CPAP in this challenging group of patients has not been written.

OTHER CARDIOVASCULAR FEATURES

Smaller studies have noted intriguing associations between cardiomyopathy and OSA and between aortic dissection and OSA. Finally, OSA has been linked to sudden cardiac death with a study showing an average SaO_2 of 93% and a lowest SaO_2 of 78% strongly predicting sudden cardiac death.

Neuropsychiatric

STROKE

SBDs are strongly associated with increased risk of stroke, independent of known risk factors. The mechanisms underlying this increased risk are multifactorial and include reduction in cerebral blood flow, altered cerebral autoregulation, impaired endothelial function and accelerated atherogenesis. There are also several overlapping risk factors for both diseases such as age, gender, hypertension, obesity, smoking and alcohol use that may

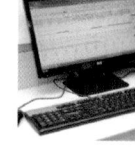

contribute to the association between OSA and stroke. Perhaps the strongest epidemiological evidence of the association between SDB and stroke comes from the Sleep Heart Health Study, which explored the cross-sectional association between SDB and risk of cardiovascular disease in 6424 individuals. This study found an odds ratio of 1.58 (1.02–2.46) for the association of stroke with SDB after adjusting for all other confounding risk factors. It is also being increasingly recognized that the association of OSA and stroke may result in unfavourable clinical outcomes after stroke including early neurological worsening, delirium, depression, poor functional status and impaired cognition. Results of CPAP treatment trials in patients with stroke have recently been published. These establish that CPAP is well tolerated and accepted in patients with stroke and OSA and this treatment may have a beneficial effect on wellbeing, depression and hypertension, post-stroke. Larger treatment trials are clearly needed to determine whether treatment improves outcome after stroke and whether treatment may serve as secondary prophylaxis preventing the risk of recurrent stroke, or death. It is suggested that all patients with stroke or transient ischaemic attack (TIA) should have a detailed sleep history enquiry with a low threshold for proceeding with PSG if there is any suspicion of OSA.

PSYCHIATRIC

Numerous studies have identified significant neuropsychological impairment in patients with OSA. These include impairments in general intellectual function, attention, memory and cognitive impairment. OSA has also been linked to depression, with a study by Mosko reporting that 58% of their OSA patients met the Diagnostic and Statistical Manual of Mental Disorders, third edition (DSM-III) criteria for major depression. Several studies have shown an improvement in many of these neuropsychiatric parameters and quality of life after treatment with CPAP.

Metabolic

TYPE 2 DIABETES

It has long been felt that central obesity which is common in Type 2 diabetes and OSA is the fundamental link between these disorders. However, rapidly accumulating data from both clinical and epidemiological studies suggest that OSA is independently associated with disturbances in glucose metabolism, and places patients at increased risk of developing Type 2 diabetes. At least nine earlier studies have all found an association between OSA and alterations in glucose metabolism consistent with an increased risk of diabetes. Frequent habitual snoring, even in the absence of OSA has itself been linked with increased risk of development of diabetes. In the largest study till date, Meslier studied 595 men referred to a sleep lab for PSG and found that Type 2 diabetes was present in 30% of OSA patients and 14% of non-apnoeic snorers. More importantly, blood sugar levels increased and insulin sensitivity decreased with rising severity of OSA, independent of body mass index (BMI). Thus while there is strong evidence to indicate that OSA and the risk of Type 2 diabetes are associated, the evidence supporting a role for OSA in the development of Type 2 diabetes is still limited. The direction of causality remains unclear; it is conceivable that diabetes may itself cause SDB as its autonomic neuropathy could indeed disturb the control of breathing. The effect of CPAP therapy on glucose metabolism has also been looked at: Several recent studies have shown that treatment with CPAP improves glucose levels and insulin sensitivity, at least when it is continued for a few months.

Thus, based on current evidence, it is noteworthy to urge clinicians to systematically evaluate the risk of OSA in Type 2 diabetic patients, and, conversely, to assess glucose tolerance in patients with known OSA. Further studies are needed to unravel the complex link between obesity, Type 2 diabetes and OSA. This need is even more pressing in a country like India with among the highest prevalence of diabetes and of OSA. Unravelling this link could have important public health consequences in these ever growing patient populations.

METABOLIC SYNDROME

Many patients with OSA have features of the metabolic syndrome; central obesity, insulin resistance, hypertension and dyslipidemia. While the clustering of OSA with these risk factors may be explained by the common link with obesity, it is also postulated that OSA may provide a stress stimulus that triggers or aggravates these metabolic factors, thus conferring independent predisposition to atherosclerosis and cardiovascular disease. The combination of Syndrome X (the metabolic syndrome) and OSA has been termed Syndrome Z by Wilcox in 1998.

Motor Vehicular Accidents

Multiple studies have linked sleep apnoea with an increased risk of having a motor vehicular accident. Such accidents are particularly dangerous because there is lack of reaction of a sleeping driver to an impending collision. These collisions are, as a consequence, often head-on and more likely to be fatal. Sleep-related accidents are most likely to occur early in the morning and late afternoon when there is a natural propensity to feel more sleepy. The risk of accidents in patients with OSA is estimated to vary from two to seven times that of the general population. Even patients with mild sleep apnoea have an increased risk of crashes in some studies, making a compelling case for treating patients with even mild OSA. It is now clear that OSA is an important preventable cause of motor vehicular accidents. Treating these patients with CPAP has been shown to reduce this accident rate. Screening and treatment for OSA has been recently recommended for commercial motor vehicle drivers in some parts of the developed world. This strategy has been shown to be cost-effective, with savings of over $6000 in total health cost per treated driver.

TREATMENT OF OSA

General Measures

The patient is encouraged to lose weight and sleep in the lateral position. Weight loss of 10% predicts a 25% reduction in the AHI. Instructions must be given to avoid sedatives, smoking and alcohol as these worsen sleep quality and may actually worsen OSA.

Continuous Positive Airway Pressure

Before the 1980s, the only effective treatment for OSA was a permanent tracheostomy; a highly effective but undesirable

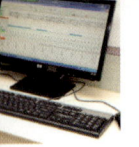

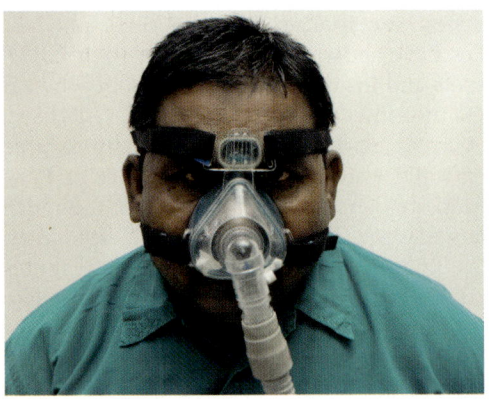

Fig 74.3: A patient using the CPAP machine.

option. In 1981, an Australian pulmonologist Colin Sullivan, in a brief report in the Lancet in 1981 described, 'reversal of obstructive sleep apnoea by continuous positive airway pressure applied through the nares' in five patients with severe OSA. Like any new idea, this took several years to catch on, but this form of therapy eventually transformed not just the treatment of OSA but also the face of sleep medicine. Continuous positive airway pressure (CPAP) is now the gold standard for moderate or severe OSA and at an appropriate pressure will be effective in almost all patients with this syndrome.

BENEFITS

CPAP therapy is gratifying to use because its benefits are almost instantly obvious. Within a single night it eliminates snoring, reverses desaturation, abolishes arousals and favourably affects EDS. When used regularly, it improves vascular risk, cognitive performance, and quality of life. In Young's cohort of 1522 patients with OSA from Wisconsin, regular use of CPAP was shown to significantly reduce mortality. Several studies show that driving risk also significantly improves after regular CPAP. A study by Douglas showed that just the saving that accrued from reduced accidents over five years would far exceed the costs of the treatment.

COMPLIANCE

Since the benefits are so obvious to the patient, compliance, even with this cumbersome form of therapy is remarkably good. Patient-reported compliance runs at around 75%, while actual objective monitoring reveals a figure closer to 50%, which is still better than the measured compliance for asthma inhalers and anti-tuberculosis drugs. Compliance can be improved by improvements in technology, with auto-CPAP machines, bi-level CPAP and humidifiers all improving compliance.

SIDE-EFFECTS

The side-effects of CPAP are generally minor and include dry mouth, ocular irritation, conjunctivitis, nasal congestion and abrasions and ulcers over the bridge of the nose due to a badly fitted mask. Advances in technology are constantly being developed to address this crucial issue of the interface between the patient and the CPAP machine. Some patients may feel very claustrophobic with a mask, and for such patients, nasal prongs or pillows may prove a more comfortable option. Rarely reported, more dangerous complications of CPAP include pneumothorax, massive epistaxis, pneumocephalus, increased intraocular pressure and tympanic membrane rupture. These are all very

rare, constituting isolated case reports. It must be stressed again that on the whole CPAP is very safe.

PRACTICAL ASPECTS

We have found that patient education goes a long way in alleviating the apprehensions most patients have regarding CPAP. A trial of CPAP for an hour or so in the daytime, prior to the first night of CPAP titration is also helpful. There is ample evidence that the patient's experience with the machine on the first night will influence his subsequent long-term acceptance (or rejection) of the treatment. This, in turn, can be affected by providing education, motivation and support to the patient.

Oral Appliances

These are established treatment options for snoring and mild OSA. They may also be considered in patients where CPAP has been tried and failed. There are two broad types of oral devices: tongue repositioning devices and mandibular repositioning devices. These devices must be designed and fitted for each individual patient by the sleep physician in close consultation with a dentist. In a recent, comprehensive meta-analysis of oral appliances, 70% of the 304 subjects had a reduction in their AHI by at least 50% from the baseline.

Surgical Options

A variety of surgical approaches have been attempted in OSA. These are listed in Table 74.3. The only one that will be discussed in detail is uvulopalatopharyngoplasty (UPPP) as it is the best studied and most frequently performed. This surgery involves excising the uvula, distal soft palate, faucial muscles, tonsillar pillars and the mucosa of the pharynx. It eliminates snoring with almost 80% success, but a recent meta-analysis by Sher showed that the mean decrease in AHI across studies was around 55%. Overall, its success rate is approximately 50% and it is less effective in patients with a BMI>30 and in those with more severe OSA. The procedure is not without morbidity and major complications have been reported, including the occasional fatality. Finally, relapses occur over time in as many as 50% of those who initially respond. Thus, this, and other forms of surgery, should never be the first-line treatment for OSA. Surgery should only be performed in special referral centres, under the supervision of experienced ENT surgeons with a special interest

Table 74.3: Surgical options for OSA
– Uvulopalatopharyngoplasty (UPPP)
– Laser assisted uvulopalatopharyngoplasty (LAUP)
– Septoplasty
– Tongue reduction
– Genioglossus advancement-hyoid myotomy and suspension (GAHMS)
– Maxillary and mandibular osteotomy (MMO)
– Tracheostomy
– Bariatric surgery

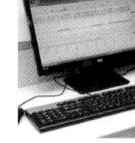

in the field. They should only be offered to patients who have tried and failed CPAP or refuse a trial of CPAP.

New and Emerging Techniques

- Temperature-controlled radiofrequency
- Nasal dilators
- Electrical stimulation of the tongue and upper airway
- Hypoglossal nerve stimulation

CENTRAL SLEEP APNOEA

CSA comprises a heterogeneous group of disorders characterized by momentary cessation of breathing in sleep due to a transient withdrawal of the respiratory drive to the muscles of respiration. Thus, in contrast to OSA, in which the respiratory drive continues during apnoea, in CSA no respiratory efforts or intrathoracic pressure swings are generated.

Aetiology

These disorders are rare and may be idiopathic or secondary. Idiopathic central hypoventilation is called Ondine's curse after a character in Greek mythology who was cursed with having to voluntarily control his automatic body functions including respiration. Secondary causes include a range of neurological conditions that cause specific damage to the neurons in the respiratory centre located in the medulla and pons. These include encephalitis, brainstem infarctions, radiation injury, bulbar poliomyelitis, multiple sclerosis and the Shy Drager syndrome.

Clinical Presentation

Central hypoventilation syndromes can go unnoticed over the years until an episode of respiratory failure develops, usually in association with respiratory infection. Indeed, many patients may have several episodes of respiratory failure before the correct diagnosis is eventually made. The disorder may be discovered in childhood, but milder forms may go undetected into adult life. These patients demonstrate awake hypoxemia and hypercapnia but can normalize gas exchange by voluntary hyperventilation. Snoring may or may not be present and is not as prominent as in patients with OSA. Morning headaches and daytime sleepiness are common. Patients may also manifest unexplained polycythemia or cor pulmonale, which are consequences of chronic hypoxemia. Pulmonary function tests and tests of respiratory muscle strength are usually normal unless the patient has coexisting lung disease or neuromuscular weakness. A further example is the obesity hypoventilation syndrome where the increased mechanical ventilatory load caused by morbid obesity may unmask an underlying weakness in the central respiratory drive resulting in alveolar hypoventilation and blood gas abnormalities that are very similar to those seen in patients with idiopathic central hypoventilation.

Impact of Sleep

Patients with central hypoventilation frequently develop severe respiratory insufficiency during sleep as a consequence of the reduction in the respiratory drive which normally occurs during sleep. The central feature is an abnormal increase in $PaCO_2$ during sleep, usually associated with severe hypoxemia. This may occur during all sleep stages but is particularly pronounced and severe during REM sleep. Apnoeas and hypopnoeas may occur in association with hypoventilation, however, central hypoventilation should only be diagnosed if the clinical sequelae can be attributed to hypoventilation distinct from the apnoeas and hypopnoeas.

Management

A number of pharmacological agents have respiratory stimulant properties. These include theophylline, progesterone and almitrine. The treatment of choice is non-invasive ventilation (NIV). This is generally delivered by a nasal or full-face mask. Several studies have reported an improvement in daytime blood gases after a night of NIV. Its mechanism includes resting of the respiratory muscles and a resetting of the respiratory drive at the chemoreceptor level. Electrophrenic pacing is an interesting form of treatment that has been in use for this condition for over two decades. The procedure involves implanting a pacing electrode around the phrenic nerve either in the cervical or high thoracic region. There are several reports of its utility in patients with central alveolar hypoventilation. Adults with central alveolar hypoventilation can often be successfully managed with a unilateral phrenic nerve pacemaker, while children generally require bilateral pacemakers by virtue of their chest wall being more compliant. Unilateral phrenic nerve pacing in children with CSA is inefficient as it results in paradoxical movement of the contralateral diaphragm and chest wall.

SUGGESTED READING

Bradley TD, Logan AG, Kimoff J et al. Continuous positive pressure for central sleep apnea and heart failure. *New Eng J Med.* 2005; 353: 2025–33.

Kryger MH, Roth T, Dement WC. *Principles and practice of sleep medicine.* Fourth edition, Elsevier Saunders.

Mosko S, Zetin M, Glen S, et al. Self reported depressive symptomatology, mood ratings, and treatment outcome in sleep disorders patients. *J Clin Psychol.* 1989; 45: 51–60.

Ng TP, Seow A, Tan WC. Prevalence of snoring and sleep breathing related disorders in Chinese, Malay and Indian adults in Singapore. *Eur Respir J.* 1998; 12: 198–202.

Peppard PE, Young T, Palta M, Skatrud J. Prospective study of the association between sleep-disordered breathing and hypertension. *New Eng J Med.* 2000; 342: 1378–84.

Reddy EV, Kadhivaran T, Mishra HK, Sreenivas V, Handa KK, Sinha S, et al. Prevalence and risk factors of obstructive sleep apnoea among middle-aged urban Indians: A community-based study. *Sleep Med.* 2009; 10: 913–18.

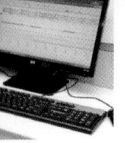

Sahar E, Whitney CW, Redline S, *et al.* Sleep disordered breathing and cardiovascular disease: cross sectional results of the Sleep Heart Health Study. *Am J Respir Crit Care Med.* 2001; 163: 19–25.

Schmidt-Nowara WW, Meade TE, Hays MB. Treatment of snoring and obstructive sleep apnea with a dental orthosis. *Chest.* 1991; 99: 1378–85.

Sharma SK, Kumpawat S, Banga A, Goel A. Prevalence and risk factors of obstructive sleep apnoea syndrome in a population of Delhi, India. *Chest.* 2006; 130: 149–56.

Stradling JR. Obstructive sleep apnea : definitions, epidemiology, and natural history. *Thorax.* 1995; 50: 683–9.

Udwadia ZF, Doshi AV, Lonkar SG, Singh CI. Prevalence of sleep disordered breathing and sleep apnea in middle aged urban Indian men. *Am J Respir Crit Care Med.* 2004; 169: 168–73.

Young T, Palta M, Dempsey J, *et al.* The occurence of sleep-disordered breathing among middle aged adults. *N Engl J Med.* 1993; 328: 1230–5.

Index

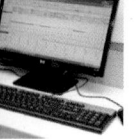

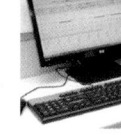

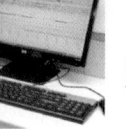

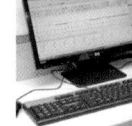

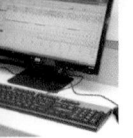

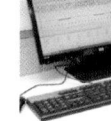

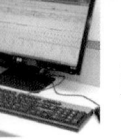

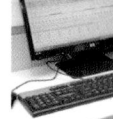

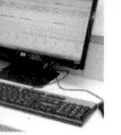

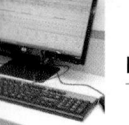

The second is a distinctive form of lymphocytic bronchiolitis observed in lung biopsies of nylon-flocking industry workers. It is probably caused by an immunological response to inhaled antigenic material.

The third is a form of chronic bronchiolitis obliterans recently described in workers at a microwave popcorn factory. Patients present with progressive dyspnoea, increasing obstructive airways disease with a normal chest radiograph. It is believed that this form of bronchiolitis is caused by exposure to diacetyl, an organic compound used to add a buttery flavour to popcorn.

A discussion on diffuse panbronchiolitis follows.

DIFFUSE PANBRONCHIOLITIS

Diffuse panbronchiolitis (DPB) is a distinct clinical entity that was first described in Japan over 40 years ago. It is an inflammatory disease of the small airways diffusely involving both lungs, the inflammation extending to all layers of the respiratory bronchioles. DPB is both a suppurative and obstructive airways' disease which if untreated leads to bronchiectasis, respiratory failure and death.

Epidemiology

Though most frequent in Japan (prevalence 11 per 100, 000) it has also been reported from other Southeast Asian countries, including Korea, China, Thailand, Malaysia and Singapore.

In Mumbai, we have encountered a few patients whose clinical and radiological features are indistinguishable from those described in DPB. Though confined almost entirely to East Asians, recently the disease has been occasionally encountered and reported in Caucasians, Hispanics and African-American populations in Europe and America.

There is no remarkable sex predominance; the disease occurs chiefly between the second and fifth decades, the average age of onset being around 40 years. Studies from Japan state that two-thirds of patients are non-smokers.

Aetiology

The aetiology is unknown but the fact that the distribution of this disease is chiefly in East Asians suggests an ethnic and genetic predisposition. This view is strengthened by the observation that many patients with DPB possessed the HLA-BW54 antigen. The HLA-Bw54 antigen is primarily confined to the Japanese, Chinese and Korean races and perhaps can be used as a marker for DPB as this antigen has a very low frequency in the general population.

Pathology

The lesions are diffuse and widespread, though the lower lobes are more involved. The pathology is centred round the respiratory bronchioles with transmural and peribronchial infiltration with lymphocytes, plasma cells and histiocytes; most of the alveoli are however unaffected. There is widespread narrowing of respiratory bronchioles, dilatation of the proximal membranous bronchioles with ultimate widespread bronchiectasis as the disease progresses.

Clinical Features

Chronic cough with expectoration of purulent sputum, dyspnoea on exertion and wheezing are the predominant clinical manifestations. Chronic paranasal sinusitis is present in over 75% of patients and may precede symptoms of chest disease by months or a few years. As the disease progresses the volume of sputum increases because of widespread bronchiectasis. An important clinical feature is the frequent isolation of *H. influenzae*, *Streptococcus pneumoniae* and in advanced cases *Ps. aeruginosa* from the sputum.

Physical findings reveal crackles all over, though more marked in the lower lobes. Airways' obstruction causes scattered wheezes on both sides. When airways obstruction is marked, wheezes may not be apparent unless the patient is asked to perform a forced expiratory manoeuvre. Clubbing is uncommon, hypoxic and still later hypoxic and hypercapnic respiratory failure occurs as the end-result of the disease.

Radiological Features

A radiographic examination of the chest reveals 2-mm nodular opacities scattered diffusely through both lungs often accompanied by hyperinflation. HRCT of the chest reveals that these nodular opacities are centrilobular in distribution with branching linear densities (tree in bud appearance). The opacities correspond to thickened dilated bronchial walls with intraluminal mucopurulent plugs. Areas of air-trapping within the lungs are often present. Bronchiectasis is observed as the disease progresses in the form of ring-shaped or tramline shadows.

Lung Function Studies

Lung functions are characterized by severe small airways obstruction with little or no reversibility following the use of an aerosolized bronchodilator. Lung volumes are often increased. Occasionally, a combined obstructive plus restrictive pattern is observed. The CO diffusion capacity may be reduced. As the disease progresses chronic hypoxic or hypoxic plus hypercapnic respiratory failure ensues.

Differential Diagnosis

Differential diagnosis from other forms of chronic bronchitis or obliterative bronchioliits may be difficult. DPB is both an obstructive and persistent suppurative disease of the small airways. The pathological distinction lies in the involvement of the respiratory bronchioles, whereas most other forms of bronchiolitis involve bronchioles proximal to the respiratory bronchioles. The frequent association of chronic sinusitis in DPB, the strongly suggestive appearances on the HRCT of the chest and the frequent isolation of *H. influenzae*, *Streptococcus pneumoniae* and in advanced stages *Ps. aeruginosa* from the sputum help in diagnosis.

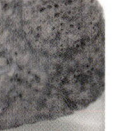

MANAGEMENT

Use of Erythromycin

Many studies in Japan have shown that 600 mg erythromycin given daily for > two years has a curative effect. There followed an improvement in symptoms, lung functions, CT appearance and survival rates.

Macrolides besides countering acute infection in the airways have other modes of action:

(a) They have an anti-inflammatory and immunoregulatory action. They do so by inhibiting the production of many pro-inflammatory cytokines such as IL-1, IL-6, IL-8. They also inhibit the formation of leukotrienes which attract neutrophils and inhibit release of superoxides.
(b) Macrolides block the release of adhesin molecules necessary for neutrophil migration. The bronchoalveolar lavage (BAL) fluid after use of erythromycin shows marked reduction in neutrophils.
(c) Macrolides cause a significant decrease in sputum volume.

The above anti-inflammatory effects lead to reduced airways infection and increased survival.

Beside erythromycin, the newer macrolides like Clarithromycin have also been successfully used in the treatment of DPB.

Use of β₂-agonist and Ipratropium or Tiotropium

Use of β_2-agonist and Ipratropium or Tiotropium through inhalation may help mucociliary clearance and bronchodilation, when there is some degree of reversibility in airways' obstruction.

Use of Corticosteroids

Though commonly used, the evidence supporting their use is lacking.

Use of Non-steroid Anti-inflammatory Drugs

These may exert non-specific anti-inflammatory effects and reduce sputum production but here again their efficacy is unproven.

Use of Antibiotics

Acute bacterial infection should be promptly treated with appropriate antibiotics, the choice of antibiotic being governed by sputum culture sensitivity reports.

SUGGESTED READING

Corris PA. Lung transplantation. Bronchiolitis obliterans syndrome. *Chest Surg Clin N Am.* 1 Aug. 2003; 13(3): 543–57.

Jay H. Ryu, Jeffrey Myers, *et al.* Bronchiolar Disorders. *Am J Resp Crit Care Med.* 2003; 168: 1277–92.

Laohaburanakit P. Bronchiolitis obliterans. *Clin Rev Allergy Immunol.* 1 Dec. 2003; 25(3): 259–74.

Poleth V, Casoni G, Chilose M, Zompatoin M. Diffuse panbronchiolitis. *Eur. Resp J.* 2006; 28, 862–41.

Scott AI. Bronchiolitis obliterans syndrome: risk factors and therapeutic strategies. *Drugs.* 1 Jan. 2005; 65(6): 761–71.

Tsang HWT. Diffuse panbronchiolitis: diagnosis and treatment. *Clin Pulmonary Med.* 2000; 7: 245–52.

CHAPTER **42** Oxygen Therapy

GENERAL CONSIDERATIONS

Cells require oxygen for their metabolic activity. Cellular hypoxia results when oxygen supply and oxygen stores within the cells do not meet the oxygen demand.

Oxygen stores are limited so that in acute respiratory failure or in cardiovascular catastrophes when oxygen supply is acutely reduced, tissue hypoxia can cause death. It is both the severity and the acuteness of hypoxia which determine the issue. However, in chronic respiratory failure (as in chronic obstructive pulmonary disease (COPD)) hypoxia evolves slowly over years, inducing metabolic changes that enable the cells to survive.

Hypoxia can be considered to be hypoxemic when associated with a fall in the oxygen saturation of arterial blood (SaO_2). Anaemic hypoxia is due to a lowered haemoglobin content which lowers the oxygen content of the arterial blood ($CaCO_2$). Hypoxia can also be due to poor supply of oxygen to the tissues vis-à-vis their demands, as occurs in low cardiac output syndromes or in shock from any cause. Histotoxic hypoxia is due to the inability of tissue cells to utilize oxygen because of an abnormality in mitochondrial cell respiration (see chapter on 'Acute Respiratory Failure in Adults').

Hypoxemia, defined as a fall in SaO_2, is nearly always associated with a fall in the arterial pressure of oxygen (PaO_2). However, the PaO_2 may remain normal even though the SaO_2 is reduced when carboxyhaemoglobin (HbCO) or methemoglobin is increased, because there is a decrease in the available functional haemoglobin. Conversely, the PaO_2 may be low in the presence of a normal SaO_2 when there is an increased affinity of haemoglobin for oxygen. This occurs when there is an intrinsic change in the structure of the haemoglobin molecule (as with variants of normal adult haemoglobin) or when there is an altered response to 2–3 diphosphoglycerate. Oxygen is used as therapy in most critically ill patients. It can be life-saving in acute respiratory failure yet can be lethal if incorrectly used. Oxygen administration aims at increasing the P_AO_2, and thereby the PaO_2 and the oxygen saturation of arterial blood. Except in some instances, it is enough to aim at a saturation of 90%; an oxygen saturation < 90% generally corresponds to a PaO_2 < 60 mm Hg, and denotes the presence of moderate hypoxia. A moderate degree of hypoxia disturbs normal cell metabolism and function; marked hypoxia results in cellular death. A PaO_2 < 20 mm Hg for a significant length of time generally produces brain death; yet a PaO_2 a little above 30 mm Hg probably maintains adequate cell function if the blood flow is adequate.

We have no means of accurately assessing cell function, and there is no doubt that the sensitivity of certain tissues (such as the brain and the heart) to lack of oxygen is far greater as compared to other tissues (e.g. skin and muscle). It is possible that even minor degrees of hypoxia which are easily tolerated in a young healthy individual, might pose problems in critically ill individuals, or in those with a poor coronary circulation, or with impaired cerebral blood flow due to diffuse cerebrovascular disease. It is important to relieve hypoxia of even mild intensity in all such critically ill patients, and preferably aim at an oxygen saturation of at least 90%, preferably even > 90%.

INDICATIONS FOR OXYGEN THERAPY

Hypoxia is the prime indication for oxygen administration. Dramatic relief with oxygen therapy is chiefly observed when arterial hypoxemia (i.e. a low PaO_2) is due to a low P_AO_2 or ventilation-perfusion mismatch within the lungs. Relief of hypoxia in such patients often brings in its wake three other effects:

(i) Decrease in the work of breathing. Hypoxia often causes increased ventilatory work and relief of hypoxia is often followed by a decrease in the work of breathing.

(ii) Decrease in myocardial work. The heart and circulatory systems are frequently involved in compensatory responses to hypoxia; once the hypoxia is reversed, these compensatory responses abate and the work of the myocardium is reduced.

(iii) Improvement in cell function involving various organ systems of the body is a welcome aspect of adequate oxygenation to the tissues.

Indications for oxygen therapy are stated below.

Hypoxemia

In an acute setting, hypoxemia (low SaO_2 with a low PaO_2) is the most important and most frequent indication for administering oxygen. These patients (particularly when hypoxemia is due to a respiratory problem) benefit the most with oxygen therapy. The following situations are included in this group.

(a) Cardiopulmonary or respiratory arrest. Administration of oxygen is of vital importance, but is of no avail unless the patient is simultaneously ventilated and cardiac resuscitation (in a cardiac arrest) is successfully performed.

(b) Anaesthetic error or accident.

(c) Hypoventilation from any cause.

(d) Respiratory diseases characterized by ventilation-perfusion mismatch, with or without impaired diffusion

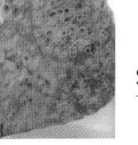

across the alveolar capillary membrane. These include severe COPD, acute severe asthma, as also interstitial lung disease. The commonest cause of hypoxemia in clinical medicine is a ventilation-perfusion mismatch. Patients who have this underlying abnormality benefit the most with oxygen therapy. In fact, if in a hypoxemic patient administration of oxygen leads to a sharp rise in the PaO_2 and SaO_2, the underlying cause of hypoxemia can be confidently attributed to a ventilation-perfusion mismatch or to hypoventilation.

(e) Respiratory diseases associated with an increase in the right to left shunt within the lungs as in acute respiratory distress syndrome (ARDS), atelectasis, and pneumonia. When there is a true right to left shunt in the lungs (desaturated blood pumped by the right ventricle perfusing totally atelectatic alveoli) there can be no relief of hypoxemia following use of oxygen. However, even in well-marked ARDS there also exists some degree of ventilation-perfusion abnormality with V/Q ratios < 1. Some degree of relief may therefore be expected. The larger the right to left shunt the lesser the relief. Patients with shunts > 20–25% may show little or no relief from administered oxygen.

(f) Respiratory distress with a respiratory rate > 24/min is an indication for oxygen therapy as per American College of Chest Physicians, NHLB Conference on Oxygen therapy. (*Ref: Fillmer JD, Snider GL. American College of Chest Physicians (ACCP). National Heart, Lung and Blood Institute (NHLBI) Conference on Oxygen Therapy. Arch Intern Med 1984; 144: 1645–55*)

Pneumothorax

High concentration of pure oxygen (fraction of inspired oxygen (FIO_2) 60%) has been shown to quicken resolution of a pneumothorax. This is related to an increase of pressure in the gases within the pleural space following use of pure oxygen at a high FIO_2, so that the increased pressure gradient between the air in the pleural space and the surrounding tissues accelerates the absorption of nitrogen from the pleural space.

Myocardial Infarction and Unstable Angina

The American Heart Association guidelines for Advanced Cardiac Life Support recommend the use of supplemental oxygen in all patients with the acute coronary syndrome regardless of the presence or absence of hypoxemia. Though undoubtedly useful in hypoxemia (as may be present in the acute stage of a myocardial infarct), the administration of oxygen in patients who are normoxic is not based on convincing data.

Decreased Oxygen Content of Arterial Blood (other than that caused by a decrease in PaO$_2$)

(a) Severe anaemia
(b) Carbon monoxide poisoning
(c) Methemoglobinemia, sulphemoglobinemia

The use of high concentration of oxygen is useful but limited in scope as the PaO_2 is generally normal in this group; it is the oxygen content which is low.

Chronic anaemia is generally well tolerated. In acute severe anaemia, use of high-flow oxygen through a non-rebreathing mask is of help, in addition to blood transfusions.

In carbon monoxide poisoning, carbon monoxide combines avidly with haemoglobin (Hb) to form a stable compound COHb, thereby sharply reducing the oxygen-carrying capacity of the blood. Management consists of administering oxygen at 10 L /min through a tight-fitting reservoir mask. The use of close to 100% oxygen provides one-third of the body requirement of oxygen through the extra oxygen dissolved in plasma. It also reduces the half-life of COHb from 4 hours to 1½ hours. Hyperbaric oxygen can further reduce the half-life to 20 minutes and can provide enough oxygen in solution to fully take care of the oxygen requirements of the body.

In acute severe methemoglobinemia, inhalation of a high concentration of oxygen is a useful temporary measure (for reasons stated above) till the methemoglobenemia is reversed.

Decreased Transport of Oxygen with Impaired Perfusion of Tissues

(a) Shock from any cause
(b) Left ventricular failure
(c) Cardiac arrhythmias causing haemodynamic instability
(d) Cardiac arrest

A fall in systolic blood pressure to < 100 mm Hg, a low cardiac output with metabolic acidosis (bicarbonate < 18 mmol/l), severe shock from any cause are indications for oxygen therapy.

A marked fall in the PvO_2 due to a fall in the cardiac output leads to a significant fall in the PaO_2. Also, many of these conditions produce an increase in the physiological dead space and/or a ventilation-perfusion mismatch. It is important to maximize both the PaO_2 (and the oxygen content), as also increase oxygen transport through an increase in the cardiac output in these patients.

Poor Uptake or Utilization of Oxygen in Tissues

Poor uptake and/or utilization of oxygen in tissues is seen in septic shock, ARDS; here again the PaO_2, oxygen content and oxygen transport or delivery to the tissue cells must be adequate if cellular and organ functions are to be well maintained.

Oxygen is not utilized by tissues in cyanide poisoning as cyanide inactivates the enzyme cytochrome oxidase within the cells. A high FIO_2 is only of marginal help; reversal of cyanide toxicity by suitable antidotes is of prime importance.

Postoperative States

General anaesthesia usually induces a decrease in the functional residual capacity, an increase in venous admixture and a slight to moderate ventilation-perfusion mismatch. This is particularly observed following thoracic surgery, coronary artery bypass graft surgery, open-heart surgery, upper abdominal surgery and any protracted surgical procedure. A mild to moderate hypoxemia results, easily relieved by administering oxygen for an appropriate period of time.

It is important to remember that even though oxygen helps in the relief of hypoxia, it does not eradicate the root

Table 42.1:
Indications for oxygen therapy
1. Hypoxemia
Cardiopulmonary or respiratory arrest
Anaesthetic error or accident
Hypoventilation from any cause
Respiratory diseases characterized by ventilation-perfusion mismatch, with or without impaired diffusion across the alveolar capillary membrane
Respiratory distress with a respiratory rate > 24/min
2. Pneumothorax
3. Myocardial infarction and unstable angina
4. Decreased oxygen content of arterial blood
Severe anemia
Carbon monoxide poisoning
Methemoglobinemia, sulphemoglobinemia
5. Decreased transport of oxygen with impaired perfusion of tissues
Shock from any cause
Left ventricular failure
Cardiac arrhythmias causing hemodynamic instability
Cardiac arrest
6. Poor uptake or utilization of oxygen in tissues
7. Post operative states

cause of hypoxia. It is therefore no substitute for adequate alveolar ventilation, neither does it solve the problem of V/Q abnormalities, nor does it abolish a right to left shunt within the lungs. Again, the oxygen content of blood is not only dependent on the PaO_2 but also on the haemoglobin concentration of the blood. The importance of an adequate cardiac output to ensure good oxygen transport cannot be overstressed. Finally, the proper uptake and utilization of oxygen by the tissue cells is necessary if tissue hypoxia is to be countered or prevented.

Important Considerations in Oxygen Administration

When uncontrolled oxygen (at high flow rates) is given to relieve hypoxia in patients with severe COPD or in patients who suffer an acute exacerbation of COPD, relief of hypoxemia may be accompanied by a sharp rise in the $PaCO_2$. Marked hypercapnia is undesirable and can cause a sharp fall in the pH of the arterial blood increasing both morbidity and mortality in these patients. The hypercapnia that results in the above circumstances is largely related to alveolar hypoventilation rather than to the inability of the respiratory centre to respond to an increasing $PaCO_2$. This has been dealt with in the chapter 'Chronic Obstructive Pulmonary Disease: Management'.

Therefore an important consideration is to use controlled oxygen therapy to relieve hypoxemia in patients with an acute exacerbation of COPD. This is achieved by administering oxygen through a Venturi mask (24.5 or 28%) or using low-flow oxygen at 2 L/min via nasal prongs. Arterial blood gas analysis should

be done prior to starting oxygen and 30–45 minutes after starting oxygen therapy. The incidence of sharply increasing hypercapnia with controlled oxygen therapy is observed only in a small percentage (13% in a recent study) of patients. If the PaO_2 during controlled oxygen therapy rises close to 60 mm Hg and the arterial pH is not lower than 7.25, controlled oxygen therapy should be continued. If however even with controlled oxygen therapy the $PaCO_2$ continues to rise so that the arterial pH falls below 7.25, or it is impossible to relieve hypoxemia (PaO_2 < 55 mm Hg) without increasing hypercapnia and a falling arterial pH, other measures such as ventilator support become necessary. The ventilator support may be non-invasive or invasive depending upon prevailing circumstances (see chapter on 'COPD: Management').

One other consideration to be remembered is that in patients who hypoventilate due to neurogenic diseases, respiratory muscle weakness, poisonings (and in other conditions where to start with the lungs are essentially normal), administering oxygen will relieve hypoxemia but will have no effects on the hypercapnia observed in these patients. Finally, it should be remembered that oxygen is a dry gas and should always be humidified before administration, particularly so when the upper airway is bypassed by the use of an endotracheal tube or a tracheostomy. Ventilation of the lungs with dry gases produces heat loss, and moisture loss from the respiratory passages, and also alters pulmonary function. Heat loss causes a fall in body temperature and increases oxygen consumption. Moisture loss leads to drying or dehydration of the respiratory mucosa. The most important effect consequent to this drying is a reduced activity of the mucociliary escalator with sputum retention. Blocked airways from inspissated respiratory secretions result in ventilation-perfusion inequalities, and may lead to or accentuate hypoxia. Thus the importance of humidifying oxygen in inspired gas cannot be overemphasized.

METHODS OF OXYGEN ADMINISTRATION

Routine Oxygen Therapy using Low-Flow Oxygen Administration Devices

A moderate rise of oxygen concentration in the alveoli suffices to relieve moderate hypoxia. An oxygen concentration of approximately 40% may be achieved by using nasal catheters, nasal prongs, or simple orofacial masks, if the flow rate is maintained between 6–8 l/min. Patients cannot ordinarily tolerate flow rates higher than 6–8 l/min through the above-mentioned devices.

NASAL CATHETERS AND NASAL PRONGS
These are the simplest and most commonly used techniques of oxygen administration. If a nasal catheter is used, its tip should be advanced to the fold of the soft palate, and then pulled back very slightly. If it is introduced too far, it can produce gaseous distension of the stomach, as oxygen finds its way into the stomach rather than into the lungs. Irritation of the nasal mucosa can be minimized by lubricating the catheter with xylocaine jelly. The catheter can be changed from one nostril to the other every 6–8 hours.

Most units prefer nasal prongs to nasal catheters. Nasal prongs (two short plastic prongs that fit into the external nares) (Figure 42.1) offer the advantage of simplicity and comfort. An

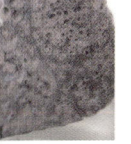

added advantage over an orofacial mask is that the administered oxygen does not have to be discontinued during eating, speaking or coughing.

When oxygen is administered through nasal prongs or a nasal catheter, at a flow rate of 1–2 l/min, the oxygen concentration is approximately 24%. At flow rates of 6–8 l/min, the oxygen concentration approximates 40%. Further increase in flow rates are poorly tolerated and produce very little additional increase in oxygen concentration.

The effect of a given flow of oxygen through a nasal catheter or prongs is dependent not only on the flow rate, but the tidal volume and minute ventilation of the patient. If the tidal volume and minute ventilation decrease, i.e. the patient hypoventilates, then the inspired oxygen concentration will rise. Precise regulation or control over inspired oxygen concentration is thus not possible with nasal prongs or catheter. Recently developed methods of administering supplemental oxygen include the use of reservoir cannulae, transtracheal oxygen delivery and pulsed oxygen delivery. Transtracheal oxygen delivery is effected via a small catheter inserted into the trachea at the base of the neck. It is totally unnecessary for intensive care unit (ICU) use though it has some benefits for patients on domiciliary oxygen therapy. Pulsed oxygen devices deliver oxygen only during inspiration. This conserves oxygen, yet provides a PaO_2 equivalent to that obtained with a continuous flow system through prongs or a face mask. Pulse type devices deliver fixed oxygen volume and flow each time a pulse is triggered. Demand devices vary the volume of oxygen delivered from breath to breath depending on the depth of inspiration.

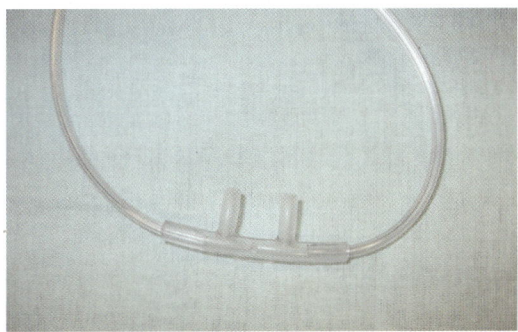

Fig 42.1: Nasal prongs.

FACE MASK

A simple oronasal plastic mask (Figure 42.2) fed with oxygen at a flow rate of 6–10 l/min, is a frequently used method for administering oxygen. The oxygen fed directly into the mask (after humidification), displaces air and creates a small oxygen reservoir. During inspiration oxygen in the mask is inhaled; room air is also entrained through the ports and through the space between the face and the mask. The oxygen concentration of inspired gas is thus much < 100%. The extent to which inspired oxygen concentration can increase depends on the size of the mask (and therefore of the oxygen reservoir), and the flow rate of oxygen. Higher flow rates are generally better tolerated through the use of a mask as compared to nasal prongs or catheters. At a flow rate of 6–10 l/min, an oxygen concentration of approximately 35–55% can be achieved.

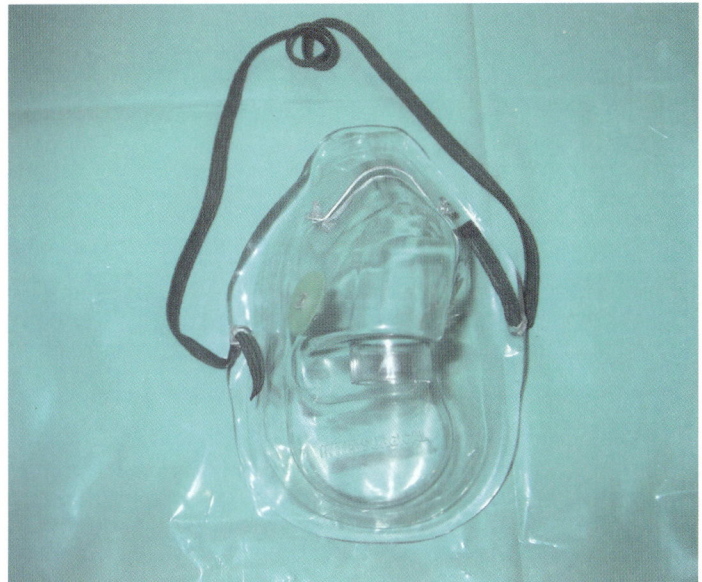

Fig 42.2: Simple face mask.

The face mask is less easy and less comfortable to wear than nasal prongs. The major disadvantage is that it has to be removed when the patient speaks, eats, drinks, coughs, or expectorates.

FACE MASK WITH RESERVOIR BAG

The addition of a reservoir bag to the face mask (Figure 42.3) increases the potential reservoir of oxygen, and allows a further increase in the concentration of inspired oxygen.

Inspired oxygen consists of oxygen from the reservoir bag of the face mask, together with some air entrained through the side ports and the small space between the mask and the skin of the face. During expiration, most of the exhaled gas passes out through the side ports, but some expired gas may return to the reservoir bag. This could lead to a fall in PO_2 and a rise in the PCO_2 in the reservoir bag, and should be avoided by a sufficiently high rate of oxygen flow to keep the bag washed

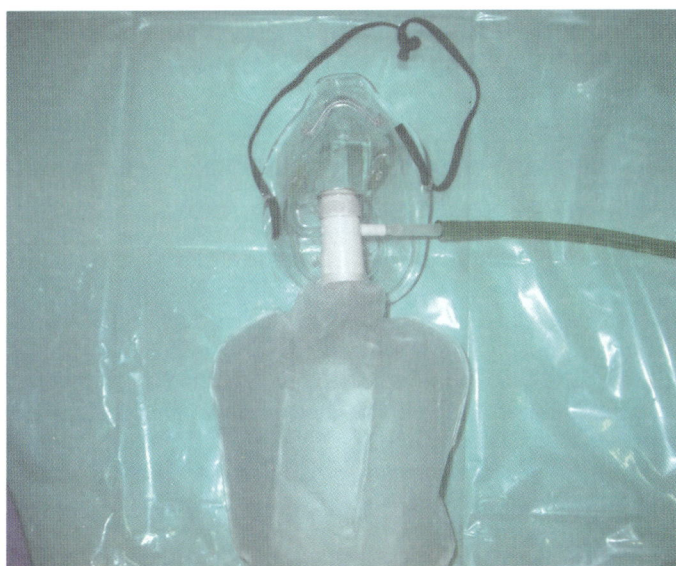

Fig 42.3: Face mask with reservoir bag.

out. Oxygen flow rates of 8–12 l/min are commonly used with this device, and can provide an inspired oxygen concentration between 50–80%. The flow rate of oxygen must be so adjusted that the reservoir bag is not emptied by more than half during inspiration.

FACE MASK WITH RESERVOIR BAG AND DIRECTIONAL VALVES

The entrainment of room air during inspiration can be almost completely prevented by covering the side ports with directional valves (Figure 42.4). Except for some air passing between the mask and the face, the entire volume of inspired gas consists of oxygen from the reservoir bag and the face mask. During exhalation, the side port directional valves open and air passes out from the mask into the atmosphere. The passage of expired air back into the reservoir bag can be prevented by a directional valve.

It is important that the flow rate of oxygen fed into the mask and reservoir bag with directional valves is in the range of 10–15 l/min. The inspired oxygen concentrations can thereby be raised in such instances to as high as 90–95%. It is also extremely important to ensure that there is no failure in oxygen supply nor a sharp fall in the flow rate, as breathing is dependent on oxygen fed into the mask-reservoir device. If the reservoir bag is inadvertently empty, asphyxia results. Table 42.2 compares the oxygen flow (l/min) and oxygen concentrations (%) obtained by using low-flow oxygen administration devices.

Controlled Oxygen Therapy

PRINCIPLES

The purpose of controlled oxygen therapy is to relieve dangerous hypoxia by producing an adequate increase in the P_AO_2

Table 42.2: Correlation between oxygen flow and oxygen concentration using low-flow oxygen administration devices		
Device	**O₂ Flow (l/min)**	**O₂ Concentration**
Nasal cannula	approx. 6	approx. 40–45%
Facial mask	approx. 8	approx. 35–55%
Mask with reservoir	approx. 10	approx. 50–80%
Mask with reservoir and directional valves	approx. 12	approx. 90–95%

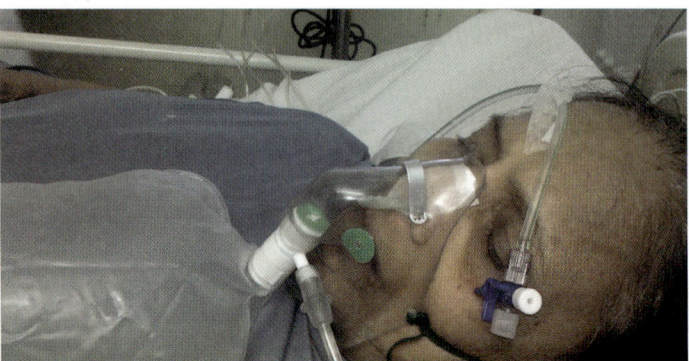

Fig 42.4: A patient breathing through a face mask with reservoir bag and directional valves.

and the PaO_2, and yet control and limit the associated rise of $PaCO_2$. This would also limit the fall in arterial pH due to respiratory acidosis.

TECHNIQUE

The concentration of inspired oxygen is controlled by using high air flows with known oxygen enrichment. The principle underlying this technique is entrainment of air with constant-pressure jet mixing. High air flows allow the immediate space or environment around the patient's face to be so thoroughly flushed, that there is no re-breathing and no contamination with room air. In this manner, the concentration of inspired oxygen can be controlled to within 2%.

VENTIMASK

The ventimask works on the Venturi principle and allows perfectly controlled oxygen administration. Oxygen is delivered to the mask through a nozzle, and the aperture of the nozzle is of set size so that as the oxygen is released through the aperture, it entrains a fixed portion of air through the side holes of the mask. Thus if an oxygen concentration of 24% is desired, the aperture of the delivery nozzle is such that 1 l of oxygen/minute will entrain 20 l of air, and 2 l of oxygen/min will entrain 40 l of air. The entrainment ratio is 1: 20, and is independent of the flow rate; the oxygen concentration of the inspired gas is thus independent of the flow rate.

Different ventimasks have different aperture size nozzles, and provide different but fixed oxygen concentrations. For example, a mask that is designed to provide an oxygen concentration of 28% will have a nozzle aperture that allows 1 l of oxygen delivered through the nozzle to entrain 10 l of air through the side holes i.e. a 1: 10 entrainment ratio, which is again independent of the flow rate of oxygen.

As mentioned at the outset, the ventimask works on the Venturi principle, and the Venturi is fairly accurate at the recommended total flow of 40 l/min (i.e. 2 l of oxygen/min for a 24% mask, and 4 l of oxygen/min for a 28% mask). The gas flow around the patient's nose and mouth flushes the mask continuously, washing out the expired carbon dioxide, and ensuring that the patient only breathes the oxygen-air mixture provided to him.

The greatest advantage of the ventimask is that the oxygen concentration it provides is independent of the flow rate, and also independent of the patient's tidal volume and minute ventilation. It can be easily used by all nurses, and requires no special adjustment. Also, the concentration of oxygen delivered is not at the mercy of faulty flow meters or reducing valves. The disadvantage as with all oronasal masks is that it has to be removed during coughing, eating, speaking, or drinking. In a seriously ill patient, removing the mask during feeds can cause a dangerous deterioration due to a sharp fall in the PaO_2 and worsening hypoxia. In severely hypoxic patients, the administration of oxygen should be continued, even when the patient is being fed, via nasal prongs at a flow rate of 1–2 l/min; this prevents the temporary but dangerous hypoxia.

Currently, other commercially available high-airflow systems have been designed to deliver oxygen concentrations varying from 24–50%, using the same principle as the Venturi mask. A jet of oxygen from a wall or tank source is passed through a precisely designed (exact size) orifice, and this

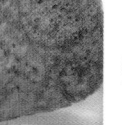

results in the entrainment of room air through the ports in the surrounding cylinder.

NASAL PRONGS

Many ICUs in Mumbai and other large cities (leave aside smaller towns all over the country), do not use ventimasks or other high-airflow oxygen-enriched delivery systems to provide controlled oxygen therapy. It is recommended that in the absence of these devices, nasal catheters or nasal prongs be used in an attempt to give controlled oxygen therapy. Oxygen at a flow rate of 1–2 l/min through nasal prongs or catheters is generally effective in providing controlled oxygen concentrations of 24–28% in inspired gas. The flow rate should be initially kept at 1 l/min; if this is well tolerated, it is increased to 2 l/min. Measurements of the PaO_2 and the $PaCO_2$ are of help, and the patient is kept under a close watch, specially as regards his ventilation. If the patient has marked hypoventilation, administration of oxygen even at 1–2 l/minute can lead to an uncontrolled or higher than desired concentration of oxygen. In such patients the flow rate should be reduced to < 1 l/min. Oxygen delivered through nasal prongs or catheters at low flow rates as stated above, is generally effective in relieving hypoxia without producing a dangerous rise in the PCO_2.

Table 42.3:
Effect of oxygen (administered through a nasal catheter at flow rate of 2 l/min) in relieving hypoxia without causing dangerous hypercapnia in 7 patients with obstructive airways disease

Patients	Before O₂ Therapy		After O₂ Therapy			
			4 hrs		24–36 hrs	
	PO_2	PCO_2	PO_2	PCO_2	PO_2	PCO_2
	(mm Hg)		(mm Hg)		(mm Hg)	
1	50	56	75	60	80	55
2	48	52	66	60	75	46
3	45	50	60	54	70	56
4	55	48	70	48	86	46
5	42	48	65	54	68	50
6	40	68	60	76	66	58
7	38	72	60	86	60	65

Source: (From Udwadia FE. *Acute Respiratory failure*. 1979. Oxford University Press, Bombay.)

Hyperbaric Oxygen

Hyperbaric oxygen is not administered in the ICU. Yet some critically ill patients under intensive care have to be transported to hyperbaric oxygen chambers in the same or distant hospitals to avail of this therapy. The administration of oxygen at higher than atmospheric pressure has certain advantages. When breathing air at atmospheric pressure, the oxygen in solution in plasma is 0.3 ml/dl; when breathing oxygen at a pressure of 2 atmospheres, it is 4.5 ml/dl. This is just a little less than the amount of oxygen taken up by tissues in unit time, and

goes a long way in aiding jeopardized tissue perfusion, and relieving tissue hypoxia. The main use of hyperbaric oxygen is in the treatment of carbon monoxide poisoning. The dissolved oxygen relieves hypoxia, and the markedly increased oxygen tension helps the quick dissociation of carbon monoxide from carboxyhaemoglobin. Hyperbaric oxygen therapy is also useful in the management of sepsis secondary to wounds contaminated by anaerobic gas-forming organisms, and in the treatment of wounds with a poor blood supply.

COMPLICATIONS OF OXYGEN THERAPY

Progressive Hypercapnia

The danger of progressive hypercapnia, particularly after uncontrolled oxygen therapy in a number of patients with hypoxia due to COPD, has already been discussed. (Also see chapter on COPD.)

Circulatory Depression

This is very rare, but has been occasionally observed in patients who have been acutely, severely hypoxic, and whose circulation is maintained by excessive sympathetic activity and excessive catecholamine discharge, induced by the severe hypoxia. Sudden relief of hypoxia abolishes this sympathetic overactivity, causing temporary hypotension, and occasionally circulatory collapse. We have observed this phenomenon following sudden relief of acute severe hypoxia in glottic or subglottic obstruction, after establishing an open airway (through a tracheotomy) and administering a high concentration of oxygen. Circulatory depression is temporary, and can be corrected by a volume load, or by an infusion containing a sympathomimetic agent.

Drying and Crusting of Secretions in the Respiratory Tract

Oxygen should always be humidified prior to administration. This is particularly imperative in patients with artificial airways. Unhumidified oxygen causes drying of secretions, and this can result in blockage of the bronchi by inspissated mucus. Partial or complete blockage of artificial airways (endotracheal or tracheostomy tube) by crusted secretions can have disastrous consequences.

Danger of Oxygen Withdrawal

Moderate or severe hypoxia warrants continuous oxygen therapy till such time as the hypoxia is relieved. Some hypoxic COPD patients may become drowsy or disoriented even on controlled oxygen therapy. To discontinue oxygen in such a situation is dangerous and wrong. If oxygen administration is stopped with the $PaCO_2$ markedly elevated, the P_ACO_2 (and consequently the PaO_2) falls to an even lower level than that prior to starting oxygen therapy. This is because the P_ACO_2 has risen to a higher level than that prevailing at the start of oxygen therapy. Such patients therefore have a worsening of their already severe hypoxic state. Intermittent oxygen therapy can be dangerous in a hypoxic patient, and is wrong on principle. It only serves to give periods of relief from hypoxia,

followed by periods of worsening and often extreme hypoxia. Oxygen, if indicated, needs to be *given continuously* till hypoxia is relieved.

Oxygen Toxicity

LUNG TOXICITY

High concentrations of oxygen over a prolonged period of time can produce changes in the lungs characterized by atelectasis, damage to the surfactant, interalveolar oedema, and interstitial thickening and fibrosis. It is generally accepted that oxygen concentrations up to 50% are safe for long periods. We have used 60% oxygen for weeks, and have observed that the patients have recovered without residual effects. We have also been forced to use 100% oxygen in two patients (who would otherwise have died of hypoxia) for as long as 24 hours, followed by 80–90% oxygen for the next four to seven days, and then 60–70% oxygen for another week. Both patients survived without any significant residual damage to the lungs. *This does not mean that very high oxygen concentrations should be used with abandon.* It does however signify that in our experience, the use of 100% oxygen is not as lethal as is often made out to be.

The practical applications to be derived from experimental and clinical studies on oxygen toxicity are summarized below:

(i) For patients with chronic hypoxemia (as in severe chronic airways obstruction), it is sufficient to use a concentration of oxygen that will correct dangerously low PaO_2 levels. A PaO_2 between 55 mm Hg to 60 mm Hg (O_2 saturation – 90%) is generally adequate in these patients.

(ii) Positive end-expiratory pressure (PEEP) should be used during mechanical ventilation if an inspired oxygen concentration > 50% fails to relieve dangerous hypoxia in patients with ARDS, atelectasis, pneumonia and interstitial lung disease.

(iii) In acute pulmonary problems with severe hypoxia, the oxygen concentration must be sufficient to allow an oxygen saturation of about 90%. If in spite of the use of PEEP, very high oxygen concentration (> 80%) is needed over a prolonged period of time to maintain an oxygen saturation of 90%, it may be permissible to allow mild to moderate hypoxia (O_2 saturation around 85%) so as to enable a reduction in the FIO_2. The degree of hypoxia one allows will depend on the patient's tolerance to hypoxia, the age of the patient, and the ability or otherwise to increase oxygen transport to the tissues.

(iv) *Life-threatening hypoxia must always be relieved, even if this requires the use of 100% oxygen for prolonged periods of time.* The fear and danger of possible oxygen toxicity is never an argument to allow a patient to irreversibly deteriorate and die of hypoxia.

(v) It is difficult, if not impossible, to detect signs of lung toxicity due to high oxygen concentrations in critically ill individuals with serious pulmonary problems. A fall in the compliance and the PaO_2 can occur due to very high oxygen concentrations, but we have found it impossible to ascertain in clinical practice, whether this is related to the disease, or is iatrogenic due to oxygen toxicity.

RETROLENTAL FIBROPLASIA

This complication occurs in the neonatal period, and is related to high P_AO_2 levels. If the inspired oxygen concentration is high enough to raise the P_AO_2 to about 160 mm Hg even for a few hours, retrolental fibroplasia can occur. Therefore in neonates, PaO_2 levels should never exceed 100 mm Hg.

CEREBRAL OXYGEN TOXICITY

This is occasionally observed when oxygen is breathed at hyperbaric pressures above one atmosphere. The syndrome is chiefly characterized by epileptic fits and is termed the Paul Bert effect, after the individual who first described it.

LONG-TERM OXYGEN THERAPY

Long-term oxygen therapy (LTOT) finds its greatest and proven use in patients who have COPD and suffer from well-marked hypoxemia. The objectives of LTOT are:

1. To relieve hypoxemia so that the PaO_2 is > 60 mm Hg (with an O_2 saturation > 90%), without inducing or increasing hypercapnia.
2. Reduction of polycythemia
3. Prevention of right heart failure
4. Improvement of quality of sleep
5. Improvement in cognition and neuropsychiatric function
6. *Most importantly, improve survival*

Accepted Indications for LTOT in COPD

The first prerequisite is that the patient should have received optimal treatment and should have stopped smoking. LTOT is then indicated in patients with COPD who have a stable PaO_2 of < 55 mm Hg breathing air. This cutoff point is chosen because it lies on the steepest part of the O_2 dissociation curve, so that any further fall would lead to severe hypoxemia.

LTOT in COPD patients is also indicated if the PaO_2 is between 55–59 mm Hg (between 7.3 and 7.8 kPa) with PCV > 55% (erythrocytosis) and right heart dysfunction –P pulmonale, pulmonary hypertension or clinical evidence of cor pulmonale, such as peripheral oedema for which there is no other cause.

The use of LTOT in COPD under the right indications has been clearly shown to improve survival rates compared to controls not on LTOT in quite a few studies. The MRC Working Party Trial showed that mortality was less when COPD patients with severe hypoxemia and CO_2 retention were treated with long-term domiciliary oxygen for 15 hours daily when compared to those who were not given oxygen.

The Nocturnal Oxygen Therapy Trial (NOTT) group in the US studied 203 patients with hypoxemic COPD being treated randomly either with nocturnal oxygen only for 12 hours daily or with continuous oxygen therapy. Results at the end of three years showed increased mortality in those being treated with nocturnal oxygen as compared to those receiving continuous oxygen.

The recommendation therefore is that hypoxemic COPD patients who satisfy the indications stated earlier should as far as possible be advised LTOT continuously through 24 hours. It is not as if nocturnal oxygen therapy is of no use. It helps survival but not to the extent of continuously administered

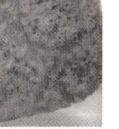

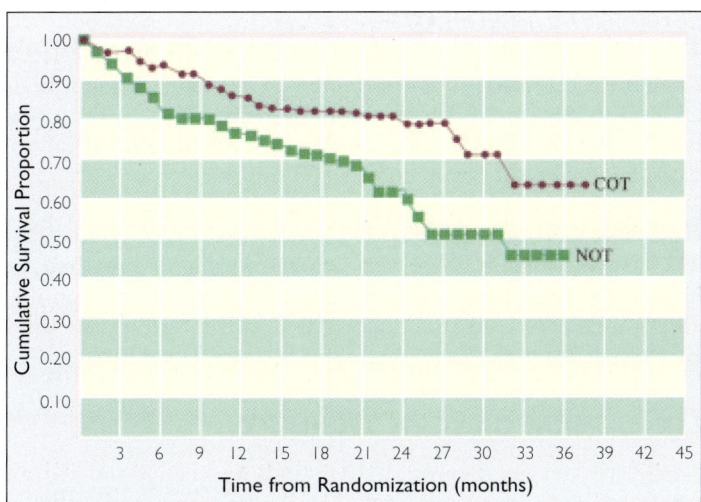

Fig 42.5: NOTT Survival Data.

Note: NOT—Noctural oxygen therapy
COT—Continuous oxygen therapy

oxygen. As a corollary it could be stated that the greater the number of hours that oxygen is administered during LTOT, the greater the survival benefit.

Possible Indications for LTOT in COPD

Oxygen is often prescribed by a number of physicians in COPD patients whose PaO_2 is $\leq$ 60 mm Hg but more than 55 mm Hg even in the absence of hypercapnia, pulmonary hypertension, polycythemia or clinical evidence of cor pulmonale. In a French study of 7770 COPD patients prescribed LTOT via the French ANTADAR network, 8.5% had a PaO_2 of 60 mm Hg or more at the start of the trial. Over an 11-year period (1984–95) the survival of these patients was reduced compared to the general population of the same age and sex, but was comparable to that of patients with a PaO_2 between 50–60 mm Hg. These findings suggest that patients with hypoxemia (at or a little above 60 mm Hg) would benefit by LTOT. However, another study by Gorecka and colleagues *(Ref: D Gorecka, K Gorzelak et al. Effect of long-term oxygen therapy on survival in patients with chronic obstructive pulmonary disease with moderate hypoxemia. Thorax 1997: 52: 674–679; doi: 10.1136/thx.52.8.674)* gave different results. A randomized study over three years on 135 COPD patients with a stable PaO_2 between 55 and 65 mm Hg, comparing air and LTOT showed no difference in survival rate. This study casts doubt on the need to use LTOT in patients with moderate hypoxemia. Many practising physicians would prefer to be on the safer side and give the benefit of doubt to the patient by prescribing LTOT when the PaO_2 is < 60 mm Hg (yet more than 55 mm Hg) or the O_2 saturation is < 90% provided the patient can afford the therapy.

LTOT and Non-invasive Ventilator Support in COPD with Severe Chronic Hypoxemic plus Hypercapnic Respiratory failure

In patients with COPD who are in chronic respiratory failure with well-marked hypoxemia plus hypercapnia, the use of non-invasive positive pressure ventilatory support in combination with LTOT controls nocturnal hypoventilation, improves quality of sleep, may lead to improved PaO_2 and $PaCO_2$ levels in the day and thereby improves the quality of life. It is impossible to give non-invasive ventilator support all through 24 hours every day. It should therefore be given all through the night and for some 4 to 6 hours during the day. Yet non-invasive ventilator support by itself is generally of little use in the above circumstances. It needs to be combined with LTOT.

Nocturnal Oxygen Only in COPD

The use of nocturnal oxygen should benefit patients with COPD (daytime PaO_2 > 60 mm Hg) who desaturate sharply at night during sleep. Severe nocturnal desaturation in these patients could a) disturb sleep; b) trigger cardiac arrhythmias, particularly in older patients with ischemic heart disease, c) perhaps cause episodes of pulmonary hypertension during periods of desaturation. The suggestion that these episodes could accelerate the evolution of permanent pulmonary hypertension and cor pulmonale though not proven, cannot be ignored.

LTOT in Chronic Respiratory Failure due to causes other than COPD

Chronic hypercapnic respiratory failure is also observed in patients with severe kyphoscoliosis, neuromuscular disease and other diseases extensively involving the lungs. If hypercapnia is not marked and if hypoxemia (PaO_2 < 55 mm Hg) can be countered by oxygen at 1–2 L/min without significant increase in the hypercapnia, then the patient can be kept comfortable on LTOT at a low flow rate. If however the hypercapnia is marked (> 60 –65 mm Hg) or is sharply increased following oxygen therapy, LTOT needs to be combined with non-invasive ventilator support for as many hours in the day and night as possible. More often than not these patients receive non-invasive support at night and for a few hours in the day.

Patients with severe restrictive disease may become increasingly hypoxic as the disease progresses. LTOT or nocturnal oxygen therapy may become necessary if the PaO_2 falls < 55 mm Hg. The same holds for severe hypoxemia caused by bilateral destructive lung disease. In end-stage disease of the nature described above, the flow rate of oxygen may need to be increased to 4 l or more per minute to counter worsening hypoxemia.

DOSAGE OF OXYGEN

Hypoxemic COPD patients satisfying the criteria stated above generally need a flow rate of 1–2 L/min. Even then, they may desaturate during sleep. Arbitrarily an increase in the flow rate by 1 L/min is administered during the night. Uncontrolled oxygen therapy can however precipitate increasing hypercapnia. Oxygen given to counter severe hypoxemia due to end-stage restrictive lung pathologies (such as interstitial lung disease) often requires a higher rate of > 2 L/min or more.

Nocturnal Oxygen Therapy in Central Sleep Apnoea in Patients with Congestive Heart Failure

Sleep disordered breathing in the form of Cheynes-Stokes respiration (CSR) and spells of central sleep apnoea (CSA)

have been frequently reported (30–100%) in patients with congestive heart failure, contributing to increasing deterioration in the cardiac condition.

The pathogenesis of Cheynes-Stoke respiration and central sleep apnoea (CSR-CSA) is believed to be related to:

(a) heightened responses of the respiratory centre to hypoxia and hypercapnia leading to an unstable respiratory centre;
(b) hypocapnia;
(c) prolonged circulation time

CSR-CSA is associated with increase in sympathetic tone, which is generally deleterious to patients in congestive heart failure. Nocturnal oxygen when administered to these patients improves CSR-CSA. This improvement was noted to correlate with increase in peak oxygen consumption during exercise, perhaps due to reduction in the sympathetic tone following the use of nocturnal oxygen.

Long-Term Oxygen Delivery System

The commonest source of oxygen for long-term oxygen therapy is the oxygen concentrator. Other systems include compressed gas or liquid oxygen. Oxygen concentrators are heavy, (about 35 lbs) require a wall current and therefore can only provide a stationary source of supplemental oxygen. Unless patients are immobilized, confined to their room or bed, mobile oxygen delivery system should also be used. Both compressed gas and liquid portable oxygen systems are available for use. Liquid oxygen containers are easier to refill when compared to high-pressure cylinders. However, liquid oxygen is not used in our country chiefly because of its expenses and difficult availability. The devices for oxygen administration chiefly include nasal prongs and cannulae. Devices to 'conserve' home oxygen include nasal reservoir nasal cannulae, electronic conserving devices and transtracheal catheter. These have already been briefly discussed earlier. Transtracheal catheter, though convenient to the patient, carry the risk of infection and is perhaps the least frequently used mode of domiciliary long-term oxygen delivery.

SUGGESTED READING

Carpagnano GE. Supplementary oxygen in healthy subjects and those with COPD increases oxidative stress and airway inflammation. *Thorax*. 1 Dec. 2004; 59(12): 1016–9.

Croxton TL, Bailey WC. Long-term oxygen treatment in COPD: recommendations for future research. An NHLBI Workshop Report. *Am J Respir Crit Care Med* [online ahead of print] 13 Apr. 2006; DOI: 10.1164/rccm.200507-1161WS. Most recent version available from: http: //dx.doi.org/10.1164/rccm.200507-1161WS.

Eastwood GM. Evaluation of nasopharyngeal oxygen, nasal prongs and facemask oxygen therapy devices in adult patients: a randomised crossover trial. *Anaesth Intensive Care*. 1 Sep. 2008; 36(5): 691–4.

Medical Research Council Working Party. Long-term domiciliary oxygen therapy in chronic hypoxic cor pulmonale complicating chronic bronchitis and emphysema. *Lancet*. 1981; 1: 681–6.

Nocturnal Oxygen Therapy Trial Group (1980). Continuous or nocturnal oxygen therapy in hypoxemic chronic obstructive lung disease: a clinical trial. *Ann Intern Med*. 93: 391–8.

Veale D, Chailleux E, Taytard A, *et al*. Characteristics and survival of patients prescribed long-term oxygen therapy outside prescription guidelines. *Eur Respir J*. 1998; 12: 780–4.

Zielinski J. Long-term oxygen therapy in COPD patients with moderate hypoxaemia: does it add years to life? *Eur Respir J*. 1998; 12: 756–8.

CHAPTER **43** # Lung Cancer and Other Lung Tumours

At the turn of the twentieth century lung cancer was considered a rare malignancy. Today lung cancer is the leading cause of cancer-related deaths in men; it has surpassed breast cancer and has also become the leading cause of cancer deaths in women. It is the most commonly diagnosed cancer with an estimated 1.35 million new cases per year and an estimated 1.1.8 million deaths every year. According to an international estimate, lung cancer is the cause of 31% of all cancer deaths in men and 27% of cancer deaths in women. In the United States (US), in 2004, 160,400 individuals were projected to die from lung cancer compared with an estimated 127,210 deaths from colorectal, breast and prostate cancer combined. It is indeed alarming that the trend of its increasing incidence with an associated increase in the number of deaths every year is likely to persist for several years.

The horrendously high incidence of lung cancer is unfortunately complemented by its high mortality, the five-year survival rate in the US and Europe being only 16%. Five-year survival rates in poor developing countries are undoubtedly less, perhaps not more than 5–7%. There are two reasons for this dismal state of affairs. First, many patients with lung cancer, even advanced lung cancer, are asymptomatic so that by the time they are diagnosed it is too late for curative therapy. Secondly, the natural history of most lung cancers is characterized by rapid intrathoracic spread and frequent metastatic spread to extrathoracic organ systems.

The chief cause of lung cancer in 85–90% of cases is smoking, a fact brilliantly proven by the excellent epidemiological studies by Doll and Hill in the early 1950s. It has been estimated that 10–15% of all smokers will develop lung cancer. Not smoking and the cessation of cigarette smoking is undoubtedly the best and the most certain method to reduce the risk of lung cancer. It is indeed a sad commentary on human affairs that a disease eminently preventable is allowed to flourish and cause so many deaths in the world.

The term lung cancer is used for cancers arising in the airways or lung parenchyma, and these are classified into two sub-groups—small cell lung cancer (SCLC) and non-small cell lung cancer (NSCLC). This distinction is important with regard to differences in the natural history, prognosis and treatment between the two groups. About 95% of all lung cancers are either SCLC or NSCLC. The remaining 5% of cancers are other tumours of comparatively rare cell-type originating in the lungs. This chapter deals chiefly with SCLC and NSCLC. The rare cancers including lung metastasis from primary sites outside the lung are dealt with briefly at the end of the chapter.

EPIDEMIOLOGY

The prevalence of lung cancer varies with the geographical area and ethnicity of the population under study. It is estimated that nearly 70% of all new cases of lung cancer in the world occur in developing countries. This may however well be an underestimate as diagnostic facilities for detection of lung cancer in the poor developing countries leave much to be desired. Also, the increasing incidence of lung cancer in developing countries, particularly in Southeast Asia, South Asia and in particular China is certain to alter the above estimate. In the year 2000, rates of lung cancer in males were 28.8 per 100,000 and 10.8/100,000 in females. There was however considerable variation in different geographic areas of the world.

Western developed countries have had both the highest number of deaths and the highest incidence of lung cancer for many years. The incidence of lung cancer in the US, Canada, Europe, New Zealand (Maori population) stands highest at 750/100,000. The state of Utah in the US is the sole exception among all other states in that it has a low incidence of lung cancer. A lesser incidence of 35–50/100,000 is observed in China, Australia, New Zealand (non-Maori), Spain, Ireland and Malta. The incidence of lung cancer in Shanghai is however more than 50 per 100,000. A low incidence of lung cancer, < 35 per 100,000, is observed in Latin America, Norway, Sweden, Iceland and most Asian countries. An age-adjusted world incidence rate of lung cancer in different countries of the world is compared in Figure 43.3.

Lung cancer all over the world is more frequent in males than in females. This risk for lung cancer varies in different geographic areas of the world. For example, the risk is believed to be less than 1% in the Indian population in Mumbai and Singapore whereas it is more than 14% in the Maori population of New Zealand. The difference in male and female incidence of lung cancer is related to smoking habits. The lower female rates are because in many countries fewer women smoke or smoke at a later period in life, or smoke less than men. However, current trends in some countries have shown an increasing trend of lung cancer in women as against a decreasing trend in men. This again is related to increasing smoking habits in females in the last decade.

Some important features of the prevalence and mortality of lung cancer in a few countries of the world are briefly discussed.

United States In the US there has been a precipitous rise in the incidence and death rate from decade to decade starting from

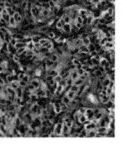

1930 onwards. In 1930, the age-adjusted lung cancer deaths in males were 5/100,00 per year and in females 3/100,000 per year. In 1987 in males they rose to 74.9/100,000 and in females to 28.5/100,000. As mentioned in the introductory remarks, today lung cancer would account for 31% of all cancer deaths in males and 27% of all cancer deaths in females.

United Kingdom The lung cancer rates in the United Kingdom (UK) are approximately 100 per 100,00 per year. The UK incidence rates in men peaked in the 1970s when it ranked highest in the world. Since then they have fallen by 10% every five years. In contrast the incidence of lung cancer increased by 5% every 10 years in women until the 1980s, following which the rise has slowed. The fall in the incidence in males and the rise in the incidence in females mirror the changing smoking trends in the country.

Europe The incidence of lung cancer in Europe standardized to the population of Europe is about 66.5 per 100,000 in men and 8.9 per 100,000 in women. Increased cigarette smoking in females between 1985 and 1995 in France led to an increase in the incidence rate by 56% in women and 5% in men under the age of 65. As expected female mortality more than doubled, while male deaths increased by just under 50%.

Asia and Africa Within Asia the standardized mortality rates were highest in China and lowest in the South Pacific Islands – 29.1 and 13.8 per 100,000 respectively. In all developing countries lung cancer in males accounts for close to three quarters of patients. The rates in females are low, except among Chinese women who have a comparatively higher rate.

In the last decade there has been a progressive increase in lung cancer in China and South Korea, mostly in men. In South Korea the age-adjusted mortality increased from 3.7/100,00 in 1980 to 17.8/100,000 in 1994 in males and from 1.4 to 7/100,000 in women. The projected average annual age-adjusted mortality in 2000–04 was 65.5 and 15.1/100,000 for males and females respectively.

Age-standardized mortalities in both North and South African regions were low – 7.9 and 11.5 /100,000 respectively in males and 3.2 and 5.3 per 100,000 in females.

The lung cancer incidence in Australia is higher compared to the UK and Canada but lower than the US. However the mortality rate for lung cancer is lower in Australia compared to the US – 32% lower than the US in males and 48% lower in women.

The increasing trend of 1 to 5% in age-related mortality rates in lung cancer is universal involving most countries of the world. Overall mortality is less in females. There is however evidence to show that in countries where women show increasing smoking habits, the rate of rise in female mortality per year is more than in males.

The Indian Scenario The incidence and mortality of lung cancer in India has shown a significant steady rise.

Lung cancer is the first and leading cause of cancer in males in the metropolitan cities of Mumbai, Delhi, Kolkata, Bhopal and Ahmedabad. The three urban registries of Bhopal, Delhi and Mumbai have registered lung cancer as the most

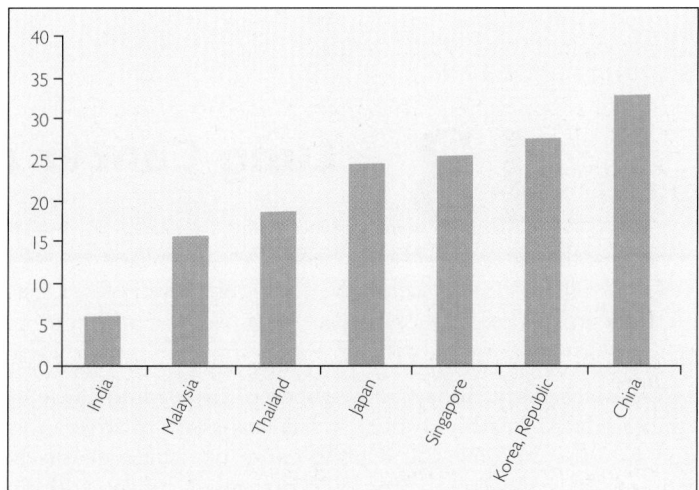

Fig 43.1: Incidence of lung cancer per 100,000 (Age-standardized rates) in Southeast Asia, Globocan, 2008.

Source: Ferlay J, Shin HR, Bray F, Forman D, Mathers C, Parkin DM. GLOBOCAN 2008, *Cancer Incidence and Mortality Worldwide: IARC CancerBase No. 1 [Internet].* Lyon, France: International Agency for Research on Cancer; 2010. Available from: http://globocan.iarc.fr

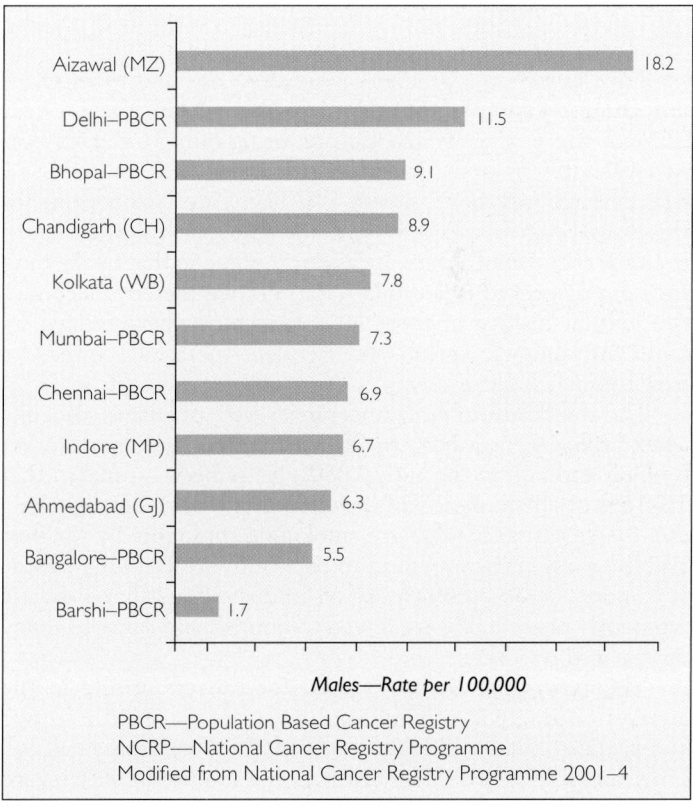

PBCR—Population Based Cancer Registry
NCRP—National Cancer Registry Programme
Modified from National Cancer Registry Programme 2001–4

Fig 43.2: Lung Cancer in India—Districtwise Comparisons of Age Adjusted Incidence Rates with that of PBCRs under NCRP (2001–4).

frequent site of cancer, constituting around 10% of cancers at all sites. It is the second leading site of cancer in Chennai and Thiruvananthapuram and the third leading site in Bangalore, Nagpur and Pune.

The National Cancer Registry Programme (NCRP) has adjudged that Aizwal in Mizoram state and Imphal in Manipur state had one and a half times the mean age-adjusted rate (MAAR) of the highest urban population-based cancer registry (PBCR)—Delhi (11.5 per 1000,00). In fact nine other districts were judged to have MAAR higher than that of–the MAAR of Delhi.

The disease though commoner in urban areas also has a grip over rural areas as evinced by rural registries from Karanagapally in Kerala where lung cancer is the most frequent of all cancers.

Population-based cancer registries show that cancer of the lung in Indian women is not as frequent a site for cancer when compared to men. Among cities the highest incidence of lung cancer in women is observed in Mumbai with age-adjusted rate of 4.2/100,000. Even this age-adjusted rate for females in Mumbai is lower than that of Indians in Singapore and other women in areas of high incidence in the world.

The influence of ethnic and genetic factors is suggested by the very low incidence of lung cancer in Parsee males living in the rural areas of Maharashtra and Gujarat. The age-adjusted incidence rate in non-Parsee males (12.6) is almost thrice the rate in Parsee males (4.2) while the rates are similar in Parsee and non-Parsee females (3.7). In Mumbai the same difference in incidence of lung cancer in the Parsee and non-Parsee population is only apparent after the age of 54 years and

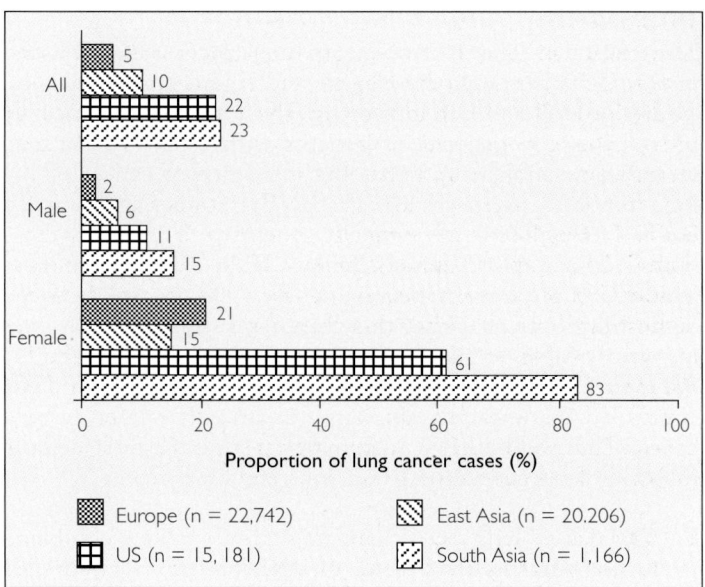

Fig 43.4: Lung cancers in never-smokers show geographic and gender variations. A review of published studies over the past 25 years included studies from the US, Europe (Germany, Sweden, Poland, Hungary, Czech Republic, Slovakia, Romania and Russia), East Asia (China, Taiwan, Korea, Japan and Singapore), and South Asia (India and Pakistan). A marked gender bias was observed whereby lung cancer in never-smokers appears to affect women more frequently than men, irrespective of geography (P <0.0001 using the Cochran-Mantel-Haenszel test). The proportion of female lung cancer cases in never-smokers is particularly high in East and South Asia.

Source: (Reprinted by permission of Macmillan Publishers Ltd: Lung Cancer in Never Smokers—AD: fberent Disease, *Nature Reviews*, vol. 7 © 2007 Nature Publishing Group October 2007.)

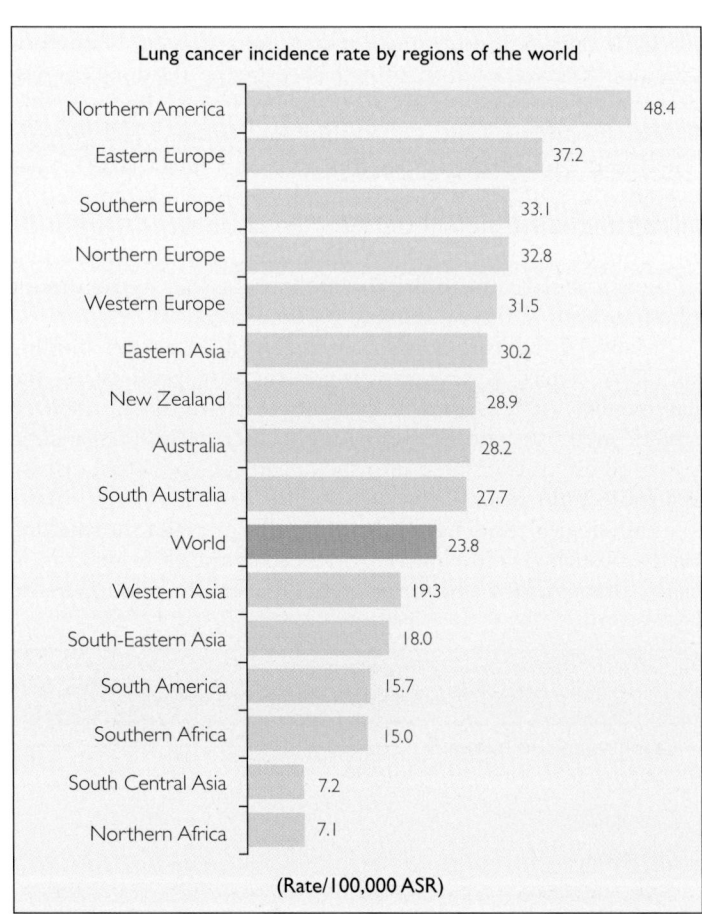

Fig 43.3: Age-adjusted lung cancer incidence rates in men worldwide in 2002.

Source: IARC, GLOBOCAN 2002 (www-dep.iarc.fr).

not before. The role of cigarette smoking and air pollution in Mumbai, in addition to ethnic and genetic factors may all be important reasons for the above findings.

The average age at the time of diagnosis of cancer is 56 years for males and 52 years for females as per the hospital-based cancer registry at Tata Memorial Hospital, Mumbai. Data from Kerala, North India and Rajasthan suggest the same average age. The male:female ratio at the Tata Memorial Hospital changed from 7.8 to 1 in 1990 to 5.5 to 1 in 1995. In North Indian studies the male to female ratio rose progressively in the 51 to 60 years age group. It was very high in smokers and was the same for all cell types.

Risk factors influencing the incidence of lung cancer have been dealt with in the section on 'Aetiology' in this chapter.

Age-adjusted world incidence ratio of lung cancer in different countries of the world is given in Figure 43.3.

AETIOLOGY AND PATHOGENESIS OF LUNG CANCER

Aetiology

Cigarette smoking is unquestionably the most important cause of lung cancer. This fact is chiefly based on epidemiological studies, supplemented by pathological findings related to the effect of cigarette smoke on bronchial mucosa.

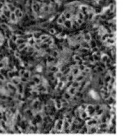

SMOKING

The relation of cigarette smoking to lung cancer was established in the 1950s through the elegant and sound epidemiological studies of Doll and Hill in the UK. These studies convincingly proved that the majority of patients with cancer of the lung were heavy smokers and that the incidence of cancer of the lung in non-smokers was low. Prospective studies again carried out by Doll and Hill, were equally conclusive. The best of these was a study on 40,000 doctors in the UK. In 1951 each of these gave details of their smoking habits. By 1964 the link between death from lung cancer in this group and smoking habits was incontrovertible. Similar results were noted in the US. The US Surgeon General's Report on Smoking and Health in 1964 concluded that cigarette smoking was causally related to lung cancer. These and other epidemiological studies established the following facts in relation to smoking and lung cancer.

1. The risk of lung cancer is increased in smokers compared to non-smokers by a factor of 10. Pipe smokers and cigar smokers have a comparatively lower incidence than cigarette smokers probably because the smoke is not inhaled into the lungs to the same degree.
2. The risk of cancer increases with the number of cigarettes smoked and increases proportionally with the time a person has smoked. The greater the number of years a patient has smoked and the larger the number of cigarettes smoked, the greater the risk of lung cancer. Current smokers smoking one pack a day for 20 years have a risk of lung cancer 10 to 15 times that of those who have never smoked. This risk increases to 25 times if two or more packs are smoked for 20 years.
3. A British study showed that in those who stopped smoking, the risk begins to decline almost immediately; it however takes 15 years for the risk to decline to a level which is still approximately twice that of those who never smoked. The Multiple Risk Factor Intervention Trial showed similar results. It is apparent that even if cigarette smoking were to cease today the current spate of lung cancer would continue for long.
4. Passive smoking by which is meant inhalation of cigarette smoke exhaled by others or smoke inhaled from smouldering cigarettes also carries a small but clear increase in risk for lung cancer. Studies showed 1.2 times risk for lung cancer in women who lived with husbands who smoked compared to women who lived in smoke-free homes. Passive smoking is estimated to give rise to 300 new cases of cancer every year in the US. The ban on cigarette smoking in many public places in many countries of the world is indeed a welcome step.

Smoking and Lung Cancer in India

Smoking in the main causative factor in India just as in the rest of the world. A history of active tobacco smoking is present in 87% of males and 85% of females. A history of passive exposure to tobacco smoke was found in only three per cent. The relative risk of developing lung cancer in bidi smokers was noted to be 2.64 whereas in cigarette smokers it was 2.23, the overall relative risk being 2.45. Studies in India further suggest that bidis are more carcinogenic than cigarettes (*Ref: Jussawalla D.J and Jain D.K: Lung cancer in Greater Bombay: correlations with religion and smoking habits. Br J Cancer. 1979 September; 40(3): 437–448*). Hookah smoking has also been associated with lung cancer.

In a recent study by Gupta D, Boefetta P et al. (*Gupta D, Boffetta P, Gaborieau V, Jindal SK. Risk factors of lung cancer in Chandigarh, India. Indian J Med Res 2001; **113**: 142–50.*), 80% of men and 33% of women among the patients were ever-smokers compared to 60% of men and 20% of women among controls. The odds ratio (OR) for ever-smoking was 5.0 (95% CI = 3.11–8.04) among the men and 2.47 (95% CT = 0.79–0.75) among women. Smoking of bidi and hookah as well as cigarettes had similar OR for cumulative consumption. The risk was noted to increase with the duration and quantity of all smoking products.

How does cigarette smoke induce lung cancer? Numerous carcinogens have been identified both in the residual fraction and the vapour phase of tobacco smoke. The acidic fraction is known to contain factors that stimulate tumour cell growth. The International Agency for Research on Cancer (IARC) has classified a number of the chemical constituents reported in cigarette mainstream smoke (MS) as carcinogens. Of the 81 compounds reported in MS, 48 IARC MS carcinogens are found in the particulate phase, the rest are found either in the vapour phase or both in the vapour and particulate phase.

Many of the carcinogens are believed to act by binding to DNA. There is probably a genetic susceptibility to the carcinogenic effects of the poisonous chemicals in tobacco smoke in those who develop lung cancer. How this genetic susceptibility is translated into the occurrence of actual disease is a subject of research.

Pathological evidence for the dangers of cigarette smoking on the bronchial epithelium is evidenced by the close association between metaplasia and atypia of mucosal cells in relation to the

Table 43.1: Relation of smoking to lung cancer	
1.	Risk of lung cancer is increased in smokers compared to non-smokers by a factor of 10.
2.	The risk of cancer increases with the number of cigarettes smoked and increases proportionally with the time a person has smoked.
3.	Risk of developing lung cancer decreases with cessation of smoking.
4.	Passive smoking is an associated risk for lung cancer.

Table 43.2: Important Carcinogens in cigarette smoke
Carcinogenic to humans
Benzene
Cadmium
Chromium
2-Naphthylamine
Nickel
Polonium-210 (Radon)
Vinyl Chloride

Table 43.3: Important carcinogens in cigarette smoke
Probably carginogenic to humans
Acrylonitrile
Benzo [a] pyrene
1,3-Butadiene
Formaldehyde
N-Nitrosodiethylamine
N-Nitrosodimethylamine
Lead
5-Methylchrysene
NNK
2-Nitropropane
ortho-Toluidine
Urethane (Ethyl Carbamate)

number of cigarettes smoked. Animal experiments lend further proof of the link between lung cancer and tobacco smoke.

Cigarette smoking can cause all histopathological types of lung cancers. The strongest association is with squamous cell carcinoma and small cell cancer which generally arise in the central airways; a weaker association exists with adenocarcinoma of the lung which generally arises in the periphery of the lung.

Smoking Habits in the World

Smoking habits in the world are a matter of considerable alarm. Smoking habits in the US have fortunately declined over the last four decades from 52% in men and 34% in women to 25% for men and 19% for women. The World Health Organization Report of 2002 mentions that about one-third of all men worldwide smoke and that approximately 15 billion cigarettes are sold daily.

Smoking habits in Europe and Asia though varying from country to country are even higher in Europe; on an overall estimate 30–40% of men and 15–30% of women smoke. Smoking rates in men in China are horrendous—close to 67% though in women it is much lower – 4%.

It is obvious that the worldwide epidemic of lung cancer due to cigarette smoking will continue to rise for decades.

Other Risk Factors

EXPOSURE TO IONISING RADIATION

Radon exposure due to ionising radiation is perhaps the most important cancer risk for non-smokers not exposed to asbestos. Radon is a decay product arising from radium which in turn is a breakdown product of uranium. Exposure to radon through ionic radiation is present in miners mining rock faces for various metals and most importantly miners mining for uranium. These miners are therefore prone to lung cancer. This has been observed for several decades in miners mining various metals in the mountains between Saxony and the Czech Republic.

Radon is also present in indoor and outdoor air and the greater the exposure, the greater the risk of lung cancer. In the US radon in the general environment has been held responsible for 10% of all lung cancers, so that it forms the second most important cause of cancer. To what extent this risk applies to other countries is not known.

ASBESTOS EXPOSURE AND OTHER OCCUPATION HAZARDS

There exists a clear link between asbestos exposure and lung cancer. The increased risk is translated into actual disease 20 or more years after initial exposure. Asbestos is chiefly used in the construction industry and for its fire-resistant properties. There are many types of asbestos fibres, some being more carcinogenic than others. The subject has been dealt with at length under Occupational Lung Disorders.

Other occupational factors reported to be associated with increased risk of lung cancer have been tabled below. Unfortunately, information on occupational risk for lung cancer in India is sadly lacking.

Table 43.4: Occupational risk factors associated with lung cancer	
Chemicals	**Occupation involved**
Arsenic	Smelter workers and vineyard workers
Asbestos	Insulation workers and shipyard workers
Nickel	Refinery workers
Radiation	Uranium mining
Chromium	Ore miners and pigment manufacturers
Chloromethyl	Industrial workers
Radon	Hematite miners
Soot, tars	Coke oven workers
Oils and coke	Gas houseworkers, rubber workers

Note: Other probable carcinogens are beryllium, cadmium, formaldehyde and silica.

AIR POLLUTION

Atmospheric pollution is also considered a risk for lung cancer. In Western countries, even allowing for smoking habits the risk of cancer is higher in the polluted urban areas compared to the less polluted rural areas. Atmospheric pollutants are mainly polycyclic hydrocarbons from the combustion of fossil fuels—wood and coal fires. These have now been given up in almost all cities of the world. The main sources of pollutants today in most countries of the world are exhausts from motor vehicles, particularly diesel smoke and emissions from factories within or close to cities.

DIETARY FACTORS

The role of dietary factors in increasing or decreasing risk for lung cancer remains unproven. Retrospective case-controlled studies suggest a protective role for fruit consumption. Vegetable consumption is reported to be associated with decreased lung cancer risk, and there are studies that support a protective role for beta carotene and vitamin C. Three randomized controlled studies have however shown that

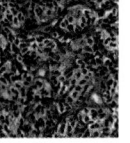

supplementation with beta carotene failed to exert a protective effect against lung cancer.

GENETICS

Inherited susceptibility for lung cancer may play a role in aetiology. A family history of lung cancer is associated with a greater risk of lung cancer even after allowing for smoking habits. Familial clustering of lung cancer has been observed particularly with squamous cell carcinoma. Inherited susceptibility theoretically should be based on genetic predisposition, though the means by which genetic predisposition increases risk is unclear.

CHRONIC OBSTRUCTIVE PULMONARY DISEASE

Recent studies suggest that chronic obstructive pulmonary disease (COPD) is a risk factor for lung cancer over and above that caused by cigarette smoking.

The Lung Health Study has supported this view based on a study of 580 patients who had mild airways' obstruction and a history of smoking. These were followed up and assessed for the effectiveness of stopping smoking and use of anticholinergic therapy. Lung cancer was the leading cause of death over a five-year follow-up. Perhaps it may well be that instead of airways' obstruction predisposing to lung cancer both airways' obstruction and lung cancer were related to the common factor—smoking.

Table 43.5:
Etiology and risk factors associated with lung cancer

1.	Smoking
2.	Exposure to ionizing radiation
3.	Asbestos exposure and other occupational hazards
4.	Air pollution
5.	Genetics
6.	COPD

PATHOGENESIS

The pathogenesis of bronchogenic carcinoma can be summarized as a step-by-step process altering normal bronchial mucosal cells into malignant cells under the influence of a carcinogenic agent. The commonest carcinogenic agents responsible for this are one or more of the many carcinogens present in cigarette smoke. Carcinogens act by inducing a genetic damage to mucosal cells so that a step-by-step progression to malignancy occurs.

The multi-step gradual evolution from normal epithelium to hyperplasia—metaplasia—dysplasia—carcinoma *in situ*—invasive carcinoma has been studied by cytopathologists in uranium miners in the US. Similar evidence demonstrating the presence of dysplasia preceding carcinoma was observed in a large autopsy study in which the whole bronchial tree was examined in several patients dying of lung cancer.

Squamous metaplasia has therefore been regarded by many as a premalignant change. This is supported by the presence of metaplasia and dysplasia frequently observed adjacent to invasive carcinoma as also by the presence of genetic abnormalities which are similar to those prevailing in adjacent invasive cancerous cells.

These premalignant changes are quite extensive and explain the high incidence of a second primary lung cancer in the same individual. It has been shown that 4% of lung cancer patients have more than one lung tumour and that a further 4–6% develop a second lung tumour later.

Atypical alveolar hyperplasia has also been noted as a focal premalignant change accompanying bronchogenic carcinoma, chiefly an adenocarcinoma of the lung. It is possible though not proven that alveolar cell carcinoma (a variant of adenocarcinoma) may perhaps evolve from these atypical hyperplastic premalignant cells.

The mechanism by which carcinogens in the smoke of cigarette smokers induce a multi-step change in the bronchial epithelial cells resulting in malignancy is poorly understood. Carcinogens in cigarette smoke probably induce a genetic change in the bronchial epithelium. Early cancers have shown a number of genetic and molecular alterations. These include mutations in the P53 tumour suppressor gene and K-ras proto oncogene as also diminished expression of P16 tumour suppressor gene because of hypermethylation.

Both NSCLC and SCLC have been known to have chromosomal abnormalities. Mutations of P53 tumour suppressor gene are present in 50% of NSCLC and 70% of SCLC. An increased expression of epidermal growth factor together with its receptor is present in about 60% of NSCLC. Identification of critical early molecular alterations may perhaps help in the early detection of cancer.

Finally, it is an accepted fact that there is a survival discrepancy between patients suffering from the same stage of cancer. This means that the biology of tumours may vary even though the disease stage is identical. The reason for this biological variation is a subject of research. Differences in outcome for tumours classified as belonging to the same stage could be related to oncogen amplification, mutations in tumours, suppressor genes, nature and level of tumour antigens and other biological factors.

The unravelling of the genetic profile of lung cancer may in the future serve two purposes—a) a better prediction of patient survival; b) tailoring patient-specific treatment (chemotherapeutic agents) to enhance survival rates.

PATHOLOGY OF BRONCHOPULMONARY CARCINOMA

The classification of lung cancer as given by the World Health Organisation (WHO) has been given below.

Although this classification includes many types of lung cancer, just four of these account for over 95% of the total. These are squamous cell carcinoma, adenocarcinoma, small cell carcinoma and large cell carcinoma. Alveolar cell carcinoma is a variant of adenocarcinoma. For clinical purposes, cancer is best divided into *non-small-cell lung cancer (NSCLC)* which in the main includes adenocarcinoma, and squamous cell carcinoma, and *small cell lung cancers (SCLC)*. It is important to distinguish between these two main types. A histopathological diagnosis is not always easy for there is a significant inter-observer variation among pathologists in identifying various subtypes of NSCLC. Though this may not be of clinical significance with regard to therapy at present, it

may prove relevant in the future if the treatment of NSCLC becomes specifically related to the subtypes.

Squamous Cell Carcinoma

The main histopathological features of squamous cell carcinoma are the presence of keratinisation and /or the presence of intercellular junctions or bridges often termed 'prickles' or desmosomes. Squamous cell carcinomas generally arise centrally in association with central airways—trachea, main stem, lobar and also with segmental bronchi. They are the least malignant of the four main types and have a high correlation with smoking history. As these cancers are usually centrally placed, they cause clinical and radiological features of obstruction to the large airways. In the very early stages, the tumour may be

radiologically occult even on a computed tomography (CT) examination of the chest.

Squamous cell carcinoma may also originate peripherally presenting as a mass lesion which may cavitate and be mistaken for a lung abscess.

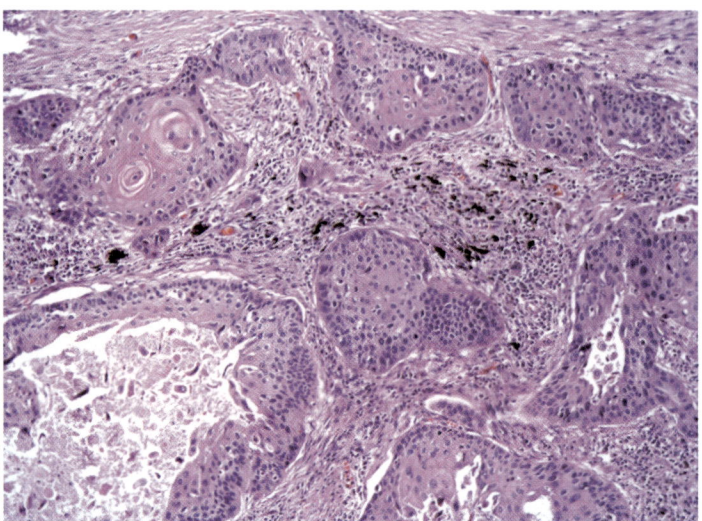

Fig 43.5: Squamous cell carcinoma of the lung. H&E microscopy image at 20 X magnification demonstrates nests of tumour cells with central keratinisation indicating a squamous cell carcinoma-lung.

| Table 43.6: |
| The New WHO/International Association for the study of lung cancer: Histological classification of tumours of the lung |

1. Squamous cell carcinoma
   • Papillary.
   • Clear cell.
   • Small cell.
   • Basaloid

2. Small cell carcinoma

3. Adenocarcinoma
   • Acinar.
   • Papillary.
   • Bronchioloalveolar carcinoma.
   • Nonmucinous.
   • Mucinous.
   • Mixed mucinous and nonmucinous or indeterminate cell type.
     – Solid adenocarcinoma with mucin.
     – Adenocarcinoma with mixed subtypes.
   • Variants.
     – Well-differentiated fetal adenocarcinoma.
     – Mucinous (colloid) adenocarcinoma.
     – Mucinous cystadenocarcinoma.
     – Signet ring adenocarcinoma.
     – Clear cell adenocarcinoma.

4. Large cell carcinoma
   • Variants.
     – Large-cell neuroendocrine carcinoma.
     – Combined large-cell neuroendocrine carcinoma.
     – Basaloid carcinoma.
     – Lymphoepithelioma-like carcinoma.
     – Clear cell carcinoma.
     – Large cell carcinoma with rhabdoid phenotype.

5. Adenosquamous carcinoma

6. Carcinomas with pleomorphic, sarcomatoid, or sarcomatous elements.
   • Carcinomas with spindle and/or giant cells.
   • Spindle cell carcinoma
   • Giant cell carcinoma. Carcinosarcoma.

7. Carcinoid tumour

8. Carcinomas of salivary-gland type.
   • Mucoepidermoid carcinoma.
   • Adenoid cystic carcinoma.
   • Others.

9. Unclassified carcinomas.

Adenocarcinoma

In the US it is the most frequent histological cell-type encountered, and its prevalence in Europe and in other Western countries appears to be clearly on the rise. It most often arises in the periphery as a peripheral nodule which grows into a mass lesion which occasionally cavitates. Most cancers identified on imaging, including a CT chest are adenocarcinomas. This is because peripheral lesions are more easily picked up on imaging studies compared to central lesions. Though closely associated with smoking, adenocarcinoma accounts for almost all lung cancers in patients who have never smoked.

The main histopathological features of an adenocarcinoma are the presence of neoplastic formation of glands, papillary structures, or a solid pattern. Mucin can be identified within the cell cytoplasm by special stains.

Alveolar cell carcinoma or bronchoalveolar cell carcinoma are variants of adenocarcinomas. The tumour grows and spreads along alveolar walls using the walls as a framework for growth, without destroying them or infiltrating into the interstitium—the so-called lipid spread. This variant of adenocarcinoma shows a variety of cytological differentiation—goblet cell, Clara cell or Type II pneumocytes.

Bronchoalveolar cell carcinoma presents as a nodule, or a mass that may be solid or have a ground glass attenuation on a CT. It may also present as multiple nodules involving one or both lungs or as-'pneumonia' involving one or more lobes of the lung.

Bronchoalveolar cell carcinomas disseminate by aerogenous spread, tumour cells being aspirated and causing satellite lesions in different parts of the lungs—initially in the ipsilateral

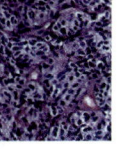

lung followed by the involvement of the contralateral lung. Aspirations have a gravitational distribution, being distributed to the lung bases, the dorsal segment of the lower lobe and the posterior segment of the upper lobe. This suggests aspiration with aerogenic spread during sleep at night. Alveolar cell carcinoma producing satellite lesions are usually of the mucus-producing variety and have the worst prognosis.

Small Cell Lung Cancer (SCLC)

SCLCs are believed to arise from neuroendocrine cells and account for about 20% of lung cancers in most series. SCLCs are strongly associated with smoking, generally occur centrally, invariably causing early metastatic mediastinal adenopathy. Imaging features usually show a large mediastinal adenopathy, the primary site of origin being unclear. SCLC is the lung cancer most frequently associated with distant metastatic spread and most frequently associated with one or more of the paraneoplastic syndrome. The latter may precede the clinical or even the imaging presence of SCLC by several months.

SCLC is considered a systemic disease, even in the limited stage, the only exception being SCLC presenting as a localized peripheral nodule without any hilar or mediastinal adenopathy.

Histologically, SCLC consist of small oval cells with little cytoplasm closely packed together, the tumour cells appearing to press on one another to produce what has been termed nuclear moulding. The cell nuclei are pyknotic with a distinct nucleolus and a dispersed granular chromatin pattern.

Large Cell Undifferentiated Carcinoma

These tumours lack either squamous or glandular differentiation, the tumour cells being arranged in sheets. The cells have a fair amount of cytoplasm, vesicular nuclei with prominent nucleoli. Large cell undifferentiated carcinomas generally present as a peripheral mass; necrosis is often present within the mass.

Some of the other rarer pathological forms of lung cancers are adeno-squamous carcinomas which partake of features of both adeno and squamous cell carcinoma, carcinoid tumours, carcinoma of the salivary gland type, mucoepidermoid carcinoma, carcinoma of the sarcomatoid and sarcomatous type, lymphomas, metastatic tumours from primaries situated outside the lungs.

Carcinoma *in situ*

The natural history of carcinoma *in situ* is not well documented. Carcinoma *in situ* has been known to progress to invasive carcinoma over months or years. Carcinoma *in situ* is not necessarily confined to the surface epithelium but can involve the ducts of the mucus glands thereby mimicking invasive carcinoma. The cells in carcinoma *in situ* show marked squamous cell differentiation. However, the invasive form of cancer that may develop shows less well-marked differentiation or may even develop into a large cell undifferentiated carcinoma or a SCLC. Adenocarcinomas do not develop from a carcinoma *in situ*.

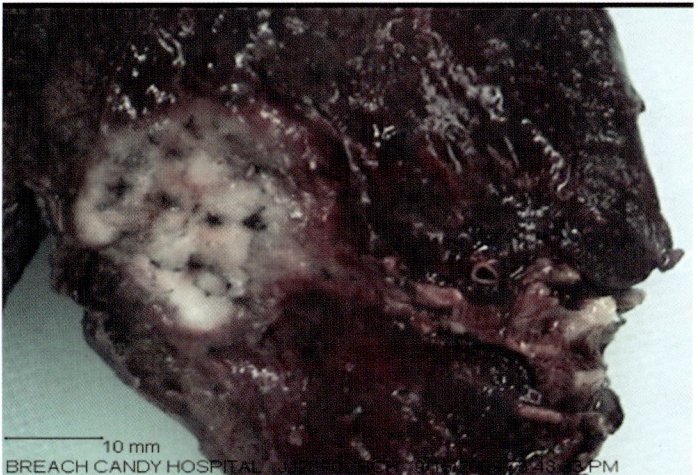

Fig 43.6: Adenocarcinoma lung. Gross lobectomy specimen demonstrates a peripherally placed solid mass lesion, fairly distant from the lobar bronchus.

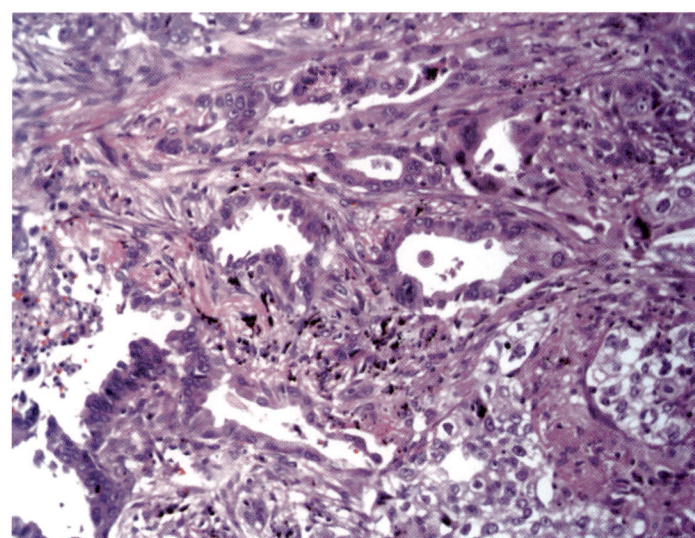

Fig 43.7: Adenocarcinoma lung. H&E microscopy at 20X magnification reveals tumour cells disposed in glandular pattern, separated by desmoplastic stroma indicative of an adenocarcinoma lung.

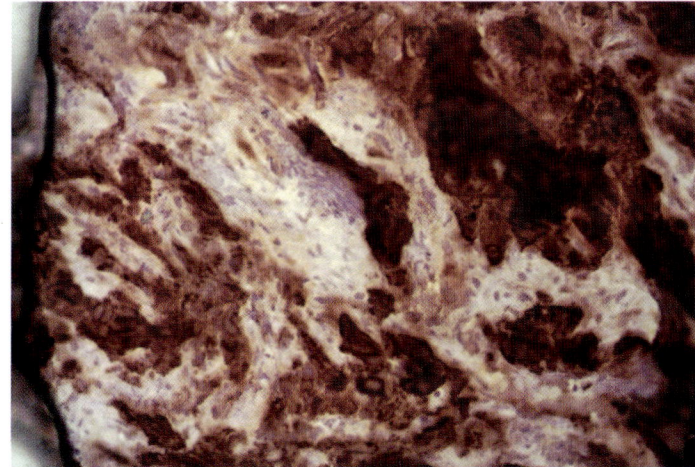

Fig 43.8: Small cell carcinoma of the lung. Immunohistochemistry using cytokeratin shows strong positivity in tumour cells.

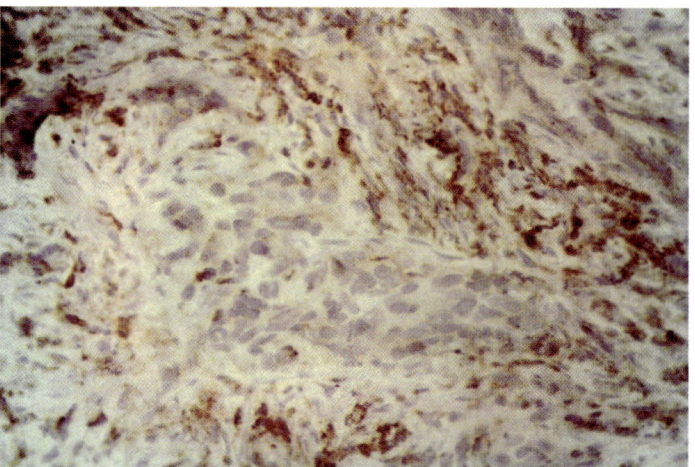

Fig 43.9: 20X. Small cell carcinoma lung. Immunohistochemistry with leukocyte common antigen (LCA). It is important to differentiate a lymphoma from small cell carcinoma. This marker helps to differentiate, as lymphoma will be positive and small cell cancer will be negative.

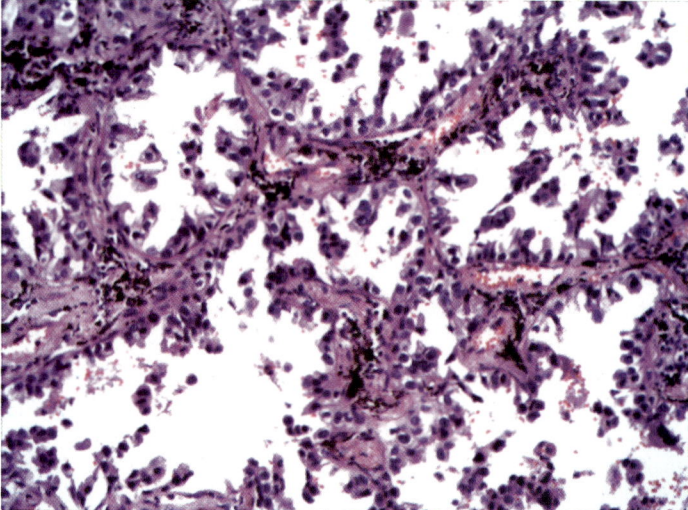

Fig 43.10: Bronchoalveolar carcinoma. Histopathology shows alveoli lined by malignant cells. The framework of the lung is preserved indicating that this is a bronchoalveolar carcinoma.

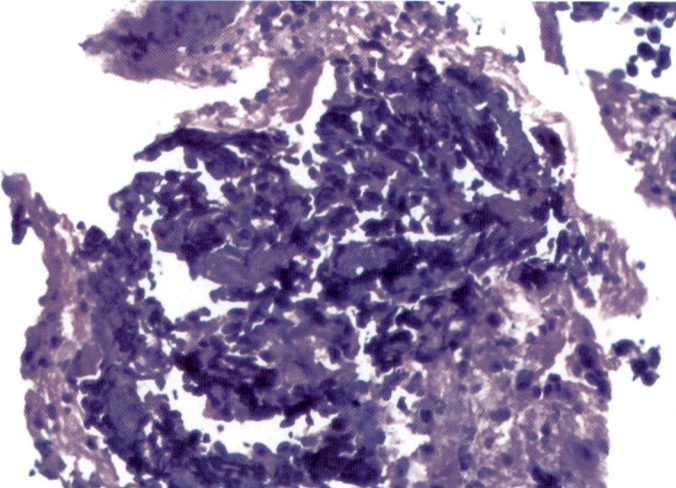

Fig 43.11: Small cell carcinoma of the lung. Nests of darkly stained small to medium-sized cells with scant indiscernible cytoplasm. Crush artifact is noted which is an important diagnostic feature.

Scar Cancer

Peripheral lung cancers, usually adenocarcinoma sometimes exhibit a central area of sclerosis resembling a scar. The question has been debated whether this scar tissue is a product of the tumour or whether the tumour has arisen from the scar. Perhaps both are possible. The diffuse scarring in usual interstital pneumonia and in some other conditions causing intersitial lung disease have a well-recognized association with the development of lung cancer. Though there are reports of this association and occurrence in the West, we have very rarely encountered a bronchogenic carcinoma arising from scar tissue in our centres.

Table 43.7: Classification of lung cancer used in clinical practice	
Type	**Incidence**
Non-small cell lung cancer (NSCLC)	75%
Adenocarcinoma • Alveolar cell carcinoma • Bronchoalveolar cell carcinoma	
Squamous cell carcinoma	
Small cell lung cancer (SCLC)	20%
Large cell undifferentiated carcinoma	
Others • Carcinoid tumours • Mucoepidermoid carcinoma • Carcinoma of the sarcomatoid and sarcomatous type • Carcinoma of the salivary gland type	

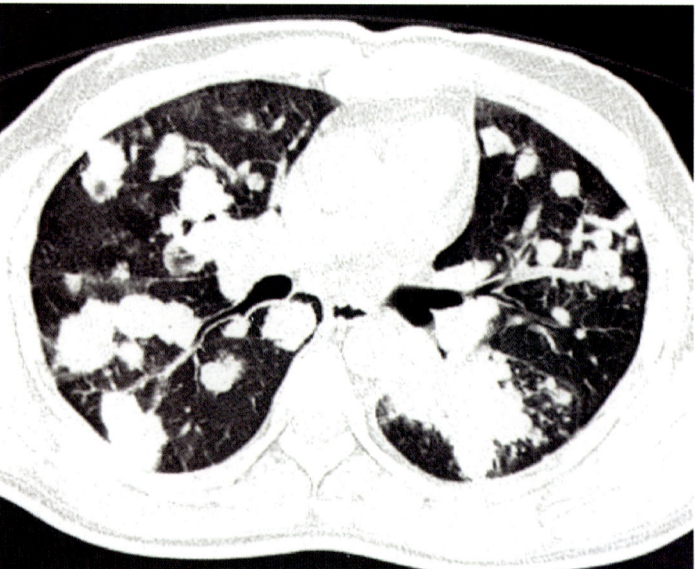

Fig 43.12: Bronchoalveolar carcinoma. CT chest demonstrates multiple well-defined lesions in both lung fields with ill-defined lesions in the right upper lobe posteriorly. CT-guided biopsy revealed a bronchoalveolar carcinoma.

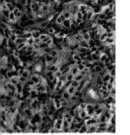

Prevalence of Histological Cell Types of Lung Cancer

The prevalence of different histological cell types is affected by the geographic areas and the population under study as also by the method in which the pathological material is obtained. There are differences in the prevalence of different cell types identified from biopsy specimens, from surgically resected specimens and from autopsy studies.

THE WORLD SCENARIO

Earlier in the Western world, squamous cell carcinoma was by far the commonest subtype of lung cancer. Close to 1980, there were twice as many squamous cell carcinomas as adenocarcinomas in men, whereas adenocarcinomas were slightly more frequent in women. By 1990, adenocarcinomas (29–37%) in the US were as frequent as squamous cell carcinomas (27–34%) and today the commonest subtype of lung cancer in the US, both in men and women is adenocarcinoma.

It thus appears that to start with, the surge of lung cancer in men was related to a marked increase in squamous cell carcinomas while the surge in women was mainly due to adenocarcinomas, there being an overall preponderance of squamous cell carcinoma. Then how does one now explain the present increase in the overall prevalence of adenocarcinoma? Wynder and Higgins believe that the change is related to the change in smoking habits. Following the introduction of filter-tipped cigarettes in the 1960s, smokers needed to take more frequent and deeper puffs to fulfil their need for nicotine. Cigarette smoke therefore reached more distally into the smaller bronchioles where adenocarcinoma occurs.

To summarize, the surge of squamous cell cancer in men before 1980 was due to smoking habits before the introduction of filter cigarettes. The surge in cancer among females after 1970 is related to smoking filter cigarettes and the change in the increased incidence from squamous to adenocarcinoma is also related (according to Wynder and Higgins) to the changeover in men to smoking filter cigarettes.

THE INDIAN SCENARIO

Studies show that in India squamous cell carcinoma is the most frequent subtype of lung cancer. But there is a slow increase in the incidence of adenocarcinoma and it is felt by oncologists in the country that as in the West, in the near future adenocarcinoma will become the most prevalent of lung cancer.

In a review article of 2004 by D Behera and T Balamugesh (Ref: Behera D, Balamugesh T: Lung cancer in India *Indian J Chest Dis Allied Sci.* 2004 Oct-Dec;46(4): 269–81. Department of Pulmonary Medicine, Postgraduate Institute of Medical Education and Research, Chandigarh, India) small cell cancer is reported to predominate under the age of 40 years. These authors report a weaker association of SCLC with smoking in contrast to Western studies and studies in Japan and all other studies which report a strong association of smoking with SCLC. A study of lung cancer in Kashmir, North India has also reported a strong association of smoking with all forms of lung cancers including SCLC (*Ref: Khan NA, et al. Profile of lung cancer in Kashmir, India: a five-year study, Indian J Chest Dis Allied Sci. 2006 Jul-Sep;48(3): 187–90).* As yet, according to the review paper of 2004 by Behera and Balamugesh, the histological cell type which has a predominant prevalence in

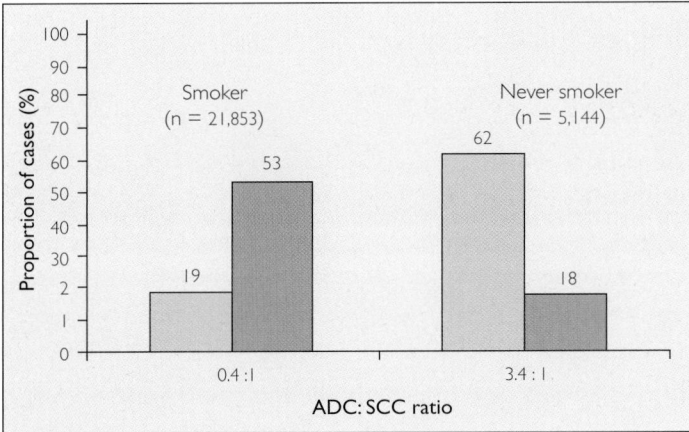

Fig 43.13: The histological distribution of lung cancers in never-smokers versus smokers was estimated using pooled data available from 17 reports published worldwide. Histological subtypes were classified as adenocarcinoma (ADC), squamous cell carcinoma (SCC) or 'other' (not shown; these included unknown histology, large cell carcinoma, mixed, not otherwise specified NSCLC and SCLC). Cases of bronchioloalveolar carcinoma (BAC) (n = 109) were combined with ADCs. The ratio of the number of ADC to SCC cases are reversed in never-smokers and smokers, reflecting the predominance of ADC in never-smokers (P <0.0001 using the Chi-square test).

Source: (Reprinted by permission of Macmillan Publishers Ltd: Lung Cancer in Never Smokers—A Different Disease. *Nature Reviews*, vol. 7 © 2007 Nature Publishing Group, October 2007.)

India is squamous cell carcinoma (45%). Small cell cancer has a reported prevalence of 20% and adenocarcinoma of 25%.

Another study by Navneet Singh, Dheeraj Gupta *et al.* on 'The Unchanging clinico-epidemiological profile of lung cancer in North India over three decades' showed that the commonest histological types of lung cancer were squamous cell (34.8%), adenocarcinoma (26.0%) and small cell (18.4%) while previously these were 34.3%, 25.9% and 20.3% respectively (*Ref: Navneet Singh, Dheeraj Gupta et al. on The Unchanging clinico-epidemiological profile of lung cancer in North India over three decades,* www.cancerepidemiology.net/article/S1877.5/abstract). However, the histological cell types reported currently by the Tata Memorial Hospital, Mumbai—the largest cancer hospital in India which drains patients of all classes from all

Table 43.8: Prevalence of histological cell types of lung cancer at the Tata Memorial Hospital		
Histology	**Male %**	**Female %**
Small cell carcinoma	10.4%	6.1%
Large cell carcinoma	1.6%	1.1%
Squamous cell carcinoma	14.6%	9.4%
Adenocarcinoma	17.3%	31.1%
Others	25.2%	22.8%
No histology	31.0%	29.4%
Total	100%	100%

Source: Annual Report, Mumbai Cancer Registry, 2006.

parts of the country are given below. The increased prevalence of adenocarcinoma in this study is worthy of note.

CLINICAL FEATURES

The clinical presentation and clinical features of lung cancer vary enormously. Ten to twenty per cent of cases are asymptomatic, being discovered fortuitously following a radiographic examination of the chest performed for a routine health check. Symptoms when they occur may be related to a gradual obstruction of one of the larger airways, or due to local spread within the lungs or the thorax. The very first clinical presentation may take the form of a distant metastatic lesion, or of multiple metastatic lesions so that the interval between the time of presentation and death is indeed very short. Finally, at times the clinical presentation and features are dominated by symptoms caused by non-metastatic (paraneoplastic) syndromes. More often than not, a combination of clinical features described above is observed. It is unfortunately a truism to state that in most patients, by the time the diagnosis of cancer of the lung has been made, treatment to alter the natural history of the disease is of little or no avail.

Local Symptoms

The cell-type of lung cancer may determine the pattern of dissemination as also the nature of problems for which the patient seeks advice. An adenocarcinoma generally arises within the lung parenchyma and may be peripherally situated. Local intrathoracic symptoms may be delayed, the disease announcing itself through one or more metastatic lesions or by a pleural effusion. On the other hand, squamous cell carcinomas tend to be confined to the thorax for a longer time so that symptoms related to the lungs and to intra-thoracic spread are more common. Small-cell lung cancers are rapidly-growing tumours, usually arising in the central airways, spreading locally and metastasising quickly so that symptoms at the time of presentation are often related both to the chest and the distant metastasis.

Cough

This is the commonest presenting clinical feature of lung cancer and is invariably present when a tumour arises in one of the central airways and tends to narrow or obstruct it. Cough is caused by ulceration of the bronchial mucosa and/or because of obstruction to the lumen of the airway. Close to 70% of lung cancers involve the major central airways—the carina, main and lobar bronchi. A tumour in any one of these situations besides causing ulceration of the mucosa and obstruction, impairs mucus clearance, thereby promoting further cough. Pneumonia—a single attack or recurrent episodes distal to a partially obstructed bronchus is a feature of bronchogenic carcinoma. Increasing bronchial obstruction can lead to atelectasis of a lobe or even a lung, causing both cough and breathlessness.

Since lung cancer occurs most frequently in cigarette smokers, cough caused by the lung cancer is often mistakenly looked upon as a smoker's cough, or attributed to chronic bronchitis, or to an upper respiratory tract infection. Persistent cough or increasing cough in a smoker merits a chest radiograph, particularly in a patient over 40 years of age. A change in the character of cough (particularly in a smoker's cough) also necessitates investigation. An ulcerating or obstructing cancerous lesion in a large bronchus often causes paroxysms of a dry brassy cough (with a metallic sound) which may be accompanied by a wheeze, noisy breathing or even stridor.

Cough is generally dry, or in a smoker may be associated with mucoid sputum; the sputum may be yellow in the presence of infection. Excessive sputum production, amounting to a bronchorrhea is occasionally seen in alveolar cell carcinoma, which is a form of adenocarcinoma that starts by lining the alveoli of one lung but often also involves the other.

Haemoptysis

Haemoptysis is the sole presenting feature in 5–10% of patients with bronchogenic carcinoma. It occurs as one among other presenting features in 30%. When it is the sole presenting feature, it prompts immediate concern and investigation. Haemoptysis is rarely profuse; more often it takes the form of streaking of sputum with blood, or sputum mixed with blood, particularly in the mornings. An X-ray of the chest is imperative; an abnormal X-ray chest necessitates further investigation. Even if the chest radiography is normal, haemoptysis, particularly in a smoker warrants a fibreoptic bronchoscopy. It needs to be however noted that the yield of endobronchial tumours following bronchoscopy in patients with haemoptysis who have a normal X-ray chest is not more than 5%. Occasionally, a bronchogenic carcinoma is diagnosed on a CT of the chest with a normal bronchoscopic study. The diagnosis of a bronchogenic carcinoma can be excluded in a patient presenting with haemoptysis, if the chest X-ray, sputum cytology, fibreoptic bronchoscopy, and a CT thorax are normal.

Dyspnoea

Dyspnoea may be a presenting symptom together with cough and sputum in 25% of patients with lung cancer. It occurs early in the natural history of this disease in over 50% of patients. Most importantly, dyspnoea occasionally may be complained of as the presenting symptom (or in association with other symptoms), even though the chest X-ray is normal. Dyspnoea in the above situation is related to progressive obstruction of a major bronchus, together with increasing obstructive emphysema of a lobe (if the lobar bronchus is involved) or the whole lung (if the main bronchus is involved). Dyspnoea may then be associated with a fixed monophonic inspiratory wheeze (Chevalier Jackson's sign) and is often mistaken for bronchial asthma. Ventilation perfusion scans have shown well-marked abnormalities disproportionate to any radiological abnormalities. A flow volume loop shows flattening of the inspiratory portion of the loop followed later by a flattened expiratory portion of the loop as well.

As the disease progresses, dypsnoea may be due to several other causes. It may be due to pneumonia distal to the obstructive lesion, due to lobar atelectasis, or due to a pleural effusion. It can also result from extensive involvement of the lung parenchyma, from left vocal chord paralysis due to pressure

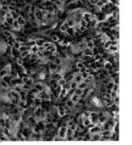
on the left recurrent laryngeal nerve and occasionally from extrinsic pressure on large airways due to extensive involvement of the mediastinum by the disease. More than one factor may be responsible for this symptom. Dyspnoea is also a prominent and distressing symptom in lymphangitis carcinomatosis and in pericardial effusion caused by malignant invasion of the parietal pericardium.

Chest Pain

Chest pain occurs in 25–50% of patients at the time of diagnosis. It is on the side of the tumour, is dull aching in character, often ill-defined and may be either intermittent or continuous. It can be related to extension of the tumour to the mediastinum, chest wall, verterbrae or pleura. Pleural involvement may cause pleuritic chest pain but not always so. Most importantly, pain due to chest wall involvement does not exclude operability as these patients, in the absence of lymph node involvement, have T3 lesions (as discussed later under Staging) and have fairly good survival rates after surgery.

Bronchogenic carcinoma arising at the apex of the lung or the superior sulcus (Pancoast's tumour) causes shoulder pain often radiating down the arm. These patients are often diagnosed as cervical spondylitis or 'arthritis', with a delay in the correct diagnosis.

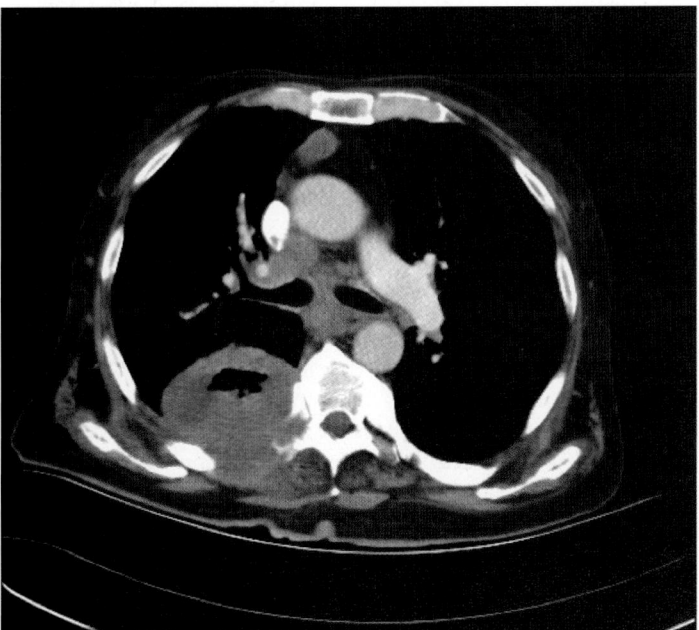

Fig 43.14: Carcinoma lung chest wall invasion: CT Chest demonstrates cavitating mass lesion in apical segment right upper lobe destroying underlying rib with chest wall involvement, as well as metastatic adenopathy to subcarinal and anterior mediastinum.

Wheezing

Wheezing as a symptom of central airways' obstruction together with cough and dyspnoea has already been mentioned earlier. It may be the presenting symptom in a few patients. The fixed monophonic wheeze should be distinguished from the polyphonic wheezes present in asthma or chronic bronchitis. Significant localized airways' obstruction (involving the main bronchus or proximal lobar bronchus) may give rise to 'noisy breathing' or even a stridor indistinguishable from that observed with an obstructed glottis. Breathlessness and a wheeze due to central airways' obstruction necessitate urgent planned treatment.

Systemic Features

Low-grade fever, lassitude, weight loss, loss of appetite may occasionally be the presenting features of lung cancer with or without respiratory symptoms.

Intrathoracic Spread

Bronchogenic carcinoma involving a central airway may involve the bronchial wall and extend outwards into the surrounding lung tissue, producing an increasing 'mass' lesion. A lesion starting within the lung parenchyma may do likewise. Spread of the tumour may extend into the mediastinum and mediastinal structures, the pleura, the pericardium, the thoracic cage and the vertebrae. The clinical presentation and clinical features may be directly related to the intrathoracic spread.

Hoarseness of the voice together with a rasping soundless cough due to left recurrent laryngeal nerve involvement as it loops round the aortic arch is a presenting symptom in close to 10% of patients. Involvement of the sympathetic trunk leads to a Horner's syndrome on the affected side, manifested by slight ptosis, a small pupil and absence of sweating on the ipsilateral affected half of the face.

The Superior Vena Caval Syndrome is characterized by obstruction and occlusion of the superior vena cava by pressure of the tumour, or by thrombosis due to slowing of blood flow through the vein due to extrinsic pressure or infiltration of the wall of the vein by tumour cells. It is invariably associated with

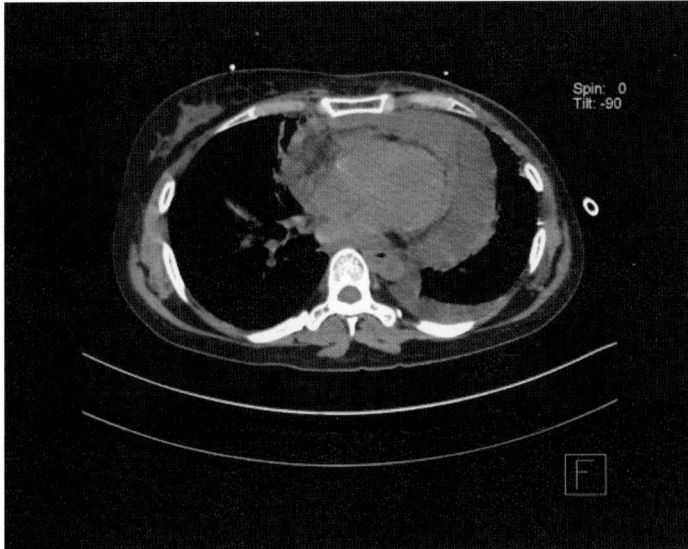

Fig 43.15: Carcinoma lung spread to pleura, pericardium. HRCT chest demonstrates left pleural and pericardial effusion. Cytology of the pleural and pericardial fluid revealed metastatic adenocarcinoma cells secondary to spread from primary lung neoplasm.

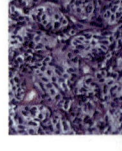

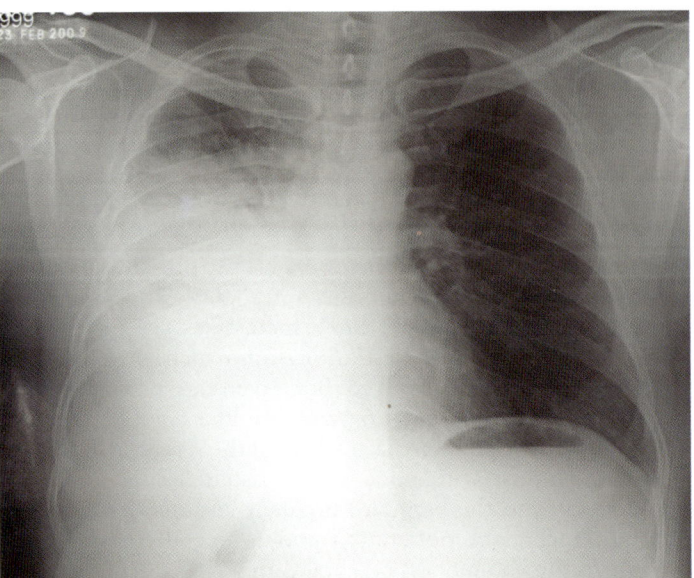

Fig 43.16: Bronchogenic carcinoma. X-ray chest demonstrates a large ill-defined opacity occupying nearly the entire right lung, there is no shift of the mediastinum even though the opacity is very large. This was due to a central bronchogenic carcinoma with associated collapse consolidation as well metastatic pleural effusion.

opening of collateral veins visible in the upper chest; these maintain adequate venous return to the heart.

Malignant mediastinal adenopathy is due to spread of tumour along lymphatics to mediastinal nodes. Malignant infiltration of the mediastinum can also occur through contiguity. Dysphagia can result from pressure of malignant nodes on the oesophagus, and rarely through direct tumour invasion and compression.

Pericardial involvement causes pericardial effusion and occasionally cardiac tamponade. Mitotic cells are not invariably recovered from the pericardial fluid.

Invasion of the chest wall by contiguity or of the vertebrae may result in chest pain, discomfort or back pain. Ribs and vertebrae are however more often involved by blood-borne metastasis.

Spread of malignant disease to the pleura by continuity or of contiguity leads to pleural effusion. Malignant pleural effusions are exudates, which may be serous, serosanguinous or frankly bloody. The presence of malignant cells in the pleural fluid points to unresectability of the tumour. Symptoms of pleural involvement are pleuritic chest pain, cough and dyspnoea.

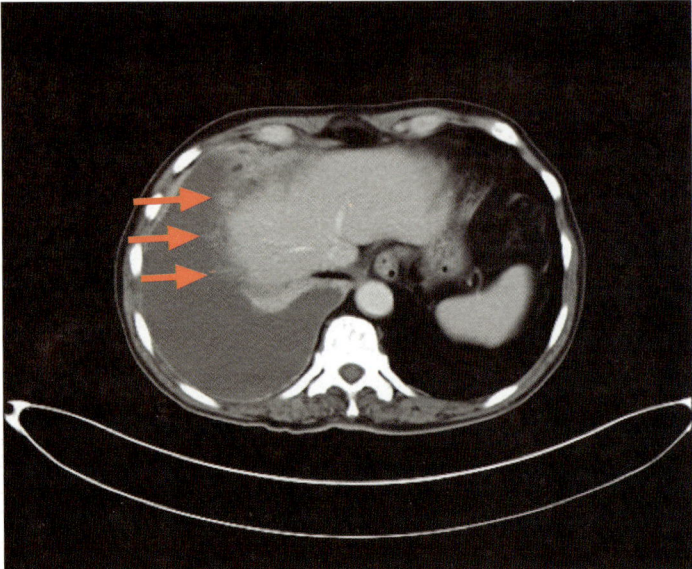

Fig 43.17: Pleural metastasis from carcinoma lung. HRCT chest reveals large right pleural effusion with multiple nodular lesions along the right diaphragmatic surface. Pleural fluid cytology revealed adenocarcinoma cells representing metastatic spread from a primary lung carcinoma.

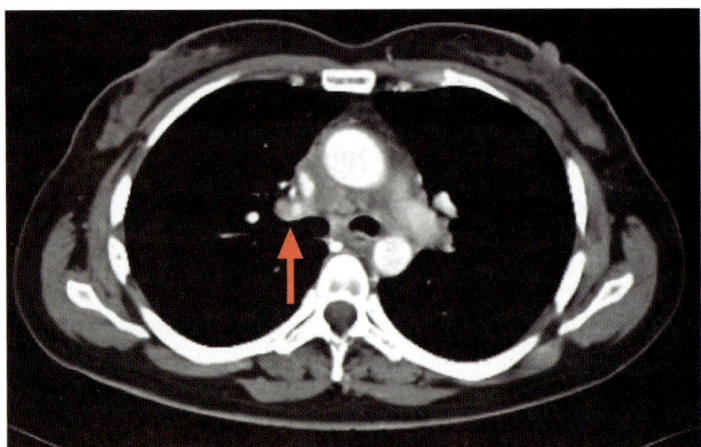

Fig 43.18a: SVC syndrome. CT chest demonstrates an ill-defined mass lesion in the mediastinum encasing the SVC. Biopsy revealed a small cell carcinoma.

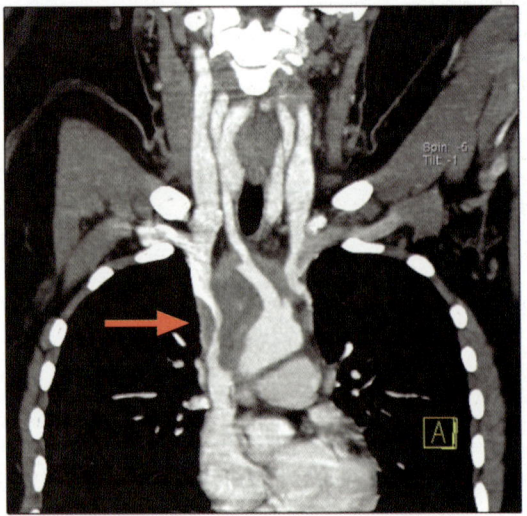

Fig 43.18b: SVC syndrome. Coronal CT reveals mass lesion encasing and narrowing the SVC.

metastatic involvement of the paratracheal glands from a tumour within the right lung. The superior vena caval (SVC) syndrome occurs most commonly with a small cell carcinoma of the lung, being a presenting feature in 10%. Patients complain of fullness of the face and neck, particularly on bending forwards. The face is puffy, plethoric with congested conjunctivae. These clinical features may take time to evolve. The presence of engorged jugular veins with absent or poorly perceptible pulsations is the first sign of this syndrome occurring well before other symptoms or signs appear. A blocked superior vena cava is associated with

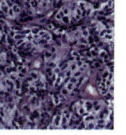
Yet close to 20% of patients with bronchogenic carcinoma with pleural effusions due to direct or metastatic spread are asymptomatic.

It is important to note that not all pleural effusions in lung cancer are malignant in aetiology. Pleural effusions could also be due to pneumonia distal to an obstructive lesion within the bronchus, due to pulmonary embolism, lymphatic obstruction, atelectasis, or coexistent heart failure. Therefore the mere presence of a pleural effusion in a patient with bronchogenic carcinoma does not always point to unresectability in the presence of an otherwise resectable tumour. Proof of a malignant pleural effusion rests in the demonstration of mitotic cells in the pleural aspirate. Unfortunately, the yield of a positive fluid cytology in malignant pleural effusions is about 65%. In retrospective studies it has been shown that this yield remains the same whether the fluid accumulation within the pleura is small or large. Blind pleural biopsy increases the yield only to a small extent. Therefore, if the initial cytology is negative, a repeat study should be done. If still negative, a video-assisted thoracoscopy allows a good look into the pleural space as also a biopsy, enabling one to make a firm diagnosis. It is important that the diagnosis of pleural metastasis is confirmed or excluded, so that the chance of a successful surgical resection of the tumour is not missed.

Involvement of the pleura can also occur from blood-borne metastasis from a bronchogenic carcinoma, or from retrograde spread of cancer cells along the lymphatics to the pleura.

Superior Sulcus Tumour (Pancoast's tumour)

The superior sulcus is a groove made by the subclavian artery on the vault of the pleura and the apex of the lung. A tumour arising at the apex of the lung presents typically with pain in the shoulder radiating to the arm down to the fingers. It is associated with erosion of the posterior portion of the first two ribs and often the seventh cervical and first, second dorsal vertebrae. Involvement of the sympathetic trunk causes Horner's syndrome and involvement of the first thoracic nerve root is often associated with wasting of the small muscles of the hand.

An X-ray of the chest in the early stages may show a faint opacity over the apex often missed as a soft tissue shadow. An HRCT however clears the diagnosis by not only revealing the tumour mass but also showing bony erosions of the ribs and vertebrae.

Distant Extrathoracic Metastatic Manifestations

Distant metastatic blood-borne spread is the presenting feature in about one-third patients. Distant metastasis can involve any organ or organ system. Bone metastases are particularly frequent—the ribs, vertebrae, the long bones such as the humerus and femur often being involved. Bone pains are present in over 20% of patients at presentation and should arouse suspicion of bony metastasis. Spontaneous fracture of the femur or a fracture after trivial injury is often due to a metastatic lesion.

Metastases to the brain are frequent and may be single or multiple. Secondary metastatic tumour generally arising from the lung is the commonest cerebral tumour occurring in adults after 40 years of age.

Small cell lung cancer has the greatest tendency to metastasize while squamous cell carcinoma has the least tendency to do so. Cranial metastasis may be asymptomatic or may produce symptoms of increased intracranial tension such as headache, vomiting, blurred vision, diplopia and/or focal signs depending on the situation of the metastatic lesion. Intacranial metastasis have been reported in 30–50% of patients with lung cancer at autopsy. Spinal chord metastasis are uncommon and when present are usually associated with cerebral metastasis.

Liver metastasis are frequent; they are generally silent except when large or multiple when they may produce an enlarged tender liver. Liver functions are not significantly disturbed, except again when the metastasis are numerous and large. Jaundice is rare except when metastatic glands at the porta hepatis press upon the bile duct.

Metastatic deposits in the suprarenal glands and in the intra-abdominal lymph nodes are common, particularly in small cell carcinomas. Adrenal metastatic lesions are a presenting

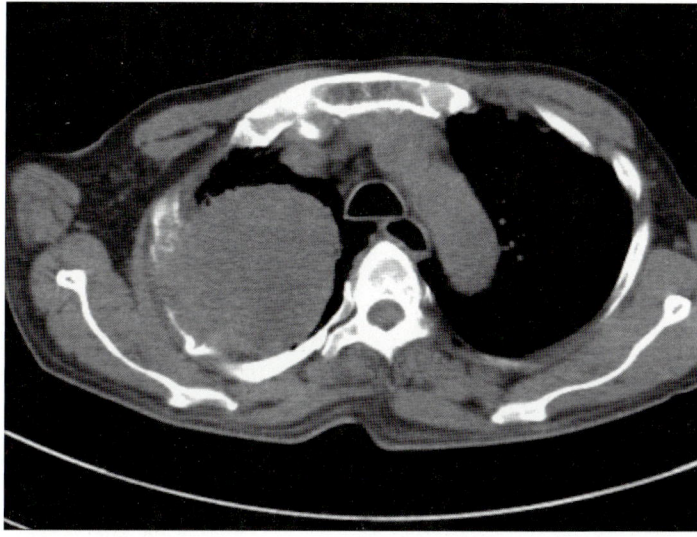

Fig 43.19: Pancoast's tumour: CT scan demonstrates large mass in the right upper lobe destroying chest wall and adjacent ribs.

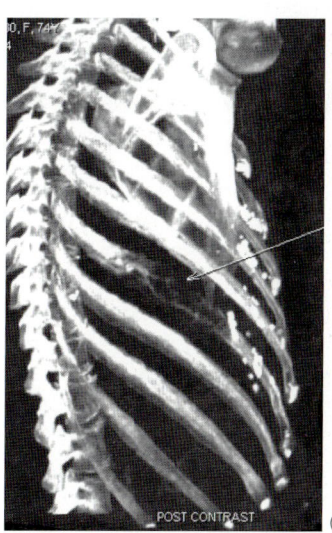
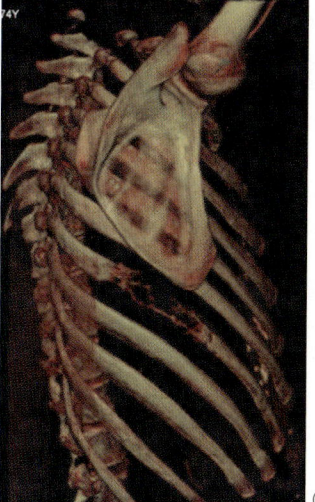

Fig 43.20a and b: Metastatic Deposit in rib: CT scan of ribs demonstrates destructive lesion of 8th rib representing a metastatic deposit.

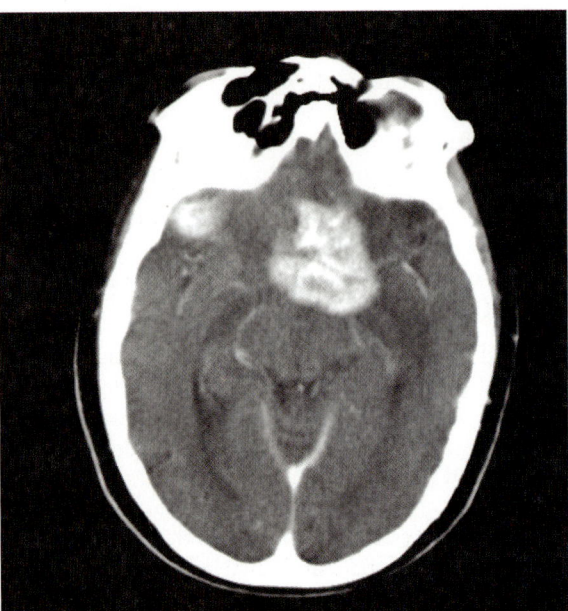

Fig 43.21: CT scan of the brain demonstrates enhancing mass lesions in the right temporal and midline frontal regions representing metastatic deposits.

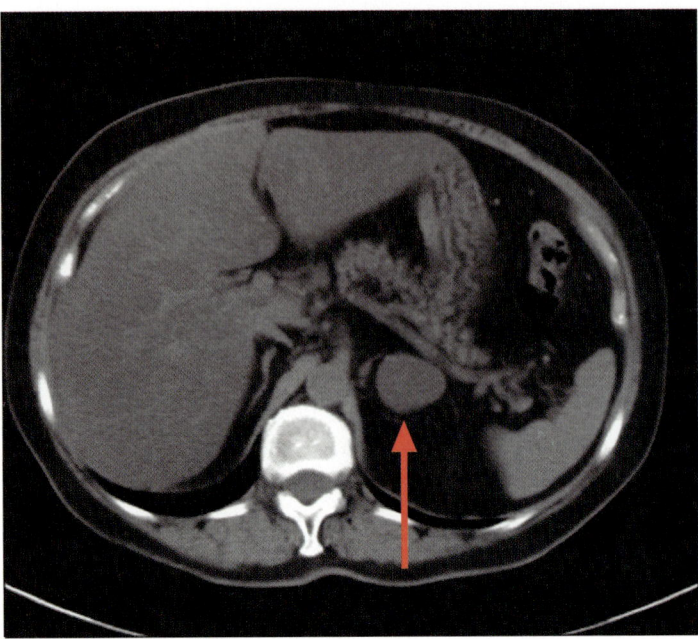

Fig 43.23: CT scan of the abdomen reveals a well-defined mass lesion in the left adrenal gland representing a metastatic deposit.

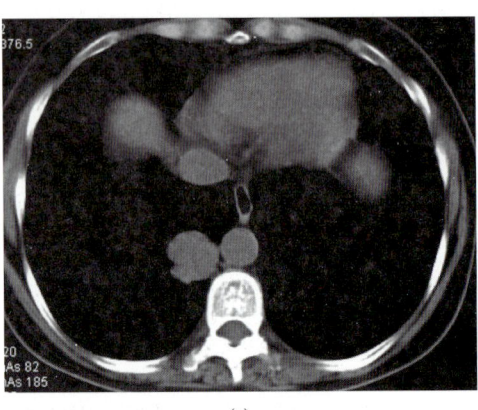

(a)

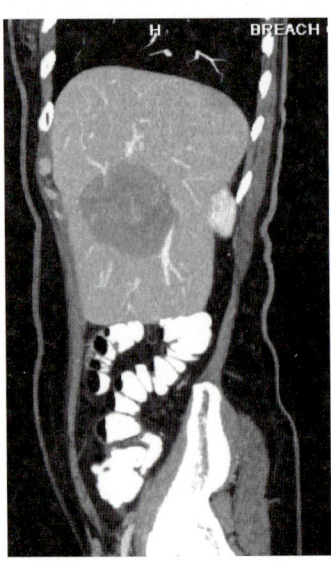

(b)

Fig 42.22: (a) CT scan of the chest demonstrates nodular right lower lobe mass with a lesion in the liver (b) Lung lesion on biopsy was the primary neoplasm, liver lesion was the metastatic deposit.

feature in close to 10% of patients with small cell carcinoma of the lung; they are less commonly observed in squamous cell carcinoma and adenocarcinoma. Destruction of the adrenal glands can lead to adrenocortical deficiency.

Spread of disease to the supraclavicular and anterior cervical lymph glands has been noted to occur in 15–30% of patients during the course of the illness.

There is no organ or organ symptom that is exempt from possible metastatic spread arising from lung cancer.

Non-Metastatic Paraneoplastic Manifestations

Paraneoplastic syndromes are related to those remote effects of lung cancer that are not caused by direct invasion or spread or metastasis. They occur in about 10–20% of patients with bronchogenic carcinoma. Paraneoplastic syndromes are most commonly (though not solely) associated with SCLC and are caused by the production of polypeptide hormones by the tumour cells. Seventy per cent of patients with SCLC and 15% of NSCLC show an elevation of one or more of these polypeptide hormones at the time of diagnosis. However, only a small minority of these present with clinical manifestations of a paraneoplastic syndrome.

Small cell lung cancers show neuroendocrine characteristics. These include cytoplasmic and membrane-bound neuro-secretory granules containing amines and polypeptide products. However 15% of non-small cell tumours also have elevated serum polypeptide levels at the time of diagnosis. Hormonal peptides are also produced by other solid tumours, lymphomas and some leukaemias. It has been postulated that all lung cancers originate from a common stem cell and that hormone production occurs at an early stage of cell development.

Ectopic hormone production is most frequently observed in SCLC, the most frequently elevated hormone being calcitonin. The adrenocorticotrophic hormone, melanocyte-producing

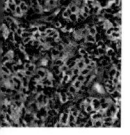

hormone, lipotropin and the antidiuretic hormone (ADH) are also frequently raised in patients with SCLC.

Polypeptides, in particular neuropeptides, have been investigated in the hope that they may serve as tumour markers of disease. The neuropeptide bombesin is often present within cells of SCLCs but the serum levels are low. However, the neurone-specific emolase present in the brain, in neuroendocrine tissue and in SCLCs shows a high serum level in patients with clinical manifestations of SCLC. The levels of elevated polypeptides fall following tumour response to chemotherapy but are not sensitive enough to predict relapse. All said and done the hope that polypeptides may serve as tumour markers in the diagnosis of lung cancer or in predicting relapse of lung cancers has so far not been fulfilled.

The paraneoplastic manifestations of lung cancer caused by the production of polypeptide hormones are briefly described below.

Hypercalcaemia

Hypercalcaemia is most frequently due to multiple bony metastases. Less commonly it is due to a parathyroid hormone-related protein (PTHP), calcitrol or other cytokines that have an osteoclastic effect. Serum parathyroid hormone levels are normal but an elevated PTHP is detected in 50% of patients. PTHP not only has an osteoclastic effect but also prevents renal reabsorption of sodium and water thereby causing polyuria. Hypercalcaemia is most often associated with squamous cell carcinomas of the lung. Generally, patients with hypercalcaemia have inoperable disease, the median survival rate after symptomatic hypercalcaemia being one month.

Clinical features of hypercalcaemia include anorexia, nausea, vomiting, lethargy, constipation, polyuria and dehydration. Confusion, drowsiness, coma and renal failure occur later. Cardiovascular effects include shortened QT interval, heart block, ventricular arrhythmias, and cardiac arrest. Various combinations of the above clinical features may be observed.

Patients with a serum Ca > 12 mg/dl require treatment. The principles of treatment are—

a) Correction of dehydration with intravenous normal saline—three or more litres of fluid need to be given.
b) Use of IV frusemide to promote diuresis, taking care that intake of fluid at least equals the increased output.
c) Inhibiting bone resorption and osteoclastic activity by the use of calcitonin and biphosphonates. Zoledronate is the most effective of the biphosphonates and is given in a dose of 4 mg intravenously over 15 min. Normal calcium levels are generally achieved within 4 to 10 days and are maintained for 30 to 40 days. Calcitonin decreases bone resorption, reduces the serum Ca level by 2 mg/dl. It is a weak agent and is given in a dose of 4 IU/kg intravenously or subcutaneously every 12 hours. It is useful to urgently bring down a high serum calcium level while waiting for the more slow-acting but more effective zoledronate to take effect. Tachyphylaxis to calcitonin generally sets in after 48 hours. Combined treatment of zoledronate with calcitonin has an additive effect in lowering serum calcium.

d) Treatment of the underlying cancer. Successful treatment (either chemotherapy or resection) is associated with a return of serum calcium levels to normal levels.

Patients with hypercalcaemia who have widespread metastatic lesions die generally within a month and are best given supportive treatment.

Syndrome of Inappropriate Anti-Diuretic Hormone Secretion (SIADH)

SIADH is due to increased secretion of the anti-diuretic hormone and is observed in about 10% of patients who have SCLC. SCLC is by the far the commonest cause of SIADH accounting for over 75% of cases of this syndrome. Diagnostic criteria of SIADH are—

1. Hyponatraemia (serum sodium less than 135 mEq/L)
2. Hypotonicity (plasma osmolality less than 280 mOsm/kg)
3. Inappropriately concentrated urine (more than 100 mOsm/kg water)
4. Elevated urine sodium concentration (more than 20 mEq/L), except during sodium restriction
5. Clinical euvolemia
6. Normal renal, adrenal, and thyroid function

Symptoms of SIADH depend on the degree of hyponatraemia and the rapidity of fall in serum sodium. A slow fall of serum sodium to < 120 mEq/L may be tolerated without untoward symptoms. Symptoms of hyponatraemia include vomiting, drowsiness, confusion, coma and seizures; these are caused by increased water content within nerve cells of the brain.

Treatment in mild to moderate cases consists of fluid restriction to ≤ 1000 ml/day. Further treatment consists of using demeclocycline 300 mg thrice daily. The drug acts by causing a nephrogenic diabetes insipidus thereby increasing water excretion. The onset of action of demeclocycline varies from a few hours to many days, so the drug is not useful for emergency action.

When central nervous system (CNS) symptoms due to marked hyponatraemia (Na < 115 mEq/L) are severe, it is best to use a titrated solution of 3% hypertonic saline 100–150 ml given intravenously over 4 to 6 hours. Hypertonic saline can be dangerous in patients with poor pump function or diastolic dysfunction and can precipitate pulmonary oedema. The serum sodium should be carefully monitored and should be increased slowly by a maximum of 8 mEq/day and not more than 16 to 18 mEq in 48 hours. A sharp rise in serum sodium can precipitate central pontine myelinosis which may manifest with drowsiness, coma, quadriparesis and even death.

Patients with SCLC who have an associated SIADH should be promptly treated with chemotherapy. Successful chemotherapy leads to improvement in SIADH within a few weeks. Relapse of the disease is invariably associated with the return of SIADH.

Ectopic Corticotropin Hormone Syndrome

This syndrome is chiefly confined to SCLC, but is occasionally observed in carcinoid tumours of the lung, thymic tumours,

neuroblastoma and medullary carcinoma of the thyroid. The syndrome is due to ectopic production of corticotropin or corticotropin-releasing hormone. Though plasma corticotropin levels may be elevated in close to a quarter to a third of patients of SCLC, the short natural history of SCLC generally does not allow the evolution of a full-fledged Cushing's syndrome. Occasionally, one encounters a partial evolution of Cushing's syndrome characterized by proximal muscle myopathy, pigmentation, hypokalaemic alkalosis and increased plasma cortisol levels which are not suppressed with dexamethasone. Marked elevation of free cortisol in the urine (> 500 µg /24 hours) and of plasma corticotropin levels (> 200 pg/ ml) are strongly suggestive of ectopic corticotropin as the cause of the partial Cushing's syndrome described above.

Ketoconazole is the drug of choice for the treatment of Cushing's syndrome in the above setting. It is given in a dose of 200 mg thrice daily, slowly increasing (in the absence of toxic effects) to 400 mg thrice daily. Liver functions should be carefully monitored. If ketoconazole does not reduce cortisol secretion effectively, metapyrone is added at 250 mg two to three times a day, increased slowly to a maximum of 4 g/day. Hypoadrenalism occasionally results with this treatment and may require the use of dexamethasone 0.25–.5 mg/day.

Appropriate treatment of SCLC with chemotherapy may help to reduce cortisol secretion and improve symptoms. Cushing's syndrome related to tumours other than SCLC is treated if possible by resection of the tumour.

Dermatomyositis, Polymyositis

Dermatomyositis and polymyositis have been reported as paraneoplastic features of an underlying malignancy, chiefly a bronchogenic carcinoma. The incidence is debatable, perhaps about 10%, though population-based studies in Australia and Sweden suggest a higher frequency of 15–25%. The risk of developing an overt malignancy is most within the first two years of the diagnosis and is more with dermatomyositis than pure polymyositis. Cancer surveillance is therefore important and should consist of a careful clinical examination together with appropriate screening, in particular mammography, X-ray chest and colonoscopy.

Finger Clubbing, Hypertrophic Pulmonary Osteoarthropathy

Clubbing of the fingers and toes is characterized by loss of the angle between the nail bed and the cuticle. The angle is first straightened and then becomes convex. Rounded nails and bulbous fingertips develop due to enlargement of the connective tissue in the distal phalanges. Clubbed nails occur in 10–30% of patients with lung cancer.

Hypertrophic pulmonary osteopathy may be preceded by clubbing and is characterized by periosteitis, painful arthropathy and often marked finger clubbing. Besides lung cancer, it has been reported in thymic carcinoma, thyroid carcinoma, chronic myeloid leukaemia, Hodgkin's disease, adenocarcinoma of the oesophagus, bronchial carcinoid tumours, and pleural fibroma. It also has been observed in a number of non-malignant conditions.

Among lung cancers, both clubbing and hypertrophic pulmonary osteopathy are most commonly associated with squamous cell carcinoma and occasionally with adenocarcinoma and large cell carcinoma. It may precede the diagnosis of lung cancer in 30% of patients. The painful periosteitis chiefly affects the distal ends of the radius, ulna, tibia and the fibula. Besides the usual painful wrists and ankles, a painful arthropathy of the knees and elbows may also occur. Radiological changes may be observed in the femur and humerus even in the absence of pain in knees and elbows. Pain may prevent walking and may restrict movements at the wrists.

The cause of hypertrophic pulmonary osteoarthropathy is unknown but it may be caused by a humoral agent. The diagnosis should be considered in a cigarette smoker when there is a short history of arthralgia or an arthropathy chiefly involving the ankles and wrists. An X-ray of the long bones in suspected hypertrophic pulmonary osteoarthropathy reveals periosteitis with periosteal new bone formation. A bone scan reveals diffuse uptake in the long bones at the site of periosteitis. Amazingly, hypertrophic pulmonary osteoarthropathy has been reported to resolve after a thoracotomy even if the cancer has not been resected. Treatment is with anti-inflammatory drugs. Recently, the use of biphosphate pamidronate has been reported to give good relief. Successful resection of the tumour leads to a regression of hypertrophic pulmonary osteoarthropathy.

Other rare paraneoplastic syndromes include hyperthyroidism (usually with squamous cell tumour), gynaecomastia, and pigmentation associated with α and β melanocyte stimulation. Somatostatin release mimicking a pancreatic tumour has also been described. Hyperglycaemia, hypoglycaemia, galactorrhoea, and growth hormone excess are some of the other rarer endocrine manifestations of the paraneoplastic syndrome.

Fever, weight loss and anaemia may be observed as the presenting features in some patients with an underlying cancer of the lung. They are considered by many as paramalignant.

Neurological Syndromes

Paraneoplastic syndromes with neurological features are most often met with in small cell cancer of the lung. The frequency of their occurrence varies; some workers estimate the frequency of any of these neurological syndromes at close to 5%. Neurological symptoms may precede the diagnosis of SCLC by months and at times as much as two years, the mean interval being about eight months.

The commonest neurological paraneoplastic feature is *a peripheral neuropathy*. It is most often a sensory neuropathy that could be painful; occasionally, a sensory motor neuropathy may occur. Other neurological syndromes include the *Lambert-Eaton myasthenic syndrome, encephalomyelopathy, cerebellar degeneration, autonomic neuropathy and impaired vision due to autoantibodies* in the serum against a specific subset of retinal neurones.

Paraneoplastic syndromes are thought to be immune-mediated because a number of autoantibodies have been identified. Two important autoantibodies that have been shown to be associated with SCLC are antinuclear neuronal antibody I (ANNA I) and ANNA II. Another recently described autoan-

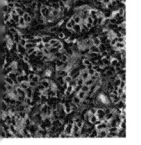
tibody termed CRMP-5 has also been found to be associated with SCLC and thymomas. An anti-Purkinje antibody (anti yo) has been recently identified; it is found to be associated in patients with ovarian cancer and breast cancer. These autoantibodies may predict the nature of the neoplasm but do not identify the nature of the paraneoplastic syndrome. More than one autoantibody may be present in a patient with SCLC.

In a review of 162 sequential patients with a positive ANNA I, 88% were found to develop lung cancer most of which were SCLCs. In the vast majority of these cases the diagnosis of SCLC was made within six months of the manifestation of the neurological syndrome; in a small minority it occurred later. Most of these patients (90%) had limited-stage disease confined to the lung and mediastinum. In another study, ANNA antibodies were again associated with limited-stage disease, good response to therapy and longer survival than patients who had SCLC without ANNA I autoantibodies.

It is important to note that in patients who present with a paraneoplastic neurological syndrome due to an underlying SCLC, the mitotic lesion may not be identified by the initial investigational workup. A careful high-resolution computed tomography (HRCT) of the chest is therefore imperative, particularly in smokers when neurological features compatible with a paraneoplastic syndrome are present. A search for autoantibodies described above should be made if the required facilities are available. PET scan is also advised; a positive PET scan may help to locate and identify the lesion, facilitating biopsy and allowing confirmation.

The *Lambert-Eaton myasthenic syndrome* is most commonly observed in association with SCLC. About 50% of patients with the Lambert-Eaton myasthenic syndrome have an underlying

malignancy, the majority of these malignancies being SCLCs. The overall incidence of this syndrome in SCLC is reported to be about 2–4%.

The syndrome is characterized by proximal muscle weakness, depressed tendon reflexes and autonomic disturbances and is related to an impaired release of acetylcholine at the motor nerve endings. This syndrome is associated with allotypes Gm2 and HLA B8 and precedes the diagnosis of lung cancer by eight months to two years.

The Lambert-Eaton myasthenic syndrome has been strongly associated with antibodies against P/Q type presynaptic voltage–gated calcium channels of peripheral cholinergic nerve endings. These autoantibodies block the release of acetylcholine at nerve endings and are present in over 90% of patients with the Lambert-Eaton syndrome. The same antibodies have also been identified in 25% of patients with SCLC who do not have Lambert-Eaton myasthenic syndrome. Diagnosis of Lambert-Eaton syndrome is based on the clinical features together with characteristic electromyography (EMG) findings.

Treatment of the cancer often induces remission of this syndrome. The use of acetylcholine esterase inhibitors has very limited value, the response to the drug often being absent or poor.

THE ASSOCIATION OF VENOUS THROMBOSIS WITH LUNG CANCER

Venous thrombosis and thrombophlebitis migrans can antedate the appearance of an adenocarcinoma of the lung. If these occur in a middle-aged or elderly smoker without obvious cause, a careful physical examination and basic screening tests for an underlying lung cancer are advisable.

Venous thrombosis also often complicates the natural history of an established lung cancer. The reason for the hypercoagulable state responsible for venous thrombosis in underlying malignancies (including lung cancer) is not known. Venous thrombosis associated with an underlying malignancy is difficult to control and may extend in spite of anticoagulants. The American College of Chest Physicians has opined that low molecular weight heparin is superior to the use of oral anticoagulants in treatment of venous thrombosis occurring in patients with malignant disease.

DIAGNOSTIC ASSESSMENT AND STAGING

Diagnostic assessment and staging are essential prerequisites for the management of lung cancers. There are three objectives that must be kept in mind. First, to establish a definite diagnosis of lung cancer, second to determine the histological cell type of lung cancer, and third to determine the degree of dissemination, both with regard to local and metastatic spread. Unnecessary investigations should be avoided in patients with obvious advanced disseminated disease unsuitable for either surgery or chemotherapy. Investigations should also be kept to a minimum in elderly people or in patients with advanced disease caused by a cell type unlikely to respond to systemic therapy. A balanced assessment is necessary before planning management.

A careful history and a meticulous physical examination is the first requisite. No routine investigation will, for example,

Table 43.9: Non-metastatic paraneoplastic manifestations of lung cancer

Endocrine System
    Hypercalcaemia
    Syndrome of inappropriate anti-diuretic hormone secretion (SIADH)
    Ectopic corticotropin hormone syndrome
    Hyperthyroidism (usually with squamous cell tumour),
    Gynaecomastia
    Pigmentation associated with α and β melanocyte stimulation
    Somatostatin release mimicking a pancreatic tumour
    Hyperglycaemia
    Hypoglycaemia
    Galactorrhoea
    Growth hormone excess

Musculoskeletal System
    Finger clubbing
    Hypertrophic pulmonary osteoarthropathy
    Dermatomyositis
    Polymyositis

Neurological features
    Peripheral neuropathy
    Lambert-Eaton myasthenic syndrome
    Encephalomyelopathy
    Cerebellar degeneration
    Autonomic neuropathy
    Impaired vision

pick up a firm gland palpable between the two heads of the sternomastoid muscle or in the supraclavicular fossa, or diagnose a slight ptosis with a smaller pupil on the affected side due to an early Horner's syndrome from involvement of the sympathetic trunk. Again, no investigation will detect a monophonic wheeze due to partial obstruction of a large airway, or detect a pleural rub, or detect clubbing with early pulmonary osteoarthropathy, or diagnose some of the neurological paraneoplastic syndromes associated with lung cancer. The importance of a thorough physical examination cannot be overemphasized.

Radiology

The chest X-ray is usually abnormal by the time symptoms appear. Radiographic abnormalities on an X-ray chest that are likely to be missed are briefly mentioned below.

OBSTRUCTION TO A LARGE AIRWAY
Lung cancers most often occur in the central airways. The earliest sign of large airways' obstruction is obstructive emphysema of the involved lobe or lung best picked up on an expiratory film. Subsequent to this there will be shrinkage of a lobe or lung as judged by a loss of lung volume with a displaced fissure or an elevated dome of the diaphragm. Complete endobronchial obstruction will manifest as a collapse of a lobe. A left lower lobe collapse can easily be missed on an X-ray because it lies behind the heart. A shrunken lobe may not cast a shadow. An abnormal hilum (an absent lower leash of vessels when the left lower lobe is collapsed or an upward shift of the hilum when an upper lobe collapses) should suggest the diagnosis.

A HILAR PATHOLOGY
A mass in the hilar region may be difficult to detect when it is small because of the superimposition of the hilar vessels. An asymmetry in size between the two hilar shadows or a difference in the densities of the two shadows should arouse suspicion.

THE SMALL PERIPHERAL NODULE
About 30–35% of lung cancers present as a peripheral lesion. A nodule must be at least 1 cm in size before it is visualized on an X-ray chest. Even then it may be difficult or impossible to recognize if it is situated behind a rib, behind the heart or in the costophrenic space.

LUNG CANCER AGAINST A BACKGROUND OF OTHER LUNG DISEASES
Lung cancer developing in a patient with asbestosis, or in interstitial pulmonary fibrosis or in systemic sclerosis (all of which have a greater incidence of lung cancer) may be difficult to detect on a radiological examination of the chest.

Sputum Cytology

Sputum cytology is a simple, inexpensive useful test in the diagnosis of lung cancer. It should always be availed of in the presence of cough with sputum. If a bronchoscopy is done the bronchoalveolar lavage (BAL) fluid should also always be sent for cytological study. Sputum cytology is generally not positive when

the disease presents as an isolated peripheral nodule. Further discussion on sputum cytology is given later in this section.

HRCT Chest

Any suspicion of bronchogenic carcinoma on radiography of the chest necessitates an HRCT of the chest. HRCT chest provides fuller detailed information not only in relation to the tumour but also about the presence or absence of obvious local spread.

Positron Emission Tomography (PET) Study

PET study when available is becoming a part of the protocol for both the diagnostic assessment and staging of lung cancers. Its usefulness is discussed later in this chapter.

Bronchoscopy

Bronchoscopy provides direct visualization of the tumour arising in the central airways. It allows a biopsy that will help determine cell type. Bronchoscopy is also important to help evaluate the patient for surgery. A tumour arising within a lobar bronchus is fit to be removed by a lobectomy. However, if the tumour extends into the main bronchus, a pneumonectomy is the answer provided the tumour is more than 1 cm away from the carina. A spread of the tumour to mediastinal structures is at times evident by the widening and fixity of the carina due to involvement of the subcarinal lymph glands or by the presence of inward pressure on the lateral wall of the bronchus or trachea

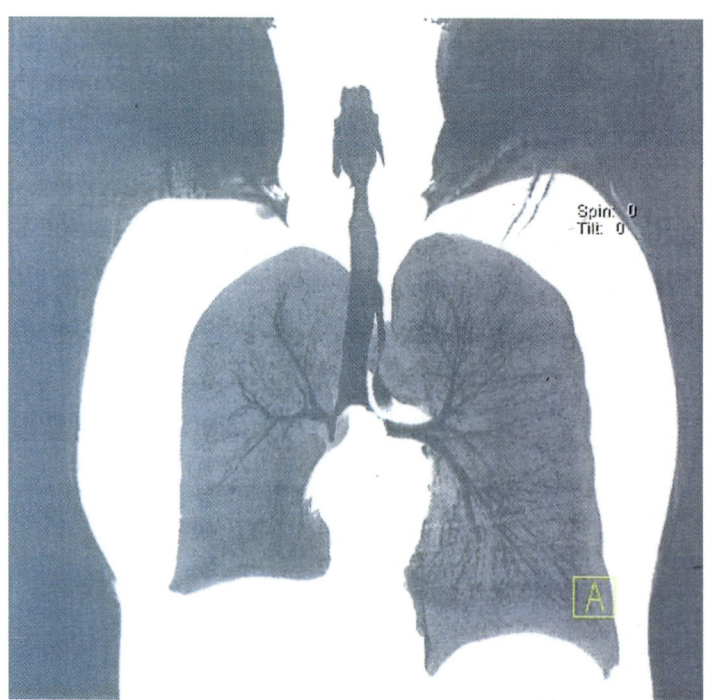

Fig 43.24: Coronal CT reconstruction reveals a subcarinal mass lesion causing encasement of the right lower lobe bronchus with resultant right lower lobe collapse and consolidation. There is extension of the lesion to involve the left lower lobe bronchus which is significantly narrowed by the mass lesion.

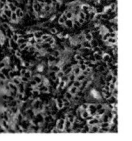

by enlarged paratracheal glands. These bronchoscopic findings often denote unresectability.

Biopsy

A confirmed diagnosis of lung cancer (except in obvious advanced disease where any specific therapy is of no use) requires histopathological proof and cytological examination.

Biopsy of a tumour in the central airways is through a fibreoptic bronchoscope. A peripherally situated 'nodule' within the lung is best approached through a CT-guided biopsy. A percutaneous aspiration needle biopsy gives a poor yield and may give misleading results. A core biopsy of a peripheral nodule has a diagnostic yield of 80–90% for a single sample and a yield of 95% for two or three samples.

Rarely, a mediastinoscopic biopsy or video-assisted thoracoscopic biopsy may be needed to confirm a diagnosis or to establish the presence and degree of dissemination.

Table 43.10: Diagnostic assessment of lung cancer
1. A careful history and a meticulous physical examination
2. Radiography of chest
3. Sputum cytology
4. HRCT of the chest
5. PET study
6. Bronchoscopy
7. Biopsy a. Transbronchial via fibreoptic bronchoscope b. CT guided biopsy c. A percutaneous aspiration needle biopsy d. Mediastinoscopic biopsy (rare) e. Videoassisted thoracoscopic biopsy (rare)

SOLITARY PULMONARY NODULE

The presence of a solitary pulmonary nodule on a plain X-ray of the chest often poses a problem in management. Is the nodule benign or malignant? That is the question!

How does one define a solitary peripheral nodule? A solitary peripheral nodule is a fairly well-circumscribed shadow within the lung parenchyma observed on a routine radiographic examination of the chest without evident hilar or mediastinal adenopathy. It may abut on the pleura, mediastinum, or diaphragm or may be completely free of these structures. It may or may not show radiological evidence of necrosis, or of cavitation or of calcification. A 'nodule' needs to be at least 1 cm in size before it can be visualized on chest radiography. Most reviews on this subject have limited the size of the nodule to 6 cm or less.

A solitary nodule can be due to several causes. Common and uncommon causes have been tabled. The prevalence of various aetiologies in different studies varies, depending on the age, ethnicity, geography and smoking habits of the patient

Table 43.11: Causes of solitary nodule detected by chest radiography
Common Causes
Metastasis
Primary bronchial carcinoma
Tuberculosis
Abscess
Pneumonia (localized)
Bronchial carcinoid
Hamartoma

Table 43.12: Causes of solitary nodule detected by chest radiography	
Uncommon Causes	
Alveolar cell carcinoma	
Lymphoma	
Bronchogenic cyst	
Pulmonary infarct	
Nocardial infection	
Wegener's granulomatosis	
Rheumatoid nodule	
Hydatid cyst	
Arteriovenous aneurysm	
Intrapulmonary lymph node	
Thymoma	
Foreign body	
Rarer tumours	Fibroma Leiomyoma Papilloma Chondroma

group under study. Even so, primary lung cancer is the cause of all nodules in 35% of most surveys; this increases to 50% in patients over the age of 50 years.

An Approach to the Assessment of a Solitary Pulmonary Nodule

HISTORY AND CLINICAL EXAMINATION

It is always best to start with a carefully taken history and a detailed physical examination, an art and a science increasingly being relegated to the background in modern medicine.

A history of past tuberculosis, a recent chest infection or a history of past malignancy is important. Malignancy can recur after several years; this is particularly so, for example, with breast cancer, a seminoma and a hypernephroma. It is important to ask for symptoms of systemic illness in the form of fever, or weight loss, or other systemic features associated

with some of the aetiological factors listed in the table above. On clinical examination one should specifically look out for peripheral lymphadenopathy, hepatosplenomegaly or physical signs of infection or underlying vasculitides. A significant polymorphonuclear leucocytosis or an ESR > 50 mm in the first hour suggests an infective or non-malignant aetiology. A strongly positive Mantoux test is in favour of a tuberculous granuloma though it does not exclude malignancy, particularly in an older man or woman who is a smoker.

REVIEW OF PREVIOUS RADIOGRAPHS OF THE CHEST

Review of previous radiographs or radiograph is perhaps the single most important investigation to obtain. A lesion that is unchanged in size over two years is almost certainly not malignant and a nodule unchanged for over one year has a higher chance of being benign. The commonest cause of a nodule that remains unchanged over two years is a healed granuloma. In parts of the world where tuberculosis has a high prevalence rate, the aetiology of the granuloma is invariably tuberculosis.

HRCT OF THE CHEST WITH CONTRAST

An HRCT of the chest gives information often not attainable on radiography. It defines the nodule more accurately, may reveal the presence of other nodules within the lung not visible on radiography, or the presence of undetected mediastinal adenopathy. If the presence of multiple nodules on the CT with or without mediastinal adenopathy suggests metastatic disease, a search for a primary through appropriate investigation and imaging studies is warranted.

The attributes of a nodule in the lung that favour malignancy are a) age over 50 years; b) a large nodule, the risk increasing if the nodule is > 2.5 cm; c) a spiculated margin of the nodule; d) a history of smoking.

Calcification within the nodule suggests a benign lesion if the calcification is laminated or centrally deposited as is seen

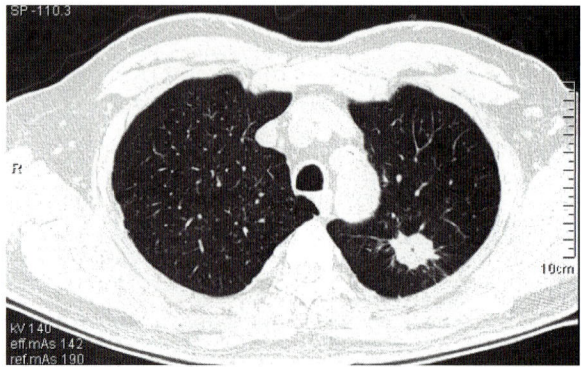

Fig 43.26: CT scan in a middle-aged smoker reveals a mass lesion in the left upper lobe with a whiskered margin and central cavitation. FNAC revealed this to be a squamous cell carcinoma.

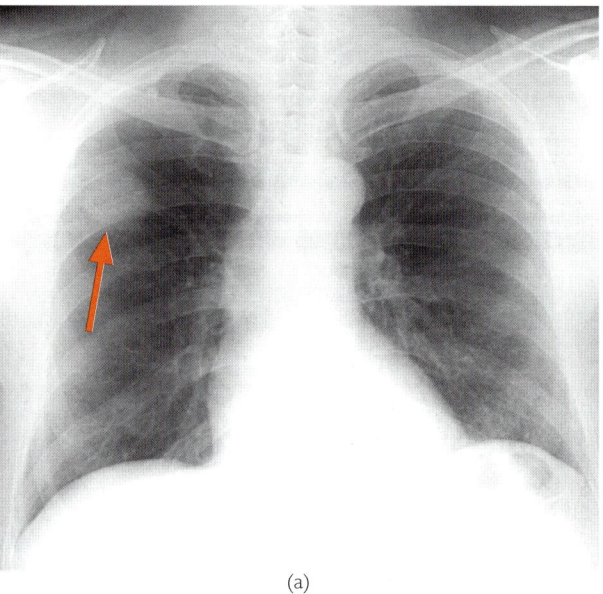

(a)

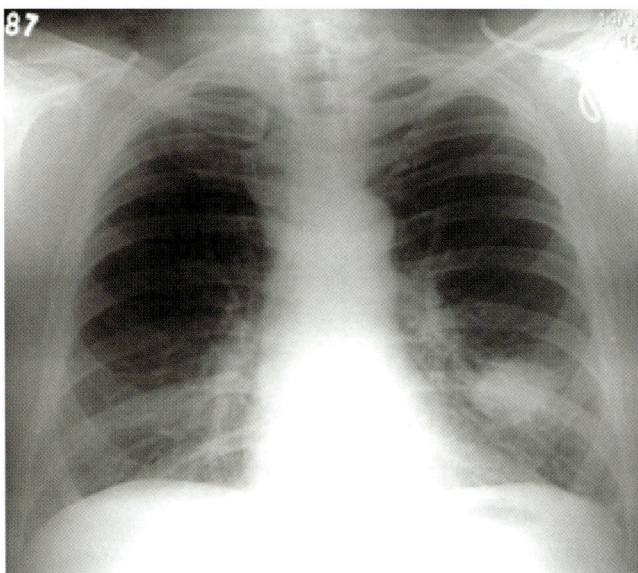

Fig 43.25: Solitary pulmonary nodule. Plain X-ray of the chest reveals a pulmonary nodule in the left lower lobe. The whiskered outline is highly suggestive of a malignancy.

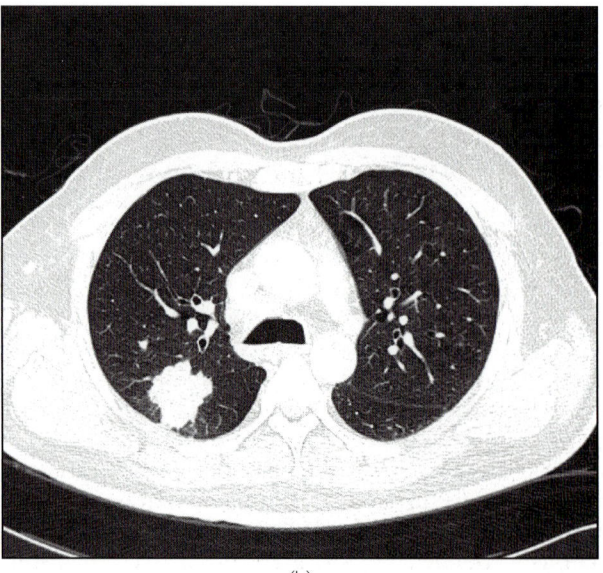

(b)

Fig 43.27: Solitary pulmonary nodule (a) CXR demonstrates a lobulated mass lesion in the right upper lobe (b) CT chest demonstrates the mass lesion to have a mildly whiskered outline raising the possibility of a neoplasm. CT guided biopsy revealed an adenocarcinoma.

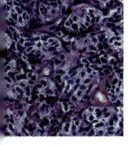

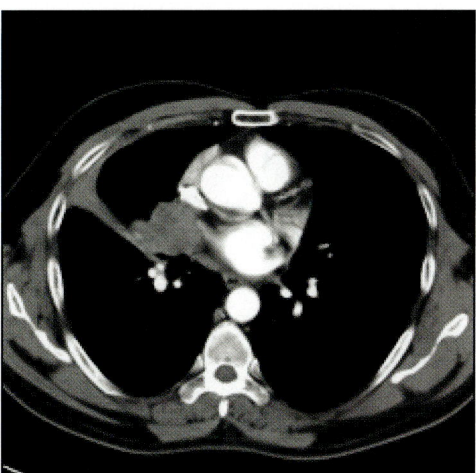

Fig 43.28: Mass lesion in right parahilar region causing segmental atelectasis of middle lobe.

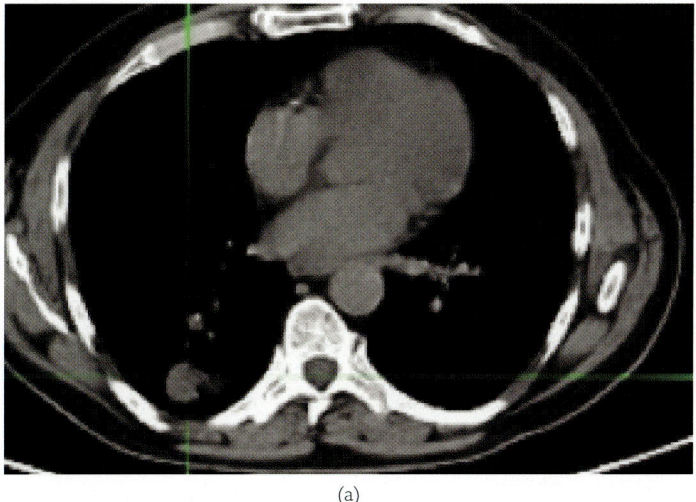

(a)

in a granuloma. A 'popcorn' pattern of calcification suggests a hamartoma. Eccentric calcification of a nodule has however been associated with malignancy. Siegelman and colleagues claimed that the characteristic of a nodule suggesting malignancy or otherwise could be determined by its' Hounsfield numbers on CT. Lack of enhancement on contrast study (< 15 Hounsfield units) was an indicator that the nodule was benign. However, other workers who used Hounsfield numbers to predict malignancy were unable to do so successfully.

PET STUDY
The use of positron emission tomography (PET) has a further advantage that it provides a diagnostic accuracy of about 90% (sensitivity 90%, specificity 95%) in lesions > 1 cm in size. The resolution limit of a nodule that can be evaluated through PET is 7 to 8 mm. An added advantage of the PET scan is its ability to detect occult metastatic disease, thereby changing the approach to management.

SPUTUM CYTOLOGY
Sputum cytology is unlikely to be contributory in the presence of a solitary peripheral nodule.

BIOPSY OF THE NODULE
If the history, physical examination, radiology of the chest, and HRCT chest on balance suggest the likelihood of a malignant lesion, a biopsy is indicated. Before doing a biopsy it is important to be doubly certain that the peripheral nodule is not due to an arteriovenous aneurysm, a hydatid cyst or a pulmonary sequestration. An arteriovenous aneurysm often presents as a single or multiple nodules (the latter may be revealed at times only on a CT of the chest). Inadvertent biopsy can cause death from profuse bleeding. Puncture of a hydatid cyst has been known to cause severe anaphylaxis. A sequestrated lobe may present as a rounded shadow generally in the left lower lobe. It often has a blood supply from an artery that arises from the abdominal aorta which then passes through the diaphragm to supply the sequestrated lobe. An inadvertent biopsy can therefore induce profuse uncontrollable bleeding.

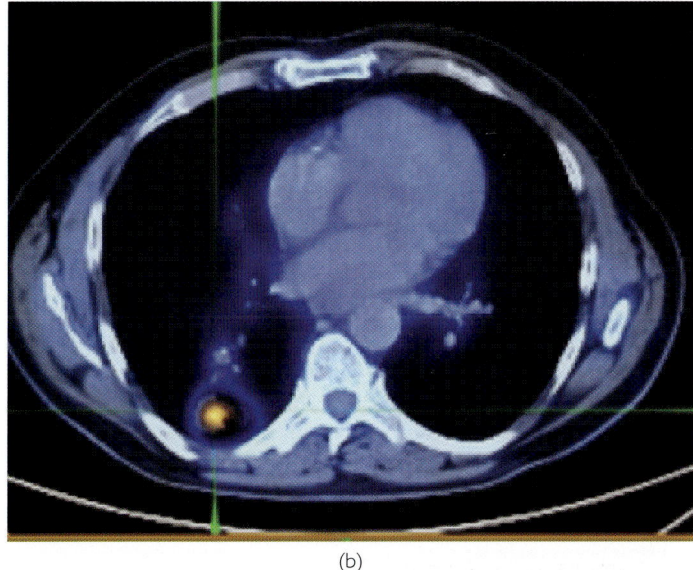

(b)

Fig 43.29: (a) CT chest demonstrates a solitary pulmonary nodule in the apical segment of the right lower lobe, FNAC revealed an adenocarcinoma (b) PET-CT done for staging revealed markedly increased uptake. No other lesions demonstrated uptake indicating a Stage 1 lesion.

A special situation that needs consideration is the presence of a peripheral nodule which on balance seems very likely to be malignant and which is associated with significant bilateral mediastinal adenopathy revealed on CT chest studies. One could presume that the malignant nodule is inoperable because of spread to both ipsilateral and contralateral mediastinal lymph nodes. This however need not always be so. The mediastinal adenopathy may be due to a different aetiology such as tuberculosis or sarcoidosis or the enlargement may be non-specific in nature. It is important through a biopsy of a mediastinal lymph node (either by a CT-guided biopsy or needle biopsy through a fibreoptic bronchoscope, or biopsy through mediastinoscopy) to determine its exact nature. If malignant, the lung nodule is often best left untouched. If not malignant the peripheral nodule is removed surgically.

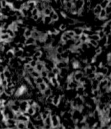

Surgical Resection of a Biopsy-Proven Malignant Nodule

This is the obvious next procedural step, provided there is no evidence of spread. A PET scan notwithstanding its few limitations is of immense value to determine this. Some patients prefer a resection without a biopsy if the nodule seems almost certainly malignant.

Table 43.13: An approach to assessment of a solitary pulmonry nodule
1. History and clinical examination
2. Review of previous radiographs of the chest if available
3. HRCT of the chest with contrast
4. PET scan
5. Biopsy of the nodule
6. Surgical resection of a biopsy proven malignant nodule

RESULTS OF SURGICAL RESECTION

Only 1–2% of solitary malignant nodules are small-cell carcinomas, most of which are resectable. About 5% of solitary malignant nodules are unresectable because of inoperable involvement of the mediastinal nodes. These are usually poorly differentiated adenocarcinomas and large-cell type of cancers.

The peri-operative mortality is about 5%, being even higher in patients above 70 years of age. The overall impact of surgery as a curative procedure is disappointing, the three-year survival rate being as low as 35%. (*Ref: Jackman RJ, Good CA et al. Survival rates in peripheral bronchogenic carcinomas up to four centimeters in diameter presenting as solitary pulmonary nodules. J Thorac Cardiovasc Surg 1969; 57:1.*)

The Indeterminate Nodule

How does one proceed if the lung nodule on tests (short of biopsy) is indeterminate—neither looks very likely to be malignant nor appears clearly benign?

1. If the size is over 2.5 cm on chest radiography, a biopsy is advised to determine the issue.
2. Nodules between 1 cm and 2.5 cm where malignancy cannot be excluded should be carefully evaluated with contrast-enhanced CT, PET study. Observation seems adequate for a PET-negative result unless the nodule shows evidence of an increase in size consistent with malignancy. In the latter instance a biopsy is advised to determine further management.

Nodules < 1 cm in size Discovered Fortuitously on CT Chest

The recommendations from the Fleischerner Society for low-risk patients (never smokers with no history of malignancy) are quoted below:

A follow-up every six months for nodules 8 mm in size. In patients who are high-risk (current and past smokers, history of malignancy) a follow-up is advised every three months. An increase in size in follow-up merits biopsy and if needs be surgical resection.

It has not been shown whether this advice has led to improved survival rates nor is such a follow-up practical in poor developing countries of the world.

Table 43.14: Diagnostic procedures in the management of solitary pulmonary nodule
1. History, physical examination
2. Characteristics of nodule on radiological examination of chest and CT chest suggest that malignancy is more likely: a. If nodule is large in size (risk increases with size > 2.5 cm)   b. Spiculated margins   c. Increased age > 50 years   d. Smoker   e. Multiple nodules present on CT suggestive of metastatic lesions

3. Biopsy (CT-guided for a peripheral nodule)
 If nodule indeterminate, advise:
 1. PET scan—if positive, biopsy is indicated. PET might also reveal occult metastatic spread.
 2. If PET negative then
    a. Observe if nodule < 2.5 cm
 If seen to grow over three to six months, biopsy is indicated
    b. Biopsy if nodule > 2.5 cm to determine management.

STAGING OF LUNG CANCER

When lung cancer is suspected on clinical findings and/or radiological examination, it is important to determine the stage of the disease and the cell-type causing cancer. The purpose of determining the stage of the disease and the cell type is to assess prognosis and to optimise treatment. *As yet treatment that best influences survival is surgery and for this staging the disease is vitally essential.* The cell-type may help the treating doctor to better understand the natural history of the disease. Two facts need to be borne in mind.

1. Two-thirds of patients with bronchogenic carcinoma at the time of diagnosis are inoperable. This may primarily be due to extrathoracic spread but could also be determined by age, very poor lung function or presence of serious co-morbid conditions.
2. Staging investigations detailed below are applicable only to NSCLCs, because almost all SCLCs at the time of presentation have intrathoracic spread, chiefly to the mediastinal nodes or extrathoracic metastatic lesions or both.

Guidelines for staging have been published by the American College of Physicians, the American Thoracic Society and European Respiratory Society. These guidelines, as expected, recommend that all patients have a careful history, detailed physical examination, basic blood chemistry, and a CT of the chest extending through the liver and adrenal glands.

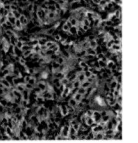

Determining presence of tumour markers is not recommended. Pulmonary function tests are absolutely necessary when the tumour is deemed resectable. Ventilation perfusion scans may help in deciding for or against surgery in patients with impaired pulmonary functions.

TNM Staging Classification on Non-Small Cell Lung Cancers

The TNM classification is based on the size, situation and local extension of the lung tumour, the presence or absence of regional lymph node involvement and if present the extent of nodal involvement, the presence or absence of distant metastasis. The classification first devised in 1975 and subsequently reviewed and upgraded in 1997 (from a database of 5319 patients assessed for surgery) remained unaltered in the sixth edition published in 2002. The classification is applicable to non-small cell lung cancers.

The Union Internationale Contre le Cancer (UICC) and the American Joint Committee on Cancer (AJCC) serve as the official bodies that define, periodically review, and refine the stage classification systems. The sixth edition of the staging system was upgraded and the seventh edition was published in 2009. The International Staging Committee (ISC) of the International Association for the Study of Lung Cancer (IASLC) collected 68,463 patients with non-small cell lung cancer and 13,032 patients with small cell lung cancer, registered or diagnosed from 1990 to 2000, whose records had adequate information for analysing the tumour, node, metastasis (TNM) classification. The T, N, and M descriptors were analysed, and recommendations for changes in the seventh edition of the TNM classification were proposed based on differences in survival.

The committee recommended the subclassification of T1 and T2 tumours according to the tumour size; the upstaging of large T2 tumours; and the downstaging of T4 and M1 tumours so described by additional nodules in the same lobe of the primary tumour or in another ipsilateral lobe, respectively, and the upstaging of pleural dissemination.

The proposed changes are given in Table 43.16.

Table 43.15: TNM staging of lung cancer (sixth edition)				
Stage	Tumour	Node	Metastasis	Definition
IA	T1	N0	M0	T1 tumour: ≤ 3 cm, surrounded by lung or pleura; no tumour more proximal than lobe bronchus
IB	T2	N0	M0	T2 tumour: > 3 cm, involving main bronchus ≥ 2 cm distal to carina, invading pleura; atelectasis or pneumonitis extending to hilum but not entire lung
IIA	T1	N1	M0	N1: involvement of ipsilateral peribronchial or hilar nodes and intra, pulmonary nodes by direct extension
IIB	T2	N1	M0	
	T3	N0	M0	T3 tumour: invasion of chest wall, diaphragm, mediastinal pleura, pericardium, main bronchus < 2 cm distal to carina; atelectasis or pneumonitis of entire lung
IIIA	T1	N2	M0	
	T2	N2	M0	
	T3	N1	M0	
	T3	N2	M0	N2: involvement ipsilateral mediastinal or subcarinal nodes
IIIB	Any T	N3	M0	N3: involvement of contralateral (lung) nodes or any supraclavicular node
IIIB	T4	Any N	M0	T4 tumour: invasion of mediastinum, heart, great vessels, trachea, esophagus, vertebral body, carina; separate tumour nodules; malignant pleural effusion
IV	Any T	Any N	M1	Distant metastasis

Table 43.16: Proposed changes for the seventh edition of the TNM classification of lung cancer	
Component of the classification	Proposed changes
T	To subclassify T1 according to tumour size in – T1a: ≤ 2 cm and – T1b: > 2 cm but ≤ 3 cm
	To subclassify T2 according to tumour size in – T2a: > 3 cm but ≤ 5 cm (or tumour with any other T2 descriptors, but ≤ 5 cm) and – T2b: > 5 cm but ≤ 7 cm
	To reclassify T2 tumours > 7 cm as T3
	To reclassify T4 tumours by additional nodule/s in the same lobe of the primary tumour as T3
	To reclassify M1 tumours by additonal nodule/s in another ipsilateral lobe as T4
	To reclassify T4 tumours by malignant pleural effusion as M1a
N	No changes
M	To subclassify M1 in – M1a: separated tumour nodule/s in the contralateral lung; tumour with pleural nodules or malignant pleural (or pericardial) effusion; and – M1b: distant metastasis

RESULTS OF CLINICAL STAGING
The survival results are indeed dismal and have shown very little improvement in the last decade. Of the 100 patients diagnosed as NSCLC, close to 65% will be deemed inoperable. Inoperability will be based on the extent of disease and its

spread based on clinical examination and on radiography of the chest and to a lesser extent on age, serious co-morbid disease and poor lung function. A further 10–15% who have a normal mediastinum on the chest X-ray will have mediastinal nodes on an HRCT of the chest or on a PET scan. In the majority, these nodes will be positive for malignancy. Finally, of the 25% operated upon, 20% will have a resectable tumour; in 5% the tumour will be inoperable on the table. Finally, of the 20% patients in whom the tumour is resected only 5% will survive for five years. A more dismal story in medicine or surgery is difficult to recount. The above scenario prevails in most centres of developing countries. In highly specialized centres the five-year survival rate has now improved to 12–15%.

Staging for Small-cell Lung Tumours

The TNM staging described above when applied to SCLC makes no difference to the prognosis. The Veterane Administration Staging system categorized SCLC into 'limited disease' and 'extensive disease'. Limited disease is limited to one hemithorax and ipsilateral cervical nodes. Extensive disease is one that has spread beyond the hemithorax—to the contralateral hilar mediastinal, cervical nodes, or to a malignant pleural effusion or to distant extrathoracic metastatic sites.

Extrathoracic Staging of Non-Small Cell Lung Cancers

Examination may help detection of obvious disease, as with the presence of palpable nodes, bony tenderness and the presence of a firm or even nodular enlarged liver. Neurological symptoms may point to metastatic spread to the nervous system or to paraneoplastic neurological syndromes. Biochemical examination of blood may show important findings such as hypercalcaemia and hyponatraemia. Hyponatraemia occurs almost exclusively in SCLCs. Hypercalcaemia may indicate bone metastasis or may be due to a paraneoplastic syndrome caused by a parathyroid hormone like peptide.

Organ screening of the liver and the adrenals is important and is provided by a CT of the chest which includes the upper abdomen. HRCT studies may reveal the presence of asymptomatic metastasis in the liver, adrenal, bone, abdominal lymph glands and the brain is some patients. It must, however, be stated that the result of CT scans of the brain and liver are usually normal in patients who have neither organ-specific features nor any non-specific features such as fever, weight loss, altered liver functions, showing metastatic spread to these organs.

Isotope bone scans are important to detect bony involvement in the presence of bone pains but many clinicians do not advise bone scans in the absence of musculoskeletal symptoms. This is because as many as 40% of bone scans may prove falsely positive, showing thereby the poor specificity of the test.

The role of PET in the evaluation of patients with known or suspected cancer is assuming increasing importance. Several studies have shown that PET may reveal unsuspected mediastinal or extrathoracic spread, so that thoracotomy is avoided in about one in five patients. Cancer cells have a high rate of glycolysis and an increased uptake of glucose by the cells because of the increased number of transport proteins compared to normal cells. The PET tracer 18-fluoro-deoxyglucose (18-FDG) is therefore selectively taken up by the neoplastic cells and accumulates within them. PET has been shown to detect distant metastatic lesions in 10–15% of patients who are thought to be operable and alter management in 40% of cases. A study that compared whole body PET scan to CT chest, CT brain, bone scan or magnetic resonance imaging (MRI) in staging lung cancer showed that PET correctly and accurately staged 83% of patients with NSCLC compared to pathological findings. Not only did PET scan pick up distant metastasis not picked up by other techniques but it also showed that lesions which were considered suspicious by other techniques but which were not PET-positive, were benign. It must however be remembered that PET scan may show false-positive reports in 10–15% of patients. It is therefore absolutely essential that a biopsy of a distant metastasis (positive on a PET scan) is obtained to decide whether the patient has truly inoperable disease.

To summarize, extrathoracic staging for metastatic lesions to start with requires a careful history, physical examination and a study of biochemical and other basic parameters. An HRCT of the chest which is essential for intrathoracic staging should include the upper abdomen so as to view possible metastasis in the liver and adrenals. PET scan of the whole body is the best investigation to detect occult metastasis. Since false-positive results are found in 10–15% of patients, biopsy of a metastatic site deemed positive by a PET study should be done for confirmation. A brain CT is not recommended as a routine screening test. However, 1–2% of asymptomatic patients have brain metastasis who would otherwise be operable. For this reason many specialized oncology centres insist on a head scan as a necessary staging investigation. Bone scanning is advised only in patients with musculoskeletal pains or in patients with non-specific symptoms such as weight loss and fever. Bone scans have a high false-positive rate; a single focal abnormality on a bone scan necessitates confirmation by CT or by a biopsy of the area concerned.

Table 43.17: Steps for extrathoracic staging of NSCLC	
1	Clinical Examination
2	Biochemical examination
3	Relevant blood tests for paraneoplastic syndromes if clinically suspected
4	CT of the chest which includes the upper abdomen (with contrast)
5	Isotope bone scan only in the presence of musculo-skeletal symptoms
6	CT brain
7	PET scan of the whole body

Intrathoracic Staging

Clinical history and examination will identify mediastinal spread from the presence of pressure symptoms such as the

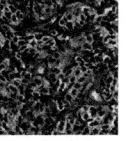

SVC syndrome, Horner's syndrome, presence of dysphagia, and hoarseness of the voice caused by recurrent laryngeal nerve palsy. The presence of mediastinal pressure symptoms or just the presence of large mediastinal lymphadenopathy on a PA and

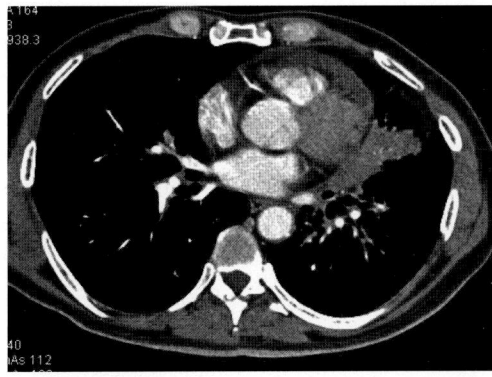

Fig 43.30a: CT scan demonstrates a mass lesion in the left lingula flush with the pericardium.

(a)

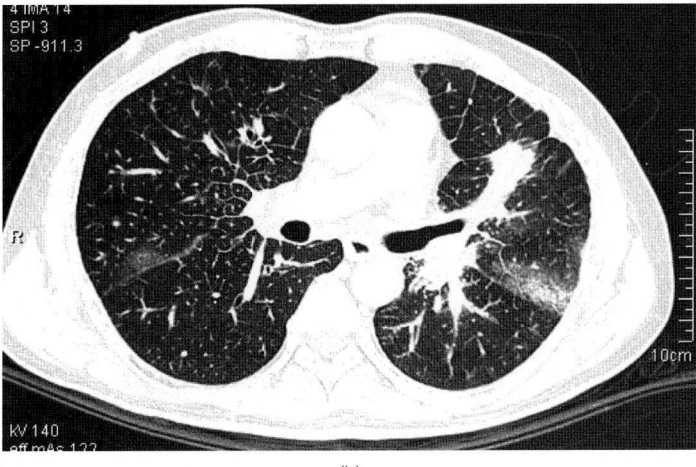

(b)

Fig 43.30b: Lung window demonstrates irregular mass lesion with adjacent lymphatic thickening as well as lymphatic thickening in opposite lung (arrows). This appearance of smooth lymphatic thickening without distortion of lung parenchyma is classical for lymphangitis carcinomatosis.

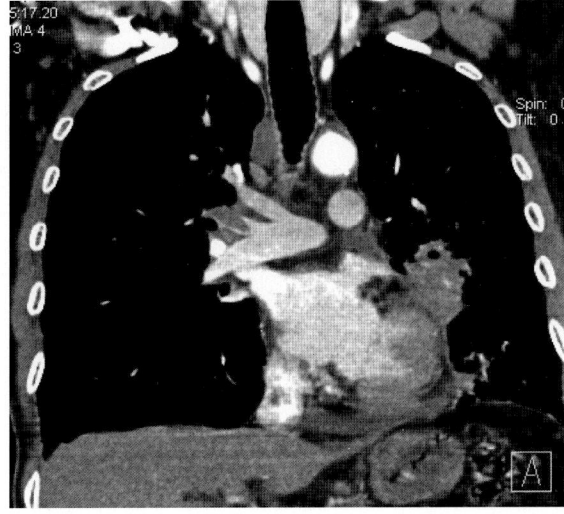

(c)

Fig 43.30c: Contrast CT demonstrates a thrombus in the right upper lobe pulmonary vessels representing thrombi.

lateral radiograph of the chest point to inoperability. Further evaluation is then unnecessary.

A pleural effusion in a proven lung cancer is due to metastatic spread, lymphatic obstruction, lymphangitis carcinomatosis and rarely due to medical causes unrelated to cancer. Pleural aspiration, repeated if necessary, reveals mitotic cells within the pleural fluid in only 75% of cases. Direct proof of malignancy can only be obtained in these instances by a video-assisted thoracoscopy which enables the thoracoscopist to view the pleura and take multiple biopsies. It is perhaps important to do so, as a non-malignant aetiology of a pleural effusion should allow surgery to proceed in an otherwise operable patient.

HRCT contrast study is essential in evaluating the extent of pulmonary disease, identifying small pulmonary nodules, detection of pleural involvement and detecting mediastinal lymphadenopathy. HRCT chest should include the upper abdomen to view possible metastasis to the liver and adrenal glands.

MRI can occasionally be more accurate in detecting invasion of mediastinal structures and involvement of the diaphragm, spine and spinal chord. On the whole it does not have significant advantage over HRCT contrast study of the chest.

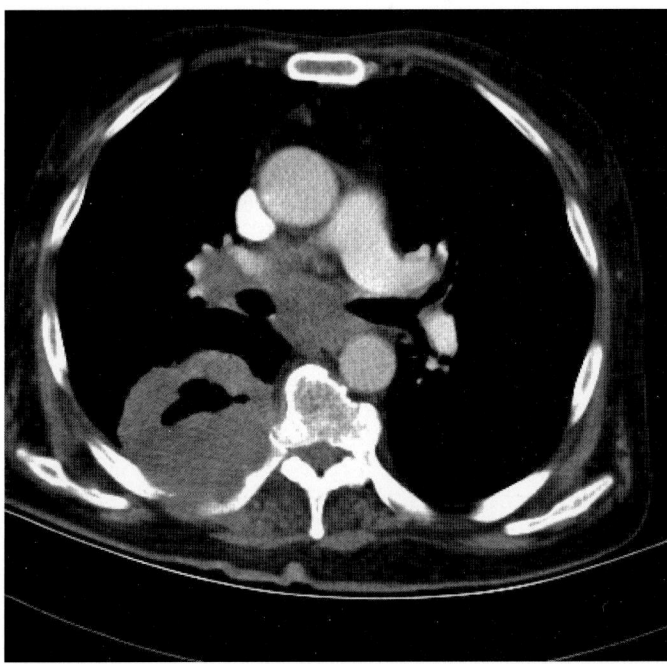

Fig 43.31: Cavitating right lower lobe posterior mass lesion involving chest wall, eroding underlying rib with metastatic mediastinal adenopathy.

Positron Emission Tomography

The value of PET in detecting distant metastasis for extrathoracic staging has already been commented upon. It is equally valuable for intrathoracic staging. PET scans detect focal pulmonary lesions with a sensitivity of 96% and specificity of 88% and has an accuracy of 94% in lesions 10 mm in size or more. It however allows for a much poorer spatial resolution so that the anatomic assessment compared to a CT is inadequate. It should be remembered that false-positive results are observed

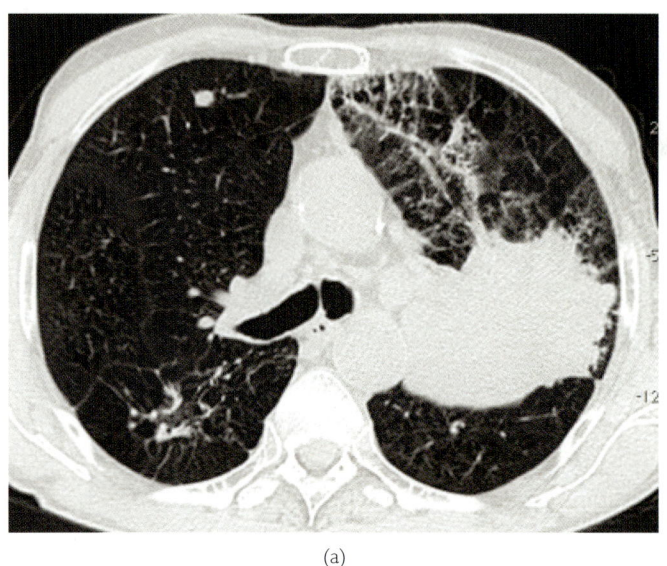
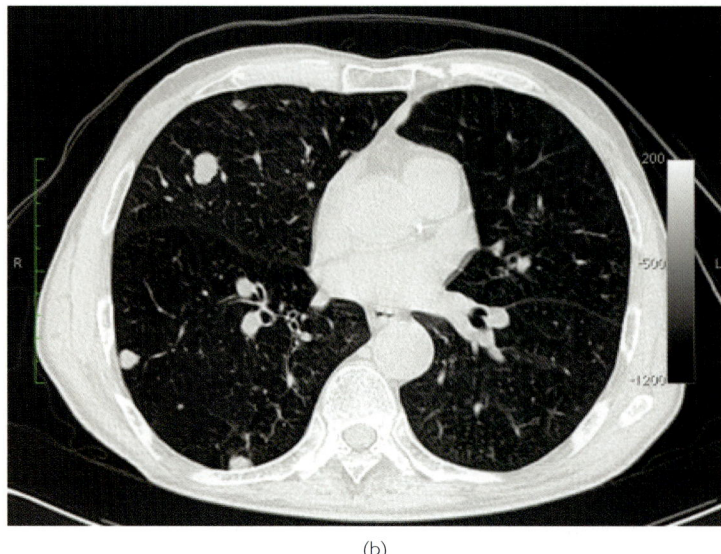

(a)   (b)

Fig 43.32: (a) Non-small-cell carcinoma. CT Chest demonstrates a large irregular mass lesion in the left upper lobe with an irregular margin representing a primary neoplasm. Biopsy showed a non-small-cell carcinoma. (b) CT chest demonstrates multiple pulmonary nodules representing metastatic deposits.

in 10–15% of patients. False-positive results have been reported in tuberculosis, fungal infection, sarcoidosis, inflammatory disorders such as cryptogenic organizing pneumonia and rheumatoid nodules. False-negative reports can occur in alveolar cell carcinoma, carcinoids and in tumours < 1 cm in size. Hyperglycaemia from whatever cause can interfere with 18-FDG uptake and can result in a false-negative scan.

A meta-analysis of the literature reveals that PET scans can identify mediastinal lymph node metastasis with an appropriate sensitivity of 90% and specificity of 85%. CT scan staging of the mediastinal lymph nodes has shown false-positive and false-negative results of about 30–40%, PET scans compare more favourably to CT scans in this regard. PET scans have also been shown to decrease nodal staging as initially determined by CT scan. The value of PET scan in both intrathoracic and extrathoracic lung cancer cannot be denied. PET study is therefore today an integral investigation in the diagnosis and staging of NSCLC.

In the final analysis, the investigation or the test chosen to diagnose and stage lung cancer depends on the site of the tumour in the lung and the degree and nature of spread. The test chosen should be one that gives the most information with the least risk.

A tumour presenting as a peripheral nodule is best diagnosed and staged through a CT-guided core biopsy as has been mentioned earlier. A biopsy through a fiberoptic bronchoscope has a very poor yield except when the CT shows a bronchus leading into the peripheral nodule.

A tumour presenting as a large central mass is often easily diagnosed by bronchoscopy. An endobronchial malignant tumour is diagnosed with 100% accuracy by a biopsy through a fiberoptic bronchoscope. The visual extent of the tumour, its relation to the carina, the fixity or otherwise of the carina also help to judge the operability or inoperability of the tumour.

When the primary tumour is not evident and the suspicion of a malignancy is aroused by the presence of a mediastinal adenopathy (identified by either CT or PET) biopsy of mediastinal lymph nodes is necessary. Biopsy of mediastinal nodes is also

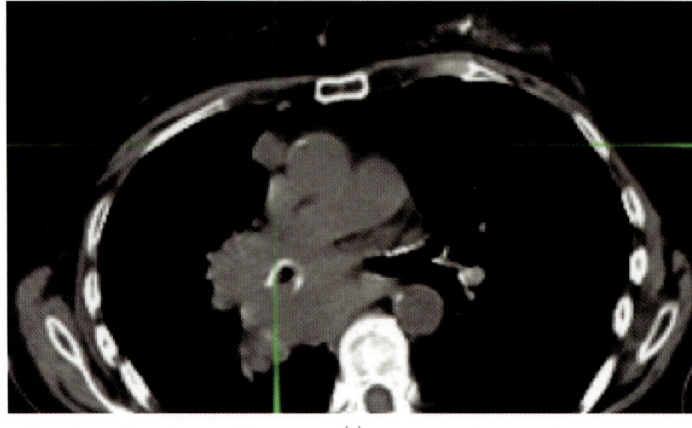
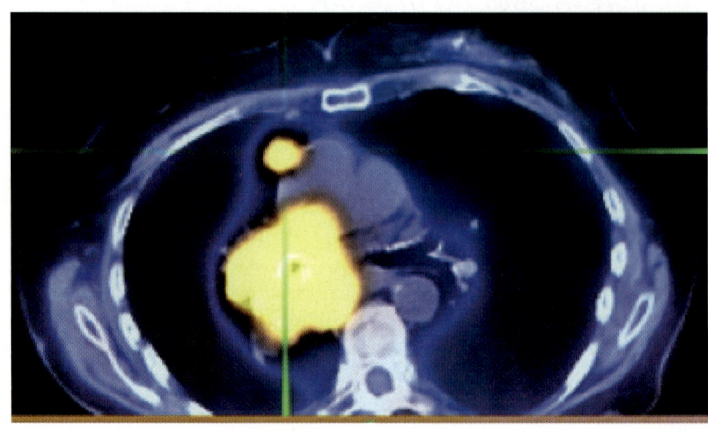

(a)   (b)

Fig 43.33: PET-CT demonstrates marked uptake by a large irregular central mass lesion in the right hilar region. There is another focus of uptake in the anterior mediastinum representing a metastatic adenopathy.

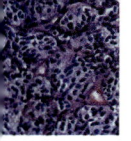

necessary for proper staging even when a tumour in the lung is visible on imaging. If a CT-guided lymph node biopsy is deemed difficult or risky, transbronchial needle aspiration through a fiberoptic bronchoscope may be used to sample lymph nodes in the paratracheal, subcarinal and hilar regions. This method may then allow both diagnosis and staging of the disease. Several studies have shown a significant improvement in the positive yield using endobronchial ultrasound (EBUS) compared to blind bronchoscopic needle aspiration. EBUS allows real-time imaging of mediastinal nodes so that the bronchoscopist can see the needle in the mediastinal node at the time of sampling. The use of EBUS obviates the need for mediastinoscopy to stage ipsilateral (N2) and contralateral nodes in lung cancer. Mediastinoscopy to sample mediastinal lymph nodes is today an increasingly uncommonly used procedure.

In advanced stage disease the test which establishes a diagnosis in the simplest and preferably noninvasive way is to be chosen. For example, rather than biopsy a mass lesion in the lung, biopsy of a fair-sized lymph node in the neck may establish the diagnosis and also prove metastasis.

When lung cancer presents as a pleural effusion, both diagnosis and staging can be accomplished by cytological examination of the pleural fluid. If positive for malignancy it establishes T4 (Stage IIB) disease.

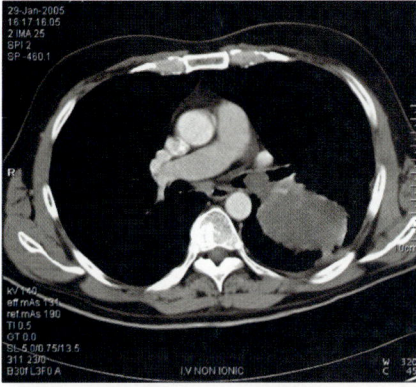

(a)

Fig 43.34a: Large left upper lobe mass lesion with left intrabronchial extension.

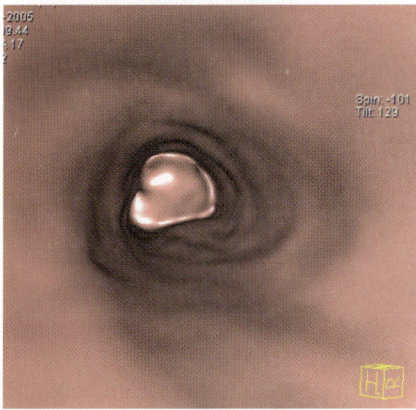

(b)

Fig 43.34b: Intrabronchial extension demonstrated on virtual bronchoscopy

Table 43.18: Approach to biopsy procedures to establish both staging and cell-type in lung cancer	
Type of lesion	**Investigation of Choice**
1. Peripheral nodule	CT guided core biopsy
2. Large central mass	Bronchoscopy
3. Endobronchial malignant tumour	Biopsy through fiberoptic bronchoscope
4. Mediastinal adenopathy	CT guided or EBUS guided transbronchial biopsy
5. Paratracheal, subcarinal, hilar nodes	Transbronchial needle aspiration

The Role of Sputum Cytology

Though mentioned last in this discussion, *sputum cytology is among the first modalities* that should be availed of in the diagnosis of lung cancer. Sputum cytological examination is cheap and when positive has a high specificity. In countries where the prevalence of tuberculosis is high, all sputum specimens sent for cytological examination should also be stained and cultured for acid-fast bacilli. The latter when present on smear or culture point to tuberculosis as the cause of a lung or mediastinal pathology. Sputum cytology is less likely to be positive when lung cancer presents as a peripheral nodule and much more likely to be positive with central tumours or large tumours, particularly large cavitating tumours. Sensitivity of a single sputum specimen for the diagnosis of cancer is approximately 50%. Repeated examination of the sputum increases sensitivity. Occasionally, a radiographically occult squamous

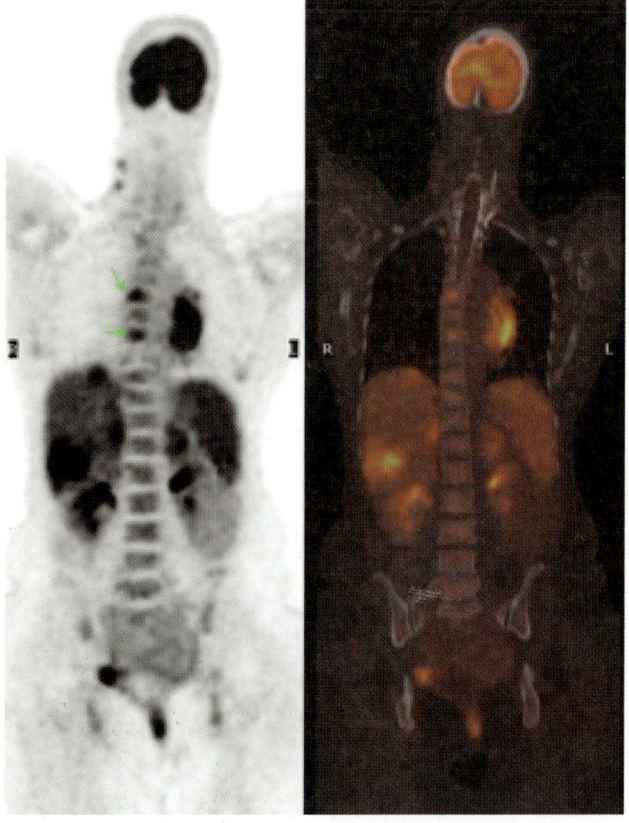

Fig 43.35: PET-CT demonstrates multiple focal lesions in the vertebrae as well as the liver representing metastatic deposits from a left parahilar primary neoplasm.

Table 43.19: Steps for intrathoracic staging	
1	Clinical history and examination; sputum cytology
2	Evaluation of a pleural effusion
3	HRCT of the chest with contrast
4	Biopsy of the tumour and/or mediastinal adenopathy
5	PET scan

cell carcinoma may be diagnosed by a sputum examination which shows mitotic squamous cells on cytology.

Management and Prognosis of Non-small-Cell Lung Cancer

Only 15–25% of patients with NSCLC present when the disease is in an early stage, so that they can be offered potentially curative surgical intervention. About 30–35% have locally advanced stage disease and need management through combined modality protocols. Close to 50% have advanced metastatic disease and can only be offered palliative treatment.

Complete staging on NSCLC is of utmost importance because the presence or absence of mediastinal lymph node involvement is the key prognostic marker in this disease. Also, the mere presence of mediastinal adenopathy in a patient with NSCLC does not always imply that the nodes are malignant. The majority of patients with NSCLC should therefore have mediastinal lymph node biopsies, either transbronchial biopsies thorough a fibreroptic bronchoscope or CT-guided biopsies or biopsies obtained thorough mediastinoscopy.

The table below gives the frequency of malignant involvement of mediastinal lymph nodes based on their size obtained on CT scans.

Table 43.20: Possibility of mediastinal lymph node involvement according to their size	
Node size (cms)	Pathological Involvement (%)
< 1 cm	13
1–2 cm	25
2–3 cm	67

The management and prognosis of NSCLC discussed below is with reference to the upgraded TNM staging classification of 2002.

All large metropolitan cities in India are now making increasing use of the PET scan in the staging of NSCLC. As mentioned earlier it is more accurate in the detection of mediastinal node involvement compared to the CT. It is however an expensive test and is unavailable in many developing countries of the world. Moreover, the sensitivity of PET in poor developing countries is not as good compared to

the West because of the high incidence of infections, notably tuberculosis in our part of the world.

Stage 0, I A/B, II A/B

The treatment of choice for Stage 0 (carcinoma *in situ*), I A/B or II A/B NSCLC is surgical resection provided there is no strong medical contraindication against surgery.

The Lung Cancer Study Group in North America carried out a prospective study in randomly assigned patients with lesions 3 cm in diameter or smaller on the role of lobectomy versus a more localised resection (segmentectomy or wedge resection) in the treatment of NSCLC. It was noted that patients who underwent segmentectomy or a wedge resection had three times as many local recurrences compared to patients who underwent lobectomy. On the basis of this trial and other reports, lobectomy is the surgical procedure of choice provided the patients have adequate pulmonary function to tolerate the procedure. In most surgical centres this involves a formal thoracotomy. However, in specialized centres, lobectomy together with dissection of nodes through video-assisted thoracoscopic surgery (VATS) has been gaining increasing acceptance.

Surgery for NSCLC should always be accompanied by sampling of mediastinal nodes from three to four different sites or by mediastinal lymph node dissection. Most surgeons today are in favour of radical dissection of mediastinal nodes than mere sampling of nodes. Failure to sample or dissect nodes leads to improper staging and hinders the decision on the role of further adjuvant therapy after surgery.

At times the situation of the tumour or its stage may necessitate a pneumonectomy. However, the frequency of performing pneumonectomy for NSCLC at major oncology centres has decreased dramatically to ≤ 5% of all operations on lung cancer.

Operative Mortality

The 30 days' operative mortality is 1–3% for a lobectomy and 5–7% for a pneumonectomy. Morbidity and mortality are chiefly due to respiratory failure, particularly in patients with borderline respiratory reserve, nosocomial pneumonia, empyema, and bronchopleural fistula. Occasionally, death can result in the postoperative period from acute myocardial infarction or pulmonary embolism.

Prognosis after surgery

Prognosis is always better in specialized oncology centres or when performed by experienced oncology surgeons in hospitals with good facilities and staff.

The five-year survival for Stage IA lung cancer is close to 70% and for IB between 50–60%. For patients with Stage II A disease, the five-year survival is 40–55% and survival for II B is close to 40%.

When long-term survival rates are analyzed in a large patient population subject to complete resection at thoracotomy, the overall results leave much to be desired. Thus 40–60% of patients who have been operated upon successfully for IB, II

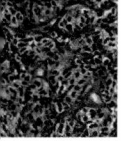
Table 43.21:
Sites of recurrence following radical surgery

Recurrence	Histology %	
	Adenocarcinoma/large cell	Squamous
Regional	17	24
Distant	79	71
Both	4	5

A/B NSCLC have a recurrence within the first five years. It is believed that this is due to a dissemination of micrometastasis to distant sites early in the natural history of the disease and/or to cancer cells left behind at the local site at the time of surgery. Modern immunohistochemical techniques on mediastinal nodes and bone marrow biopsies have demonstrated the presence of disseminated cytokeratine-positive cells. The sites of recurrence following radical surgery are given in Table 43.21.

Adjuvant therapy is therefore invariably recommended in patients after surgical resection. Postoperative radiotherapy does not seem to improve survival; it may do more harm than good. However, a number of studies from Europe, North America and other countries including India have shown increased survival rates in patients who have undergone total resection for IIA, IIB and even IIIA disease, and have received four cycles of adjuvant cisplastin-based chemotherapy when compared to those who after resection received no adjuvant chemotherapy. There are a number of oncologists who would prefer to follow up successful surgical resection on IA and IB patients also with adjuvant chemotherapy provided no contraindication for chemotherapy exists.

Stage IIIA and IIIB

The presence of metastatic involvement of mediastinal lymph nodes is a marker of Stage IIIA disease. No longer is this considered an absolute contraindication to surgery. Two randomized prospective trials included patients with IIIA disease treated with surgery alone, and patients treated with preoperative chemotherapy followed by surgery. The results showed statistically significant increased survival rates in patients given preoperative chemotherapy followed by surgery.

There have been a number of other trials using neoadjuvant preoperative treatment with two to three cycles of chemotherapy with or without radiotherapy to the affected region followed by surgical resection. Most of these trials include IIIA patients but there were some carefully selected within the IIIB group as well. Surgery in these patients often involved a pneumonectomy and there was 10% treatment-related mortality in some series.

A comparison of neoadjuvant treatment (chemotherapy with or without radiation therapy) followed by surgical resection vis-à-vis definitive treatment with chemotherapy and radiation therapy has also been done. The results proved interesting in that there was overall no statistically significant difference in survival rates between the two groups. Interestingly, patients who underwent a pneumonectomy after chemoradiation therapy had a worse survival that those who were treated with chemoradiotherapy alone. Yet patients who underwent just a lobectomy after induction therapy had better survival rates than those treated with just chemoradiation therapy.

Tumours arising at the apex of the lung or in the superior sulcus (Pancoast's tumour) are rarely resectable. When considered resectable, prior radiotherapy followed by surgical resection is the treatment of choice allowing a 'five-year survival rate of 25–30%'.

A multi-centre trial in the West as also a Japanese trial treated patients with Pancoast's tumour without involvement of mediastinal nodes with chemotherapy (two cycles of etoposide and cisplatin) and concurrent thoracic radiotherapy, followed three to five weeks by surgical resection. The five-year survival was around 40%.

Inoperable Stage IIIA, IIIB

Unresectable Stage IIIA, IIIB tumours are best treated with chemotherapy and thoracic radiation provided the patient is considered to be fit to withstand the treatment. Combination therapy is better than just radiotherapy alone. A seven-year follow-up study of combined chemotherapy + radiation versus radiation alone showed that the former group had a five-year survival of 17% versus 6% for the group who received only radiotherapy.

Stage IV

These patients have metastatic lesions. Treatment is aimed at palliation plus possible control of the disease. Numerous combinations of chemotherapy regimes have been tried in these patients. Many show no response; those who do respond have an extended average survival of just six to nine months. The disease returns and death is inevitable. Before very briefly dealing with results of chemotherapy in this group, the question that should be asked particularly with regard to Stage IV disease in developing countries is this—should one rest content with palliation or should one advise and use chemotherapeutic regimes in addition to palliation? The 'pros' of using a chemotherapeutic regime is that the patients may live some months longer. The points against the use of chemotherapy, particularly in a poor country is the cost of therapy that often spells financial ruin to the patient and his family, the side-effects of treatment which may well be worse than the disease itself and very often, the poor quality of life which can be made even poorer with chemotherapeutic regimens during the very short period of extended survival. Each patient should be considered separately in his or her own right with the pros and cons explained in detail.

The physician should, however, be aware of the results of chemotherapeutic regimens at Stage IV. A large meta-analysis of 700 patients with Stage IV disease showed an absolute improvement in survival of 10% at one year in the chemotherapy group compared to the group treated with palliative therapy alone. A number of newer chemotherapeutic agents like **gemcitabine, irinotecan, pemetrexed, doxetacel** and others have been introduced and compared with cisplatin and carbiplatin. None of the newer drugs have been shown to be clearly superior to the platinum-based combinations. The use of the latter combinations has been reported to lead to a median survival time of eight to nine months with about 35% of survival at the end of one year. Patients who respond

to chemotherapy generally do so within two to three cycles of treatment. It is pointless using more than four to six cycles. If disease appears to progress, the choice lies between using a second-line chemotherapeutic agent and opting for palliation.

TARGET DRUGS FOR STAGE IV NSCLC

There is now an increasing emphasis on the use of targeted drugs for lung cancer. The first class of these neo-agents is the epidermal growth factor receptor (EGFR) tyrosine kinase inhibitor. It has shown a survival benefit when used in Stage IV NSCLC. The drug in use belonging to this class is erlotinib; it has been approved as second and third line treatment of Stage IV NSCLC. The EGFR tyrosine kinase inhibitors are of no benefit when added to standard chemotherapy.

The second class of new drugs involving targeted therapy is the anti-angiogenesis drug **bevacizumab**. This drug is an antivascular endothelial growth factor monoclonal antibody shown to increase survival in Stage IV non-squamous NSCLC. Severe bleeding at times with fatal results is a known complication following use of this drug.

In conclusion, though chemotherapeutic regimens may prolong survival to a small extent do they improve quality of life during the small extended period to any significant extent? Assessment of quality of life is difficult; it is conditioned not only by physical discomfort but by mental attitudes to bodily discomfort and to impending dissolution. Measurements of quality of life by various questionnaires such as the Quality of Life Index or the Functional Living Index Cancer Instrument are to our mind of very dubious value.

THE USE OF THE BRONCHOSCOPE IN THE TREATMENT OF LUNG CANCER

The main use of bronchoscopy is to help stage lung cancer. Bronchoscopy also had limited use in the treatment of lung cancer through photodynamic therapy (PDT), laser therapy, brachytherapy and through the use of airway stents in patients where an endobronchial growth is obstructing a large airway. PDT can only be used in NSCLC (in particular squamous cell carcinoma) if the tumour is within the reach of a flexible fiberoptic bronchoscope, if the lesion is smaller than 3 cm in surface area and does not extend more than just a few mm into the bronchial wall. Superficial squamous cell carcinoma or carcinoma *in situ* not evident on radiographic examination can be successfully treated by this method. Seventy to eighty per cent have a good response; there is a recurrence rate of 15–20%. Even so, in the above situation surgical resection is the treatment of choice if the patient is operable, PDT being reserved for patients who are unfit for surgery because of poor lung function or co-morbid states.

Laser Therapy

Laser therapy is for palliative use in lung cancers obstructing central airways. The maximum clinical experience is with the neodymium:ytrium aluminum garnet (Nd:YAG) laser. Laser produces its effects by causing tissue necrosis + photocoagulation. Indications for use are: a) lesions obstructing the central airways, particularly the trachea or main stem bronchi; b) presence of a visible bronchial lumen and of functioning lung tissue beyond

the obstructing cancerous lesions; c) patients unresponsive to other modalities of treatment.

Relief of symptoms follows promptly on successful laser resection but median survival after this palliative treatment is generally not more than six months.

Brachytherapy

Brachytherapy is again a form of palliative therapy used to relieve both luminal obstruction of large airways and obstruction of large airways from extrinsic pressure. It is most often used in patients who have already received external beam radiation. Brachytherapy consists of an application of a titrated radiation dose applied through a nylon catheter placed into the lesion endoscopically. Successful and significant relief of an obstructed airways is observed in about 50% of patients, but median survival rate after brachytherapy does not extend beyond a few months.

Use of Prosthetic Stents

Bronchoscopic placement of airway stents is again a palliative treatment to relieve airways' obstruction involving large airways or lobar bronchi. The largest experience is with silastic stents and metal stents. Combination of metal plus silastic and other materials in the stent have also been used. Stent insertion is done through either a flexible or rigid bronchoscope. Prompt relief of obstructive symptoms is observed after successful placement of the stent. Complications of the use of a stent are: a) migration of the stent; b) obstruction of the stent by secretions; c) granulation tissue formation.

Table 43.22: Management of NSCLC
Stage 0, IA/B, IIA/B
Surgery for NSCLC with mediastinal lymph node dissection
Adjuvant chemotherapy for IIA, IIB and even IIIA disease; can be given in IA and IB as well
Stage IIIA
Neoadjuvant treatment (chemotherapy with or without radiation therapy) followed by surgical resection
Stage IIIB
Generally considered inoperable but in some cases surgery involves a pneumonectomy
Pancoast's tumour without involvement of mediastinal nodes
Treated by chemotherapy (two cycles of etoposide and cisplatin) and concurrent thoracic radiotherapy followed 3–5 weeks later by surgical resection.
Inoperable stage IIIA, IIIB
Combination therapy of chemotherapy and thoracic radiation
Stage IV
Palliative treatment plus possible control of the disease
Newer chemotherapeutic agents like gemcitabine, irinotecan, pemetrexed, doxetacel have been introduced
Target Drugs for Stage IV NSCLC—erlotinib, bevacizumab

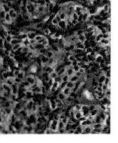

Table 43.23: Prognosis of NSCLC (with appropriate management)		
1.	The 5-year survival for stage	IA – 70% IB – 50–60% IIA – 40–55%' IIB – 40%
2.	Pancoast's tumour	25–30%
3.	Inoperable stage IIIA, IIIB	17%

Table 43.24: Palliative treatment for NSCLC	
1.	PDT
2.	Laser therapy
3.	Brachy therapy
4.	Use of prosthetic stents

An advantage of the silastic stent over the metal stent is that the former can be removed; while the latter can became incorporated within the bronchial wall and is then not removable. Even when a stent is appropriately placed, in time to come the growth can extend proximal or distal to the stent, again leading to airway obstruction.

SMALL-CELL LUNG CANCER

Close to 15–20% of lung cancers are SCLCs and about one-third of patients who have SCLC have limited stage disease. SCLC has an 80% response to present-day conventional therapy, a clinical remission being obtained in about 50% of patients. Unfortunately, relapse is frequent, the median survival time being 18 to 20 months, with a two-year survival rate of 30–40% and five-year survival of 15–20%.

Surgery in SCLC

Surgery even today has indeed a very limited role in SCLC. Before the era of chemotherapy, surgery was the only modality of treatment with the sad five-year survival rate of just 1–2%.

Effective chemotherapy was discovered in the 1960s and since then surgery for SCLC was given up. In recent years (a little over the past decade) the role of surgery has been re-examined. SCLC presenting as a localized solitary nodule when surgically resected has a five-year survival rate of 25–35%.

Less than 5% of SCLC present as a solitary peripheral nodule. The survival rate mentioned above can only be achieved if successful surgery for SCLC presenting as a solitary peripheral nodule is followed up with four cycles of standard chemotherapy and radiotherapy to the thorax given sequentially. It is important that SCLC presenting as a peripheral nodule should be evaluated thoroughly prior to surgery. Evaluation should include CT chest and abdomen, MRI of the head or contrast HRCT of the head, and isotope scan or PET scan to exclude distant metastasis. Some oncology centres advocate a mediastinoscopy to ensure that the mediastinal lymph nodes are negative for metastatic spread.

Surgery, however, has no role in the management of all other forms of limited-stage SCLC. A randomized prospective trial on limited-stage SCLC was carried out by the Lung Cancer Study Group in the United States. All patients first received chemotherapy in the form of five cycles of cyclophosphamide, doxorubicin and vincristine. Patients who showed even a partial response were randomized to either throracotomy and surgical resection or no surgery. Both groups were given radiotherapy. There was no difference in survival rates between the two arms of the study, suggesting that surgery was not indicated in the usual patient with limited-stage SCLC.

Chemotherapy and Radiation in Limited-Stage SCLC

Chemotherapy plus radiation therapy is the standard treatment for all forms of limited-stage SCLC other than those presenting as an isolated peripheral nodule where surgery also plays a role. The current recommendation is the use of etoposide and cisplatin or etoposide and carboplatin with radiotherapy to the thorax administered early in the treatment protocol. Randomized trials have shown that four to six cycles of chemotherapy suffice. Additional cycles do not improve long-term survival and only add to toxic side-effects. Complete remission with two-year and five-year survival rate of 40% and 20% respectively is observed with the above combination therapy. Unfortunately, patients who experience 70–75% of complete remissions relapse within two years. Second-line chemotherapeutic agents for SCLC have overall poor results.

Extensive-Stage SCLC

More than two-thirds and not uncommonly three quarters of all SCLCs present as extended-stage disease. The treatment is with standard chemotherapy outlined for limited-stage SCLC. A response to chemotherapy occurs in over 60% of patients, complete clinical remission being seen in about 20%. Yet the disease recurs so that the median survival time is 8 to 10 months with a two-year survival of less than 10%. No patient survives for five years. Identical response rates and identical survival rates are observed with etoposide and cisplatin, etoposide and carboplatin, etoposide, ifosfamide and cisplatin, or cyclophosphamide, doxorubicin and etoposide.

The poor survival rates have led to the trial of primary new chemotherapeutic agents in the treatment of SCLC. Two new agents that have been tried are pacitaxel and topotecan. However, no newer agent nor any combination therapy involving newer agents has been shown to be of more benefit than standard chemotherapy.

Relapse in SCLC

Once relapse occurs in SCLC, the median survival rate is just three to four months. Second-line therapy in the treatment of relapse is by and large unsatisfactory, particularly if relapse has occurred within three months of initial therapy or if the patient has failed to respond adequately to initial therapy. If initial therapy did not include a platinum-based regime, the

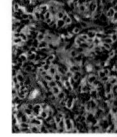

	Table 43.25: Management of SCLC
Solitary peripheral nodule	
Surgical resection followed by four cycles of standard chemotherapy and radiotherapy given to the thorax sequentially	
Limited Stage SCLC	
Chemotherapy plus radiotherapy	
Extensive Stage SCLC	
Chemotherapy	

patients should be given the benefit of treatment with etoposide and cisplatin or etoposide and carboplatin. A 50% response is often observed.

If response to initial first-line therapy has been good so that there has been a remission for over six months then a subsequent relapse is best treated with the same chemotherapeutic regime used initially.

CLINICAL COURSE OF LUNG CANCER

Many aspects of the clinical course have been covered in the earlier discussion on lung cancer. The following points are however briefly summarized and are worthy of note:

1. The overall five-year survival in patients who have lung cancer even today is just 15% in good experienced oncology centres. In the average surgical centres and in most centres in developing countries, the five-year survival is even more dismal—around 5–7%.
2. The most important prognostic determinant is the tumour stage. As mentioned earlier, NSCLC Stage IA after successful surgical resection has a five-year survival rate of 50–60% compared to 10% survival rate in patients with NSCLC–Stage–IA cancer who are not operated upon either because they are unfit or refusing surgery.
3. Patients detected with lung cancer (at various stages) who are asymptomatic have a 35% long-term survival vs. 10% survival in those detected with the presence of symptoms.
4. Squamous cell cancer of the lung, and younger patients have a better prognosis. Surgically unresectable NSCLC and SCLC have a poor prognosis.
5. Squamous cell cancer of the lung has a greater incidence of local recurrence and lower rate of metastatic lesions compared to adenocarninoma and large cell carcinoma.
6. Patients with SCLC have the highest rate of metastatic spread.
7. Genes may influence survival. A study has shown that the presence of genes DUSP 6 MMD, STAT1, ERBB3 and LK was an independent predictor of five-year plus overall survival in a cohort of resected NSCLC patients.
8. Functional state has been shown to be an important predictor of survival. A number of performance status scales have been devised to assess functional state. A patient who is unable to carry out normal activities but is confined to his home and manages to care for himself is an example of an independent predictor of poor survival. Significant weight

loss of > 10% and the male gender are also independent predictors of shortened survival in unresectable disease.
9. After successful surgical resection of lung cancer at any stage of the disease, Western literature has reported a second primary lung cancer developing in 2–3% per year. This suggests that patients successfully treated for lung cancer should be closely followed up for at least five years and preferably 10 years. Follow-up, however, has not been shown to improve overall survival. No reliable and comprehensive Indian data with regard to the incidence of second primary lung cancers is available.

	Table 43.26: Clinical course of lung cancer
1.	Overall 5-year survival in patients – 15%
2.	The most important prognostic determinant is the tumour stage.
3.	Asymptomatic patients diagnosed with lung cancer have a better long-term survival rate compared to symptomatic patients
4.	Squamous cell cancer of the lung and younger patients have a better prognosis. Surgically unresectable NSCLC and SCLC have a poor prognosis.
5.	Squamous cell cancer of the lung has a greater incidence of local recurrence and lower rate of metastatic lesions.
6.	Small cell lung carcinoma have the highest rate of metastatic spread.
7.	Genes may influence survival.
8.	Functional state has been shown to be an important predictor of survival.
9.	After surgical resection of lung cancer, second primary lung cancer may develop in 2–3% per year.

OTHER LUNG TUMOURS

Pulmonary Metastasis

A pulmonary metastatic lesion from a primary cancer arising outside the thorax may present as a single solitary nodule or multiple nodular lesions. These are generally evident on an X-ray chest and are often asymptomatic. Occasionally, an HRCT of the chest may reveal single or multiple pulmonary metastatic lesions not picked up by routine radiography.

The lung is a common site of metastatic deposits. Sources of primary cancer causing frequent blood-borne metastasis to the lungs include the breast, kidney thyroid, colon, stomach and head and neck cancers. Melanomas also metastasize frequently to the lung as do sarcomas. Besides metastatic pulmonary nodules, metastasis may involve the pleura and result in lymphangitis carcinomatosis. The latter is particularly frequently observed with breast and stomach cancers. Endobronchial secondary deposits may also occur.

The diagnosis of a pulmonary metastasis depending on the size and situation of the lesion can be made by a CT-guided biopsy or a transbronchial biopsy through a fiberoptic bronchoscope. A video-assisted thoracoscopic biopsy may

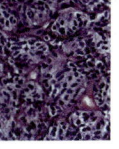

occasionally be necessary to establish a definite diagnosis. A video-assisted thoracoscopy may also be necessary to confirm or refute the diagnosis of a metastatic pleural effusion. Multiple metastases need requisite systemic chemotherapy depending on the source or site of the primary cancer.

Though randomized trials are not available, an isolated single pulmonary metastatic lesion from a primary arising form the kidney, breast, colon or from a sarcoma may be resected with perhaps improved survival provided distant metastatic lesions are not present in other organ systems.

presence of nodal metastasis; it is even further reduced with liver metastasis.

Atypical carcinoids are so termed if histology reveals necrosis or increased mitosis. These tumours tend to recur, have a higher rate of metastasis to regional lymph nodes and are usually larger at the time of diagnosis. Surgery if possible is still the optimal line of treatment, the five-year survival rate being 60%. Carcinoid tumours respond poorly to radiotherapy or chemotherapy compared to NSCLC.

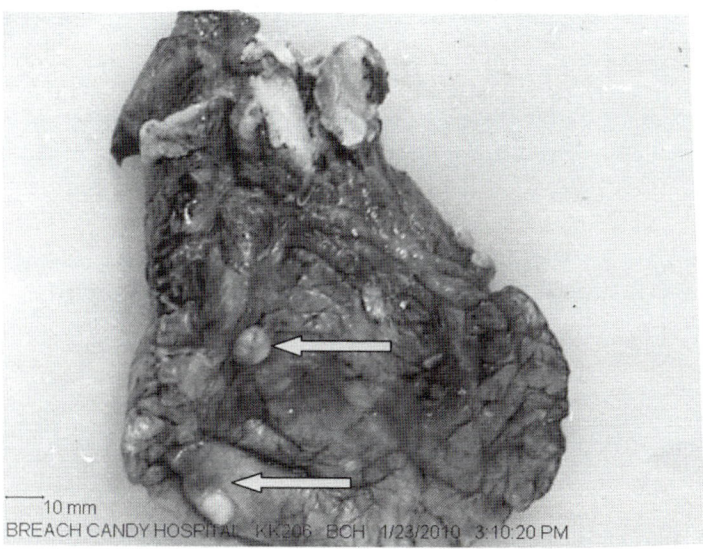

Fig 43.36: Gross lobectomy specimen which demonstrates multiple subpleural well-defined homogenous rounded nodules. These represented metastatic deposits from a chondrosarcoma of the rib.

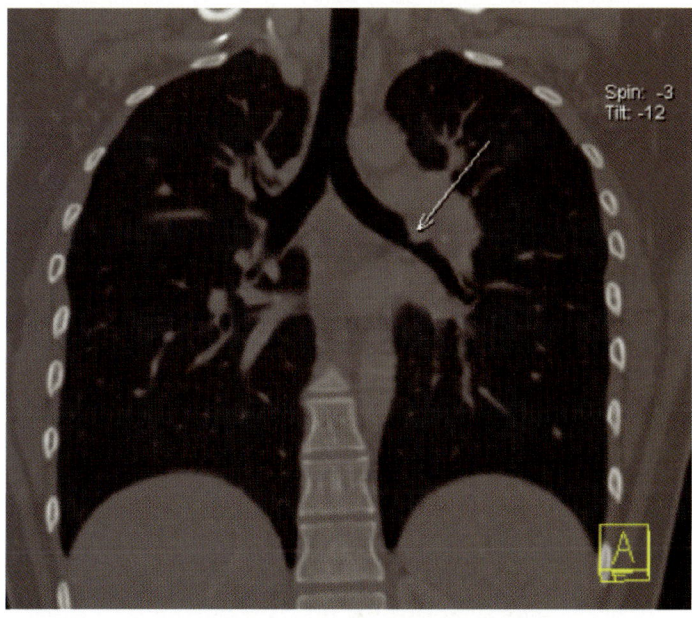

Fig 43.37: Carcinoid tumour. Coronal image demonstrates a nodular mass protruding into the left main bronchus representing a carcinoid tumour.

Carcinoid Tumours

Carcinoid tumours are low-grade malignant neoplasms consisting of neuroendocrine cells. They constitute 1 to 2% of lung tumours.

Patients with carcinoid tumours may be asymptomatic, the tumour being discovered as a solitary nodule on chest radiography. Carcinoid tumours are often endobronchial; the presentation then is with cough, haemoptysis and features of partial or complete bronchial obstruction. These include clinical features of pneumonia distal to the tumour or of atelectasis of a lobe or lung when the obstruction to the airway is complete.

Though a carcinoid tumour is composed of neuroendocrine cells, the carcinoid syndrome characterized by episodes of flushing, urticaria, diarrhoea, and hypotension is rare and generally occurs in carcinoids that have metastasized to the liver.

Diagnosis is made by bronchoscopy as these tumours are often endobronchial. A carcinoid within the lung parenchyma can be diagnosed through a CT-guided biopsy. These tumours are often vascular and biopsy at times leads to significant bleeding.

Surgical resection of the tumour is curative in the absence of any nodal or extrathoracic spread (chiefly to the liver). The 10-year survival rate in such patients is well over 90%. Survival rates are reduced if the carcinoid is > 3 cm in size, or in the

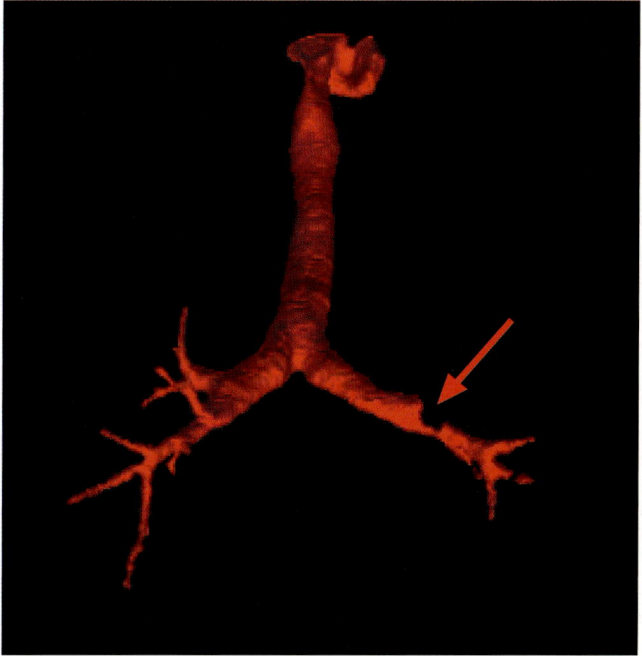

Fig 43.38: Carcinoid tumour. CT volume-rendered image of the tracheobronchial tree reveals the intrabronchial extension of the carcinoid tumour.

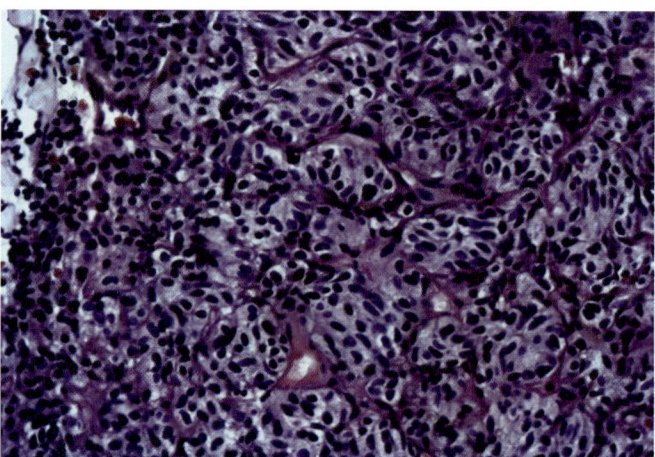

Fig 43.41: Carcinoid tumour of the lung. H&E 20X magnification microscopy demonstrates discrete nests of tumour cells with uniform oval nuclei in a carcinoid tumour of the lung.

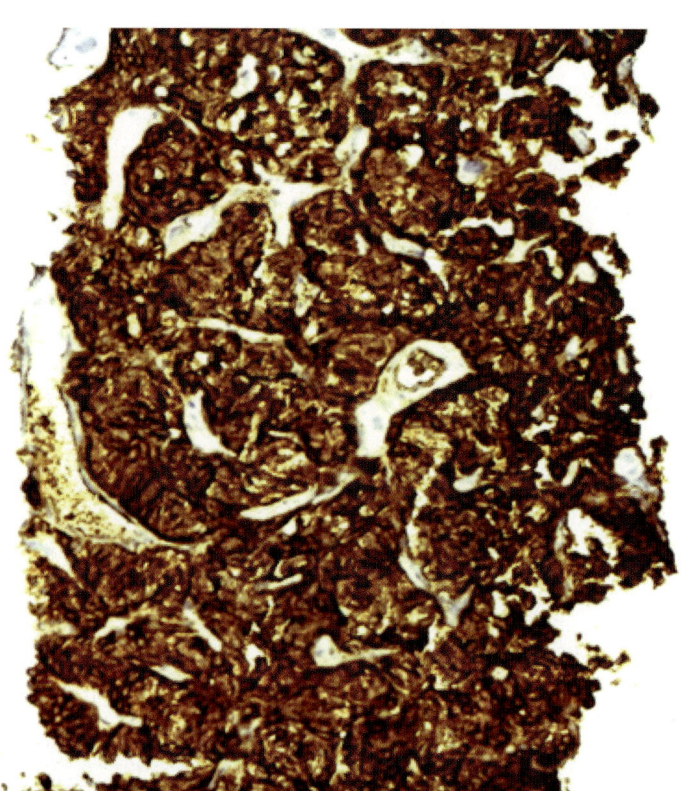

Fig 43.39: 10 X. Carcinoid tumour-immunohistochemistry for neuroendocrine marker synaptophysin. Strong cytoplasmic positivity is noted.

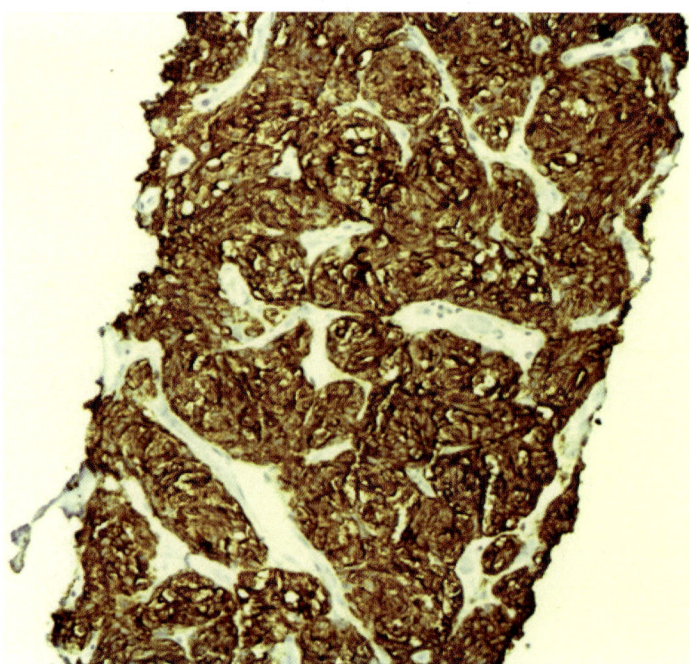

Fig 43.40: 10 X. Carcinoid tumour-immunohistochemistry for neuroendocrine marker chromogranin. Strong cytoplasmic positivity is noted.

Pulmonary Lymphoma

Pulmonary lymphomas are invariably of the non-Hodgkin's variety and form less than 1% of all tumours. The diagnosis is generally made on a CT-guided biopsy. It is uncommon to come

across a non-Hodgkin's lymphoma solely involving the lung. A clinical plus other investigational search for involvement of lymph glands and other organ systems should be made. Surgical resection for a single, isolated non-Hodgkin's lymphoma may be curative. Chemotherapy is indicated in patients with more extensive pulmonary or disseminated disease.

Microepidermoid Carcinoma

Microepidermoid carcinomas are rare tumours involving the large airways—the trachea or the proximal bronchi. They arise from salivary gland tissue within the large airways. Being endotracheal or endobronhcial, they present with cough, haemoptysis, dyspnoea, stridor and obstructive symptoms. They are low-malignancy tumours but may metastasize to lymph nodes.

Treatment is by surgical resection if this is feasible—complete resection is rewarded with an excellent prognosis.

Adenoid Cystic Carcinoma

Adenoid cystic carcinoma is a salivary gland tumour arising from the trachea, main stem or lobar bronchi, constituting less than 1% of all lung tumours. Rarely, it arises peripherally. Presenting symptoms, because of its endobronchial situation, are cough, haemoptysis, dyspnoea and obstructive clinical features distal to the obstruction.

The treatment of choice is surgical resection though this is often incomplete. Local recurrence as well as metastasis is observed.

Hamartoma

Hamartoma is the commonest benign neoplasm of the lung with the highest frequency of occurrence in the fifth or sixth decade. A hamartoma is invariably asymptomatic and is detected as a well-defined nodule either on chest radiography or CT of the chest. Histologically, a hamartoma consists of mixed tissue, a combination of cartilage, muscle, fat, connective tissue and respiratory epithelium. Calcification is often noted; it may take the form of popcorn calcification in about 25% of patients. The radiographic

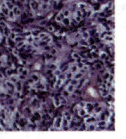

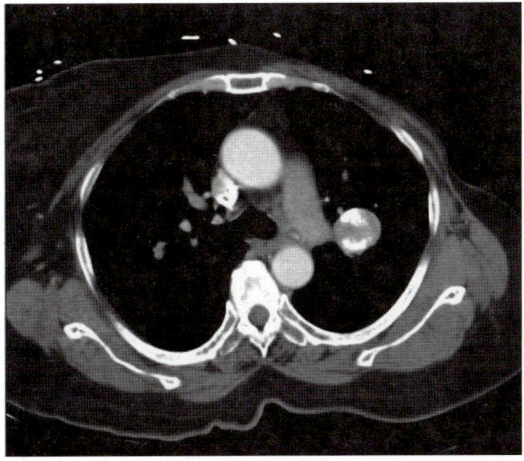

Fig 43.42: CT chest confirms the irregular internal calcification indicative of a hamartoma.

appearance is generally typical and no treatment is advised other than periodic observation. A radiographically doubtful or indeterminate nodule however warrants surgical resection.

PREVENTION

Avoidance of smoking (never-smoking) and stopping smoking are the prime preventive measure considering the fact that 85% of lung cancers occur in smokers or former smokers. Tobacco is addictive and smoking cessation proves difficult. Motivation through repeated meetings with the physician often helps—but only to a small extent. Use of supplemental nicotine patches, hypnosis, group therapy, and acupuncture has at various times led to one year abstinence rates of 20% or more. The drug varenicline, a nicotine agonist has been shown to be superior to bupropion in stopping cigarette smoking in randomized trials. The cessation rate for smoking at 12 weeks is 44% with varenicline, 29.5% with bupropion and 17.7% with placebo. In our opinion, in addition to what is mentioned above, patients addicted to cigarette smoking can give up cigarettes only if they are sufficiently motivated from within to do so. The incidence of lung cancer would indeed fall precipitously if smoking of tobacco is declared a dreadful poison and is banned all over the world.

SUGGESTED READING

Alberg AJ. Epidemiology of lung cancer. *Chest*. 1 Jan. 2003; 123(1 Suppl): 21S–49S.

Bryant A. Differences in epidemiology, histology, and survival between cigarette smokers and never-smokers who develop non-small cell lung cancer. *Chest*. 1 Jul. 2007; 132(1): 185–92.

Detterbeck FC. The new lung cancer staging system. *Chest*. 1 Jul. 2009; 136(1): 260–71.

Erasmus JJ. CT, positron emission tomography, and MRI in staging lung cancer. *Clin Chest Med*. 1 Mar. 2008; 29(1): 39–57, v.

Ginsberg MS. Lung Cancer. *Radiol Clin North Am*. 1 Jan. 2007; 45(1): 21–43.

Hahn O. Novel therapies in lung cancer. *Hematol Oncol Clin North Am*. 1 Apr. 2005; 19(2): 343–67, vii.

Jett JR. Treatment of non-small cell lung cancer, stage IIIB: ACCP evidence-based clinical practice guidelines (second edition). *Chest*. 1 Sep. 2007; 132(3 Suppl): 266S–276S.

Kelley MJ. Prevention of lung cancer: summary of published evidence. *Chest*. 1 Jan. 2003; 123(1 Suppl): 50S–59S.

Khuder SA. Effect of smoking cessation on major histologic types of lung cancer. *Chest*. 1 Nov. 2001; 120(5): 1577–83.

Molina JR. Advances in chemotherapy of non-small cell lung cancer. *Chest*. 1 Oct. 2006; 130(4): 1211–19.

Robinson LA. Treatment of non-small cell lung cancer-stage IIIA: ACCP evidence-based clinical practice guidelines (second edition). *Chest*. 1 Sep. 2007; 132(3 Suppl): 243S–265S.

Scott WJ. Treatment of non-small cell lung cancer Stage I and Stage II: ACCP evidence-based clinical practice guidelines (second edition). *Chest*. 1 Sep. 2007; 132(3 Suppl): 234S–242S.

Simon GR. Management of small cell lung cancer: ACCP evidence Seo, 2007; 132(3 Suppl): 324S–339S.

Socinski MA. Treatment of non-small cell lung cancer, stage IV: ACCP evidence-based clinical practice guidelines (second edition). *Chest*. 1 Sep. 2007; 132(3 Suppl): 277S–289S.

Subramanian J. Molecular genetics of lung cancer in people who have never smoked. *Lancet Oncol*. 1 Jul. 2008; 9(7): 676–82.

Tanoue LT. Treatment of lung cancer in older patients. *Clin Chest Med*. 1 Dec. 2007; 28(4): 735–49, vi.

Travis WD. Pathology of lung cancer. *Clin Chest Med*. 1 Mar. 2002; 23(1): 65–81, viii.

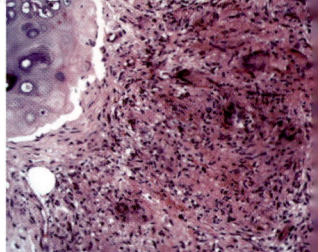

CHAPTER 44 Interstitial Lung Disease—Idiopathic Interstitial Pneumonia

Interstitial lung diseases (ILDs) are a group of diffuse lung diseases that affect not just the interstitium of the lung but also the airspaces, peripheral airways and vessels along with their respective epithelial and endothelial linings. Diffuse parenchymal lung diseases (DPLD) may hence be a more accurate description of these disorders.

The ILDs may be classified as those secondary to a known cause or disease state like drugs or collagen vascular disease or granulomatous conditions like sarcoidosis or rarer diseases like Langerhans cell histiocytosis or pulmonary alveolar proteinosis. At last count there were at least 150 diseases which were known to present with ILD. Many of these have been discussed in different parts of this text. More often than not, the cause of the ILD remains unknown despite a detailed history, physical examination and investigation. Osler first described the generic 'chronic interstitial pneumonia' over a century ago but these idiopathic forms of ILD are currently called Idiopathic Interstitial Pneumonias (IIPs).

The first modern classification schema was proposed in 1969 by Liebow and Carrington who described five distinct histopathological patterns in patients with IIP: usual interstitial pneumonia (UIP), desquamative interstitial pneumonia (DIP), lymphocytic interstitial pneumonia (LIP), bronchiolitis obliterans organizing pneumonia (BOOP) and giant cell interstitial pneumonia. Each of these patients had a distinct clinical profile suggesting that they represented separate diseases.

Katzenstein and Myers revised Liebow and Carrington's classification in 1998, excluding BOOP (felt to represent an intraluminal rather than an interstitial process), LIP (as it was a lymphoproliferative disorder) and giant cell interstitial pneumonia (felt to be a hard-metal pneumoconiosis). They instead divided IIPs into five groups, maintaining UIP and DIP, but adding three newly recognized entities: respiratory bronchiolitis-associated interstitial lung disease (RB-ILD), acute interstitial pneumonia (AIP, formerly Hamman-Rich syndrome) and non-specific interstitial pneumonia (NSIP).

Most recently, the American Thoracic Society (ATS) and European Respiratory Society (ERS) convened a consensus panel of clinicians, radiologists and pathologists to establish a uniform set of criteria for diagnosis of IIPs. They combined the two earlier classifications into the current schema with seven distinct disease entities now falling under the umbrella of IIP. This classification is outlined in Table 44.1 which describes the clinical entity and its corresponding histopathological pattern.

Table 44.1: ATS/ERS consensus classification of IIP's	
Histopathological Pattern	Corresponding Clinical Diagnosis
Usual interstitial pneumonia	Idiopathic pulmonary fibrosis
Nonspecific interstitial pneumonia	Nonspecific interstitial pneumonia
Organizing pneumonia	Cryptogenic organizing pneumonia
Diffuse alveolar damage	Acute interstitial pneumonia
Respiratory bronchiolitis	Respiratory bronchiolitis—associated ILD
Desquamative interstitial pneumonia	Desquamative interstitial pneumonia
Lymphocytic interstitial pneumonia	Lymphocytic interstitial pneumonia

EPIDEMIOLOGICAL SPECTRUM AND DISTRIBUTION OF ILD IN INDIA

In India, the ILDs remain significantly under-diagnosed and under-reported. This is probably due to the lack of awareness and lack of easy availability of computed tomography (CT) scanning and surgical centres offering open and video-assisted lung biopsy. The considerable expenses involved in these special investigations are also a deterrent for the Indian patient with ILD. Finally, the overwhelming burden of tuberculosis (TB) in India tends to dominate respiratory medicine in this country. TB can mimic some of the ILDs, especially sarcoidosis, and leads to diagnostic errors and delays. Nevertheless, in the last few decades, ILDs and DPLDs have been increasingly recognized in India. The surge in the recognition of ILD in India corresponds to the turn of the century when high-resolution computed tomography (HRCT) scanning became more readily available as a primary diagnostic aid. Most of the earlier reports on ILDs in the 1980s and 1990s generally referred to the diffuse interstitial involvement that occurred in systemic diseases like connective tissue disorders. In that era there were very few reports on idiopathic pulmonary fibrosis (IPF) in the Indian literature. At one of our hospitals, a tertiary referral centre in Mumbai, we analyzed 274 biopsy-proven cases of DPLD over a seven-year period. In this series, IPF constituted the single largest disease group, accounting for 43% of all patients encountered. The spectrum of secondary causes was no different from that seen in Western countries. Drug-induced DPLD, pneumoconiosis, sarcoidosis, extrinsic allergic

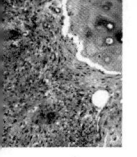

alveolitis, histiocytosis X, Wegener's granulomatosis, pulmonary alveolar proteinosis and lymphomatoid granulomatosis were all encountered. (*Sen T, Udwadia ZF. Retrospective study of ILD in a tertiary care centre in India. Indian J Chest Dis Allied Sci. In Press*). Another retrospective study from the same centre looked into the clinical features, radiology, pulmonary function test (PFT) and follow-up of 117 biopsy-proven cases of IPF over seven years. We found that 6% of these cases had familial IPF. Another comprehensive retrospective review revealed 34 cases of biopsy-proven cryptogenic organizing pneumonia (COP) encountered from 2000–05, establishing that COP was not uncommon in India although the majority of cases were initially mislabelled as TB before the final diagnosis was made. There are several smaller Indian case series of ILDs secondary to different connective tissue diseases with recent Indian studies pointing out the presence of ILD in 65% of patients with systemic sclerosis and 25% of patients with rheumatoid arthritis. Thus, to conclude, the epidemiology of ILDs in India is no different from that seen in the West. IPF remains the most common diagnosis but the entire spectrum of secondary causes is encountered as can be seen from the data published from a tertiary centre with the facilities to correctly diagnose these cases. What is needed are larger prospective, population-based epidemiological studies so that the prevalence of ILD and IIP in the Indian context can be determined.

DIAGNOSIS OF ILD

1. **History:** The patient's age, gender and smoking status often provide the initial clues in the history. Patients with IPF are usually more than 60 years old. Indeed, it is essential to rule out a secondary cause before labelling a young patient as having IPF. Patients with IIP of the NSIP variety are usually less than 60 years old. Sarcoidosis usually occurs at a younger age. Lymphangioleiomyomatosis (LAM) is exclusively a disease of women, while pulmonary Langerhans cell granulomatosis (also called Histiocytosis X or eosinophilic granuloma) occurs in young cigarette-smoking males. A family history of ILD in parents, siblings or children raises the possibility of familial IPF. A detailed environmental and occupational history is essential and may provide vital clues to the aetiology of the ILD. At-risk occupations include farmers (extrinsic allergic alveolitis), miners (pneumoconiosis), workers in nuclear, aerospace, computer or electronics industries (berylliosis), and shipyard workers, mechanics and electricians (asbestosis). Hobbies such as bird breeding or pigeon feeding as is common in this country and exposure to pets like budgerigars or parakeets may also be relevant and must be specifically inquired for. Several drugs are known to cause ILD; the use of amiodorone, methotrexate, penicillamine and chemotherapeutic agents must be checked for.
2. **Symptoms:** The two cardinal symptoms of ILD are cough and dyspnoea. Though these are non-specific symptoms, a careful teasing out of these symptoms can often provide clues to ILD being the underlying cause. The cough is always dry and non-productive. Unlike the dry cough caused by asthma which is intermittent and often nocturnal, the cough of patients with IPF shows no diurnal variation. It does not

wax and wane and can be incessant. It may worsen (as the dyspnoea does) with exertion. It is a disabling and distressing symptom for the patient and one which is often mislabelled asthma or bronchitis by the physician, especially in the early stages. It is often refractory to all therapies. The other cardinal symptom is dyspnoea. In the early stages this may be present only on undue exertion like climbing stairs and absent at rest or with routine activity. It is relentlessly progressive however and there is no more crippling symptom than the dyspnoea of advanced IPF. As the disease progresses it occurs with trivial activity and eventually at rest. It is relieved to some extent by oxygen, but eventually persists despite high-flow oxygen. Other respiratory symptoms are rare and if present may provide important clues to the aetiology or complications. Thus, for example, haemoptysis points to underlying alveolar haemorrhage which may complicate the ILD of collagen vascular disorders like systemic lupus erythematosus (SLE) or raise suspicions of pulmonary embolism or malignancy, both known complications of ILD. Pleuritic pain should raise the possibility of the occurrence of a pneumothorax. Wheeze may occur in ILD related to sarcoidosis or extrinsic allergic alveolitis (both being ILDs with frequent airway involvement). Symptoms outside the lungs like fever and joint pains raise the possibility of sarcoidosis or collagen vascular disorder.

3. **Signs:** Crackles are the distinctive physical finding. The crackles are typically dry or Velcro-like and heard in the very bases of the lung during end-inspiration. In the early stages they are very subtle and must be carefully auscultated for with the patient instructed to lean forward and breathe very deeply. They are different in character from those heard in bronchiectasis and do not change with coughing. Once heard they are almost pathognomonic and must never be ignored even if the patient has few symptoms and a normal chest radiograph at the time. The only condition which produces similar crackles is interstitial pulmonary oedema. While crackles are heard in all the ILDs they are relatively less common in granulomatous ILDs like sarcoidosis. Squawks and wheeze may be heard in EAA and occasionally in sarcoidosis with airway involvement. Finger clubbing is another common sign. It is more commonly seen in IPF and is rare in sarcoidosis, collagen vascular disease-associated ILD and BOOP. Signs of pulmonary hypertension must be carefully assessed and are not uncommon in advanced ILD, often portending a grave prognosis. Finally, extra-pulmonary signs like erythema nodosum (sarcoidosis), Raynaud's phenomenon and sclerodactyly (systemic sclerosis), subcutaneous nodules (rheumatoid arthritis) and café au lait spots (underlying tuberous sclerosis and associated LAM) must be carefully checked for.

4. **Chest Radiography:** The chest radiograph remains an integral part of the workup of a patient with suspected ILD. However, the chest radiograph has shortcomings with regard to sensitivity and specificity which must be borne in mind. Various limitations of the chest radiograph can be listed;
    a. The range of patterns on a chest radiograph is obviously limited even when the ILD is obvious.
    b. About half the lung volume is obscured on a frontal chest radiograph by the mediastinum and diaphragm making early ILD often impossible to pick. The sensitivity of

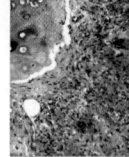

Table 44.2:
Clinical features of idiopathic interstitial pneumonia
Symptoms
1. Cough
2. Dyspnoea
3. Wheeze in case of sarcoidosis or extrinsic allergic alveolitis (EAA)
4. Extra-pulmonary features suggests association of collagen vascular disease or sarcoidosis
Signs
Crackles-dry or 'velcro' crackles
Wheeze in sarcoidosis or EAA
Finger clubbing
Signs of pulmonary hypertension
Extra-pulmonary signs like erythema nodosum (sarcoidosis), Raynaud's phenomenon and sclerodactyly (systemic sclerosis), subcutaneous nodules (rheumatoid arthritis) and café au lait spots (underlying tuberous sclerosis and associated LAM)

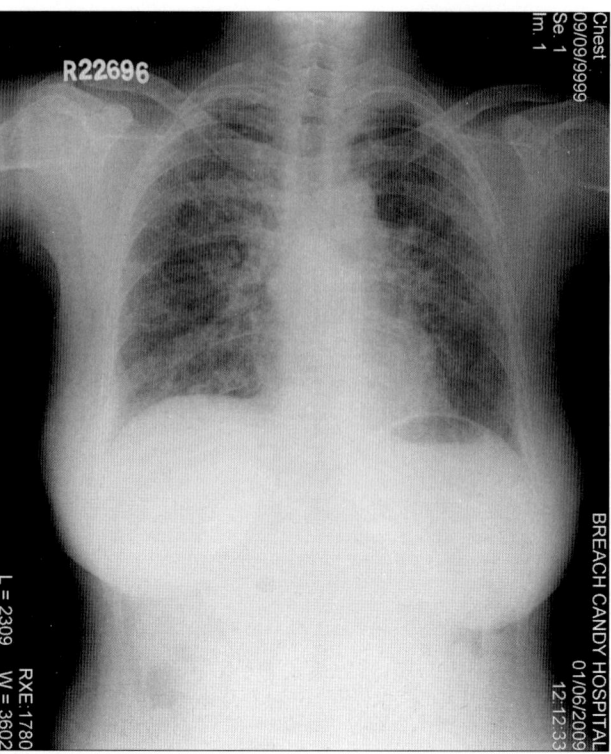

Fig 44.1: IPF. X-ray chest demonstrates reticular opacities in both lung fields, particularly the right lung base. HRCT chest confirmed presence of reticular opacity in a case with a UIP pattern.

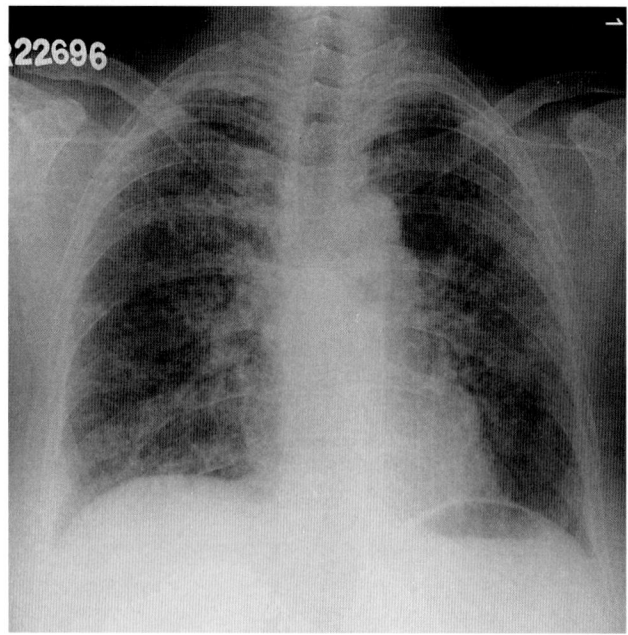

Fig 44.2: IPF. X-ray chest demonstrates reticular opacities in both lung fields, particularly the right lung base with evidence of loss of lung volume. HRCT demonstrated extensive UIP with destructive change.

chest radiography is difficult to gauge but one historical series showed that at least 10% of cases with biopsy-proven ILD had an apparently normal radiograph.

c. A diagnosis made on chest radiograph is seldom confident. In a large series by Mathieson, (*Mathieson JR, Mayo JR, Staples CA, Muller NL. Chronic diffuse infiltrative lung disease: comparison of diagnostic accuracy of CT and chest radiography. Radiology 1989; 171; 111–116.*) a confident diagnosis could be made in less than a quarter of the cases by experienced radiologists and this diagnosis correctly matched the histological diagnosis in only 77%.

d. The chest radiograph cannot determine disease activity or whether the disease is likely to be reversible or not.

Having pointed out these limitations, the chest radiograph has a number of advantages;

a. It is useful for pattern recognition; for example, the bilateral hilar adenopathy and upper lobe preponderance of sarcoidosis or the lower lobe honeycombing of IPF.

b. It is widely used for serial monitoring of progress (along with PFT) as it is impractical to use HRCTs too frequently in this role.

c. It is more than adequate to detect complications such as pneumothorax or superadded infection.

Thus, in summary, chest radiography though inferior to the HRCT scan remains a pivotal screening tool. Because of its ready availability it is often the first and only tool in parts of the developing world.

5. **High-Resolution Computed Tomography (HRCT):** HRCT provides cross-sectional images of the lungs that possess spatial and contrast resolution such that sub-millimetre structures in the lung are clearly visible.

a. *Sensitivity of HRCT:* The sensitivity of HRCT for ILD is believed to be in the vicinity of 95%. This is much higher than that of chest radiography but is not yet 100%. Thus, it is possible on rare occasions to have biopsy proof of ILD with a normal HRCT. In one series of biopsy-proven IPF

by Orens et al., CT appearances were considered normal in three of 25 cases (i.e. 12%). The clinical significance of such subtle and early ILD is unclear.

b. *Specificity of HRCT:* Many reports have shown that HRCT is significantly more accurate than chest radiography in

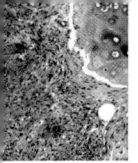
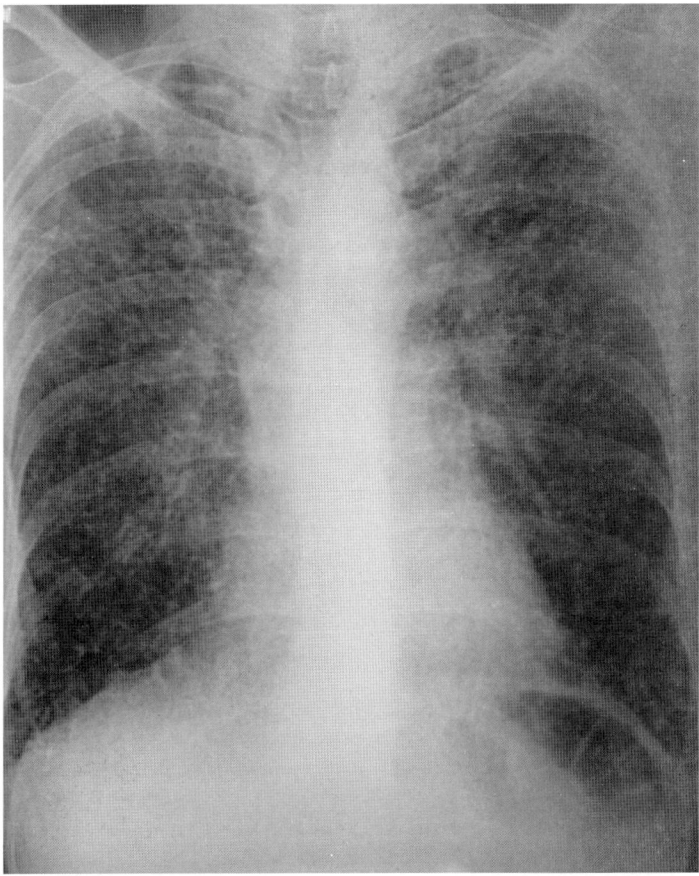

Fig 44.3: ILD. X-ray chest demonstrates reticulonodular opacities in the upper and mid-zones. The reticulonodular opacities indicate ILD. In view of the upper and mid-zone involvement, the possibility of an IPF is less likely. HRCT chest revealed peribronchial interstitial thickening as a result of chronic hypersensitivity pneumonitis.

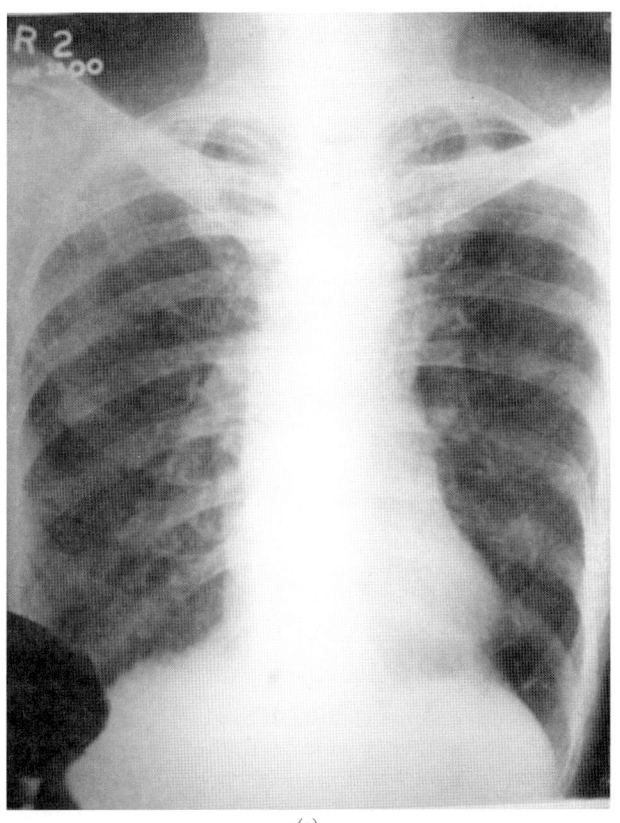

(a)

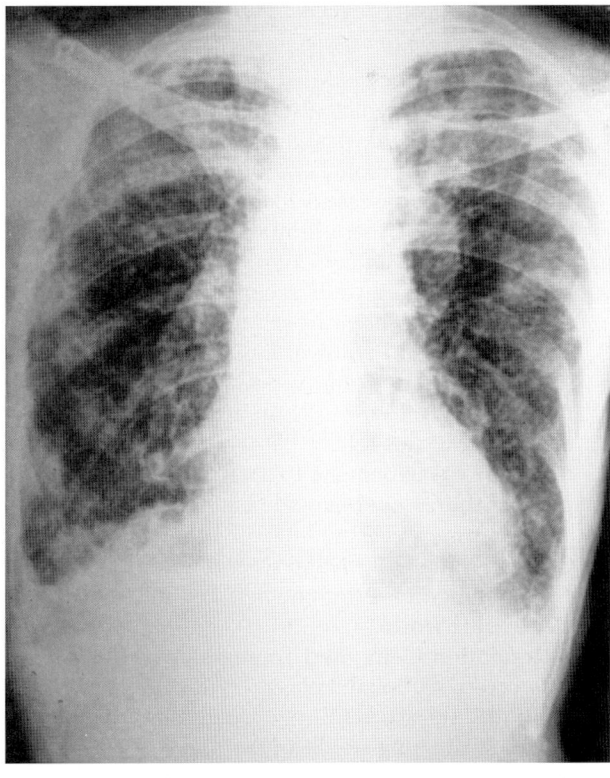

(b)

Fig 44.4: (a) Chest X-ray reveals reticular opacities in a patient with IPF. (b) Follow-up X-ray after six years demonstrates progression of disease process. The chest X-ray has a low specificity and sensitivity in diffuse lung diseases but is an easy and cheap modality to assess progression of the disease.

diagnosing individual ILDs. In the study by Mathieson referred to earlier, a confident diagnosis was reached more than twice as often with CT than with chest radiography. This diagnosis was correct in 93% of cases compared with 77% of cases of first-choice radiographic diagnosis. If clinical features, chest radiography and HRCT are combined there is an exponential increase in diagnostic accuracy to 66–80% of patients with ILD. It must be noted that the diagnostic accuracy of HRCT is highly disease-dependent. Thus, when the HRCT appearance is typical of UIP, the diagnosis is correct > 90% of times. On the other hand, the wide range of HRCT patterns of NSIP makes this a difficult diagnosis to accurately make on CT.

c. *Observer variations* amongst thoracic radiologists to make a histo-specific diagnosis are not uncommon and inter-observer variation is especially divergent in NSIP.

d. *HRCT and Biopsy:* HRCT may make a biopsy unnecessary. A typical HRCT pattern of UIP in an elderly male with the classic history is diagnostic of IPF so often that a biopsy is not indicated in this situation. More and more centres are relying on typical CT features to help them decide which patients need not undergo biopsy, thus sparing these elderly patients from undergoing an

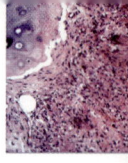

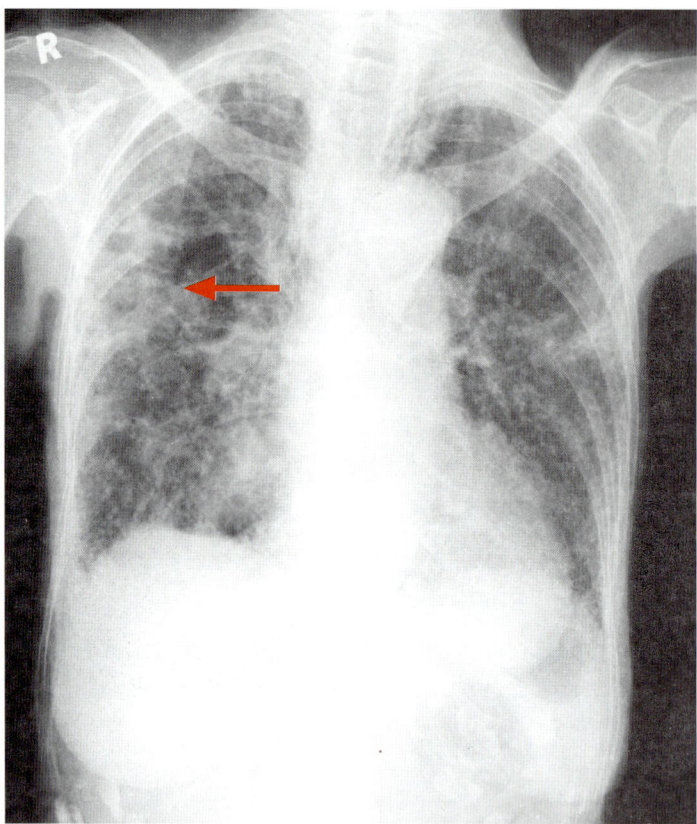

Fig 44.5: IPF with opportunistic infection. Chest X-ray reveals reticular opacities in both lung fields as a result of IPF, ill-defined areas of consolidation with cavitation in right upper lobe. Patient was on long-term treatment with immunosuppresants for IPF, developed cough with expectoration and fever. The right upper lobe consolidation with cavitation was due to an opportunistic infection. Sputum was positive for acid-fast bacilli (AFB).

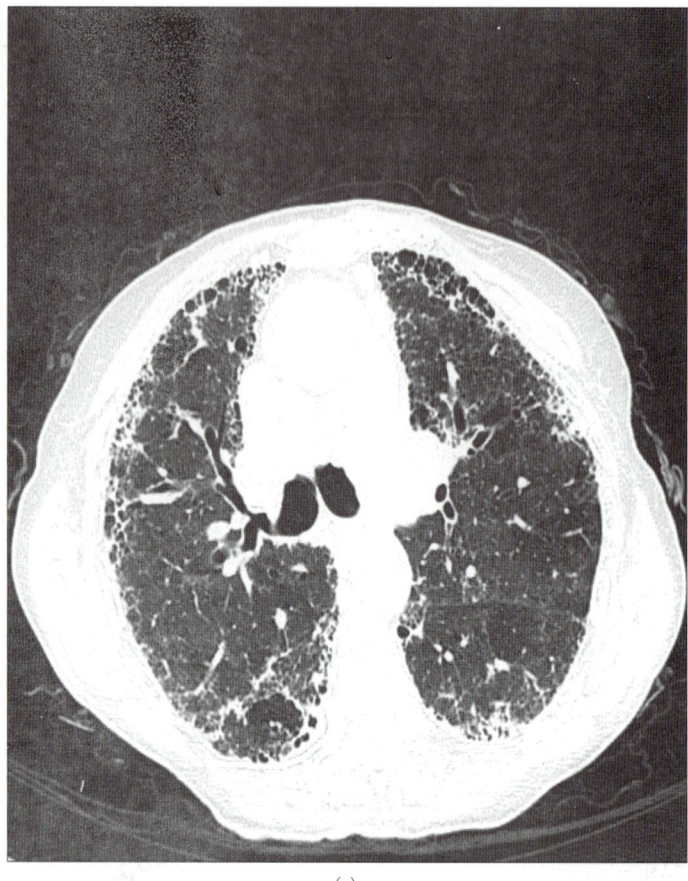

(a)

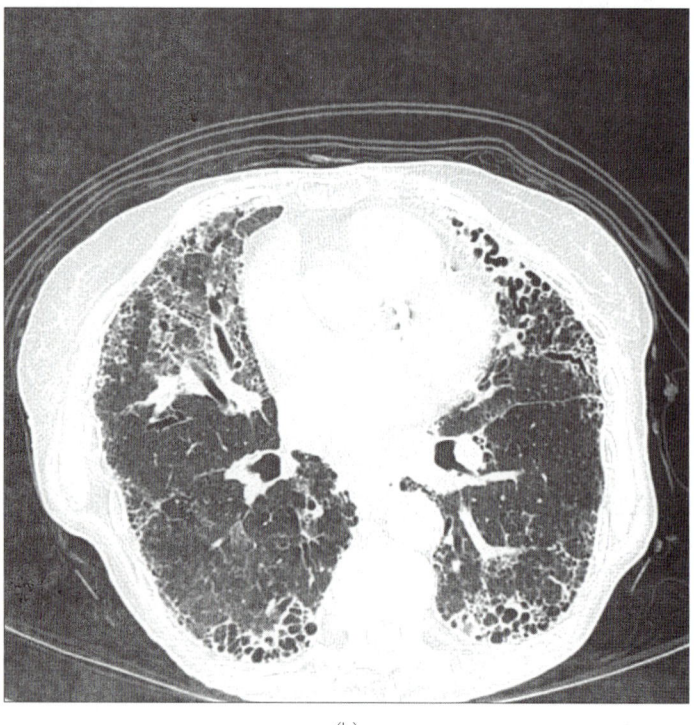

(b)

Fig 44.6: UIP: (a and b) HRCT chest demonstrates thin-walled honeycomb cysts in a subpleural location, especially with adjacent septal thickening involving the subpleural interstitium. These features favour a diagnosis of usual interstitial pneumonia (UIP), there is no significant involvement of the peribronchovascular interstitium or ground-glass densities to suggest a diagnosis of NSIP.

invasive procedure. Conversely, if the CT findings are atypical in any way then a biopsy should be ideally performed. An HRCT may also provide invaluable information to the surgeon on which lobes or segments of the lung he should sample for biopsy.

e. *HRCT and Disease Reversibility*: A ground-glass pattern on HRCT predicts the response to treatment and increased survival compared to patients in whom the predominant CT type is reticulation. The HRCT pattern of honeycombing is highly predictive of an irreversible pattern that is unlikely to respond even with high doses of immunosuppressive therapy.

f. *HRCT and Detecting Complications*: HRCT is an accurate way of picking up complications of an ILD in a patient faring poorly. TB is an important opportunistic infection and may be impossible to pick up on traditional chest radiography in a patient with pre-existing fibrosis. An HRCT may, on the other hand, pick up a cavity or infiltrate that can be a useful pointer to TB. A septal carcinoma is another complication that can be picked up more accurately on CT scanning compared to chest radiography.

6. **Pulmonary Function Testing (PFT):** A restrictive defect is the most frequent ventilatory abnormality in patients with ILDs. A drop in the transfer factor may be the only

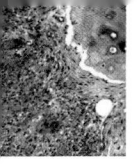

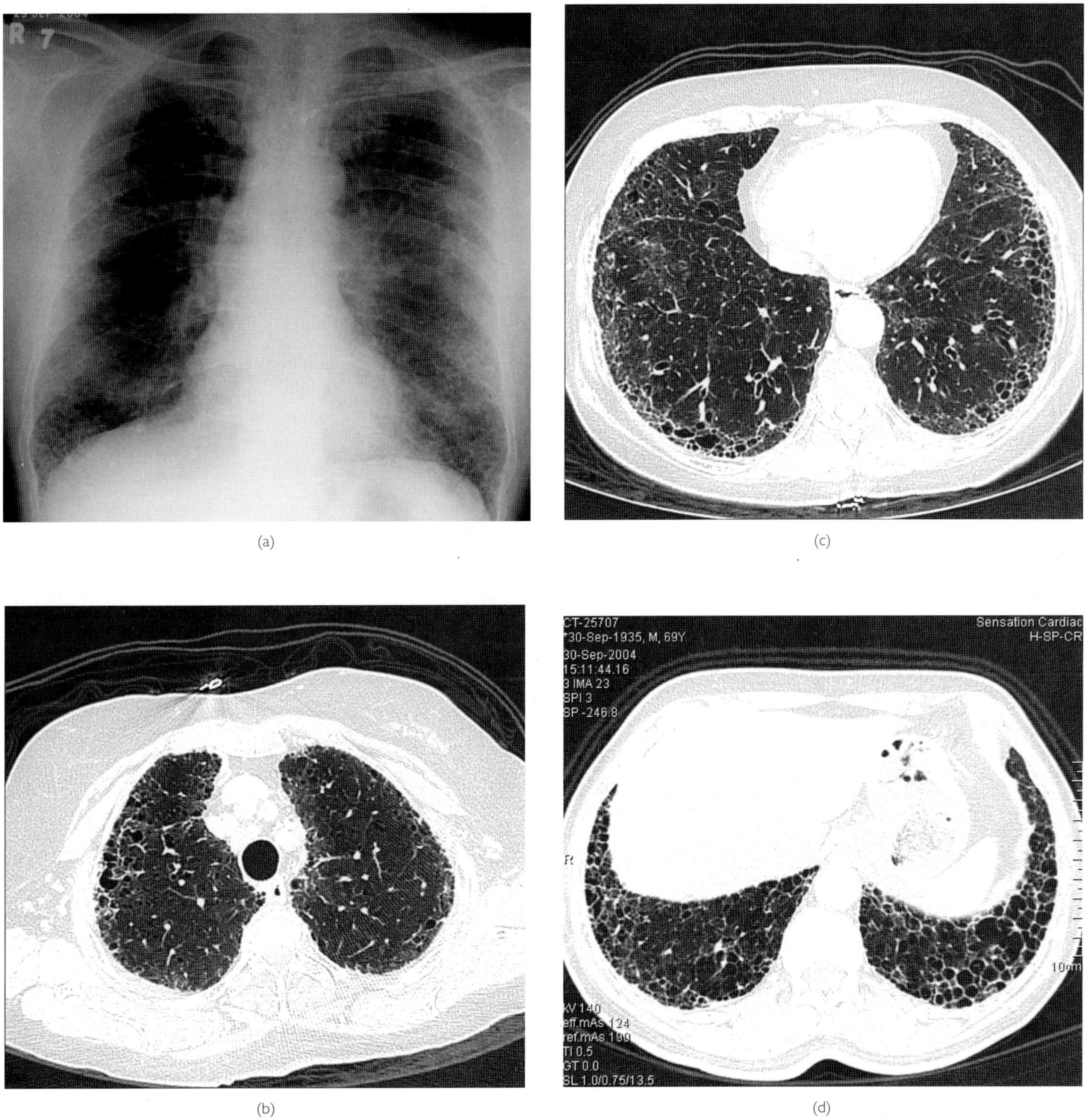

(a)

(b)

(c)

(d)

Fig 44.7: UIP: (a) Chest X-ray demonstrates reticular and honeycomb changes in both lung fields, especially lung bases. HRCT chest (b, c, d) demonstrates similar appearances of honeycomb cysts with septal thickening in subpleural regions. No ground-glass densities are seen indicating UIP pattern of interstitial pneumonia.

abnormality in patients with ILD; spirometry may be normal in early stages. Some ILDs such as LAM and Histiocytosis X have a mixed picture, with evidence of gas trapping with increased lung volumes and an increased RV/TLC ratio. Patients with ILD who smoke and have concomitant

emphysema have even more severely reduced transfer factors than non-smokers with ILD.

The aims of lung function testing in ILD are to quantify disease severity, monitor disease progression and, ideally, to identify variables that predict mortality.

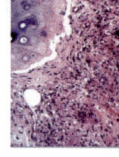

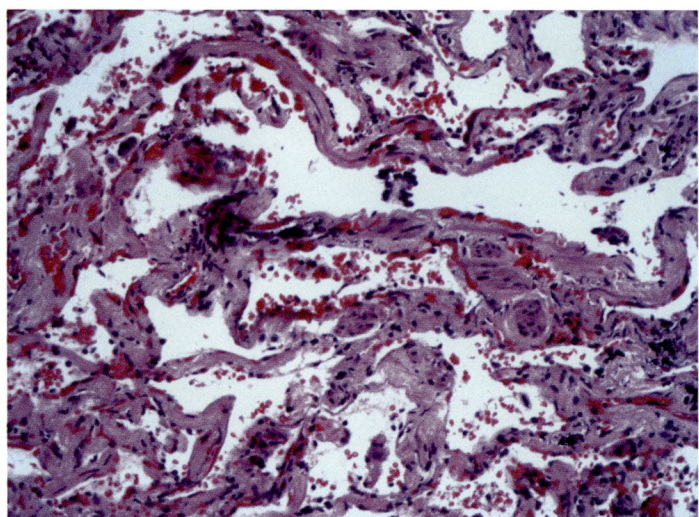

Fig 44.8: Usual interstitial pneumonia, markedly thickened, widened fibrotic interstitial septae.

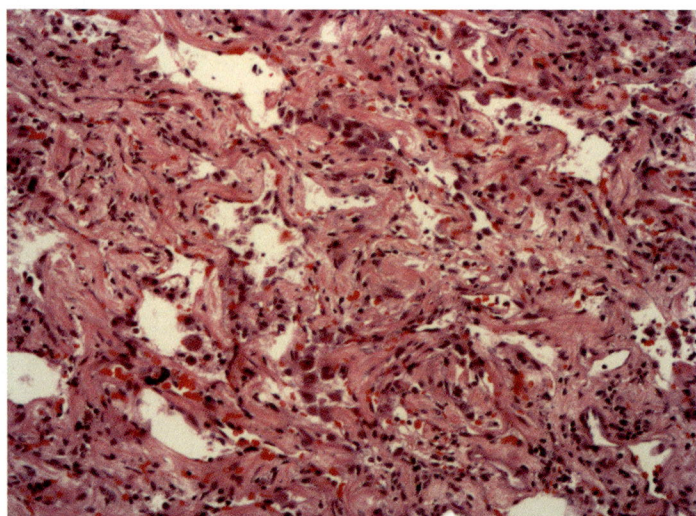

Fig 44.9: Usual interstitial pneumonia, late stage. Marked fibrotic thickened interstitial septae with collapse of alvelae.

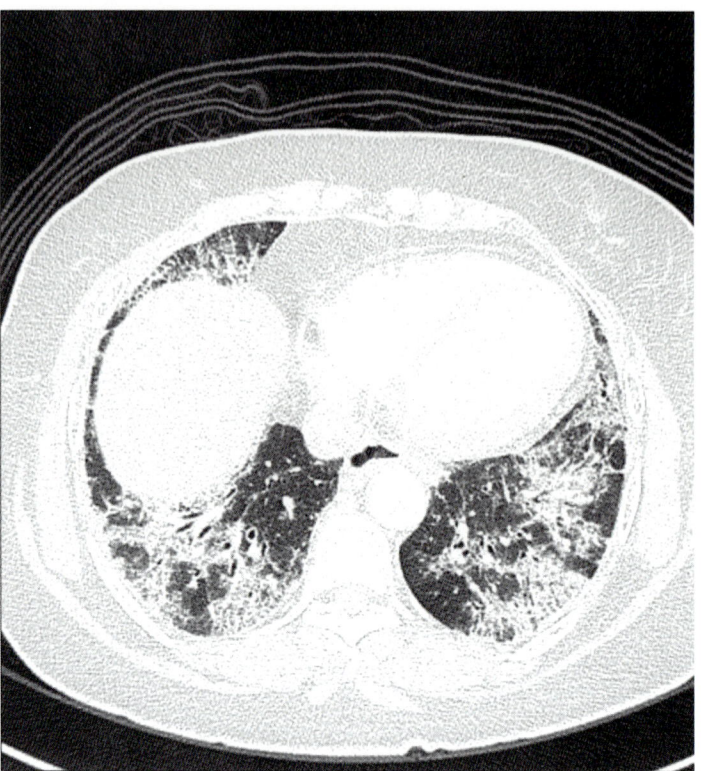

Fig 44.10: NSIP. HRCT chest demonstrates ill-defined ground-glass densities in both lung bases in a peribronchovascular and subpleural location, there are no honeycomb changes. These features are indicative of NSIP pattern of interstitial pneumonia.

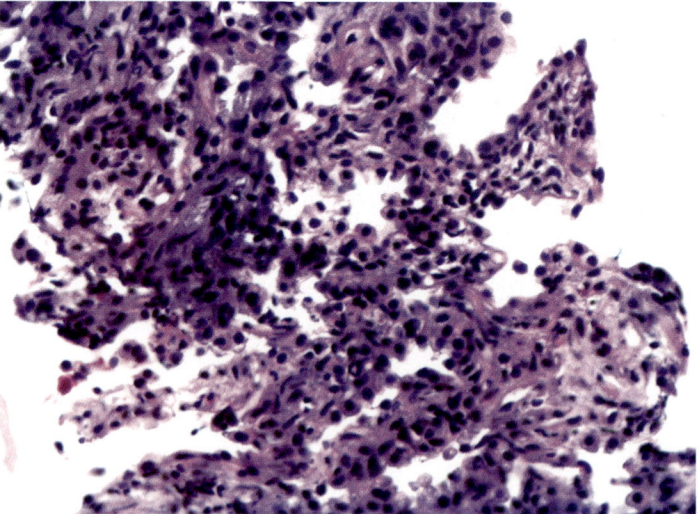

Fig 44.11: NSIP. H &E 40x. NSIP, cellular phase. Diffuse uniform interstitial inflammatory infiltrate is present in the interstitium, composed predominantly of lymphocytes. The alveoli show hyperplasia of Type II pneumocytes. Temporal uniformity is noted. Fibrosis is indiscernible.

Several studies have shown that the worse the PFT at presentation the worse the outcome. A Transfer Factor of the lung for carbon monoxide (TLCO) < 35% was associated with a mean survival of only 24 months with no difference in the outcome between IPF and NSIP. Thus the severity of IPF is best staged by TLCO estimation.

Serial lung function is a simple, non-invasive and easily reproducible way to monitor disease progression. Change in Forced vital capacity (FVC) and TLCO have emerged as the serial PFT measurements most consistently predictive of mortality. A decline in FVC of 10% and a decline in TLCO of 20% from their baseline values are predictive of a 2.4-fold increase in mortality. A study by Latsi et al. showed that serial FVC trends are even more reliable than serial TLCO trends in predicting poor survival. Even more interestingly, his study showed that the histological diagnosis is irrelevant once lung function

changes over 12 months have been taken into account. (*Latsi PL, du Bois RM, Nicholson AG et al. Fibrotic idiopathic interstitial pneumonia: the prognostic value of longitudinal functional trends. Am J Respir Crit Care Med 2003; 168; 531–537*)

Desaturation during exercise is a sensitive but not specific test for diagnosing ILD. The six-minute walk test (6MWT)

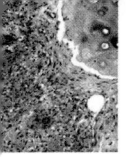

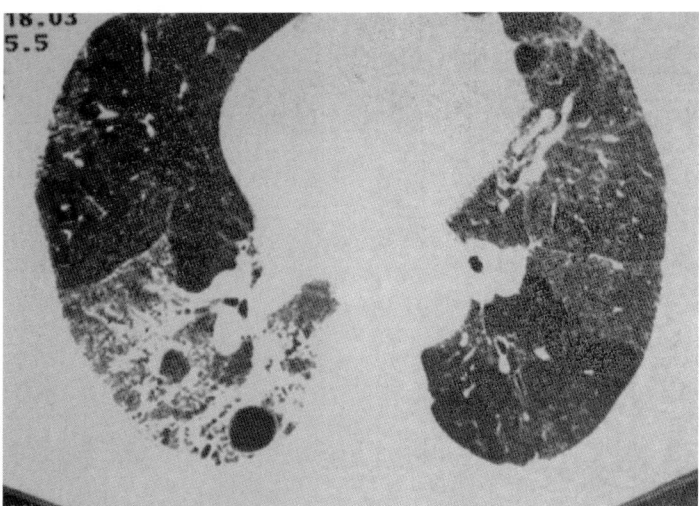

Fig 44.12: Desquamative interstitial pneumonia. HRCT chest demonstrates diffuse ground-glass densities in both lung fields, particularly in the right lung base. There are thin-walled cysts seen in the right lung base as well as the left lingula. The patient was a chronic smoker. These features of ground-glass densities with lung cysts are typical in smokers, representing desquamative interstitial pneumonia.

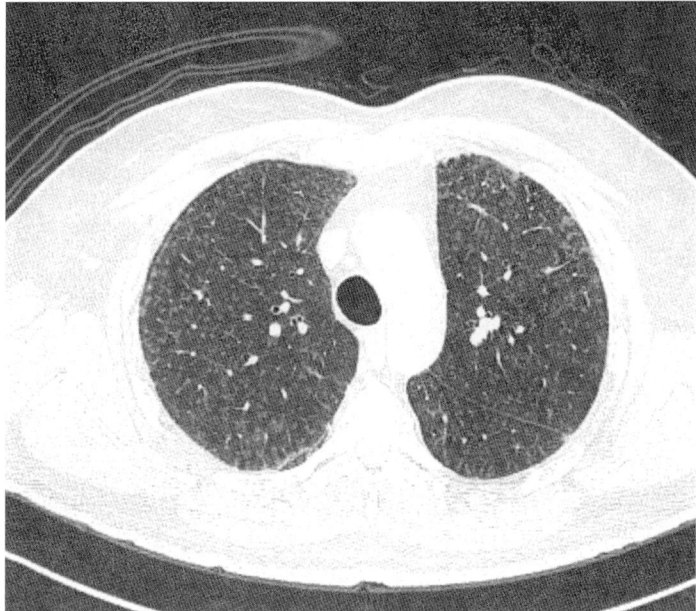

Fig 44.14: Respiratory bronchiolitis. HRCT chest in a chronic smoker demonstrates small centrilobular nodules in both lung fields. These are small with ill-defined margins representing respiratory bronchiolitis.

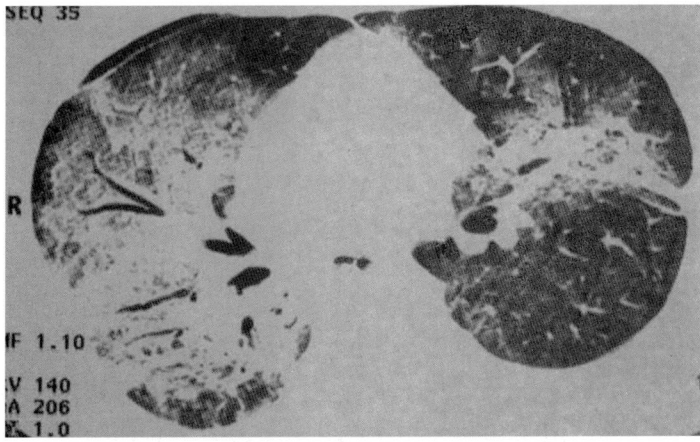

Fig 44.13: Acute interstitial pneumonia. HRCT demonstrates diffuse ill-defined ground-glass densities/consolidation with airbronchograms in both lung fields. Patient presented with acute onset of respiratory failure. This represents acute interstitial pneumonia, patient responded well to corticosteroid therapy.

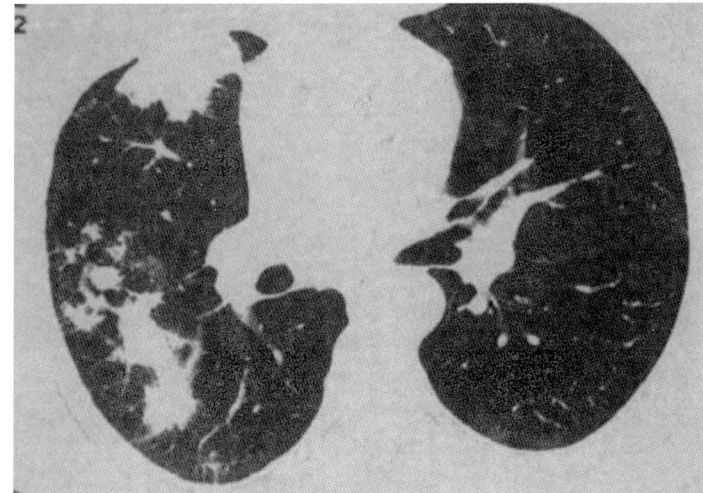

Fig 44.15: COP. HRCT chest demonstrates ill-defined subpleural and peribronchovascular consolidations in the right lung. Patient had a high ESR, biopsy of subpleural consolidation revealed COP. Patient had an excellent response to oral corticosteroid therapy.

has only recently been applied to ILD but has provided powerful prognostic information in four studies of IPF. Indeed, desaturation to 88% in a baseline 6MWT either during or at the end of the walk has emerged as a much more powerful predictor of mortality than resting lung function tests. A recent study concluded that desaturation < 88% was associated with a survival of 3.2 years compared to median survival of 6.6 years in those patients who maintained saturation > 88%. Two recent studies have also confirmed the prognostic significance of distance walked in the 6MWT in IPF patients. Those walking < 212 meters had a significantly lower survival than those walking further distances. The distance walked may also be of prognostic value. Attempts to formulate a combined measure of desaturation and distance covered may represent a novel and useful marker of disease severity and prognosis. Serial 6MWT is also useful in following up disease progression. Thus 6MWT is a cheap, simple, reproducible but underutilized monitoring tool in patients with ILD. It requires no equipment apart from an oximeter and a clock and can be done even in smaller centres without facilities for measuring transfer factor.

The ATS/ERS have published a set of clinical criteria supporting the diagnosis of IPF. These are summarized below: (*American Thoracic Society/European Respiratory Society Idiopathic pulmonary fibrosis: diagnosis and treatment. International Consensus Statement. Am J Respir Crit Care Med 2000; 161; 646–664.*)

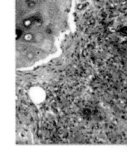

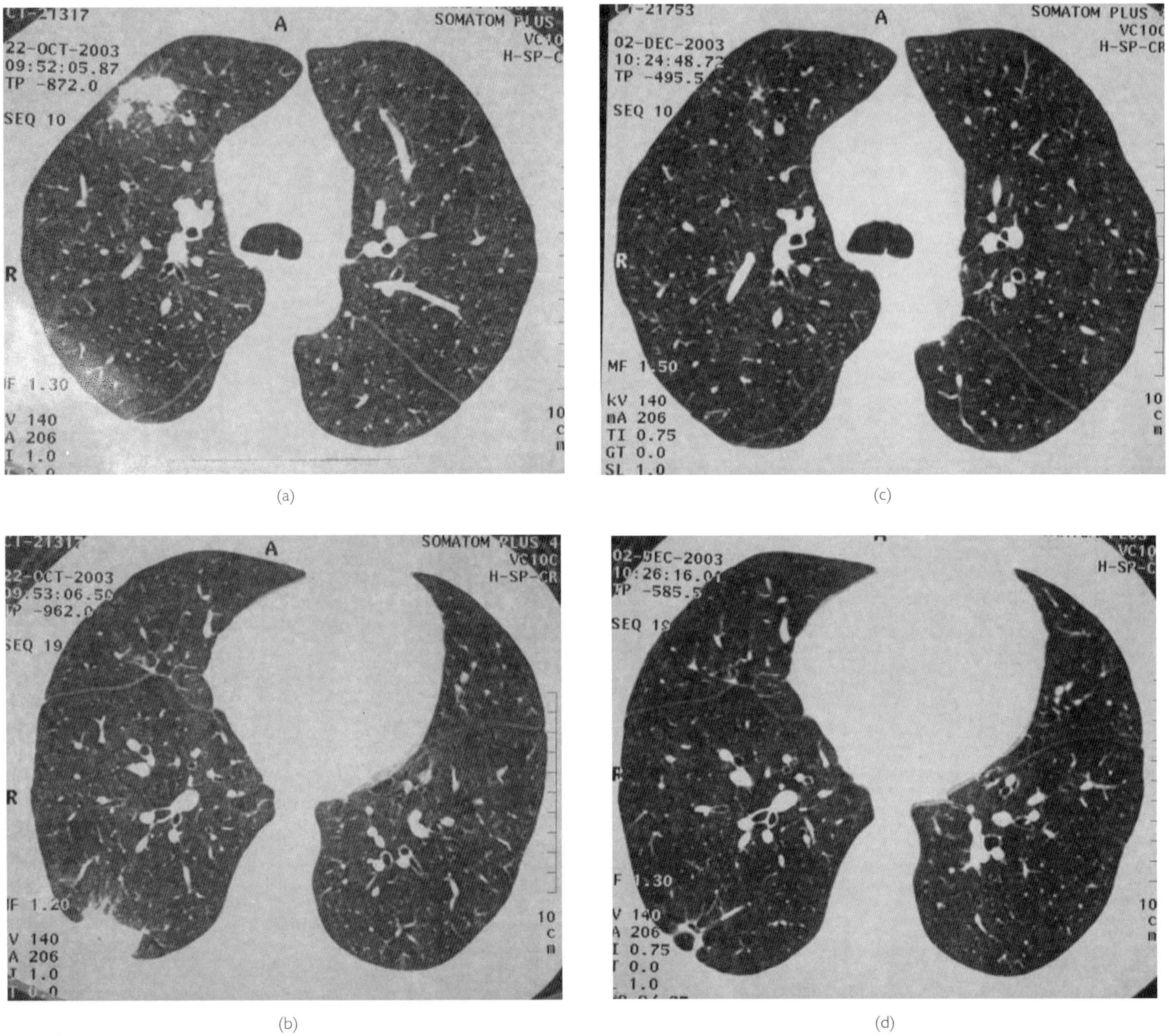

(a)

(b)

(c)

(d)

Fig 44.16: Middle-aged man with a right upper zone opacity treated with antibiotics and antitubercular drugs. Opacity in right lung upper zone persisted. HRCT chest revealed ill-defined peribronchial and subpleural consolidation (b) right lower zone lesion (c) right upper zone lesion resolves (d) right lower zone lesion also resolves. Patient had a high ESR, biopsy revealed COP; after treatment all lesions resolved (c) (d).

7. **Bronchoscopy, Bronchoalveolar Lavage (BAL), and Transbronchial Lung Biopsy (TBLBx):** Bronchoscopy and BAL are likely to add diagnostic value in only a few situations. BAL is useful if a secondary infection like TB is suspected in a patient with ILD. BAL may also be of value in rarer ILDs with eosinophilia or in pulmonary alveolar proteinosis when proteinaceous PAS positive material may be of diagnostic value. Outside these settings, BAL remains a research tool. BAL lymphocyte ratios (CD4/CD8) are raised in sarcoidosis but lowered in EAA. Other BAL cell fractions have been studied as well: BAL neutrophilia is believed to be linked to the extent and severity of disease, while BAL eosinophilia is linked to disease progression. However, these generalizations are not discriminatory enough for us to recommend BAL in the routine workup of a patient with ILD.

Transbronchial lung biopsy cannot replace a surgical biopsy. It cannot determine the type of IIP encountered. Having said this, it may be of great diagnostic value in sarcoidosis, EAA, BOOP and occasionally in PAP. We recently reported a series of over 30 cases of BOOP all of whom had been diagnosed on TBLBx thus sparing the patient the need for open lung biopsy.

8. **Open lung biopsy:** An open biopsy is the only way to accurately determine which of the seven types of IIP a

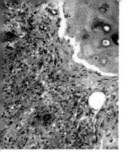

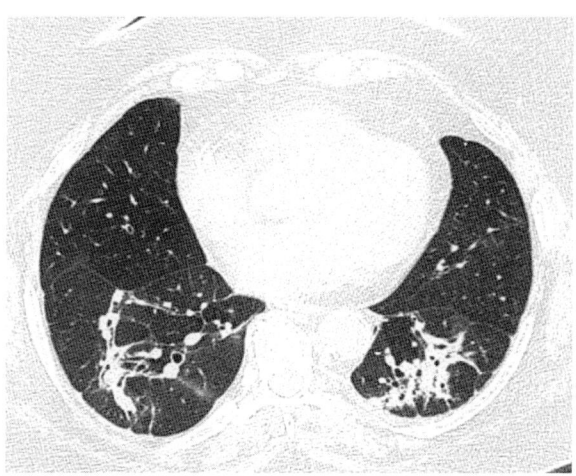

Fig 44.17: COP. HRCT demonstrates ill-defined peribronchial consolidations and fibrotic lesions. Biopsy revealed COP. The peribronchial and subpleural location is an important indicator to the diagnosis of COP.

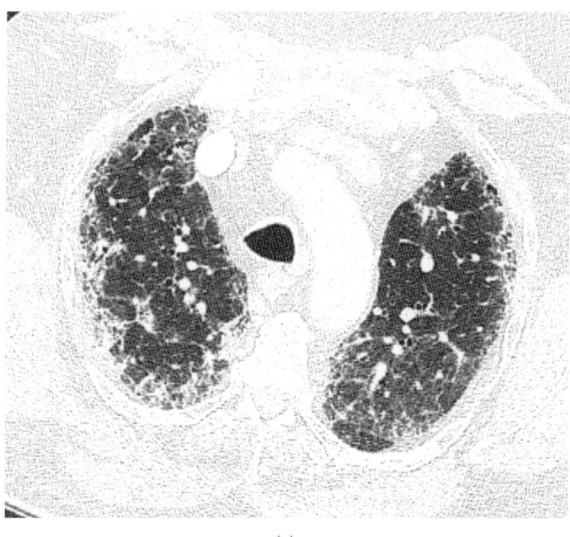

(a)

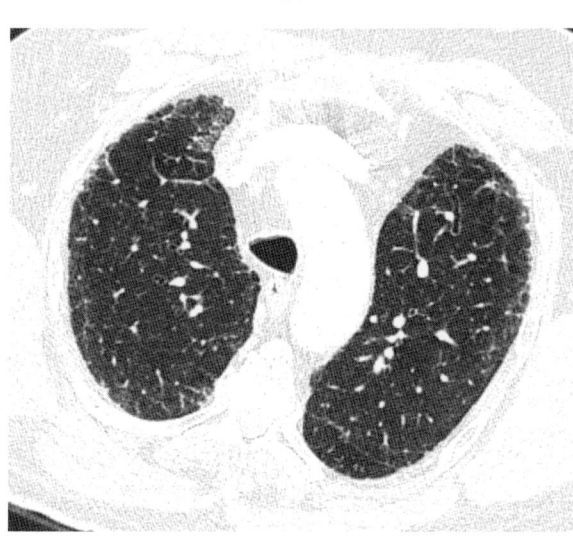

(b)

patient has. It is also often the only way to make a definitive diagnosis in patients with many of the rarer DPLDs. There is a natural reluctance in the minds of many physicians to subject their patients to an invasive procedure like an open lung biopsy. These patients are often elderly, have impaired lung function and multiple comorbidities. Furthermore, it is often argued that since there are limited effective therapies for IPF, pathological diagnosis does little to change overall management. As a result the frequency with which a surgical lung biopsy is performed is very low.

A number of questions need to be asked:

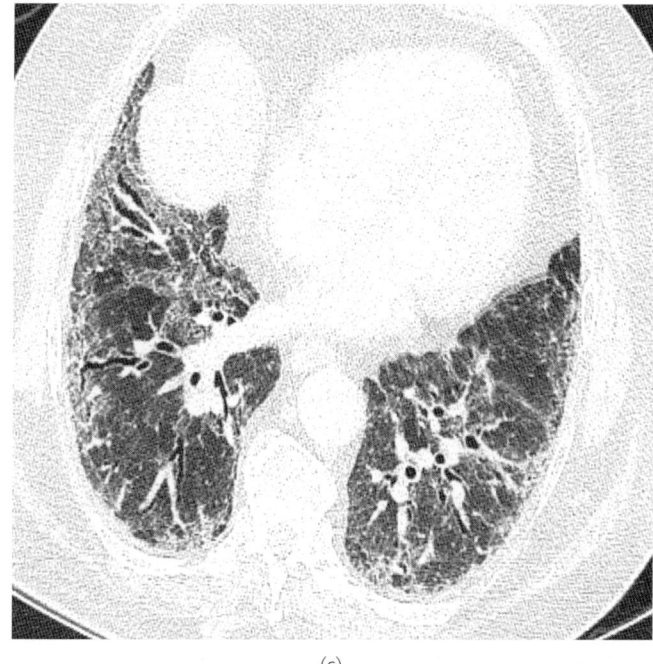

(c)

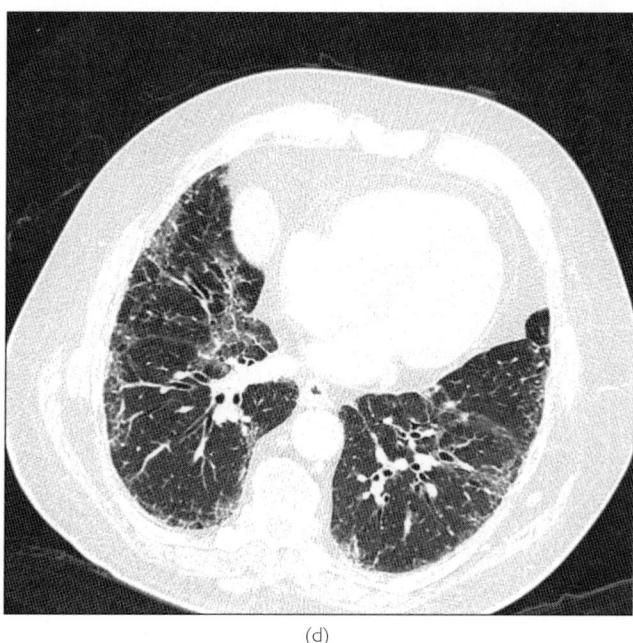

(d)

Fig 44.18: NSIP. HRCT demonstrates ill-defined ground-glass densities in a peribronchovascular and subpleural location with associated traction bronchiectasis (a, c). No significant honeycomb changes are visualized. These features are of NSIP. Follow-up CT studies (b, d) after treatment reveal resolution in ground-glass densities with residual traction bronchiectasis.

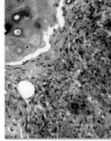

Table 44.3:
ATS/ERS criteria for diagnosing IPF
Major Criteria (mandatory)
1. Exclusion of other causes of ILD
2. Abnormal PFT
3. Bi-basal reticular abnormalities with minimal ground glass opacities on HRCT
4. BAL or transbronchial biopsy excluding all other alternative diagnosis
Minor criteria (3 of 4 mandatory)
1. Age > 50 years
2. Insidious onset of otherwise unexplained dyspnoea on exertion
3. Duration of illness of > 3 months
4. Bi-basal, inspiratory, dry crackles

a) *With advances in HRCT, is a biopsy still needed?*
HRCT is a critical element in the diagnosis of IIP but unfortunately often cannot be relied on to make an accurate diagnosis. When the classic findings of reticulonodular opacities at the bases and peripheries of the lung, with associated traction bronchiectasis and honeycombing are present, the diagnostic accuracy of CT approaches 90–100% and can then obviate the need for a biopsy. Unfortunately these features are found in only 50% or less of patients with IPF. For the non-UIP subtypes, radiographic specificity drops even further. An elegant study asked how frequently combined clinical and HRCT data can confidently diagnose IPF making open lung biopsy unnecessary. (*Hunning-hake GW, Zimmerman MB, Schwartz DA et al. Utility of a lung biopsy for the diagnosis of idiopathic pulmonary fibrosis. Am J Respir Crit Care Med. 2001; 164: 193–196.*)
When expert pulmonologists and radiologists agreed on a core diagnosis of IPF with high clinical confidence, the positive predictive value approached 90%. Unfortunately a confident clinical diagnosis can be achieved in only 50% of these patients. The accuracy decreased even more when the diagnosis was less certain and especially in non-UIP subtypes. Thus often an open lung biopsy remains the only way to obtain a definite diagnosis.

b) *Is it safe*: In experienced hands a surgical biopsy is safe. Advances in anaesthesia and surgical techniques have made the procedure much safer. A study for risk factors showed that advanced age, low diffusion capacity, need for oxygen therapy and pulmonary hypertension are all independent risk factors for complications and mortality after a surgical biopsy. Video-assisted thoracoscopic surgery (VATS) has revolutionized the procedure and the 30-day mortality is no more than 1–3% when these high-risk patients are excluded.

c) *Technical considerations*: Biopsies should be ideally taken early in the disease not only because this is safer but because when end-stage fibrosis has developed little further histological information can be gleaned.

Biopsy should be taken after careful discussion with the radiologist, from more than one lobe (preferably both upper and lower) to improve the overall yield. When discordant findings are obtained in samples from different sites (for example, UIP in one lobe and NSIP in another), these patients must be presumed to have UIP for their prognosis is comparable to concordant UIP.

d) *What advantages are there from obtaining a surgical biopsy?* A definite label of UIP on biopsy allows a patient to be labelled a definite case of IPF. This has great prognostic value and such information is useful for patients and their families. Novel therapies are constantly being developed and such patients can ideally be enrolled in trials with these new agents armed with the knowledge that their survival with routine immunosuppressives alone is likely to be dismal.

e) *So who should it be done on?* Even the most aggressive-minded physician would agree that there is little to be gained in subjecting an 80–year-old male with gross clubbing and distinctive crackles who has an HRCT showing classical basal and peripheral honeycombing to an open lung biopsy. However, in younger patients or those with atypical features on HRCT a surgical biopsy would be ideal and might provide useful insights into the patients' further course and outcome.

9. **Putting it all together:** In no other branch of respiratory medicine is close coordination between physician, radiologist and pathologist more important than in the ILDs. Even an expert pathologist will be lost without the input provided by the clinician and radiologist. This multidisciplinary approach is recommended so that the patient has the benefit of a unified clinicopathological diagnosis.

Major Criteria (must have 4)

1. Exclusion of other known causes of ILD such as drugs, environmental exposures etc.
2. Abnormal PFT which includes evidence of restriction (reduced VC with normal FEV_1/FVC ratio) and impaired gas exchange (increased alveolar-arterial oxygen gradient at rest or with exercise or decreased TLCO).
3. Bi-basal reticular abnormalities with minimal ground-glass opacities on HRCT.
4. Transbronchial lung biopsy or bronchoalveolar lavage (BAL) showing no features to support an alternative diagnosis.

Minor Criteria (must have at least 3 of 4)

1. Age > 50 years
2. Insidious onset of otherwise unexplained dyspnoea on exertion.
3. Duration of illness of > 3 months
4. Bi-basal, inspiratory, dry crackles.

TREATMENT

Patients with newly diagnosed IPF currently have a mean life expectancy of 2.9 to 5 years. No current drug or regime has the ability to check the relentless decline in lung function that characterizes this condition. The heterogeneous group of

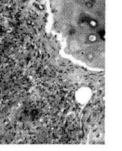

Table 44.4:
Radiology and histopathological features of various interstitial pneumonias

Type of Pneumonia	Radiology	Histopathology
UIP	Reticular abnormality, honey combing, basal peripheral predominance, often patchy with intervening normal lung	Heterogenous areas of young connective tissue, scarring, honeycomb changes, normal lung
NSIP	Ground-glass abnormality. Reticular shadows, traction bronchiectasis, basal predominance with or without subpleural sparing	Alveolar septal thickening by inflammation/fibrosis Spatially and temporarily homogenous
DIP	Ground glass, basal peripheral pre-dominance with or without cysts	Diffuse macrophage accumulation within alveolar spaces, mild interstitial thickening. Homogenous involvement
RBILD	Centrilobular nodules Ground-glass attenuation Diffuse/upper lobe predominance	Bronchogenic accumulation of alveolar macrophages. Mild bronchiolar fibrosis
AIP	Ground glass consolidation, organizing architectural distortion, traction bronchiectasis.	Acute oedema, hyaline membrane, interstitial inflammation, airspace organization
LIP	Ground glass, septal thickening, cysts, diffuse or lower lung distribution	Diffuse alveolar Infiltration by lymphocytes Infrequent lymphoid Hyperplasia
OP	Consolidation in peribronchial/subplueral distribution	Intraluminal organizing fibrosis in bronchioles, alveolar ducts and alveoli. Temporarily homogenous patchy distribution

Table 44.5:
Diagnosis of ILD

1. History—dry cough, dyspnoea

2. Clinical examination—Dry 'velcro' crackles, specific features related to ILD secondary to a known cause (e.g. connective tissue disease)

3. Chest radiography—Useful for diagnosis, pattern recognition and for serial monitoring

4. HRCT chest—Sensitivity of 95% for diagnosis, ground-glass pattern predicts reversibility, detects complications

5. Pulmonary function test—Restrictive pattern. Reduced transfer factor; reduced FVC; reduced lung volumes. Some ILDs have a mixture of obstructive + restrictive pattern. Helps monitor disease

6. Bronchoscopy, Bronchoalveolar lavage (BAL)—Adds diagnostic value in just a few situations

7. VATS/Open lung biopsy—Only way for a definitive diagnosis in the rarer forms. Not required in the typical UIP.

patients with NSIP and other non-typeable IIPs has a better outcome and there are significant numbers of patients who seem to at least stabilize with treatment. Hence although the outcome for the classic IPF is bleak, treatment should always be offered after a careful and realistic discussion of the benefit of treatment versus the potential side-effects of the drugs. The following treatment options will be discussed:

1. **Steroids**: Steroids in the earlier decades were the standalone treatment of choice for IPF. Large doses of up to 1 mg/kg prednisolone were recommended and major side-effects were encountered in this usually elderly population of patients. Steroids in these doses ended up doing more harm than good and objective improvement occurred in no more than 12% of those who received them. The earlier studies have

been subjected to current scrutiny, and an elegant Cochrane review by Richeldi recently concluded that there is no role for steroids alone in the management of IPF. (*Richeldi L, Davies HRHR, Spagnolo P, Luppi F Cochrane Database of Systematic Reviews 2009, Issue 2. Art. No.: CD002880.*) Currently, low doses of steroids in combination with other immunosuppressives are the treatment of choice as we shall discuss later.

2. **Azathioprine**: is a purine analogue which inhibits DNA synthesis and has widespread immunosuppressive effects. No study has looked at this as the sole drug in IPF but two prospective studies have evaluated its effects in combination with steroids. There was some survival benefit documented in one study but no improvement in lung function. This drug is felt to have a steroid-sparing effect, is generally well

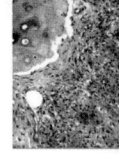

tolerated and has hence along with steroids become the current immunosuppressive regimen of choice.

3. **N-acetylcystine (NAC)**: The clinical observation that lung epithelial lining fluid from patients with IPF had depleted glutathione laid the foundation for clinical trials of NAC. A landmark study called the IFIGENIA study published in the NEJM added NAC in a dose of 600 mg thrice a day or placebo to 155 patients with confident or probable diagnosis of IPF. (*Demedts M, Behr J, Buhl R, et al. High dose acetylcystine in idiopathic pulmonary fibrosis. N Engl J Med 2005; 353; 2229–2242.*) The results were encouraging with the patients who received NAC having a slower decline in lung function than those not receiving it. NAC was postulated to have a synergistic effect with steroid and azathioprine. Trials of NAC alone versus placebo are urgently needed to tease out how much of this benefit was due to NAC alone.

Based on our current knowledge the current recommended treatment of IPF is a triple combination of low-dose steroid, azathioprine and NAC.

4. **Interferon-γ-1b (IFNγ-1b)**: is a Th 1 cytokine that has been shown to downregulate collagen gene expression and suppress the effects of profibrotic growth factors. An initial study by Ziesche *et al.* caused great excitement in the field when it was reported that nine patients who received steroids and IFNγ-1b showed stabilized or in some cases, even improved lung function compared to patients on steroids alone. However, this remains a highly controversial study with doubts raised about whether these patients had true IPF. (*Ziessche R, Hofbauer E, Wittmann K et al. A preliminary study of long term treatment with interferon gamma-1b and low dose prednisolone in patients with idiopathic pulmonary fibrosis. N Engl J Med 1999; 341; 1264–1269.*) Subsequent studies including a large Phase 3 randomized study of IFNγ-1b in 330 patients could not confirm these results and concluded that IFNγ-1b did not have any beneficial effect on PFT in patients with IPF and the drug cannot currently be recommended.

5. **Cyclophosphamide**: is an alkylating agent with powerful immunosuppressive properties. It is much more toxic than azathioprine and except in patients with scleroderma-related ILD where it may be the drug of choice it has no added benefit over azathioprine in IPF.

6. **Pirfenidone**: is a pyridine which inhibits fibroblast proliferation and collagen synthesis. This drug, currently only marketed in Japan, may have some effect on IPF progression and recent publications have been promising. More specifically, it is believed to prevent acute exacerbations, a dangerous complication of IPF.

7. **Newer drugs and experimental agents**: Bosentan, an endothelin receptor blocker, etanercept, a tumour necrosis factor blocker are two drugs currently undergoing trials. Other drugs that have been considered are statins, sildenafil, thalidomide, imatinib mesylate and angiotensin inhibitors.

8. **General supportive measures**: Sadly, in the vast majority of patients with IPF, the disease continues to follow a relentlessly aggressive course. In these patients, all the caring physician can hope to provide is the best supportive care possible.

Cough is a disabling symptom and oral codeine in intractable cough and in end-stage disease even oral opiates have been tried. Gastro-oesophageal reflux can worsen cough and this should be treated with proton pump inhibitors.

Supplemental oxygen and treatment of breathlessness: Unlike in COPD, there is no evidence that oxygen therapy influences long-term survival in patients with IPF. However, breathlessness is the most distressing symptom for patients with IPF and oxygen undoubtedly provides symptomatic relief and improves quality of life. Initially, the IPF patient may be provided oxygen only during or after exertion or activity, but as the disease worsens and the PaO2 drops below 55 mm Hg, long-term oxygen via cylinders or concentrators may be the only 'drug' that provides these unfortunate patients some relief. Nebulized morphine has been tried but had no effect on the breathlessness of six patients with IPF. Oral opiates may provide some relief from this crippling symptom in end-stage patients.

Pulmonary rehabilitation: There is much less data on the role of pulmonary rehabilitation in ILD than in COPD.

Table 44.6: Treatment of ILD
1. Steroids
2. Azathioprine
3. N-acetylcystine (NAC)
4. Interferon-γ-1b (IFNγ-1b)
5. Cyclophosphamide
6. Pirfenidone
7. Newer drugs: Bosentan, etanercept, statins, sildenafil, thalidomide, imatinib mesylate and angiotensin inhibitors
8. General supportive measures like cough suppression, supplemental oxygen and pulmonary rehabilitation
9. Lung transplantation

Table 44.7: ATS/ERS recommendations for treatment of IPF
Corticosteroid (prednisolone):
0.5 mg/kg body weight orally for 4 weeks
0.25 mg/kg body weight for 8 weeks
Taper to 0.125 mg/kg/day on alternate days
PLUS
Azathioprine:
2–3 mg/kg/day—Start dosing at 25–30 mg/day with 1–2 weekly increment of 25 mg until the maximum dose is achieved. (Maximum dose—150 mg/day)
OR
Cyclophosphamide:
2 mg/kg/day—Start dosing at 25–50 mg/day with 1–2 weekly increment of 25 mg until the maximum dose is achieved. (Maximum dose—150 mg/day)

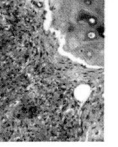

However, several recent observational studies show that it does improve quality of life.

9. **Lung Transplantation**: Lung transplantation is often the only option for the younger patient (less than 65 years) with advanced IPF. It is one of the commonest indications for lung transplantation in most centres. The actuarial survival following lung transplantation for IPF is 75% at one year and 50% at five years. The optimal timing for transplantation is unclear and varies from centre to centre. What is clear is that the measurement of TLCO has proved to be a dependable measure for predicting survival in patients with IPF and hence is a useful guide to timing of referral for transplantation. A TLCO < 35% has consistently been shown to be a marker of poor survival in patients, irrespective of histological type. Sadly, there are still no centres in India performing lung transplantation.

COMPLICATIONS OF ILD

1. **Acute exacerbations of IPF**: Some patients with IPF have an atypically precipitous course in which an acute deterioration follows a period of relative stability. When infectious causes of worsening are excluded by endotracheal aspiration or BAL, other causes of worsening like acute LVF and PE are ruled out, and when the HRCT shows bilateral ground-glass abnormality superimposed on the background of reticulation or honeycombing, the patient can be said to have an acute exacerbation. Disease severity does not predict the risk of acute exacerbation. Surgical biopsies are sometimes implicated as risk factors. The mortality may be as high as 90% but large pulses of steroids have been tried more in desperation than in the belief that they will help.

2. **Opportunistic infections**: Opportunistic infections are frequent in these immunosuppressed patients. TB is the most frequent in the Indian setting. It is difficult to diagnose and the clinician must have a high index of suspicion if he is not to miss it completely.

3. **Bronchial carcinomas** are not uncommon. In a review of the causes of death in 550 patients with IPF, 10% of all deaths were due to bronchial carcinoma. These are usually scar carcinomas arising from diffuse areas of scarring. They are most often localized adenocarcinoma or alveolar cell carcinomas. They are again difficult to diagnose and can only be treated palliatively as these patients are generally not candidates for resection or chemotherapy.

4. **Heart failure and ischemic heart disease**: Pulmonary hypertension and right heart failure are almost inevitable in advanced ILD and may contribute to mortality. These patients are usually elderly hence coexisting ischemic heart disease and LV dysfunction are also common.

5. **Pulmonary embolism**: has been reported to cause 3–7% of deaths in IPF. The real incidence may be higher because most of these patients are bedridden in the late stages of this disease.

6. **Pneumothorax**: can complicate fibrotic lungs. If it occurs it is often difficult to treat since the lung is stiff and difficult to expand. Prolonged intercostal tube drainage may be required as these patients are usually too unwell to undergo thoracoscopic intervention.

Table 44.8: Complications of ILD
1. Acute exacerbations of IPF
2. Opportunistic infections
3. Bronchial carcinomas
4. Heart failure and ischemic heart disease
5. Pulmonary embolism
6. Pneumothorax

A study by Panos looked at the causes of death in 550 patients with IPF. Mean survival ranged from 3.2 to 5 years. Respiratory failure (39%), heart failure (14%), bronchogenic carcinoma (10%) and ischemic heart disease (10%) were the four commonest causes of death in this series. (*Panos RJ, Mortenson R, Niccoli SA, King TE Jr. Clinical deterioration in patients with idiopathic pulmonary fibrosis. Causes and assessment. Am J Med 1990; 88; 396–404.*)

FEATURES OF ILD SPECIFIC TO INDIA

1. **Overlap with TB**: Because of the very high burden of TB in India, most patients with pulmonary symptoms and diffuse radiological opacities are invariably initially labelled TB. In our series of 134 patients of biopsy-proven sarcoidosis at the Hinduja Hospital, Mumbai, over a third (37%) were initially labelled TB and received several months of inappropriate anti-TB therapy before the correct diagnosis was confirmed. Another series of biopsy-confirmed BOOP from the same institution revealed that 10% were mislabelled TB and received inappropriate anti-TB therapy. Additionally, pulmonary infections like TB continue to remain frequent causes of pulmonary fibrosis. In a follow-up study of patients with newly diagnosed TB, residual fibrosis was seen in 40% of patients at three months and in 25% at 12 months. In all these patients follow-up HRCT scans showed evidence of fibrosis with irregular linear opacities. There is a tendency to over-diagnose such post-tubercular fibrosis as ILD. Post-tubercular fibrosis is neither progressive nor active. It usually affects the upper lobes and is limited to the site where the active TB originally occurred. A careful review of old chest radiographs should make the diagnosis of post-TB scarring obvious.

2. **Limitations of chest radiography**: In a resource-limited setting like India, the chest radiograph is per force given undue weightage for the diagnosis or exclusion of any condition. In a series of 117 biopsy-proven cases of IPF from the Hinduja Hospital in Mumbai, the chest radiograph was reported normal in as many as 27% of patients though subsequent CT scans showed them to have fairly advanced disease. Thus overdependence on chest radiographs for the diagnosis of DPLD may result in delays in diagnosis with large numbers of patients remaining undiagnosed or misdiagnosed till advanced fibrosis sets in.

3. **HRCT scanning in India**: The first attempts at HRCT scanning of the chest began in 1991, in centres in Mumbai and New Delhi. Currently, India has a CT scanner base of

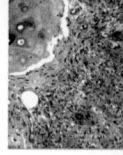

3000 machines which works out to 1 scanner per million population. This penetrance is considered very low when compared to other countries in the region: Korea and Japan have 31 and 92 per million population respectively. Besides the numbers it would not be unfair to claim that no more than a handful of radiologists countrywide would have an interest in chest imaging and using the correct end-inspiratory breath-holding techniques needed to obtain good-quality images.

4. **Lung function testing in India**: Only a few tertiary referral hospitals in the country have the equipment to perform diffusion capacity studies. 6MWTs although not requiring any specialized equipment are under-utilized.

5. **Surgical biopsy**: VATS is underutilized. Countrywide there are no more than 15 thoracic surgeons capable of performing this procedure. This results in delays in making a definitive diagnosis.

6. **Treatment issues in India:**
   a) *TB reactivation*: ILD patients on steroids and immuno-suppressants are prone to develop opportunistic infections of which TB is the most common. In a country where the rates of LTBI are as high as 50–70%, reactivation of TB is a constant worry in patients on immunosuppressants. In a study from the Hinduja Hospital, of 146 patients with systemic lupus erythematosus (SLE) who received steroids in a median cumulative dose of 7.5 mg for a median duration of 12 months, 17 patients went on to develop active TB. Ideally a tuberculin skin test or one of the IGRAs (interferon-gamma release assays) should be done prior to starting immunosuppressives, and isoniazid prophylaxis offered to those with a positive result. However, there is no consensus on the protective effect of isoniazid in this setting and care must be taken to rule out active disease prior to starting a single drug.
   b) *Diabetes flare-up*: India has the largest diabetic population in the world (30 million) and many patients with ILD will have pre-existing diabetes prior to starting steroids, while several will go on to develop it after commencement. It is vital to aim for tight control of diabetes in these patients on steroids.
   c) *Transplant*: Sadly, in a country of over 1 billion there is not a single centre performing lung transplantation. Large numbers of young DPLD patients thus have no recourse to this important intervention.

   The way ahead in this country involves increasing awareness amongst physicians, pulmonologists, radiologists and pathologists and establishing countrywide centres of excellence with special interest in these fascinating but neglected diseases.
   (*Udwadia ZF, Sen T, Jindal SK. Interstitial lung diseases in a resource-limited setting: the case of India. In Interstitial Lung Diseases. European Respiratory Monograph 46. December 2009. Editors: du Bois R, Richeldi L.*)

BRONCHIOLITIS OBLITERANS ORGANIZING PNEUMONIA

In 1983, Davidson described a clinicopathological entity which he called cryptogenic organizing pneumonia (COP). Two

Table 44.9: Features of ILD specific to India
1. Overlap with tuberculosis
2. Chest radiography is the main diagnostic tool but has significant limitations
3. Scarcity of HRCT machines (1 scanner per million population)
4. Lung function tests—only a few tertiary centers can perform CO diffusion studies
5. Surgical biopsy using VATS is underutilized
6. TB reactivation on treatment, increase in or precipitation of diabetes with treatment of the disease
7. No lung transplant facilities in India

years later Epler reported the same condition but labelled it bronchiolitis obliterans organizing pneumonia (BOOP). These two terms for the same disease, from different sides of the Atlantic have stood the test of time. COP probably is a better descriptor as it captures the clinical and radiological profile which is that of an alveolar rather than an airway disease. This is the term that will be used in the rest of this discussion. BOOP is the more commonly used term however, but care must be taken not to confuse it with 'bronchiolitis obliterans' which is a completely different and unrelated entity.

Aetiology

Organizing pneumonia can occur secondary to a number of diseases including infection, drug toxicity and connective tissue disorders. When it occurs in the absence of any of these known aetiologies it is termed cryptogenic. It can, on occasion, be found accompanying other histological patterns seen in patients with IIPs, such as UIP and NSIP in which case it is considered to be a secondary phenomenon. Thus when organizing pneumonia is found on lung biopsy, a careful search for other underlying pathology patterns and clinical conditions should be performed.

Clinical Features

COP often has a mean age of presentation of 50–60 years but has been reported at an age range of 20–80 with no gender predilection. Patients present acutely or subacutely with fever, malaise, cough and dyspnoea. It mimics a viral infection or a community-acquired pneumonia and most patients are labelled as such and receive multiple courses of antibiotics. Spontaneous remissions can occur in up to 50% of patients and in correctly treated patients the outcome is usually good with prompt resolution of symptoms and a slower improvement in radiology. Relapses are common but unpredictable and occur as the steroid dose is reduced with a 58% relapse rate being reported in a recent European cohort.

An acute fulminant variant of COP is also recognized without pulmonary fibrosis, presenting as an acute respiratory distress syndrome (ARDS). These patients are extremely ill and require mechanical ventilation but have an excellent and

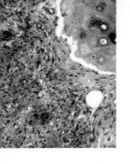

rapid response to steroids even at this stage. Fibrosing COP is another variant with this subtype having extensive fibrosis which can progress to a fatal outcome despite treatment. Finally, a unifocal form of COP occurs in about 10% of patients. Such forms present as a solitary pulmonary nodule (SPN) and undergo resection with the correct diagnosis being made only after histopathology is available.

HRCT

HRCT in COP shows a number of distinctive features. There are bilateral, patchy, air space consolidations with a subpleural or peribronchial distribution often with ground-glass opacities. Shadows sometimes resolve spontaneously on serial radiographs only to reappear in another area. Honeycombing is rare.

Other Tests

These patients often have a leukocytosis making the distinction from community-acquired pneumonia even more difficult. The ESR is almost always markedly elevated. BAL shows increased lymphocytes and foamy macrophages.

Pathology

COP can be definitively diagnosed only after a tissue biopsy. While earlier authors stressed the need for an open lung biopsy, our experience and that of others suggests that this is one IIP that can often be diagnosed by transbronchial lung biopsy. The characteristic lesion of COP is granulation tissue which proliferates within the distal air spaces, occluding the terminal bronchioles and alveolar ducts and spaces. These buds are called Masson's buds and are the pathological hallmark of BOOP.

MANAGEMENT AND OUTCOME

COP responds very well to steroids. It is, in fact, the most steroid-responsive of all the IIPs with a favourable response in more than 80% of cases. Rarely, especially if COP is diagnosed late, it can continue to progress despite steroids. These patients then behave like an NSIP. Treatment with steroids in COP needs to continue for at least 6–12 months and relapses are not uncommon, especially as the steroid dose is tapered. Second-line immunosuppressives are sometimes needed. Recent case reports have shown a beneficial effect of macrolides in COP probably due to their anti-inflammatory effect.

Indian Data on COP

The first Indian case of COP was described from our institution. We recently published the only large case series from this country where we reported on 34 cases of biopsy-proven COP from a single centre from 2000–05. This study provides the first detailed analysis of the clinical and radiological presentation of COP from India. This is a good-sized cohort from a single centre and shows that COP is not uncommon in India but under-recognized. Our patients had almost all received multiple courses of antibiotics and often prolonged anti-TB chemotherapy before the correct diagnosis was eventually made. Because of these long delays, as many as 21% of our patients responded sub-optimally to steroids. Other distinctive features in our patients was female preponderance with females being affected three times as frequently as males. Transbronchial lung biopsy yielded the correct diagnosis in all our patients thus making surgical biopsy unnecessary. (Sen T, Udwadia ZF. Cryptogenic organizing pneumonia: clinical profile in a series of 34 admitted patients in a hospital in India.)

SUGGESTED READING

Cordier JF. Cryptogenic organizing pneumonia. *Clin Chest Med.* 1 Dec. 2004; 25(4): 727–38, vi–vii.

Davies G. Respiratory bronchiolitis associated with interstitial lung disease and desquamative interstitial pneumonia. *Clin Chest Med.* 1 Dec. 2004; 25(4): 717–26, vi.

du Bois RM. Evolving concepts in the early and accurate diagnosis of idiopathic pulmonary fibrosis. *Clin Chest Med.* 1 Mar. 2006; 27(1 Suppl 1): S17–25, v–vi.

Leslie KO. Pathology of interstitial lung disease. *Clin Chest Med.* 1 Dec. 2004; 25(4): 657–703, vi.

Lu BS. Lung transplantation for interstitial lung disease. *Clin Chest Med.* 1 Dec. 2004; 25(4): 773–82, vii–viii.

Noth I. Recent advances in idiopathic pulmonary fibrosis. *Chest.* 1 Aug. 2007; 132(2): 637–50.

Patel NM. Pulmonary hypertension in idiopathic pulmonary fibrosis. *Chest.* 1 Sep. 2007; 132(3): 998–1006.

Pipavath S. Imaging of interstitial lung disease. *Clin Chest Med.* 1 Sep. 2004; 25(3): 455–65, v–vi.

Vourlekis JS. Acute interstitial pneumonia. *Clin Chest Med.* 1 Dec. 2004; 25(4): 739–47, vii.

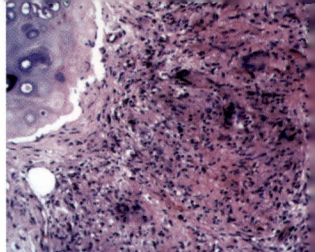

45   Sarcoidosis

GENERAL CONSIDERATIONS

Sarcoidosis is a disease of worldwide distribution characterized by the presence of non-caseating epitheloid granulomas in affected organs or organ systems; it is caused by an immune response to an unknown antigen in genetically susceptible individuals.

Sarcoidosis is a multisystem disease that can involve any organ in the body. The lungs and intrathoracic nodes are, however, most frequently involved. The mere presence of non-caseating granulomas is not proof of the disease. Preferably, there should be granulomatous lesions in more than one organ system and it is important that other causes of non-caseating epitheloid granulomas have been excluded. Unfortunately, as yet there is no test of sufficient sensitivity and specificity to help in the diagnosis, which therefore is based not just on histological evidence but on clinical and imaging features compatible with the disease.

Clinical, epidemiological and familial studies have stressed the role of genetic susceptibility in the occurrence of the disease. Sarcoidosis has a variable clinical presentation and clinical course, and though corticosteroids form the cornerstone of treatment, there is as yet no specific cure for the disease.

EPIDEMIOLOGY

Sarcoidosis has a worldwide distribution though it is commoner in some parts of the world compared to others. Prevalence rates are underestimated even in the West and the US because a large number of people have asymptomatic disease and are therefore unaware of it. The highest prevalence rates are in Sweden, Denmark and in African Americans. African-Americans (particularly African-American women), are three and a half times more commonly affected, with a reported age-adjusted incidence of 35.5/100,000 compared with 10.9/100,00 in whites. The overall prevalence rates in the US, Southern Europe and Japan are reported as 10–40 per 100,000.

In the West, the disease occurs most frequently in the age group of 20–40 years with a second peak in women after the age of 50 years. The disease is more common in women than in men.

Geography and ethnicity often determine clinical presentation and severity of the disease. Erythema nodosum and Löfgren's syndrome are frequent clinical presentations in Scandinavian countries. They are comparatively less frequent in the US and Europe and infrequent in blacks and Japanese. However, cardiac involvement with sarcoidosis is more commonly observed in the Japanese than in any other race or country.

African-Americans and Africans are more likely to have severe disease, carrying a higher morbidity and mortality compared to Europeans or the white population in US. In South Africa, skin lesions such as lupus pernio, nodules, plaques, and psoriasis-like lesions are more common, often leading to a misdiagnosis of leprosy. In the United Kingdom, Southern Europe, US and in most other countries of the world, mortality is most often due to progressive pulmonary sarcoidosis. However, in Sweden and Japan, cardiac involvement is the leading cause of death in sarcoidosis. The overall mortality of sarcoidosis as judged from Western figures is 1–5%.

INDIA AND SOUTHEAST ASIA

In the fifties and sixties sarcoidosis was considered a rare disease in India. It is now accepted that the disease is not uncommon, there being reports of fairly large series from western India, eastern India and northern India. The disease appears to be more frequent over the age of 40 years, partly because of lack of awareness of the problem among physicians and partly because the disease is often wrongly diagnosed and treated for a long time as tuberculosis. SK Gupta, working on sarcoidosis in Kolkata was able to trace 640 proven cases of sarcoidosis in India, published in 11 series up to December 2001. This number will probably have more than doubled now. The disease seems to be commoner in Kolkata and Bengal than in any other part of India. Interestingly, in Kolkata and Bengal the disease is commoner in the ethnic Rajasthani patients (Rajasthani migrants who have migrated from Rajasthan in northwest India to Kolkata and Bengal) than in the local Bengali population. Many patients seeking advice in our units in Mumbai are also Rajasthanis living in Bengal and Rajasthanis from Rajasthan. Ethnicity and perhaps geography are responsible for this case selection. The true prevalence rate of sarcoidosis in any part of India (leave aside the whole country) is however undetermined. The differences in clinical phenotypes of sarcoidosis as reported in the West and in studies from India are probably determined by geography and ethnicity. These are given later in the chapter.

Sarcoidosis is an uncommon disease in Southeast Asia, with the exception of Japan. Luo Wei and colleagues have reported just 223 patients (59% women) with histological evidence of sarcoidosis from the many different provinces of China.

The disease is barely seen in Hong Kong; in Korea sarcoidosis is believed to be very rare. However, a nationwide survey in Korea between 1992 and 1999 reported 309 biopsy-proven cases from 58 hospitals, the incidence of sarcoidosis being 0.125/100,000.

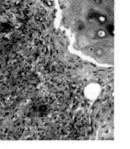
The incidence of sarcoidosis is significantly more in Japan than in all other Southeast Asian countries. In 2004, a large study of 1027 patients enrolled from a cluster encompassing 79.4% of the entire Japanese population was designed using the National Epidemiological Survey, with the objectives of determining clinical phenotypes in sarcoidosis and the incidence of the disease. The study revealed an average incidence rate of 1.01 per 100,000 inhabitants (0.73 for males and 1.28 for females). The female to male ratio was shown to have increased from 1.12 in 1973–77 to 1.82 in 2004. *(Ref: T. Morimota, A. Azuma et al. Epidemiology of Sarcoidosis in Japan. Eur Resp J 2008; 31: 372–379)*

The increased incidence of cardiac sarcoidosis in the Japanese has already been commented upon. In a comparative study of cardiac sarcoidosis in the Japanese, African-Americans, and US Caucasians, by Iwai and co-workers, the incidence of cardiac sarcoid granulomas was 67.8 %, 21.2 % and 13.7 % respectively. *(Ref: Iwai K, Sekigutti M et al. Racial difference in cardiac sarcoidosis incidence observed at autopsy. Sarcoidosis 1994;11–26–31)*

AETIOLOGY

The aetiology of sarcoidosis, in spite of a great deal of research, is still unknown. It is probably the interaction between an unknown antigen in the environment, the host response and genetic factors that results in disease.

Non-caseating granulomas are the essential and characteristic features of sarcoidosis. Granulomas can be caused by mycobacteria, fungi, viruses, other microorganisms and by inorganic agents. None of these have been consistently or convincingly demonstrated in sarcoid tissue. The occasional demonstration of one or the other does not prove causality. Also, a microorganism may trigger the disease and then could be destroyed by the host immune response. The immune response may, however, continue to be directed against undegradable antigenic protein products of the microorganism. Alternatively, an autoimmune response may be induced by the host- antigen reaction thereby perpetuating the inflammatory disease. In either case it could be impossibly difficult to identify the antigen triggering the disease.

The link between environmental exposure and sarcoidosis is suggested by the seasonal clustering of the disease in winter and early spring months, both in the Northern and Southern hemispheres. The ACCESS (A Case Control Etiological Study of Sarcoidosis) is a recent multi-centred US-based study of over 700 newly diagnosed biopsy-proven patients with sarcoidosis compared to age-sex-race-matched controls. The results of this study showed an absence of environmental or occupational exposure positively linked to sarcoidosis (Odds ratio > 2 and exposure prevalence > 5%). Weak positive associations (Odds ratio 1.5) were found for insecticide use at work, mould/mildew exposure at work and musty odours, suggesting a possible role of microbial-rich environment. The ACCESS study found a negative association between smoking and risk for sarcoidosis. The study demonstrated that there was no single dominant environmental exposure responsible for the disease, again suggesting the importance of the interaction between the gene, the environment and the host response in initiation of the disease.

The possibility of an infectious agent causing sarcoidosis has been considered and researched upon for several years. There are reports of systemic sarcoidosis developing in transplant recipients following transplant of donor organs of patients with active sarcoidosis. This clearly suggests a transmissible agent as the likely cause of sarcoidosis.

American, European and Japanese researchers have demonstrated mycobacterial DNA in a number of biopsy specimens; however, similar DNA were present in a number of controls using the sensitive polymerase chain technique. Recently, Japanese investigators have found Propionibacterium acnes DNA in over 80% of sarcoid tissue specimens from Japan and Europe, but also in 0–60% in controls. Other organisms implicated in the aetiology of sarcoidosis are Chlamydia, Rickettsia and lymphotropic DNA viruses (cytomegalovirus, Epstein Barr virus and human herpes virus Type 6) and the human T-cell lymphotropic virus (HTLV1) virus.

Recently, Maller DB and his colleagues have detected the mycobacterial catalase–peroxidase protein (mkatG) in over 50% of sarcoid tissue specimens. IgG antibodies were also present in 50% of patients with sarcoidosis. Perhaps mkatG antigen may be responsible for a subset of patients with sarcoidosis. There is always the possibility that more than one antigen (maybe multiple different antigens) could perhaps trigger the disease. Other mycobacterial antigens causing the disease may well be identified in future.

In clinical practice there does seem to be some relation between *Mycobacterium tuberculosis* and sarcoidosis. Besides clinical similarities, patients with sarcoidosis may occasionally develop proven tuberculosis (TB) and very occasionally patients with proven TB may in later years develop biopsy-proven sarcoidosis. In the last situation there is no response to anti-TB drugs but a good response to corticosteroids. Yet it needs to be stated that though different mycobacterial proteins may perhaps cause sarcoidosis, *Mycobacterium tuberculosis* does not cause this disease. The fact that anti-TB drugs are ineffective in sarcoidosis is sufficient proof of this.

GENETIC FACTORS

Familial clustering and racial differences in incidence and in clinical presentation point to the importance of genetics in the aetiology of sarcoidosis. Studies in the West have shown that familial clustering of the disease occurs in 3–14% of patients, more in the blacks than in the whites. The US ACCESS study found siblings of patients with sarcoidosis having a higher relative risk (Odds ratio approximately 5.8) compared to parents (Odds ratio approximately 3.8). The US ACCESS study also suggests that genetic factors have a greater influence in susceptibility to sarcoidosis in whites than in blacks.

Genetic studies have examined the role of human leukocyte antigen (HLA) alleles (both Class I and Class II) and non-HLA genes in relation to sarcoidosis.

The Role of Genetics in Sarcoidosis

The differences in the incidence of sarcoidosis in various ethnic groups as also disease clustering in families suggests that genetics may well play an important role in the etiology of sarcoidosis. The importance of ethnicity has already been

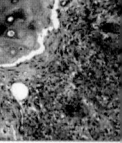

mentioned, specifically with African-Americans who are three-and-a-half times more commonly affected than the rest of the population in the United States. Worldwide, familial sarcoidosis occurs in 3–14% patients. The ACCESS study (A Case-Control Etiological Saroidosis Study) showed that cases were five times more likely than control subjects to report an affected sibling or parent.

The current advances in genetic marker maps and genotyping technology make present-day investigations and exploration of genes linked to sarcoidosis both exciting and challenging.

Human Leucocyte Antigens

Human leucocyte antigens (HLAs) play an important role in antigen presentation. The search for a link between HLAs and sarcoidosis began several years ago. Early reports revealed an association of acute sarcoidosis with HLA Class I antigen HLA-B8, and noted that HLA-B8/DR3 genes were inherited as a sarcoidosis risk haplotype, a haplotype which is also associated with autoimmune disease in whites. Studies in HLA Class I antigens were followed by studies on HLA Class II antigens. The current belief is that both HLA Class I and II genes work together in the evolution of the pathophysiology of sarcoidosis.

Though current work on the genetics of sarcoidosis is in a state of flux, some important observations from genetic research on this subject are worth noting.

1. The HLA-DRB1 is associated with sarcoidosis, with variations of the HLA-DRB1 gene affecting both susceptibility and prognosis of sarcoidosis.
2. A consistent finding across populations is that the HLA-DQB1*0201 allele is associated with decreased risk and lack of disease progression.
3. Several different HLA class II genes acting in concert or independently predispose to sarcoidosis.
4. The linkage disequilibrium (LD) within the major histocompatibility complex (MHC region) limits the ability to exactly identify the HLA genes.

An important negative finding is the lack of association of sarcoidosis with HLA-DPB1*0201, the allele that carries glutamate in amino-acid position 69 (Glu69). This allele has been consistently associated with berylliosis, a disease very similar to sarcoidosis.

Non-HLA Canditate Genes

Genes that influence antigen processing, antigen presentation, macrophage and T-cell activation, cell recruitment are considered sarcoidosis candidate genes. Numerous such genes have been investigated in relation to sarcoidosis. Some of the candidate genes investigated in relation to sarcoidosis include the following:

Angiotensin converting enzyme, CC chemokine receptor + a receptor for monocyte chemoattractant protein; CCR5 which serves as a receptor for macrophage inflammatory proteins and for monocyte chemotactic protein 2. Other candidate genes investigated include Clara cell 10-kD protein, Heat Shock Protein A1L, interleukins IL-1, IL-4R, IL-18, IFN-α and Vascular Endothelial Growth Factor. Not one of these or several others that have been investigated show a significant

or consistent association with sarcoidosis. For a fuller review on this subject, the reader is referred to the article: *Michael C. Iannuzzi and Benjamin A. Rybicki. Genetics of Sarcoidosis. Am Thorac Soc* Vol 4, pp. 108–16, 2007.

In conclusion, sarcoidosis probably results from an interaction of environmental factors and alleles of many genes. A genetic association has been extensively researched upon in the hope that identifying alleles and candidate genes influencing risk and phenotype will increase our understanding of the disease. A few HLA genes have been shown to be associated with sarcoidosis. No convincing association has been found with candidate genes. Unfortunately many of the reported associations have not been corroborated by different groups of researchers.

Future research in this field holds promise. Profiling gene expression in BAL fluid and blood at the time of presentation may perhaps help to predict disease progression, resolution, and response to treatment. Functional analysis of candidate genes identified by linkage analysis in conjunction with genome association studies may throw greater light upon the pathogenesis of this disease.

IMMUNOPATHOGENESIS

Non-caseating granulomas within affected tissue is *the* characteristic feature of sarcoidosis. These granulomas are a result of a cell-mediated immunological response of the host to an unidentified antigen. Though the immunological mechanisms and the molecular biology of the immune response are now better elucidated, the interaction between antigen, host response and genetic factors that ultimately causes sarcoidosis is poorly understood.

The initial or primary event in the immunopathogenesis is an alveolitis due to the accumulation of activated CD4+ T helper cell lymphocytes within the alveoli. Bronchoalveolar lavage (BAL) studies show a marked increase in the CD4:CD8 ratio. An increase beyond 3.5 to 4 is considered to be highly specific for sarcoidosis. In fact, in acutely presenting sarcoid the CD4:CD8 ratio may exceed 10 and may be as high as 30.

The activated CD4+ T helper cells seem to be derived from the blood, the lymphocytes from the blood being trapped and then compartmentalized within the lung. The T4 lymphocyte count in the blood is thereby reduced. The migration of T4 lymphocytes from the blood into the lungs is due to increased production of cytokines and chemokines. Two active chemokines that attract peripheral lymphocytes into the lungs are IP-10 and RANTFS. These are present in a high concentration in patients with active sarcoidosis. The increased number of CD4 cells within the lungs is also due to the local proliferation of lymphocytes within the lung, probably a response to an antigen.

The depletion of CD4 cell lymphocytes within the blood is responsible for the depressed cell-mediated immunity present in patients with sarcoidosis. This is evinced by a negative tuberculin test as also by a depressed immune response to viral and fungal antigens.

Alveolar macrophages also proliferate (in addition to CD4+ helper lymphocytes) within the lungs. These are derived from mononuclear cells within the blood as also from local proliferation. Alveolar macrophages are activated, are monocytic in appearance and have two functions. They are antigen-processing and antigen-presenting cells and produce proinflammatory

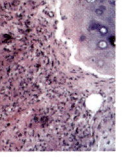

cytokines that induce further proliferation and activation of T4 cells and alveolar macrophages. The characteristic inflammatory response in sarcoidosis is of the Th1 type with the production of Th1_-associated cytokines, IL-2, interferon (IFN)-γ and TNF α. The production of IL-12 by activated alveolar macrophages intensifies Th1 response as it induces production of TNF α by T cells and natural killer (NK) cells. Another cytokine produced by activated macrophages and lymphocytes is IL-18, which acts in synergy with IL-12 to increase the production of IFN-γ by T cells and NK cells. Both IL-12 and IL-18 are present in increased concentrations in patients with sarcoidosis.

The above-described T cell-mediated immune response directed against an unknown but perhaps persistent antigen is responsible for the characteristic sarcoid granulomas. TNF α, IFN-γ, interleukins, in particular IL-1 are necessary for the formation and persistence of these granulomas. Under the influence of chronic cytokine influence and stimulation, alveolar macrophages differentiate into epitheloid cells. Some of these epitheloid cells fuse to form giant cells. The cluster of lymphocytes and mononuclear cells forming the granuloma may be encased by fibrous tissue laid down by fibroblasts.

Research is directed towards the identification of markers associated with an increased risk of fibrosis. It is possible that a switch from a Th$_1$ inflammatory profile to a Th2 inflammatory profile may contribute to fibroblasts and fibrosis. IL-4 production is a feature of the Th$_2$ inflammatory profile and IL-4 is chemotactic for fibroblasts stimulating them to lay down fibrous tissue. Other fibrogenic factors are insulin-like growth factor binding protein (IGFBP), platelet-derived growth factor, IGF1 and granulocyte-macrophage colony stimulating factor (GM-CSF).

Though the immunopathogensis of sarcoidosis is chiefly T-cell-mediated, there is also a polyclonal activation of B cells in this disease. This leads to presence of antibodies to numerous viral antigens and to the formation of immune complexes which are associated with and which may be responsible for erythema nodosum. It has been postulated that increased B cell activity may contribute to arthralgia, uveitis and erythema nodosum seen in sarcoidosis.

PATHOLOGY

The classic feature of sarcoidosis is the well-defined non-caseating granulomas without the presence of micro-organisms on staining or even on tissue culture. The granuloma consists of epitheloid cells, T-lymphocytes of the CD4 kind, and a few macrophages, and multinucleated Langhan's giant cells. The giant cells may contain inclusion bodies of calcium carbonate or form asteroid bodies. There is an outer peripheral layer of CD8 T cells, monocytes and B lymphocytes. Both CD4$^+$ and CD8$^+$ T cells carry the αβ form of the T cell receptor (TCR). T cells carrying γδ-TCR are rarely observed within or at the periphery of the granulomas.

Fibroblasts with collagen and fibrous tissue are often present surrounding the granuloma. In the lungs the granulomas are distributed peribronchially, perivascularly and are noted to 'dot' the fissures. The granulomas may resolve, persist, or coalesce to destroy lung tissue and ultimately lead to progressive fibrosis, which chiefly involves the upper lobes.

It is to be noted that non-caseating granulomas are not specific for sarcoidosis. They may occur in tuberculosis,

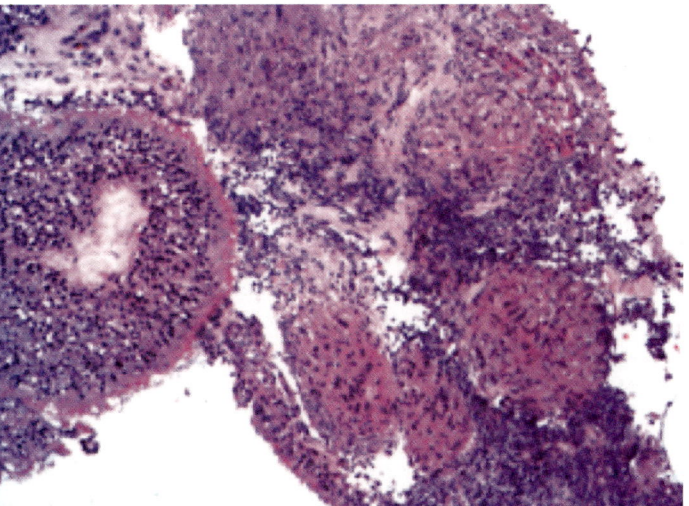

Fig 45.1: H&E. Transbronchial biopsy of the lung. Presence of non-caseating granulomas consistent with sarcoidosis is noted.

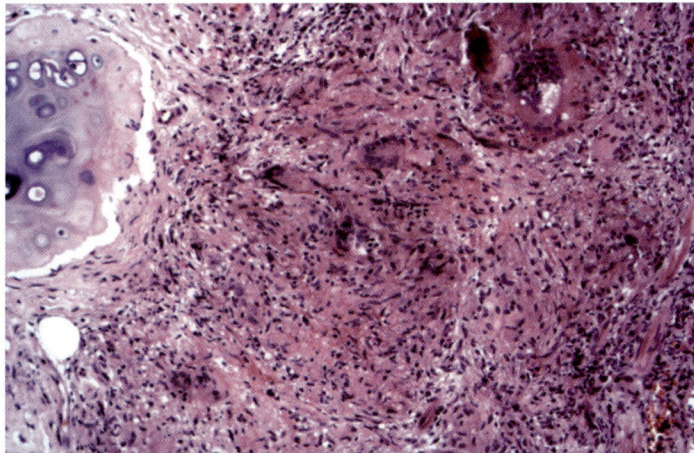

Fig 45.2: 20X H&E. Sarcoidosis. Transbronchial biopsy of the lung. Presence of non-caseating granulomas, replete with Langhan's and foreign body type giant cells.

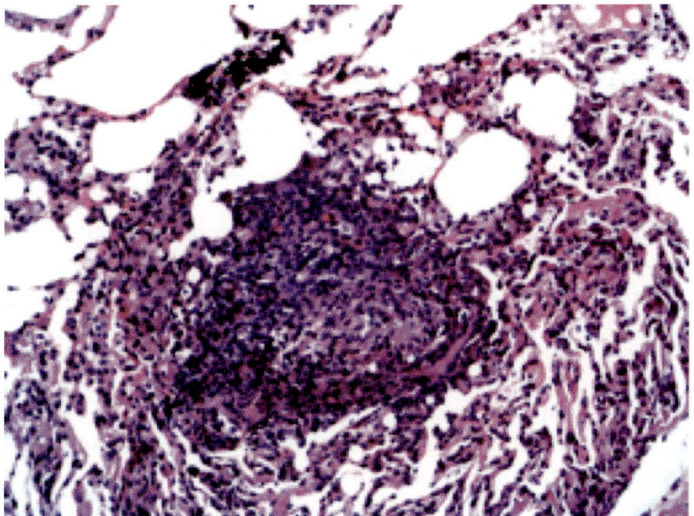

Fig 45.3: 20X H&E. Sarcoidosis. Transbronchial biopsy of the lung. Presence of non-caseating granulomas in the interstitium is noted.

berylliosis and extrinsic allergic alveolitis and can be caused by a number of other micro-organisms.

The epitheloid cells in the granuloma secrete angiotensin-converting enzyme (ACE) so that serum levels of ACE are often though not always elevated in sarcoidosis. The ACE level in the serum is used as a nonspecific marker of the total granuloma burden and of sarcoid activity. Another product secreted by the sarcoid granuloma is vitamin D_3 which when secreted in excess leads to increase in serum calcium levels. The vitamin D receptor gene has two allele variants; the B allele of the vitamin D receptor gene is believed to be associated with sarcoidosis.

CLINICAL PRESENTATION

Sarcoidosis is a multi-organ disease; any one or more organs or organ systems can be involved. The clinical presentation, the clinical features and the course of the disease therefore vary considerably. Patients with symptomatic disease may seek advice from an internist or from any one of the different medical specialities depending on which organ or organ system is clinically involved.

The following section first deals with the overall clinical presentation, clinical features of pulmonary sarcoidosis and extrapulmonary sarcoidosis. It then gives a brief description of sarcoidosis in the Indian scenario.

Close to two-thirds of patients are asymptomatic and have sarcoidosis diagnosed accidentally following a routine chest radiograph on the basis of a bilateral hilar adenopathy. When symptoms do occur, the most frequent presentation is that of a dry cough and exertional dyspnoea. This is because the lungs and/or intrathoracic lymph nodes are involved in over 90% of patients with sarcoidosis. Exertional dyspnoea when present suggests that the disease has probably been in existence for some months. In the ACCESS study more than half the patients were initially seen with pulmonary symptoms.

Constitutional symptoms in the form of fever, malaise, lassitude, weight loss and arthralgias occur in 20% of patients in most Western reports. These can occur in association with clinical features of any organ involvement or may occur as the sole presenting feature. Pyrexia of unknown origin is not an uncommon presentation of sarcoidosis.

Ethnicity plays an important role in the clinical presentation of the disease. African-Americans are noted to develop more severe constitutional and respiratory symptoms compared to Caucasians. Uveitis is commoner in the Japanese. Lupus pernio characterized by disfiguring lesions of the cheek and nose is more commonly observed in elderly women of the Afro-Caribbean race.

The disease may present acutely or may be subacute or insidious in onset and progress. The two well-recognized acute forms of the disease are Löfgren's syndrome and Heerfordt's syndrome. Löfgren's syndrome is described later under 'Clinical Features'. Heerfordt's syndrome is characterized by fever, parotid gland enlargement, uveitis, xerostomia and unilateral or bilateral facial nerve palsy.

A classification scheme given by Fishman (Systemic Sarcoidosis; Fishman's *Pulmonary Diseases and Disorders*) based on the initial presentation of patients with sarcoidosis is as follows: asymptomatic, acute sarcoidosis with or without erythema nodosum, intermediate sarcoidosis with symptoms

or signs of pulmonary disease for less than two years, chronic pulmonary sarcoidosis of more than two years and predominately extrapulmonary sarcoidosis. Patients who have persistent disease for more than two years, usually, though not always have persistent long-term disease.

CLINICAL FEATURES

The clinical features are best described under the following heads—asymptomatic sarcoidosis, acute sarcoidosis with or without erythema nodosum, pulmonary sarcoidosis, extrapulmonary sarcoidosis.

Asymptomatic Sarcoidosis

As mentioned under 'Clinical Presentation', up to two-thirds of patients are asymptomatic, the diagnosis being made on the basis of a radiographic examination of the chest which shows bilateral hilar adenopathy. Pulmonary infiltrates may be occasionally present in some patients; these are more evident on a high-resolution computed tomography (HRCT) of the chest.

Acute Sarcoidosis With or Without Erythema Nodosum (Löfgren's Syndrome)

Löfgren's syndrome is manifested by acute onset of high fever, bilateral hilar adenopathy, eyrthema nodosum, polyarthritis often associated with uveitis. Erythema nodosum is characterized by painful reddish nodules, several centimetres in diameter, chiefly involving the lower limbs. The nodules change colour to a dull brown with time, may disappear, but often return in crops. Biopsy of the nodules reveals a panniculitis. Occasionally, the nodules also involve the thighs and the upper limbs. The polyarthritis is very painful, chiefly involving the ankles and knees, and occasionally the wrists and elbows as well. Variants of this syndrome are important to recognize. The chest radiograph is normal in 10% of patients; an HRCT of the chest may reveal a hilar adenopathy in these patients. Some patients manifest fever, constitutional symptoms, bilateral hilar adenopathy, polyarthritis, but have no erythema nodosum. This syndrome either in its full form or its variants has a good prognosis. Eighty per cent of patients enjoy a remission in weeks or months. Recurrence generally does not occur.

In Scandinavia one-third of patients with sarcoidosis may present with Löfgren's syndrome; the incidence is lower in the Caucasian race, and still lower in African-Americans, Africans, and in India and South-East Asia.

Pulmonary Sarcoid

Dry cough is an early symptom. Dyspnoea on exertion is observed as the disease progresses. Dyspnoea progressively worsens and in late stages of the disease is present even at rest. Dyspnoea is due to airways' obstruction or due to restrictive lung disease or more often due to both airways' obstruction plus restrictive lung disease. Occasionally, enlarged mediastinal lymph glands pressing on large airways may contribute to or be chiefly responsible for dyspnoea. With advanced pulmonary disease leading to pulmonary fibrosis and bronchiectasis, cough is associated with expectoration. Haemoptysis may

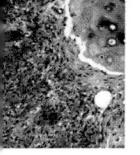

also then occur. Wheezing is common in patients with endobronchial disease causing airways' obstruction or in patients with late fibrocystic disease. Bronchodilators may offer relief only to patients with increased bronchial hyper-reactivity. Vague chest pain, the cause of which is uncertain, is a frequent complaint. Though diffuse endobronchial involvement may be present, segmental atelectasis or localised bronchial or tracheal stenosis is rare. In the late stage of pulmonary sarcoid characterized by fibrocystic disease and bronchiectasis, an aspergilloma may form in a cystic space or in a bronchiectatic cavity. This may remain silent or may cause profuse haemoptysis at times.

PHYSICAL FINDINGS

Physical findings are sparse. Rhonchi may be heard in patients with airways' obstruction only on forced expiration. Crackles are infrequent being present in less than 20% of patients. Clubbing is rare; it is generally absent.

IMAGING STUDIES

An X-ray chest is abnormal in over 90% of patients with sarcoidosis and to an extent has prognostic implications. The chest radiograph should be used as the basis for a grading or staging system. The stages range progressively from Stage 0 to Stage IV.

Stage 0 Stage 0 is characterized by a normal chest radiograph. A normal chest radiograph is found in 5–10% of patients with sarcoidosis, invariably in those with extrapulmonary sarcoidosis.

Stage I Stage I is characterized by bilateral hilar adenopathy and is present in about 40% of patients. This may be associated with a right paratracheal adenopathy, and in some patients there may also be a subcarinal, and pretracheal adenopathy.

Stage II Stage II is characterized by hilar adenoapthy with or without mediastinal adenopathy and with the presence of pulmonary infiltrates. This is seen initially in 30–50% of patients. Pulmonary infiltrates take the form of perivascular or peribronchial reticulonodules in the upper and mid-zones of the lungs. Discrete nodules may also be seen along the fissures of the lungs. Radiographic findings may also take the form of fluffy alveolar shadows resembling small areas of consolidation. Rarely, a miliary pattern resembling miliary TB is observed. Calcification of lymph nodes may be observed in longstanding cases.

Stage III Stage III is characterized by the presence of pulmonary infiltrates without hilar or mediastinal adenopathy. Pulmonary infiltration takes the form of reticulonodular shadows or alveolar shadows chiefly involving the upper and mid-zones of both lungs.

Stage IV The radiograph of the chest in Stage IV shows extensive fibrosis. The hila are pulled up; there is extensive fibrocystic disease, bronchiectasis, together with small and large bullae and honeycombing of the lungs chiefly involving the upper lobes, the lingula and the right middle lobes. There is also a significant loss of lung volume. The radiological features are

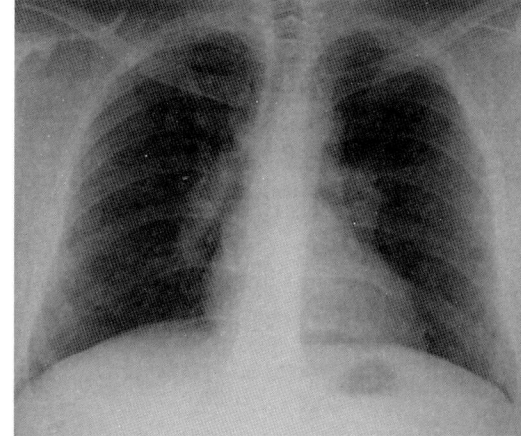

Fig 45.4a: 33-year-old man at a routine pre-employment health check. Chest X-ray demonstrates bilateral hilar adenopathy due to Stage I sarcoidosis.

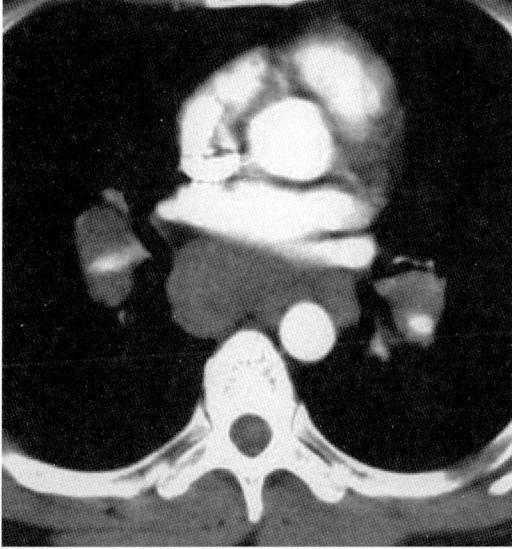

Fig 45.4b: Stage I sarcoidosis—contrast-enhanced CT scan demonstrates large bilateral hilar adenopathy and large subcarinal adenopathy. No necrosis is seen in the adenopathy.

akin to longstanding bilateral burnt-out TB involving the upper lobes of both lungs.

Unusual radiographic findings in sarcoidosis include the presence of a mycetoma in one of the cystic spaces or in a bronchiectatic cavity, an isolated nodule, or nodules, pleural involvement in the form of a pleural effusion or rarely, a pneumothorax.

HRCT of the chest may reveal details, particularly in relation to an adenopathy not visible on plain X-ray. HRCT of the chest also reveals the exact nature and distribution of pulmonary infiltrates; these are generally centrally distributed, peribronchially, perivascularly and along lung fissures. Ground glass opacities and honeycombing not present on an X-ray chest may be seen on an HRCT examination. CT of the chest is often useful a) in the evaluation of suspected sarcoidosis presenting with extrapulmonary manifestations but with a normal chest X-ray; b) prior to planned biopsy of enlarged mediastinal nodes; c) to evaluate uncommon X-ray appearances in sarcoidosis; d) to evaluate the degree of fibrocystic disease or bronhiectasis, or detect the presence of a mycetoma in a patient with sarcoidosis who has well-marked haemoptysis.

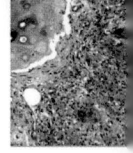

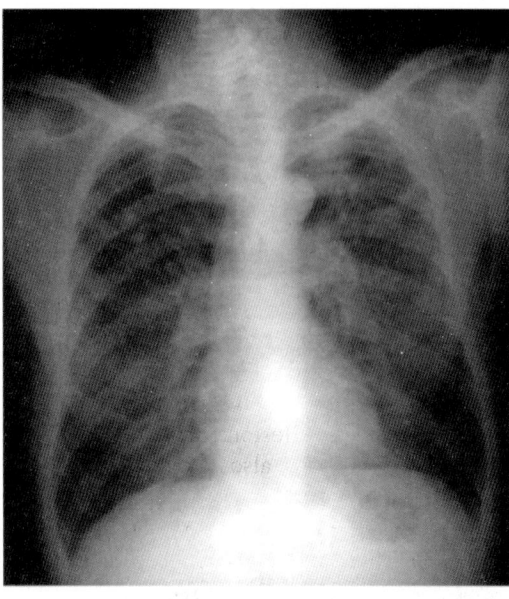

Fig 45.5: Stage 2 sarcoidosis: Chest X-ray demonstrates enlarged hilar adenopathy as well as extensive bilateral interstitial lesions.

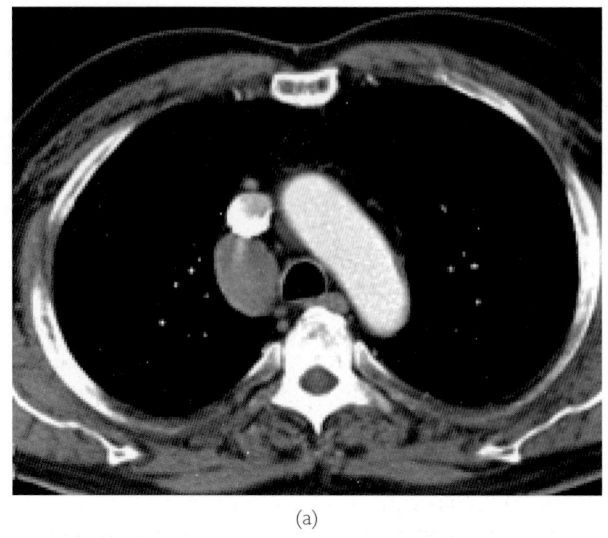

(a)

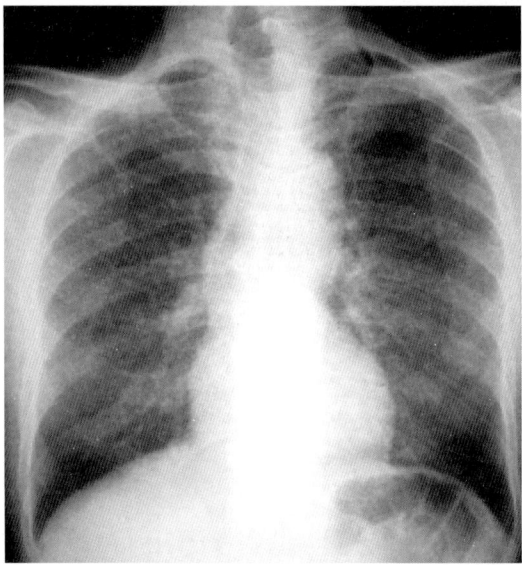

Fig 45.6: Stage 3 sarcoidosis. Chest X-ray demonstrates extensive interstitial nodules in both lung fields. No significant mediastinal adenopathy.

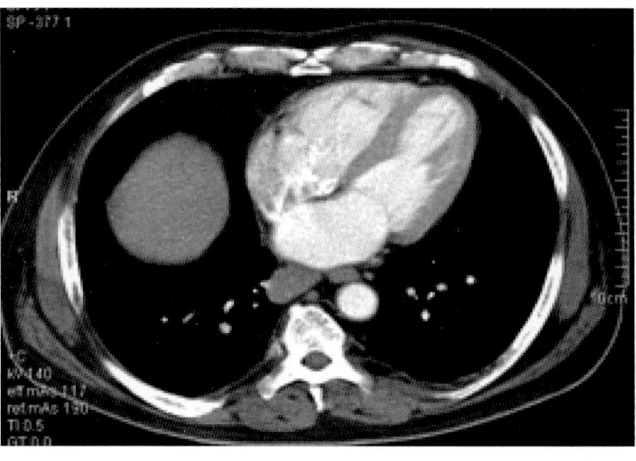

(b)

Fig 45.8a and b: Chest CT reveals large right paratracheal adenopathy as well as moderate-sized subcarinal adenopathy, no necrosis is seen in the adenopathy.

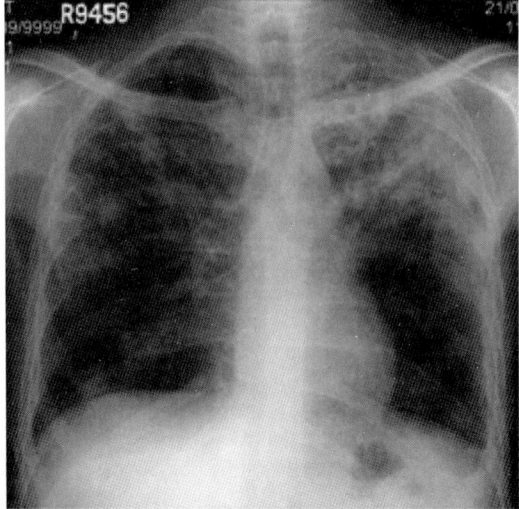

Fig 45.7: Stage 4 sarcoidosis. Chest X-ray demonstrates extensive fibrotic and interstitial opacities in the upper zones due to burnt-out sarcoidosis.

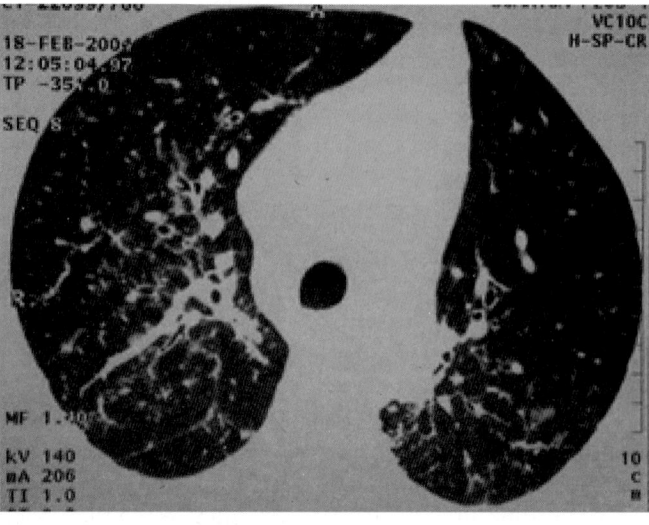

(c)

Fig 45.8c: HRCT reveals multiple small interstitial nodules as well as peribronchial interstitial thickening due to sarcoidosis.

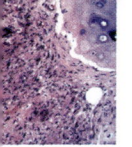

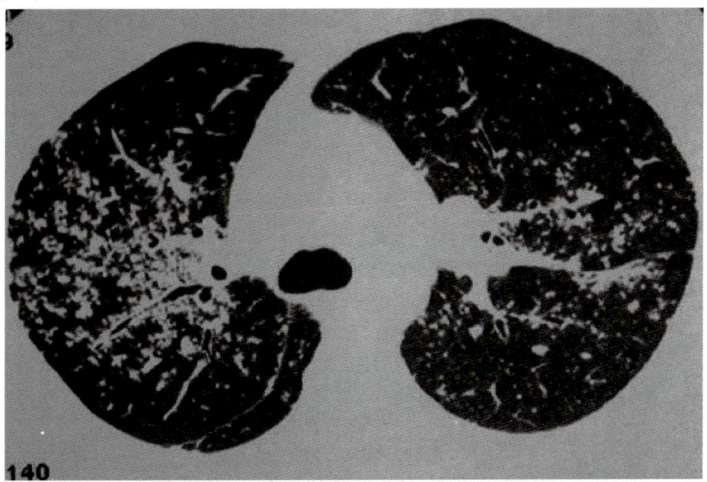

Fig 45.9: Extensive sarcoid granulomas on an HRCT chest demonstrating multiple nodules along the fissures, subpleurally as well as along bronchovascular structures, typical location for interstitial nodules.

Table 45.1: Approximate frequency of different stages in radiological examination of the chest on presentation as reported in the West and in western India		
	Western Figures	**Mumbai**
Stage I	40%	43%
Stage II	30–50	36%
Stage III	15%	21%

LUNG FUNCTIONS

Lung functions may show a restrictive pattern, an obstructive pattern and more often, as the disease progresses, features of both airways' obstruction and a restrictive ventilatory pattern. It needs to be remembered that lung functions may be normal even when there are pulmonary infiltrates on an X-ray chest.

The earliest features of a restrictive ventilatory defect are a fall in CO diffusion with a decrease in the total lung capacity. Later, there is a fall in the forced vital capacity, the residual volume and the functional residual capacity. Obstructive lung disease is typically characterized by decreased forced expiratory volume in the first second, forced vital capacity, FEV$_1$/FVC ratio and by reduced expiratory flow rates. Typical features of combined obstructive + restrictive patterns are a reduced CO diffusion, reduced FVC, reduced lung volumes, with a significant reduction in the expiratory flow rates and in the FEV$_1$/FVC ratio.

Bronchial hyper-reactivity may contribute to airways' obstruction in a small subgroup of patients. These patients may respond to aerosolized bronchodilators.

Resting hypoxemia is observed in some patients with Stage IV disease in the presence of well-marked airways' obstruction and restriction. Further oxygen desaturation occurs with exercise. We have seen two patients of sarcoidosis with miliary mottling of both lungs developing respiratory failure with well-marked hypoxemia. There was dramatic response to corticosteroid therapy. CO$_2$ retention does not occur except in the presence of advanced pulmonary disease.

Necrotising Sarcoid Granulomatosis

Necrotising sarcoid granulomatosis is a rare disorder characterized by the presence of one or more solid non-caseating granulomas involving pulmonary arteries and veins without evidence of systemic vasculitis. The condition has similarities to Wegener's granulomatosis but is considered to be a variant of sarcoidosis. The patient may be asymptomatic or may present with constitutional symptoms, chest pain and dyspnoea. Chest radiography demonstrates solid, generally multiple, non-cavitatory nodules resembling metastatic lesions. Pleural effusion has been reported in a majority of these patients and should lend suspicion to a possible correct diagnosis. A thoracoscopic biopsy is imperative to confirm the diagnosis of this rare variant of sarcoidosis. The lesions have been reported to improve spontaneously; there is also a rapid response to corticosteroid therapy.

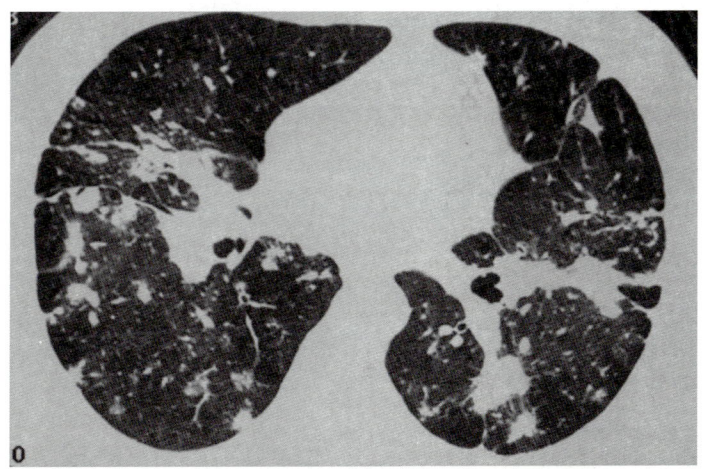

Fig 45.10: Necrotising sarcoidosis—HRCT demonstrates large nodules in both lung fields in a peribronchovascular location bilaterally. Transbronchial biopsy revealed necrotising granulomas.

EXTRAPULMONARY MANIFESTATIONS OF SARCOIDOSIS

Some patients have sarcoid involvement of one or more organ systems either in addition to pulmonary involvement or without evidence of pulmonary disease. The incidence of involvement of different organs or organ systems in extrapulmonary sarcoidosis depends on the geography as also the ethnicity of the population studied; it clearly varies in different parts of the world. The incidence of the involvement of different organ systems, as reported in the West and as reported in studies from the Indian subcontinent is given later in this section.

Cutaneous Sarcoid

In Indians, the skin is the most frequently involved organ system outside the lungs and intrathoracic lymph nodes. The incidence would perhaps be greater than that reported if a meticulous search for skin sarcoid is made on every patient with pulmonary sarcoid. Skin involvement takes the form of small yellowish papules, plaques, subcutaneous nodules and

erythema nodosum. Typically, the lesions are noted along the hairline, nose, ears, extensor surfaces of the arms and legs and the back. Lupus pernio is a disfiguring skin lesion of the face characterized by dull red or reddish-brown plaques on the nose (the tip and the alae nasi in particular), the cheeks and the skin below the eyes. The lesions disfigure the nose and the face.

Sarcoid nodules have a propensity to form in scar tissue (an operation scar, for example). The diagnosis of sarcoid is at times made when a 'tumour' removed from within and below an operation scar is noted on histology to be a non-caseating granulomatous mass.

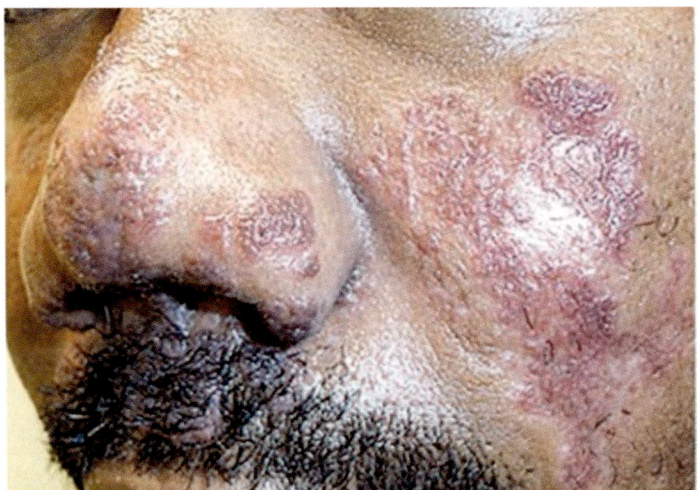

Fig 45.11: Lupus pernio. Sarcoid involvement of nose, alae nasi, cheek, nasolabial folds characterized by destructive lesions.

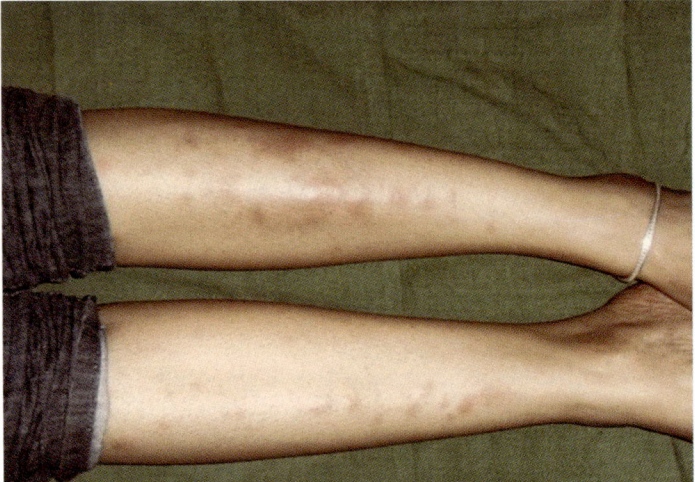

Fig 45.12: Erythema nodosum. Reddish nodules on the skin of both lower limbs, more marked on the extensor surface. This was associated with severe pain in the ankles and knees.

Ocular Sarcoid

Ocular sarcoid typically takes the form of an anterior uveitis affecting one or both eyes. It is often associated with a hilar adenopathy but may occur in isolation. Though uveitis is known to occur as a manifestation of TB, it is far more frequently observed with sarcoid. Rarely, optic neuritis or chorioretinitis may occur causing a dramatic loss of vision. Conjunctivitis can also result from sarcoid involvement of the conjunctiva.

Lymph Glands

Sarcoid involvement of the lymph glands outside the thorax is often mistakenly diagnosed as TB. The lymph glands generally show mild to moderate enlargement, are mobile and non-tender. Any group of lymph glands including those within the abdomen may be involved.

Liver and Spleen Involvement

The incidence of hepatosplenomegaly varies in different geographic areas. Splenic involvement is being increasingly observed with the advent of HRCT studies of the abdomen. Though generally asymptomatic, involvement of the spleen on CT studies is manifest in the form of one or multiple hypoechoic lesions. The spleen may be palpable in a few of these patients.

Granulomatous hepatitis may cause an asymptomatic rise in liver enzymes, chronic cholestasis and very rarely has been reported to result in cirrhosis with portal hypertension.

An important presentation of sarcoid is pyrexia of unknown origin with hepatomegaly or hepatosplenomegaly. A liver biopsy shows non-caseating granulomas and the splenomegaly if present shows hypoechoic lesions on a CT of the abdomen. There is a dramatic response to corticosteroids. It is to be noted that similar clinical findings and CT appearances may also occur with TB.

Neurosarcoid

Neurosarcoid is not as rare as is believed and we have dealt with a number of patients either in association with pulmonary involvement or occurring without pulmonary disease. The most important and frequent symptom is persistent headache. Change in the mental state, confusion and seizures may also occur as presenting symptoms. Cranial neuropathy chiefly involving one or both facial nerves is an important feature of neurosarcoid.

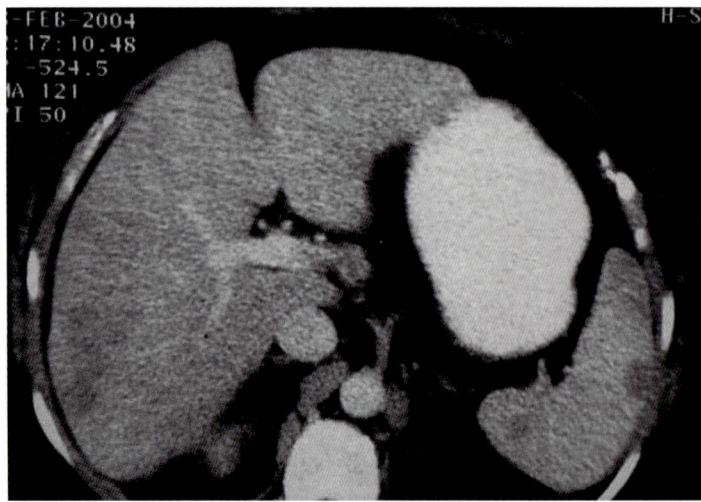

Fig 45.13: Abdominal CT reveals multiple focal hepatic and splenic lesions. Biopsy revealed non-caseating granulomas.

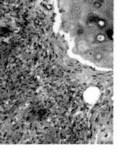

Other cranial nerves may be involved; optic neuritis can cause blurred vision, field defects and blindness. Sarcoid deposits in the hypothalamus and/or in the pituitary gland can cause hypothalamic and/or pituitary dysfunction. Aseptic meningitis, and spinal chord sarcoid deposits causing transverse myelitis are also a feature of neurosarcoid. The imaging findings on an MRI are fairly characteristic showing dural thickening over the convexity of the cerebral hemispheres and dural thickening in the tentorial area. Lesions obstructing the third ventricle can cause obstructive hydrocephalus.

Sarcoid Involvement of the Heart

This disorder is again not as uncommon as supposed and probably occurs in about 5% of patients. The classical presentation is that of a dilated or congestive cardiomyopathy with a fall in systolic ejection fraction to at times as low as 15–20%. Left ventricular failure followed by congestive heart failure occurs. Echocardiographic findings often show focal hypokinesia. Gallium studies show a positive pickup of gallium by sarcoid tissue within the heart muscle. Another classic presentation is the presence of heart block—either a bundle branch block or complete heart block, or the presence of arrhythmias. An important aetiology of dangerous ventricular arrhythmias in young individuals between 20 and 40 years of age, for which there is no obvious cause, is sarcoidosis. An HRCT of the chest showing hilar or mediastinal adenopathy in such a patient should strongly suggest this diagnosis. A therapeutic trial with high-dose corticosteroids is often rewarding. Electrophysiological studies with high-frequency ablation of ectopic foci and the use of an implantable defibrillator is the treatment of choice today. Death has occurred during such procedures even in excellent specialized clinics.

Hypercalcaemia

Hypercalcaemia is an infrequent observation in our units. Sarcoid granulomas result in increased conversion of 1-hydroxy-vitamin D3 to 1,25 hydroxyvitamin D3. Increased absorption of calcium from the gut occurs, leading to hypercalcemia. Renal stones and nephrocalcinosis may result. Non-caseating granulomatous lesions may occur in the kidneys. They may occasionally cause serious renal dysfunction. Significant renal dysfuntion in the presence of granulomatous lesions (as seen on renal biopsy) is more likely to be related to Wegener's granulomatosis than to sarcoidosis.

Other Organs and Organ Systems

Any organ or organ system may be involved. Sarcoid involvement of the upper respiratory tract may cause epistaxis, nasal congestion, sinusitis; involvement and destruction of the nasal septum can cause a saddle deformity of the nose. Laryngeal sarcoid can cause stridor, hoarseness and marked upper airways obstruction.

Granulomatosis involvement of the parotid, submandibular or lachrymal glands can lead to xerostomia and dry eyes. The association of bilateral parotid enlargement, facial palsy, fever and uveitis has been mentioned earlier.

Muscle pains and muscle weakness may be observed, the clinical picture resembling polymyositis. Muscle biopsy often

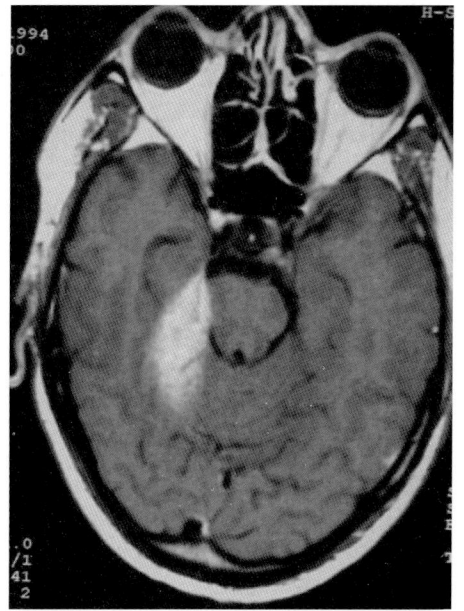

(a)

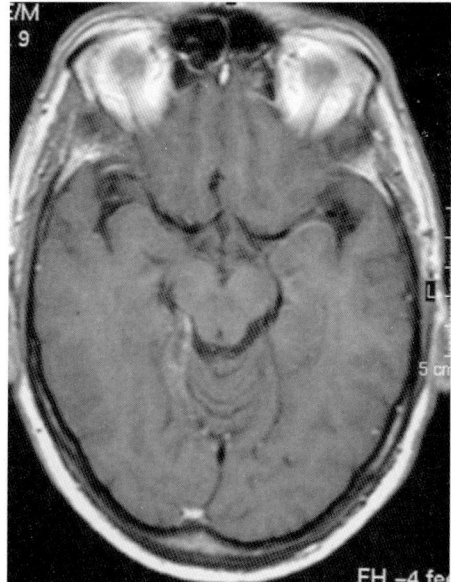

(b)

Fig 45.14: 43-year-old man with biopsy-proven pulmonary sarcoid presented with blurring of vision and headaches. On examination, the only positive finding was papilloedema. (a) Contrast-enhanced MRI demonstrates plaque-like enhancement along the dura. Intracranial sarcoid often manifests as dural mass lesions. After treatment (b) MRI demonstrates nearly total disappearance of dural mass lesion.

shows the presence of sarcoid granulomas. Punched out bony lesions with cystic changes and loss of trabeculae may be observed, particularly in the metacarpophalyngeal and interphalangeal joints. Lytic bony lesions involving the spine or long bones have been reported but in our experience these lesions in patients with proven sarcoid involving the lungs are invariably related to separate metastatic disease than to sarcoid.

Haematogenous involvement may lead to granulomatous lesions in the bone marrow, peripheral lymphopenia and hypersplenism.

THE INDIAN SCENARIO

It is worth briefly highlighting the clinical features of sarcoidosis in India, so as to enable comparison with observations on the disease in the West.

	Table 45.2: Approximate frequency of commonly occurring organ involvement in the West as compared to western India (Mumbai)	
Organ Involved	**Western Studies**	**Western India (Mumbai)**
Lung	> 90% (on conventional X-ray)	> 90% (on conventional X-ray)
Respiratory symptoms (cough, dyspnoea)	40–60%	64%-cough; 43%-dyspnoea
Constitutional symptoms	20–25%	> 35%
Cutaneous	25%	17%
Ocular	20–30%	13%
Peripheral lymphadenopathy	35%	< 10%
Hepatic Sarcoid	65% (on biopsy) Much less frequent with regard to clinical manifestation	< 5% Frequency on liver biopsy undetermined
Musculoskeletal system (including arthralgia)	25%	25%
Neurosarcoid	5–10%	5–7%
Cardiac sarcoid	5–10%	5%
Exocrine gland sarcoid	10%	< 2%
Haematogenous sarcoid	< 5%	< 2%

Note: Studies from eastern India (Kolkata) showed a greater frequency of hepatomegaly (43.5%), splenomegaly (31.5%), peripheral lymphadenopathy (12%) and hypercalcaemia compared to a study in western India (Mumbai).

A study of 135 patients with biopsy-proven sarcoidosis over a seven-year period (1994–2001) from one of our units in Mumbai showed that the disease presented at a mean age of 48.5 years with a male to female ratio of 1:1.4. The commonest presenting symptoms were cough (64%), exertional dyspnoea (43%), fever (36%), weight loss (35%), and arthralgia (25%). There appears to be an increase in the incidence of constitutional symptoms compared to Western figures. Skin involvement (17%) and ocular symptoms (13%) were commonly seen. On the other hand hepatosplenomegaly, peripheral lymphadenopathy, and parotid enlargement were infrequent clinical manifestations. Contrary to the above, studies from eastern India (Kolkata, Bengal) show an increased incidence of hepatomegaly (43.5%) and splenomegaly (32.5%) and peripheral lymphadenopathy (22%). Hypercalcaemia, uncommon in the study from Mumbai, was much more frequent in eastern India. These differences between eastern and western India are probably related to geography and difference in ethnicity. Other clinical features as observed in the subcontinent of India are worthy of comment. The acute form of sarcoidosis, characterized either by Lofgren's syndrome or Heerfordt's syndrome is rarely observed. Sarcoid involvement of the heart and neurosarcoid though not common, do occur. In fact, any and every organ has been seen to be involved just as in the West. Table 45.2 above gives the frequency of organ involvement as reported in the West and as observed in India.

The multisystem involvement in sarcoidosis is illustrated by the brief case report given below.

A 40-year-old man had a bladder neck obstruction requiring transurethral resection of the prostrate. Histological study of the prostate showed non-caseating granulomas compatible with sarcoid. A CT and MRI study of the abdomen and pelvis and chest done subsequent to this procedure showed enlarged seminal vesicles which also showed granulomatous lesions on a CT-guided biopsy. Abdominal lymphadenopathy, hypoechoic lesions in the liver and spleen and Stage II sarcoid on imaging of the chest were also present. The serum ACE (SACE) level was markedly elevated. The patient refused treatment, preferring ayurveda to allopathy. He returned six months later, very ill, with increased sarcoid involvement of all systems mentioned above, together with sarcoid epidydimitis and sarcoid of the skin, muscles and joints. He also had hypersplenism manifested as an enlarged spleen, anaemia, leukopenia, and thrombocytopenia. Bone marrow biopsy showed the presence of multiple sarcoid granulomas. After admission to hospital he developed an acute cholecystitis necessitating emergency surgery. The wall of the gall bladder on histology showed non-caseating sarcoid granulomas. His response to corticosteroids given in a dose of 40 mg/day was excellent except for a persistent severe hypersplenism. A splenectomy brought relief with the blood count and platelet count returning to normal. It is over five years since the onset of his disease and he now has a persistent low-grade sarcoid activity in many of his organ systems; he is on a maintenance dose of 10 mg prednisolone/day + azathioprine 100 mg/day.

DIAGNOSIS AND DIAGNOSTIC APPROACH

Diagnosis of sarcoid needs to fulfil three requisites—a compatible clinical picture, presence of non-caseating granulomas on biopsy and the exclusion of other causes of non-caseating granulmomas. Two important causes of non-caseating granulomas are TB and fungal infections. Other causes of non-caseating granulomas include brucellosis, Hansen's disease, Wegener's granulomatosis, and Churg-Strauss syndrome. Occupational diseases or work-related diseases such as berylliosis, extrinsic allergic alveolitis and drug-related lung diseases should also be considered. It is therefore imperative that non-caseating

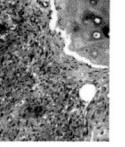

granulomas in biopsy material should be stained for all relevant organisms, particularly for TB and fungal infection. Culture of biopsy material, in particular for *Mycobacterium tuberculosis* is also advisable. Negative staining for acid-fast bacilli, negative culture and a negative polymerase chain reaction (PCR) for acid-fast bacilli strengthens the diagnosis of sarcoidosis in a patient with a clinical picture compatible with the disease. In poor, developing countries TB remains the main differential diagnosis as non-caseating granulomas can occur in TB and acid-fast bacilli are not necessarily always present on staining. A negative Mantoux skin test in the above circumstances favours the diagnosis of sarcoidosis.

Chronic berylliosis, an occupational hypersensitivity disorder due to exposure to beryllium is indistinguishable from sarcoidosis. Exposure to beryllium occurs in nuclear, aerospace, computer and electronic industries. The disease is characterized by non-caseating granulomas in the affected organs, chiefly the lungs and the skin. The diagnosis is made by a careful occupational history and demonstrating sensitivity to beryllium by a positive beryllium lymphocyte proliferation test. Chronic berylliosis is generally resistant to corticosteroid treatment. If undiagnosed, in the presence of continued exposure the mortality is as high as 25%. Resolution of the disease has been reported after cessation of exposure to beryllium.

As a rule, biopsy to confirm the clinical suspicion of sarcoidosis should be performed from a site which is most easily accessible and which is least traumatic. Thus if pulmonary sarcoidosis is also associated with skin involvement or peripheral lymphadenopathy or enlargement of the parotid or lachrymal glands, a biopsy of the skin lesion or an excision biopsy of a lymph gland or lachrymal gland biopsy may give the diagnosis with the least trauma.

Isolated pulmonary sarcoidosis needs a fiberoptic bronchoscopy with a transbronchial biopsy. The diagnostic yield in a patient with hilar or mediastinal adenopathy varies from 60–90% if at least four to six biopsies are taken, depending on the experience and expertise of the bronchoscopist. It is even higher if hilar or mediastinal adenopathy is associated with pulmonary infiltrates on radiography or a chest CT. Intrathoracic lymph nodes can be sampled when technically feasible through a transbronchoscopic needle aspiration biopsy or through a CT-guided biopsy. These procedures in combination with a transbronchial lung biopsy increase the diagnostic yield to over 90%. Bronchial mucosal biopsies may yield positive results in over 50% of patients even in the absence of endobronchial involvement as judged by the naked eye. It needs to be remembered that transbronchial biopsy in Stage IV of pulmonary sarcoidosis has a low yield.

BAL studies show a CD4:CD8 ratio greater than 3.5 in sarcoidosis; this test has a high specificity but a low sensitivity and is not recommended for diagnostic purposes.

Mediastinoscopy with mediastinoscopic biopsy may have to be resorted to when fiberoptic transbronchial biopsy or a CT-guided biopsy fails to give definite results, provided the intrathoracic lymphadenopathy is accessible through a mediastinoscope.

Rarely, a video-assisted thoracoscopic biopsy becomes necessary to establish a diagnosis, particularly in rare manifestations of pulmonary sarcoidosis—as with solid lesions due to necrotising sarcoid granulomatosis.

It is to be noted that though bilateral hilar adenopathy, fever, polyarthritis and erythema nodosum occurring in Lofgren's syndrome are typically due to sarcoidosis, they also occur with TB in countries where TB is strongly endemic and in histoplasmosis and other fungal infections in areas of the world endemic to these infections. A diagnostic hilar or mediastinal gland biopsy may not be necessary in Lofgren's syndrome in Western countries but is on occasion advisable in poor developing countries of the world, particularly if use of corticosteroids is contemplated. A strongly positive Mantoux test in a patient with erythema nodosum, arthralgia and hilar plus mediastinal adenopathy is invariably due to TB; a biopsy is generally neither indicated nor necessary.

Asymptomatic bilateral hilar adenopathy with a negative Mantoux skin test, in our opinion, does not need a diagnostic biopsy. It invariably points to sarcoidosis, though TB and very rarely a lymphoma may enter into the differential diagnosis. A close follow-up is however warranted.

Sarcoidosis presenting as a mediastinal adenopathy needs to be differentiated from all other causes of such adenopathy—notably TB, Hodgkin's and Non-Hodgkin's lymphoma, and metastatic involvement of mediastinal lymph nodes. The presence of well-marked necrosis of lymph glands on an HRCT of the chest invariably points to TB. Lymphadenopathy due to sarcoid involvement does not show necrosis. Lymphomas and metastatic lymphadenopathy though generally non-necrotic may occasionally show necrosis. A CT-guided biopsy, a transbronchial biopsy through a fibreoptic bronchoscope or if necessary a biopsy obtained through a mediastinoscopy should give the correct diagnosis.

Diagnosis of sarcoidosis involving other organ systems without pulmonary involvement may be difficult. Fortunately, more often than not, one or more of the organ systems involved are accessible to a biopsy procedure. Neurosarcoid has fairly characteristic though not absolutely specific imaging findings. Very rarely, a brain biopsy becomes necessary to exclude malignant or infectious disease.

Sarcoidosis involving the heart is suggested by clinical features stated earlier, by suggestive echocardiographic findings and by a positive gallium scan. Endomyocardial biopsy is not advised as the diagnostic yield is less than 10–20%.

For organ involvement which is difficult to biopsy, imaging techniques such as gallium 67 scan or ^{18}F-fluorodeoxyglucose positron emission tomography (FDG-PET) may help to pick up areas of occult inflammation that could then allow easy biopsy for confirming the diagnosis. It has been suggested that a gallium 67 scan showing an uptake in bilateral hilar and right paratracheal glands (lambda sign) together with an uptake in the parotids, submandibular, and lachrymal glands' regions (panda sign) is pathognomic of sarcoidosis. PET scanning is associated with much less radiation exposure, provides excellent resolution and will probably replace gallium scan to help locate sites of inflammation which are not clinically evident.

Other laboratory tests may be necessary to exclude other diseases. There is no laboratory test that is specific for sarcoidosis. Serum angiotensin converting enzyme (SACE) levels are elevated in 40–80% of cases with clinically active disease. Elevated SACE levels are, however, also seen in TB, other granulomatous disease, lymphoma, hepatitis, thyroid disorders, Hansen's disease and a few others. In our experience we have found the

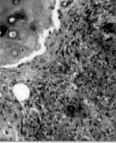

SACE level elevated in close to 80% of active sarcoidosis. The test, however, lacks the specificity to allow a diagnosis on this basis alone, more so as the test is not infrequently positive in TB and lymphoma—two conditions that need to be specially considered in the differential diagnosis of sarcoidosis. In a histologically proven case of sarcoid an elevated SACE level is a fairly good marker of the activity of sarcoidosis. A fall is consistently though not always observed in clinical remission. A subsequent rise often heralds a recurrence of the disease. The test is however variable and has no prognostic value.

PROGNOSIS

The ACCESS study has given valuable information with regards to the natural history of sarcoidosis in patients living in the West. The following features are of note—

1. Organ involvement is defined early in the natural history of the disease. Only 23% of patients in the ACCESS study were noted to have a new organ involvement during a two-year follow-up.
2. Patients who undergo remission generally do so within two to three years. Sarcoidosis rarely recurs after a prolonged period of remission. Notable exceptions are neurosarcoidosis and sarcoid uveitis.
3. Patients who do not show remission continue with chronic sarcoidosis and these patients constitute 30–50% of all known patients with sarcoidosis. These patients have progressive organ involvement, the rate of progression varying from patient to patient.
4. Acute presentation of sarcoidosis as in the Lofgren's syndrome is associated with a good prognosis, the remission rate being 70–80%.
5. Patients presenting with Stage I chest radiograph have a spontaneous remission rate of 60–90%. Those presenting with a Stage II chest radiograph have a poorer outcome with a spontaneous remission rate of 40–70%. Patients presenting with a Stage III chest X-ray have a remission rate of 10–20% and those with Stage IV chest radiographs showing extensive pulmonary fibrosis do not undergo remission.

Death when it occurs is generally due to progressive pulmonary fibrosis causing chronic hypoxemic or hypoxemic plus hypercapnic respiratory failure. Pulmonary hypertension and cor pulmonale are end-stage phenomena.

Occasionally, TB occurs as a complication, particularly in countries where the prevalence rate of TB is high. Pneumothorax can complicate sarcoidosis in rare instances, particularly when the radiograph of the chest is at Stage IV level.

Secondary infection with gram-positive or gram-negative organisms in the fibrocystic stage of the disease is also observed. An aspergilloma is not an uncommon complication in patients with severe fibrocystic disease and bronchiectasis. Aspergillomas can cause exsanguinating bleeds.

TREATMENT

Many patients with sarcoidosis have a good prognosis; some indeed have an excellent prognosis. For example, asymptomatic or mildly symptomatic patients presenting with Stage I disease

(with reference to radiological examination of the chest) may show remission rates as high as 90%. These patients require a follow-up but no specific therapy, even if the glands are large. Patients with Stage II radiographic findings who have minimal or no symptoms, very little pulmonary infiltrates on an X-ray chest and who have normal lung functions may also be closely observed to determine if there is evidence of remission or progression. Clear evidence of progressive pulmonary infiltration or the presence of impaired lung function or of disturbing symptoms warrants systemic therapy. The mild form of Löfgren's syndrome either in its full form or a variant form responds to rest and non-steroidal anti-inflammatory drugs. The severe form of this syndrome characterized by high fever, painful arthropathy and painful erythema nodosum warrants systemic corticosteroid therapy. The presence of uveitis, even in mild Löfgren's syndrome, is an indication for corticosteroid therapy.

As a general principle, systemic corticosteroids are indicated—

a. When there is significant disturbance of organ function in the organ or organs affected by sarcoidosis;
b. When there are constitutional symptoms in the form of persistent fever, weight loss, lassitude, arthralgias or painful arthropathy.

Table 45.3: Indications for systemic corticosteroids
Chronic pulmonary sarcoid which is invariably associated with symptoms and deteriorating lung function
Severe form of Löfgrens syndrome
Neurosarcoidosis or sarcoidosis involving the heart
Persistent hypercalcemia
Renal or hepatic dysfunction
Uveitis not responding to topical corticosteroids or showing frequent relapse while on topical corticosteroids
Palpable spleen with multiple hypoechoic areas on imaging studies—hypersplenism
Disfiguring skin sarcoids
Persistent disabling constitutional symptoms in the form of fever, weight loss, tiredness, arthralgias

Systemic Therapy

Use of corticosteroids: Corticosteroids form the mainstay of therapy for sarcoidosis. They provide prompt symptomatic relief and reverse organ dysfunction. The extent to which organ dysfunction is reversed depends on the degree of damage to organ structure already present and in particular to the degree of fibrosis before starting therapy. Most clinical trials conclude that the use of corticosteroids favourably influences the outcome in chronic pulmonary sarcoidosis.

There is however some controversy as to whether steroids significantly influence the long-term natural history of the disease. Many authorities are of the view that they neither influence the natural history nor improve the ultimate survival. Comparative studies of patients receiving corticosteroid

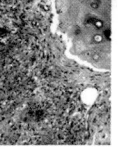
treatment for 18 months and those not receiving corticosteroids suggest that though steroid therapy improved symptoms and suppressed granulomas, there was no evidence of improvement in long-term prognosis.

The British Thoracic Society Sarcoidosis Study was conducted on a multi-centre basis to determine the long-term effects of corticosteroids in pulmonary sarcoidosis. A group of 58 patients was treated for one and a half years starting with 30 mg /day for a month; 20 mg daily for the next month; 10 mg daily to complete a year, following which the drug was very slowly tapered and stopped after a further six months. Another group of 31 patients was offered selective treatment; in these, treatment was offered only if there was a development of symptoms or there was deteriorating lung function. The initial dose of prednisolone was 30 mg/day and this was tapered and stopped after six to nine months. The average follow-up of the two groups was five years. The group on prolonged one and a half years' treatment with the arm of optimizing radiographic appearance of the chest showed significantly better long-term functional outcome, though in the final analysis the difference between the two groups though significant, was not very large.

Regardless of the controversy, corticosteroids should be given in pulmonary sarcoidosis in presence of significant or worsening symptoms or if there is deteriorating lung function.

DOSAGE OF CORTICOSTEROIDS

The optimal dose and duration of therapy has not been determined by prospective randomized controlled trials. Treatment is therefore individualized depending on the organ or organs involved, the severity of symptoms, the degree of organ dysfunction and the patient's response to therapy.

Initial treatment is generally started with 30 to 40 mg prednisolone per day in an average-sized adult. Sarcoid involving the heart, neurosarcoid, involvement of the kidneys or the presence of hypersplenism may warrant a dose of 60 mg/day to start with. The dose is slowly tapered every three to four weeks to a maintenance dose of 5 to 10 mg/day. Treatment should preferably be continued for at least 12 months since tapering the dose completely before this period generally leads to a relapse. Some patients require a maintenance dose of prednisolone for two to three years or even indefinitely to keep the disease under control. Inhaled steroids may offer symptomatic relief in patients who have airways' obstruction and hyper-reactive airways. They do not replace oral steroids in the management of pulmonary sarcoidosis.

Corticosteroid dosage in patients presenting with severe life-threatening neurosarcoidosis or with severe ocular involvement with impending blindness (as with acute optic neuritis or chorioretinitis) needs to be larger than that stated above. Pulse therapy of IV methylprednisolone 0.5 g to 1 g daily for three to four days is followed by 60 mg prednisolone daily. Immunosuppressive therapy (discussed later) is often used for its steroid-sparing effect, as therapy may need to be continued for years.

Alternative Therapy

Alternative therapy which has an immunomodulatory or immunosuppressive effect may be used in patients who respond poorly to corticosteroids, in corticosteroid-resistant patients or for their steroid-sparing effect.

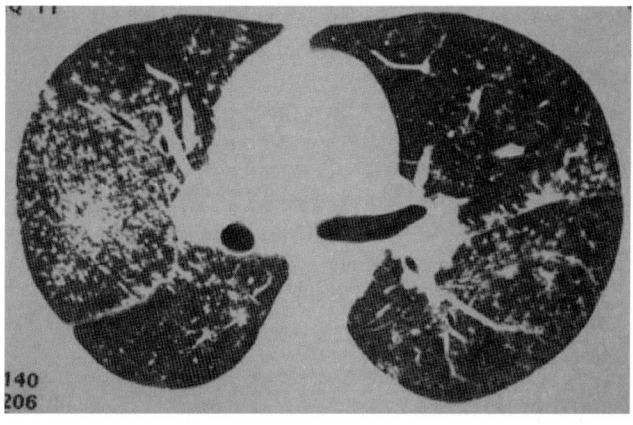

(a)

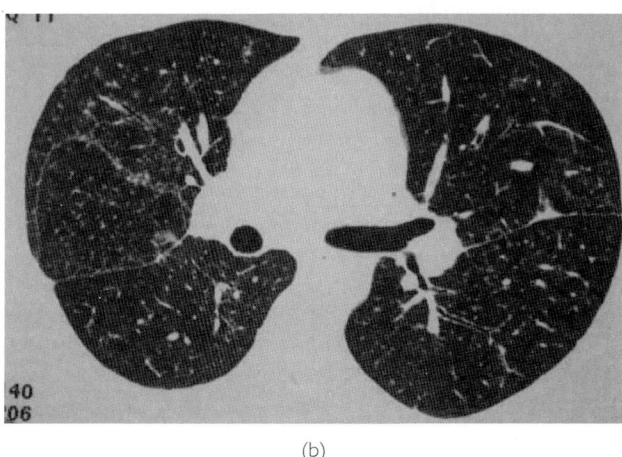

(b)

Fig 45.15: Extensive interstitial nodules. (a) Interstitial nodules seen (b) After 6 months of treatment nearly all nodules have disappeared.

HYDROXYCHLOROQUINE

Hydroxychloroquine is perhaps the most frequently used drug after corticosteroids. It is particularly useful in skin sarcoidosis and in neurosarcoidosis. It is believed to have a direct effect on sarcoid granulomas and does not just act through a non-specific anti-inflammatory mechanism. The drug can cause a retinitis and should not be used in the presence of a sarcoid uveitis. A three- or six-monthly ophthalmic check is recommended.

TETRACYCLINE

Doxycycline, minocycline may prove useful in patients with skin sarcoid; they are not effective in sarcoid involving other organ systems.

PENTOXIFYLLINE

Pentoxifylline, a phosphodiesterase inhibitor has anti-inflammatory effects and has been found to be effective in early pulmonary sarcoidosis in one study. By and large most authorities feel the drug has little to offer in the treatment of the disease.

AZATHIOPRINE, METHOTREXATE, LEFLUNOMIDE, MYCOPHENOLATE MOFETIL, CYCLOPHOSPHAMIDE

Methotrexate is often the first drug to be tried in steroid-resistant sarcoidosis. Studies suggest that the drug benefits 50–70% of patients though a response may be observed only after six

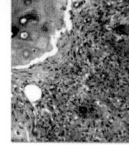

months. Unfortunately, hepatic, renal and pulmonary toxicity limits its use. Methotrexate can also be used as a steroid-sparing drug allowing a reduction in the maintenance dose of corticosteroids. Leflunomide, an analogue of methotrexate may have the same effect with less pulmonary toxicity.

Azathioprine or cyclophosphamide has been found useful in some patients with severe corticosteroid-resistant sarcoidosis.

Mycophenolate mofetil has been tried recently with reportedly good effects in neurosarcoid, ocular, hepatic and corticosteroid-resistant pulmonary sarcoidosis.

Cyclophosphamide has not proved useful with the possible exceptions of a few patients with neurosarcoidosis.

ANTI-TNF THERAPY

TNF is an important factor in the formation and persistence of sarcoid granulomas. Anti-TNF therapy has therefore a scientific basis. A recent multi-centred trial with infliximab found the drug effective with regard to several end-points, including improvement in FVC after six months of therapy. Etarnercept in a similar trial was ineffective. Anti-TNF therapy carries inherent risks and it is better for the present to await the results of further trials before prescribing this therapy.

Symptomatic Therapy

1. Profuse haemoptysis from an aspergilloma in advanced fibrotic pulmonary sarcoidosis may need embolisation of culprit bronchial or pulmonary vessels. Surgery is usually contraindicated in view of very poor lung function in these patients.
2. Hypoxemic respiratory failure in advanced cases requires continues oxygen at 1 to 2 L/min if PaO_2 at rest is < 55 mm Hg.
3. Pulmonary hypertension and cor pulmonale require symptomatic treatment. The role of currently available drugs (such as Bosentan) in these patients is not known.
4. Sarcoidosis involving the heart and manifesting with arrhythmias necessitates the use of appropriate anti-arrhythmic drugs and if needs be the insertion of an automatic implantable cardioverter + defibrillator. Congestive cardiomyopathy needs conventional treatment in the form of diuretics, after-load reducing agents, digoxin, aldactone and the judicious use of a β blocker. These patients require larger doses of corticosteroids initially and may also need a higher maintenance dose of 15 mg to 20 mg/day for many months.

Lung Transplant

In specialized centres in the West, lung transplantation is an important option in patients with advanced pulmonary sarcoidosis who show severe impairment of pulmonary function refractory to medical therapy. Timing of transplantation is both difficult and challenging. Mortality rates in Western countries for patients with sarcoidosis awaiting transplants are high (27–53%). There are as yet no clear guidelines even in the West for candidate selection as there are, for example, in patients with idiopathic pulmonary fibrosis. For the present, it has been suggested that selection of patients with sarcoidosis for lung transplantation should be based on an extrapolation of prevalent guidelines for lung transplantation in patients with severe idiopathic pulmonary fibrosis. These guidelines are:

a. Forced Vital Capacity (FVC) of less than 50% of predicted;
b. Diffusion Capacity (DLCO) less than 50% of predicted;
c. Hypoxemia at rest or hypoxemia induced by exercise;
d. Deteriorating lung function on optimal medical therapy.

Special risk factors associated with mortality in patients on Lung Transplant Waiting List as observed in the West are:

1. Elevated right atrial pressure (> 15 mm Hg)
2. Pulmonary hypertension
3. Increased quantity of supplemental oxygen used
4. The African-American race

It is to be noted that after lung transplantation, recurrent sarcoidosis in the lung allografts can occur though this does not affect survival or the risk of complications.

In India and other developing countries where lung transplantation is yet to take off, advanced sarcoidosis will continue to be treated on medical lines. It would be of relevance to study the life expectancy of advanced pulmonary sarcoidosis

Table 45.4: Drugs used in the treatment of sarcoidosis		
Systemic Therapy		
Corticosteroids	Start with 30 to 40 mg prednisolone/day Cardiac sarcoid, neurosarcoid, involvement of the kidneys or the presence of hypersplenism - 60 mg/day	Taper till maintenance dose of 5–10 mg/day is reached in 12 months
	Pulse doses with intravenous methyl prednisolone 0.5–1 g/day for 4 days are needed in severe neurosarcoidosis or with severe ocular involvement with impending blindness	Switch to oral prednisolone 60 mg/day and taper slowly
Systemic side-effects of corticosteroids should be periodically monitored and prophylactically treated if possible		
Systemic Therapy		
Hydroxychloroquine	Skin sarcoidosis and in neurosarcoidosis	
Pentoxifylline	Early pulmonary sarcoidosis 400 mg TDS or QID	
Doxycycline Minocycline	Skin sarcoid—200 mg/day	
Azathioprine	Severe corticosteroid resistant sarcoidosis 50 mg/day for 2 weeks, increase up to 100 mg/day	
Methotrexate	Sterioid resistant sarcoidosis 10–20 mg/week	
Leflunomide	Steroid resistant sarcoidosis—20 mg/day	
Mycophenolate mofetil	Neurosarcoid, ocular, hepatitic and corticosteroidresistant pulmonary sarcoidosis	
Cyclophosphamide	Rarely tried in neurosarcoidosis.	
Anti TNF therapy— Infliximab	Experimental	

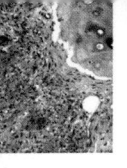

in Indian and other Asian patients who are hypoxemic at rest or on a standard six-minute walk, and whose FVC and CO diffusion capacity are < 50% of predicted, while continuing optimal medical therapy which includes supplemental oxygen.

SUGGESTED READING

Badgwell C. Cutaneous sarcoidosis therapy updated. *J Am Acad Dermatol.* 1 Jan. 2007; 56(1): 69–83.

Baughman RP. Treatment of sarcoidosis. *Clin Chest Med.* 1 Sep. 2008; 29(3): ix–x, 533–48.

Chen ES. Etiology of sarcoidosis. *Clin Chest Med.* 1 Sep. 2008; 29(3): vii, 365–77.

Gupta Samir Kumar. *Sarcoidosis: A Journey through 50 years.*

Gupta SK, Gupta S. Sarcoidosis in India: A Review of 125 Biopsy Proven Cases from Eastern India. *Sarcoidosis.* Mar. 1990; 7(1): 43–9.

Kim JS. Cardiac sarcoidosis. *Am Heart J.* 1 Jan. 2009; 157(1): 9–21.

Mihailovic-Vucinic. V-Pulmonary sarcoidosis. *Clin Chest Med.* 1 Sep. 2008; 29(3): 459–73, viii–ix.

Nagai S. Outcome of sarcoidosis. *Clin Chest Med.* 1 Sep. 2008; 29(3): 565–74.

Rose AS. Hepatic, ocular, and cutaneous sarcoidosis. *Clin Chest Med.* 1 Sep. 2008; 29(3): 509–24, ix.

Sharma OP. Sarcoidosis around the world. *Clin Chest Med.* 2008; 29: 357–363.

Sharma SK. Uncommon manifestations of sarcoidosis. *J Assoc Physicians India.* 2004 Mar; 52: 210–14.

Stern BJ. Neurologic presentations of sarcoidosis. *Neurol Clin.* 1 Feb. 2010; 28(1): 185–98.

CHAPTER **46**

Pulmonary Langerhans' Cell Histiocytosis

GENERAL CONSIDERATIONS

Pulmonary Langerhans' cell histiocytosis is characterized by the monoclonal proliferation and infiltration of Langerhans' cells in the small bronchioles and interstitium of the lungs. The earlier designation was histiocytosis X and eosinophilic granuloma. The term histiocytosis X was coined in 1953 by Lichtenstein for a group of three clinical entities, each with a differing clinical spectrum, but having as a common feature, the proliferation of a histiocytic-appearing cell. The three clinical entities considered by Lichtenstein under histiocytosis X were—

1. Letterer–Siwe disease—an aggressive, lethal disorder of young children, characterized by multi-system involvement
2. Hans-Schuller Christian Syndrome—generally occurring in children and young adults, characterized by multiple focal bone lesions (invariably involving the skull bones), exophthamous and diabetes insipidus
3. Eosinophilic granuloma of the bone or the lungs—focal lesions involving one or more bones or lesions involving both lungs.

The underlying offending proliferating histiocytic-appearing cell present in all these three clinical entities was later identified as the 'Langerhans' cell'. Therefore Langerhans' cell histiocytosis is now preferred to the term histiocytosis X and pulmonary involvement in histiocytosis X is termed Pulmonary Langerhans' cell histiocytosis.

Table 46.1 Simplified system of classification of Langerhans' cell histiocytosis in audults
Single-organ involvement
Lung (occurs in isolation in > 85% of cases with lung involvement)
Bone
Skin
Pituitary
Lymph nodes
Other sites: thyroid, liver, spleen, brain
Multi-system disease
Multi-organ disease with lung involvement (5–15% of cases with lung involvement)
Multi-organ disease without lung involvement
Multi-organ histiocytic disorder

Though Langerhans' cell histiocytosis is characterized by a clonal proliferation of the Langerhans' cell, it is considered (even in the more aggressive form) to be a reactive disease rather than a malignant disease. The current classification of Langerhans' cell histiocytosis is given below.

EPIDEMIOLOGY AND AETIOLOGY

Pulmonary Langerhans' cell histiocytosis is a smoker's disease occurring in young adults generally between 20–40 years of age. Tobacco smoke is the causative factor; no other environmental or occupational factor has been incriminated. Though previously thought to have a male preponderance in the West, current literature suggests equal distribution between males and females or even a predominance in females, perhaps related to the increasing smoking habit of women in the West. A smoking history is obtained in more than 90% of patients. We have seen a patient in his early teens who was a non-smoker, but passive smoking may have played a role in this patient as the father was a heavy smoker. There is no evidence of a genetic predisposition though familial clustering in children has been reported in Western literature.

Pathogenesis

The pathogenesis is not well understood. The disease is thought to be caused by an abnormal immune response to cigarette smoke initiated and perpetuated by Langerhans' cells. Animal studies have shown that mice exposed to cigarette smoke developed granulomatous lesions indistinguishable from those seen in human Langerhans' cell histiocytosis. When exposure to cigarette smoke was stopped, the density of Langerhans' cells in these mice decreased to that observed in controls.

Langerhans' cells probably function as antigen-presenting cells and stimulate lymphocyte proliferation in the interstitium and the bronchial wall. Both Langerhans' cells and lymphocytes are attracted and become attached to the lesions due to elaboration of various cytokines which include granulocyte—macrophage colony-stimulating factor (GM-CSF), tumour necrosis factor α (TNFα), interleukin, and transforming growth factor (TGF-β) expressed in the granulomas as also by the altered epithelium within the airways of smokers. It has been hypothesized that activated Langerhans' cells induce an exaggerated T-lymphocytic cell stimulation, thereby causing and perpetuating the granulomatous lesions observed in the disease. The role of other cells in the granulomas, notably the eosinophils that may be present is unclear.

The antigen that initiates this immune response is not definitely known. Neuroendocrine cells are increased within the lungs of cigarette smokers and cigarette smoke is known

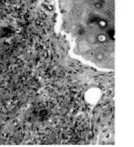

to induce the secretion of bombesin-like peptides from these neuroendocrine cells. It has been suggested that the bombesin-like peptides may act as antigens, stimulating cytokine production by macrophages which in turn activate and stimulate Langerhans' cells within the lungs.

Glycoprotein, a constituent of cigarette smoke is an immunostimulant and has also been implicated in the pathogenesis of this disease.

Finally, a third concept is that new antigens are expressed by the altered epithelium of the airways in smokers and that these antigens trigger an altered immune response to cause the disease.

Pathology

The characteristic infiltrate and granulomas consist typically of Langerhans' cells. On light microscopy these cells are usually mononuclear with abundant acidophilic cytoplasm and highly characteristic nuclei. The nuclei are irregular, elongated with prominent grooves and folds traversing in all directions. Eosinophils are also frequently present as are a few lymphocytes and plasma cells. As the lesions heal, fibrosis occurs; Langerhans' cells and eosinophilis are scarce or even absent in fibrotic lesions, being replaced by lymphocytes, macrophages and plasma cells. Fibrosis may lead to marked honeycombing of the lungs, most marked in the upper lobes where the disease is more marked from the very beginning.

On electron microscopy the Langerhans' cell has a characteristic appearance. Within its cytoplasm can be found typical granules termed the Birbeck granules. Birbeck granulas are rod-shaped with zipper-like striations and sometimes have a bulbous racket-shaped end. Immunostaining shows CD1 antigen on the cell surface and S100 protein in the cytoplasm.

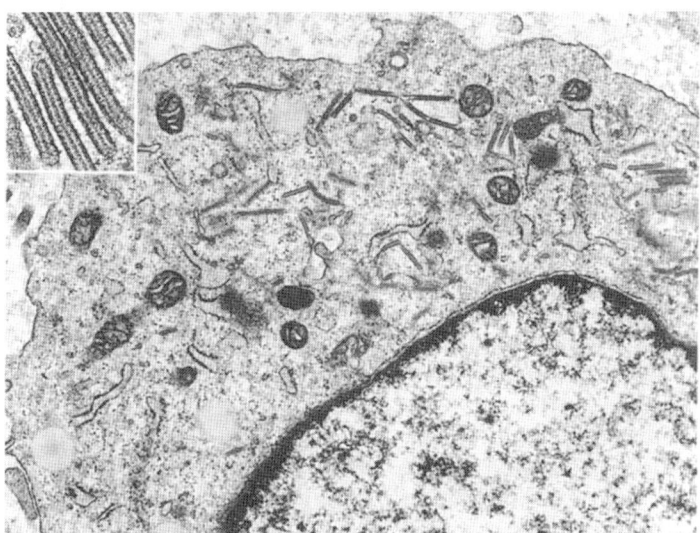

Fig 46.1: Ultrastructurally the Langerhans' cells contain Birbeck granules, which are seen in the cytoplasm of the cell and in the inset.

CLINICAL FEATURES

The clinical presentation varies. A history of cigarette smoking is important.

1. The patient may be asymptomatic (10–25% of patients), the disease being discovered on a routine X-ray chest which shows small nodular lesions chiefly in the upper and mid-zones of both lungs. At times the X-ray appears indistinguishable from miliary tuberculosis (TB) and is treated for a time as such. The absence of any change in the miliary lesions after treatment prompts an open lung biopsy which reveals the true nature of the pathology.

2. The two important respiratory symptoms are cough and dyspnoea on exertion. Increasing dyspnoea is observed when there is progression of the disease.

3. The first manifestation of the disease may be a spontaneous pneumothorax which may recur on the same side or may occur after a varying interval on the other. We have observed a patient with spontaneous pneumothorax occurring simultaneously on both sides causing acute respiratory distress and failure.

4. Constitutional symptoms include low-grade fever, weight loss, and fatigue occurring in 20% of patients. A mistaken diagnosis of miliary TB is frequent when these patients also have small nodular shadows in the lungs.

5. Rarely (in perhaps 5% of patients) extrapulmonary manifestations in the form of cystic, solitary or multiple bone lesions or diabetes insipidus may be present. They may be the presenting feature and the diagnosis of pulmonary Langerhans' cell histiocytosis is only made on an investigation of the respiratory system.

Physical Findings

There may be no physical finding on examination of the chest. Clubbing of the nails is uncommon. Some patients have rhonchi on auscultation, others may have fine crackles, particularly in the upper lobes and a few have both rhonchi and crackles.

In patients who show progression of the disease, increasing pulmonary fibrosis produces hypoxic respiratory failure, pulmonary hypertension, cor pulmonale and congestive heart failure.

Natural History

The natural history is variable. In 25% of patients, there is complete spontaneous remission. In 50% of patients, the disease stabilizes after mild to moderate progression. There is however always the possibility of the disease resuming activity after a varying period of stabilization. In 25% of patients there is progressive deterioration. In the last group the end-result is chronic hypoxic cum hypercapnic respiratory failure and increasing pulmonary hypertension with cor pulmonale and congestive heart failure; the median survival is reported to be 13 years. The natural history can be punctuated at any point in time by pneumothorax. Pulmonary infection or systemic sepsis from any other cause is an important complication, particularly in those on corticosteroids and /or cytotoxic drugs.

Investigations

CHEST RADIOGRAPHY

An X-ray of the chest shows micronodular lesions, at times miliary lesions, chiefly involving the upper and mid-zones of both lungs, with a sparing of the costophrenic angles. The lesions on a careful examination are often superimposed on cystic

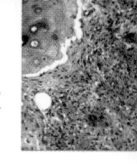

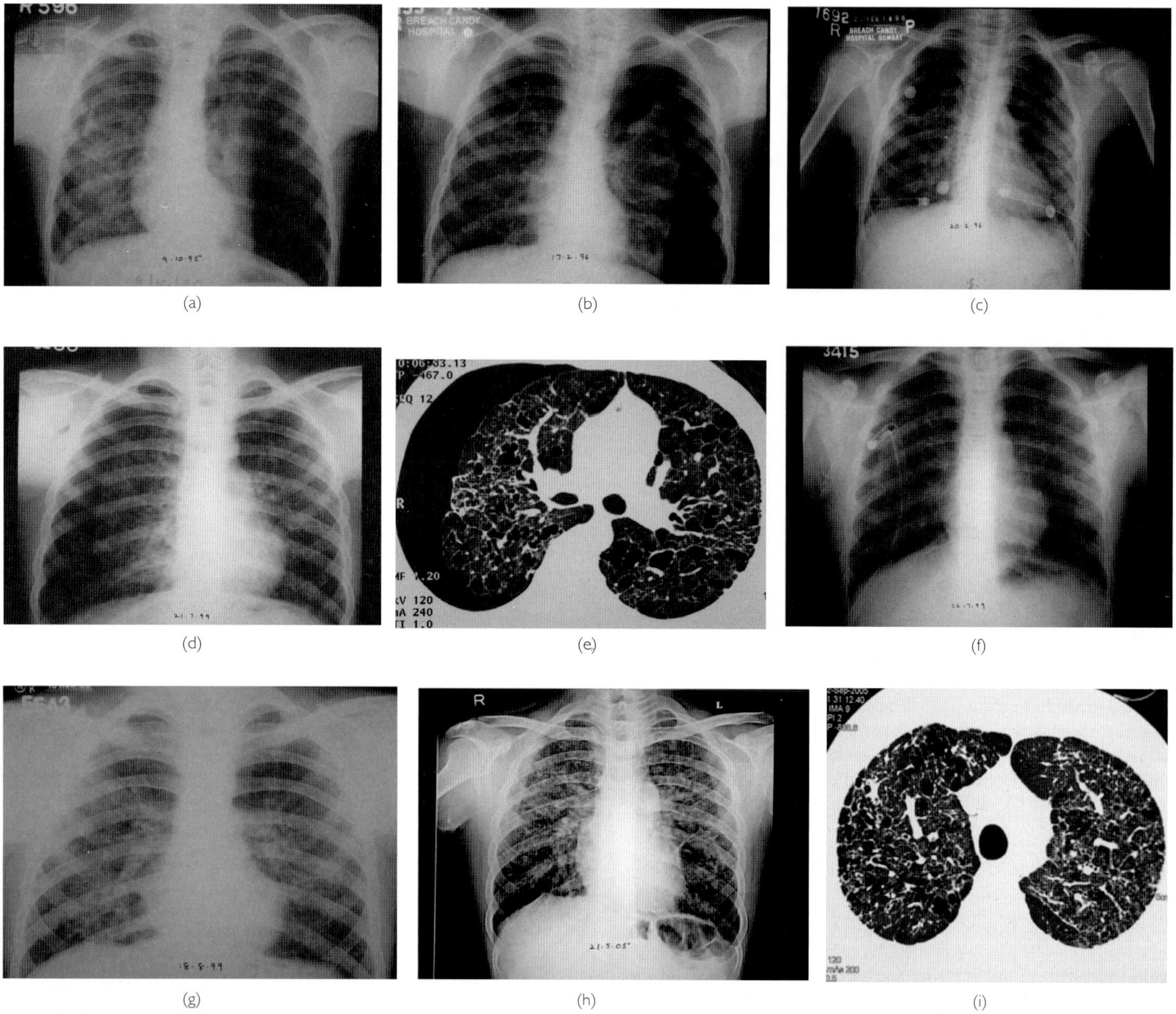

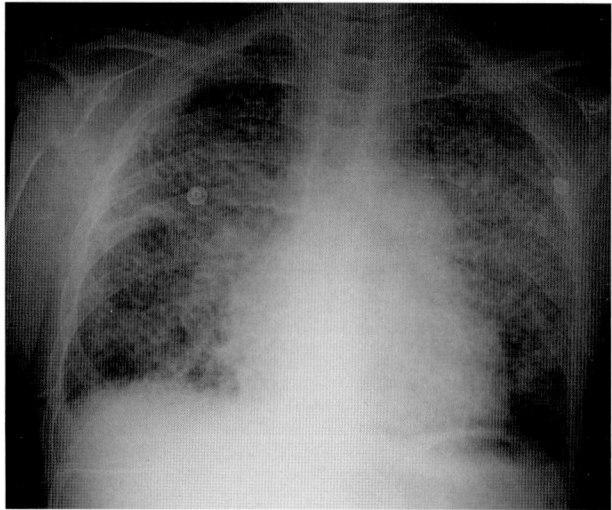

Fig 46.2a–j: Pulmonary Langerhans' cell histiocytosis.' An 11-year-old boy presented with sudden onset chest pain, breathlessness. (a) Chest X-ray revealed bilateral pneumothorax, larger on the left side. Pneumothorax resolved with intercostal tube drain (ICD) insertion (b) Four months later, he developed bilateral pneumothorax again (c) Treated with bilateral ICD and subsequently left pleurodesis done (d) Three years later developed recurrence of right pneumothorax. Visualized lung parenchyma reveals reticulonodular lesions in both lung fields (e) HRCT chest reveals cysts which are bizarre in shape with abnormal intervening parenchyma, a typical finding of Langerhans' cell histiocytosis (f) Subsequently, right pleurodesis done (g) Post pleurodesis X-ray reveals extensive reticulonodular lesions in both lung fields (h, i) Follow-up X-ray and CT chest, 10 years after the first pneumothorax reveals bilateral reticulonodular opacities which have considerably increased, CT chest at this point reveals progression in size, shape and extent of the cysts. Note presence of nodules indicating that the disease is still active (j) Chest X-ray a short while later demonstrates extensive bilateral pulmonary opacities denoting acute respiratory distress syndrome (ARDS) related to overwhelming bacterial sepsis. Note enlarged cardiac silhouette with dilated pulmonary artery denoting chronic cor pulmonale at the end stage of the disease.

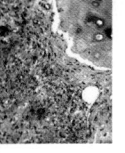
ring shadows 5–10 mm in diameter; the cystic ring shadows represent cavitation of the nodular lung lesions. As the disease progresses there is increasing fibrosis; the smaller cyst lesions merging to form larger thin-walled cysts and bullae. Well-marked honeycombing of the lungs is evident with progression of the disease. Very importantly the lung volumes on a chest X-ray remain normal, unlike what is observed in interstitial pulmonary fibrosis.

HIGH-RESOLUTION COMPUTED TOMOGRAPHY (HRCT) OF THE CHEST

An HRCT of the chest in the early stages shows nodules in the upper and mid-zones of both lungs. Serial CTs over time show a progression from nodular lesions to cavitation and cystic lesions. Increasing fibrosis leads to honeycombing of the lung, most marked in the upper and middle lobes.

The above typical pattern is not always present. Ground-glass attenuation may accompany the typical changes noted above. Also, at times, large cysts and bullae may be formed all over, including the lower lobes.

It has been shown that nodular lesions on an HRCT chest are an indication of active disease. Cystic lesions cannot however be considered inactive, as it is impossible to distinguish inactive cysts from cavitating granulomas.

LUNG FUNCTION TESTS

Lung function tests show typically a mixture of an obstructive plus restrictive pattern. At times one pattern predominates over the other. A fall in the diffusing capacity of carbon monoxide may be an early finding. A standard six-minute walk may show a fall in oxygen saturation. In the presence of increasing airways obstruction, the forced expiratory volume in one second/ forced vital capacity (FEV_1/FVC) is progressively reduced and there is an increased ratio of residual volume to total lung capacity.

BRONCHOALVEOLAR LAVAGE

The presence of > 5% Langerhans' cells in the bronchoalveolar lavage (BAL) fluid is considered to be diagnostic of the disease. However, the BAL may be negative with regard to Langerhans' cells in more than 50% of patients. A lower proportion of Langerhans' cells (<4%) can be seen in interstitial lung disease, bronchiolitis, and bronchoalveolar carcinoma.

LUNG BIOPSY

Transbronchial lung biopsy generally affords a poor yield of 10–40%. A thoracoscopic or open lung biopsy is the diagnostic procedure of choice. Even here the diagnosis may not be proven because of sampling errors since the lesions are focal and sampling of a cystic area may show no evidence of active disease.

DIAGNOSIS

The diagnosis should be suspected in young adults who are smokers and who have nodular lesions in the upper and mid-zones of both lungs. The HRCT chest appearances should be compatible with those described earlier. In the typical patient with the expected clinical features and typical imaging findings, a BAL study and/or a lung biopsy may not be necessary. A BAL study, failing which a lung biopsy, is indicated when the imaging findings are atypical; as for example in symptomatic patients where the shadows are purely nodular or to distinguish lymphangiomyomatosis from Langerhans' cell histiocytosis. A differential diagnosis of TB, extrinsic allergic alveolitis and sarcoidosis may need to be entertained in some patients with Langerhans' cell histiocytosis.

TREATMENT

The patient should be instructed to stop smoking. The disease has been then known to regress or at least stabilize in some but not all patients.

If a period of observation shows that the lung disease is progressive, corticosteroids are indicated. Prednisolone in a dose of 40 mg/day is given for four weeks; reduced by 5 mg every three to four weeks to a maintenance dose (preferably not > 10 mg/day) that controls the disease.

In rapidly progressive disease uncontrolled by corticosteroids, cytotoxic drugs such as cyclophosphamide, methotrexate, chlorambucil have been tried. Their effect on the natural history of progressive disease is undetermined. In disseminated disease, a combination of corticosteroids and cytotoxic drugs is advocated from the very beginning.

In rapidly progressive systemic disease bone marrow transplantation has been successfully performed. Advanced pulmonary disease with respiratory failure or pulmonary hypertension has been treated with lung transplantation. The disease may however recur in the transplanted lung.

Complications such as pneumothorax, pulmonary or any other systemic infections need requisite treatment.

SUGGESTED READING

Brown RE, Arico M, Nichols KE, Danesino C, O'Regan AW, Brophy MT, Miller WT, Vassallo R, Ryu JH, Limper AH. Pulmonary Langerhans' Cell Histiocytosis. *NEJM*. 2000; 343: 1654–6.

Mendez JL, Nadrous HF, Vassallo R, Decker PA, Ryu JH. Pneumothorax in Pulmonary Langerhans Cell Histiocytosis. *Chest*. 2004; 125: 1028–32.

Sundar KM, Gosselin MV, Chung HL, Cahill BC. Pulmonary Langerhans Cell Histiocytosis: Emerging Concepts in Pathobiology, Radiology, and Clinical Evolution of Disease. *Chest*. 2003; 123: 1673–83.

Tazi A. Adult pulmonary Langerhans' cell histiocytosis. *Eur Respir J*. 2006; 27: 1272–85.

Vassallo R, Ryu JH, Schroeder DR, Decker PA, Limper AH. Clinical Outcomes of Pulmonary Langerhans' Cell Histiocytosis in Adults. *NEJM*. 2002; 346: 484–90.

CHAPTER **47**

Pulmonary Lymphangioleiomyomatosis and Other Rare Diffuse Lung Diseases

GENERAL CONSIDERATIONS

Pulmonary lymphangioleiomyomatosis (LAM) is a rare, generally progressive disease affecting women in the childbearing age, characterized by infiltration of the lung by an unusual form of smooth muscle cell (termed LAM cells) causing extensive cyst formation and destruction of lung tissue. It is characterized clinically by dyspnoea, cough, recurrent pneumothorax, chylous pleural effusion and in most patients progression to respiratory failure. Some patients with pulmonary LAM show the presence of benign angiomyolipomas in the kidneys and/or enlargement of the axial retrocrural and retroperitoneal lymphatics.

The pulmonary manifestations of LAM predominate, but rarely, the disease may present exclusively within the abdomen, or the extrapulmonary abdominal presentation may precede involvement of the lungs.

Therapy for this disease is unsatisfactory but advances in molecular biology have identified several potential targets for future clinical trials with appropriate drugs.

EPIDEMIOLOGY

The prevalence in the UK, France and USA is about 1 per million of the population. It is also met with as a rare disease in India and other countries but the prevalence is unknown. The mean age of onset as judged from several studies is 35 years. Though almost exclusively occurring in females of childbearing age, there are reports of this disease in post-menopausal women receiving hormonal therapy.

There are two forms of LAM: sporadic LAM (S-LAM) and LAM occurring in association with tuberous sclerosis (TSC-LAM). Both are associated with mutations of tuberous sclerosis genes which regulate pathways that control energy supply and nutrients to cells. Global estimates indicate that the prevalence of TSC-LAM is probably five times more than S-LAM. However, women with S-LAM form > 85% of the 1300 patients registered by the LAM foundation, suggesting that TSC-LAM may perhaps be a milder disease than S-LAM. It has been estimated that 30–40% of women with TSC may have high-resolution computed tomography (HRCT) finding consistent with LAM.

GENETICS—MOLECULAR PATHOGENESIS OF LAM

LAM and TSC both are caused by mutations of either the hamartin (TSC-1) gene on chromosome 9 or the tuberin (TSC-2) gene on chromosome 16. These are tumour suppressor genes which form a complex that has a negative regulatory effect on the cell cycle. These genes control cell growth and survival through the rapamycin-signalling pathway. Deficiency or dysfunction of the encoded proteins hamartin or tuberin results in a loss of regulatory cell control. The consequent activation of the mTOR kinase and S-6 kinase leads to increased protein synthesis, cellular proliferation, migration and invasion.

It is believed that mutation and loss of hetrogenicity in the TSC-2 gene, or less commonly in the TSC-1 gene is responsible for sporadic pulmonary LAM. Pulmonary LAM cells and cells of angiomyolipomas in the kidney in sporadic LAM have been shown to possess the same TSC-2 gene mutation, not present in normal cells. There is evidence to suggest that LAM cells can metastasize. When a lung transplant performed for this disease shows a recurrence of pulmonary LAM in the transplant, the same TSC-2 mutation is observed in LAM cells of the recurrent disease as is present in the LAM cells of the original disease.

The mechanism whereby the mutations described above are translated into the clinical features of pulmonary LAM is uncertain. It is possible that factors in addition to mutations in the TSC-2 gene may be necessary for the development of LAM. The disease is limited to women, is exacerbated by the administration of oestrogen and may regress after menopause. Also LAM cells have oestrogen and progestrone receptors. These findings suggest that female sex hormones, in particular oestrogens may have a role in the evolution of the disease.

PATHOLOGY

The macroscopic appearance is of numerous cysts distributed all through the lungs. Microscopically, there is a proliferation of LAM cells. Proliferation within the wall of the airways leads to airways obstruction and airflow limitation; proliferation within the lymphatic walls leads to lymphatic obstruction; and proliferation within vessel walls leads to obstruction and rupture of vessels with intra-alveolar haemorrhage.

LAM cells appear to be a type of smooth muscle cells as they express actin, desmin and vimentin. The cells are however not typical of smooth muscle cells as they contain electron-dense membrane-bound vesicles. The cells stain with HMB-45, a feature useful for diagnosis in biopsy specimens of patients suspected to have this disease. LAM cells express receptors for oestrogens and progesterone. The oestrogen receptors are associated with antiapoptotic protein BCL-2. It is likely that suppression of apoptosis by oestrogen may be the mechanism underlying hormonal dependence in this disease.

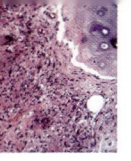

CLINICAL FEATURES

Pulmonary LAM presents most frequently with cough, and progressive breathlessness on exertion. The breathlessness may be associated with a wheeze. Haemoptysis though less common may also occur. An important presentation is with pleural chest pain caused by a pneumothorax. Pneumothorax may occur on either or both sides, may be recurrent and can occur at any time in the natural history of the disease. An important and often classical clinical feature is the presence of a unilateral or bilateral chylous pleural effusion, which recurs promptly on tapping and which may be occasionally associated with chyloptysis. A chylous pleural effusion may be the presenting clinical feature or may occur later in the course of the disease.

Rarely, extrapulmonary symptoms may be the presenting features. Extrapulmonary features include angiomyolipoma, abdominal lymphadenopathy, abdominal LAM and chylous ascites. Angiomyolipomas are within the kidneys (very rarely outside, within the abdomen); they are generally small and

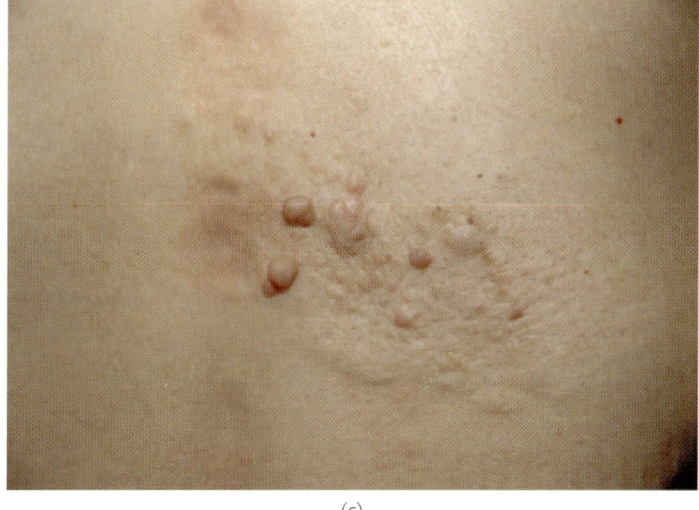

(c)

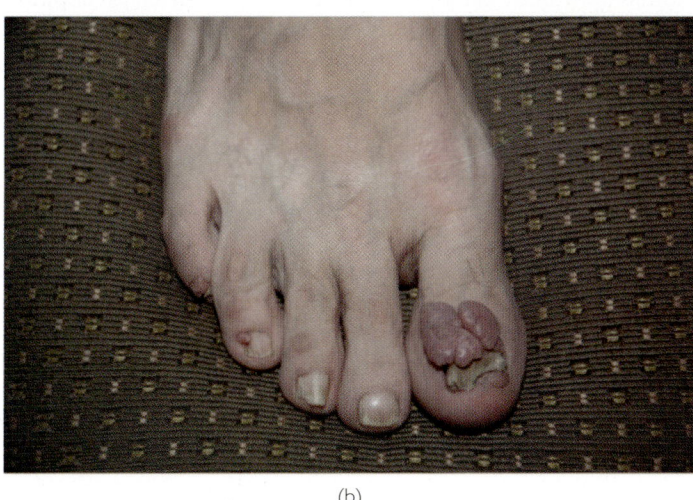

(a)

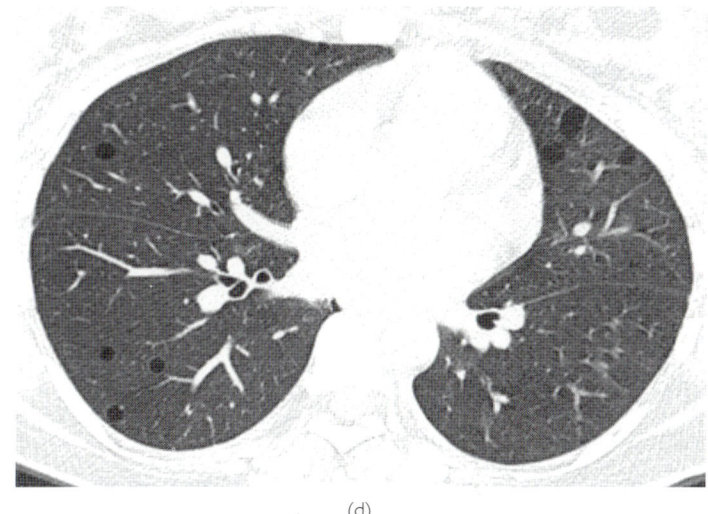

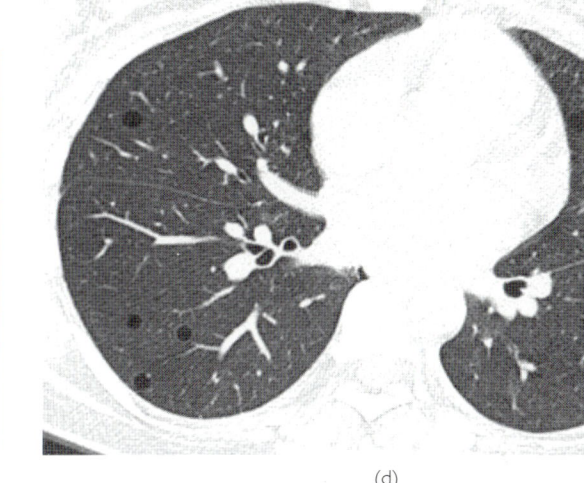

(d)

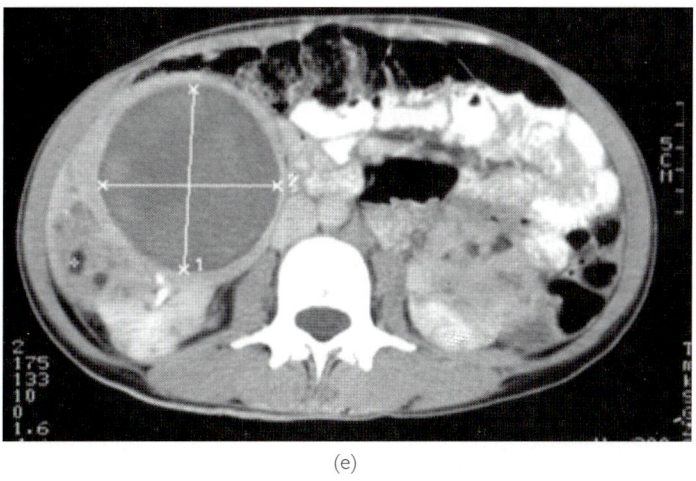

(b)

(e)

Fig 47.1: Lymphangioleiomyomatosis: A 40-year-old lady with a past history of generalized tonic clonic seizures since the age of two, no history of mental retardation, lived with a diagnosis of neurofibromatosis for 38 years, with extensive erythromatous maculopapular lesions over the face. In the seventh month of pregnancy she had a pneumothorax, intercostal tube drain (ICD). Note (a) facial angiofibroma (b) Ungual fibroma (c) Shagreen patch (d) Post-pleurodesis HRCT chest reveals multiple thin-walled cysts in both lung fields. The intervening lung parenchyma is normal. These are not as a result of centrilobular emphysema as they are in the lower zones, the centrilobular vessels are on the periphery of the cyst and patient denied a history of smoking. The cysts are thin-walled and rounded as compared to Pulmonary Langerhans' cell histiocytosis cysts which are thick-walled and irregular in shape (e) CT of the abdomen reveals a well-defined mass lesion which is relatively homogenous in consistency with internal hyperdensities representing haemorrhage. Surgical excision revealed an angiomyolipoma.

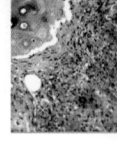

asymptomatic, but occasionally are large and may bleed. Mediastinal and abdominal lymphadenopathy is a frequent feature. LAMs are large, lobulated generally retroperitoneal masses containing chylous fluid. They can cause abdominal pain and chylous ascites.

The clinical features of tuberous sclerosis should always be sought because of the clear association between LAM and this disease. Pulmonary and extrapulmonary features of LAM are listed below:

Table 47.1: Pulmonary and extra pulmonary features of LAM	
Pulmonary	**Extrapulmonary (during course of the disease)**
Dyspnoea	Angiomyolipoma (generally renal, rarely extrarenal)
Cough	Lymphadenopathy
Chest pain	Lymphangioleimyomas
Haemoptysis	Chylous ascites
Pneumothorax	
Chylous effusion	

NATURAL HISTORY

In most, but not all cases, pulmonary LAM is a progressive disease chiefly producing airways obstruction but often a combination of obstruction plus restriction. It leads to progressive hypoxic or hypoxic + hypercapnic respiratory failure. The natural history is punctuated by pneumothorax which is often recurrent and by chylous pleural effusion. Life expectancy from the onset of symptoms is reported at 4 to 16 years. Currently, the median survival is around 10 years though patients with milder disease and slower progression may live longer. The disease may regress after menopause.

DIAGNOSIS

The major differential diagnosis is Langerhans' cell histiocytosis occurring in a female. Langerhans' cell histiocytosis invariably has a smoking history, chiefly involves the upper and mid-zones and spares the costrophrenic region. The cysts occur against the background of small nodules in the lung, are thicker walled, more irregularly shaped and often not as symmetrical as in pulmonary LAM.

Airflow limitation due to emphysema with luscent cysts on imaging studies is another important differential diagnosis. More often it is pulmonary LAM which is mistaken for emphysema than vice versa. Cystic spaces in emphysema have no clear defining walls in contrast to LAM. Other diseases that can mimic LAM are cavitating metastatic lesions, extrinsic allergic alveolitis, bronchiolitis, bronchopulmonary dysplasia and the Birt-Hogg-Dube (BHD) syndrome. The latter is a very rare tumour suppressor syndrome characterized by spontaneous pneumothorax, skin lesions, pulmonary cysts and inherited renal cell cancer.

INVESTIGATIONS

Chest Radiography

As the disease progresses, radiography of the chest shows reticular shadowing with thin-walled cysts distributed all over. Septal Kerley-B lines are visible. Cysts may merge to form larger cysts. Pneumothorax or chylous pleural effusion may be present. The cystic changes in the lung may become more evident and discernible when a pneumothorax produces a partial collapse of the lung. An important feature is that the lungs are normal-sized or often hyperexpanded, and not small in volume as is observed in the honeycombed lungs of interstitial pulmonary fibrosis.

HRCT

An HRCT of the chest very often strongly suggests the correct diagnosis. The following features are noted—

a. The presence of evenly distributed thin-walled cysts in both lung fields with normal intervening parenchyma. The cysts vary in size, generally from 2 to 20 mm but may merge to form much larger cysts of 5 to 10 cm. The cysts even when large invariably have discernible thin walls unlike in emphysema where they do not have discernible walls.
b. Ground-glass densities may be present and represent recent pulmonary haemorrhage.
c. Hilar and retrocrural lymphadenopathy may be present.

HRCT of the abdomen often reveals extrapulmonary features which may be silent and asymptomatic. These include angiomyolipomas recognized by the presence of areas of fat density (< 10 Hounsfield units); lymphadenopathy along the course of the axial lymphatics in the retrocrural, retroperitoneal and pelvic regions may also be present. LAMs are visible as large cystic, retroperitoneal masses with thick well-defined walls.

Lung Function Tests

In the early stages the lung functions may be normal. As the disease progresses an increasingly obstructive pattern is observed on spirometry. Very often the ventilatory pattern is characterized by both obstructive and restrictive changes. Reduced CO transfer occurs early in the disease. Arterial blood gases show increasing hypoxemia as the disease progresses. Hypercapnia often occurs later in the course of the disease.

MANAGEMENT

Hormonal Therapy

Treatment for this disease is unsatisfactory. Since the disease was thought to be hormone-dependent, attempts at treatment were directed towards oestrogen depletion or blockade. Though earlier reports on the use of progesterone (orally or intramusccular depot preparation) suggested that the drug may be of some benefit, a retrospective meta-analysis by Taveria-Da Silva et al., showed that progesterone did not prevent a decline in forced expiratory volume in one second (FEV_1) and appeared to accelerate the decline in diffusion lung capacity for carbon

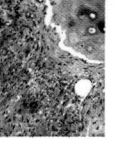

monoxide (DLCO) compared to untreated patients. The early enthusiasm for progesterone treatment has therefore waned.

Oopherectomy was earlier recommended as a method of causing oestrogen depletion. There is however no evidence that oopherectomy is of any use and currently this treatment has also fallen out of favour.

Current Clinical Trials

The Cincinnati Angiolipoma Sirolimus Trial involved 20 patients with angiomyolipomas including 11 with LAM. After one year of receiving the drug, angiomyolipomas decreased by almost 50% and FEV_1 and forced vital capacity (FVC) increased by 5–10%. This improvement waned after the drug was stopped. Even so targeting the mTOR pathway may hold promise in the treatment of LAM. The drug also has a number of untoward side-effects.

A large three-year randomized controlled trial called the Multicenter International LAM Efficacy of Sirolimus (MILES) trial, opened in 2006. The primary outcome to be measured in the trial is the FEV_1.

Symptomatic Treatment of Airways Obstruction in LAM

The use of bronchodilators in the form of inhaled or nebulised β_2 agonists may afford some relief to patients with some degree of reversibility to their airflow limitation.

Oxygen affords a degree of relief to those who are increasingly dyspnoeic and in those who have hypoxic respiratory failure.

Pneumothorax

Pneumothorax is associated with a fair degree of morbidity, more so as it recurs in over 50% or more of patients. Pleurodesis may be necessary but this may increase complications for future lung transplantation. Lung transplantations with current techniques have however been successful even in patients with pleurodesis.

Chylous Effusions

Chylous effusions are due to rupture of subpleural lymphatics or blockage of the thoracic duct. Management consist of—

a. use of octreotide which reduces the production of lymph through reduction of splanchnic blood flow;
b. a low-fat diet which reduces production of lymph;
c. aspiration of fluid when the chylous effusion is symptomatic. Repeated aspirations may however lead to significant loss of fat and protein.
d. Surgical measures when conservative methods fail. These include pleurodesis, pleurectomy, thoracic duct ligation, pleuroperitoneal shunt.

Angiomyolipomas

Angiomyolipomas in the kidney if large can cause bleeding, which may be severe. Surgical treatment should be aimed at conserving as much renal tissue as possible. A close follow-up of angiomyolipomas by frequent three to six-monthly ultrasound examination is important.

Lung Transplantation

Lung transplantation is the only available and effective treatment for advanced disease. The presence of marked dyspnoea, hypoxemia and a significantly reduced DLCO is an indication for considering lung transplantation even when airflow obstruction is not critical. Dyspnoea with severe airflow obstruction as judged by FEV_1 near 30% of its predicted value is in itself an indication for lung transplantation. The cumulative survival rate for patients with pulmonary LAM who had lung transplantation in the United States is 65% at five years which is better than the survival rate for other lung diseases requiring transplant surgery. Many centres prefer double-lung transplants to single-lung transplants even though survival rates are similar, because double-lung transplants are associated with lower rates of bronchiolitis obliterans and greater improvement in the FEV_1.

PULMONARY AMYLOIDOSIS

Amyloidosis is characterized by the homogenous extracellular deposition of material that stains with Congo-red and that has an apple-green birefringence under polarized light. Amyloid is laid down in the form of fibrils 7–10 mm in diameter and these can be generated from a number of precursor proteins in the blood. The two major amyloid proteins are AL and AA proteins. The AL protein is derived from the light chains of immunoglobulins and is associated with primary amyloidosis, amyloidosis complicating multiple myeloma and in isolated tracheobronchial and nodular pulmonary amyloidosis. The AA is derived from a protein normally found in serum and is present in secondary amyloidosis, occurring in patients with chronic inflammatory disorders and rheumatoid arthritis.

Amyloid involvement of the lung takes three forms.

1. Pulmonary involvement in primary systemic amyloidosis. The pulmonary parenchyma or the alveolar septa or both show amyloid infiltrates. The frequency of pulmonary involvement in primary systemic amyloidosis is 36–60%. The mean age is around 60 years, both sexes being equally affected. It is often discovered on imaging studies and generally produces few or no symptoms. X-ray of the chest shows a diffuse reticular infiltrate or reticulonodular infiltrates. The prognosis is poor being related to the primary systemic amyloidosis of which pulmonary amyloidosis is just a part. The median survival rate is generally not more than 1.5 years.
2. Pulmonary involvement in secondary amyloidosis. Amyloid deposition in the lung is rare in secondary amyloidosis. It is generally limited and clinically silent.
3. Isolated pulmonary amyloidosis. This is a rare disease and can present in three forms—tracheobronchial amyloidosis, nodular amyloidosis and diffuse parenchymal amyloidosis.

Tracheobronchial Amyloidosis

Tracheobronchial amyloidosis is characterized by the deposition and infiltration of amyloid deposits in the tracheobronchial tree.

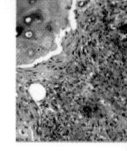

The presentation may be in the form of one or more strictures in the trachea or the large airways due to local and focal deposits of amyloid.

Clinical presentation could also be related to a more diffuse deposition of amyloid involving the entire or greater part of the tracheobronchial tree causing bronchial constriction.

Rarely, amyloid deposits may take the form of endobronchial or tracheal polypoid or tumour-like lesions.

The amyloid deposits in tracheobronchial amyloidosis are of the AL type and are generally deposited in the submucosa. Calcification and even ossification within deposits may be observed.

CLINICAL FEATURES

Cough, wheezing and breathlessness on exertion are the most frequent symptoms; these may be indistinguishable from the clinical features observed in chronic obstructive pulmonary disease (COPD). If strictures form in the trachea or large bronchi, noisy breathing or stridor is observed. Haemoptysis is not frequent. Bronchial strictures could cause atelectasis, repeated episodes of pneumonia and ultimately bronchiectasis of the affected segment or lobe. Hilar and mediastinal adenopathy due to amyloid deposits may occur.

The differential diagnosis is from COPD and asthma. Atelectasis or lobar collapse due to a bronchial stricture may raise the possibility of lung cancer, particularly in the presence of hilar and mediastinal adenopathy.

DIAGNOSIS AND TREATMENT

Diagnosis is by bronchial biopsy through a fibreoptic bronchoscope. Bronchoscopic appearance is that of shiny pale plaques with areas of focal narrowing. The biopsy material stains positive with Congo-red. Focal strictures or lesions can be generally resected by laser therapy. Solitary polypoid masses can be resected with excellent results. Diffuse amyloid tracheobronchitis has a poor prognosis. Breathlessness and airways obstruction progress, leading to death from respiratory failure. In one series, 30% patients died within four to six years. Haemoptysis is frequent in diffuse tracheobronchial disease and can be fatal.

Nodular Parenchymal Amyloidosis

Isolated nodular parenchymal amyloidosis is rare, occurs generally after 60 years of age with an equal sex distribution. The amyloid is of AL type.

The disease is characterized by the presence of one or multiple amyloid nodules within the lung parenchyma, the size of the nodules varying from 0.5 to 5 cm. Larger nodules may also be present. Calcification or cavitation has been reported in one-third of the nodules. Mediastinal and/or hilar adenopathy may occur when there is multinodular involvement. Multiple nodules can cause cough and breathlessness.

The differential diagnosis is chiefly from a metastatic lesion, and from tuberculosis (TB) or other granulomatous diseases.

Diagnosis is generally made on examination of a solitary nodule removed at surgery. A thoracoscopic biopsy of a nodule gives the diagnosis when there is multinodular involvement of the lung. The multinodular form of the disease cannot be cured surgically; even so the prognosis is good, far better than for the tracheobronchial form of the disease.

Diffuse Parenchymal Amyloidosis

Isolated diffuse parenchymal amyloidosis is extremely rare, amyloid being deposited in the alveolar septa and in the media of the blood vessels.

In contrast to parenchymal lung involvement occurring as a feature of primary systemic amyloidosis, patients with isolated diffuse lung involvement with amyloid are always symptomatic, with cough, progressive dyspnoea leading to progressive hypoxemia and respiratory failure. End-inspiratory crackles are generally present as with other interstitial lung diseases. Death generally occurs within two years of the diagnosis.

Imaging studies involving both chest X-ray and high-resolution computed tomography (HRCT) show progressively increasing reticulonodular infiltrates; hilar and mediastinal nodes may be enlarged in some cases. The imaging features are indistinguishable from other pathologies causing interstitial lung disease.

Corticosteroids and/or immunosuppressive drugs have not been shown to be of any use.

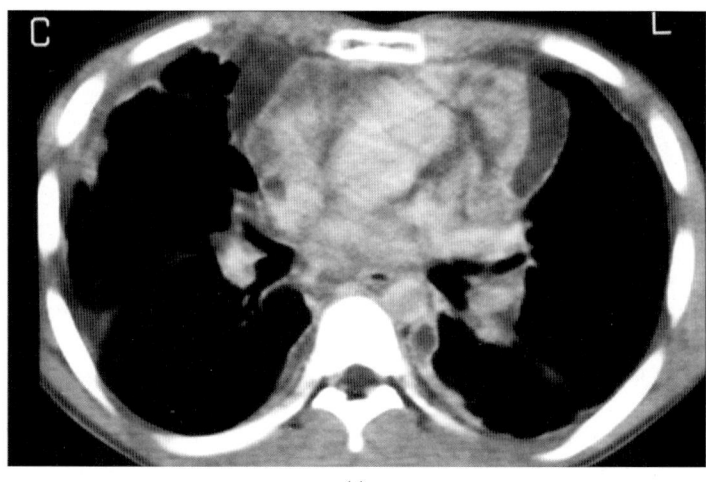

(a)

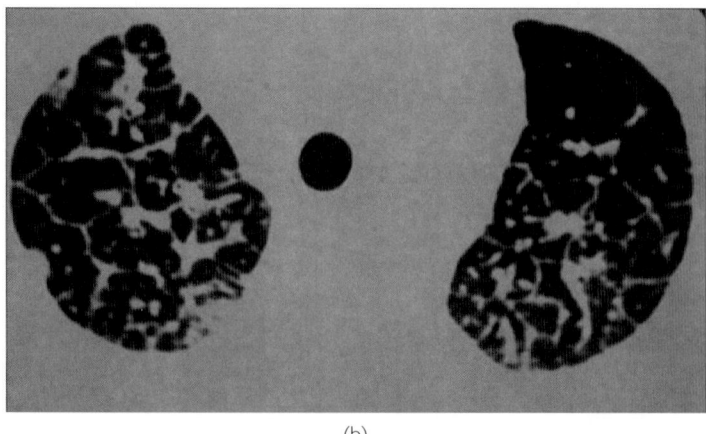

(b)

Fig 47.2a and b: Amyloidosis: CT chest reveals a small pericardial effusion with bilateral pleural thickening. HRCT chest reveals septal thickening with nodules along the septa. The lung architecture is preserved; such an appearance may be seen in lymphangitic carcinomatosis. Transbronchial biopsy revealed amyloidosis.

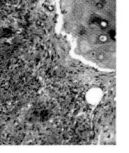

PULMONARY ALVEOLAR PROTEINOSIS

Pulmonary alveolar proteinosis is a disease diffusely involving the alveoli and sparing the interstitial structures of the lung, characterized by the accumulation of proteinaceous material in the alveoli. This proteinaceous material consists of lung surfactant and protein components.

Alveolar proteinosis can be

1. Idiopathic or primary
2. Secondary to other lung pathologies; these include-
   a. Inhalation exposure to silica and other metal dusts, chemicals (insecticides);
   b. Lymphomas, leukaemia and other malignancies;
   c. Infections—Infections reported to be associated with alveolar proteinosis are fungal infection (cryptococcal infection, histoplasmosis, mucormycosis), mycobacterial infection, nocardosis, pneumocystis infection (in both HIV and non-HIV patients) and HIV disease.

Most of the conditions listed above are associated with impairment of either local or systemic defence mechanisms.

Congenital pulmonary alveolar proteinosis has been rarely reported in infants and children. It is fatal and is due to a genetic mutation that results in a surfactant protein B deficiency.

Pulmonary alveolar proteinosis is also reported in a rare genetic disorder, lysurinic protein intolerance, which results in impaired cellular aminoacid transport.

Epidemiology

Alveolar proteinosis is a rare disease occurring predominately in men (male–female ratio 3:1). We have encountered five proven patients as yet. There is an increased incidence in smokers. The peak age of onset as judged by reviews is between 30–50 years. However, it has also been reported in neonates, infants and children. Familial incidence is rare but reported.

Pathophysiology

Surfactant and surfactant-like material consisting of phospholipids and apoproteins diffusely fill the alveoli. This suggests that the above abnormality is related either to increased or excessive secretion of surfactant, or to its poor degradation, or to the failure to reuse the normally secreted surfactant. Surfactant is normally secreted by Type II alveolar cells, being released in the form of lamellar bodies, which are converted to tubular myelin. After use, surfactant is taken up by Type II alveolar cells, 50% of the surfactant being recycled in this manner. The rest of the surfactant is cleared through phagocytosis by macrophages and by the lymphatics. Recycling of the surfactant is believed to be mediated by receptors for surfactant apoprotein A present in Type II alveolar cells. If re-uptake of the surfactant by Type II alveolar cells is decreased there is an accumulation within the alveoli. The macrophages then need to engulf large quantities of surfactant to help clearance. This leads to several defects in the function of the overburdened macrophages, contributing thereby to pulmonary infection in patients with this disease. The above description remains an attractive hypothesis that has not been proved.

Recent animal experiments and data on human disease have suggested a role for granulocyte—macrophage—colony stimulating factor (GM-CSF) in the pathogenesis of alveolar proteinosis. The assumption is made for the following reasons—

a. GM-CSF binds to alveolar macrophages through specific receptors, this being an essential step for phagocytosis and degradation of surfactant by macrophages. Primary alveolar proteinosis is presumed to be caused by autoantibodies to GM-CSF thereby hindering the clearance of surfactant. Decreased stimulation of macrophages through lack or deficient GM-CSF could perhaps also cause functional defects in the macrophages predisposing the patient to pulmonary infection. Experiments on mice show that mice lacking GM-CSF or the GM-CSF βc receptors develop alveolar proteinosis resembling human disease. Also, aerosolized GM-GSF inhalation corrects alveolar proteinosis in mice.
b. Patients with congenital alveolar proteinosis have been shown to have a defect in the GM-CSF/Interleukin (IL)-3/IL-5 receptors or common β chain expression. No such receptor defect has however been reported in adults.
c. Bronchoalveolar lavage (BAL) fluid in patients has been shown to contain an autoantibody that inhibits GM-CSF production. This has again not been corroborated by other studies.
d. Administration of GM-CSF has been shown to improve gas exchange in humans with primary alveolar proteinosis. This contention has yet to be proven by more extensive study.

Clinical Features

The disease to start with is often silent and is then only discovered by imaging studies. Presenting features chiefly include increasing breathlessness on exertion and cough. Low-grade fever, haemoptysis and vague chest discomfort may also be present.

Physical examination in some patients is essentially normal. Crackles on end inspiration may be heard in 50% of patients. Mild to moderate clubbing is observed in one-third of patients. Extensive or advanced pulmonary alveolar proteinosis may present with cyanosis, hypoxic respiratory failure and cor pulmonale.

Though the disease is invariably insidious in onset and has a fair degree of chronicity before it is diagnosed, very rarely, a subacute onset presenting with low-grade fever, increasing shadows in both the lungs (resembling ARDS), increasing hypoxemia and respiratory failure necessitating ventilator support may occur. The clinical picture is often mistaken to start with for ARDS. We have encountered one such patient, but this presentation must indeed be very rare.

An important complication of alveolar proteinosis is a complicating infection, in particular by nocardia, mycobacteria and fungi. These complications are rare if therapeutic lavage is offered appropriately. In rare instances interstitial pulmonary fibrosis results as a sequel to longstanding alveolar proteinosis.

Investigations

Chest X-ray shows diffuse bilateral alveolar shadows, generally more marked centrally and less marked peripherally. This distribution gives rise to 'bat-wing' shadows resembling

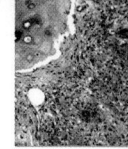

pulmonary oedema. Air bronchograms are clearly visible through these shadows.

Occasionally, atypical findings are present, consisting of focal or diffuse asymmetrical shadows, consolidation or reticulonodular shadows.

HRCT of the chest is often diagnostic and shows the following features—

1. Ground-glass opacification with a sharp differentiation from the normal lung;
2. Marked septal thickening with the formation of polygonal shapes—crazy pavement pattern;
3. Areas of consolidation with air bronchograms. These may be surrounded by ground-glass densities.

LUNG FUNCTIONS

Lung function shows a restrictive pattern with well–marked reduction in the diffusion capacity. With progressive disease there is increasing hypoxemia which increases with exercise.

There are no specific laboratory markers for this disease. The lactate dehydrogenase (LDH) is raised; it declines after therapeutic lavage. The levels of surfactant protein A and D may be increased but this again is not specific to this disease. Serological diagnostic testing for GM-CSF autoantibodies is yet not available.

Diagnosis

The diagnosis of alveolar proteinosis should be suspected in patients with varying degree of dyspnoea who on an X-ray of the chest show alveolar shadows resembling the bat—wing appearance of pulmonary oedema. The HRCT findings are often typical in this disease though rarely atypical features may be present. The chief diagnostic tool is a BAL study, the BAL fluid having a characteristic milky appearance. Examination of BAL fluid on light microscopy shows—

a. Acellular globules that stain positive with PAS and are basophilic with the May-Giemsa stain;

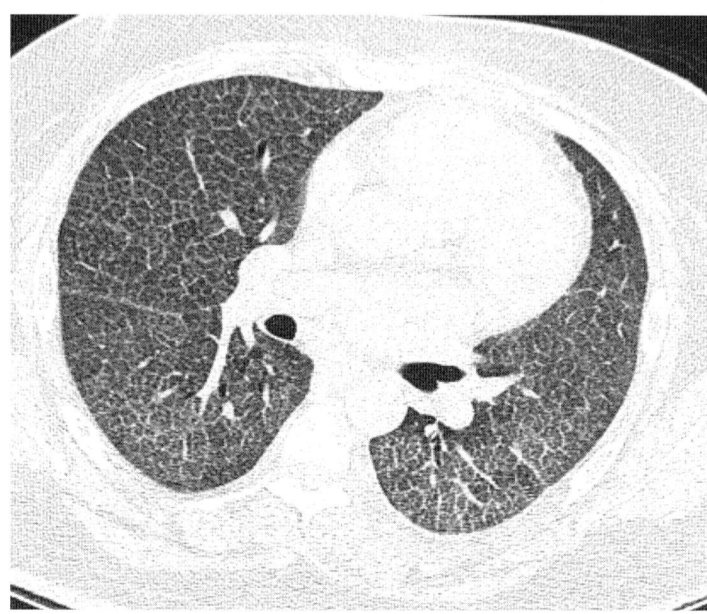

Fig 47.4: Pulmonary alveolar proteinosis. HRCT chest demonstrates diffuse ground-glass densities with septal thickening indicative of a crazy pavement appearance. These features are fairly diagnostic of pulmonary alveolar proteinosis.

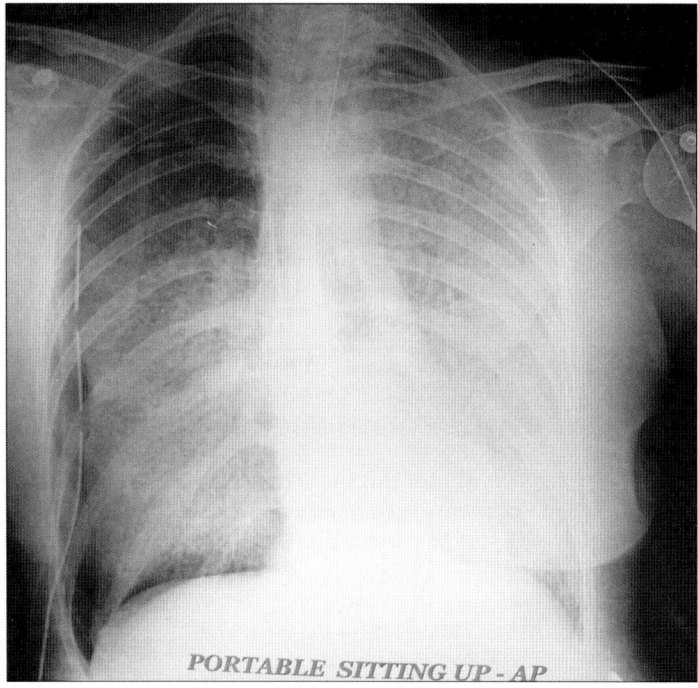

Fig 47.3: Pulmonary alveolar proteinosis. Chest X-ray demonstrates diffuse ground-glass densities in both lung fields. Thoracoscopic biopsy revealed pulmonary alveolar proteinosis. Intercostal tube drain (ICD) in situ, right side following the thoracoscopic biopsy.

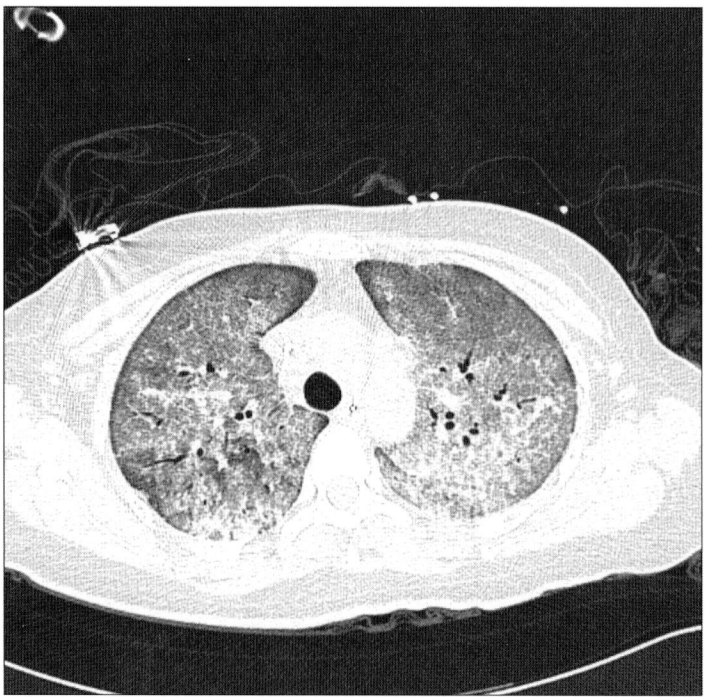

Fig 47.5: Pulmonary alveolar proteinosis. HRCT chest demonstrates diffuse ground-glass densities in both lung fields with a thin dark subpleural line; this is due to the proteinaceous material being compressed away from the chest wall.

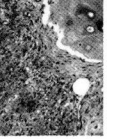
b. presence of few macrophages

c. cell debris which also shows a positive though weak PAS stain. Electron microscopy of BAL fluid is unnecessary for diagnosis. An examination of the BAL sediment through electron microscopy shows myelin-like multilamellated structures and lamellated bodies.

DIFFERENTIAL DIAGNOSIS

Alveolar shadows on imaging may occur in the following situations—pulmonary oedema, intraalveolar haemorrhage, bronchoalveolar carcinoma, chronic eosinophilic pneumonia, exogenous lipid pneumonia, microlithiasis.

An overall assessment of the clinical features and imaging studies, in particular the HRCT of the chest allow a definite diagnosis is most instances. The appearance of the BAL fluid is pathognomic in alveolar proteinosis.

Table 47.2: Differential diagnosis of alveolar shadows on imaging
• Pulmonary oedema
• Intraalveolar haemorrhage
• Bronchoalveolar carninoma
• Chronic eosinophilic pneumonia
• Exogenous lipid pneumonia
• Microlithiasis

Management

The disease does not continue to progress in all patients. In fact, spontaneous remission occurs in one-third of patients. Patients should be offered treatment if symptoms are bothersome enough to interfere with the quality of life or when pulmonary functions deteriorate.

The only effective treatment is lung lavage with normal saline. This should only be done by an experienced team with constant monitoring of O_2 saturation, electrocardiography (ECG) and blood pressure. The lung more severely affected is lavaged first. If both are equally affected then the left lung is first lavaged as the right has a larger volume and greater ventilatory capacity compared to the left.

Whole lung lavage is done under general anaesthesia after intubating the patient with a double-lumen, endotracheal tube (Carlen's tube). Both lungs are first oxygenated with 100% oxygen for 15 minutes, to wash out nitrogen. This is then followed by a single-lung lavage. The volume used for each filling is 500–1000 ml. The lavage fluid is then allowed to drain out by gravity, helped by mechanical chest percussion. Filling of the lung with isotonic saline followed by drainage of the lavage fluid is done repeatedly till the effluent loses its milky appearance and is virtually clear. This may require 10–30 litres of isotonic saline lavage.

At each cycle there should be a careful record of the inflow fluid into the lung and the outflow fluid out of the lung. The inflow and outflow should match. If fluid retention exceeds 1.5 to 2 litres, the procedure should be stopped and

leakage into the pleural space or contralateral lung should be suspected. The procedure is generally well tolerated. Complications include pneumonia, hydropneumothorax and bronchoconstriction.

Whole lung lavage of the other lung should be done three to seven days after the first. If the patients are too ill for whole lung lavage, partial lavage of segments or a lobe through a fibreoptic bronchoscope may provide a degree of relief. In very ill patients whole lung lavage has been performed with the help of extra-corporeal membrane oxygenation.

Whole lung lavage produces a permanent remission in 25–50% of patients with marked clearing of radiological shadows, relief of symptoms and marked improvement in lung function. In the others, the disease returns and the lavage procedure may have to be repeated as and when necessary, often at intervals of three to six months.

Currently, GM-CSF administration in patients with alveolar proteinosis has shown a favourable response in 40–50% of patients. These are small studies; more extensive studies need to be undertaken to determine the overall efficacy of the drug. The dose of GM-CSF advocated in these small studies is 5–20 ug/kg/day subcutaneously or 250–500 ug/kg/day aerosolized twice every alternate week. Corticosteroids produce no benefit in this disease.

NEUROFIBROMATOSIS AND PULMONARY ALVEOLAR MICROLITHIASIS

Neurofibromatosis

Neurofibromatosis (NF) is an autosomal disorder with various clinical presentations. NF Type 1 is related to the NF1 gene on chromosome 17 which codes for neurofibromin. NF Type 2 is related to the NF2 gene which codes for merlin.

Pulmonary involvement takes the form of intrathoracic neurofibroma, meningocele, and parenchymal lung disease with fibrosis. Kyphoscoliosis is also a feature observed with NF. A large earlier series suggested that 7–23% of patients with NF had parenchymal lung involvement. A more recent study of 156 patients of NF at the Mayo Clinic revealed parenchymal involvement in only 1.9% of patients. All the rest with parenchymal disease had other causes for pulmonary infiltrates such as smoking-related lung disease, rheumatoid disease, and recurrent pneumonia. The true incidence of parenchymal involvement in NF is perhaps therefore much less than what was reported earlier.

PULMONARY ALVEOLAR MICROLITHIASIS

Pulmonary alveolar microlithiasis is characterized by the diffuse deposition of concentrically laminated calcium phosphate particles in the form of microliths within the alveoli of both lungs.

The diffuse deposition of microliths within the alveoli produces distinctive calcific micronodular shadows in both lung fields, likened to a 'sand-storm' appearance. The mean age at diagnosis reported in studies is in the mid-thirties. The disease however can occur at any age. The disease is an autosomal recessive disorder with a familial presence in about one-third of

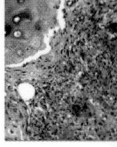

patients. It is due to a mutation on the gene (SCL34A2) present on chromosome 4. This gene is strongly expressed in Type II alveolar cells and its function is to encode a sodium phosphate co-transporter thereby preventing its accumulation within the alveoli. A mutation of this gene prevents this function—hence the accumulation of microliths within the alveoli.

A recent large review revealed that more than 50% of patients were asymptomatic in spite of the frightening appearance of the lung on radiographic examination. The others had cough, dyspnoea and chest pain. Progress of the disease was slow; death from progression was due to cardiorespiratory failure.

Diagnosis can be confirmed by transbronchial lung biopsy and by the increased uptake during [99m]technetium scanning of the lungs. There is no therapy, though attempts at lung transplantation have been made. Calcific microliths have been reported to regress in paediatric patients treated with biphosphonate.

IDIOPATHIC PULMONARY HEMOSIDEROSIS

Idiopathic pulmonary hemosiderosis is a very rare disease of unknown aetiology characterized by a single or by recurrent episodes of diffuse alveolar haemorrhage, each episode typically presenting with dyspnoea, haemoptysis, anaemia and bilateral acinar infiltrates, generally in the parahilar and lower zones of the lungs. The disease occurs chiefly in children and adolescents with an equal male-female ratio. It is also observed in adults generally under 30 years of age, but has been reported in older individuals as well.

Pathogenesis

The aetiology is unknown. The current belief is that idiopathic pulmonary hemosiderosis has an immunological basis. This assumption is based on the following:

1. Its association with other autoimmune diseases, such as haemolytic anaemia, thyrotoxicosis, celiac disease.
2. Idiopathic pulmonary hemosiderosis is known to occur in children who show hypersensitivity to cow's milk. The disease improves when cow's milk is struck off the diet.
3. Treatment with immunosuppressive drugs has been successful in several cases.

Pathology

There is intra-alveolar haemorrhage together with an accumulation of hemosiderin-laden macrophages within the alveoli. The alveolar capillaries are often dilated; various other structural abnormalities of the alveolar capillaries have been reported. As a consequence of repeated haemorrhage the alveolar walls are thickened with increased interstitial connective tissue. In patients with a longstanding history there is well-marked interstitial pulmonary fibrosis.

Immunological studies do not show the presence of either immmunoglobulin or complement deposition. Microscopic examination may reveal various abnormalities in the basement membrane of the capillaries. These are non-specific in nature and are more severe in children than in adults.

Clinical Features

Intra-alveolar haemorrhage occurs episodically and each episode is characterized by dyspnoea, cough, and haemoptysis. Low-grade fever is often present. A single severe episode or frequent episodes cause iron deficiency anaemia. Icterus with an increase in unconjugated bilirubin may be present following the release of bile pigments from the blood in the alveoli. Physical findings during an episode of intra-alveolar bleed include tachycardia, tachypnoea, pallor and fine crackles generally over the mid-zones and bases. Severe episodes cause arterial hypoxemia, the degree of hypoxemia being directly related to the severity of the intra-alveolar haemorrhage. Hepatosplenomegaly and generalized lymphadenopathy have been observed in chronic cases.

When intra-alveolar haemorrhage is mild but fairly frequent, the presenting feature is that of an iron deficiency anaemia of obscure origin. The chief complaints are fatigability, weakness and breathlessness on exertion.

Repeated intra-alveolar haemorrhage leads to interstitial pulmonary fibrosis, characterized by increasing breathlessness on exertion, end-inspiratory crackles over the bases and arterial hypoxemia. Mild to moderate clubbing may occur. Progressive fibrosis can lead to hypoxemic respiratory failure.

Imaging Findings

An episode of intra-alveolar haemorrhage leads to bilateral basal and parahilar alveolar shadows. Rarely, the shadows may be unilateral or may involve just one lobe. Once the alveolar bleed subsides the shadows clear over a week or two. Repeated bleeds produce interstitial fibrosis with characteristic reticulation chiefly involving the lung bases. HRCT of the chest is more sensitive in picking up intra-alveolar bleeds and later the presence of interstitial pulmonary fibrosis.

LUNG FUNCTION TESTS

Lung function tests show a restrictive ventilatory defect which becomes more pronounced with increasing fibrosis. During an active bleed, particularly in the early part of the natural history of the disease, CO diffusion may be more than normal, the CO being picked up by the haemoglobin within the alveoli.

BLOOD EXAMINATION

The peripheral blood shows all the features of iron deficiency anaemia—a low serum iron, high iron-binding capacity, a low iron saturation. Mild peripheral eosinophilia may be present; cold agglutinins have been reported in half the patients.

Differential Diagnosis

The diagnosis of idiopathic pulmonary hemosiderosis can only be made if all other causes of intra-alveolar haemorrhage have been excluded. These causes have been listed in the chapter on 'Pulmonary Vasculitis'.

In longstanding cases the condition is often mistaken for interstitial pulmonary fibrosis of undetermined origin or related to one of the interstitial pneumonias.

When iron deficiency anaemia together with hepatosplenomegaly is a presenting feature, the diagnosis is often missed.

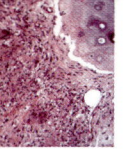

BRONCHOALVEOLAR LAVAGE

Bronchoalveolar lavage shows bloody or pink-tinged BAL fluid during an acute episode. Microscopic examination during a fresh bleed shows free RBCs and phagocytosed erythrocytes within macrophages; a few days later hemosiderin-laden mcrophages are observed.

LUNG BIOPSY

Transbronchial biopsy may show hemosiderin-laden macrophages within the alveoli with thickened alveolar walls and an increase in interstitial connective tissue.

A thoracoscopic lung biopsy may be necessary in longstanding cases who present with interstitial lung fibrosis or when it is important to exclude with certainty other causes of intra-alveolar haemorrhage.

Natural History

The disease may take the following courses:

1. Spontaneous remission even after many years;
2. Recurrent episodes over many years of typical intra-alveolar bleeds, leading to chronic interstitial pulmonary fibrosis.

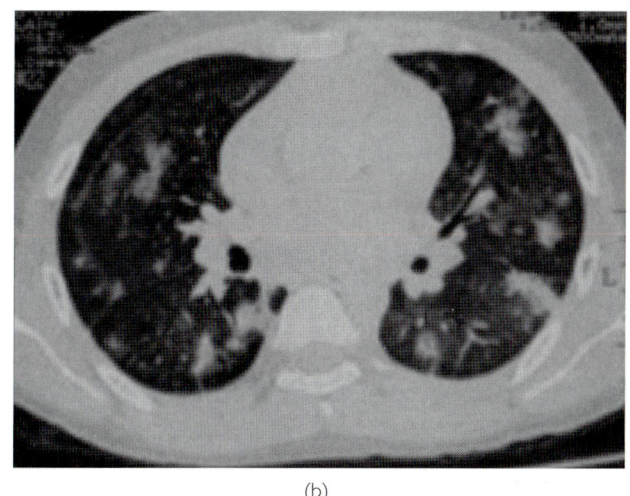

(b)

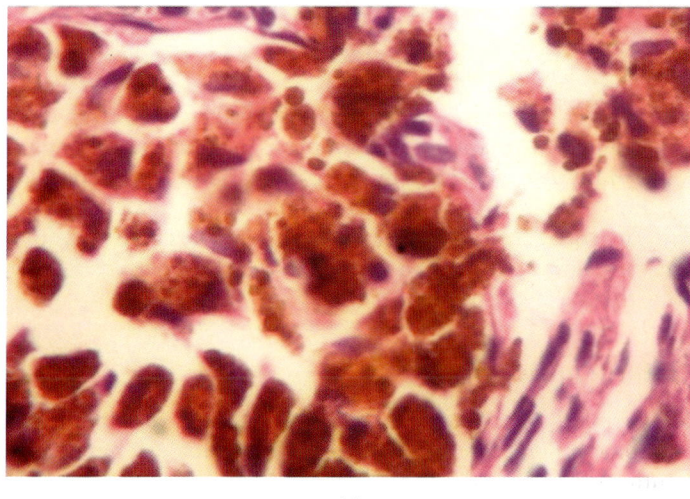

(c)

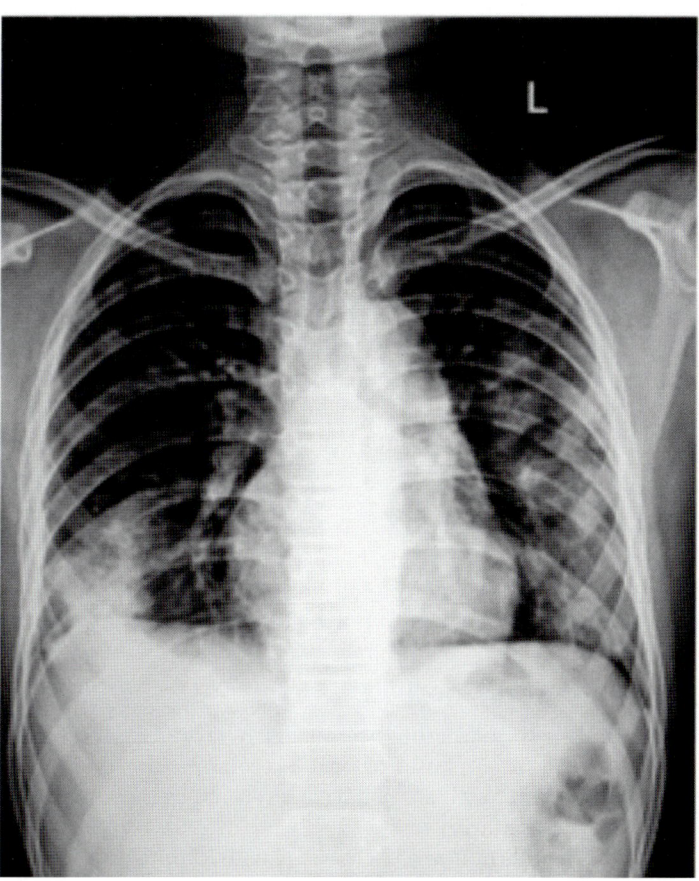

(a)

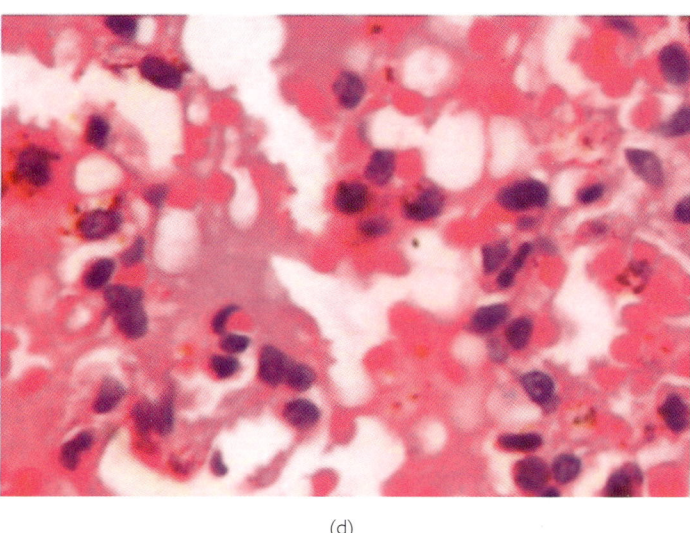

(d)

Fig 47.6: Idiopathic pulmonary hemosiderosis: A 13-year-old boy presented with history of repeated episodes of haemoptysis over the last 9 months. (a) Chest X-ray reveals diffuse alveolar opacities in both lower zones as well as the left mid-zone (b) HRCT revealed ill-defined ground-glass densities in the subpleural regions of both lung fields. Thoracoscopic biopsy was performed (c, d) Histopathology revealed mild bronchiolitis with fresh and old intra-alveolar haemorrhage, and clusters of hemosiderin pigment-laden macrophages in many of the alveolar spaces. No evidence of granulomas, capillaritis or vasculitis.

Hypoxemic respiratory failure and chronic cor pulmonale may result;

3. Mild disease with occasional haemoptysis, iron deficiency anaemia, and a varying degree of interstitial pulmonary fibrosis;

4. Rapid progression, with death from massive diffuse intra-alveolar haemorrhage.

Treatment

Prednisolone 0.75–1 mg/kg together with azathioprine are believed to help control episodes of acute intra-alveolar bleed and prevent recurrence. They are also perhaps useful in patients who develop interstitial pulmonary fibrosis.

Massive intra-alveolar bleeds need packed RBC transfusions, and hemodynamic support. Endotracheal intubation accompanied by ventilatory support is often necessary.

SUGGESTED READING

Berk JL. Persistent pleural effusions in primary systemic amyloidosis: etiology and prognosis. *Chest*. 1 Sep. 2003; 124(3): 969–77.

Collard HR. Diffuse alveolar hemorrhage. *Clin Chest Med*. 1 Sep. 2004; 25(3): 583–92, vii.

Engel PJ. Pulmonary hypertension in neurofibromatosis. *Am J Cardiol*. 15 Apr. 2007; 99(8): 1177–8

Glodstein LS, Kavier MS, Curtis-McCarthy, *et al*. Pulmonary alveolar proteinosis clinical features and outcomes. *Chest*. 1998; 114: 1357–62.

Johnson S, Tattersfield A. Clinical experience of lymphangioleiomyomatosis in the UK. *Thorax*. 2000; 55: 1052–7.

Johnson SR, Cordier JF, *et al*. European Respiratory Society guidelines for the diagnosis and management of lymphangioleiomyomatosis *Eur Respir J*. 1 Jan. 2010; 35: 14–26.

Kavuru Ms, Sullivan EJ, Precink, *et al*. Exogenous granulocyte-macrophage colony stimulating factor administration for pulmonary alveolar proteinosis. *Am J Respir Crit Care Med*. 2000; 161: 1143–8.

Lachmann HJ and Hawkins PN. Amyloidosis and the lung. *Chronic Respiratory Disease*. 1 Nov. 2006 3: 203–14.

Lauta VM. Pulmonary alveolar microlithiasis: an overview of clinical and pathological features together with possible therapies. *Respir Med*. 1 Oct. 2003; 97(10): 1081–5.

McCormack FX. Lymphangioleiomyomatosis: A Clinical Update. *Chest*. 2008; 133: 507–16.

Michaud G. Whole-lung lavage for pulmonary alveolar proteinosis. *Chest*. 1 Dec. 2009; 136(6): 1678–81.

Presneill JJ. Pulmonary alveolar proteinosis. *Clin Chest Med*. 1 Sep. 2004; 25(3): 593–613, viii.

Righ JH Mos, *et al*. The NHLN lymphaigioleimyomatosis registry characteristics of 250 patients at enrollment. *Am J Respir Crit Care Med*. 2006; 73: 105–11.

Seijmour JF, Presneill JJ. Pulmonary alveolar proteinosis: progress in the first 44 years. *Am J Respiratory Crit Care Med*. 2002; 160: 215–35.

Stewart DR. Is pulmonary arterial hypertension in neurofibromatosis type 1 secondary to a plexogenic arteriopathy? *Chest*. 1 Sep. 2007; 132(3): 798–808.

Tachibana T. Pulmonary alveolar microlithiasis: review and management. *Curr Opin Pulm Med*. 1 Sep. 2009; 15(5): 486–90.

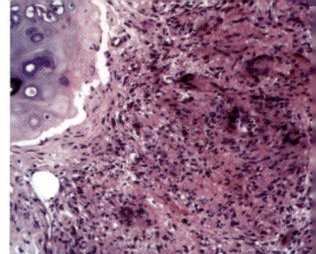

INTERSTITIAL LUNG DISEASES AND OTHER DIFFUSE LUNG DISEASES

CHAPTER **48**   # Extrinsic Allergic Alveolitis

Extrinsic allergic alveolitis (EAA) also called Hypersensitivity Pneumonitis constitutes a group of immunologically mediated diseases characterized by an inflammatory response of the alveoli, bronchioles and the interstitium of the lung to the repeated inhalation of a wide variety of antigen-containing organic dusts.

Extrinsic allergic alveolitis is often an occupational, work-related disease though it can occur from exposure to specific antigenic dust in the home or in the outside environment. Only a minority of the many people exposed to environmental or work-related antigens develop EAA. Risk factors are governed to an extent by the antigen concentration, duration, frequency and intermittency of exposure, as also by the local seasons, climate and the use of respiratory protective devices. Farmer's lung for example is most frequently seen in the monsoon when damp harvested hay is stocked in poorly ventilated enclosures. Bird fancier's lung occurs with greater frequency in the hot summer months, when exposure to avian antigen is increased. In Japan EA is most frequently seen in the hot, wet summer months and is associated with microbial contamination of damp indoor furnishings. Host factors which increase susceptibility must also play an important role. The nature of these factors is poorly understood.

AETIOLOGY

Numerous antigenic dusts when inhaled have been shown to cause EAA. The list has grown over the years and presumably will continue to grow. An important common feature of all antigenic dusts causing EAA is that the particle size of the antigenic dust must be less than 3 um so that is reaches the periphery of the lungs.

Antigenic dust or particles causing EAA can be broadly divided into microorganisms (which serve as antigen) in dust, animal proteins, chemicals and drugs. In a number of instances the antigen responsible for EAA remains undetected or is unknown. A list of important causes of EAA is tabled below.

Perhaps the commonest antigens responsible for EAA are the thermophilic actinomycetes, which are ubiquitous, found in soil, decaying vegetable matter and compost. A survey of clinically important thermophilic actinomycetes covering numerous soil samples from different sites in Delhi, Punjab, Uttar Pradesh, and Jammu and Kashmir (North India) revealed that *Thermoactinomycetes vulgaris* was the commonest species occurring in 56% of the samples. This was followed by *Saccharomonospora viridis* (29%), *Thermoactinomycetes thalpophilus* (27%), *Saccharopolyspora rectivirgula* (21%) and *Thermoactinomycetes sacchari* (40%). The commonest substrate for *S. rectivirgula* was hay, yielding 44% of its isolates. This survey carried out by the V P

Patel Chest Institute, Delhi, showed the widespread environmental presence of thermophilic actinomycetes suggesting the propensity for frequent exposure of humans to these antigenic microorganisms. (*Ref: Medical Mycology in India (1957–2007): Contributions by the VPCI Mycoses Group* H.S. Randhawa and Anuradha Chowdhary Department of Medical Mycology, Vallabhbhai Patel Chest Institute, University of Delhi, Delhi, India; Indian J Chest Dis Allied Sci 2008; 50: 19–32)*

Antigens present in fungi such as the Aspergillus species or animal proteins (e.g. from birds) or in certain chemicals have also been shown to cause EAA.

All over the world, the commonest form of EAA is farmer's lung caused chiefly by exposure to mouldy hay. The antigen was initially named *Micropolyspora polyspora*, classified as a mould. It was then termed *Micropolyspora faeni*. The current classification is *Saccharopolyspora rectivirgula*. T vulgaris and Aspergillus species are also contributory antigens.

An exploratory prevalence study of farmer's lung carried out by the V P Patel Chest Institute in Delhi showed that 30% of 197 farmers (who formed the test subjects) with respiratory complaints related their symptoms to exposure to wheat straw, thresher's dust or other vegetable matter in their environment. There was an overall prevalence of 13.2% precipitating antibodies against clinically important thermophilic actinomycetes. Of these Saccharopolyspora rectivirgula accounted for 55% of the positive reactors. Based on clinical history, imaging studies, lung functions and serum precipitation antibodies to *Saccharopolyspora rectivirgula*, farmer's lung was diagnosed in four workers. (*Ref: Medical Mycology in India (1957–2007): Contributions by the VPCI Mycoses Group* H.S. Randhawa and Anuradha Chowdhary,, Vallabhbhai Patel Chest Institute, University of Delhi, Delhi, India; Indian J Chest Dis Allied Sci 2008; 50: 19–32)*

Obviously, a large epidemiological study is warranted in view of the huge farming population in our country.

Another important cause of EAA is exposure to avian antigen. The antigens are glycoproteins with Immunoglobulin A (IgA) activity and are present in bird droppings, serum and bloom from the feathers of several birds. These include pigeons, parrots, chicken, ducks, geese and turkeys.

In large metropolitan cities of India, exposure to pigeon droppings and bloom from feathers is an important cause of EAA. This is because pigeons abound and feeding pigeons (which gather en masse at certain places in the city) with grain is a semi-religious custom. Pigeons also frequently dirty the window sills and terraces of buildings. Heavy exposure to avian antigen is to be anticipated in these circumstances.

Exposure to mouldy pressed sugarcane can lead to a form of EAA termed bagassosis. This is common in the sugarcane belt

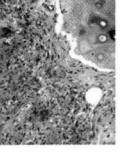

in the province of Maharashtra, the offending antigens being *T. sacchari* and *T. vulgaris.*

Inhalation of antigen-contaminated grain and grain dust is another important cause of the both allergic asthma and EAA in many cities of India where the grinding of grain in poorly ventilated shops leads to exposure to a great deal of grain dust.

Occasionally, low-molecular-weight chemicals can react with protein in the airways to form antigens causing EA. These chemicals include trimellitic anhydride and phthalic anhydride used in plastic, and causing plastic worker's lung. Diisocyanates such as toluene diisocyanate have also been reported to cause EAA.

Free-living amoeba and nematodes contaminating water and ventilation systems have been thought to be responsible for 'humidifier lung' and 'air-conditioner lung'. Drugs such as amiodarone, gold, procarbazine have also been reported to cause EAA.

PATHOPHYSIOLOGY

EAA is a hypersensitivity response to an inhaled antigen. It is believed that both Type III and Type IV hypersensitivity responses as defined by Coombs and Gel are involved.

Table 48.1:
Causes of EAA

Plant proteins	Exposure
• Farmer's lung	Mouldy hay
• Bagassosis	Mouldy pressed sugarcane
• Mushroom-worker's lung	Mouldy compost and mushroom
• Malt-worker's lung	Contaminated barley
• Compost lung	Compost
• Tobacco-worker's lung	Mould on tobacco
• Wood pulp worker's lung	Contaminated wood pulp or dust
• Summer-type HP	Contaminated house furnishings
Animal proteins	
• Bird-fancier's disease Exposure to pigeon dust	Pigeons, parrots, chickens, parakeets, geese, ducks
Insect proteins	
• Miller's lung	Contaminated grain
Chemicals	
• Chemical worker's lung	Polyurethane foams, spray paint, glues
• Epoxy resin lung	Heated epoxy resin
• Thatched roof lung	Dried grasses and leaves
• Humidifier lung; air conditioner lung	Contaminated humidifiers and air conditioners
Others	
• Coffee-worker's lung	Coffee-bean dust
• Tea-grower's lung	Tea plants

Table 48.2:
Probable antigens associated with various conditions

• Farmer's lung	Saccharospora rectivirgula, T.vulgaris
• Bagassosis	T.sacchari, T.vulgaris
• Mushroom-worker's lung	Saccharospora rectivirgula T.vulgaris
• Malt-worker's lung	Aspergillus clavatus
• Compost lung	Aspergillus spp, T.vulgaris
• Tobacco-worker's lung	Aspergillus spp.
• Humidifier lung; air conditioner lung	Amoebae, nematodes
• Wood pulp worker's lung	Alternaria spp.
• Thatched roof lung	Saccharomonospora viridis
• Summer-type HP	T. cutaneum
Animal proteins	
• Bird-fancier's disease Exposure to pigeon 'dust' and 'dust'	Avian droppings, serum, feathers
Insect proteins	
• Miller's lung	Sitophilus granarius
Chemicals	
• Chemical worker's lung	Diisocyanates, trimellitic anhydride
• Epoxy resin lung	Phthalic anhydride

Type III response is characterized by the formation of antigen-antibody immune complexes which excite a hypersensitivity response in the lung through activation of the complement system. Though IgG antibodies predominate, IgM and IgA antibodies are also found. There in an elevation of C1q, C3, C5a levels in the bronchoalveolar lavage (BAL) fluid of affected patients. Immune complexes release pro-inflammatory cytokines, notably tumour necrosis factor α (TNFα) and interleukins which can induce inflammatory changes within the lungs.

Type IV reaction plays an equally important role in the pathogenesis of EAA. BAL fluid in the initial stages shows the presence of neutrophils; this is soon followed by activated lymphocytes, there being an increase in CD_8 lymphocytes so that the CD4:CD8 ratio is reduced. Histological studies show the presence of granulomas, a feature observed in Type IV response, as also the presence of activated lymphocytes and macrophages in the alveolar and interstitial cellular infiltrates in the lungs.

Though EAA is chiefly an antigen-dependent and anti-gen-driven disease, there is a suggestion that non-antigenic factors may also perhaps play a role. Inhaled dust particles themselves can cause a degree of inflammation. Also, organic dust may contain toxins such as myco or endotoxins and histamine-releasing substances that are directly or indirectly toxic to alveolar cells. There are also a number of protein antigens that have immunological adjuvant effects which can activate macrophages and the complement system. The above view has been based on animal experiments. To what extent these non-antigen challenges to the lung play a role in EAA in conjectural.

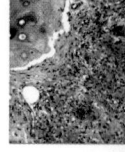

Finally, host factors in the pathogenesis of EAA play a significant role. After all, only a small number of individuals who inhale antigen-containing dust develop EAA. There are obviously host-protective factors that come into play. The nature of these protective factors is undetermined except that smoking surprisingly has a protective role.

Genetic factors that influence the occurrence of EA are poorly understood. A number of alleles and haplotypes of the MHC Class II alleles seem to confer susceptibility or resistance to bird fancier's lungs. Thus polymorphisms in 5' promoter regions of the TNFα gene increase susceptibility. On the other hand a recent study suggested that variants in tissue inhibitor of metalloproteinase–3 (TIMP–3) protected against susceptibility to this disease.

Histopathology

The main histopathological features of EAA are: a) the presence of small scattered granulomas which may be poorly defined; b) a mononuclear and lymphocytic alveolar cum interstitial infiltrate; c) a bronchiolitis. Granulomas are a distinguishing feature, which help to differentiate EAA from interstitial pneumonia. Unfortunately, they are not always present.

CLINICAL FEATURES

EAA may present in an acute, subacute or chronic form. In the classic acute form symptoms are observed 4–12 hours after antigenic dust exposure. Constitutional symptoms observed are fever, chills, myalgia, and prostration. Respiratory features include cough, breathlessness, tachypnoea, basal crackles and in rare instances hypoxemia severe enough to cause cyanosis. The symptoms generally peak within 6 to 24 hours and subside even without treatment within two to four days if antigenic exposure has ceased. In many patients antigenic exposure remains unsuspected and the condition is often diagnosed as an acute infection, particularly when peripheral blood examination reveals polymorphonuclear leucocytosis with a raised ESR.

In the subacute and particularly in the chronic form, the relation between antigenic dust exposure and clinical presentation is not often apparent. Dyspnoea which is gradually progressive, cough with or without expectoration, fatigability, and malaise are present. Digital clubbing may occur in the chronic form. Progressive fibrosis occurs in the chronic form if antigenic exposure continues, the clinical picture being that of interstitial pulmonary fibrosis. An important distinguishing feature from some of the other forms of interstitial lung disease is predominant involvement of the upper and middle lobes of the both lungs. The interstitial pulmonary fibrosis consequent to the chronic form of EAA may progress to result in chronic hypoxemic respiratory failure and cor pulmonale. It is likely that after a certain stage is reached the disease not only fails to regress but may continue to progress even after exposure to the offending antigen ceases.

Lung Functions

Acute EAA is characterized by a restrictive ventilatory defect—a low forced vital capacity (FVC) with a low CO transfer factor.

Some degree of small airways obstruction as evinced by reduced expiratory flow rates may be observed.

Subacute and chronic forms show a restrictive pattern with a loss of lung volume. Arterial hypoxemia on exercise, later even at rest, may be present. Mixed ventilatory defects may also be observed, there being a combination of obstruction to small airways (reduced mid-expiratory flow rates) and restriction (reduction in FVC, total lung capacity (TLC) and CO diffusion). Some patients show well-marked airways obstruction with hyper-reactive airways.

Imaging Studies

CHEST X-RAY

A normal X-ray does not exclude acute or even subacute EAA. Abnormalities if present take the form of diffuse ground-glass shadowing and reticulonodular infiltrate. Radiographic examination of the chest in chronic EAA shows bilateral upper lobe fibrosis with upward retraction of the hila, volume loss chiefly affecting the upper and middle lobes. Reticular opacities may be present.

High-resolution computed tomography (HRCT) is often far more revealing than a chest X-ray. The following features are observed—

1. Centrilobular nodules. Centrilobular nodules which are small in size (between 2 to 4 mm) are frequent, chiefly occurring in the middle and lower lobes. Their close relation to bronchioles (bronchocentric) probably corresponds to an underlying bronchiolitis.
2. Ground-glass opacities. These are hazy confluent opacities which may dominate the imaging findings in acute EAA. But they also occur in varying degrees in the subacute and chronic forms. They probably indicate an alveolitis related to ongoing antigenic exposure. Rarely, consolidation may be observed in the acute form of the disease, resolving spontaneously or with treatment.
3. Expiratory air-trapping. Expiratory air-trapping leads to a mosaic appearance of portions of the lung fields. The portion of the lung where air is trapped during and following expiration appears dark and lucent compared to its surrounding areas. This imaging feature is best viewed on HRCT cuts taken at end-expiration; it represents small airways obstruction caused by bronchiolitis.
4. Fibrosis. Chronic EAA leads to fibrosis characterized by linear reticular opacities, volume loss, traction bronchiectasis and ultimately in honeycombing of the lung. Fibrosis chiefly involves the upper and middle lobes but the lower lobes may also be involved. CT features may at times be indistinguishable from those observed in non-specific interstitial pneumonia. Greater involvement of the upper lobes and the presence of discernible centrilobular nodules help in correct differentiation.
5. Emphysema. Recent studies in chronic Farmer's lung suggest that emphysema is more frequent than fibrosis. The distribution of emphysema is more in the upper lobes, similar to that observed in smoking-related emphysema. Emphysema probably results from obstruction to the small airways due to ongoing bronchiolitis.

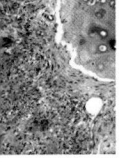

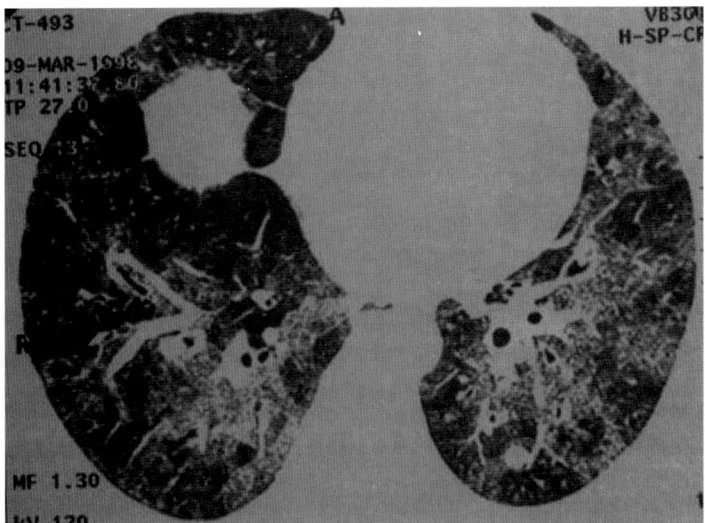

Fig 48.1: HRCT chest reveals diffuse ground-glass densities in both lung fields in a geographical pattern with small nodules within the areas of ground-glass density. There is presence of mosaic perfusion as evidenced by areas of reduced lung attenuation interspersed in these areas of ground-glass density.

BAL STUDIES

BAL fluid shows a lymphocytosis with CD8 predominance. In chronic EAA there may be increase in the CD4 cells. Abnormalities in BAL fluid may persist after clinical symptoms abate and have no correlation with clinical features, or lung function abnormalities.

Diagnosis

There is no single diagnostic test (including lung biopsy) which clinches the definite diagnosis of EA. Diagnosis should be made taking several factors into consideration—history, exposure to an antigenic dust known to cause EAA, pulmonary function tests, imaging features, particularly an HRCT of the chest and the demonstration of antigens contained in the dust, together with precipitating antibodies within the blood to these antigens.

Recent diagnostic criteria proposed by the Hypersensitivity Pneumonia Study Group include the following—

1. Exposure to a known antigen;
2. Precipitating antibodies;
3. Recurrent respiratory symptoms;
4. Inspiratory crackles
5. Symptoms 4 to 8 hours after exposure;
6. Weight loss.

The diagnostic sensitivity is believed to be 80%, with specificity also of 80%, if all six variables are present. In clinical practice one rarely encounters patients who satisfy all the above criteria. A clinical diagnosis is often necessary on lesser evidence. Imaging studies are of significant help in an overall assessment.

The two important differential diagnoses for acute EAA are an acute chest infection and the organic dust toxic syndrome (ODTS). The latter is a toxic syndrome related to exposure to organic dust; it is characterized by high fever, chills, but little or no dyspnoea. Lung functions and chest X-ray are normal.

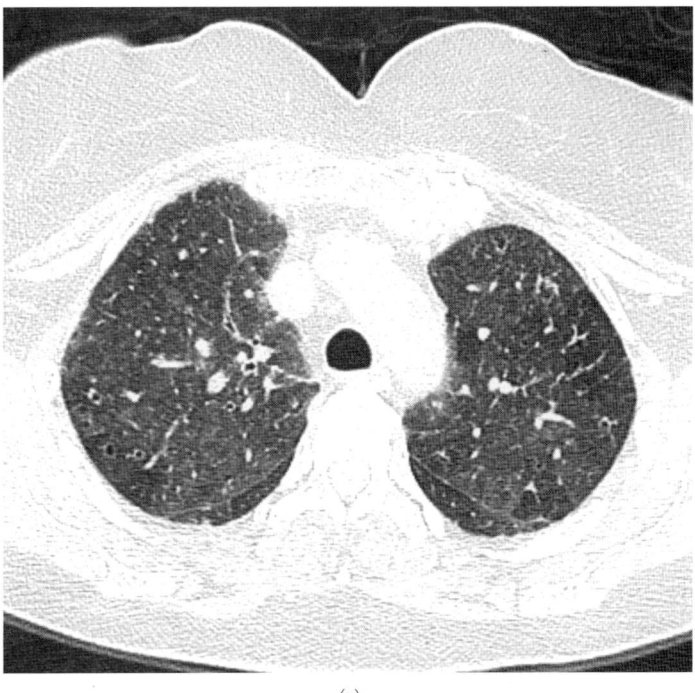

(a)

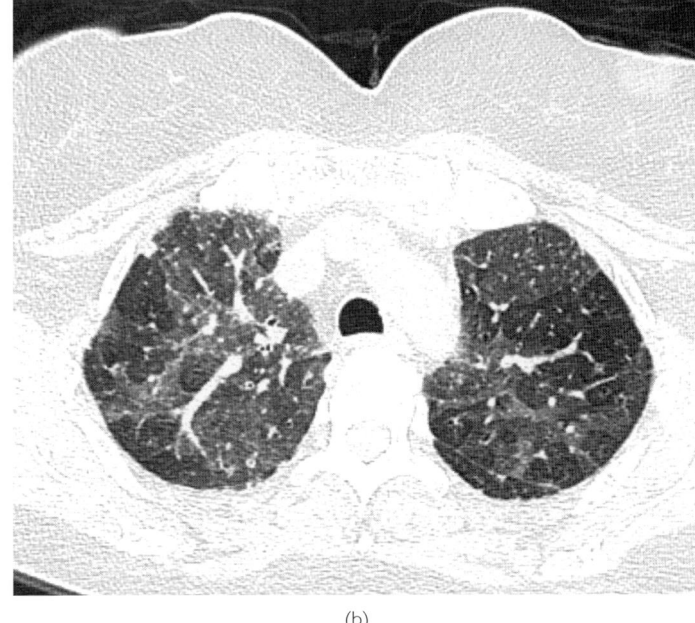

(b)

Fig 48.2: (a) HRCT chest demonstrates diffuse ground-glass densities in both lung fields with presence of mosaic perfusion as evidenced by areas of reduced attenuation interspersed in the areas of ground-glass density. The vasculature in these areas of reduced attenuation has small-sized vessels. On the expiratory image (b) there is evidence of air trapping as the areas of mosaic attenuation are further accentuated.

The differential diagnoses of chronic EAA include sarcoidosis, tuberculosis, and other pathologies causing interstitial pulmonary fibrosis, notably idiopathic interstitial pneumonia.

In patients who have some degree of airways obstruction, the differential diagnosis includes chronic bronchitis and asthma. It

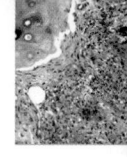

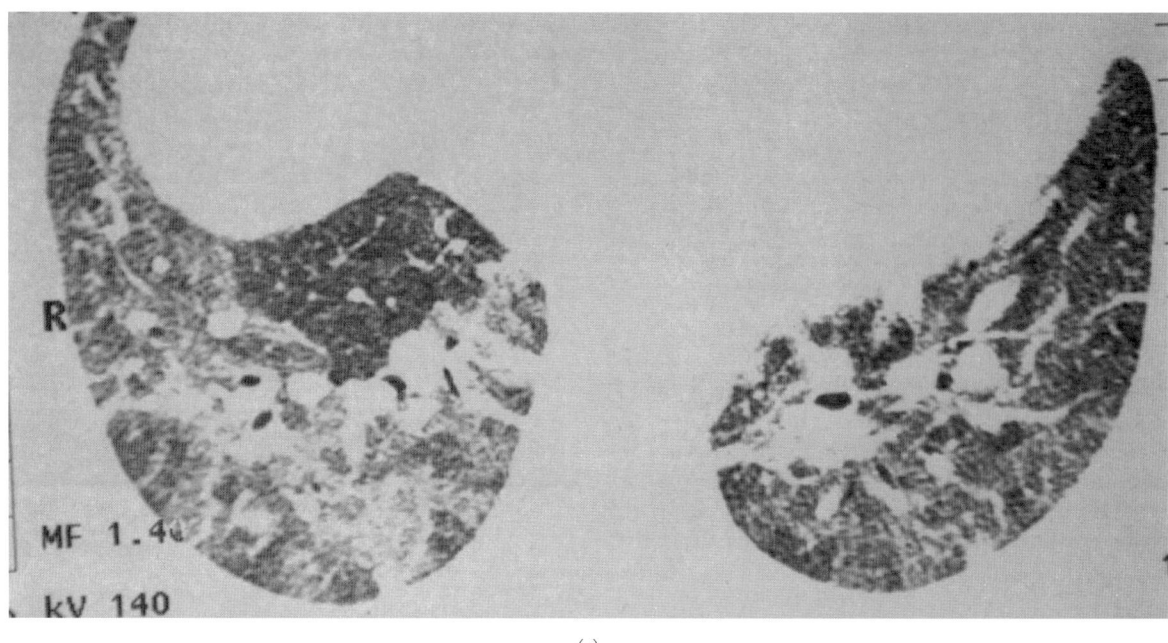

(a)

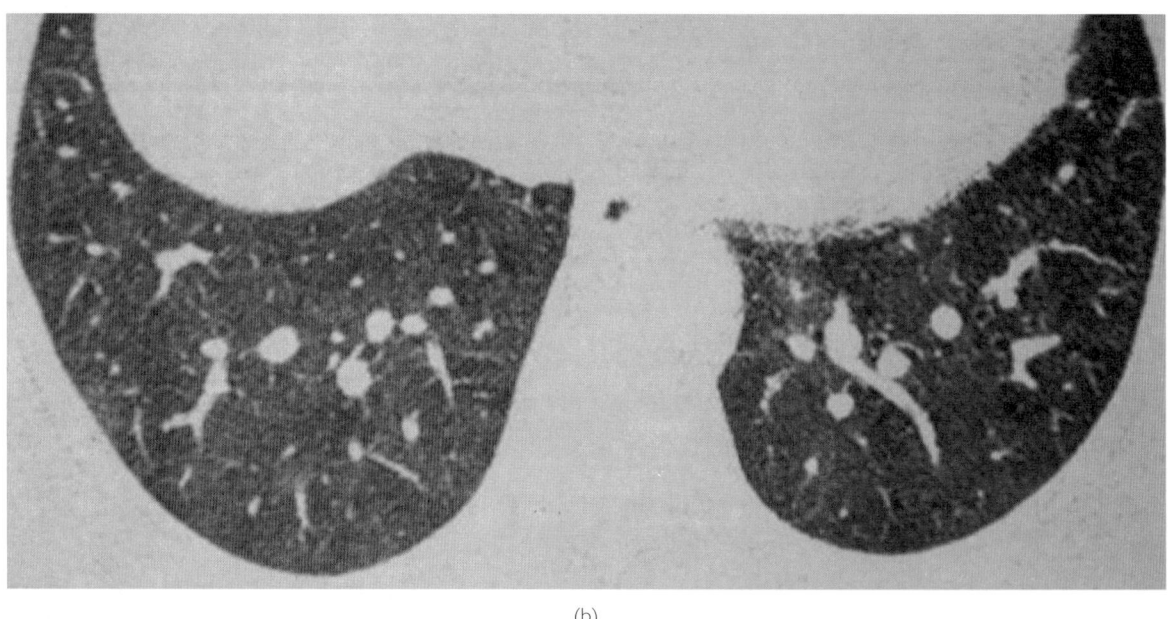

(b)

Fig 48.3: (a) HRCT chest reveals diffuse ground-glass densities in a middle-aged female with a history of hypersensitivity to cat hair representing hypersensitivity pneumonitis. Follow-up HRCT (b) after the cat was given away and a short course of steroids reveals clearing up of all lesions.

needs to be remembered that allergies known to cause EAA can also cause allergic asthma.

Management

The mainstay of treatment is to avoid exposure to the offending antigen. At times, particularly in poor developing countries this may be impossibly difficult. Avoidance of exposure to the offending antigen in farmer's lung requires precautionary measures such as dust masks with filters, improved ventilation, adequately improved storage facilities, mechanization of

farming processes, all of which are often beyond the reach of most farmers in poor developing countries.

As mentioned earlier, EAA due to exposure to pigeon dust and pigeon droppings is largely preventable. There are religious groups in India (notably Jains) who feed large flocks of pigeons which gather at certain sites in the large cities of India. Antigen exposure in this setting can be overwhelming and if avoided completely can prevent EAA and afford relief to those patients in whom EA is due to such exposure.

Removing pet birds from the home is of vital importance if an inmate is found to have EAA even if precipitins of avian antigen

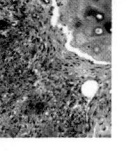
are absent, provided there is no evidence of any other antigenic exposure. This should be followed by a thorough cleaning of the apartment as dust containing avian antigen may persist in the environment long after the birds have been removed.

A detailed occupational history and a history of a specific environmental exposure are of help in identifying possible antigens. Not uncommonly, at least in our experience no such incriminating antigen can be identified.

Corticosteroids are often used in the treatment of acute EAA, though the acute episodes are known to resolve spontaneously without treatment. A placebo controlled therapeutic trial by Kokkarinen *et al.* on farmer's lung showed that those treated with steroids showed significant improvement in physiological parameters, particularly in the diffusion capacity at the end of two months, compared to placebo-treated patients. There is however no documented improvement in long-term prognosis. Steroids when used should be given in a dose of 40–60 mg per day for three to four weeks slowly tapered over the next three to four months. A maintenance dose of 5 to 10 mg may be necessary in subacute disease. Patients who show evidence of airways obstruction should be given the benefit of inhaled β_2-agonist and steroids. Patients with EAA need a careful follow-up, both clinical and with regards to lung function tests.

Chronic EAA may continue to progress to pulmonary fibrosis even if antigen exposure is absent. These patients should also be given the benefit of corticosteroid therapy on the lines used for idiopathic interstitial pneumonia and interstitial pulmonary fibrosis. Cytotoxic therapy using azathorpine or cyclophosphamide has been added to corticosteroids in poorly controlled patients with chronic EAA. Their efficacy with regard to outcome has not been proven.

Table 48.3: Management of EAA
1. Avoid exposure to the offending antigen
2. Acute EAA is self-limiting. In severe episodes use corticosteroids
3. Steroids and cytotoxic therapy in chronic EAA

SUGGESTED READING

Cormier Y, Brown M, Worthy S, Racine G, Müller NL. High-resolution computed tomographic characteristics in acute farmer's lung and in its follow-up. *Eur Respir J*. 2000; 16: 56–60.

Glazer CS and Rose CS. Clinical and radiologic manifestations of hypersensitivity pneumonitis. *J Thoracic Imaging*. 2002; 17: 261–72.

Lacasse Y, Selman M, Costabel U, Dalphin JC, Ando M, Morell F, Erkinjuntti-Pekkanen R, Muller N, Colby TV, Schuyler M, Cormier Y. Clinical diagnosis of hypersensitivity pneumonitis. *Am J Respir Crit Care Med*. 2003; 168: 952–8.

Medical Mycology in India (1957–2007): Contributions by the VPCI Mycoses Group* H.S. Randhawa and Anuradha Chowdhary, Vallabhbhai Patel Chest Institute, University of Delhi, Delhi, India. *Indian J Chest Dis Allied Sci*. 2008; 50: 19–32.

Selman M. Hypersensitivity pneumonitis: a multifaceted deceiving disorder. *Clin Chest Med*. 1 Sep. 2004; 25(3): 531–47, vi.

Spurzem JR. Agricultural lung disease. *Clin Chest Med*. 1 Dec. 2002; 23(4): 795–810.

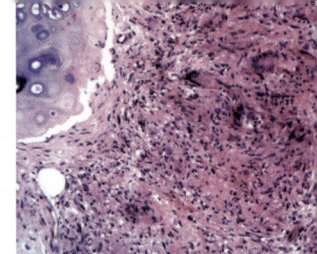

CHAPTER 49 **Eosinophilic Pneumonia**

Eosinophilic pneumonia is a consolidation of a portion of the lung due to the filling of alveoli with inflammatory cells, which are predominately eosinophils. This is usually but not always accompanied by peripheral eosinophilia. In clinical practice, a diagnosis of eosinophilic pneumonia is often made in the presence of a pulmonary shadow accompanied by peripheral eosinophilia, without a tissue diagnosis. This may be incorrect for several reasons—a) peripheral eosinophilia is very common in the tropics, chiefly due to past parasitic infection. The lung pathology may be unrelated to the peripheral eosinophilia; b) peripheral eosinophilia has been occasionally noted to occur in pulmonary tuberculosis, Hodgkin's disease and lung cancer.

Eosinophilic pneumonia has also been variously termed Loeffler's syndrome or pulmonary infiltration with eosinophilia syndrome (PIE syndrome) or pulmonary eosinophilia.

PATHOLOGY

Gross pathologic features of the lung are similar in spite of different aetiologies. The lung tissue involved appears solid, airless and grey. Microscopic examination reveals alveoli filled with eosinophils; mononuclear cells, chiefly macrophages are also present. The eosinophilic infiltration often extends to the interstitial tissue and may involve the bronchial walls. There is a perivascular inflammation noted around the vessels but no actual infiltration of the vessel wall.

A classification of eosinophilic pneumonia is given below. There is a certain degree of overlap in the conditions described in an individual patient. For example, the prevasculitic phase of Churg-Strauss syndrome may be difficult to distinguish form cryptogenic eosinophilic pneumonia or from asthmatic pulmonary eosinophilia.

Classification of Eosinophilic Pneumonia

1. *Parasitic causes* (particularly in the tropics) (See section on 'Tropical Infections Involving the Lungs').
2. *Other known and unknown antigens.* These include drugs, in particular non-steroidal inflammatory drugs, pollen, and other agents. Pulmonary infiltrates with peripheral eosinophilia have been described in patients in contact with nickel, following sensitization to ivy, rarely in brucella infections and in the early stages of the Spanish Toxic Oil syndrome. These conditions may or may not be associated with airways obstruction.
3. *Allergic bronchopulmonary aspergillosis.*
4. *Pulmonary vasculitis—Churg-Strauss syndrome.*
5. *Unknown causes*
   a. *Associated with asthma* (Intrinsic, Extrinsic)
   b. *Acute eosinophilic pneumonia*
   c. *Cryptogenic chronic eosinophilic pneumonia.*
6. *Hypereosinophilic syndrome.*

Eosinophilic pneumonia (also called pulmonary eosinophilia) due to parasitic causes has been dealt with in the section on Tropical Infections Involving the Lung. Allergic bronchopulmonary aspergillosis has been considered in the section on 'Airway Diseases' while Churg-Strauss Syndrome has been considered in the chapter on 'Pulmonary Vasculitis'.

This chapter will deal with just 5 and 6 of the classification described above.

ASTHMATIC PULMONARY EOSINOPHILIA

Asthmatic pulmonary eosinophilia is a rare condition and in large series in the West was found in just 0.4% of patients with asthma. It is probably related to more than one cause; there are two groups of patients—one with extrinsic asthma and the other with intrinsic asthma.

Pulmonary Eosinophilia in Extrinsic Asthma

These patients are generally atopic children often less than 10 years of age. The Immunoglobulin E (IgE) levels are significantly raised and there is a close resemblance to allergic bronchopulmonary aspergillosis. However, the skin test to aspergillus antigen is negative and precipitins to aspergillus are absent in the peripheral blood. The condition probably arises from unidentified inhaled antigens in atopic children.

Segmental atelectasis due to mucus plugging in children with extrinsic asthma is often mistaken for eosinophilic pneumonia.

Pulmonary Eosinophilia in Intrinsic Asthma

The onset of intrinsic asthma in these patients is rapidly followed by diffuse bilateral mottling. The condition is generally observed in the third and fourth decade. There is no history of atopy and the IgE levels are normal. The peripheral eosinophilia is generally mild to moderate

A radiological examination shows bilateral shadows more often peripherally distributed. The response to corticosteroids is dramatic. It is impossible in a given patient to distinguish the above entities from the prevasculitic phase of Churg-Strauss syndrome. The histopathology shows eosinophils filling alveoli and involving the interstitial tissue, which again is indistinguishable from the prevasculitic phase of Churg-Strauss syndrome. Upper lobe involvement needs to be distinguished

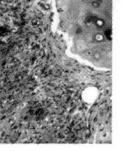

from allergic bronchopulmonary aspergillosis, in which the skin-prick test to aspergillus antigen is positive.

A follow-up of these rare patients after steroids have been stopped may clarify the diagnosis.

Acute Eosinophilic Pneumonia

Acute non-infectious pneumonia characterized by alveoli filled predominantly with eosinophils and with a few macrophages has been described since 1989. The patient generally presents with a 10 to 30-day illness, which is characterized by fever, progressive dyspnoea, mottled lung fields, again chiefly involving the peripheries. Hypoxic respiratory failure requiring ventilatory support is invariably present. The response to corticosteroids is excellent, the mottled shadows clearing within one to two weeks. Generally, there is no recurrence on withdrawal of the corticosteroids.

Cryptogenic Chronic Eosinophilic Pneumonia

This entity was first described by Carrington and his associates. It is characterized by eosinophilic pulmonary infiltrates generally involving both lungs, with peripheral eosinophilia. Asthma may be associated but not always so. Subsequently the same entity was described by Turner Warwick (who used the term cryptogenic eosinophilic pneumonia) as also by Pearson and Rosenov.

Cryptogenic eosinophilic pneumonia is more common in women, generally occurring in the third decade. The clinical picture has the features of a systemic illness with fever, weight loss, night sweats, and anaemia together with respiratory symptoms of cough and breathlessness. In addition to peripheral eosinophilia, there is often a polymorphonuclear leucoytosis, an erythrocyte sedimentation rate (ESR) which is often as high as 100 mm/hour and a raised C-reactive protein. The IgE may be just slightly raised, quite disproportionate to the degree of peripheral eosinophilia present. Rarely, pulmonary eosinophilia may not be associated with peripheral eosinophilia. This renders diagnosis doubly difficult.

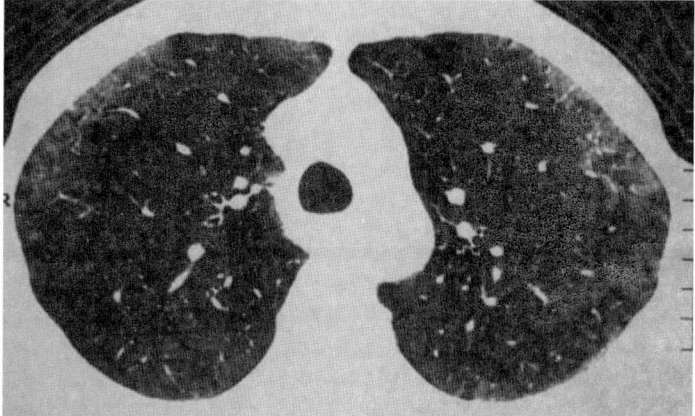

Fig 49.2: HRCT chest demonstrates ill-defined peripheral subpleural ground-glass densities. Patient presented with low-grade fever, cough and well-marked peripheral eosinophilia. A video-assisted thoracoscopic biopsy revealed eosinophilic pneumonia. Good response to corticosteroid theapy.

The radiograph of the chest shows bilateral shadows generally peripherally placed and this distribution should arouse suspicion as to the nature of the lesion. Lung functions show a restrictive pattern or features of both obstruction and restriction.

Diagnosis is best proven by a video-assisted thoracoscopic (VAT) biopsy which reveals typical eosinophilic consolidation of alveoli.

Treatment is with corticosteroids 0.5 to 1 mg/kg. There is dramatic improvement starting within a few days and being complete with regard to symptoms, pulmonary infiltrates, and peripheral eosinophilia within about two weeks. However, after steroid withdrawal, there is a tendency for the eosinophilic pulmonary infiltrates to return, often at the same sites within the lungs as where they first appeared. A maintenance dose of corticosteroids is preferably given for a year. Even then the disease may recur several months after stoppage of corticosteroids.

The Role of the Eosinophils in Eosinophilic Pneumonia

The role of eosinophils in eosinophilic pneumonia continues to be a subject of research. Type I IgE-mediated responses probably initiate the eosinophilic syndrome. Mast cells release an eosinophilic chemotactic factor which attracts eosinophils to the site of reaction. IgE levels in blood generally mirror the degree of disease activity though IgE levels in chronic cryptogenic eosinophilic pneumonia are not significantly elevated.

Eosinophils have a protective function and yet can also cause tissue damage. Their protective function is conceivably related to the presence of lysosomal enzymes which include sulphatase, aryl sulphatase, ≤ glucoronidase, and histamine. These enzymes help to neutralize products secreted by the mast cells. Their protective action extends to attenuating Type I regain-mediated hypersensitivity reactions. Eosinophils can phagocytose immune complexes, and mast cell granules. In pulmonary eosinophilia due to parasitic infection, the eosinophil is a warrior of distinction, particularly in pulmonary eosinophilia associated with filarial infection. The microfilaria trapped in the lungs are destroyed chiefly through the action of eosinophils which secrete certain proteins such as major basic protein, eosinophilic

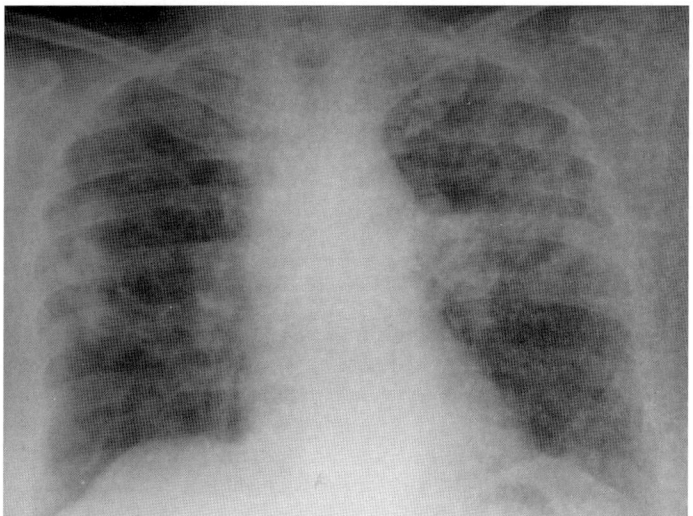

Fig 49.1: Chest X-ray demonstrates ill-defined consolidations in the upper and mid-zones in a predominantly peripheral location.

cationic protein, each of which is toxic to parasites within the lung. Yet these very secretory products are also toxic to normal lung tissue—to alveolar cells, bronchial epithelium and to the vascular endothelium. Tissue damage therefore results.

HYPEREOSINOPHILIC SYNDROME

This is a multisystem disorder involving the heart, the lungs, the central and peripheral nervous system, other organs and is associated with a very high peripheral eosinophilia. Eosinophilia is marked, with mean eosinophil levels of 20×10^9/L going as high as $160–200 \times 10^9$/L. The eosinophils in the peripheral smear show increased vacuolation and degradation.

Clinically, this syndrome is characterized by systemic features of fever, weight loss, anorexia, and hepatosplenomegaly. The cardiovascular system is involved in the majority of patients. Involvement takes the form of arrhythmias, heart failure, thrombosis within the cardiac chambers with thromboembolic episodes, and finally to gross subendocardial fibrosis which causes mitral cum tricuspid incompetence and resultant recalcitrant congestive heart failure.

Respiratory involvement is characterized by cough, focal or diffuse lung consolidation and eosinophilic pleural effusions. Generally, asthma is not a feature of the disease.

Central nervous system (CNS) involvement takes the form of focal lesions in the brain, either caused by focal arteritis or thromboembolic episodes. Peripheral neuropathy, in particular mononeuritis multiplex may be observed.

Other features include skin rashes, abdominal pain, proteinuria, hypertension, muscle weakness and polyarthropathy.

Thromboembolic episodes punctuate the natural history of the disease. Bone marrow examination shows massive eosinophilic infiltration, with masses of eosinophils in all stages of maturity. The serum IgE level may be raised but not unduly so.

Diagnosis

Diagnosis is based on the clinical features of multisystem involvement, together with marked peripheral eosinophilia for which there is no obvious cause. When the main brunt of the disease is on the lungs causing well-marked eosinophilic pneumonia, the differential diagnosis is from Churg-Strauss syndrome. The latter is hardly ever associated with the degree of peripheral eosinophilia seen in the hypereosinophilic syndrome. Also, the Churg-Strauss syndrome is characterized by a significant degree of arteritis.

Treatment

Prednisolone often produces a remission, especially in the presence of pulmonary eosinophilia, heart failure and raised serum IgE level. Hydroxyurea and vincristine have been reported to be of help. Plasmapheresis has been used but with indeterminate results. The presence of marked mitral and tricuspid incompetence causing heart failure may prompt valve replacement surgery.

Remissions are associated with relief of symptoms and with a fall in the peripheral eosinophilia. Nevertheless the disease has a high morbidity and mortality.

SUGGESTED READING

Guillevin L, Cohen P, Gayraud M, Lhote F, Jarsousse B, Casassus P. Churg-Strauss Syndrome. Clinical Study and long-term follow-up of 96 patients. *Medicine* (Baltimore). 1999; 78: 26–37.

Janz DR. Acute eosinophilic pneumonia: A case report and review of the literature. *Crit Care Med*. 1 Apr. 2009; 37(4): 1470–4.

Keogh KA, Specks U. Churg-Strauss Syndrome. *Semin Respir Crit Care Med*. 2006; 27: 148–57.

Roufosse F, Goldman M, Cogan E. Hypereosinophilic Syndrome: lymphoproliferative and myeloproliferative variants. *Semin Respir Crit Care Med*. 2006; 27: 158–70.

Savani DM. Eosinophilic lung disease in the tropics. *Clin Chest Med*. 1 Jun. 2002; 23(2): 377–96, ix.

Udwadia FE. Tropical Eosinophilia: a review? *Respiratory Medicine*. 1993; 87: 17–21.

Udwadia FE. Eosinophilic Lung Disease and Tropical Pulmonary Eosinophilia in *API Textbook of Medicine*. 2008; (eighth edition), 390–3

Wechsler ME. Pulmonary eosinophilic syndromes. *Immunol Allergy Clin North Am*. 1 Aug. 2007; 27(3): 477–92.

CHAPTER **50** **Pulmonary Vasculitis**

Pulmonary vasculitis is characterized pathologically by destruction of the blood vessel wall, cellular inflammation and tissue necrosis. The pulmonary vessels may be involved as part of a systemic vasculitis or primarily affected as the sole site of involvement. Thus vasculitis may be classified as primary idiopathic, primary immune complex-mediated and secondary vasculitis. Further classification of the primary idiopathic vasculitis is also possible based on the size of the vessel affected into small, medium or large vessel vasculitis. A comprehensive classification is given in Table 50.1.

As a group the pulmonary vasculitides pose many diagnostic dilemmas. They are rare, with Wegener's granulomatosis

Table 50.1: Classification of vasculitis
CLASSIFICATION:
1. PRIMARY IDIOPATHIC VASCULITIS:
A) Small vessel:
1. Wegener's granulomatosis
2. Churg-Strauss syndrome
3. Microscopic polyarteritis
4. Idiopathic pauci-immune rapidly progressive glomerulonephritis
5. Isolated pauci-immune pulmonary capillaritis
B) Medium vessel:
1. Polyarteritis nodosa
2. Kawasaki disease
C) Large vessel:
1. Giant cell arteritis
2. Takayasu's arteritis
2. PRIMARY IMMUNE COMPLEX-MEDIATED VASCULITIS:
1. Goodpasture's syndrome
2. Henoch-schonlein purpura
3. Beçhet's disease
4. IgA nephropathy
3. SECONDARY VASCULITIS:
1. Autoimmune disease: SLE, RA, Polymyositis, Scleroderma
2. Essential cryoglobulinemia
3. Miscellaneous: Drugs (propylthiouracil, diphenylhydantoin)

affecting 20/million and Churg-Strauss syndrome affecting 2/million population. They are multifaceted with variable presentations and overlapping symptoms and signs with many common diseases like infections (tuberculosis) and malignancy. Therefore the average diagnostic delay is 3–12 months.

The most common primary idiopathic small vessel vasculitis syndromes that involve the pulmonary vessels are Wegener's granulomatosis, Churg-Strauss Syndrome and microscopic polyarteritis. These are all antineutrophilic cytoplasmic antibodies (ANCA) +ve vasculitis affecting small vessels.

WEGENER'S GRANULOMATOSIS

Wegener's Granulomatosis (WG) is the prototype of an ANCA +ve vasculitis. It was first described by Friedrich Wegener, a young German pathologist in 1936. It was not till 1985 that the link between WG and ANCA was established and only in 1990 that the antigen responsible was identified as PR3, a 29 kd serine proteinase called proteinase 3. WG was considered a uniformly fatal disease in 1955 when Churg reviewed the available data. It was only in 1973 when Fauci treated 18 WG patients with steroids and cyclophosphamide that it was realized that sustained remissions could be achieved in this disease once thought uniformly fatal.

WG is characterized by a triad of findings; necrotizing granulomatous inflammation of the upper and/or lower respiratory tract, generalized focal necrotizing vasculitis of the lungs and other organs, and focal necrotizing glomerulonephritis. All findings may not be apparent at the time of diagnosis although up to 90% of patients will ultimately manifest renal disease.

The initial clinical features vary from the mild and non-specific (fever, arthralgia, myalgia and malaise) to the dramatic (massive haemoptysis) depending on the site of involvement. The American College of Rheumatology criteria for diagnosis of WG include: nasal or oral inflammation, abnormal chest radiographs, abnormal urine sediment and granulomatous inflammation on biopsy. If biopsy is not available, haemoptysis can be substituted as the fourth criterion. This definition has a diagnostic sensitivity of 88% and specificity of 92%. The important organ-specific manifestations will now be discussed.

Pulmonary

The lung is the most commonly affected organ. There is evidence of lung involvement in more than 80% of patients with WG at some stage of their disease. Indeed, 90% of patients with WG will first seek medical attention for pulmonary or upper airway involvement. Whilst lung involvement is part of

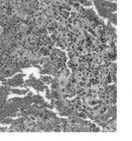
multi-system involvement in most patients, the lung may be the only organ affected in 10% of patients (Limited Wegener's Granulomatosis).

Spectrum of respiratory system involvement in WG: Every part of the respiratory system may be affected:

1. Nasal involvement with congestion, crusting and epistaxis is frequent and perforation and saddle deformity may be observed. Sinusitis and bony destruction is not infrequent.

2. Tracheobronchial: Subglottic stenosis may be the presenting symptom of WG and the patient may present with dyspnoea and stridor which may initially be misdiagnosed as asthma. The subglottic area is the most common site of tracheobronchial involvement as it is a watershed area of the microcirculation. Bronchial stenosis and endobronchial granulomatous occluding lesions are also described.

   Subglottic stenosis is reported to occur in 16–23% of patients with WG. It has been reported to occur more commonly in females than males and the median age at diagnosis is 26 years. Patients with WG who develop subglottic stenosis tend to have more sinus involvement and saddle-nose deformity and less pulmonary involvement than other WG patients. Subglottic stenosis can present and progress in the absence of any other systemic involvement. Thus in any patient with subglottic stenosis an ANCA test should be mandatory. In a series of patients with WG and subglottic stenosis, only 57% initially showed a positive ANCA. Interestingly, 85% of the cohort became positive at a later date emphasizing the need to perform serial ANCAs if there is diagnostic uncertainty. A spirometry will show characteristic, box-like flattening of the flow-volume loop in the inspiratory and expiratory portions and dynamic computed tomography (CT) with tracheal reconstruction may outline the extent of the stenosis. A laryngoscopic examination is the definitive procedure needed to document the subglottic stenosis and grade the severity of circumferential narrowing by the Cotton-Myer classification. Biopsies of the subglottic stenosis are usually not sensitive for the diagnosis of WG with only 10% of subglottic biopsies revealing changes consistent with WG. In contrast, nasal biopsies on a similar cohort of patients yield a positive biopsy in 80% of patients.

3. Pulmonary involvement: Symptoms from pulmonary involvement include cough, dyspnoea, chest pain and haemoptysis. A variety of radiological abnormalities have been described including infiltrates (63%), nodules (31%), infiltrates with cavitation (8%) and nodules with cavitation (10%). The nodules are rounded, range in size from a few millimetres to several centimetres and are commonly bilateral. Overall, 50% of nodules will cavitate. Solitary nodules are seen in 40% of all patients. Another important radiographic pattern is alveolar filling shadows secondary to alveolar haemorrhage. Unusual appearances include lymphadenopathy, consolidation and large pleural effusions. Chest CT may pick up more than radiography and frequently reveals nodules and ground-glass opacification not apparent on chest radiography.

   Diffuse alveolar haemorrhage (DAH) is another distinctive, potentially life-threatening manifestation of WG and can on occasions (10%) be a presenting feature.

It occurs with an incidence of 7–45% in WG and 10–30% in microscopic polyangiitis. It is rare in Churg-Strauss syndrome (CSS), though it has been reported. It is a major cause of morbidity and mortality in vasculitis with the acute mortality from vasculitis and DAH being six times that of vasculitis alone. DAH is recognized by the diagnostic triad of anaemia, haemoptysis and pulmonary infiltrates. The haemoptysis may be massive and exsanguinating. On the other hand, one-third of patients with DAH may not report significant haemoptysis but may have alveolar haemorrhage. This group is more difficult to diagnose and a sudden drop in haemoglobin accompanied by alveolar filling shadows should alert the physician to possible DAH even in the absence of overt haemoptysis. An increase in the corrected transfer factor (KCO), due to increased Hb-CO binding, to more than 30% above baseline may be another clue. Diagnosis of DAH is often made by fibreoptic bronchoscopy which demonstrates diffuse bleeding throughout the bronchial tree. Hemosiderin-laden macrophages can be stained by Prussian blue stain and are often of diagnostic value. Transbronchial or open lung biopsy is rarely required and often not possible in these very sick and hypoxic patients. If performed they reveal pauci-immune haemorrhagic necrotizing alveolar capillaritis without evidence of granulomatous inflammation.

4. Pleural: Pleural effusions are not common but have been reported in WG. They are more common in CSS when they may be rich in eosinophils.

5. Pulmonary artery: Pulmonary vessel involvement in WG chiefly involves the small and medium-sized vessels but pulmonary hypertension has been reported in scattered case reports, presumably secondary to larger vessel involvement.

Renal

The renal involvement in WG takes the form of a rapidly progressive crescentic necrotizing glomerulonephritis with little or no immune deposits. These changes are not specific for WG and can also be seen in other vasculitides such as microscopic polyangiitis and CSS. They also occur in idiopathic necrotizing crescentic glomerulonephritis without evidence of extra-renal vasculitis. The proportion of patients with renal involvement at presentation has varied from < 20% to 80% but invariably increases to 80–94% during follow-up. The presence of renal involvement in WG heralds a more severe outcome.

Other Systems

Other systems that may be involved include joints, eyes, skin, nervous system, heart and gastrointestinal tract. Almost any and every organ has been reported to be involved in WG. Skin involvement is frequent and takes the form of vasculitic necrotic ulcers, nodules, and palpable purpura. Peripheral neuropathy, mononeuritis multiplex are often seen. Central nervous involvement also occurs.

Pyrexia of unknown origin may present for weeks and rarely for months before involvement of the respiratory or renal system is observed.

The clinical manifestations in 26 patients of proven WG have been tabled below.

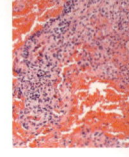

Table 50.2: Study of 26 patients with proven Wegener's granulomatosis	
Organ/Organ system involved	**No. of patients**
Upper Respiratory tract and subglottic	
Sub-glottic	3
Sub-glottic + larynx	2
Limited Wegener's (Lungs only)	
Nodular	4
Multiple solid lesions	3
Cavitatory	2
Full blown Wegener's (Lungs { L} + Renal {R} +/- any other organ system involvement	
L + R	5
L + R + Peripheral neuropathy + Skin	3
L + R + sinusitis	2
L + R + sinusitis + nasal bones + septum	1
L + R + sinusitis with orbital extension	1
Total	26

DIAGNOSIS OF WG

1. Routine tests include complete blood count (CBC), urine analysis (proper microscopy, not dipstick), creatinine, other antibodies like ANA and anti-GBM antibody.
2. ANCA: Anti neutrophilic cytoplasmic antibody. Two distinct staining patterns have been identified: cytoplasmic or c-ANCA and perinuclear or p-ANCA. C-ANCA primarily recognizes the enzyme proteinase 3 (PR3) hence is also called pr3-ANCA, while p-ANCAs interact with a number of distinct antigens, but most commonly antimyeloperoxidase antibody (MPO) and are also called MPO-ANCA.

A positive ANCA is highly sensitive and specific for WG. C-ANCA is positive in about 90% of patients with active generalized WG and in 40–60% of those with limited WG. A p-ANCA is positive in less than 10% of patients with WG but in the majority of patients with microscopic polyangiitis and CSS.

Specificity is however not absolute and a positive c-ANCA may be found in tuberculosis, HIV, infective endocarditis and monoclonal gammopathy of unknown significance (MGUS). Hence, a positive ANCA supports the diagnosis of WG but is not a replacement for tissue diagnosis. We have seen inappropriate administration of powerful cytotoxics to patients with suspected WG based on a positive ANCA with disastrous consequences as the ANCA was falsely positive due to tuberculosis.

Much interest has also focused in recent years on the role of ANCA in diagnosing relapses of WG. This disease remits with appropriate treatment but relapses are common. There is some evidence that changing ANCA titres can mirror these relapses. A meta-analysis by Cohen showed that 81 of 157 relapses were preceded by a rise in ANCA titre. Overall, this meta-analysis showed that a rising ANCA titre had a sensitivity of 85% and specificity of 52% in diagnosing relapses. The pragmatic

conclusion that can be reached from this is that while a rising ANCA titre may herald a flare and justify heightened vigilance, it cannot be the sole basis for acceleration of therapy.

Pathogenic role of ANCAs in vasculitis ANCAs are not just a diagnostic test, they play an important role in the pathogenesis of WG and other vasculitis. The close association between MPO-ANCA and PR3-ANCA and WG suggests they play an important role in the pathogenesis of vascular damage in WG. These antibodies are directly pathogenic with ANCA activating cytokine primed neutrophils, thereby reducing changes in the neutrophil actin cytoskeleton, which favour adhesion to small vessel endothelium. Only when adhering to endothelium can ANCA-activated neutrophils release reactive oxygen species and lytic enzymes including MPO and PR3 that damage vessel walls.

3. Biopsy: A biopsy is usually needed to confirm the clinical suspicion of vasculitis. Tissue must be obtained from an involved but accessible organ or site. Lung, upper-airway lesions, skin and kidney are all potential biopsy sites. Biopsy yield is best from the lung (>90%). A firm diagnosis can rarely be made from a trans-bronchial biopsy or a CT-guided biopsy of a lung lesion. An open lung or video-assisted thoracoscopic surgery (VATS) biopsy is usually needed to make a definitive diagnosis. Biopsy should show the distinctive triad of: necrotizing granulomatous inflammation, necrotizing vasculitis and micro-abscesses. This is not always realized. Depending on the site of disease that is biopsied, some biopsies may show only granulomatous inflammation, or only a vasculitis. Biopsy findings should be considered in relation to the overall clinical picture and results of the ANCA test. Biopsy specimens are always stained and at times cultured to exclude infective aetiologies.

Sub-glottic stenosis, airway lesions and skin have a low yield, while sinus and nasal mucosa have a higher yield. Percu-

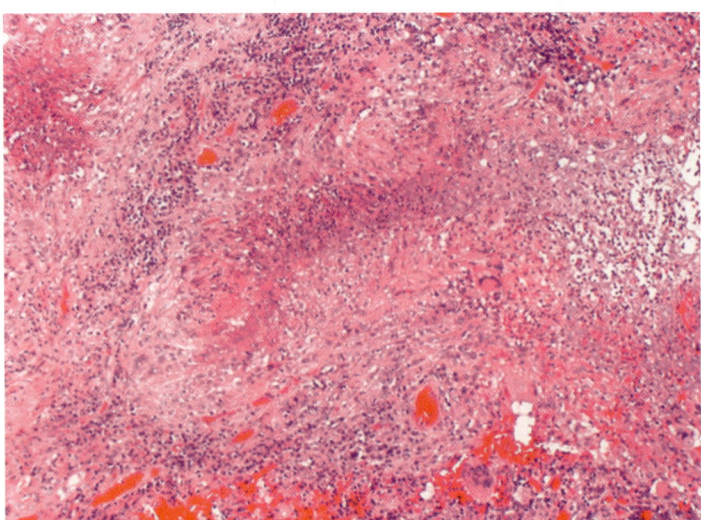

Fig 50.1: Wegener's granulomatosis involving the lungs. Necrotizing granulomas, the central necrosis contains amorphous pink material, nuclear debris and inflammatory cells and is surrounded by palisaded histiocytes and giant cells. c-ANCA done prior to the biopsy was strongly positive.

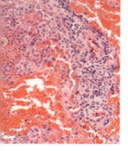

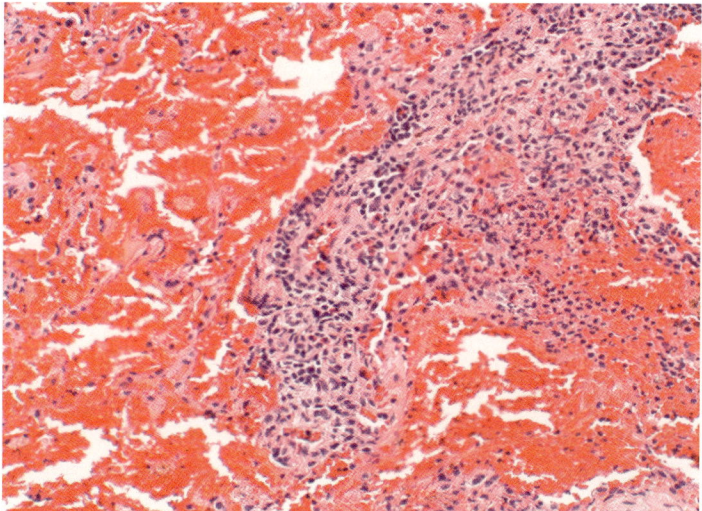

Fig 50.2: Wegener's granulomatosis. Intra-alveolar haemorrhage with marked perivascular inflammatory infiltrate.

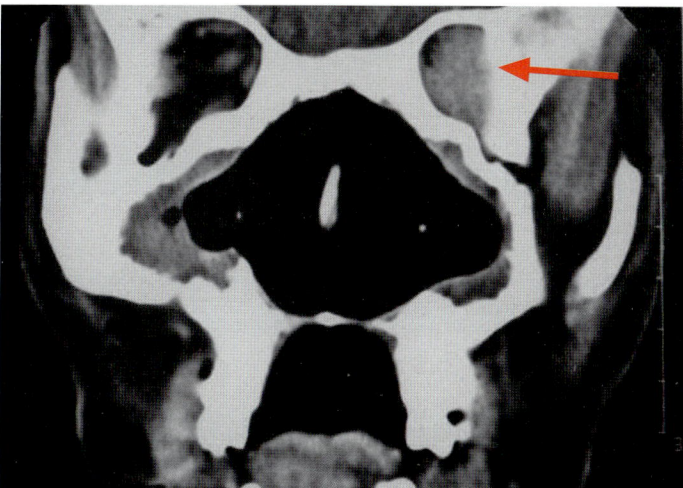

Fig 50.3: Wegener's granulomatosis. Paranasal sinuses (PNS) CT demonstrates near-total destruction of nasal cavity. Note soft tissue in the left orbit. Biopsy revealed Wegener's granulomatosis.

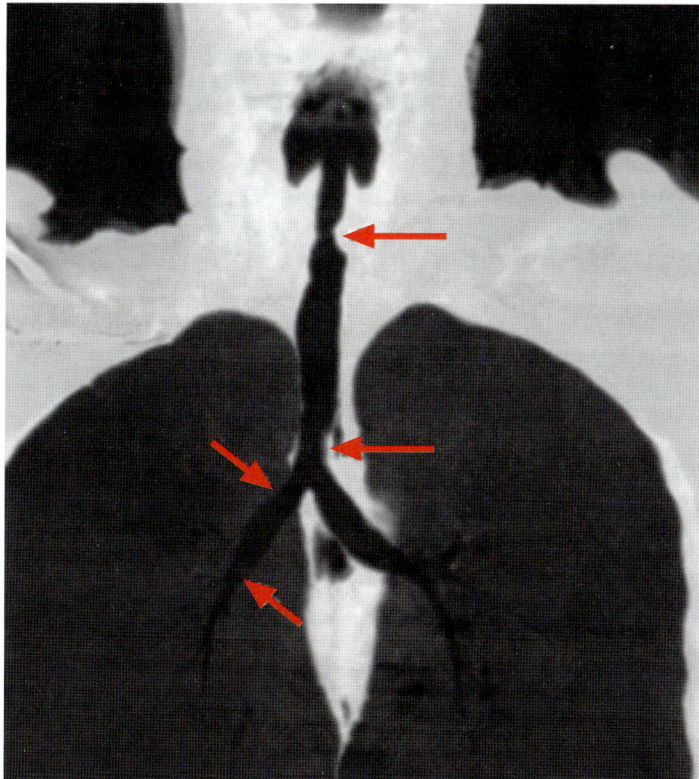

Fig 50.4: Sub-glottic stenosis. 3D CT using maximum intensity projection (MIP) of tracheobronchial tree demonstrates multifocal strictures in trachea—sub-glottic region, distal trachea, proximal right bronchus and distal right bronchus.

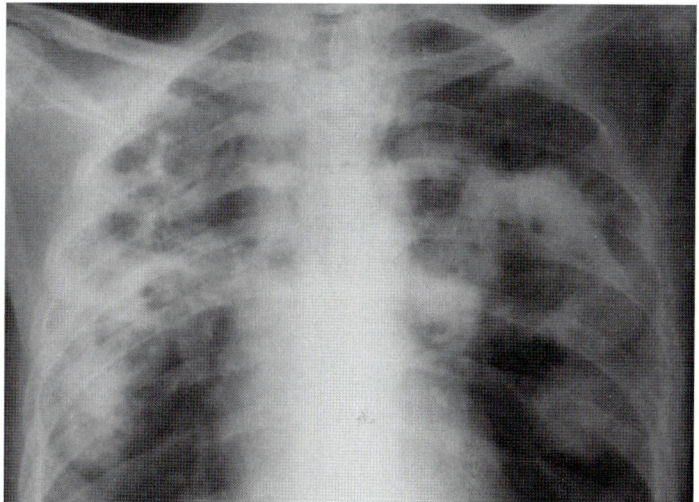

Fig 50.5: Wegener's granulomatosis. Chest X-Ray reveals multiple nodular conglumerative lesions bilaterally with cavitation. Biopsy revealed Wegener's granulomatosis.

taneous renal biopsy may be indicated if glomerulonephritis is suspected, though kidney biopsy is seldom diagnostic.

TREATMENT

The principles of therapy are:

1. Induction of remission
2. Maintenance of remission
3. Prevention of relapse
   - All of which should be undertaken with:
     - minimal morbidity and mortality either from the disease itself or the therapy.

Modern treatment has transformed WG from a near uniformly fatal rapidly progressive disease to a chronic relapsing one with a five-year survival of around 80%. This has however come at the cost of significant treatment-related morbidity.

Table 50.3: Diagnosis of wegener's granulomatosis
1. CBC, urine analysis, creatinine
2. ANA and anti-GBM antibody
3. ANCA—pANCA and cANCA
4. Biopsy—Tissue biopsy from skin, lung, kidney, upper airway Open lung or VATS biopsy for a definitive diagnosis

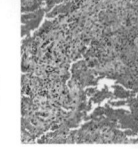

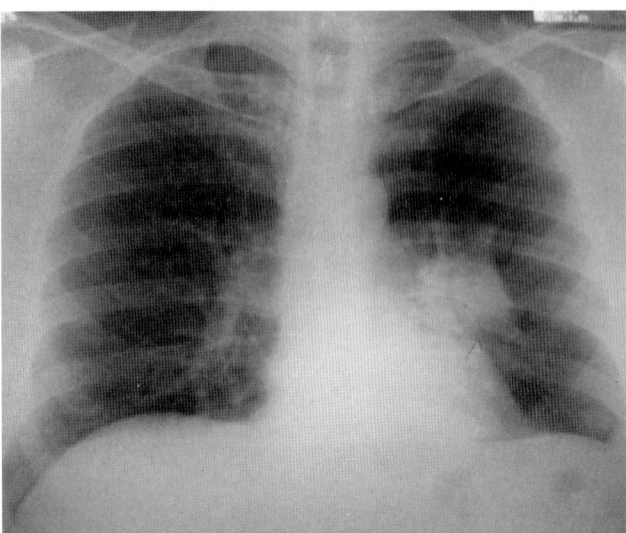

Fig 50.6: Wegener's granulomatosis. Chest X-ray reveals a well-defined mass lesion in the left infrahilar region. WG may present as just a consolidation or mass indistinguishable on X-ray from a pneumonia or neoplasm.

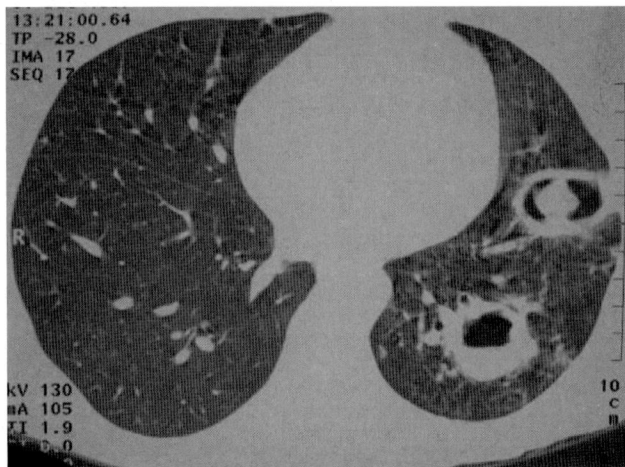

Fig 50.7: Wegener's granulomatosis. CT chest reveals thick-walled cavitating lesions in the left lower lobe with solid lesions and air-fluid levels in the lesions.

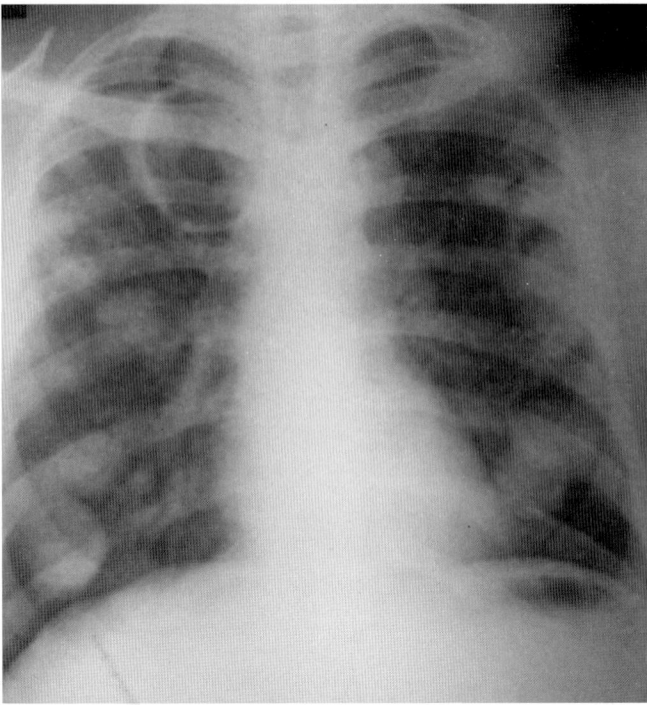

Fig 50.8: Wegener's granulomatosis. X-ray chest demonstrates multiple well-defined nodular lesions in both lung fields with a large thin-walled cystic lesion in the right upper lobe.

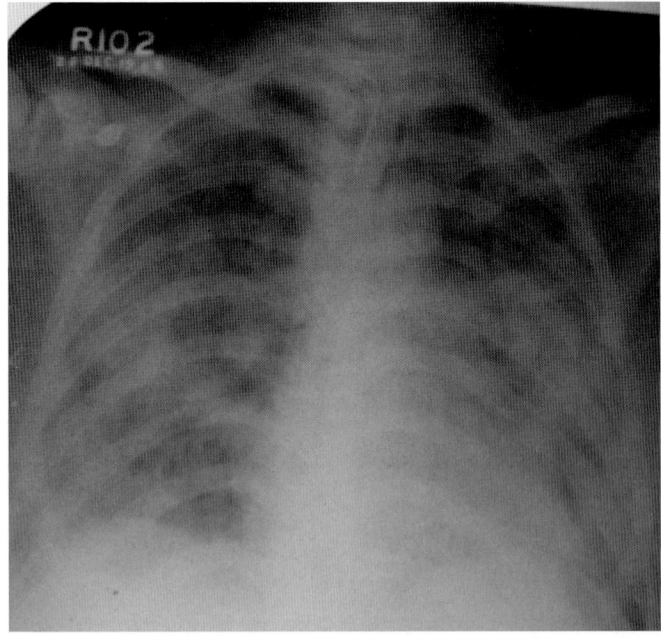

Fig 50.9: Wegener's granulomatosis. X-ray demonstrates ill-defined nodular lesions in both lung fields as a result of intra-alveolar haemorrhage.

The PRINCIPLES of therapy are:

- Induction phase to achieve remission.
- Maintenance phase, where treatment is carefully deescalated.
- Assessment of disease activity with dose titration.
- Careful monitoring for drug toxicity.
- Monitoring for opportunistic infections.
- Add-on therapies in failures.

1. Induction Phase: For active, severe, generalized disease, steroid and cyclophosphamide remain the gold standard. Oral prednisolone can be used in a dose of 1 mg/kg and cyclophosphamide in a dose of 2mg/kg daily. There is some evidence that intravenous monthly cyclophosphamide pulses are as effective as and less toxic than oral cyclophosphamide. A steroid plus cyclophosphamide regimen will achieve remission in 90% of patients.

Special situations:

a) In patients with mild indolent disease localized to the upper and or lower airways, trimethoprim/sulfamethoxazole in a dose of 160/180 mg twice daily may be tried. Such patients must be carefully monitored and if there is any evidence of other organ involvement stronger immunosuppressants must be started.

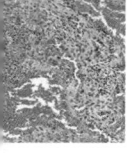

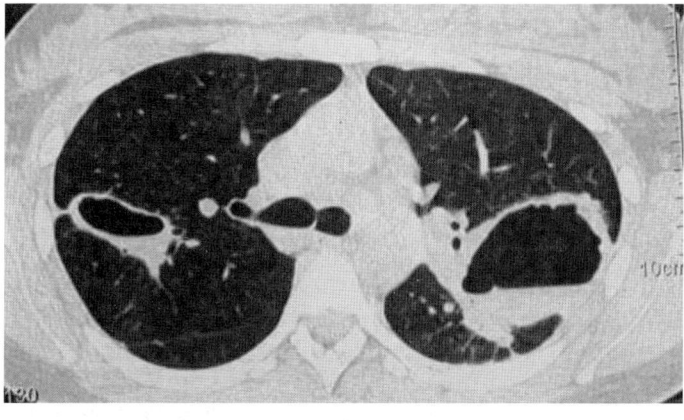

(a)

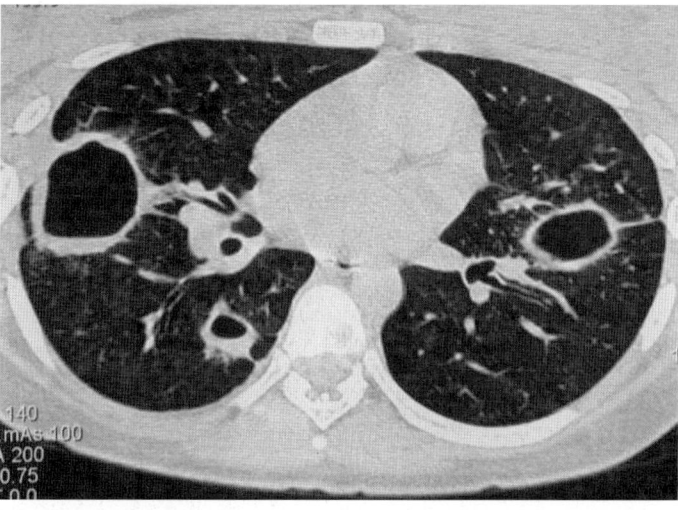

(b)

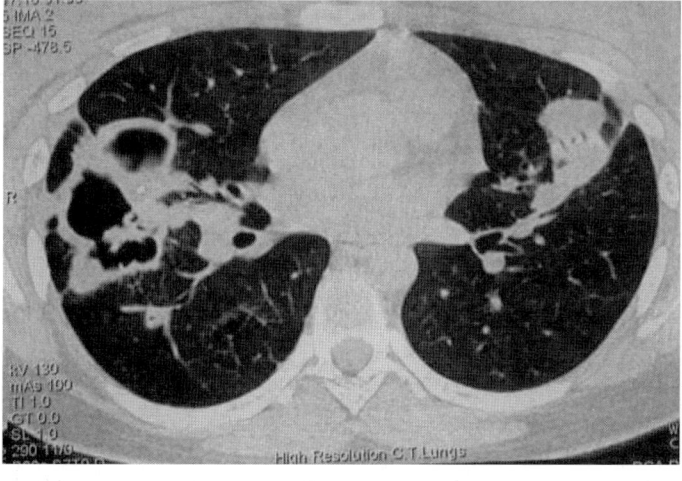

(c)

Fig 50.10: Wegener's granulomatosis in a young girl who presented with haemoptysis with systemic features of weight loss, fever and anaemia. CT chest at intervals showed cavitation and consolidation in both lung fields, most importantly, changing areas of consolidation and changing cavities. (a) done in June '02 shows a cavity with a fluid level in the left lung and another cavity in the right lung (b) done in May '03 shows disappearance of the cavity in the left lung and appearance of fluid-filled cavity in the right lung. Note other multiple cavities (c) done in November '03 shows cavitatory lesions in the right lung and nodular consolidation in the left lung. This is a typical feature of Wegener's granulomatosis where the lesions appear and disappear or change in size spontaneously.

b) Limited WG or patients with early generalized disease without renal involvement can receive methotrexate in a dose of 20–25mg /week. This milder immuno-suppression avoids the more serious toxicity of cyclophosphamide and is equally effective in this group of patients.

c) Rapidly progressive fulminant disease, diffuse alveolar haemorrhage, and rapidly progressive renal failure are best treated with pulses of methyl-prednisolone in doses up to 1 g/day for three days. A large recent study, the MEPEX trial (methyl prednisolone versus plasma exchange) showed that two weeks of plasma exchange was clearly superior to pulses alone in terms of renal recovery. Recombinant Factor VII A and desmopressin have also been tried to control torrential haemorrhage in patients with diffuse alveolar haemorrhage.

d) Sub-glottic stenosis: Sub-glottic lesions are generally unresponsive to systemic therapy. Success rates of medical therapy in relieving the obstruction run at 20–25%. Intralesional steroids have been used with some success, methylprednisolone being injected in a four-quadrant, submucosal pattern. The steroid injections are best combined with endoscopic dilatation or cold knife lysis. Lasers have been used but may result in extensive scarring making such patients more difficult to manage later. The use of airway stents to maintain airway patency is also controversial. Most experts feel that the long-term safety of these stents has not been well established; stent fracture, migration, excess granulation tissue and even death have been reported. A number of surgical techniques involving laryngotracheal reconstruction have been described and involvement of a skilled ear, nose and throat (ENT) surgeon is mandatory in all such cases. Tracheostomy is of course the procedure of choice when the airway is critically compromised or in an emergency setting.

2. Maintenance Therapy: Once remission has been successfully achieved with prednisolone and cyclophosphamide, treatment can be deescalated to a less toxic agent than cyclophosphamide to maintain remission. Agents used at this stage include azathioprine, methotrexate, mycophenolate mofetil, cyclosporine and trimethoprim/sulfamethoxazole. The timing of the transition is controversial. While traditional teaching was that steroids and cyclophosphamide be tapered down over a year, a study by Jayne D, Rasmussen N et al (*Ref: Jayne D, Rasmussen N et al, A randomized trial of maintenance therapy for vasculitis associated with antineutrophil cytoplasmic autoantibodies. N Engl J Med. 2003 3 Jul.; 349(1):36–44.*) suggested that the switch from cyclophosphamide to azathioprine could be made in three to six months with no increased risk of relapse.

3. Monitor for Toxicity. Cyclophosphamide is a very toxic agent and careful monitoring of blood counts is essential. The optimal dose is one that reduces the lymphocyte count but maintains the total WBC count over 3500/mm^3. To avoid bladder toxicity the patient must be advised to take the entire dose in the morning and drink plenty of water. Regular checks of urine are also advised. Steroid-related side-effects must also be monitored and every attempt made to get down to alternate day maintenance doses to

minimize toxicity. Concomitant calcium, Vitamin D and bisphosphanates are also recommended in most patients on steroids to prevent osteoporosis.

4. Monitor for Opportunistic Infections (OIs): OIs like tuberculosis or pneumocystis pneumonia (PCP) are common after immunosuppression and must be carefully monitored for. In our setting tuberculosis is of special importance and is difficult to diagnose as the clinical and radiological features may mimic flare-up of WG. The role of isoniazid prophylaxis in patients of WG with positive tuberculin skin tests (latent TB) has not been established. Trimethoprim-sulfamethoxazole (Tmp/ Smx) prophylaxis against pneumocystis infection is recommended in all patients receiving cyclophosphamide or methotrexate for remission induction or maintenance.

5. Treatment of patients refractory to treatment: Patients who have not responded to cytotoxic agents, high-dose steroids, or plasma exchange are deemed to have refractory disease. Novel therapies considered in this small but critically ill group of patients include tumour necrosis factor (TNF) blockers (etanercept, infliximab) and rituximab. A large study showed no efficacy of etanercept when added to standard therapy. In fact such patients had a higher incidence of malignancy. On the other hand an open-label trial of rituximab conducted by Keogh showed promising results. All 10 patients with refractory WG in whom this drug was used achieved remission with improvement in renal function. Rituximab is a chimeric monoclonal antibody directed at CD 20, an antigen expressed exclusively on B lymphocytes. It is a drug used in oncology for non-Hodgkin's B-cell lymphoma. B lymphocytes play an important role in autoimmune disease and produce antibodies including ANCA. Based on this study a large multicentre trial is currently underway evaluating this drug as a possible alternative to cyclophosphamide as a remission-inducing agent.

CHURG-STRAUSS SYNDROME

Definition

The Chapel Hill Consensus Conference defines Churg-Strauss Syndrome (CSS) as an eosinophil-rich and granulomatous inflammation involving the respiratory tract, and a necrotizing vasculitis involving the small to medium vessels, with associated asthma and eosinophilia.

Background

The syndrome was first described in 1951, in an article in the American Journal of Pathology, by Churg and Strauss in 13 patients with asthma, eosinophilia, granulomatous inflammation, necrotizing systemic vasculitis and necrotizing glomerulonephritis.

Diagnosis

The American College of Rheumatology (ACR) has proposed six criteria for the diagnosis of CSS. These include:

1. Asthma
2. Eosinophilia (>10% in the peripheral blood)
3. Paranasal sinusitis
4. Pulmonary infiltrates (often transient)
5. Histological evidence of vasculitis with extravascular eosinophils
6. Mononeuritis multiplex or polyneuropathy.

The presence of four or more criteria helps diagnose CSS with a sensitivity of 85% and a specificity of 99.7%.

Epidemiology

The incidence of CSS in the US is one to three cases per 100, 000 adults per year. Globally, the incidence is similar at 2.5 cases per 100, 000 adults per year. There is no Indian data but scattered case reports abound and it is likely that many patients with CSS might be missed and labelled "Tropical eosinophilia". The disease occurs in all ages from 15–70 years with a mean age of approximately 38 years. Several case reports and small series describe CSS in paediatric populations as well. CSS is slightly more common in males.

Pathophysiology

CSS is a granulomatous small-vessel vasculitis. It is an idiopathic disorder though recent reports have reported this condition secondary to a number of agents.

The report that has excited the greatest attention is the association of CSS with the use of leukotrine receptor antagonists. These cases initially led to a general warning on the possible link between CSS and leukotrine receptor antagonists. However, careful analysis of all reported cases suggests that CSS develops primarily in those patients taking these medications

Table 50.4: Management of wegener's granulomatosis
Induction of remission
Oral prednisolone can be used in a dose of 1 mg/kg + cyclophosphamide in a dose of 2 mg/kg daily
Maintenance Therapy
Azathioprine, methotrexate, mycophenolate mofetil, cyclosporine and trimethoprim/sulfamethoxazole
Monitor for Toxicity
Monitor for Opportunistic Infections like tuberculosis or PCP
Treatment of patients refractory to treatment
TNF blockers (etanercept, infliximab) and Rituximab
Management of special situations:
Mild indolent disease localized to the upper and or lower airways, trimethoprim/sulfamethoxazole—150/180 mg twice daily
Limited WG or patients with early generalized disease—20–25 mg/ week
Rapidly progressive fulminant disease—methyl-prednisolone in doses up to 1 gram/day for 3 days
Subglottic stenosis—Intralesional steroids plus endoscopic dilatation or cold knife lysis. Laser therapy, airway stents and surgical procedures like laryngotracheal reconstruction and tracheostomy

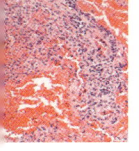

who almost certainly had an underlying eosinophilic disorder which was being masked by corticosteroids. Administration of the leukotrine receptor antagonists improved asthma control, permitted steroids to be tapered and stopped, and hence served to unmask the underlying CSS.

The same reasoning helps explain the link reported in small series with inhaled corticosteroids. Again, it is believed that the inhaled steroids improved asthma control sufficiently to permit reduction/withdrawal of systemic steroids thus unmasking the active vasculitis. These links between leukotrine antagonists and inhaled corticosteroids merely emphasize the importance of monitoring patients carefully when severe asthma is controlled with any substance allowing withdrawal from systemic steroids.

Other drugs believed to be implicated in CSS include mesalazine, propylthiouracil, and freebase cocaine (in a solitary case report).

Clinical Features

CSS has three phases:

- Prodromal phase: of allergic rhinitis and asthma
- Eosinophilic phase: of infiltrative disease such as eosinophilic pneumonia or gastroenteritis
- Vasculitic phase: Systemic small to medium-vessel vasculitis with granulomatous inflammation

The three phases are not seen in all patients and do not necessarily appear in this order.

Asthma is a cardinal feature of CSS, being present in 98% of patients. In general, asthma precedes the vasculitis by three to ten years and may be well-controlled and even forgotten by the time the vasculitic phase announces itself. Less frequently, asthma may coincide with the appearance of the vasculitis. The asthma in CSS is usually persistent and hence these patients are often on maintenance doses of steroids for their 'persistent, chronic asthma'. This might mask other features of the syndrome.

Sinusitis: Paranasal sinusitis is a feature in around 60% of patients with CSS. Allergic rhinitis is also frequent. Unlike WG, necrotizing and destructive lesions of the upper airways are not seen.

Pulmonary: In addition to asthma, important pulmonary manifestations include transient lung infiltrates, haemoptysis secondary to alveolar capillaritis, and pleural effusions which are typically eosinophilic. Consolidation and cavitation have also been reported.

Skin manifestations: are frequent in the vasculitic phase and include nodules, palpable purpura, urticarial rash, livideo reticularis, necrotic bullae, digital ischemia, skin necrosis and gangrene.

Rheumatological manifestations: joint pains are common but arthritis is rare.

Renal: Renal involvement takes the form of a pauci-immune glomerulonephritis which is seldom as frequent or severe as that observed in WG.

Gastrointestinal (GI): symptoms related to vasculitis of the GI tract are distinctive and include abdominal pain and bloody diarrhoea. Abdominal crisis as in Henoch Schonlein purpura may occur and the skin and GI manifestations of these two vasculitides are similar.

Peripheral neuropathy: mononeuritis multiplex occurs in as many as 77% of patients, and, like polyarteritis nodosa, this vasculitis is an important cause of neuropathy.

Cardiac manifestations: are important causes of morbidity and mortality in this condition. Myocarditis and myocardial infarction can be fatal. Pericarditis has also been reported.

Investigations/Laboratory Workup

Blood and biochemistry: Peripheral eosinophilia is always seen. The levels vary from a minimum of 10% to strikingly high eosinophil counts. Mild anaemia, elevated ESR and C-reactive protein (CRP) are inevitably found. Immunoglobulin E (IgE) levels are usually elevated. Serum creatinine must always be checked along with routine urine microscopy for proteinuria, casts and microscopic haematuria. ANCA is positive in approximately 40% of patients with CSS. The pattern of staining is usually perinuclear-ANCA (p-ANCA) positive (antimyeloperoxidase antibodies).

Radiology

Pulmonary infiltrates are found in up to 75% of cases of CSS. Transient infiltrates which are often bilateral are common. Localized nodular or patchy opacities may be seen which may cavitate on occasion. Extensive air-space consolidation should suggest intra-alveolar haemorrhage, especially if this is accompanied by drop in haemoglobin levels and haemoptysis. Eosinophilic pleural effusions are observed in 10–30%.

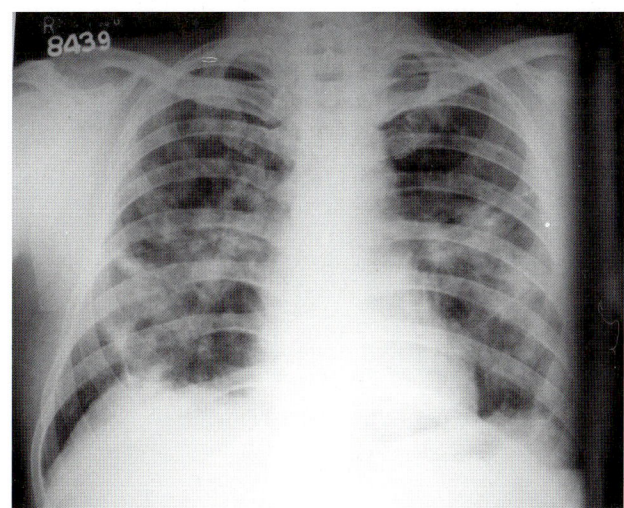

Fig 50.11: Churg-Strauss syndrome. X-ray demonstrates ill-defined-nodular areas in both lung fields.

Other organ-specific tests that may be needed depending on the organ involved include: electromyography and nerve conduction studies, ECHO and Holter monitoring for cardiac involvement, and GI endoscopy for GI bleeding.

Biopsy Proof

Pathological proof through a biopsy is helpful but not essential in confirming the diagnosis. Depending on the site of organ

involvement, biopsies can be taken from skin, lung (ideally VATS or open-lung biopsies), kidney, nerves or muscle. The characteristic pathological findings include small, necrotizing granuloma, and vasculitis affecting the small arteries and venules. The granulomas have a eosinophilic centre and are surrounded by epitheloid giant cells and macrophages. Kidney biopsies usually reveal a focal and segmental glomerulonephritis.

Differential Diagnosis

CSS must be considered in the differential diagnosis of any asthmatic with more than the expected peripheral eosinophilia. If vasculitic manifestations occur in any asthmatic when oral steroids are tapered or stopped, often with the aid of inhaled steroids or leukotrine antagonists, CSS must be the first disorder to be considered. It must be considered in any asthmatic with any evidence of multi-organ involvement or when asthma is accompanied by transient pulmonary shadows. Allergic bronchopulmonary aspergillosis (ABPA) and chronic eosinophilic pneumonias are close differentials. Other causes of pulmonary eosinophilia, especially hypereosinophilic syndromes and drug-induced eosinophilias must be distinguished from CSS. Other vasculitis syndromes like WG and microscopic polyarteritis must also be distinguished. When the GI system is primarily affected, the differential includes Henoch-Schonlein purpura (HSP), mesenteric ischemia and eosinophilic gastroenteritis. Other causes of acute glomerulonephritis including polyarteritis nodosa and Goodpasture's syndrome must be considered when the kidneys are primarily affected. Multi-system diseases like infective endocarditis, systemic lupus erythematosus (SLE) and essential cryoglubulinemia may share a few features with CSS.

Treatment

Steroids are the drug of choice in CSS and are usually the sole immunosuppressive therapy needed. They are usually given orally in a dose of 1 mg/kg/day (around 40–60 mg) of prednisolone. Life-threatening organ involvement like alveolar haemorrhage should be treated initially with a pulsed dose of 1g IV methyl prednisolone daily for three days followed by oral prednisolone. No more than 20% of patients with CSS will need additional immunosuppressives. Drugs that have been used include azathioprine, cyclophosphamide, IV immunoglobulin, interferon alpha, infliximab and rituximab. Plasma exchange has been tried but does not have the dramatic effect seen in WG and is probably not helpful in this condition.

Prognosis and Outcome

The five-year survival in untreated CSS is 25%. Treatment with systemic steroids improves survival rates to 70% at five years. The commonest cause of mortality in CSS is myocarditis and myocardial infarction secondary to coronary arteritis. Other causes of death reported in some series include alveolar haemorrhage, renal failure, GI bleeding and status asthmaticus.

MICROSCOPIC POLYANGIITIS

Microscopic Polyangiitis (MPA) was for several decades been grouped together with polyarteritis nodosa (PAN). It was only in 1944, that the Chapel Hill Consensus Conference recognized MPA as an entity in its own right, distinguishing it from PAN and WG, the diseases with which it had been confused over the years and with which it has considerable overlap. MPA affects small and medium-sized vessels and is a disease of middle-aged patients. It is the commonest cause of pulmonary renal involvement. Pulmonary involvement takes the form of diffuse alveolar haemorrhage secondary to pulmonary capillaritis and occurs in approximately 12% of patients with MPA. Renal involvement occurs in more than 80% and results in glomerulonephritis with distinctive RBC casts in urine. GI involvement is much more common in MPA than in WG where it is rare. General non-specific symptoms like fever, malaise and weight loss are common as are skin lesions and peripheral neuropathy which occur in 60% of cases. The histology is indistinguishable from WG except that granulomatous inflammation is not a feature. The ANCA is usually positive and is of the p-ANCA variety, reacting with MPO. Treatment is as for WG.

The table below gives the distinguishing features of MPA, WG and PAN.

OTHER PULMONARY VASCULITIDES

Takayasu's Arteritis

This is a large-vessel vasculitis predominantly affecting the aorta and its major branches. It results in intimal fibroproliferation of the aorta, great vessels, pulmonary arteries, and renal arteries and results in segmental stenosis, occlusion, dilatation, and aneurysmal formation in these vessels. Of the four types of Takayasu's arteritis, the most common is Type III, which is found in as many as 65% of patients. The most commonly involved vessels include the left subclavian artery (50%), the left common carotid artery (20%), the brachiocephalic trunk, and the renal arteries. The pulmonary arteries are affected in significant numbers of patients with Takayasu's arteritis. This leads to pulmonary hypertension and pulmonary stenosis. Fistula formation between branches of the pulmonary artery and bronchial arteries has been reported as has non-specific interstitial lung disease. The link with mycobacterial infection remains unproven. Steroids have been tried with variable results. There are recent reports of antitumor necrosis factor agents being useful.

Giant Cell Arteritis

Giant cell arteritis is a vasculitis affecting large and medium-sized arteries. While the common symptoms are headaches, jaw pain and blurred vision, respiratory symptoms are reported in a quarter of cases. Cough, hoarseness, and throat pain have all been reported and on occasion can be the presenting symptoms. Occasional cases of pleural effusion associated with giant cell arteritis have been reported. A strikingly high ESR is common and the response to steroids is generally dramatic.

Beçhet's Disease

Beçhets disease is an immune complex vasculitis that affects arteries and veins of all sizes. It is characterized by aphthous oral and genital ulcers in combination with uveitis, cutaneous nodules or pustules and meningoencephalitis. The distinctive feature when the lungs are affected is haemoptysis. This can be

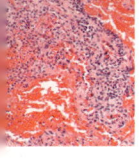

Table 50.5: Distinguishing featurs of MPA, WG and PAN			
	MPA	**MPA**	**PAN**
Blood Vessel Size	Small to Medium	Small to Medium	Medium
Blood Vessel Type	Arterioles to venules, and sometimes arteries and veins	Arterioles to venules, and sometimes arteries and veins	Muscular Arteries
Granulomatous Inflammation	No	Yes	No
Lung Symptoms	Yes	Yes	No
Glomerulonephritis	Yes	Yes	No
Renal Hypertension	No	No	Yes
Mononeuritis Multiplex	Common	Occasional	Common
Skin Lesions	Yes	Yes	Yes
GI Symptoms	No	No	Yes
Eye Symptoms	Yes	Yes	No
ANCA-Positivity	75%	65–90%	No
Constitutional Syptoms	Yes	Yes	Yes
Necrotizing Tissue	Yes	Yes	Yes
Microaneurysms	Rarely	Rarely	Typical

Source: John Hopkins Vasculitis Center, rheumatology@jhmi.edu.

massive and even fatal, and occurs secondary to rupture of pulmonary artery aneurysms that some of these patients develop.

Idiopathic Pauci-immune Pulmonary Capillaritis

This condition is diagnosed when the patient presents with alveolar haemorrhage and the biopsy shows capillaritis in the absence of any other detectable systemic disorder. It is a diagnosis of exclusion and the histology is indistinguishable from that of an ANCA-positive vasculitis. Treatment is with immunosuppressives as for Wegener's granulomatosis.

SUGGESTED READING

Frankel SK. Vasculitis: Wegener's granulomatosis, Churg-Strauss syndrome, microscopic polyangiitis, polyarteritis nodosa, and Takayasu arteritis. *Crit Care Clin*. 1 Oct. 2002; 18(4): 855–79.

Frankel SK. Update in the diagnosis and management of pulmonary vasculitis. *Chest*. 1 Feb. 2006; 129(2): 452–65.

Gómez-Puerta JA. Antineutrophil cytoplasmic antibody-associated vasculitides and respiratory disease. *Chest*. 1 Oct. 2009; 136(4): 1101–11.

Keogh KA. Churg-Strauss syndrome: clinical presentation, antineutrophil cytoplasmic antibodies, and leukotriene receptor antagonists. *Am J Med*. 1 Sep. 2003; 115(4): 284–90.

Polychronopoulos VS. Airway involvement in Wegener's granulomatosis. *Rheum Dis Clin North Am*. 1 Nov. 2007; 33(4): 755–75, vi.

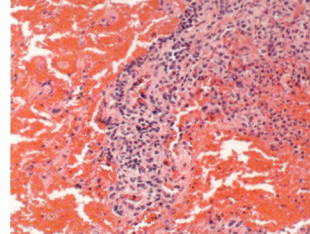

CHAPTER **51** **Pulmonary Hypertension**

INTRODUCTION

The pulmonary circuit is embedded in the matrix of the lung and interposed between the two sides of the heart. Though it plays a pivotal role in gas exchange and oxygen transport it is not the exclusive domain of either the cardiologist or the pulmonologist and hence has been relatively ignored by both sets of specialists. Tremendous advances have occurred in the last few decades in our understanding of the pathogenesis of pulmonary hypertension (PH) and its treatment which have served to redress the centuries of neglect in this field. Primary idiopathic PH is a devastating disease; without effective treatment; it is rapidly progressive and inevitably fatal. Indeed the outlook for a patient with primary PH and NYH 4 (breathless at rest) is worse than that for a patient with lung cancer, with a median survival of nine months.

DEFINITION

Pulmonary hypertension (PH) is defined as an increase in mean pulmonary artery pressure > 25 mmHg at rest as assessed by right heart catheterization. The normal pulmonary artery pressure at rest is 14 +/− 3 mmHg with an upper limit of no more than 20 mm and the level of 25 mmHg has been chosen to maintain consistency in all trials and registries of PH.

MILESTONES IN THE HISTORY OF PH

The pulmonary circulation was first described in the 16th century but it took another 400 years for the first clinical description of PH. In the 1950s this coincided with the advent of cardiac catheterization. In the 1960s an epidemic of PH secondary to appetite suppressants (fenfluramine) helped rekindle interest in the disease and this culminated in the first World Health Organization (WHO) meeting on PH in Geneva in 1975. In 1981 the National Institutes of Health (NIH) began a registry on all patients with PH in the US, so data on their natural history and course became available. Two further landmark WHO meetings on PH took place over the next few years in Evian and Venice; the current classification of PH was established at the Venice meeting in 2003. In terms of therapy, exciting developments were also occurring. After centuries of neglect, in 1991 the first Food and Drug Administration (FDA)-approved drug apoprostenol emerged and it was only after 2000 that sildenafil and its derivatives and the endothelin receptor blockers (bosentan) were developed.

AETIOLOGY

A wide range of common and rare disorders can result in PH. Primary PH is now called Idiopathic Pulmonary Arterial Hypertension. This is a prototype of PH but is a diagnosis of exclusion. Other broad headings the chest physician should always exclude before labelling a patient "Idiopathic" include: PH secondary to left heart disease, PH secondary to lung diseases and hypoxia and pulmonary veno-occlusive disease. Chronic thromboembolic disease is a rare but surgically reversible cause of PH which should always be actively considered and ruled out. It results from recurrent thromboemboli or thrombi in the pulmonary vasculature, leading to increasing obliteration of the pulmonary vasculature. PH with right ventricular hypertrophy and failure are the presenting features, the true cause of which is often missed. Finally, PH could be secondary to a number of rarer haematological, systemic and metabolic disorders which should be considered before labelling a patient as idiopathic PH.

A detailed classification based on the Dana Point consensus is outlined below.

PATHOGENESIS OF PH

Idiopathic PH has a complex aetiology. Of singular importance is the excessive vasoconstriction these individuals develop due to abnormal expression of potassium channels in the smooth muscle cells and due to endothelial dysfunction. Endothelial dysfunction leads to impaired production of vasodilator and anti-proliferative agents like nitric oxide (NO) and prostacyclin. This is accompanied by overexpression of vasoconstrictor and proliferative substances such as endothelin-1. As a consequence vascular remodelling and proliferation occur. Prothrombotic abnormalities have also been demonstrated and small distal thrombi in pulmonary arterioles are known.

When PH occurs in a familial context mutations in the bone morphogenetic protein receptor 2 gene have been detected in 70% of cases. Mutations of this gene have been detected in around 10–40% of cases, with apparently sporadic cases thus representing the major genetic predisposing factor for PH.

PH due to lung disease A number of pathophysiological factors are involved in this group including hypoxic vasoconstriction, mechanical stress of hyperinflated lungs, loss of capillaries and inflammatory and toxic effects of cigarette smoke. Endothelium-derived vasoconstrictor-vasodilator imbalance may

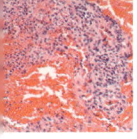
Table 51.1:
Updated clinical classification pulmonary hypertension

1.	**PAH**
1.1	Idiopathic
1.2	Heritable
1.2.1	BMPR2
1.2.2	ALK-1, endoglin (with or without hereditary haemorrhagic telangiectasia)
1.2.3	Unknown
1.3	Drugs and toxins induced
1.4	Associated with
1.4.1	Connective tissue diseases
1.4.2	HIV infection
1.4.3	Portal hypertension
1.4.4	Congenital heart disease
1.4.5	Schistosomiasis
1.4.6	Chronic haemolytic anaemia
1.5	Persistent pulmonary hypertension of the newborn
1′:	**Pulmonary veno-occlusive disease (PVOD) and/or pulmonary capillary haemangiomatosis (PCH)**
2.	**Pulmonary hypertension due to left heart disease**
2.1	Systolic dysfunction
2.2	Diastolic dysfunction
2.3	Valvular disease
3.	**Pulmonary hypertension due to lung diseases and/or hypoxia**
3.1	Chronic obstructive pulmonary disease
3.2	Interstitial lung disease
3.3	Other pulmonary diseases with mixed restrictive and obstructive pattern
3.4	Sleep-disordered breathing
3.5	Alveolar hypoventilation disorders
3.6	Chronic exposure to high altitude
3.7	Developmental abnormalities
4.	**Chronic thromboembolic pulmonary hypertension (CTEPH)**
5.	**PH with unclear and/or multifactorial mechanisms**
5.1	Haematological disorders; myeloproliferative disorders, splenectomy
5.2	Systemic disorders: sarcoidosis, pulmonary Langerhans' cell histiocytosis, lymphangioleiomyomatosis, neurofibromatosis, vasculitis
5.3	Metabolic disorders: glycogen storage disease, Gaucher disease, thyroid disorders
5.4	Others: tumoral obstruction, fibrosing mediastinitis, chronic renal failure on dialysis

BMPR2: bone morphogenetic protein receptor, type 2; ALK-1: activin receptor-like kinase 1; PAH: pulmonary arterial hypertension.

Source: Reprinted from Simonneau G, Ivan M, *et al*. Classification of Pulmonary Hypertension, *Journal of the American College of Cardiology*, 2009; 54: S43–54.

also contribute. Seotonin gene polymorphism may determine the severity of PH in hypoxemic patients with chronic obstructive pulmonary disease (COPD).

PREVALENCE OF PH

Pulmonary Arterial Hypertension is not a common disease. Data from recent registries in Europe and Scotland show the prevalence of PH and IPH are 16 and five cases per million respectively. In the French registry 39% of patients had IPAH of which around 4% had a family history of PH. PH secondary to chronic lung disease and hypoxia is of course much more common. The incidence of significant PH in COPD patients

with at least one prior admission for acute exacerbation is around 20%. In advanced COPD, PH is highly prevalent (around 50%). In interstitial lung disease (ILD) the prevalence of PH is around 30–40%. In the subset of patients with a combination of emphysema and ILD the prevalence and severity of PH is even higher. There is no available data on the prevalence or epidemiology of PAH from India but with the ready availability of some of the newer drugs there are growing calls for maintenance of a national drug registry.

CLINICAL FEATURES

The clinical features of PH may be subtle and non-specific and the earliest symptom is often an unexplained dyspnoea on exertion. This may indeed be the sole symptom in the first few years of presentation and patients often visit multiple doctors before the diagnosis is made. In a young patient this is often passed off as secondary to physical deconditioning or even anxiety and hyperventilation. Other early non-specific symptoms include fatigue and palpitation. In more advanced cases, syncope (usually exertional), anginal pain, oedema of the feet and free fluid in the abdomen may be noticed.

The earliest physical sign is also subtle and easily missed. It is an accentuation of the pulmonary component of the second heart sound. As the PH worsens the patient may develop a pansystolic murmur of tricuspid regurgitation often with an accompanying right-sided S3 gallop. A diastolic Graham Steele murmur of pulmonary regurgitation may also be heard. In advanced cases the patient presents with right heart failure with distended neck veins, congestive hepatomegaly and ascites and/or oedema of the feet.

Examination should include attempts at determining the aetiology of PH. Thus gross clubbing may denote congenital cyanotic heart disease; telangectasia and sclerodactyly point to scleroderma as the cause of PH. If PH is secondary to COPD there is obvious evidence of airflow limitation; the fine Velcro-like dry crackles of ILD causing PH may be missed unless carefully auscultated for.

Table 51.2:
Clinical features of pulmonary hypertension

a)	Early unexplained dyspnoea on exertion
b)	Syncope (usually exertional), anginal pain, oedema of the feet; accentuated P2 with progression of the disease
c)	Right ventricular enlargement
d)	Dilated PA
e)	Tricuspid incompetence
f)	Graham Steele murmur of pulmonary incompetence
g)	JVP +; prominent 'a' wave
h)	Oedema feet, free fluid in the abdomen
i)	Enlarged tender liver

DIAGNOSING PH

Once PH is suspected from history or examination it is incumbent on the clinician to:

– Confirm the diagnosis of PH
– Determine its severity
– Check for an underlying secondary cause before labelling the patient Idiopathic Pulmonary Arterial Hypertension.

The following tests are useful:

1. *Chest radiograph*   In the early stages the chest radiograph may be normal but in 90% of patients with IPAH the chest radiograph is abnormal at the time of diagnosis. Findings include central pulmonary artery dilatation, peripheral pruning and evidence of right atrial and ventricular enlargement. If present, radiographic features of ILD or emphysema may give a clue to secondary causes of PH.

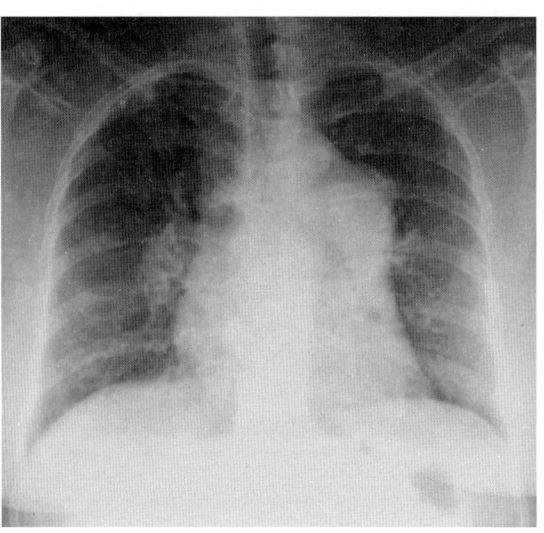

Fig 51.1: Pulmonary hypertension. X-ray chest reveals a markedly dilated main pulmonary artery visualized as a well-defined opacity in the left paracardiac region just below the aortic arch. The right pulmonary artery is also dilated as seen by the prominence of the right hilum.

2. *Electrocardiography* (ECG)   The ECG has insufficient sensitivity (55%) and specificity (70%) to be a screening tool for diagnosing PH. However, evidence of RV hypertrophy and strain may be seen in advanced cases. Atrial fibrillation if present carries a bad prognosis and invariably leads to further clinical deterioration.

3. *Pulmonary function test* (PFT)   A mild to moderate reduction in the diffusion capacity may be the sole abnormality directly due to the PH itself. The main role of PFT is to rule out an airway or an interstitial cause of PH.

4. *Arterial blood gas* (ABG)   ABG analysis is usually normal till advanced PH sets in. It may however show a mild hypoxia, and desaturation after exercise is a subtle and sensitive (but not specific) pointer to PH. Hypocapnia is often present secondary to alveolar hyperventilation. If COPD is the cause of the PH patients may have hypercapnia.

5. *Polysomnography*   A history of snoring and excessive daytime sleepiness must be enquired from every patient with PH. Obstructive sleep apnoea may present with PH and right heart failure and can only be diagnosed by overnight polysomnography.

6. *Echocardiography*   Is an indispensable test to determine the presence and severity of PH. It may also be of value in picking up a hitherto undetected cardiac shunt responsible for the

PH. The pulmonary artery pressure can be estimated based on the peak velocity of the tricuspid regurgitation jet. When tricuspid regurgitation is difficult to measure or cannot be measured, contrast echocardiography with agitated saline significantly increases the Doppler signal allowing proper measurement of peak tricuspid regurgitation velocity. Pulmonary artery measurements on echocardiography cannot be made for mild cases and do not always correlate with degree of PH determined on pulmonary angiography. A study based on echocardiographic screening of a tricuspid regurgitant jet in symptomatic patients with scleroderma determined that 45% of patients with echocardiographic diagnosis of PH were actually falsely positive. Exercise echocardiography has been used in patients with PH only on exercise.

7. *Ventilation Perfusion Scanning*   The ventilation perfusion scan is a good screening test for chronic thromboembolic PH and ideally should be performed on all patients before labelling them idiopathic. A normal or low-probability V/Q scan effectively rules out chronic thromboembolic PH with a sensitivity of 90–100% and a specificity of 94–100%.

8. *CT scanning*   High-resolution computed tomography (HRCT) scanning is a useful way to rule out ILD or emphysema as a cause of PH. Pulmonary venoocclusive disease (PVOD) also has a specific HRCT appearance with interstitial oedema, central ground-glass opacification and thickening of interlobular septa. Contrast CT of the pulmonary artery helps determine if there is evidence of surgically amenable chronic thromboembolic pulmonary hypertension (CTEPH). CT features of CTEPH include blockages, webs, bands and intimal irregularities.

9. *Pulmonary angiography and right heart catheterization*   This is an underutilized procedure, chiefly because of fears of safety in patients with severe PH. When performed in an experienced centre it carries a morbidity of no more than 1% and mortality of 0.05%. Pulmonary angiography remains the gold standard when it comes to diagnosing PH and assessing the severity of the haemodynamic derangement it produces. Right heart catheterization is also useful to test the vaso-reactivity of the pulmonary circulation. Vasoreactivity testing is again seldom performed but invaluable to

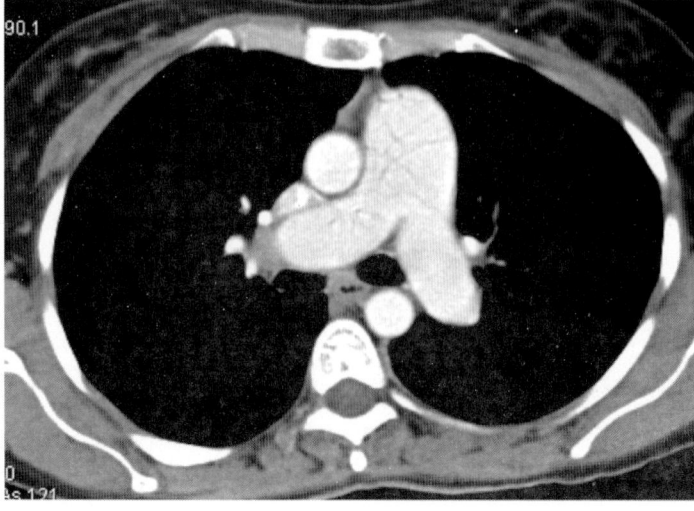

Fig 51.2: Pulmonary hypertension. CT Chest reveals markedly dilated main and right/left pulmonary arteries.

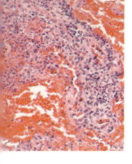

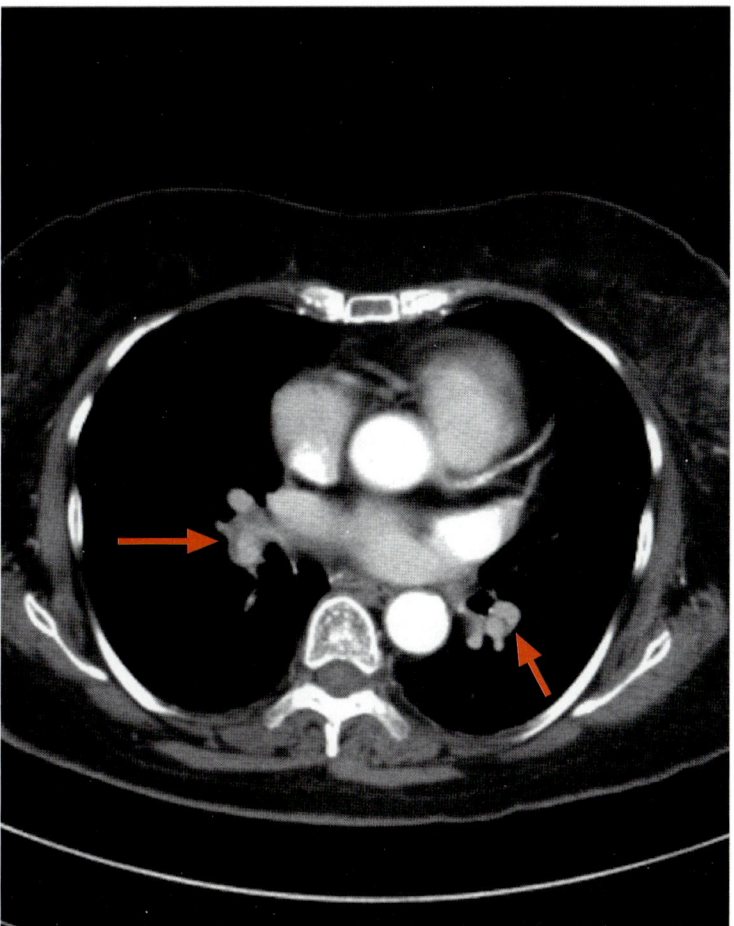

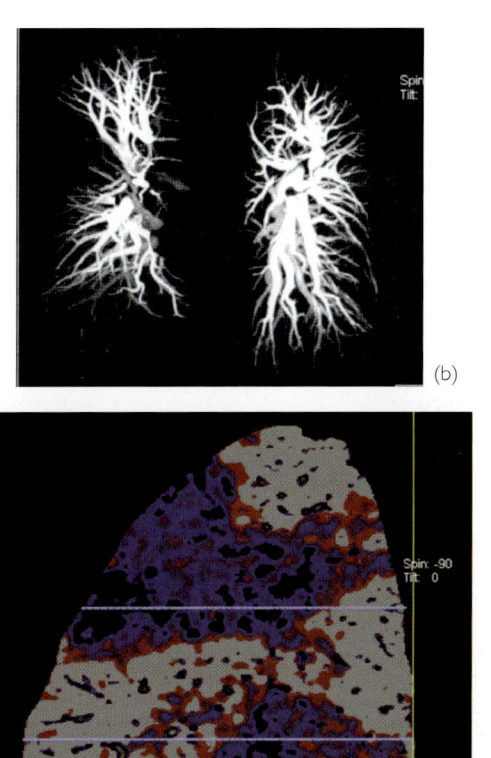

Fig 51.3: (a) CT angiography demonstrates linear bands in the descending left pulmonary artery indicating chronic pulmonary emboli (b) Maximum intensity projection (MIP) of CT pulmonary angiography demonstrates a large wedge-shaped area of no vascularity in the right upper zone due to segmental occlusion (c) Dual-energy CT pulmonary angiogram perfusion image demonstrates multiple wedge-shaped areas of reduced perfusion indicative of chronic pulmonary embolism.

determine which patients with PH will respond to long-term therapy with calcium channel blockers. It should ideally be performed at the same time as right heart catheterization. The agents currently used in vasoreactivity testing are inhaled nitric oxide, intravenous epoprostenol or intravenous adenosine. An acute responder is defined as one whose mean pulmonary artery (PA) pressure declines > 10 mmHg to reach an absolute value of < 40 mmHg with an increased or unchanged cardiac output. Unfortunately, only around 10% of patients with IPAH will meet this definition of acute responders. These acute responders are the only ones likely to show a sustained response to long-term calcium channel blockers and these are the only patients in whom these drugs may safely be used in large doses. Only 50% of patients who are acute responders are likely to have a sustained long-term response to these drugs and these are the only patients in whom they should be continued.

Evaluation of Severity

A number of parameters predict poor survival.

1. *Clinical parameters* WHO Class III or IV, extremes of age, syncope, haemoptysis or RV failure, are all clinical markers of severity.

Table 51.3: Investigations of pulmonary hypertension
a) Chest Radiograph
b) ECG
c) Pulmonary function testing
d) Arterial blood gases
e) Polysomnography
f) Echocardiography
g) Ventilation perfusion scanning
h) CT chest
i) Pulmonary angiography and right heart catheterization

2. *Echocardiographic markers* of poor survival include pericardial effusion, indexed right atrium area, and RV Doppler index. Interestingly, estimated systolic pulmonary arterial pressure (PAP) is not prognostic.

3. *Right heart catheterization parameters* are also useful in determining prognosis. These include PA oxygen saturation, right atrial pressure, pulmonary vascular resistance and cardiac output. PAP is less reliable, as with the advent of

right ventricular failure in the advanced stage of the disease, pulmonary artery pressure falls.

4. *Six-minute walk test (6MWT)* is an inexpensive, reproducible and well-standardized test. Walking distance < 250 meters and desaturation > 10% indicate poor prognosis in PH.

5. *Biochemical markers* Over the last decade a number of biochemical markers have emerged. Brain natriuretic peptide (BNP) levels, pro-BNP levels and elevated cardiac Trop T levels have all been shown in several studies to correlate with survival. Exact cut-off points of each of these markers have not been established as yet. Increases or decreases in these markers when serially measured over time also correlate well with response or lack of response to treatment. Newer markers like H-FABP and GDF-15 are also being looked at.

Table 51.4:
Estimating severity of pulmonary hypertension

a) Clinical parameters: WHO class III or IV, extremes of age, syncope, haemoptysis or RV failure

b) Echocardiographic markers like pericardial effusion, indexed right atrium area, and RV Doppler index

c) Right heart catheterization parameters like PA oxygen saturation, right atrial pressure, pulmonary vasular resistance and cardiac output.

d) 6 minute walk test (6MWT)

e) BNP levels, pro-BNP levels and elevated cardiac Trop T levels

---

THERAPY OF PH

The last decade has seen great advances in the treatment of PH. A position of helplessness with no drug options has been transformed to one of hope with the current availability and regulatory approval of eight drugs and further molecules at trial stage in the pipeline. Although PH remains a chronic disease without a cure, modern drug therapy leads to significant improvement in the patients' symptomatic status and a slower rate of clinical decline.

Therapeutic options include:

General Measures

Once diagnosed the patient is advised about certain lifestyle changes that must be made. These patients are generally young: strenuous activity and pregnancy must be avoided. Pregnancy carries a 30–50% mortality in patients with PH. Barrier methods of contraception are to be preferred to hormonal methods like contraceptive pills. Travel should be curtailed unless essential and the need for supplemental oxygen on flights must be clarified.

Supportive Therapy

Oral anticoagulants are advised in all patients with IPH unless there is a specific contraindication. Diuretics and digoxin are useful if there is evidence of a decompensated right ventricle. Oxygen is required in many patients with severe PH who are hypoxemic at rest or with exertion. It should be titrated to

maintain SaO_2 > 90%. Long-term oxygen has been shown to partially reduce the progression of PH in COPD.

Calcium Channel Blockers

Only a small fraction of patients with PAH will benefit from calcium channel blockers. As discussed earlier, these should ideally be identified by acute vasodilator challenge testing at the time of right heart catheterization. The drugs used include nifedipine, diltiazem and amlodipine. Relatively high doses are needed for them to be effective (120–240 mg for nifedipine and 240–720 mg for diltiazem). This underscores the importance of not using them in patients who have not undergone a vasoreactivity study or have a negative study because of the potential of major side-effects like hypotension and syncope.

Prostanoids

A number of prostacyclin derivatives have been used in the treatment of PH. These include epoprostenol, iloprost, treprostinil and beraprost. Epoprostenol has a very short half life (3–5 minutes) and is stable at room temperature for only eight hours. It is therefore administered by means of a syringe pump via a permanent tunnelled catheter. This is not practical on a long-term basis and this drug is usually reserved as a bridge to transplant. Iloprost is available by the intravenous, oral and inhaled routes and is well tolerated, though oral iloprost has been associated with flushing and jaw pain. Treprostinil is usually given by continuous subcutaneous infusion by a microinfusion pump and a small subcutaneous catheter. Infusion site pain is a limiting side-effect. Beraprost is the first chemically stable and orally active prostacyclin derivative and recent studies have shown an improvement in exercise capacity that unfortunately persists for only six months. None of the drugs in this group are available in India.

Phosphodiesterase Type-5 Inhibitors

Since the pulmonary vasculature contains substantial amounts of phosphodiesterase Type-5, the potential benefit of these agents in PH has been studied. Sildenafil and tadalafil, both drugs used to treat erectile dysfunction have been shown to cause significant vasodilatation with peak effects observed after 60 and 90 minutes respectively. A number of smaller uncontrolled studies first reported the favourable effects of sildenafil in pulmonary hypertension in IPH, PH secondary to connective tissue disease, in congenital cyanotic heart disease-associated PAH and in chronic thromboembolic pulmonary hypertension, (CTEPH). A large randomized controlled trial (RCT) of 278 PH patients treated with sildenafil called the SUPER-1 trial confirmed its favourable effects at different doses on symptoms, exercise capacity and haemodynamics. The approved dose is 20 mg three times a day but doses as high as 80 mg three times a day have been safely used. Side-effects are mild and are mainly linked to vasodilatation (headache, flushing, epistaxis). Tadalafil has the convenience of a once daily dose. A recent RCT called the PHIRST study on 406 PH patients showed good effects on symptoms, exercise capacity, haemodynamics and time to clinical worsening using the largest dose which was 40 mg once a day.

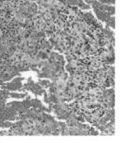

Endothelin Receptor Antagonists

Activation of the endothelin system has been consistently demonstrated in plasma and lung tissue of patients with PH. Endothelin exerts its effect by binding endothelin A and B receptors. Bosentan is an oral active dual endothelin-A and B receptor antagonist. It represents a breakthrough in PH because it is the first molecule in a new class of drugs specifically designed to treat this disorder. Its effect was established in five RCTs that have each shown improvement not just in functional class and exercise capacity, but also in hemodynamic and echocardiographic variables. Between them these studies have established its use in not just IPH but also PH secondary to connective tissue disease, cyanotic heart disease and CTEPH. Bosentan is initiated in a dose of 62.5 mg twice a day orally and then increased if tolerated to 125 mg twice a day after four weeks. Elevation of hepatic transaminases occurs in a dose-dependent manner in up to 10% of patients on this drug and hence monthly monitoring of liver function is mandatory. Sitaxentan and Ambrisentan are two other molecules in the same class that are also in use. Both cause less frequent elevation of liver transaminases compared to bosentan.

Combination Therapy

Combination therapy has become the standard of care in many centres. More than one PH-specific class of drugs are used in conjunction. These include prostanoids, endothelin receptor antagonists and phosphodiesterase inhibitors. The choice of combination agents, the optimal timing, when to switch and when to combine are all unclear and should prove fertile research opportunities for clinicians in the field.

Balloon Atrial Septostomy

The creation of an inter-atrial right to left shunt can decompress the right heart chambers, and increase left ventricular (LV) preload and cardiac output. In addition this improves systemic oxygen transport despite arterial oxygen desaturation. The recommended technique is graded balloon atrial septostomy. This is often a last resort measure in patients on transplant lists, buying them some time while they await their transplant.

Pulmonary Embolectomy

Surgical pulmonary endarterectomy is the treatment of choice for patients with CTEPH. Patients should be carefully selected and surgery should be done in a centre with experience in this form of surgery. In India, Narayana Hrudayalaya Health City in Bangalore has had the maximum experience, with excellent results with surgical removal of thromboemboli from blocked pulmonary vessels in patients with CTEPH. This is the only form of PH where one can talk of cure. Surgery can transform a patient disabled by breathlessness, on continuous oxygen and in right heart failure into normalcy. A dramatic fall in pulmonary vascular resistance and near normalization of haemodynamics can occur in even the most severe cases if properly selected and operated on by an experienced surgeon.

Transplantation

Transplantation is a real option in patients with severe PH who fail to respond to all available medical measures. Some forms of PH like pulmonary venoocclusive disease have a worse prognosis and these patients should be referred to a transplant centre as soon as they are diagnosed. Currently, either heart-lung or bilateral lung transplantation are offered for PH. The overall five-year survival following transplantation for PH stands at 50% in the best centres. The quality of life post-transplant is excellent. Sadly there are no centres in India performing lung transplantation.

Table 51.5:
Therapy for pulmonary hypertension
a) Lifestyle changes
b) Supportive therapy with oral anticoagulants, diuretics and digoxin
c) Calcium channel blockers—nifedipine, diltiazem and amlodipine
d) Prostanoids—epoprostenol, iloprost, treprostinil and beraprost
e) Phosphodiesterase type-5 inhibitors—sildenafil and tadalafil
f) Endothelin receptor antagonists—bosentan, sitaxentan and ambrisentan
g) Combination therapy with prostanoids, endothelin receptor antagonists and phosphodiesterase inhibitors
h) Balloon atrial septostomy
i) Pulmonary embolectomy
j) Transplantation—heart-lung or bilateral lung transplantation

SUGGESTED READING

Fishman AP. Clinical classification of pulmonary hypertension. *Clin Chest Med.* 1 Sep. 2001; 22(3): 385–91, vii.

Kim NH. Diagnosis and evaluation of the patient with pulmonary hypertension. *Cardiol Clin.* 1 Aug. 2004; 22(3): 367–73, v–vi.

McArdle JR. Pulmonary hypertension in older adults. *Clin Chest Med.* 1 Dec. 2007; 28(4): 717–33, vi.

McCrory DC. Methodology and grading for pulmonary hypertension evidence review and guideline development. *Chest.* 1 Jul. 2004; 126(1 Suppl): 11S-13S

McGoon MD. The assessment of pulmonary hypertension. *Clin Chest Med.* 1 Sep. 2001; 22(3): 493–508, ix.

Nauser TD. Diagnosis and treatment of pulmonary hypertension. *Am Fam Physician.* 1 May 2001; 63(9): 1789–98.

Rubenfire M. Pulmonary hypertension in the critical care setting: classification, pathophysiology, diagnosis, and management. *Crit Care Clin.* 1 Oct. 2007; 23(4): 801–34, vi-vii.

Voelkel NF. Pathology of pulmonary hypertension. *Cardiol Clin.* 1 Aug. 2004; 22(3): 343–51, v.

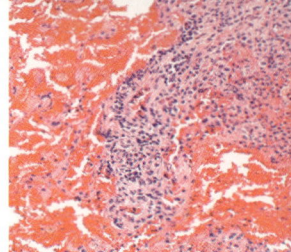

CHAPTER **52** **Pulmonary Embolism**

INTRODUCTION AND IMPORTANCE

Pulmonary embolism (PE) is the third most common cause of mortality after coronary artery disease and stroke. It is the commonest cause of death in the puerperium and postoperative period. Despite its importance it remains under-diagnosed and hence in a sense neglected. Indeed, up to 80% of pulmonary emboli found at autopsy have not been suspected ante-mortem. This must be one of the most staggeringly poor diagnostic rates for any disease in all of medicine. Despite all the advances in diagnosis this appalling diagnostic rate has not changed over the last four decades. Sadly, physicians cannot diagnose what they do not suspect and this is the crux of the problem with PE as we shall discuss later in the chapter.

PE is believed to affect 600, 000 patients annually in the US. Of these, 200, 000 die from their PE. It is responsible for at least 15% of all hospital deaths in some hospital mortality series from the US. Its true incidence is unknown because its many non-specific clinical features make it one of the most difficult diagnostic challenges in all of medicine. A study by Stein and colleagues in the mid-nineties from the Henry Ford Heart and Vascular Institute in Detroit showed PE occurred with an incidence of 1% of 51, 000 hospitalized patients over a 21-month period. It however accounted for 14% of all autopsies, thus emphasizing the fact that most cases were only being diagnosed post-mortem.

EPIDEMIOLOGY IN INDIA, CHINA AND SOUTH-EAST ASIA

INDIA

A study from a large private hospital in Mumbai showed that only 0.14% of 42, 000 in-patients were given the diagnosis of PE. This does not mean that PE is uncommon in India; it is just a reflection of the extent of under-diagnosis. In one of our critical care units, the incidence of PE was very close to that in the West.

In Chandigarh (North India), of 700 autopsies performed between 1964–80, the incidence of PE was 3.1%, lower than the West and similar to the low incidence in Africa. Yet in 2006, Kapadia SR and colleagues from Sir Ganga Ram Hospital, New Delhi (*Ref: Parakh R, Kapadia SR et al, Pulmonary embolism: a frequent occurrence in Indian patients with symptomatic lower limb venous thrombosis. Asian J Surg.2006 Apr; 29 (2):86–91*) noted that PE occured in as many as 40% of 1552 consecutive Indian patients with symptomatic deep vein thrombosis (DVT); 47% of patients with PE in this study (judged from a high-probability lung perfusion scan) were asymptomatic. Considering that many patients with DVT are asymptomatic, the incidence of both DVT and PE would be much higher than is apparent to-day. Increasing awareness will perhaps provide a much clearer idea about the prevalence of venous thromboembolism in India, which is certainly much higher than what is generally believed.

CHINA AND SOUTH-EAST ASIA

There have been several reports on DVT and PE in the Chinese population in the recent years; they cite a prevalence of DVT of 2.6–17%. A similar figure has been reported from Malaysia and Thailand. Data from a study performed in Hong Kong between 1990–94 showed an increased prevalence of 4.7% of pulmonary thromboembolism (PTE) (*Ref: Chau KY, Yuen ST, Wong MP. Clinicopathological pattern of pulmonary thromboembolism in Chinese autopsy patients: comparison with Caucasian series. Pathology 1997; 29:263–6*). These figures are within the lower range of the prevalence of PTE in Caucasian patients; reported rates of significant PTE from all autopsies are 3.4–9.0% in the United States and 12.8% in the United Kingdom.

Irrespective of the exact numbers, the impact of PE is considerable. PE has been described as the most important preventable cause of hospital deaths. In a recent study of 13, 000 admissions to six trauma centres, 17% of preventable deaths were caused by PE.

AETIOLOGY

LINK BETWEEN DVT AND PE

PE and DVT are intimately related. The perils posed by DVT are most sharply forced into focus when it culminates in a life-threatening PE. Dissimilar at first sight, they are in reality, two sides of the same coin, twin partners in crime, part of the same pathological process. DVT is by far the most common cause of PE. Indeed, PE is not a disease, but most often a complication of DVT. Exploring the link further, 40% of DVT patients without symptoms of PE will have positive (high probability) ventilation/perfusion (V/Q) scans. From another angle, 30% of PE patients without symptoms of DVT will have a positive venous Doppler. DVT is not more universally found because leg thrombi have often already embolised and because Doppler as a screening test has limitations, which will be discussed later.

Venous thromboembolism is a multigenic disease. Virchow's triad of venous stasis in the lower limbs, a hypercoagulable state and damage to the venous endothelium still hold good today though they were formulated at the end of the 19th century.

Genetic Determinants

There have been major advances in our knowledge of the molecular markers of thrombophilic states. The two most

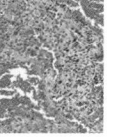

important are the Leiden mutation of Factor V, which confers a resistance to activated protein C and the G20210A mutation of prothrombin. Both these occur in about 4% of the Caucasian population. Other rarer genetic defects include: antithrombin deficiency (0.02%), protein C deficiency (0.2%), and protein S deficiency (0.1%). Similar data from Indian populations are needed but at present lacking. Intriguingly, Factor V Leiden and prothrombin mutation are stronger risk factors for DVT than PE. Occasional patients are heterozygous for two of these anomalies and then carry a much greater thrombotic risk. Conversely, certain genetic traits offer protection. These include: the O blood group which appears to reduce the risk of DVT even in carriers of Factor V Leiden. Elevated levels of homocysteine are also independent risk factors though the genetics of transmission are not as yet clear. A detailed genetic prothrombotic screen should be mandatory in patients with a history of DVT or PE occurring without any other traditional risk factor, in those with a positive family history, those with recurrent episodes of thrombosis, patients with their initial thrombotic episode at a young age, and in patients with arterial and venous thrombosis or thrombosis in unusual sites.

Environmental and Acquired Determinants

These traditional risk factors are well-known and are summarized in Table 52.1.

Only a few of these factors will be discussed here. The pulmonologist must not forget chronic obstructive pulmonary disease (COPD) as an important cause of DVT and PE. The prevalence of DVT in COPD patients requiring hospitalization for acute exacerbations in the West is in the range of 10–12%, though some studies quote rates as high as 20%. Indian data is limited but in a study conducted by us from the Hinduja Hospital in Mumbai, we looked for Doppler evidence of DVT in 100 patients admitted for exacerbations and found 9% had DVTs. Two patients in this series died of fatal PE.

Malignancy and DVT

Neoplastic cells are capable of activating the coagulation cascade either directly, by activation of thromboplastin, or indirectly by stimulating macrophages to synthesize procoagulant molecules. The risk of discovering a cancer in the first year after an episode of DVT is increased fourfold. The value of initiating a detailed workup for an occult carcinoma in a patient presenting with DVT is however still uncertain.

Newer Risk Factors

Recent data from the Nurses' health study have identified heavy smoking and hypertension as new, independent risk factors for DVT.

The PE Spectrum

Not all PEs are fatal. The outcome following a PE is a function of the size of the PE and the underlying cardiopulmonary status. A small PE may be poorly tolerated and tip the balance in a patient with advanced COPD while an otherwise fit young person might tolerate the effects of a larger PE without

Table 52.1: Environmental and acquired risk factors
Acquired thrombophilia
Lupus anticoagulant
Antiphospholipid antibody syndrome
Surgery
Major abdominal, pelvic surgery
Hip, knee surgery
Trauma
Fractures
Spinal cord injury
Immobilization
Hemiplegia
Paraplegia
Obstetrics
Pregnancy
Puerperium
Hormonal treatment:
Oral contraceptives
Hormone replaclement therapy
Tamoxifen, raloxifen
Cardiorespiratory
Congestive cardiac failure
Myocardial infarction
COPD
Malignancy
Abdominal, pelvic
Advanced, metastatic
Concurrent chemotherapy
Inflammatory bowel disease
Nephrotic syndrome

compromise. There is a spectrum in the size of the PE, from mild to massive. At one end, the patient with mild PE may remain asymptomatic with the PE detected incidentally. In the Prospective Investigation of Pulmonary Embolism Diagnosis (PIOPED) study, there were 20 such patients who had mild PE which was not initially diagnosed and hence not treated. The mortality in these patients, untreated, was only 5%. At the other end of severity is a massive PE which can cause almost immediate cardiorespiratory arrest. A massive PE is one that results in haemodynamic instability. Overall, these PEs are rare; in the PIOPED series, only 10% of all PEs could be classified as massive. The mortality in this group was however 3–7% higher. The majority of PEs fall in between these two groups. This category includes sub-massive PE. These are patients with a sizeable clot burden, no haemodynamic instability when they first present, but show echocardiographic evidence

of right heart dysfunction. These patients will be discussed in more detail later.

CLINICAL FEATURES: PE SYNDROMES

The symptoms of PE are non-specific and include dyspnoea, chest pain, fever, cough, haemoptysis and apprehension.

The signs are equally non-specific and include: tachypnoea, tachycardia, crackles, a pleural rub and an accentuated pulmonary component of the second heart sound. Evidence of an associated DVT must be carefully looked for, though this is often not clinically obvious. Because the symptoms and signs are non-specific, attempts have been made to combine them into scoring systems. The best validated is that of Wells which can immediately be applied at the bedside when first seeing a patient. It gives the patient points based on: previous PE/DVT, heart rate > 100/min, recent surgery or immobilization, clinical signs of DVT, alternative diagnosis less likely than PE, haemoptysis and cancer. This scoring system can be applied to in—and outpatients and has recently been externally validated. Adding on D-dimer further increases the accuracy of this clinical prediction system.

Table 52.2: Wells Clinical Prediction Rule for pulmonary Embolism (PE)	
Clinical feature	Points
Clinical symptoms of DVT	3
Other diagnosis less likely than PE	3
Heart rate greater than 100 beats per minute	1.5
Immobilization or surgery within past 4 weeks	1.5
Previous DVT or PE	1.5
Haemoptysis	1
Malignancy	1
Total	
PE = pulmonary embolism; DVT = deep venous thrombosis.	
Risk score interpretation (probability of PE): • > 6 points: high risk (78.4%); • 2 to 6 points: moderate risk (27.8%); • < 2 points: low risk (3.4%)	

The following pulmonary syndromes should be kept in mind.

1. *Pulmonary infarction syndrome* This occurs due to peripheral pulmonary emboli causing pulmonary infarction. The hallmark of this syndrome is pleuritic chest pain and haemoptysis. Radiologically, the classic wedge-shaped pleural-based shadow is seen. Only about 20% of all PEs will present in this fashion.

2. *Isolated dyspnoea syndrome* A high index of suspicion is needed if this form of PE is not to be missed. It is often mis-diagnosed and mislabelled as asthma or anxiety-related hyperventilation. An accompanying tachycardia may often be present. Another clue may be that these patients though

having a normal SaO_2 at rest often desaturate when made to walk for a few minutes or climb a flight of stairs.

3. *Syndromes associated with massive PE* The following manifestations singly or in combination may be observed.
   a. Sudden death—This may occur without apparent reason or typically follows straining over a bedpan.
   b. Shock and/or prolonged syncope—Shock characterized by hypotension, tachycardia, sweating, and cold clammy extremities with or without substernal chest pain is a feature of massive PE. The clinical picture may be indistinguishable from an acute myocardial infarct.
   c. Acute right heart failure may be the presenting feature, with engorged neck veins, a prominent 'a' wave in the neck, a right ventricular diastolic gallop and an accentuated pulmonary component of the second heart sound. The liver may be palpable and tender.
   d. Acute respiratory failure with tachypnoea, hypoxia associated at times with cyanosis and dyspnoea.
   e. Rarely, severe bronchospasm and pulmonary oedema have also been reported. We have witnessed the former but not the latter.
   f. Features of b, c, d, e are often combined in massive PE—various combinations are observed depending on the interval after acute embolism. Shock often predominates in the earlier phase and is associated with a raised central venous pressure, hypotension and hypoxemic respiratory failure. If recovery ensues, features of pulmonary hypertension (PH) are more evident.

Pulmonary embolism, particularly small often multiple emboli occurring in already critically ill individuals may show very subtle features. These include any one or more of the following–unexplained tachycardia, increasingly unstable circulatory state, supraventricular tachycardia, unexplained tachypnoea, postural hypotension or syncope, unexplained low-grade fever, icterus, and a marked rise in the erythrocyte sedimentation rate (ESR). There may be an unexplained fall in the PaO_2 or an increase in an already existing hypoxia. Sometimes a rapid deterioration in the clinical state is related to a silent PE. All these features described

Table 52.3: Syndromes associated with pulmonary embolism
Pulmonary infarction syndrome
Isolated dyspnoea syndrome
Syndromes associated with massive pulmonary embolism manifesting as:
i. Sudden death
ii. Shock and/or prolonged syncope
iii. Acute right heart failure
iv. Acute respiratory failure
v. Severe bronchospasm and pulmonary oedema
vi. Combination of ii, iii, iv, v
Subtle features like unexplained tachycardia, increasingly unstable circulatory state, supraventricular tachycardia, unexplained tachypnoea, postural hypotension or syncope

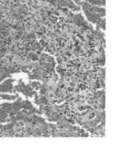
above, as mentioned earlier, lack specificity and sensitivity. They could well be related and interpreted as being due to the critical illness per se, rather than to complicating pulmonary emboli rendering a correct diagnosis doubly difficult.

DIAGNOSTIC TESTS

1. *Chest Radiograph* The chest radiograph can be normal though this is rare with massive PE. In the PIOPED series of massive PE, only 16% of patients had a normal chest radiograph. Focal oligemia, if carefully looked for, will be noted in 40–80% of patients. Plate-like atelectasis, basal wedge-shaped shadows and pleural effusions are other distinctive but non-specific radiological manifestations. The presence of preexisting cardiopulmonary disease makes appreciation of these features even more difficult. The chest radiograph is also invaluable in patients with PE for differential diagnosis of other conditions like pneumonia, left ventricular failure (LVF) or pneumothorax.

2. *Electrocardiogram (ECG)* The ECG is usually normal in smaller PE. In massive PE a normal ECG is uncommon but did occur in as many as 30% of PIOPED patients with major PE. Transient ST-T changes are the commonest ECG manifestation and may occur in 50–70% of patients. A $S_1Q_3T_3$ pattern may be seen, along with transient right bundle branch block (RBBB) or atrial fibrillation. Anterior lead T wave inversion is the pattern that best correlates with the severity of the PE, occurring in 90% of massive compared to 20% of non-massive PE.

3. *D-dimer* is a breakdown product of cross-linked fibrin and is a sensitive marker of acute thrombosis. A normal D-dimer in a low clinical probability setting is an accurate way of ruling out PE. On the other hand, though the D-dimer is very specific for fibrin, the specificity of this test for PE is poor because fibrin is produced in a variety of conditions including inflammation, infection, necrosis, and cancer. Hence a D-dimer above 500 ug/L has a poor positive predictive value for PE and cannot reliably rule in the disease. But a D-dimer level below this cut-off value reliably rules it out, especially in a low probability setting. Nuclear scanning or spiral CT angiography may not be needed in this group. There are presently four different assays available and it is important to use the highly sensitive enzyme-linked immunosorbent assay (ELISA) or automated turbidimetric assay to get the most sensitive results. Results are generally available at the bedside in an hour, making this a cost-effective and useful screening test.

4. *Lower limb venous compression ultrasonography* In studies using venography as the gold standard for detecting proximal DVT, lower limb venous compression ultrasonography, an entirely non-invasive test, had a sensitivity of 97% and a specificity of 98% for symptomatic, proximal DVT. The absence of full compressibility of the deep vein on applying pressure through the ultrasound probe is the single best validated diagnostic criterion. The advantage of this test is that it is non-invasive and can be performed at the bedside. The finding of DVT by ultrasonography in a patient with suspected PE is sufficient evidence to commence anti-coagulant therapy without any further testing. Approximately 50% of PE suspects will have evidence of

DVT on sonography and further invasive and costly tests are not required in these patients. The exact position of ultrasonography in the diagnostic algorithm of PE is still being refined.

5. *Arterial blood gases* Hypoxia is usual but not universal following a major PE. Approximately 20% of patients with proven PE will have a normal arterial oxygen pressure and alveolar-arterial oxygen gradient.

6. *Echocardiography* is an enormously useful test to detect the presence and severity of right ventricular (RV) pressure overload. RV dysfunction (RV dilatation, dyskinesia) on ECHO helps in stratification of these patients. If present it denotes > 30% obstruction to the pulmonary circuit. Other echocardiographic findings include: increased RV/LV diameter ratio, paradoxical septal motion, pulmonary artery dilatation and evidence of tricuspid regurgitation. The sensitivity of these signs which are often combined is between 40–70% in patients with clinically suspected PE and their specificity approaches 90%. Thus, echocardiography has emerged as a first-line test in patients with suspected massive PE. It is extremely useful in the differential diagnosis of shock due to massive PE from cardiogenic shock, cardiac tamponade, valvular heart disease and aortic dissection. Indeed, absence of PH and/or right ventricular dilatation and hypokinesia makes PE as the cause of shock unlikely. In a small subset of patients with PE, transthoracic echocardiography allows a direct visualization of the clot in the right heart chambers or in the right main pulmonary artery.

7. *Ventilation/Perfusion lung scintigraphy* The landmark PIOPED study showed us that V/Q scanning retains its importance. The perfusion scan is done by injection of albumin macroaggregates labelled by technetium-99m. The macroaggregates are trapped in approximately 0.1% of the pulmonary capillary circuit and may be imaged by a gamma camera. Any disease that narrows the airways or fills the alveoli will result in hypoxic pulmonary vasoconstriction, hence this pattern is not highly specific for PE. If the perfusion defect is large or segmental it makes the diagnosis more likely. The addition of ventilation scintigraphy by xenon-133 or aerosolized technetium-99m further increases the specificity. This so-called mis-matched defect, i.e. perfusion defect with normal ventilation, is highly predictive of PE. Based on revised data from the PIOPED study, lung scans are currently classified into normal, high probability and non-diagnostic. The high negative predictive value of a normal lung scan has been confirmed by several studies including a large outcome study. Equally useful is the positive predictive value of a high probability scan (around 90%) and this is sufficient evidence to rule in PE and proceed with treatment without subjecting the patient to further testing. Recent evidence suggests that a chest radiograph may replace the ventilation scan and be combined with a perfusion scan to give excellent overall agreement of 88% and positive predictive value of 86% for a scintigraphic mismatch. Unfortunately, in the latest study from Wells and his group, only 41% of all V/Q scans fell into the normal or high probability group. The majority were non-diagnostic. These scans carry a 30% likelihood of PE and hence the majority (around 60%) of patients who

undergo V/Q scanning will need to undergo further tests to rule in or rule out suspected PE.

8. *Helical CT Pulmonary Angiography* This non-invasive test offers excellent imaging of the pulmonary vasculature. It has by and large replaced V/Q scanning as a diagnostic modality for PE and has nearly (if not completely) eliminated the need for invasive pulmonary angiography.

Newer and still evolving technology used in helical CT pulmonary angiography has further increased the sensitivity and specificity for detecting PE, the sensitivity ranging from 83–100% and specificity from 89–97%. This sensitivity and specificity favours comparably with that observed in invasive pulmonary angiography.

The advantages of CT angiography when compared to V/Q screening and invasive pulmonary angiography are summarized below.

   (i) CT angiography is non-invasive, convenient and can be performed safely and quickly in critically ill patients, particularly those in shock and/or in acute right heart failure.

  (ii) Studies comparing CT angiography to V/Q scanning suggest that CT angiography is a better test because of more frequent definitive confirmation of pulmonary emboli.

 (iii) In a critically ill individual, there is often a large differential diagnosis to PE. A CT angiography offers evidence of other causes as well as that of PE, which neither a V/Q scan nor invasive pulmonary angiography can provide.

 (iv) CT angiography of the legs and pelvis could be performed with the same contrast injection used to image the pulmonary vasculature. Detection of DVT in the femoro-popliteal veins was as accurate as with ultrasonography. This procedure could also detect clots in the iliac, renal and caval veins which are ultrasonographically inaccessible.

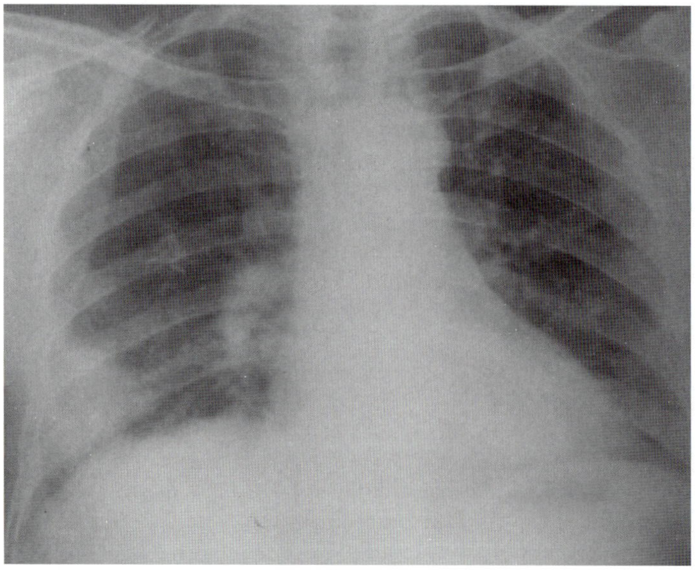

The major limitation of helical CT pulmonary angiography is the inability to diagnose sub-segmental branch emboli, with sufficient certainty. However, invasive pulmonary angiography also has significant limitations in detecting isolated sub-segmental emboli. The only other major limitation of helical CT pulmonary angiography compared to V/Q scanning is the need to use contrast material, precluding its use in patients with renal failure and in patients allergic to the dye. It is also inadvisable to use this modality in pregnant women.

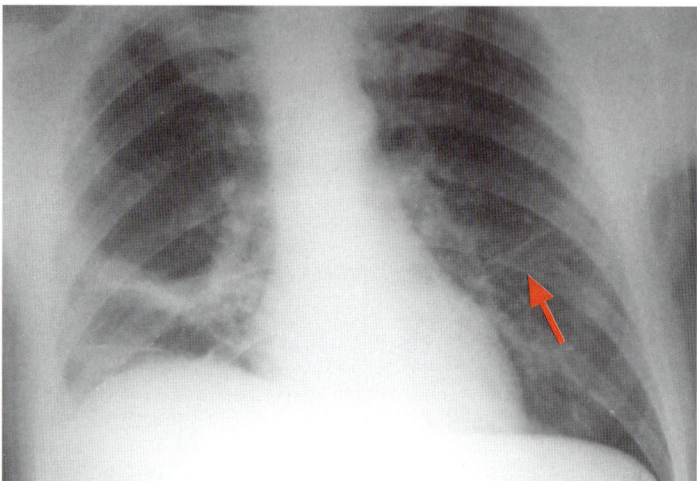

Fig 52.2: Pulmonary infarct. Chest X-ray demonstrates a linear band in the right lower zone with an elevated right dome of diaphragm. The linear band represents an infarct with elevation of the right dome due to underlying volume loss. An atelectatic band is also seen in the left lower zone representing an infarct.

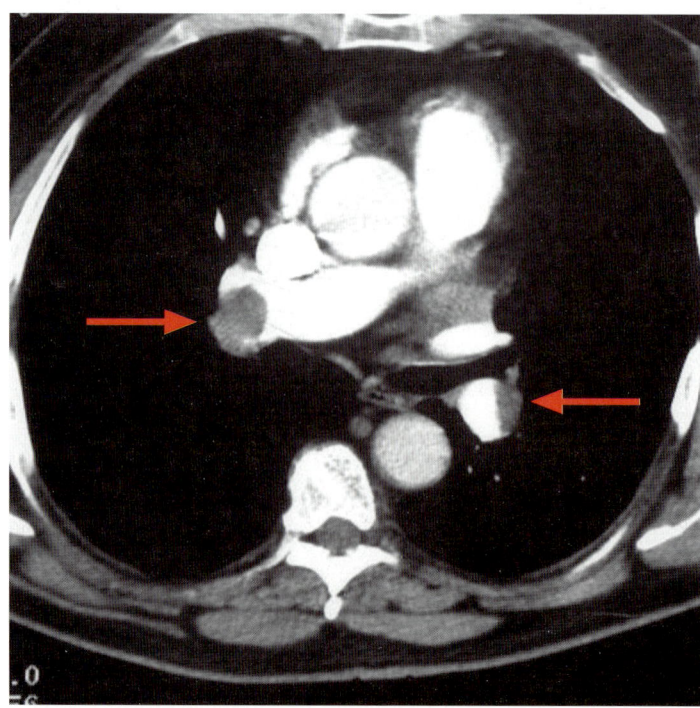

Fig 52.3: Bilateral pulmonary emboli. CT angiography demonstrates pulmonary emboli in both pulmonary arteries.

Fig 52.1: Chest X-ray demonstrates a wedge-shaped opacity in the right lower zone with its apex pointing to the hilum representing a pulmonary infarct. Note the enlarged and prominent right pulmonary artery (Westermark sign).

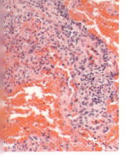

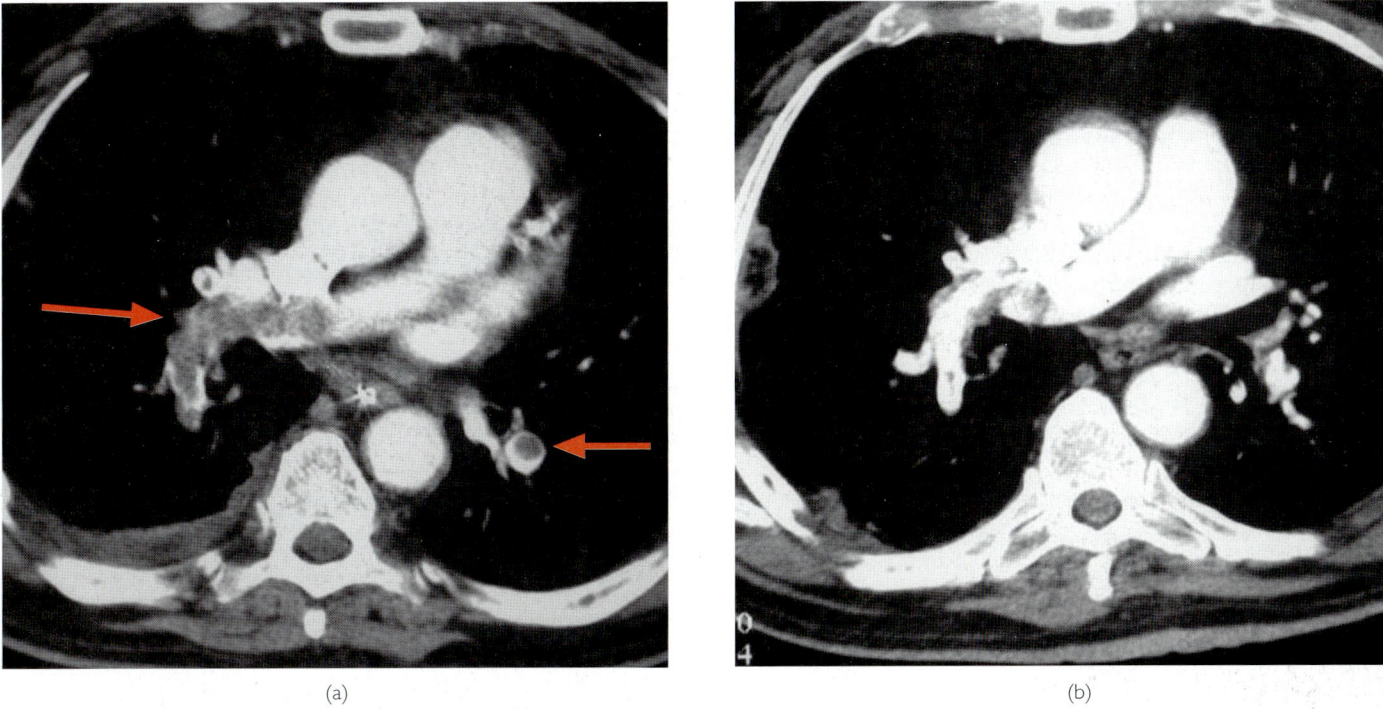

(a)　　　　　　　　　　　　　　　　　　(b)

Fig 52.4: (a) Pulmonary emboli. CT angiography demonstrates a large embolus in the right pulmonary artery and a smaller embolus in the left pulmonary artery (b) CT angiography following anticoagulation therapy demonstrates considerable resolution in the thrombi.

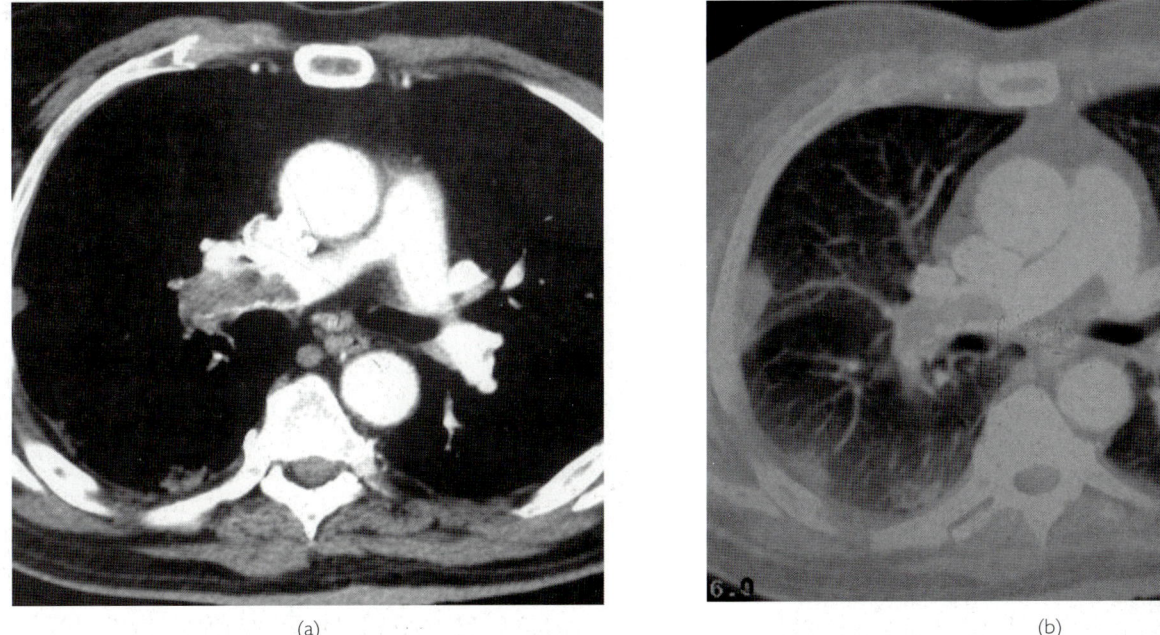

(a)　　　　　　　　　　　　　　　　　　(b)

Fig 52. 5: (a) Pulmonary emboli with pulmonary infarcts. CT angiography demonstrates a large embolus in the right pulmonary artery (b) Lung window setting demonstrates multiple wedge-shaped subpleural soft tissue density lesions representing pulmonary infarcts.

9. *Pulmonary Angiography* The role of pulmonary angiography in the diagnosis of PE is now sharply reduced. Perhaps a helical pulmonary CT angiography might miss out on sub-segmental pulmonary emboli which an invasive CT angiography would detect. But is it necessary to diagnose with certainty sub-segmental emboli? Data from three large studies suggests that under-diagnosing sub-segmental emboli by avoiding pulmonary angiography does not affect the clinical outcomes of recurrent embolism or death. A clinical outcome approach is as safe as the PIOPED approach, less

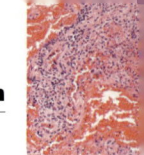

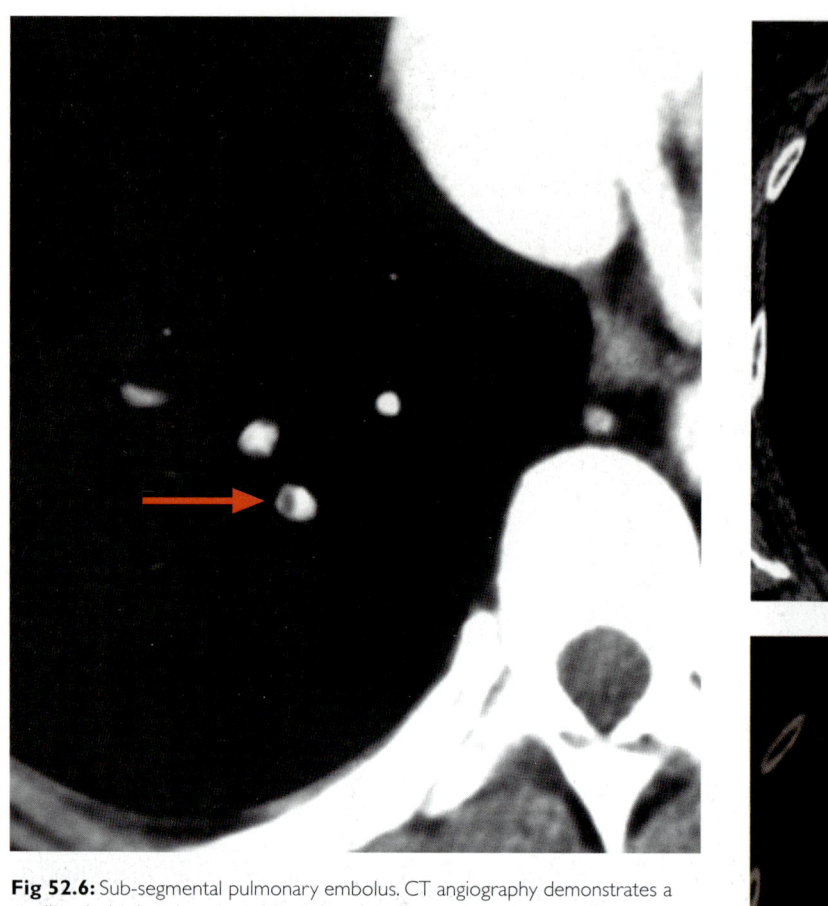

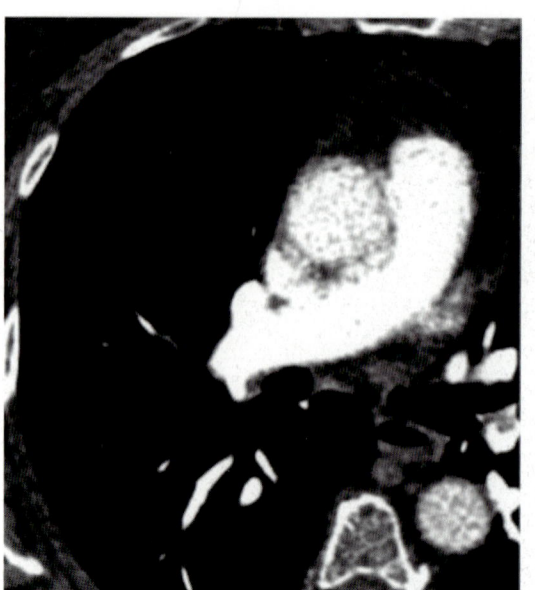

(b)

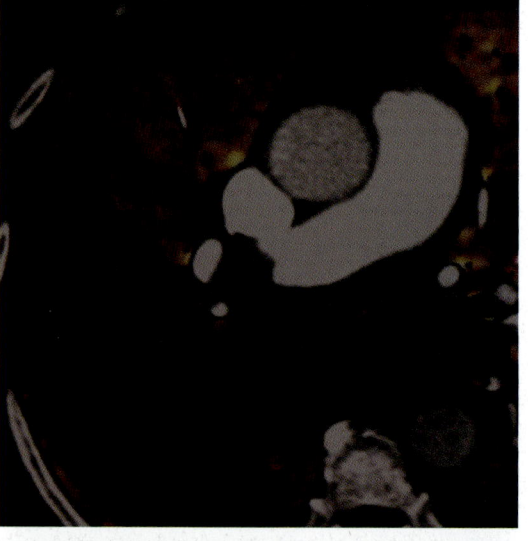

(c)

Fig 52.6: Sub-segmental pulmonary embolus. CT angiography demonstrates a small embolus in sub-segmental pulmonary arteries.

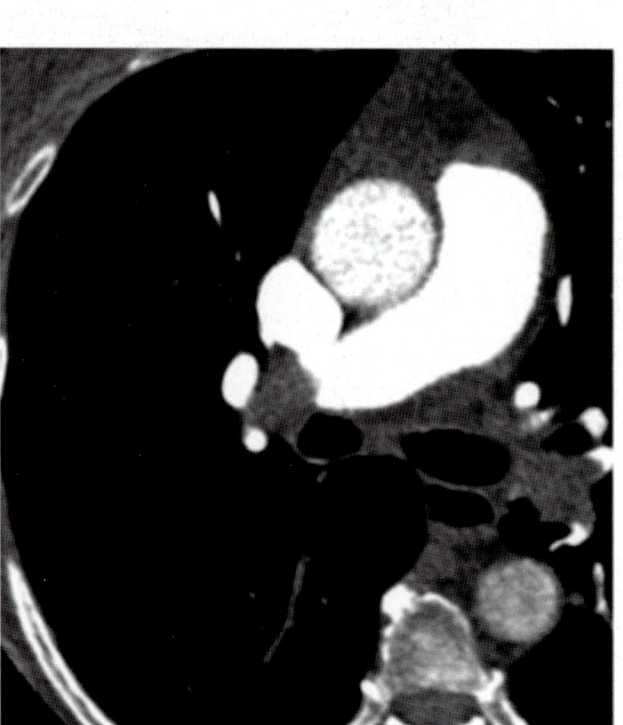

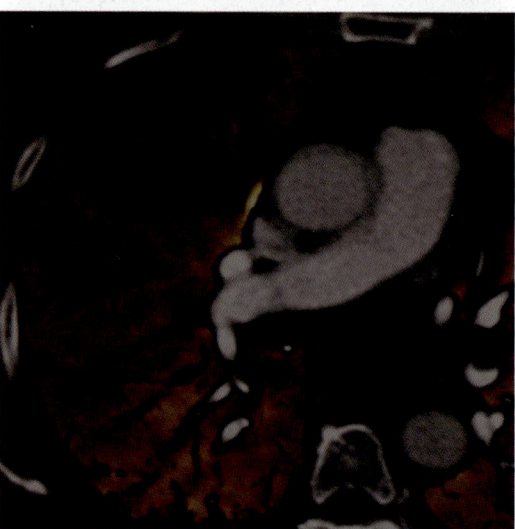

(a)

(d)

Fig 52.7: Pulmonary embolism. (a) CT angiography demonstrates a thrombus in the right pulmonary artery (b) dual-energy CT angiography reveals perfusion defect secondary to thrombus (c, d) Follow-up CT angiography after thrombolysis reveals resolution of thrombus in right pulmonary artery, corresponding dual-energy CT angiography reveals resolution of perfusion defect.

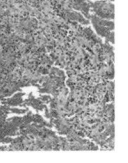

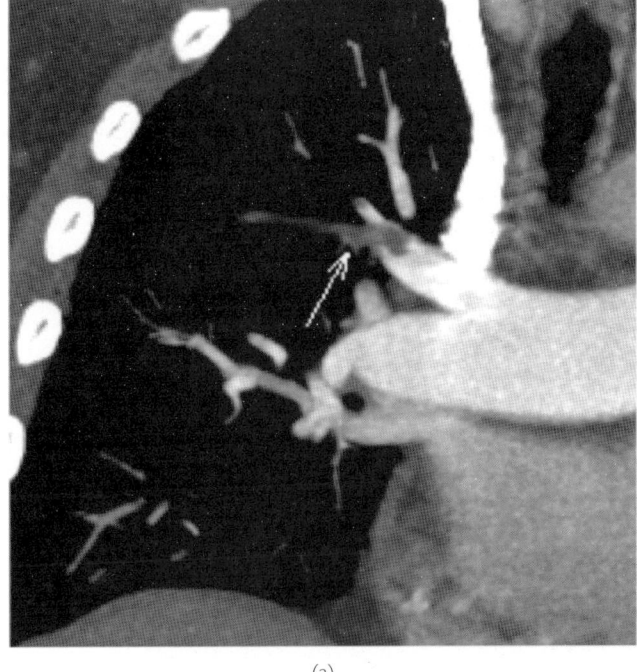

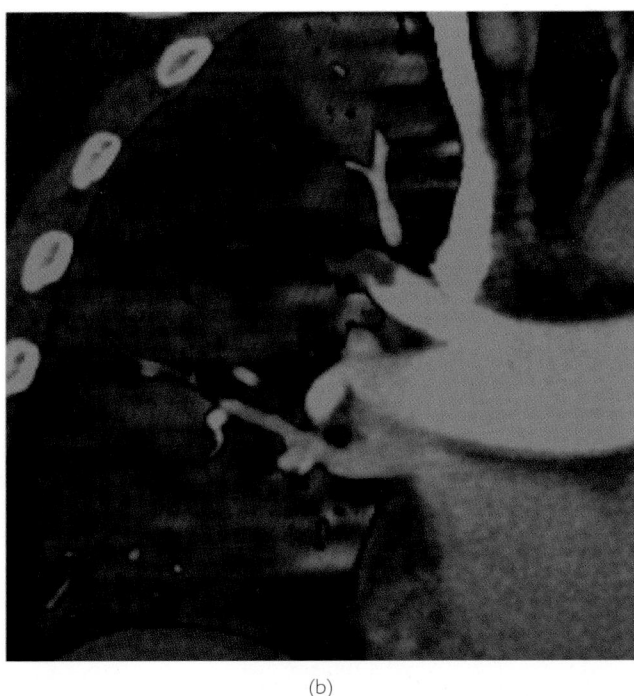

(a)

(b)

Fig 52.8: (a) CT angiography reveals a segmental embolus, in the right upper lobe pulmonary arterial branch (b) corresponding dual-energy CT perfusion images reveal a segmental perfusion defect.

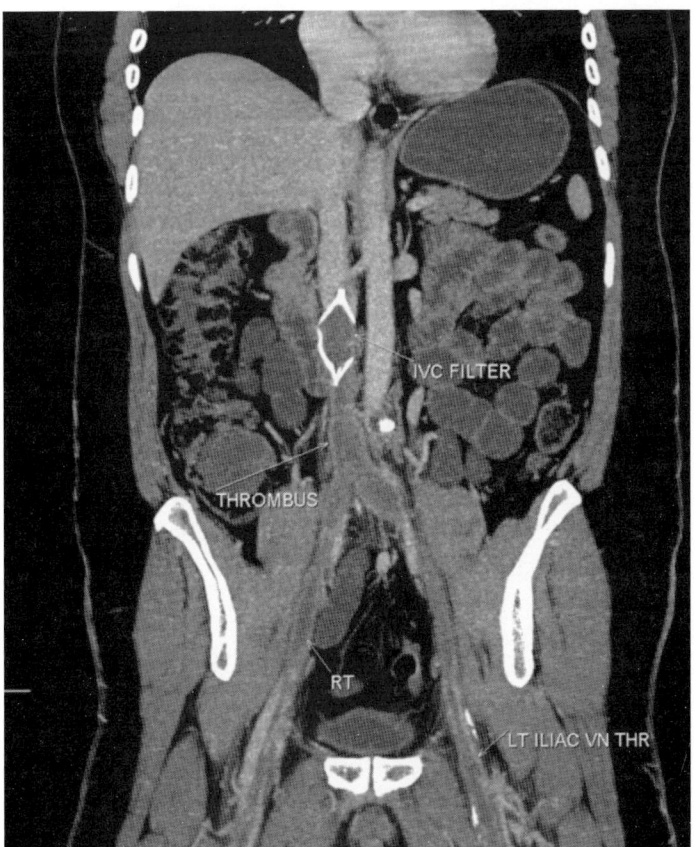

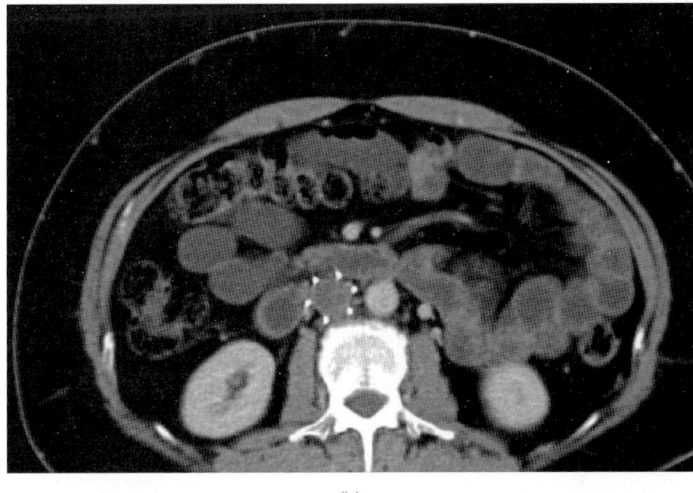

(b)

(a)

Fig 52.9 (a and b): IVC Filter. CT angiography following placement of IVC filter demonstrates IVC filter in situ with extensive thrombosis of IVC and iliac veins distal to the IVC filter.

expensive, more convenient, less fraught with immediate risks to the patient and more acceptable to the patient and the physician.

MORTALITY OF PE

The International Cooperative Pulmonary Embolism Registry (ICOPER) enrolled 2454 consecutive PE patients from 52 hospitals in seven countries with the specific purpose of establishing the three-month all-cause mortality rate and to identify factors associated with death. The results are important

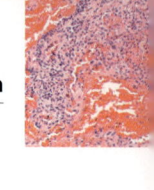

Table 52.4: Diagnostic tests for PE
i.   Chest radiograph
ii. ECG
iii. D-dimer
iv. Lower limb venous compression ultrasonography
v.   Arterial blood gases
vi. Echocardiography
vii. Ventilation/Perfusion lung scintigraphy
viii. Helical CT pulmonary angiography
ix. Pulmonary angiography

enough to discuss here. The all-cause mortality rate was 17.4% at three months. Importantly, most patients who succumbed died of their PE, not of other co-morbidities like cancer. Age greater than 70 years increased the likelihood of death by 60%. Other risk factors which independently increased the likelihood of death by two to threefold included cancer, congestive cardiac failure (CCF), COPD, hypotension (systolic BP<90 mmHg), tachypnoea (respiratory rate > 20/min) and evidence of right ventricular hypokinesia on echocardiogram.

MANAGEMENT OF PE

1. *Anticoagulation with unfractionated or low molecular weight heparin (LMWH).* LMWH has several pharmacokinetic and practical advantages over unfractionated heparin. These are summarized below.

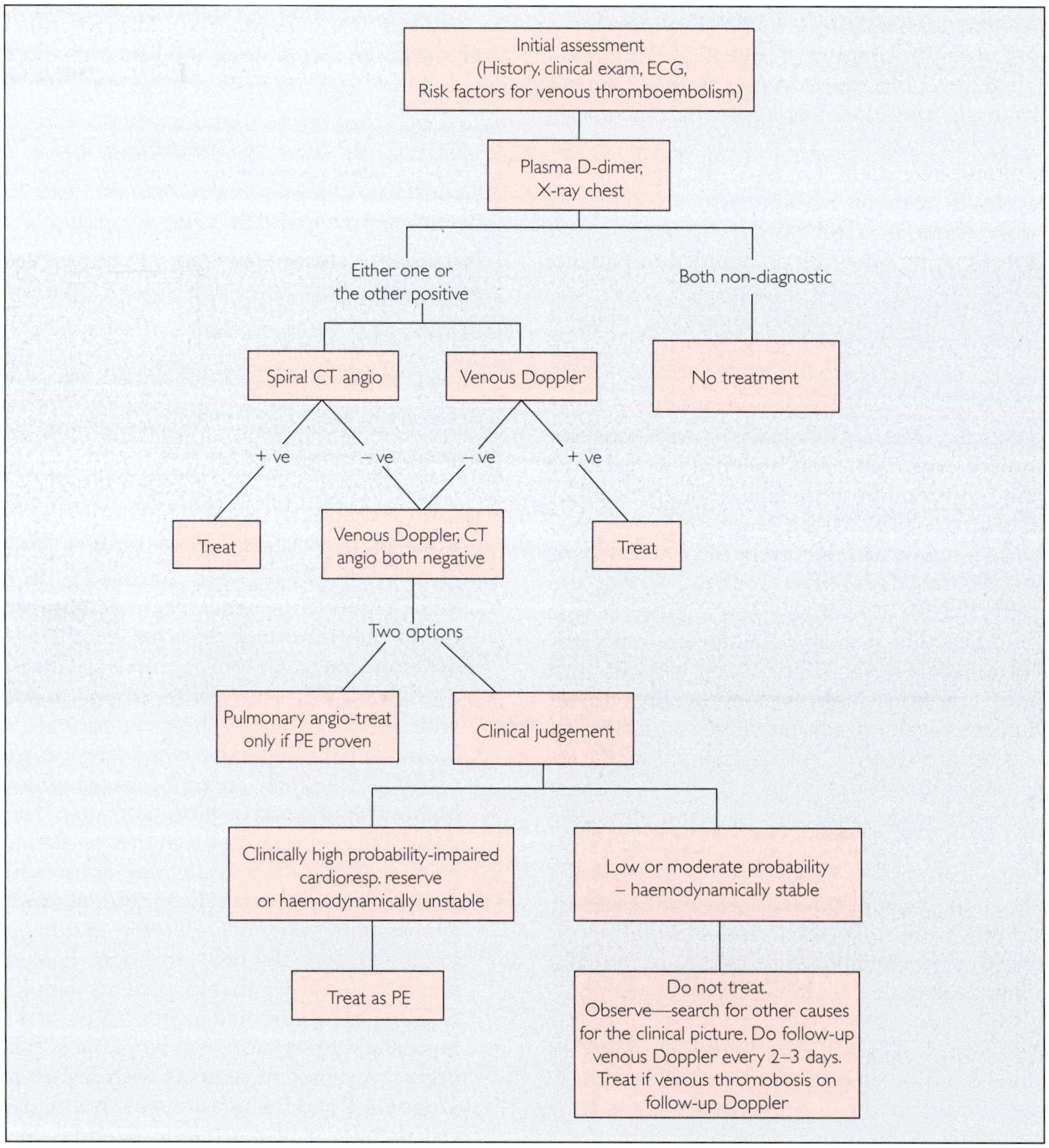

Initial assessment
(History, clinical exam, ECG,
Risk factors for venous thromboembolism)

Plasma D-dimer,
X-ray chest

Either one or the other positive

Both non-diagnostic

Spiral CT angio — Venous Doppler

No treatment

+ ve – ve   – ve + ve

Treat

Venous Doppler, CT angio both negative

Treat

Two options

Pulmonary angio-treat only if PE proven

Clinical judgement

Clinically high probability-impaired cardioresp. reserve or haemodynamically unstable

Low or moderate probability – haemodynamically stable

Treat as PE

Do not treat.
Observe—search for other causes for the clinical picture. Do follow-up venous Doppler every 2–3 days. Treat if venous thrombosis on follow-up Doppler

Fig 52.10: Algorithm for a diagnostic work-up of pulmonary embolism.

- Ease of use without need for routine monitoring of prothrombin time or International Normalized Ratio (INR).
- More predictable anticoagulant response.
- Standard dose irrespective of weight apart from chronic renal failure (CRF) and morbid obesity.
- Longer half life which permits once or twice daily dosing.
- Facilitates earlier discharge and in some stable patients even home treatment.
- Lower risk of heparin-induced thrombocytopenia (HIT).
- Less binding to osteoblasts hence less osteopenia.

A meta-analysis of over 3000 patients who participated in DVT treatment studies showed that those receiving LMWH had lower mortality rates, less recurrence and suffered fewer complications including reduced HIT. All this was achieved at lower cost compared to unfractionated heparin. A pivotal study by Levine showed that enoxaparin, a LMWH administered twice daily reduced mean hospital stay from 6.5 to 1.1 days with fewer deaths and fewer bleeding complications. As a result of this and similar trials, the FDA has approved enoxaparin (1mg/kg twice a day) and tinzaparin (175 units/kg once daily) for outpatient or home treatment for patients who present with symptomatic DVT with or without associated PE. As opposed to this data, there is as yet no data to suggest that out-patient treatment can be safely recommended in patients with PE alone.

Whether LMWH or unfractionated heparin is used, it serves as a bridge for five to seven days till anti-coagulation with warfarin takes over.

2. *Oral anticoagulation* Oral anticoagulation with warfarin is the mainstay of treatment and the dose is adjusted according to the prothrombin time. This is standardized by reporting results as the INR with a target INR of 2 to 3 being aimed for. In patients with recurrent PEs or underlying thrombophilic states the target INR is raised to 3–4. Warfarin is not reliably effective for at least five days after it has been commenced. During this period patients are especially vulnerable to thrombosis hence concomitant heparin must be administered. If warfarin is used as monotherapy without heparin it will paradoxically result in hypercoagulability by decreasing the level of Protein C, resulting in a higher rate of recurrent venous thromboembolism.

Warfarin interacts with a number of commonly used drugs and even with the Vitamin K in green leafy vegetables resulting in wide fluctuations of INR. In addition some patients (2–3% of the general population) have a genetic defect (polymorphisms in the cytochrome P450 CYP2C9) which makes them slow metabolizers and prone to major bleeding complications with even lower doses of warfarin.

The current American College of Chest Physicians (ACCP) guidelines on optimal duration of anticoagulation after a DVT/PE is ideally three months, if the patient had an underlying precipitating factor which is no longer applicable. In patients with a first episode of idiopathic DVT/PE a 6–12 month initial period of anticoagulation is recommended. A study called the PREVENT trial showed that after six months of warfarin, lower intensity dosing, so as to target an INR of 1.5–2 resulted in a further significant reduction in the risk of recurrences by 64%. In patients who have documented anti-phospholipid antibodies or an underlying thrombophilic state, indefinite anticoagulation therapy is recommended.

Recurrent thrombosis The five-year incidence of recurrent venous thromboembolism off anticoagulants is approximately 30%. Well-documented factors for recurrent thrombosis include an initial unprovoked DVT or PE, advancing age, male sex, race (higher in blacks), presence of active cancer, obesity, an elevated serum d-Dimer prior to stopping warfarin or two months after stopping warfarin, and ongoing immobility.

Complications of warfarin include bleeding, skin necrosis, alopecia and rashes. When patients present with very high INRs as a result of warfarin, the majority will be asymptomatic even with INR values > 5. Most can be managed with fresh frozen plasma if they are bleeding or low oral doses of Vitamin K. The usual injectable dose of 10 mg of Vitamin K will result in patients being resistant to further anti-coagulation with warfarin for at least a week and hence should be avoided.

Table 52.5: Contraindications to anticoagulant therapy
Recent major surgery/ocular surgery/neurosurgery
Diastolic BP > 110 mm Hg
CNS haemorrhage
Recent trauma/head injury
Recent cerebrovascular accident/transient ischaemic attack
GI bleeding or other haemorrhagic diathesis
Concomitant hepatic/renal failure

3. *Thrombolysis* Thrombolysis can be a potentially lifesaving measure in patients with massive PE. In patients with PE who present with haemodynamic compromise, there is little doubt that thrombolysis is indicated and can dramatically lower mortality. A more controversial decision is whether to extend the indications of thrombolysis to include patients with sub-massive PE. These are patients with PE who are haemodynamically stable when seen but who have evidence of RV dysfunction on echocardiography putting them at higher risk of a bad in-hospital course. The presence of RV dysfunction is a warning sign that escalation of therapy may be required or that death may occur with a conservative "hands off" approach. Even though these patients may appear stable they may develop ensuing cardiopulmonary instability over the next 48 hours. Pooled data from four studies have shown that PE patients with RV dysfunction on ECHO have a nine-fold higher risk of death than those with normal RV function. Other biomarkers that also attempt to predict a subset of patients with higher mortality include Troponin T and I which are sensitive markers of myocardial cell damage, and natriuretic peptides like BNP and NT-pro-BNP which are sensitive indicators of ventricular dysfunction. A limitation of both sets of biomarkers is that

they have low positive predictive value but high negative predictive value with regard to death or poor outcome.

Thrombolytic agents such as TPA act on plasminogen by cleaving the peptide bond between arginine at position 560 and valine at position 561, thereby converting plasminogen to plasmin and dissolving the embolus. They help dissolve the clot at source in the pulmonary vessels and perform a "medical embolectomy", preventing the downward spiral into right heart failure. They may also help in dissolution of clot at its source in the pelvic and deep veins of the leg. The only FDA-approved regimen is alteplase 100 mg as a continuous infusion over two hours, however, streptokinase and urokinase-based regimens are probably equally efficacious and a lot cheaper. Thrombolytics can be administered within a two-week time window from the onset of PE and dramatic results have been reported in patients with massive PE even in patients in shock and circulatory arrest. The evidence of their role in sub-massive PE is also emerging, initially from small case studies in the 1960s, then from eight smaller randomized Level 2 studies in the next two decades and finally from the study by Konstantinides in the New England Journal of Medicine in 2002. In this landmark randomized, double-blind controlled study in 49 German centres, 256 patients who met strict inclusion criteria of sub-massive PE (no haemodynamic instability but RV dysfunction on echocardiography) were randomized to heparin plus recombinant-tissue plasminogen activator (r-TPA) or heparin plus placebo. Although this study could not demonstrate any difference in mortality between the two groups, the clinical deterioration was significantly higher in those that did not receive alteplase. The 30–day event-free survival was also significantly higher in the alteplase group so that patients not receiving alteplase were significantly more likely to need escalation of treatment. On the basis of this study, most experts would consider using thrombolytic therapy in patients with sub-massive PE. Samuel Goldhaber a leading authority in the field remarks: "I believe on the basis of this trial that we should consider expanding the indications for thrombolysis to include this group of patients."

Complications of thrombolysis include bleeding but in a pooled analysis of 896 patients enrolled in every PE thrombolysis study, the overall risk of intracranial bleed was 1.2%. It is best not to use heparin and thrombolytic therapy simultaneously as this can cause uncontrollable bleeding and death.

4. *Cardiorespiratory Support* This is imperative in major or massive PE. Shock should be promptly treated. An intravenous infusion of isoproterenol (1–2 mg in 500 ml dextrose) is very useful as it dilates the pulmonary vasculature. If possible, the patient should have a central venous line inserted and it is advisable to keep the central venous pressure (CVP) between 12–14 mm Hg in order to ensure an adequate right ventricular stroke volume. This is best achieved by infusing 500 ml Dextran or Haemaccel, which besides raising right atrial pressure, also expands the pulmonary vascular bed, and thereby reduces pulmonary vascular resistance. If the patient does not respond to isoproterenol, or has marked tachycardia to start with, it is best to use dobutamine. Dopamine may need to be used in addition to dobutamine. The use of digoxin is disappointing, but it may be used in a dose of 0.25 mg intravenously to start

with, and repeated six-hourly till a digitalizing dose of 1 mg is given over 24 hours.

Oxygen is administered at 6–8 l/minute. Ventilator support is invariably required in the presence of acute cardiorespiratory failure. Morphine or pethidine is used for the relief of pain and/or restlessness.

5. *Surgical embolectomy* Open surgical embolectomy is the most effective procedure for emergent removal of large amounts of thrombus due to acute PE. Surgery is especially useful in those in whom thrombolysis is contraindicated and who have not yet deteriorated to the point of cardiorespiratory arrest or shock. In this setting, when used in patients with anatomically extensive PE and concomitant moderate to severe RV dysfunction, Goldhaber and colleagues report impressive 89% survival rates. Impressive survival rates have been reported even in patients taken up in extremis after suffering cardio-pulmonary arrest following massive PE.

Transvenous catheter embolectomy in the catheter laboratory offers a less invasive alternative to open surgical embolectomy. A number of devices including the Greenfield embolectomy device, the Amplatz Thrombectomy Device, the Angiojet device and the Hydrolyser Thrombectomy catheter are available.

Table 52.6:
Management of pulmonary embolism
1. Anticoagulation with unfractionated or low molecular weight heparin (LMWH)
2. Oral anticoagulation
3. Thrombolysis
4. Cardiorespiratory Support
5. Surgical embolectomy

PREVENTIVE MEASURES

Prevention of venous thrombosis with the associated risk of PE, is a major objective in the management of critically ill patients in the intensive care unit (ICU). These patients often form a high-risk group as a consequence of bed rest, serious infections or trauma.

Prevention of venous thrombosis in high-risk patients reduces morbidity. High-risk patients include the old and obese, those who are poorly mobile or are confined to bed, patients with myocardial infarction or a stroke, or those with atrial fibrillation and congestive heart failure. Postoperative patients are also at high risk, particularly after orthopaedic surgery (particularly hip replacement or hip fracture), gynaecological surgery and other major surgery. Low molecular weight heparin like enoxaparin given in a dose 40 mg or 60 mg (depending on body weight and renal function) once daily offers good prophylaxis against DVT. Compression stockings over lower limbs, movement of the lower limbs at the ankles and knees, pneumatic compression of the lower limbs, all help to prevent DVT. Any form of heparin is contraindicated in certain patients—as after trauma, following surgery on the brain and spinal cord, or in patients with an acute peptic ulcer or a bleeding diathesis. In this group

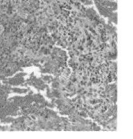

one can only offer pneumatic compression of the lower limbs, with active and passive movements at the ankles and knees as prophylaxis.

Once venous thrombosis is detected low molecular weight heparin in a dose of 40 or 60 mg of enoxaparin twice daily is given. Warfarin is started on the third or fourth day. It takes about a week of warfarin to take effect; heparin should be continued till such time as the INR is > 2. As mentioned earlier, a 6–12 month period of anticoagulants is advised after the first episode of DVT/PE for which there is no apparent cause.

Transvenous Insertion of a Filter in the Inferior Vena Cava

This is achieved by the placement of a filter in the inferior vena cava generally below the renal veins. The procedure is done by a vascular surgeon or an interventional radiologist through the transveonous route. The filter stops emboli from the lower limb or pelvic veins from reaching the lungs. Specific indications for vena caval interruption include the following:

(a) Pulmonary embolism in patients in whom anticoagulants are absolutely contraindicated—as in the neurosurgical patient, or in those with active bleeding.
(b) Recurrent thromboembolism in spite of adequate anticoagulation.
(c) Patients who have survived a massive embolism, but who are haemodynamically unstable, and in whom the risk of a fresh embolism is ever present.
(d) Patients with septic pulmonary embolism from thrombi in the lower limbs or pelvis, who have shown an unsatisfactory response after 48 hours of antibiotic plus anticoagulant therapy.
(e) Prophylaxis in high-risk patients, as in—
   (i) extensive or progressive venous thrombosis;
   (ii) in conjunction with catheter-based or surgical pulmonary embolectomy;
   (iii) in patients with active cancer with extensive venous thrombosis of the pelvic or leg veins.

Vena caval interruption in the last four groups should be accompanied by the use of heparin in the dosage recommended earlier.

Though IVC filters reduce the incidence of short-term embolic recurrence and reduce short-term (90 days) mortality, this benefit may be lost over a prolonged period of time. In fact there appears to be a long-term increase in the incidence of venous thromboembolism following the use of IVC filters. For this very reason, retrievable IVC filters have been introduced. However, since these filters are endotheliased at the point of vascular contact retrievability may be difficult after a lapse of time.

FAT EMBOLISM

Fat embolism is a dramatic form of embolism which occurs when neutral fat gains entry into the vascular system. The precipitating factor is a fracture of a long bone, the incidence increasing with multiple fractures. Fat embolism has been

Table 52.7:
Specific indications for vena caval interruption
Pulmonary embolism in patients in whom anticoagulants are absolutely contraindicated
Recurrent thromboembolism in spite of adequate anticoagulation
Hemodynamically unstable patients who have survived a massive embolism
Patients with septic pulmonary embolism
Prophylaxis in high risk patients

also noted to occur after orthopaedic procedures and rarely following liposuction. It generally occurs 24 to 72 hours after these precipitating factors.

Pathophysiology

Fat embolism produces two effects—1. Blockage of vessels by neutral fat, and 2. The release of fatty acids due to the action of lipase on neutral fat. Liberated fatty acids cause a vasculitis with increased permeability of pulmonary, cerebral and other vascular beds.

Clinical Features

The clinical picture is characterized by the sudden onset of dyspnoea, increasing hypoxemia and mental confusion. Acute lung injury or acute respiratory distress syndrome (ARDS) may occur as a result of increased permeability of pulmonary capillaries. Seizures or even focal signs may be present. About 30–50% have petechiae on the skin, chiefly on the upper half of the body.

There is no test which is diagnostic of fat embolism. Fat may be present in the serum of patients with fat embolism.

Treatment

Treatment is generally supportive as no specific treatment has proved effective. Ventilatory support is invariably necessary. Use of corticosteroids in the prevention of fat embolism following an inciting factor is controversial.

AIR EMBOLISM

An important form of non-thrombotic embolism is venous air embolism. The possibility of air embolism has increased with numerous invasive medical and surgical procedures in practice today. These include the use of central venous catheters, surgery on the neck, thorax, and use of positive pressure ventilation with high positive end expiratory pressure (PEEP). Two important causes are allowing a large bolus of air to enter a central vein by failing to notice that an infusion through the vein is over, and removing the central venous catheter in the sitting position.

Air bubbles enter the pulmonary vascular bed, blocking it; some bubbles go through microvascualar pulmonary shunts to enter the systemic circulation.

Clinical Features

Clinical features include severe chest pain, dyspnoea, hypoxia, syncope. Pulmonary oedema and altered sensorium are observed if death has not already occurred. Symptoms are related to widespread blockage of the pulmonary circulation and of systemic capillaries by air and by platelet fibrin aggregates causing diffuse microthrombi.

TREATMENT

Treatment consists of—

1. Placing patient in the **Trendelenburg position** with the left side down.

2. Removing air through a central venous catheter or direct needle aspiration, thereby promoting blood flow.
3. Cardiorespiratory resuscitation.
4. Promoting absorption of air by using 100% oxygen and when possible hyperbaric oxygen.

OTHER FORMS OF EMBOLISM

These include tumour embolism, septic thromboembolism, catheter embolism (a cut off segment of a central venous catheter) and thrombotic complications caused by intravenous use of drugs meant to be taken orally, as is met with in some drug addicts.

SUGGESTED READING

Bounameaaux H, de Moerloose P, Perriwer A, *et al.* D-dimer testing in suspected venous thromboembolism. *Q J Med*. 1997; 90: 437–42.

Carlbom DJ. Pulmonary embolism in the critically ill. *Chest*. 1 Jul. 2007; 132(1): 313–24.

Cummings KW. Multidetector computed tomographic pulmonary angiography: beyond acute pulmonary embolism. *Radiol Clin North Am*. 1 Jan. 2010; 48(1): 51–65.

Fengler BT. Fibrinolytic therapy in pulmonary embolism: an evidence-based treatment algorithm. *Am J Emerg Med*. 1 Jan. 2009; 27(1): 84–95.

Goldhaber SZ, Viani L, De Rossa M. Acute pulmonary embolism: clinical outcomes in the International Cooperative Pulmonary Embolism Registry (ICOPER). *Lancet*. 1999; 353: 1386–9.

Goldhaber SZ. Thrombolysis in pulmonary embolism: a debatable indication. *ThrombHaemost*. 2001; 86: 444–51.

Konstantinides S, Geibel A, Heusel G, *et al.* Heparin plus alteplase compared with heparin alone in patients with submassive pulmonary embolism. *N Engl J Med*. 2002.

Kuriakose J. Acute pulmonary embolism. *Radiol Clin North Am*. 1 Jan. 2010; 48(1): 31–50.

Mullins MD, Brecker DM, Hagspiel KD, *et al.* The role of spiral volumetric computed tomography in the diagnosis of pulmonary embolism. *Arch Intern Med*. 2000; 160: 293–8.

Peacock AJ, Rubin LJ. (ed.) *Pulmonary Circulation*. 2004, Arnold Press, London.

Stein PD, Henry JW. Prevalence of acute pulmonary embolism among patients in a general hospital and at autopsy. *Chest*. 1995; 108: 878–981.

Stein PD. Challenges in the diagnosis of acute pulmonary embolism. *Am J Med*. 1 Jul. 2008; 121(7): 565–71.

The PIOPED Investigators. Value of the ventilation-perfusion scan in acute pulmonary embolism. *JAMA*. 1990; 263: 2753–9.

Wells PS, Ginsberg JS, Anderson DR, *et al.* Use of a clinical model for safe management of patients with suspected PE. *Ann IntERN Med*. 1998; 129: 997–1005.

CHAPTER

53 Acute Respiratory Failure in Adults

GENERAL CONSIDERATIONS

Acute respiratory failure is an important and frequently encountered problem in intensive care units all over the world. The usual or traditional definition of respiratory failure is the inability of the respiratory system to maintain the normal homeostasis of arterial blood gases, so that the oxygen tension in arterial blood (PaO_2) is < 60 mm Hg, and/or the carbon dioxide tension in arterial blood ($PaCO_2$) is 50 mm Hg or greater.

Respiratory failure may be acute or chronic depending on the onset and duration of the failure. An acute exacerbation may at times prevail on a background of chronic respiratory failure (acute on chronic failure).

Respiratory failure is mainly of two types. Type I or hypoxic respiratory failure is due to a failure of oxygenation with a PaO_2 < 60 mm Hg; Type II or hypercapnic respiratory failure (ventilatory failure) is due to hypoventilation and is characterized by a $PaCO_2$ > 50 mm Hg. Hypoxaemic and hypercapnic respiratory failure may both occur in the same patient. Some intensivists also consider Type III and Type IV failure.

Type III respiratory failure is that occurring peri-operatively and is largely due to basal atelectasis. Cardiothoracic surgery and/or major upper abdominal surgery splint the diaphragm and induce an abnormal mechanics of the abdominal muscles. These factors cause a fall in the functional residual capacity and an increase in the closing volume of the lungs. The end result is increasing atelectasis of the dependent alveoli, 'small lungs' with a high diaphragm, respiratory distress and hypoxaemia.

Type IV respiratory failure is that associated with shock—a poorly functioning circulatory system with a low cardiac output is the main cause of hypoxaemic failure in this situation. Both Type III and Type IV failure merely constitute hypoxaemic failure or both hypoxaemic and hypercapnic failure occurring against specific background conditions.

The above traditional definition of acute respiratory failure evolved when measurements of arterial pH and arterial blood gas tensions were first introduced into clinical medicine. This definition is useful in that (i) it focuses attention on abnormalities of gas exchange due to disturbances in lung function; (ii) it stresses the importance and need for a laboratory diagnosis of respiratory failure; (iii) it emphasizes the difficulty and often the impossibility of either diagnosing acute respiratory failure, or gauging its severity on clinical grounds. Yet, this traditional definition ignores the role of the cardiovascular system in gas exchange, and above all in oxygen transport to tissues. In a critical care setting, this is of particular concern. It is vital to look upon the circulatory and respiratory systems as a single interrelated unit whose purpose is to supply oxygen to the tissues.

A broad definition of respiration would be an exchange of oxygen and carbon dioxide between man and his environment. It can be divided into the following sequential steps:

(i) *Ventilation*—in which an exchange of oxygen and carbon dioxide occurs between the lungs and the atmosphere.

(ii) *Gas exchange*—this occurs across the alveolar-capillary membrane within the lungs, mixed venous blood being oxygenated, and carbon dioxide being removed during its transit through the lungs.

(iii) *Gas transport*—the transport of oxygenated arterial blood to the tissues, and of venous blood (with a high carbon dioxide content), to the lungs.

(iv) *Gas exchange within the tissues*—release of oxygen, oxygen uptake and utilization by the tissues, and release of carbon dioxide by the cells for transport back to the lungs.

In critical care medicine, it is a great advantage to look upon acute respiratory failure as an acute impairment of any one or more of the steps described above. We shall briefly consider (I) acute ventilatory failure; (II) acute failure in gas exchange or acute hypoxaemic failure; (III) a combination of (I) and (II); (IV) a failure of oxygen transport; (V) a failure of tissue oxygenation.

Acute Ventilatory Failure

DEFINITION
Acute ventilatory failure occurs when alveolar ventilation cannot adequately remove the carbon dioxide produced by cell metabolism, via the lungs.

RELATION BETWEEN PaO_2 AND $PaCO_2$ IN VENTILATORY FAILURE
Ventilatory failure always results in a rise in $PaCO_2$ and a fall in PaO_2, and as mentioned earlier is also termed hypercapnic respiratory failure. The relation between PaO_2 and $PaCO_2$ is defined by the alveolar gas equation

$$P_AO_2 = P_IO_2 - PaCO_2 \times \frac{1}{R}$$

where P_AO_2 is the alveolar oxygen tension, P_IO_2 the inspired oxygen tension corrected for water vapour, and R is the respiratory exchange ratio (see section on 'Lung Physiology'). Once the P_AO_2 is calculated from the above equation, the PaO_2 can be determined if the alveolar-arterial oxygen gradient is known. In ventilatory failure due to central nervous system (CNS) causes or due to neuromuscular disease, the alveolar-arterial gradient is normal (i.e. 10–20 mm Hg), so that the

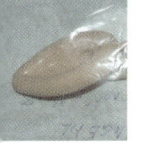

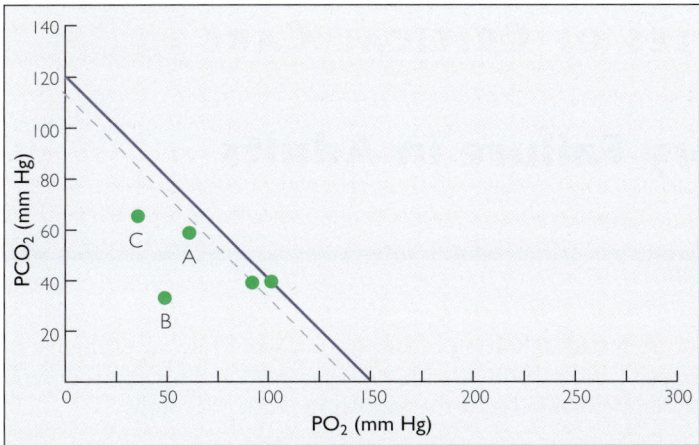

Fig 53.1: O_2–CO_2 diagram. The continuous line represents the relation between alveolar PO_2 and alveolar PCO_2 with an RQ of 0.8 and when breathing air (PIO_2 = 149 mm Hg). The circle marked on this line represents the normal P_AO_2 and P_ACO_2. The broken line represents the normal relation between PaO_2 and P_ACO_2 (or $PaCO_2$) when breathing air. It takes into consideration the slight venous admixture occurring in normal lungs so that the PaO_2 may be 10–15 mm less than P_AO_2. The circle marked on the broken line represents the normal PaO_2 and PCO_2. Points A, B and C illustrate blood gas readings in different types of respiratory failure: A. Ventilatory failure: $PaCO_2$ 60 mm Hg; PaO_2 65 mm Hg. The point falls on or is very close to the broken line. B. Hypoxaemic failure: $PaCO_2$ 38 mm Hg; PaO_2 45 mm Hg. The point is markedly to the left of the broken line. The large alveolar-arterial gradient is chiefly due to a ventilation-perfusion imbalance and/or an increase in the true venous admixture. C. Hypoxaemic and ventilatory failure: $PaCO_2$ 70 mm Hg. Note high $PaCO_2$ indicating ventilatory failure and PaO_2 less than what can be predicted from the $PaCO_2$ reading. The point is again to the left of the broken line

Source: Udwadia FE. 1979. *Diagnosis and Management of Acute Respiratory Failure*, Oxford University Press, Mumbai.

PaO_2 is 10–20 mm Hg less than the P_AO_2. The oxygen-carbon dioxide diagram (Figure 53.1) gives the value of P_AO_2 and PaO_2 for any given value of $PaCO_2$. The arterial blood gas tensions of oxygen and carbon dioxide fall on this line in pure or isolated ventilatory failure.

Physiopathology of Ventilatory Failure

The carbon dioxide produced by tissue metabolism ($\dot{V}CO_2$) is removed by the lungs. Normally, the alveolar carbon dioxide tension (P_ACO_2) and the arterial carbon dioxide tension ($PaCO_2$) are maintained around 40 mm Hg by adjusting alveolar ventilation to balance the $\dot{V}CO_2$. Thus an increase in the latter is met by a proportionate increase in alveolar ventilation. The relationship between P_ACO_2, $\dot{V}CO_2$ and alveolar ventilation, can be stated as follows:

$$P_ACO_2 = PaCO_2 = \frac{\dot{V}CO_2}{\dot{V}_A} \times \text{a constant } (0.86)$$

$\dot{V}_A$ or the alveolar ventilation is the difference between minute ventilation ($\dot{V}_E$) and the physiological dead space ventilation ($\dot{V}_D$) within the lungs—i.e. the ventilation that does not participate in gas exchange. The above equation can thus be rewritten:

$$P_ACO_2 = PaCO_2 = \frac{\dot{V}CO_2}{\dot{V}_E - \dot{V}_D}$$

Thus a rise in $PaCO_2$ due to ventilatory or hypercapnic respiratory failure can occur under the following conditions: (i) A fall in $\dot{V}_A$ or alveolar ventilation—this could be due to (a) a fall in $\dot{V}_E$ or minute ventilation or (b) a rise in physiological dead space ventilation ($\dot{V}_D$), without a concomitant increase in minute ventilation ($\dot{V}_E$). (ii) A rise in carbon dioxide production ($\dot{V}CO_2$) without a proportionate increase in alveolar ventilation ($\dot{V}_A$).

Important Causes of Acute Ventilatory or Hypercapnic Respiratory Failure in an Intensive Care Unit

1. *Hypoventilation in lungs which are normal to start with.* This occurs in patients with a depressed ventilatory drive or in neuromuscular disease. A depressed ventilatory drive is observed in poisonings with narcotics, sedatives, antidepressants, coma from other causes, in head injuries, encephalitis, increased intracranial tension, and other pathologies depressing the respiratory centre. Important neuromuscular diseases causing hypoventilation include acute poliomyelitis, acute infective polyneuritis (Guillan Barré syndrome), tetanus, myasthenia gravis, botulism and snakebite poisoning. Other causes of respiratory muscle weakness and/or decreased respiratory muscle endurance include severe myopathy, amyotrophic lateral sclerosis, polymyositis, critical illness polyneuropathy/myopathy, malnutrition, severe electrolyte disturbances, notably hypokalaemia, hyperkalaemia, hypomagnesaemia, prolonged ventilator dependence, disorders of the phrenic nerve, respiratory muscle fatigue from any cause.

2. Rarely, hypoventilation can occur following large airways obstruction. In an intensive care unit (ICU) setting, this is chiefly observed in tracheal or subglottic stenosis, when an artificial airway has been in place for many weeks, or has been incorrectly managed. Upper airways obstruction with hypoventilation can also occur in children with acute epiglottitis, in obstructive sleep apnoea, vocal cord paralysis, and foreign bodies including dentures, clots, secretions, soft tissue tumours or inflammation, obstructing the upper airway.

3. Poor expansion of the thoracic cage with ventilatory failure can occur following trauma to the thorax (as in flail chest), in patients who are severely obese, or have marked kyphoscoliosis, or in those with well-marked pleural disease (as in bilateral pleural effusion or pneumothorax).

   It is important to realize that in most of the above-mentioned conditions, the lungs are normal to start with. However, if hypoventilation is not promptly recognized and correctly managed (and this is most important in hypoventilating comatose patients), secretions accumulate within the large and small airways producing areas of atelectasis. As a result of secondary changes within the lungs, gas exchange due to ventilation-perfusion imbalance is further impaired.

4. Hypoventilation can also occur in lungs which are abnormal. This is most frequently seen in severe airways obstruction—either acute severe asthma, or an acute crisis in chronic bronchitis emphysema. In these patients hypoventilation is due to a decrease in $\dot{V}_E$, and/or an increase in physiological

dead space. Extensive thromboembolic disease within the lungs can rarely produce a sufficient rise in dead space ventilation (V_D), so as to cause a fall in alveolar ventilation. Severe late (almost terminal) stage restrictive disease can also be associated with hypoventilation and hypercapnic respiratory failure.

5. Increase in carbon dioxide production, at times cannot be countered by an increase in alveolar ventilation. Marked increase in carbon dioxide production can occur in high fever, hypermetabolic critical illnesses, severe hyperthyroidism, frequent seizures, and uncontrolled tetanus. In patients with respiratory muscle fatigue, or in those with mechanical limitations to breathing (as in chronic bronchitis), alveolar ventilation cannot keep pace with carbon dioxide production, and hypercapnic respiratory failure is observed. Hyperalimentation with increased caloric intake through carbohydrates or a high-carbohydrate diet given by the enteral route also results in an increase in VCO_2. An increase in V_A is imperative if this excess CO_2 is to be removed. In critically ill patients, carbon dioxide retention may occur as respiratory muscle fatigue may prevent a proportionate rise in alveolar ventilation.

The important causes of hypercapnic respiratory failure are listed in Table 53.1.

HYPOXAEMIC RESPIRATORY FAILURE

Acute hypoxaemic respiratory failure results from poor gas exchange of oxygen within the lungs leading to a low PaO_2. The $PaCO_2$ may be normal or even less than normal.

Table 53.1:
Important causes of hypercapnic respiratory failure in the ICU

1. Patients with normal lungs to start with (decrease in $\dot{V}_E$)

  • Depressed ventilatory drive
    – Poisoning e.g. narcotics, antidepressants, sedatives
    – Head injury, encephalitis, increase in intracranial tension

  • Neuromuscular diseases
    – Acute poliomyelitis, acute infective polyneuritis, polymyositis, critical care neuropathy/myopathy, amyotrophic lateral sclerosis
    – Tetanus, myasthenia gravis, botulism
    – Snake bite poisoning
    – Respiratory muscle weakness or fatigue from any cause

  • Large airways obstruction
    – Tracheal/subglottic stenosis, obstructive sleep apnoea, vocal cord paralysis, foreign bodies

2. Patients with abnormal lungs (decrease in $\dot{V}_E$ and/or increase in V_D)

  • Acute severe bronchial asthma
  • Acute crisis in chronic bronchitis, emphysema
  • Extensive thromboembolic disease
  • Severe terminal stage restrictive lung disease

3. Patients with increased production of CO_2

  • High fever, hypermetabolic critical illness
  • Frequent seizures, uncontrolled tetanus
  • Hyperalimentation with increased carbohydrate intake

Physiopathology

The normal alveolar ventilation ($\dot{V}_A$) is about 4–5 l, and the normal perfusion (Q) around 5 l, the $\dot{V}_A$/Q ratio being approximately 0.8–1. Even in the normal lung, there are regional differences in ventilation—perfusion ratios, but by and large the ventilation-perfusion ratios are even and range from 0.8–1.2. For explanatory purposes, the lung can be compartmentalized into the following divisions:

1. Alveoli with normal ventilation and perfusion—normal V/Q ratios.
2. Alveoli with increase in ventilation-perfusion ratios, the V/Q ratios being > 1. The capillaries leaving these alveoli have a normal or slightly increased PaO_2 but a reduced $PaCO_2$.
3. Alveoli with a decrease in ventilation-perfusion ratios; blood after perfusing these alveoli has a lowered PaO_2, and an increased $PaCO_2$. The lower the V/Q ratio, the lower the PaO_2 of the blood leaving these alveoli.
4. Alveoli that are ventilated, but have no perfusion. The V/Q ratio is infinity, and such alveoli contribute significantly to increased physiological dead space.
5. Alveoli which are atelectatic but continue to be perfused. These alveoli contribute to a right to left shunt within the lungs. The blood leaving the alveoli has the same PaO_2 as mixed venous blood i.e. 40 mm Hg.
6. Alveoli which are neither ventilated nor perfused. These are 'resting' alveoli, and probably come into physiological action only when ventilatory or respiratory demands increase.

Acute hypoxaemic respiratory failure occurs when: (a) there is a ventilation-perfusion mismatch characterized predominantly by low ventilation-perfusion ratios in the lungs; (b) there is a significant increase in the right to left shunt due to perfusion of atelectatic alveoli; (c) both the above factors are present; (d) there is a marked decrease in the diffusion of oxygen across the alveolar capillary membrane.

LOW VENTILATION-PERFUSION (V/Q) RATIOS

Alveoli which have a perfusion in excess of ventilation (i.e. low $\dot{V}_A$/Q ratios), will have a reduced P_AO_2, and therefore a reduced PaO_2, as well as a reduced oxygen content of blood leaving the alveoli. When the poorly oxygenated blood mixes with the blood perfusing the alveoli that have $\dot{V}_A$ which is normal in proportion to the perfusion, or $\dot{V}_A$ even in excess of the perfusion, the resultant blood stream has a lower oxygen content, and a lowered PaO_2. Increased V/Q ratios in some alveoli cannot therefore compensate for sharply lowered V/Q ratios in other alveoli. After all, the oxygen saturation of arterial blood in the presence of normal V/Q ratios is close to 100 per cent. A further increase in the V/Q ratio may increase both the P_AO_2 and the PaO_2, but because of the plateau shape of the upper part of the oxygen-haemoglobin dissociation curve, there will be no appreciable increase in oxygen saturation or content, of blood leaving such alveoli. This is illustrated in Figure 53.3.

INCREASE IN RIGHT TO LEFT SHUNT WITHIN THE LUNGS

A shunt refers to the proportion or fraction of venous blood that enters the systemic arteries without coming into contact

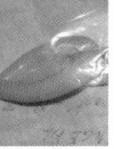

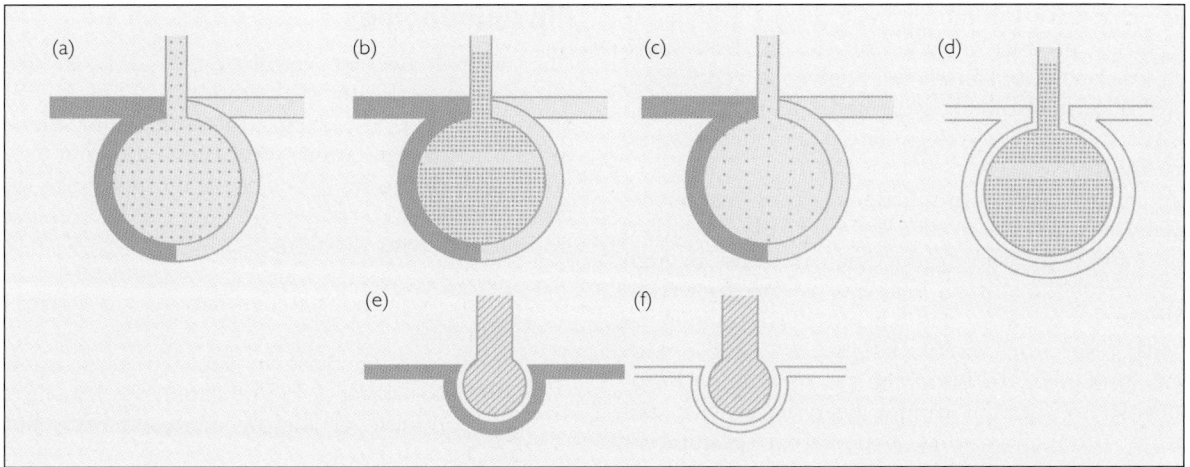

Fig 53.2: Various gas exchange units in the lung (a) Normal unit-alveoli with normal V/Q ratios (b) Hyperventilated unit-alveoli with increase in V/Q ratios (> 1) (c) Hypoventilated unit-alveoli with decrease in V/Q ratios (d) Dead Space unit-alveoli are ventilated, but have no perfusion (e) Shunt unit-alveoli are atelectatic but have good perfusion (f) Silent unit-alveoli are neither ventilated nor perfused (Modified from Udwadia FE. 1979. *Diagnosis and Management of Acute Respiratory Failure*. Oxford University Press, Mumbai).

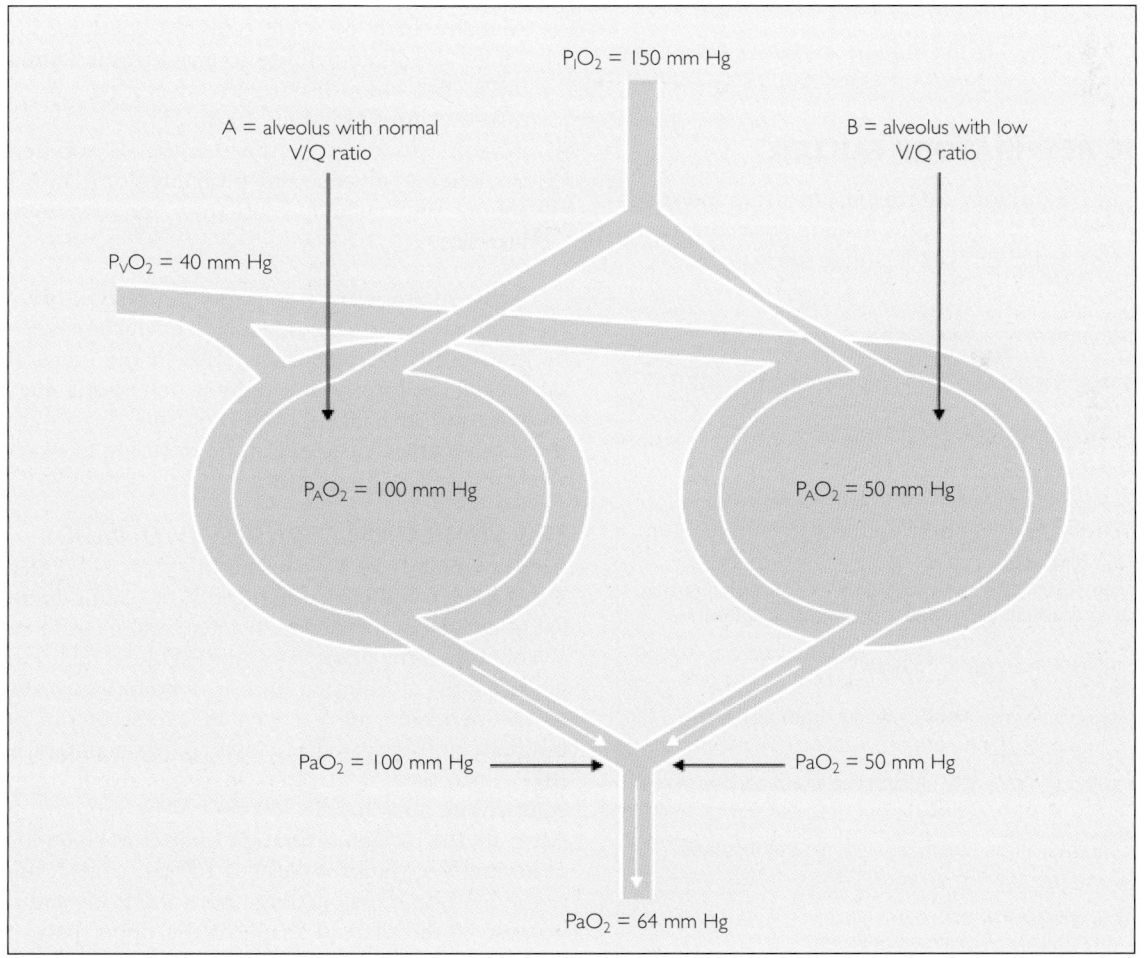

Fig 53.3: The PaO_2 of blood leaving A (alveolous with normal V/Q ratio) is normal; the PaO_2 of blood leaving B (alveolus with reduced V/Q ratio) is reduced. When this poorly oxygenated blood mixes with well-oxygenated blood from alveoli with normal or high V/Q ratios, the resultant PaO_2 is still lower than normal. This shows that increased V/Q ratios in some alveoli cannot compensate for markedly lowered V/Q ratios in other alveoli.

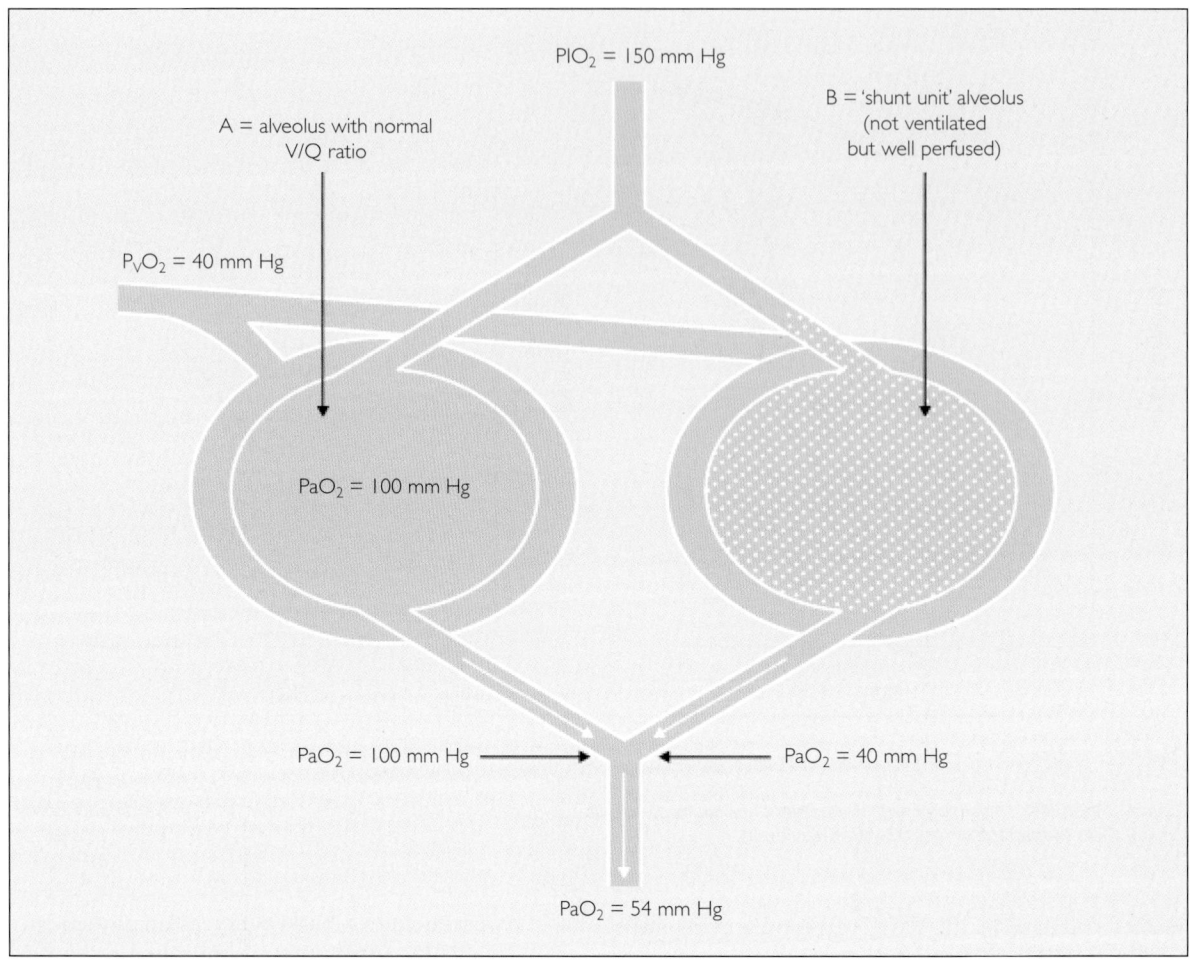

Fig 53.4: The PaO_2 of blood leaving A (alveolus with normal V/Q ratio) is normal. The mixed venous blood perfusing B (shunt unit alveolus) is not oxygenated at all. When this blood mixes with well-oxygenated blood perfusing a normal alveolus, the resultant PaO_2 is still very low.

with gas exchanging areas of the lungs. The present discussion is not concerned with right to left shunts in the heart or the larger vessels due to congenital defects or anomalies. Right to left shunts within the lungs due to perfusion of atelectatic alveoli constitute the most important cause of refractory acute hypoxaemic respiratory failure. It is to be remembered that there is a small right to left shunt even in normal lungs. This is because of bronchial venous blood draining directly through pulmonary veins into the left atrium, and a small amount of coronary venous blood that drains via the thebesian veins directly into the left ventricle. The normal shunt averages not more than 5 per cent. In patients with a right to left shunt due to perfusion of atelectatic alveoli, the shunt fraction may be as high as 30–50 per cent. The higher the right to left shunt within the lungs, the greater the degree of hypoxaemia, and lower the PaO_2.

The effect of a right to left shunt within the lungs is illustrated in Figure 53.4.

COMBINATION OF LOW V/Q RATIOS AND INCREASED SHUNT

Most lung diseases causing acute respiratory failure are characterized by a pathology in which there are areas of low V/Q ratios, high V/Q ratios, and increase in the right to left shunt.

Patients in whom disturbance in gas exchange is predominantly due to an increase in the shunt have the gravest prognosis.

IMPAIRMENT IN DIFFUSION OF OXYGEN

A diffusion abnormality does exist in several lung diseases, but it almost never is the chief cause of a low PaO_2 at rest. All patients with diffusion abnormalities have regional variations in compliance resulting in uneven and low ventilation-perfusion ratios.

Effect of an Increasing Inspired Oxygen Content (FIO$_2$) on V/Q Abnormalities

Increase in the FIO$_2$ rapidly produces an increase in the PaO_2 and the oxygen content of blood leaving the alveoli with low V/Q ratios. The hypoxaemia of acute respiratory failure in patients with low V/Q ratios is thus easily corrected. The improvement in PaO_2 depends upon the degree of perfusion to areas with poor ventilation. Except where the V/Q ratios are extremely low, a satisfactory PaO_2 of about 60 mm Hg, with an oxygen saturation of 90% is achieved by using an FIO$_2$ of < 0.6. Even in alveoli with extremely low V/Q ratios, as long as there is some ventilation present, an FIO$_2$ of 100% will always

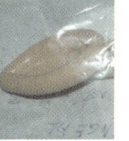

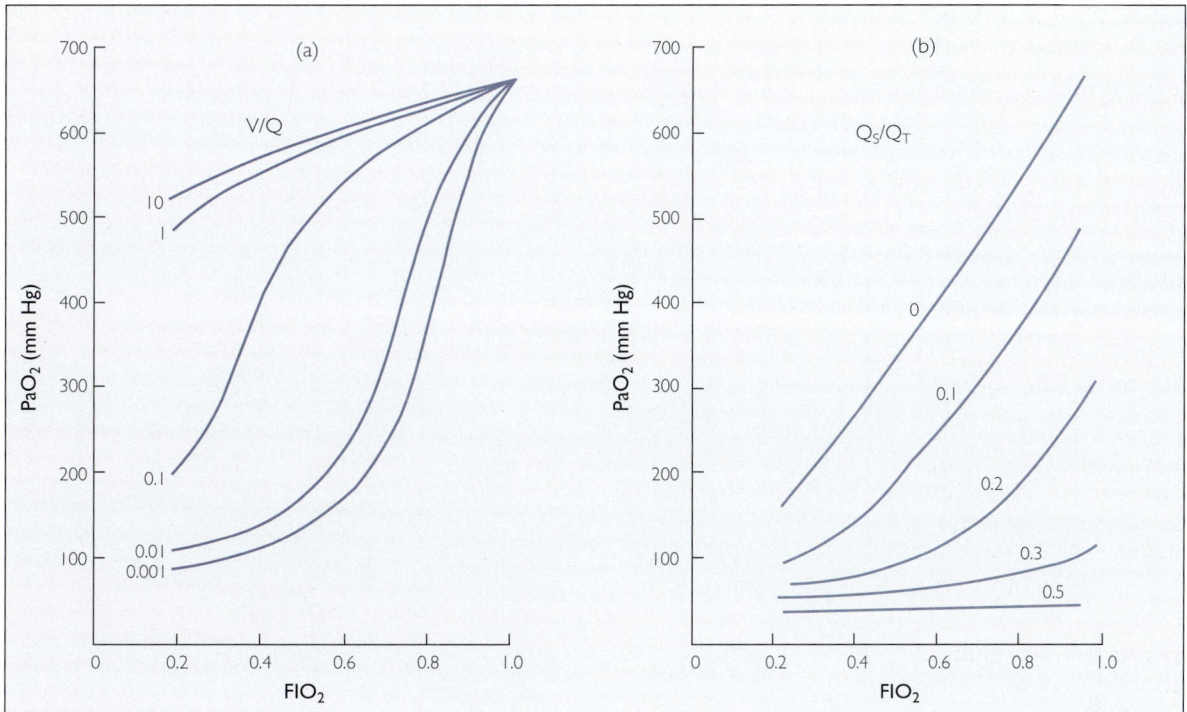

Fig 53.5: (a) PaO$_2$ improves with increasing FIO$_2$ in patients with a V/Q mismatch. When the FIO$_2$ is increased to 1 (100%), the PaO$_2$ reaches 600 mm Hg even if the V/Q ratio is very low (b) Note that with increase in Q$_S$/Q$_T$ beyond 0.3, increasing FIO$_2$ has little or no effect on the PaO$_2$.

Source: Albert RK. *Physiology and Mangement of Failure of Arterial Oxygenation.* 1988 in Fallat RJ, Luce JM. eds *Cardiopulmonary Critical Care Management*, pp. 37–59. Elsevier, Inc.

produce a marked increase in the PaO$_2$ of blood leaving such alveoli. This is illustrated in Figure 53.5a.

Effect of an Increased FIO$_2$ on the Shunt

It is obvious that the treatment of hypoxaemia due to a severe right to left shunt within the lungs is difficult, because increasing the FIO$_2$ improves the oxygen content to a very slight extent. The greater the shunt, the poorer the response in PaO$_2$ to a rise in FIO$_2$ (Figure 53.5b.). Fortunately, acute hypoxaemic respiratory failure solely due to a marked increase in the right to left shunt within the lungs is rare. Even in patients with severe acute respiratory distress syndrome (ARDS), though there are many areas of shunt which do not respond to an increase in FIO$_2$, there are some areas of V/Q mismatch which respond to such an increase.

CLINICAL PROBLEMS CAUSING ACUTE HYPOXAEMIC RESPIRATORY FAILURE

These can be broadly divided into three groups:

(i) Those characterized chiefly by airways' obstruction causing uneven ventilation and V/Q inequalities—an acute crisis in chronic bronchitis emphysema, and acute severe asthma are classic examples. In some of these patients there is an element of acute ventilatory failure in addition to hypoxaemic respiratory failure. This is due to mechanical limitations which prevent increased ventilatory demands from being adequately met, due to alveolar hypoventilation

consequent to a marked increase in physiological dead space ventilation, or due to a diminished respiratory drive. One or more of these factors may contribute to an associated ventilatory failure.

(ii) Restrictive lung diseases. Examples of these include acute pulmonary oedema, acute pulmonary infections, acute lung injury (ARDS), and major atelectasis within the lungs.

(iii) Acute thromboembolic lung disease. This is characterized by V/Q inequalities and increase in the dead space resulting in acute hypoxaemic respiratory failure.

The important causes of acute hypoxaemic respiratory failure are listed in Table 53.2.

Table 53.2:
Important causes of acute hypoxaemic respiratory failure
Obstructive airways disease
• Acute crisis in chronic bronchitis, emphysema • Acute severe bronchial asthma
Restrictive lung disease
• Acute pulmonary edema • Acute pulmonary infection • Acute lung injury (ARDS) • Major pulmonary atelectasis
Trauma to the chest
Acute thromboembolic lung disease

A Combination of Acute Ventilatory and Hypoxaemic Respiratory Failure

This is seen in intensive care medicine in four groups of patients.

(a) Acute severe asthma.
(b) Acute on chronic respiratory failure due to a respiratory crisis in patients with chronic airways obstruction.
(c) Muscle fatigue involving muscles of respiration in patients with acute respiratory failure due to severe lung disease.
(d) Advanced or late stage interstitial lung disease.

Failure of Oxygen Transport

A satisfactory gas exchange at the alveolar level must be accompanied by an adequate transport of oxygenated blood to the tissues. This requires an adequate cardiac output, a normal oxygen content of arterial blood and good tissue perfusion. A low output state, or shock from any cause can also indirectly lower the PaO_2 in the following ways:

(i) A low cardiac output results in increased oxygen extraction from the blood by the tissues. This leads to a fall in the mixed venous oxygen pressure (PvO_2). The lowered PvO_2 in the mixed venous blood reaching the alveoli will lead to a lowered PaO_2. This can be even more marked if the cardiac output falls in a patient who already has a right to left shunt within the lungs (Figure 53.6).

(ii) A low output state leads to a low pressure of perfused blood in the pulmonary vessels; perfusion is more in the dependent alveoli of the lungs. This results in an increase in the physiological dead space involving non-dependent alveoli, and in low V/Q ratios within the dependent alveoli of the lungs, thereby contributing to a fall in PaO_2.

(iii) Respiratory muscle fatigue is an important factor in low output states. Hypotension and shock lead to poor perfusion of respiratory muscles and quick, easy fatigability. Respiratory muscle fatigue can cause hypoventilation, can increase ventilation-perfusion inequalities, and can thereby further reduce the PaO_2.

RESPIRATORY MUSCLE FATIGUE

The importance and role of muscle fatigue in acute respiratory failure (also see section on 'Lung Physiology') in critically ill patients cannot be overemphasized and is best considered at this stage. As with other muscle groups in the body, excessive work performed by the muscles of respiration leads to fatigue. Increasing fatigue results in increasingly poor function and hypoventilation; ultimately the patient literally stops breathing. Increasing respiratory fatigue explains the abrupt stoppage of breathing with resulting disaster, in patients with acute severe asthma, or in patients with a very low pulmonary compliance due to acute alveolar oedema. Difficulties in weaning patients off ventilator support are also frequently related to respiratory muscle fatigue brought on by the inability to cope with the work of breathing.

The second major factor predisposing to respiratory muscle fatigue is the gravity or critical nature of an illness. The more critically ill the patient, the easier and quicker fatigue arises in respiratory muscles. Tachypnoea and an unstable circulation,

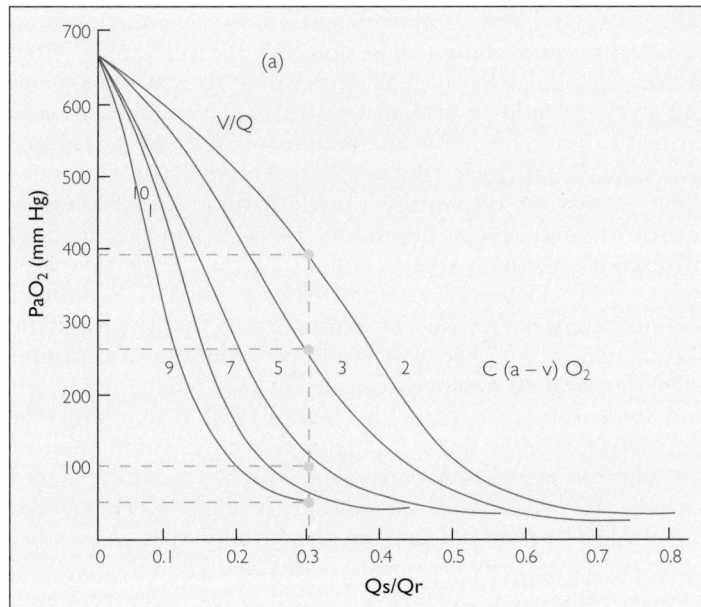

Fig 53.6: Dependence of PaO_2 on the oxygen extraction C (a–v) and the shunt fraction. If the shunt fraction is 30%, the PaO_2 varies from 100 to 400 mm Hg, as the C (a–v) O_2 narrows. The patient may have a high PaO_2 if he has a high cardiac output and a decreased C (a–v) O_2 of 3, even if his shunt fraction is as high as 0.3. However if the patient's oxygen consumption increases without a corresponding increase in the cardiac output, the C (a–v) O_2 widens to 9, and the PaO_2 falls to 50 mm Hg.

Source: Albert RK. *Physiology and Mangement of Failure of Arterial Oxygenation*. 1988 in Fallat RJ, Luce JM. eds *Cardiopulmonary Critical Care Management*, pp. 37–59. Elsevier, Inc.

hypotension with poor perfusion of the respiratory muscles, electrolyte disturbances, probably all play a role in muscle fatigue in these individuals.

The clinical recognition of respiratory muscle fatigue is difficult, and may occasionally be impossible to detect till the patient very nearly has a respiratory arrest. A voiced complaint by an ill patient that he or she is tired and cannot continue to breathe for long should always be taken seriously, particularly in a patient with severe airways' obstruction. Tachypnoea with a rate > 35/min, always predisposes to fatigue, particularly in obese individuals or very ill patients. Poor chest excursions, irregular breathing and above all apnoeic spells, all point to fatigued respiratory muscles. Respiratory alternans, in which intercostal muscles and diaphragmatic contractions alternate, is also observed at times. Fatigued muscles also occasionally cause a paradoxical respiratory movement, with the lower part of the chest and the upper abdomen being drawn in, instead of being pushed out during inspiration.

Objective measurements are also of use. As a rough guide, spontaneous breathing can be easily sustained if the effort involved in each spontaneous breath is less than one-third of the maximal respiratory effort that can be achieved. The maximum inspiratory pressure (MIP) is a good guide to the respiratory muscle power. An MIP of < 30 cm H_2O generally denotes muscle fatigue. Similarly a tidal volume (measured by a Wright's spirometer) of < 300 ml, or a vital capacity (VC) less than three times the tidal volume, suggests respiratory muscle fatigue under appropriate clinical conditions. A minute ventilation > 10–12 l/min is difficult to sustain indefinitely in critically ill

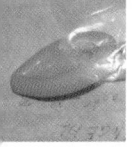

individuals, and often ultimately leads to hypoventilation from respiratory muscle fatigue. The objective measurements stated above when judged against an appropriate clinical background can give only indirect evidence of probable respiratory muscle fatigue. It has to be admitted that unequivocal direct evidence of contractile fatigue has not yet been demonstrated. The major determinants of respiratory muscle fatigue are inspiratory muscle strength, mean inspiratory pressure and the duration of inspiration, which when combined form the tension time index (TTI). However, interpretation of the TTI is difficult and often misleading. Recent work suggests that the magnetic stimulation of the phrenic nerve (a procedure far less painful than electrical stimulation) can detect diaphragmatic fatigue, and measuring changes in the oesophageal twitch pressure, can detect ribcage muscle fatigue. Magnetic stimulation of the phrenic nerve is however a research procedure in our setting. *Medicine need not always be evidence-based.* For the present we should act on the premise that respiratory muscles (particularly if they are weak) can, like other skeletal muscles experience fatigue if subjected to excessive work for a prolonged period of time.

The clinical features of respiratory muscle fatigue are listed in Table 53.3.

Table 53.3:
Features of respiratory muscle fatigue
Complaint of fatigue in relation to breathing
Respiratory rate > 35/min
Poor chest excursions, irregular breathing, apnoeic spells
Respiratory alternans, paradoxical respiratory movements
MIP < 30 cm H_2O
TV < 300 ml; VC < 3 × TV; MV > 10–12 l/min

Respiratory muscle fatigue causing or contributing to acute respiratory failure should be managed by resting the respiratory muscles by mechanical ventilation. During the period of rest, the acutely depleted glycogen stores of the respiratory muscles are replenished, and lactic acid and other metabolites associated with muscle fatigue are washed out. Aminophylline is believed to preserve muscle strength and contraction of the diaphragm; however, it is doubtful if this drug has a clinical role in patients with severe respiratory muscle fatigue.

Failure of Oxygen Uptake

Despite good ventilation, normal exchange of blood gases at the alveolar level, and good oxygen transport, oxygen uptake may be deficient at the tissue level. The main purpose of the cardiorespiratory system is then defeated. Thus cyanide poisoning is characterized by an arrest of intracellular respiration due to the inactivation of an intracellular enzyme, cytochrome oxidase. A patient with cyanide poisoning has a normal PaO_2, SaO_2, CaO_2 and oxygen transport, but cannot utilize oxygen at the tissue level. Blood after perfusing tissues shows severe lactic acidosis and has a high PvO_2 and SvO_2. The patient literally dies of 'strangulation' or hypoxia at the tissue level.

The most important clinical problem associated with failure of oxygen uptake is septic shock, often associated with ARDS. To many physicians it may seem inappropriate to consider failure of oxygen uptake by tissues in acute respiratory failure. Yet, it is ultimately the oxygen supply to, and oxygen uptake by tissues (in particular tissues of vital organs), which are of crucial importance. In the final analysis, acute cardiorespiratory failure is a failure to adequately oxygenate the tissues.

CLINICAL FEATURES OF ACUTE RESPIRATORY FAILURE

In the presence of a background disease known to cause acute respiratory failure, the only sure way to diagnose the latter is by estimating the arterial blood gases. One should never rely only on clinical features to diagnose acute respiratory failure. Clinical features may, however, be present. These include the presence of disease known to cause acute respiratory failure, and the features associated with hypoxia and hypercapnia. Many, though not all patients also show respiratory distress.

Hypoxia

Hypoxia is the basic underlying feature in every patient with acute hypoxaemic respiratory failure. Increasing hypoxia depresses cell function, induces metabolic acidosis, and if marked and unrelieved leads to cellular death. It may be impossible to detect hypoxia on clinical grounds in critically ill patients. The only sure way of detecting hypoxia is by measuring the arterial PaO_2. The importance of this fact cannot be overemphasized.

The only pathognomonic manifestation of hypoxia is central cyanosis. Nevertheless, well-marked arterial hypoxaemia may exist in the absence of clinical cyanosis, so that to await the development of cyanosis before diagnosing acute respiratory failure, is to court disaster. Cyanosis can only be clinically evident if the mean capillary concentration of reduced haemoglobin exceeds 5 g/dl. It is evident that a patient with severe anaemia (Hb < 7 g/dl), may die of severe arterial hypoxaemia before cyanosis can become clinically manifest. A hypermetabolic state with a hyperdynamic circulation characterized by a quick blood flow through the peripheries, also renders the clinical recognition of cyanosis difficult. The presence of anaemia together with a quickened circulatory flow therefore constitutes a formidable combination which prevents the clinical appearance of cyanosis in spite of marked hypoxia.

Mental confusion, restlessness, and acute anxiety are early manifestations of hypoxia. The ghastly pitfall of dubbing the anxiety and restlessness of early hypoxia in acute respiratory failure as 'functional' should be guarded against.

COMPENSATORY MECHANISMS INDUCED BY HYPOXIA

Hypoxia triggers compensatory mechanisms which are easily recognized, and are therefore of diagnostic value. The main compensatory mechanism is sympathetic stimulation which causes tachycardia and hypertension. Increase in the respiratory rate is another compensatory mechanism produced by stimulation of the chemoreceptors in the carotid body and aorta. Increase in the respiratory rate will not occur if the respiratory centre is markedly depressed, or if there is weakness or paralysis of the respiratory muscles. However, tachycardia and

hypertension are important signs of hypoxia. They should be sought for, and their significance recognized in situations that can lead to acute respiratory failure. These signs depend on the integrity of the sympathetic nervous system. In the old and feeble, in diabetics with a neuropathy involving the sympathetic nerves, or in patients who have received drugs affecting the autonomic nervous system, sympathetic response to hypoxia may be absent or feeble. With severe increasing hypoxia, the clinical hallmarks are progressive bradycardia, hypotension, lactic acid acidosis, arrhythmias, circulatory failure and death.

The myocardium has no oxygen reserve so that hypoxia depresses myocardial function, and increases ectopic irritability. Bradycardia and hypotension result from the direct depressant effect of hypoxia on the myocardium. Arrhythmias arise due to increased ectopic irritability. Atrial flutter and fibrillation are often observed; severe hypoxia ultimately results in ventricular tachycardia, fibrillation and arrest.

Hypercapnia

Hypercapnia may also be impossible to detect on clinical grounds. The $PaCO_2$ should therefore always be estimated in any disease which can conceivably produce carbon dioxide retention.

Carbon dioxide has a local depressant effect on the cardiovascular system. It thus produces generalized vasodilatation except in the pulmonary circulation. Generalized vasodilatation manifests as *cutaneous flushing, warmth, sweating, and a bounding pulse.*

The depressant effect of carbon dioxide on the central nervous system leads to confusion, disturbance in behaviour, a reversal in the sleep rhythm, and increasing drowsiness that may lead to deep coma (carbon dioxide narcosis). Carbon dioxide narcosis is an important metabolic cause of coma, and can be often missed if the $PaCO_2$ is not measured. Wing flap tremors of the outstretched hands are often observed with CO_2 retention. They are indistinguishable from those observed in hepatic failure. Wing flap tremors are not consistently present. At times, even a slight rise in the $PaCO_2$ induces wing flap tremors; at other times, a marked rise in $PaCO_2$ may not be associated with 'flaps'. However, increasing levels of $PaCO_2$ produce increasing disturbance of consciousness. Marked confusion and drowsiness occur by the time $PaCO_2$ rises to between 80–100 mm Hg, and the patient is generally unconscious when the $PaCO_2$ is well over 100 mm Hg. Coma in CO_2 narcosis is associated with loss of the deep reflexes, and urinary incontinence. The plantars are generally not elicitable or are flexor; rarely, they may be extensor.

High levels of $PaCO_2$ can produce headache, muscle twitchings, seizures and papilloedema. The combination of drowsiness, headache and papilloedema closely simulates an intracranial tumour.

An increasing $PaCO_2$ stimulates the respiratory centre, producing an increase in the respiratory rate and tidal volume. Nevertheless, a depressed centre or a centre with a reduced or absent sensitivity to increasing $PaCO_2$ will not permit an increased respiratory drive to materialize.

Hypercapnia also produces a central stimulation of the sympathetic nervous system, resulting in tachycardia and hypertension. The pattern of symptoms in a patient will depend on the balance between the depressant action on the cardio-vascular system, and the stimulant effects on the sympathetic nervous system.

Respiratory Distress or Dyspnoea

Many patients in acute respiratory failure are uncomfortably aware of a difficulty in breathing. This unpleasant awareness of respiration, and difficulty in breathing is termed dyspnoea. Dyspnoea is a subjective phenomenon, and its correlation with the degree of respiratory failure is difficult. In fact, breathlessness and respiratory failure are not synonymous. Many patients who are breathless are not in respiratory failure, and a number of patients in respiratory failure are not breathless. Nevertheless, in a patient with chronic lung disease, increasing impairment of lung function and increasing respiratory failure are invariably associated with increasing dyspnoea.

The important clinical features of hypoxia and hypercapnia are listed in Table 53.4.

Table 53.4: Important clinical features of hypoxia and hypercapnia	
Hypoxia	Hypercapnia
Cyanosis	Flushing, warmth, sweating, bounding pulse
Mental changes, restlessness, anxiety	Headache, wing flap tremors
Tachycardia, hypertension	Drowsiness, confusion, coma
Rhythm disturbances	Muscle twitching, seizures, papilloedema
Metabolic acidosis	
Bradycardia, hypotension, circulatory failure, when hypoxia is marked	

MANAGEMENT OF ACUTE RESPIRATORY FAILURE

A number of diseases produce acute respiratory failure for which there is no specific cure. The patient then needs respiratory care and support till such time as the disease resolves. There are other diseases producing acute respiratory failure for which specific therapy is available. Prompt diagnosis and specific treatment in such instances can quickly reverse respiratory failure. The general principles involved in the management of acute respiratory failure include: (i) maintenance of a clear airway; (ii) maintenance of adequate ventilation; (iii) use of oxygen; (iv) treating the cause of acute respiratory failure, in so far as this is possible; and (v) the use of mechanical ventilation when indicated—if the cause of acute respiratory failure cannot be treated, or if despite treatment the patient is hypoxic or hypercapnic, ventilatory support is indicated.

Maintenance of a Clear Airway

Obstruction of the airways due to retained secretions, mucus plugs or foreign matter (invariably food particles), worsen respiratory failure. Secretions obstructing airways can lead to hypoventilation with a further fall in the PaO_2. Mucus plugs within the airways contribute to uneven and poor distribution

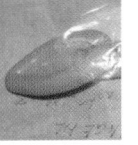

of inspired gas to the alveoli within the lungs, and also produce areas of atelectasis. Uneven ventilation accentuates V/Q inequalities, while increasing areas of atelectasis worsen or produce a right to left shunt within the lungs. The net effect is increasing hypoxia and worsening respiratory failure. Undrained secretions or mucus plugs also form a nidus for infection, which may ultimately lead to pneumonia or bronchopneumonia. Maintaining a clear airway is therefore, vital. This is often lost sight of in a comatose patient who may have normal lungs to start with, but who develops a quickly worsening respiratory failure due to undrained secretions plugging the airways.

METHODS TO CLEAR SECRETIONS

(1) *Liquefy Secretions* Undrained secretions can dry and form crusts which obstruct the airways. Such crusted secretions can be removed only with great difficulty; therefore drying of secretions should be prevented, and their liquefaction promoted by:

(a) proper hydration of the patient, if necessary with intravenous fluids. A severely ill, distressed, breathless patient generally does not drink enough water on his own.

(b) humidification of inspired gas. This is of utmost importance when the nasal and upper respiratory passages are bypassed, and the patient is breathing through an endotracheal or tracheostomy tube. Lack of humidification in such patients besides causing drying and crusting of secretions in the trachea, the large and the small airways, can also result in inspissated secretions that block the endotracheal or tracheostomy tube with disastrous consequences.

(c) use of N saline. We often instil N saline (2–5 ml at a time) through an endotracheal or tracheostomy tube, to help liquefy inspissated mucus secretions. This is particularly of value in patients with acute severe asthma on ventilator support.

Acetylcysteine is also a good liquefactant of inspissated mucus, but is a strong irritant. It can produce severe bronchospasm even in a dose as small as 0.5 ml. The drug can also markedly increase the volume of secretions in the tracheobronchial tree, necessitating very frequent suction. We use this drug very rarely in our unit.

(2) *Promotion of Cough* Cough, in a patient with acute respiratory failure should always be assisted and promoted, and never suppressed. When pain prevents cough (as after thoracic, open-heart or upper abdominal surgery, or in crush injuries), analgesics need to be given, taking care to use a dose that does not produce respiratory depression. Physiotherapy is vital to enable secretions to be brought up and coughed out. The patient may need to be postured to drain his secretions. *In critically ill patients who retain secretions within the respiratory tract, good physiotherapy often spells the difference between survival and death.*

(3) *Removal of Secretions by Suction* When secretions gather in the mouth and the upper respiratory passages, and the patient is too ill to spit or cough them out, frequent suction should be done to keep the upper airways patent, and to prevent the possibility of aspiration of the secretions into the lungs. Secretions around the larynx can be sucked

Table 53.5:
Management of acute respiratory failure

1. Maintenance of clear airways

- Clear secretions
  - Liquefy secretions
  - Promote cough—good physiotherapy
  - Suctioning of secretions
  - Use of an airway—oropharyngeal airway, other airways, endotracheal intubation/tracheostomy

2. Maintenance of adequate ventilation

- Artificial ventilation with AMBU bag in emergency, till mechanical ventilator support is organized
- Use of respiratory stimulants (in rare situations)

3. Use of oxygen

4. Treat cause of acute respiratory failure whenever possible

5. Use mechanical ventilator support if cause cannot be treated, or if patient hypoxic or hypercapnic despite above measures

with the aid of indirect laryngoscopy. Suction stimulates cough in an obtunded patient, and this is of added help. It is important never to roughly touch or 'hit' the tip of the catheter to the pharynx or larynx during suctioning, as this can traumatize the pharyngeal or laryngeal mucosa, induce bleeding and sloughing, and further worsen the problem of maintaining a clear airway. The tip of the suction catheter should lie on the posterior portion of the tongue, preferably not touching the pharynx during suctioning. The floor and sides of the mouth should be suctioned; the nasal cavity and the pharynx can also be conveniently suctioned through a catheter inserted through the nares.

(4) *Endotracheal Intubation* (Also see chapter on 'Airway Management') If the upper airway cannot be kept clear and open by the methods indicated above, or by the use of a simple oropharyngeal or nasopharyngeal airway, the patient should be intubated. Endotracheal intubation is an invaluable aid to maintain a clear airway as it allows easy access to secretions in the trachea and the large airways.

The main indication for endotracheal intubation is upper airways obstruction and the inability of the patient to handle upper respiratory secretions. The latter feature is frequently observed in unconscious patients, and is invariably so in comatose patients. It also occurs when the cough reflex is poor or the patient is just too ill or feeble to cough. Paralysis of the palate and pharynx will also prevent the patient from handling his upper respiratory secretions because of difficulty in swallowing. This could lead to aspiration of accumulated secretions, as also to aspiration of regurgitated stomach contents. The four common conditions in critical care medicine wherein an endotracheal tube serves to maintain an open airway, are poisoning by respiratory depressants, cerebrovascular accidents, coma from any cause, and following major surgery. Endotracheal intubation is also indicated when the patient is to be put on mechanical ventilator support.

Maintenance of Adequate Ventilation

ARTIFICIAL VENTILATION

When respiration is feeble or the patient is apnoeic, immediate resuscitation is aimed at ensuring adequate ventilation. Initially mouth to mouth respiration may be necessary, followed within seconds by a mask fitted to an AMBU or anaesthetic bag, fed with 100% oxygen. This should be quickly followed by endotracheal intubation, mechanical ventilation being carried out either through an AMBU bag or by a mechanical ventilator.

THE USE OF RESPIRATORY STIMULANTS IN ACUTE RESPIRATORY FAILURE

The role of respiratory stimulants in acute respiratory failure in ICUs is very limited and to many nonexistent. No respiratory stimulant acts specifically and solely on the respiratory centre; all such drugs in addition to stimulating the respiratory centre, also act as analeptics, in that they awaken the patient, and thereby enable him to ventilate and cough better. In fact, almost certainly the analeptic effect is clinically more important than the specific stimulating effect on the respiratory centre. Good physiotherapy should always be given during an analeptic phase, so that secretions within the lungs are mobilized, and either coughed up or removed through suction. Unfortunately, all respiratory stimulants and analeptics frequently produce vomiting as a side-effect, and if the dose is large, or the drug is administered rapidly, localized twitchings or generalized seizures can result. If alveolar hypoventilation due to a depressed respiratory centre is sufficiently severe to produce well-marked hypoxia and hypercapnia, it is far better to use non-invasive ventilation or to intubate and ventilate the patient, rather than waste time in administering respiratory stimulants. We have stopped using respiratory stimulants in our units.

Perhaps the only valid use of respiratory stimulants is (a) to tide over a critical period in a patient with acute respiratory failure, while he awaits transfer to an ICU; (b) in patients with hopelessly crippling chronic obstructive pulmonary disease (COPD) who on balance, are not given ventilator support. Respiratory stimulants could then be tried along with the other far more important conservative measures.

The respiratory stimulant with probably the least side-effects is doxapram. It is given intravenously at a rate of 1–3 mg/min, and can be continued till a maximum dose of 600 mg is reached. The risk of seizures is low with doxapram. The infusion can however cause hypertension and cardiac arrhythmias as the drug can stimulate the release of epinephrine from the adrenals. It should therefore be avoided in hypertensive patients, and in those with ischemic heart disease.

Use of Oxygen

The prompt administration of oxygen is crucial in the management of acute respiratory failure. This is considered in a separate section (See section on 'Airway Diseases').

Treatment of the Cause of Acute Respiratory Failure Whenever Possible

Treatment is individualized depending upon the aetiological factor operating in a patient. The following examples are illustrative and worthy of mention:

(i) Treatment of infection. This is the commonest cause that precipitates acute respiratory failure in patients with chronic lung disease. Infection can also occur later as a complication in the natural history of acute respiratory failure due to other causes.

(ii) Removal of air in a tension pneumothorax, and tapping of a massive unilateral pleural effusion or moderate-sized bilateral effusions.

(iii) Removal of a foreign body obstructing the larynx, trachea, or a large bronchus.

(iv) Expanding an atelectatic lobe or lung with physiotherapy or bronchoscopic suction.

(v) Use of prostigmine in myasthenia gravis, and of antivenin in snakebite poisoning.

(vi) Use of naloxone in narcotic poisonings.

(vii) Use of nebulized beta-2 agonists, intravenous aminophylline, and oral or intravenous corticosteroids in acute severe asthma.

There are many situations where the cause of acute respiratory failure cannot be promptly treated. This particularly holds true for the numerous conditions which produce ARDS, severe tetanus, severe head injuries and other CNS problems, and poisonings due to sedatives and tranquillizers. The doctor in charge of the ICU has then to rely on the general principles of management outlined above, till such time as the illness causing acute respiratory failure resolves over a period of time.

Mechanical Ventilation

When well-marked and in particular life-threatening hypoxia and/or hypercapnia are uncorrected by the general principles above, the patient needs mechanical ventilator support to aid in more effective gas exchange within the lungs. This is dealt with in a separate chapter.

SUGGESTED READING

Hill NS. Noninvasive ventilation in acute respiratory failure. *Crit Care Med.* 1 Oct. 2007; 35(10): 2402–7.

MacIntyre NR. Current issues in mechanical ventilation for respiratory failure. *Chest.* 1 Nov. 2005; 128 (5 Suppl 2).

Rogovik A. Permissive hypercapnia. *Emerg Med Clin North Am.* 1 Nov. 2008; 26(4): 941–52, viii–ix.

Sevransky JE. Respiratory failure in elderly patients. *Clin Geriatr Med.* 1 Feb. 2003; 19(1): 205–24.

CHAPTER **54** **Airway Management**

ESTABLISHING THE AIRWAY

Nothing is more critical in emergency respiratory care than ensuring a patent airway and then maintaining it. An obstructed airway can lead to death within a few minutes. In patients with cardiac arrest, inability to secure a patent airway generally renders all efforts at cardio-pulmonary resuscitation ineffective.

UPPER AIRWAYS OBSTRUCTION

Upper airways obstruction may result from 'soft tissue' obstruction or from laryngeal obstruction.

'Soft tissue' obstruction is probably the commonest airway emergency. It results from the encroachment on the patency of the upper airway by soft tissues of the pharynx or by tissue in close relation to the pharynx. Upper airways obstruction is thus seen in comatose patients when the pharynx loses it tone or in patients with lower cranial nerve palsies when the pharynx is paralyzed. It also occurs in angioneurotic oedema, inflammation, retropharyngeal abscess and can be caused by bleeding and soft tissue tumours within that area. Foreign bodies, dentures, vomitus, blood clots, thick oropharyngeal secretions can also block the upper airway. The common factor underlying all these causes of upper airways obstruction is the absent or the markedly diminished patency between the base of the tongue and the pharyngeal wall.

Obstruction at the larynx can be caused by laryngeal spasm as in tetanus, by a bilateral vocal cord abductor palsy, by inflammatory or neoplastic lesions above or within the larynx or by laryngeal oedema. A foreign body or food (such as a piece of meat) may also obstruct the larynx and cause severe asphyxia and death.

Partial upper airways obstruction is characterized by noisy breathing, akin to snoring. Partial upper airways obstruction can be easily missed, particularly in comatose patients who in addition often hypoventilate due to a depressed respiratory centre. Laryngeal or tracheal obstruction gives rise to a high-pitched inspiratory sound termed 'stridor'.

Complete or almost complete airways obstruction results in marked inspiratory efforts with little or no movement of air into the lungs. There is severe retraction of the intercostal spaces, the sternum and epigastrium, together with strong contraction of the accessory muscles of respiration during inspiratory efforts. The patient, to start with, is extremely distressed, restless, anxious and becomes increasingly cyanosed. Tachycardia or a bradyrhythm is related to hypoxia. Death ensues if hypoxia is unrelieved.

Management

The treatment obviously is to relieve soft tissue obstruction by simple basic manoeuvres.

NECK EXTENSION WITH FORWARD AND UPWARD CHIN THRUST

This should be the first manoeuvre to be attempted as it can promptly relieve mild to moderate obstruction by increasing the patency between the back of the tongue and the pharynx.

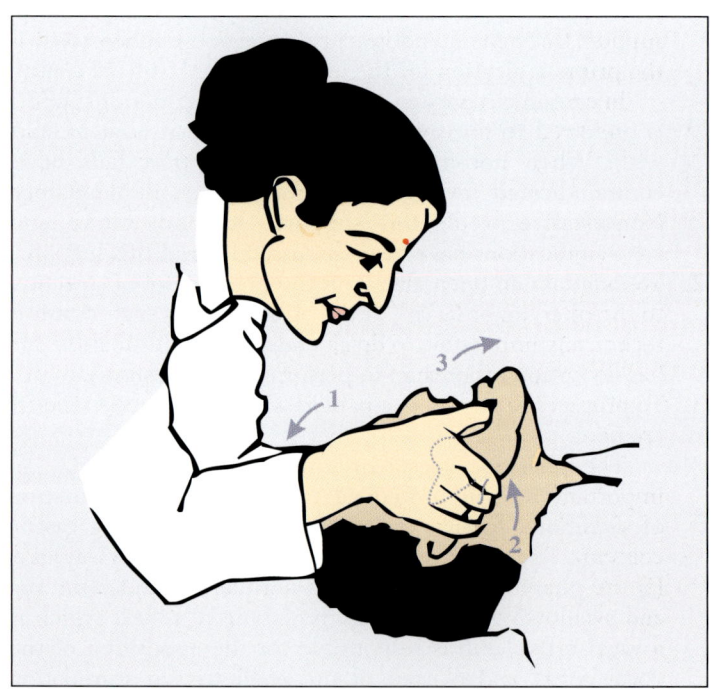

Fig 54.1: Maintaining a clear airway by triple airway manoeuvre (1) Tilt head backwards (2) Lift mandible forwards (3) Open the mouth and try to remove any foreign body.

Careful suction of secretions, blood, and vomitus from the pharynx may be necessary, as also the removal of dentures or a foreign body that may be obstructing the airway.

The Oropharyngeal Airway

This device is a conduit inserted along the top of the tongue until the teeth or gums limit its insertion. It is positioned

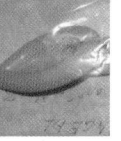

between the base of the tongue and the pharynx (separating the two) thereby maintaining a patent airway. The airway should be inserted with its curve up initially and rotated into position when the end reaches the base of the tongue. It is designed to permit a suction catheter to pass through it, and allow suction of secretions in the pharynx and upper larynx.

An oropharyngeal airway is chiefly suited for comatose patients and that too for limited periods of time. As it rests at the base of the tongue, it stimulates the gag reflex, and can induce excessive salivation, vomiting and even laryngospasm in the conscious patient.

ARTIFICIAL AIRWAYS

An artificial airway is a conduit or tube inserted into the trachea bypassing the pharynx and larynx which no longer form part of the total airway. In essence, this means endotracheal intubation or tracheostomy.

Indications

1. Hypoxia and/or hypercapnia (due to acute respiratory failure) severe enough to necessitate invasive ventilator support through an endotracheal tube or a tracheostomy is the prime indication for the insertion of an artificial airway.

   In certain circumstances non-invasive ventilator support is preferred to invasive ventilator support at least to start with. When non-invasive ventilator support fails or is contraindicated invasive ventilator support is mandatory. Non-invasive ventilator support, its indications and contraindications have been discussed later in this section.

2. To maintain an open airway in the presence of obstruction to the pharynx or larynx. If the obstruction is such that it is technically impossible to do an endotracheal intubation one has no option other than to perform a tracheostomy.

3. To protect the airway in a patient whose protective reflexes are poor.

   The pharynx, vocal cords and the epiglottis play an important role in protecting the airway from aspiration of secretions, foreign matter, food or regurgitating gastric contents. The reflexes that normally protect the airways are: (i) the pharyngeal reflex, which normally includes the gag and swallowing reflexes; (ii) the laryngeal reflex, which is a vagal reflex, and is responsible for the apposition of the vocal cords, and closure of the epiglottis on stimulation of the larynx by secretions or by foreign matter; (iii) the tracheal reflex, which is a vagal reflex causing cough when the trachea is stimulated by some irritant or foreign matter; (iv) the carinal reflex, which is a vagal reflex causing cough and irritation of the carina.

   The protective reflexes are generally obtunded from above downwards, irrespective of whether the cause of obtundation is due to drugs, disease or a deepening state of unconsciousness. When these reflexes return in a recovering patient, they recover from 'below' 'up'. The preservation of the pharyngeal reflex (gag reflex) therefore suggests preservation of the laryngeal and tracheal reflexes. However, the gag reflex is believed to be diminished or inelicitable in

10% of the normal population. Therefore, absence of this reflex does not always indicate absence of other protective reflexes. Clinically, the inability to handle secretions in the upper airway and to swallow in a coordinated manner, denotes a loss of protective airway reflexes and necessitates the establishment of an artificial airway. In such patients, the artificial airway also seals the respiratory from the alimentary tract, thereby preventing aspiration of gastric contents into the tracheobronchial tree.

4. To facilitate suction of secretions (from within the tracheobronchial tree), which the patient is incapable of coughing up and expectorating. This could be because the secretions are copious, the cough reflex is poor, or the patient is just too feeble to cough and expectorate. Although it is possible to insert a suction catheter through the vocal cords for suctioning tracheal secretions, it is not advisable to do so except on rare occasions. Laryngeal oedema and obstruction, and precipitation of fatal arrhythmias in critically ill patients can occur following such attempts. The establishment of an artificial airway allows easy, safe and direct suctioning of the tracheobronchial tree.

Table 54.1: Indications for artificial airway
1. Acute respiratory failure necessitating invasive ventilator support
2. To maintain an open airway in the presence of obstruction to the pharynx or larynx
3. To protect the airway when protective reflexes are lost
4. To facilitate suction of secretions within the tracheobronchial tree which the patient is unable to cough up and expectorate

The Disadvantages of Artificial Airways

The establishment and maintenance of an artificial airway (endotracheal intubation or tracheostomy) has its hazards and complications depending on the expertise with which it is established, the quality of after care, and the nature and degree of the critical illness in the patient. These complications are dealt with later. However, there are some inherent universal drawbacks of artificial airways which need to be considered.

1. An artificial airway bypasses the normal defence mechanisms which counter bacterial contamination of the airways. The airways and lungs are more prone to nosocomial infection.

2. An endotracheal tube removes the effectiveness of cough because the vocal cords are non-functional; a tracheostomy bypasses the cords.

3. An artificial airway prevents the patient from communicating vocally. This can be frustrating and frightening, and it is important, in a conscious patient, to provide a pad and a pen to help the patient communicate in writing.

4. In a conscious patient, there is often a feeling of a loss of dignity and a loss of control over one's self due to tubes which prevent the patient from speaking or breathing normally.

ESTABLISHING AN EMERGENCY AIRWAY

An emergency airway is one that must be established immediately, with utmost urgency, as it involves a matter of life and death. The chief indications for an 'immediate' airway are:

(i)   Severe life-threatening upper airways obstruction.
(ii) Cardiac or respiratory arrest—or impending cardiorespiratory arrest.
(iii) Fulminant pulmonary oedema.

The emergency airway of choice is an oral endotracheal intubation, with the aid of direct laryngoscopy. In an intensive care unit (ICU) or in any setting where the expertise and the necessary equipment is promptly available, oral endotracheal intubation can be performed in a matter of minutes. However, emergency endotracheal intubation may prove difficult even in experienced hands, and at times, may fail. In such circumstances, an alternative airway needs to be established urgently.

OTHER EMERGENCY AIRWAYS

The Laryngeal Mask Airway

The laryngeal mask airway (LMA) can secure the airway in an emergency, in a situation where endotracheal intubation fails, or in a situation where experienced personnel to intubate are unavailable. A properly placed LMA not only secures the airway, but allows ventilatory support and reduces the risk of gastric aspiration. A standard adult LMA consists of a 12-mm internal diameter tube fused at a 30° angle to an elliptical spoon-shaped cuff with an inflatable rim. The cuff is soft and when inflated adapts to the shape of the larynx forming an airtight seal over it. The tube opens into the concavity of the cuff ellipse through a fenestrated aperture. The LMA should be placed with the patient placed in sniffing position—neck flexed and head extended. The cuff is deflated and lubricated prior to insertion. The patient's mouth is opened and with the distal aperture of the cuff positioned anteriorly, the tip of the cuff is applied against the hard palate and advanced by the index finger of the right hand over the back of the tongue till it meets resistance when it abuts on the upper oesophageal sphincter. The cuff is inflated with 10–30 ml air so that the cuff centres on the laryngeal inlet. Studies show that the procedure is easily learnt by nurses and that adequate ventilation could be provided in 87% of cases. Studies in mannequins suggest that the LMA decreased gastric distension compared to the AMBU and could be more easily placed than the combitube.

The Intubating Laryngeal Mask Airway

The standard LMA can allow intubation with the aid of a fibreoptic bronchoscope. However, the size of the endotracheal tube that can be inserted through the LMA is necessarily small. The intubating LMA consists of an anatomically curved rigid tube with a metal-guided handle and a distal silicone laryngeal cuff. The floor of the cuff aperture has an epiglottis-elevating bar and guiding ramp which permits a specially designed endotracheal tube (8 mm in diameter) to be directed towards the glottis and inserted blindly into the trachea. The intubating LMA can be placed without moving the patient's head or neck. This is of definite advantage to patients who have sustained an injury to the cervical spine or to those who have an unstable cervical spine—situations where spinal flexion is best avoided.

The major concerns in the use of the LMA are: (i) the risk of gastric aspiration, (ii) the possibility of ineffective ventilation because of suboptimal positioning over the larynx, (iii) the inability to generate high inflation pressures in patients with increased airway resistance or low lung compliance.

Cricothyroidotomy

A cricothyroidotomy with insertion of a tube or a conduit into the trachea may serve as a life-saving temporary emergency procedure. A cricothyroidotomy should be replaced by an appropriate airway as soon as possible.

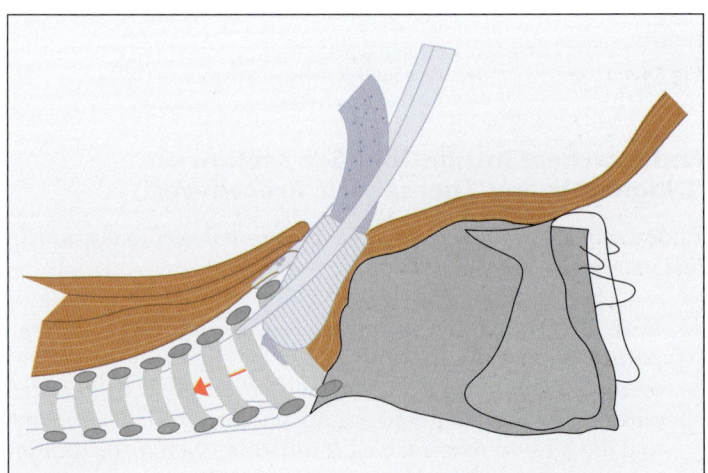

Fig 54.3: Procedure for cricothyroidotomy. Tracheostomy tube advanced behind the clamp and trachea pulled up by clamp.

Emergency Tracheostomy

An emergency tracheostomy can be performed by an experienced surgeon in 15 minutes.

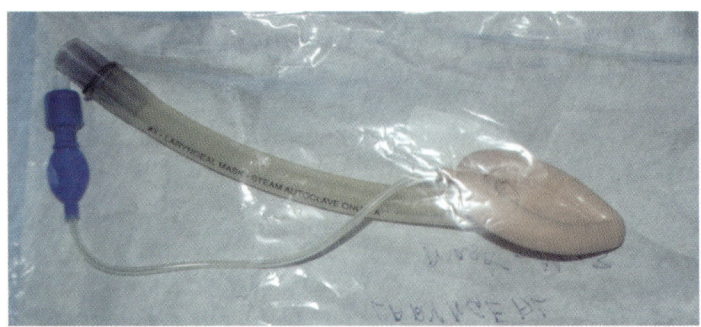

Fig 54.2: Laryngeal mask airway.

Percutaneous Tracheostomy (See section on 'Diagnostic and Therapeutic Procedures')

A percutaneous tracheostomy can be carried out by an experienced intensivist or surgeon in perhaps even lesser time.

Till such time as an emergency airway is ultimately secured, it is vital to continue to ventilate the patient with a bag-mask using 100% oxygen and to ensure that at least the upper airway (above the vocal cords) is patent.

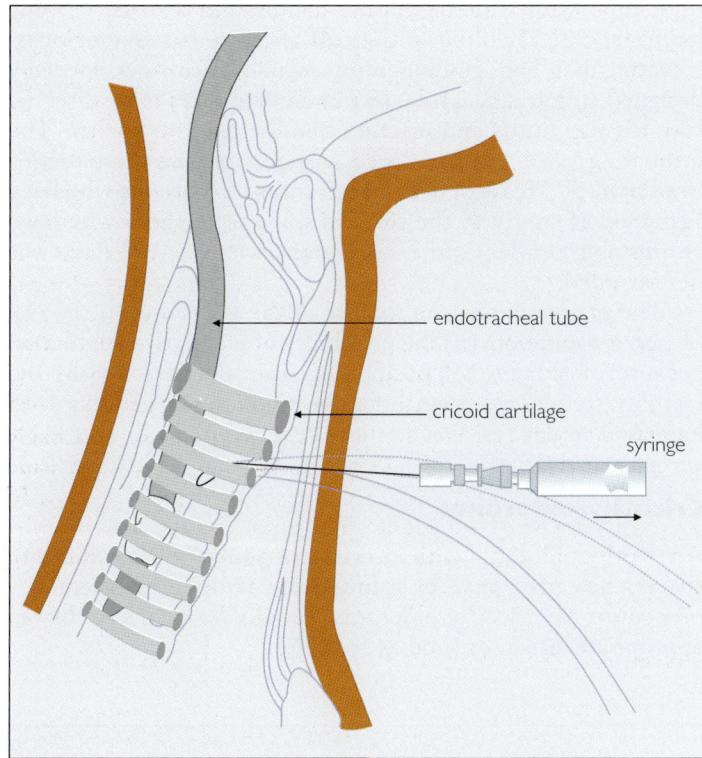

endotracheal tube

cricoid cartilage

syringe

Fig 54.4: Procedure for percutaneous dilatational tracheostomy (PDT).

Endotracheal Intubation (See section on 'Diagnostic and Therapeutic Procedures')

Endotracheal intubation is often performed electively and in less emergent situations. It can be performed

1. **With the Patient Awake** This is very unpleasant for the patient but has the great advantage that it allows the patient to ventilate and oxygenate himself or herself. It is preferred particularly in patients with difficult airways. The approach may be a blind nasotracheal intubation or endotracheal intubation using topical anaesthesia and direct laryngoscopy to visualize the larynx, or endotracheal intubation through the use of a fibreoptic bronchoscope.
2. **With the Patient Sedated** Sedative agents such as midazolam or propofol are administered as a bolus. The patient though sedated, maintains spontaneous ventilation. Endotracheal intubation is then done with the aid of direct laryngoscopy, or if needs be with the help of a laryngoscope or a bronchoscope. If a laryngeal mask airway has been introduced earlier, intubation can be done via a fibreoptic bronchoscope passed through the larynx.

3. **After Inducing Neuromuscular Paralysis** This is the method most frequently used when performing endotracheal intubation with the aid of direct laryngoscopy. Muscle paralysis with relaxation of the masseters and paralysis of the pharynx generally allows a good view of the larynx with the aid of a laryngoscope and allows quick intubation. However, respiratory muscle paralysis abolishes spontaneous ventilation and the physician must therefore obtain immediate airway control or failing this ensure effective bag-mask ventilation till spontaneous ventilation returns. Also, in a difficult intubation, the larynx if situated anteriorly may not be visualized even after neuromuscular paralysis, so an alternative plan to secure the airway and maintain ventilation should be promptly available.

A standard rapid sequence method is followed when using neuroparalytic agents prior to endotracheal intubation in patients at risk for aspiration of gastric contents.

1. The patient is oxygenated with 100% oxygen for some minutes through a bag and full-face mask.
2. A sedative (midazolam) is administered as a bolus followed immediately by the administration of the neuroparalytic agent.
3. At the same time an assistant exerts pressure on the cricoid using the Selick's manoeuvre which occludes the oesophagus and reduces the risk of aspiration.
4. Endotracheal intubation is quickly performed, the pressure on the cricoid being relieved only after the airway has been secured.

The major disadvantage of neuromuscular paralysis is that effective spontaneous respiration may not return for several minutes so that a failed intubation can turn into a disaster.

The procedure for endotrancheal intubation has been described in the section on 'Diagnostic and Therapeutic Procedures'.

MANAGEMENT OF ASPIRATION DURING BAG-MASK VENTILATION

Danger of aspiration is significant in high-risk patients—those with a full stomach, patients with a hiatus hernia or gastro-oesophageal reflux, obese individuals and in pregnancy. Aspiration should be countered by maintaining pressure over the cricoid cartilage (thereby closing the oesophageal lumen), putting the patient promptly in the Trendelenberg position and suctioning the gastric contents. If possible intubation should be prompt with the help of direct laryngoscopy. The airway should be secured and the cuff of the endotracheal tube inflated before resuming positive pressure ventilation.

DIFFICULT AIRWAY

A difficult airway is a clinical situation in which an anaes-thesiologist or an intensivist experiences difficulty with mask ventilation, or difficulty with tracheal intubation or both. Difficult mask ventilation implies an inability to maintain an O_2 saturation > 90% using 100% oxygen and positive pressure mask ventilation. Difficult intubations are those requiring three or more attempts using conventional laryngoscopy. In an ICU

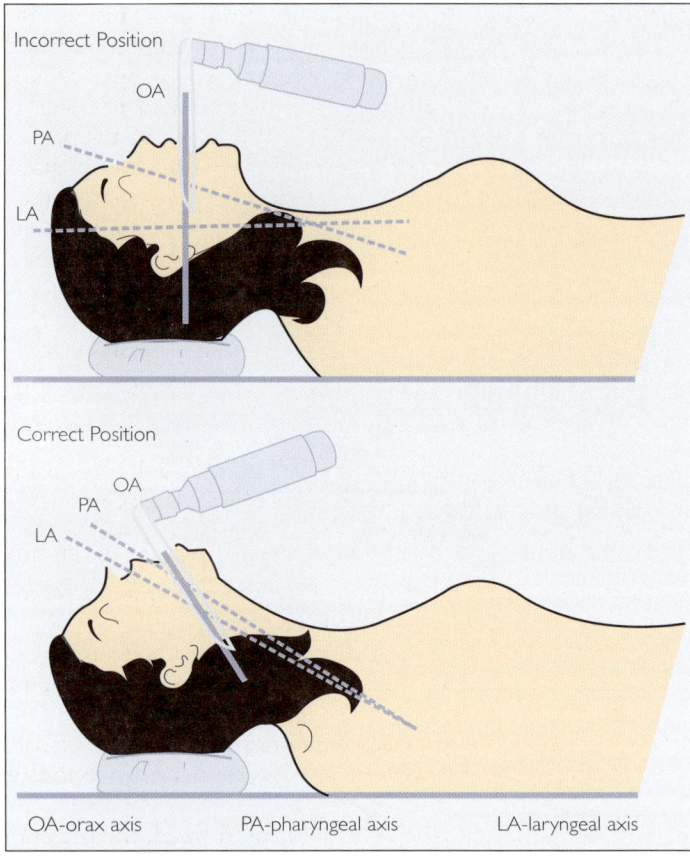

Fig 54.5: The position of the head and neck for endotracheal intubation.

laryngoscopic endotracheal intubation by noting the degree of visibility of the faucial pillars and the uvula, with the patient seated, mouth wide open and the tongue fully protruded. Patients were classified into three classes according to the difficulty experienced in intubation.

Class I—clearly visible fauces, uvula, with a wide oropharynx—easy intubation.

Class II—less clearly visible fauces and uvula, with a smaller opening of the oropharynx—intubation not as easy as in Class I.

Class III—poorly visible fauces, uvula with a small oropharynx, encroached upon by the above structures—intubation could prove difficult. This pre-intubation evaluation correlated with the laryngoscopic visualization of the larynx—in Class I the larynx being well visualized and in Class III, the larynx being poorly visualized. Samson and Young added a Class IV to Mallampati's classification;

Class IV—is characterized by the inability to see the fauces, uvula and the oropharyngeal opening (patient seated, tongue protruded, mouth wide open). The vocal cords are not visualized on direct laryngoscopy, and intubation in these patients is generally unsuccessful.

In an emergency setting in the ICU, there is no time for elaborate pre-intubation evaluation. Patients requiring intubation are often hypoxic, restless, uncooperative and haemodynamically unstable. The simplest predictor of a likely successful intubation at the bedside in an emergency is the 'Rule of Threes'. If the intensivist can place three finger breadths (6 to 7 cm) between the upper and lower teeth, between the mandible and the hyoid bone and between the thyroid cartilage and the sternal notch, intubation is usually successful.

Difficult Intubation in the Critical Care Unit

It is important not to make several attempts at intubation as this traumatizes the pharynx, larynx and makes a subsequent successful intubation doubly difficult. More than two attempts are associated with increased morbidity and an increased risk of cardiac arrest. Patients who are hypoxic are rendered even more hypoxic with all the attendant risks. Patients who to start with are hypotensive, haemodynamically unstable, or are in shock from any cause, or who are on vasopressors to maintain perfusion are at grave risk from pre-intubation death following repeated failed attempts at intubation. Sudden fluctuations in blood pressure and heart rate consequent to repeated attempts at intubation are dangerous in patients with aneurysms or in patients with unstable angina or myocardial infarction.

The management of failed endotracheal intubation attempts in a critical care setting should be considered under two heads.

1. Failed intubation attempts in patients in whom securing an airway and establishing effective ventilation is a matter of extreme urgency, a matter of life and death—e.g. cardiac arrest, respiratory arrest, extreme obstruction to the airway.

The following emergency measures need to be followed:

i. Call for help.
ii. Continue bag-mask ventilation with 100% oxygen. Two individuals can perform this more effectively than one. One individual ensures that the mask fits tightly over the nose and mouth, preventing any air leak; the other squeezes the AMBU bag fed with 100% oxygen. The intensivist or

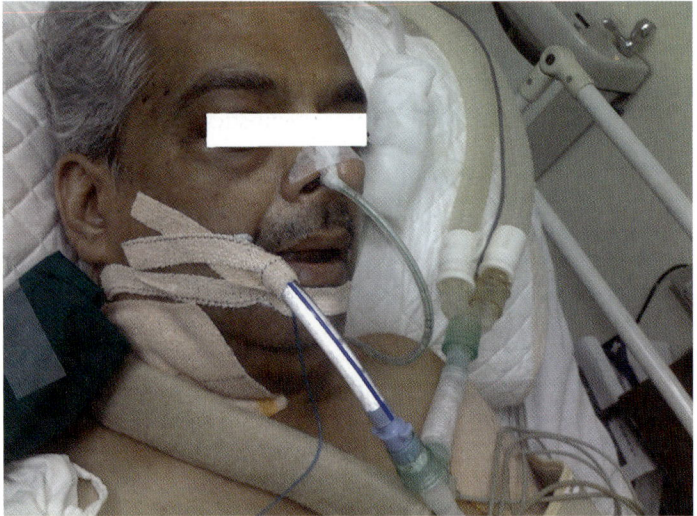

Fig 54.6: Endotracheal intubation.

setting, a difficult-to-intubate airway may be apparent on a pre-intubation evaluation or becomes manifest only on attempted intubation. A markedly receding jaw, prominent incisors, macroglossia, soft tissue lesions obstructing the oropharynx or the entrance to the larynx, a rigid spine as in ankylosing spondylitis or a very anteriorly placed glottis can make intubation difficult or impossible.

Mallampati assessed the ability to perform a direct

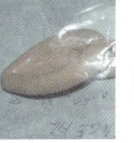

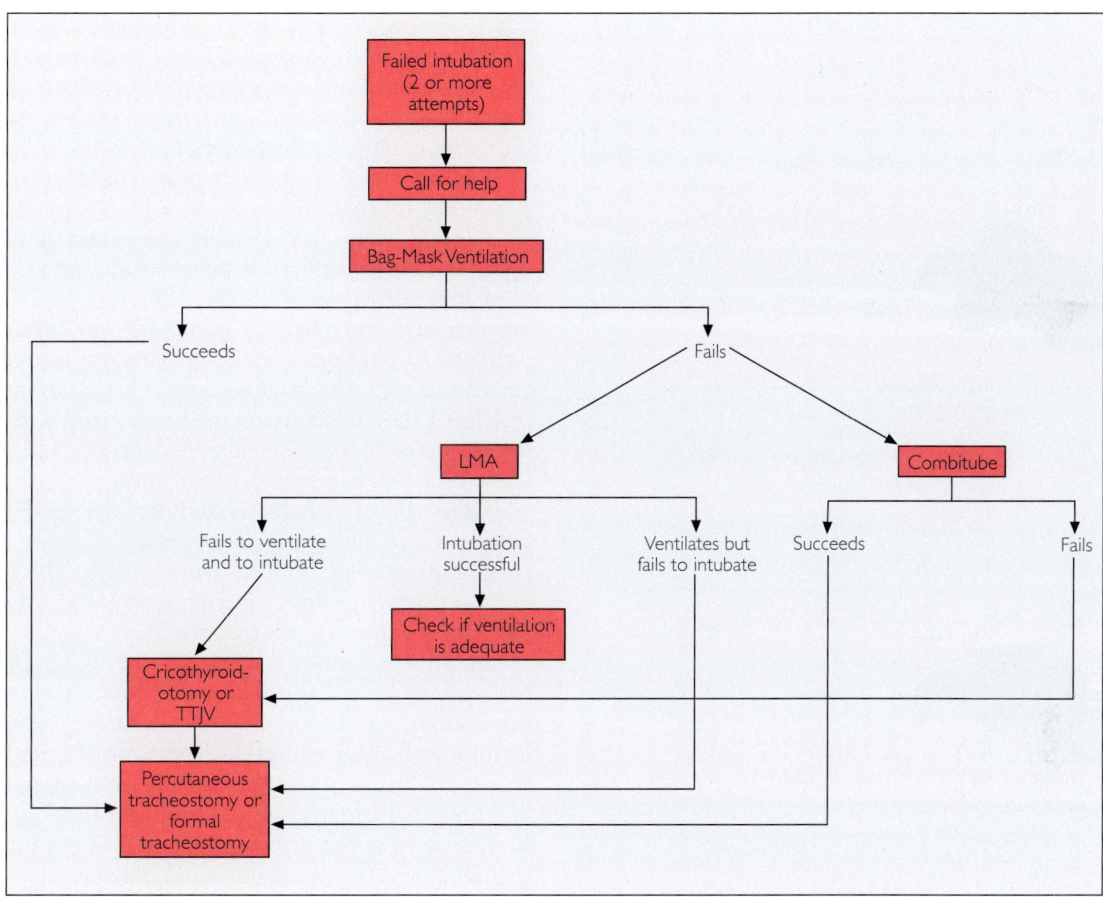

Fig 54.7: Algorithm for the management of difficult airway and ventilation (in the ICU) in a life and death emergency.

physician should note whether the bag-mask ventilation is effective, as judged by good breath sounds over both lungs and by an oxygen saturation ≥ 90 per cent. Difficulties in bag-mask ventilation are likely if any two of the following are present—age > 55 years, edentulous patient, obesity (body mass index > 26 kg/m²), beard, history of snoring.

iii. If a bag-mask ventilation fails or is ineffective, the situation is indeed very critical ('cannot intubate—cannot ventilate' scenario).

Insert a laryngeal mask airway (LMA) or even better (if available), an intubating laryngeal mask airway (I-LMA) and ventilate the patient via this airway. If the intubating LMA is in place, attempt to intubate blindly using the specially designed endotracheal tube that goes with the I-LMA. *Intubation (with a small-sized endotracheal tube) can also be attempted through a plain LMA with the aid of a fibreoptic bronchoscope.*

If effective ventilation through an LMA or a combitube fails, and intubation via the LMA or via the I-LMA is unsuccessful, the quickest way of securing ventilation and preventing death from hypoxia, is by performing a cricothyroidotomy. A cricothyroidotomy should be promptly followed by an emergency percutaneous tracheostomy or by an emergency formal tracheostomy.

iv. Even if either bag-mask ventilation or ventilation through an LMA is successful, a more permanent and secure artificial airway is mandatory if spontaneous effective breathing

has not returned. This is achieved either by a percutaneous tracheostomy or a formal tracheostomy. In expert hands, this can be performed within 10 to 15 minutes.

v. If a pre-intubation clinical evaluation suggests that bag-mask ventilation or LMA ventilation cannot possibly be successful (as in extreme obstruction to the oropharynx, facial, neck injuries), proceed straight to a cricothyroidotomy, or a percutaneous tracheostomy, or a formal tracheostomy depending on the degree of the urgency of the situation.

vi. Transtracheal jet ventilation (TTJV) is an alternative to a surgical airway in a 'cannot intubate–cannot ventilate' situation. After stabilizing the larynx, a 12–16-gauge catheter-over-needle (attached to a syringe particularly filled with saline) is directed caudally through the cricothyroid membrane into the trachea. Tracheal entry is confirmed by aspiration of air bubbles. The catheter is now advanced (up to the hub), over the needle into the trachea with the aid of a small skin incision. The placement is confirmed by aspiration of air. The hub of the catheter is connected to a jet ventilation system. Care should be taken to stabilize the catheter and prevent any air leak at the incision site. We are not familiar with TTJV but it has been performed in all age groups and is the preferred surgical airway in children below 12 years. Airway obstruction below the larynx or complete upper airway obstruction can render expiration impossible and

is a contraindication to TTJV. Complications with TTJV include subcutaneous emphysema, oesophageal puncture, bleeding, and barotraumas. TTJV is an emergency measure and is continued only till such time as a definitive airway has been secured.

2. Failed intubation attempts in situations which are emergent but which still allow some time to the intensivist for establishing an airway.

In the above circumstance, the intensivist should use one or more of the other intubation techniques:

(a) Direct laryngoscopy with topical or local anaesthesia (if topical anaesthesia has not been already used);
(b) Use of a stylet, preferably a lighted one, to help guide the endotracheal tube into the trachea;
(c) A flexible fibreoptic scope to aid nasal or oral intubation;
(d) Blind nasal intubation;
(e) Intubation through an LMA;
(f) Retrograde intubation (in very rare circumstances).

Retrograde intubation is attempted by first puncturing the cricothyroid membrane with an 18-gauge introducer needle with catheter. A guide wire is threaded through the needle cephalad into the oropharynx and is then pulled out under vision using Magill's forceps. The guide wire is then placed directly in the lumen of the endotracheal tube. The latter is then guided along the guide wire through the glottis into the trachea. The guide wire is now pulled out through the proximal end of the endotracheal tube and the endotracheal tube fixed in proper position. This procedure requires practice and is more difficult than it appears; we have as yet never attempted retrotracheal intubation in our units.

TRACHEOSTOMY

A tracheostomy is in our opinion the most satisfactory artificial airway, particularly when the airway needs to be maintained for over 7 to 10 days. It completely bypasses the upper airway and the glottis, thus preventing any potential complications in that area. It causes less resistance to airflow (vis-à-vis the endotracheal tube), reduces dead space, allows easy and efficient suction of the tracheobronchial tree, and is easy to fix and stabilize. The conscious patient can eat freely, is not bothered by oropharyngeal secretions commonly observed with endotracheal tubes and tolerates the tracheostomy without undue discomfort. When performed by a skilled, experienced surgeon, the overall mortality (procedural with the tube in situ, or after removal) is around 1.5% (range 0–5%). This holds even when the procedure is done in critically ill patients.

Endotracheal Tube vs. Tracheostomy

There is still a controversy as to when to continue with an endotracheal tube and when to opt for a tracheostomy. The decision to do a tracheostomy or persist with the endotracheal tube rests on the intensivist's perception of optimal patient care, available nursing care and the unit's experience and record of complications with each of the two artificial airways.

We prefer to do an elective tracheostomy after first intubating the patient, whenever we are convinced that the disease

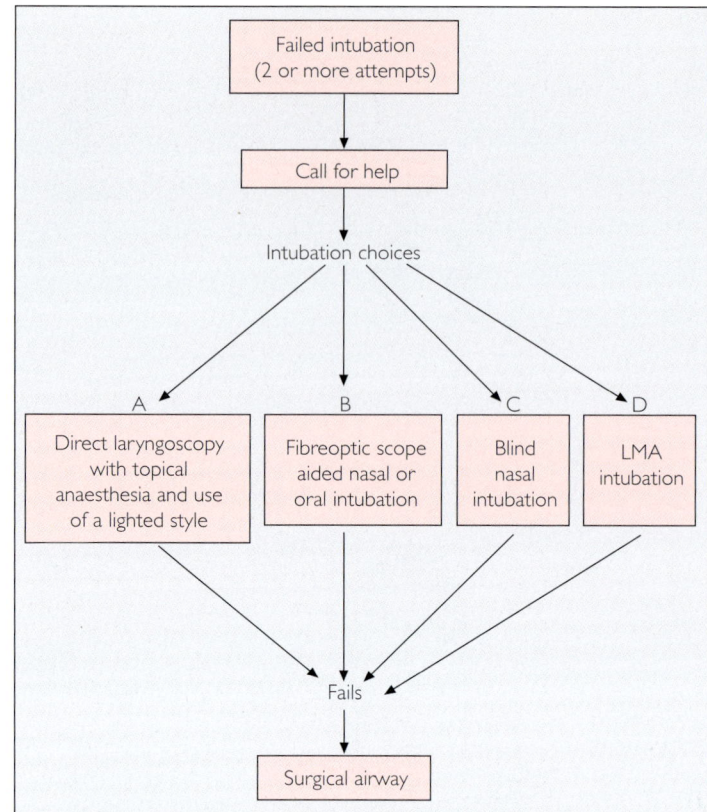

Fig 54.8: Algorithm for the management of difficult airway and ventilation (in the ICU) in failed laryngoscopic attempts in less emergent situations.

will necessitate the use of an artificial airway for more than 7 days. If it is difficult to gauge the time duration required for the artificial airway, we persist with the endotracheal tube for about 7 to 10 days, and then change over to a tracheostomy. Probably each unit has its own preferences. We base our preferences on the fact that our unit has had few complications with tracheostomies, and that tracheobronchial toilet with suction of secretions is far easier through a tracheostomy than through an endotracheal tube. We have also noticed a significant incidence of subglottic oedema and stenosis whenever an endotracheal tube has been in place for more than 7 to 10 days, prompting us to switch to a tracheostomy if we feel that an artificial airway is required beyond that period of time. However, there are many units in the West who persist with an endotracheal tube for as long as three weeks without encountering significant complications.

COMPLICATIONS

The inability to secure a patent airway or the inability to perform bag-mask ventilation so as to provide oxygenation can lead to cardiac arrest with hypoxic brain damage.

Endotracheal intubation can lead to damage to teeth, to the mucosa of the airways and to the larynx, sometimes causing life-threatening haemorrhage. These risks are increased in patients with coagulopathy and in those with markedly inflamed mucosa of the air passage. The tracheotomy tube may be misplaced outside the trachea causing severe subcutaneous emphysema and life-threatening hypoxemia. Similarly, an endotracheal tube may be misplaced in the oesophagus; attempts at ventilation

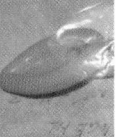

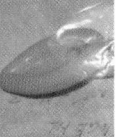

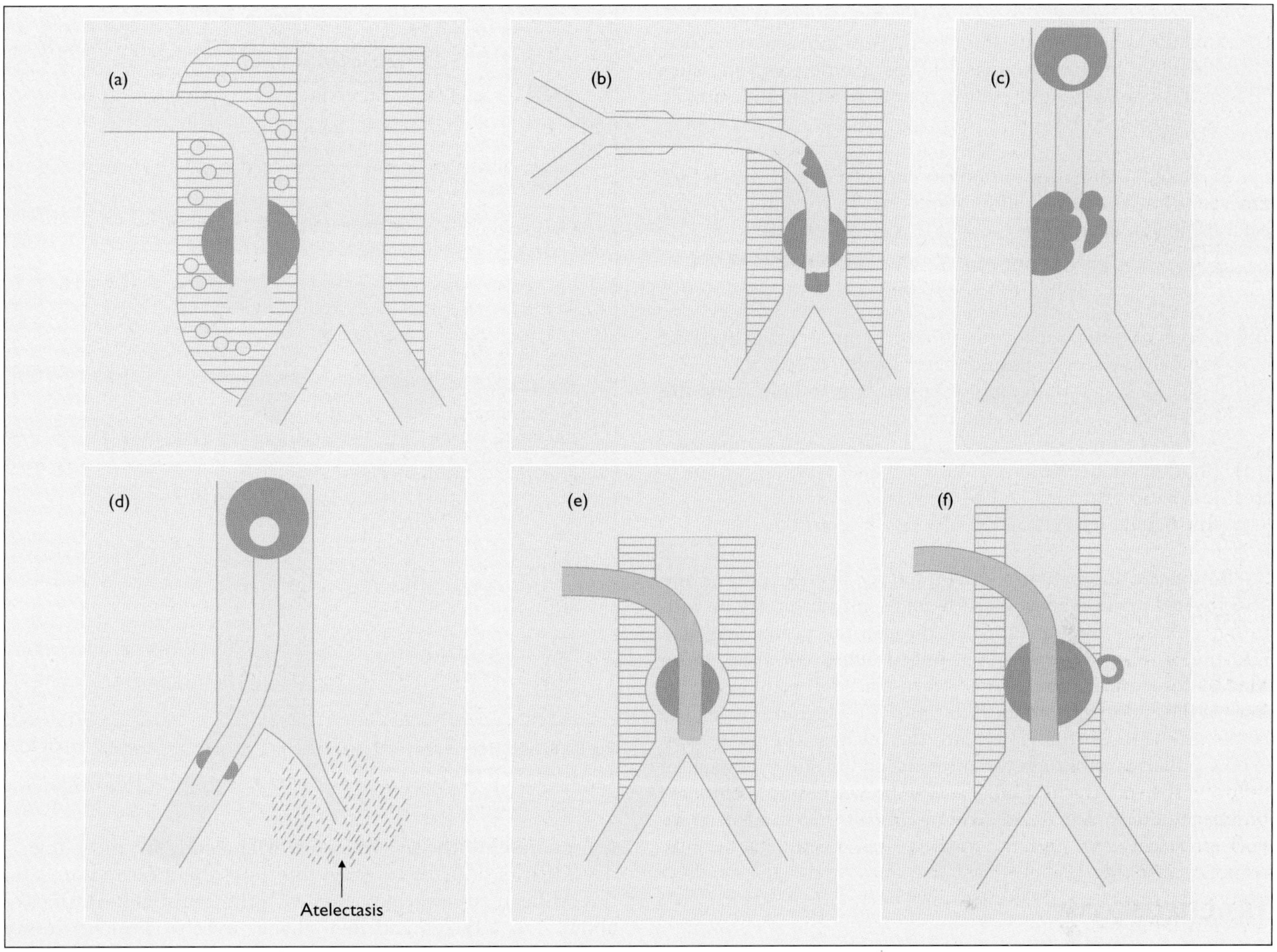

Fig 54.9: Complications of tracheostomy (a) Tube in pretracheal fascia-resulting in surgical emphysema of face and neck and sometimes of the mediastinum (b) Blocked tube (c) Overinflated cuff slipping over the end and blocking it (d) Tube slipping into right main bronchus, preventing ventilation to the left lung (e) Damage to trachea, either due to a very tight-fitting tube with an overinflated cuff, or injury to the posterior wall-end result, dilatation (as in the figure) or stricture (f) Erosion of the posterior wall of the trachea, and rarely erosion of the innominate artery.

Source: Udwadia FE. (1979). *Diagnosis and Management of Acute Respiratory Failure*. Oxford University Press, Mumbai.

would then cause acute gastric dilation and worsening of pre-existing hypoxia.

The endotracheal tube instead of being above the carina may lie in the right main bronchus resulting in ventilation of the right lung and collapse of the left. Position of endotracheal and tracheostomy tubes should be checked by an X-ray to ensure correct placement.

Tracheostomies can lead to bilateral pneumothorax because of the proximity of the apices of the lungs. Damage to neck veins during the surgical procedures can cause uncontrollable haemorrhage.

MAINTAINING THE ARTIFICIAL AIRWAY

It is not enough to establish and secure the airway. It is equally important to maintain, manage and care for the artificial airway,

if the hazards and complications involving the use of artificial airways are to be minimized.

Tracheostomy Care

A high tracheostomy is always preferable as it enables the tip of the tube to lie well above the carina. It is best to use the largest tube that can be comfortably accommodated by the trachea. Small tubes should be avoided as they tend to get blocked, and they offer resistance to airflow. This is particularly unwelcome in those patients with acute respiratory failure who have well-marked airways obstruction, or who have a low compliance due to 'stiff lungs'. The tube should have an even inflated cuff. High residual volume (low-pressure) cuffs should be always used; high-pressure cuffs have no place in modern respiratory care. Even when using high-

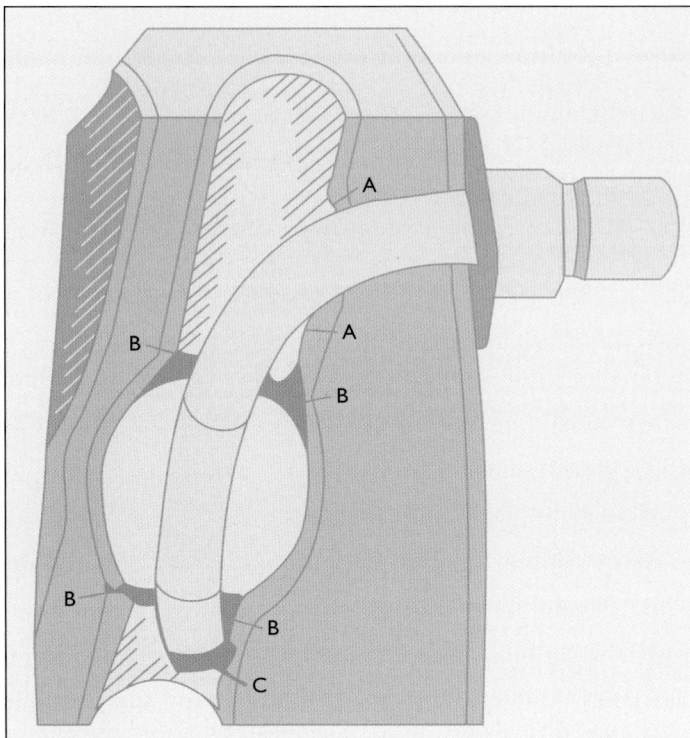

Fig 54.10: Sites for occurrence of post-extubation tracheal stenosis. A—site of tracheostomy, B—cuff site (commonest), C—where tip irritates tracheal wall.

Table 54.2: Salient points in tracheostomy care
Use sterile gloves for handling tracheostomy tube
Care of cuff
– Use minimal occluding volume for inflating cuff—minimal leak techniques
– Measure cuff pressure daily, and keep this within acceptable limits (14–24 cm H_2O)
– Deflate cuff periodically, except when this is contraindicated for specific reasons
Care over suction of secretions
– Use 'no-touch' sterile technique
– Pre-oxygenate (with high FIO_2) a haemodynamically unstable patient before suction
– Do not suck for more than 10 seconds
– Do not use a very large bore catheter for suction
– If possible, suck through an adaptor so that ventilator support on high-flow oxyen is not interrupted
– Stop suction if bradycardia or hypotension occur
– Increase FIO_2 to 100 per cent for a short time
– Liquefy viscid secretions; use physiotherapy
– Humidify inspired gas
Care of tracheostomy tube
– Ensure that tube is central in position and does not tilt and slip into one bronchus
– Ensure that tube does not get blocked
– Change tube every 4–7 days
Care of tracheostomy wound
– Use sterile dressing and antibiotic ointment
– Be alert to possible complications of tracheostomy

volume, low-pressure cuffed tubes, the cuff pressure should be checked daily and kept within acceptable limits. Excessive cuff pressures can induce tracheal injury and subsequent stenosis, particularly if the tracheostomy has been in use over several days or weeks. Salient points in tracheostomy care are given in Table 54.2.

SPECIAL CONSIDERATIONS IN AIRWAY MANAGEMENT

Cervical Spine Injury

A patient with polytrauma, who requires intubation should be presumed to have a cervical spine injury. In the absence of severe maxillo-facial trauma or cerebrospinal rhinorrhoea, a nasal intubation can be attempted. However, if urgent intubation is required as in the apnoeic or hypoxic patient, oral intubation should be done. During oral endotracheal intubation, a colleague or assistant should hold the neck in position, ensuring axial stability and preventing any flexion or anterior movement of the neck for fear of damaging the spinal cord.

Increased Intracranial Tension

Intubating patients with head injury who have a rise in intracranial pressure may be difficult for several reasons—change in mental state, difficulty in opening the mouth, associated facial trauma. Further rise in intracranial pressure should be avoided as far as possible during intubation. Also, cervical spine trauma should always be suspected in a patient with head injury. The anaesthetic agent used for intubating these patients should ideally preserve cerebral perfusion, and lower cerebral blood volume while maintaining haemodynamic stability. Thiopental offers neuroprotection but cerebral hypoperfusion may result from its depressant effect on the myocardium and because of peripheral vasodilatation. Etomidate is preferred in haemodynamically unstable patients. If a neuroparalytic agent needs to be used for intubation, vecuronium (0.25 mg/kg) or rocuronium (1.2 mg/kg) is to be preferred.

In patients with polytrauma including head injury with raised intracranial pressure, it may at times be impossible to perform a laryngoscopic endotracheal intubation. The airway may need to be secured by alternative means.

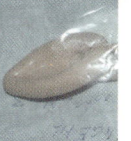

SUGGESTED READING

Blanda M. Emergency airway management. *Emerg Med Clin North Am.* 1 Feb. 2003; 21(1): 1–26.

Idris AH. Advances in airway management. *Emerg Med Clin North Am.* 1 Nov. 2002; 20(4): 843–57, ix.

Mace SE. Challenges and advances in intubation: rapid sequence intubation. *Emerg Med Clin North Am.* 1 Nov. 2008; 26(4): 1043–68, x.

Marco CA. Airway adjuncts. *Emerg Med Clin North Am.* 1 Nov. 2008; 26(4): 1015–27, x.

Vissers RJ. The high-risk airway. *Emerg Med Clin North Am.* 1 Feb. 2010; 28(1): 203–17, ix–x.

Walz JM. Airway management in critical illness. *Chest.* 1 Feb. 2007; 131(2): 608–20.

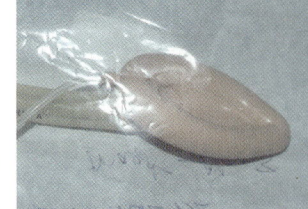

CHAPTER **55** # Mechanical Ventilation

Mechanical ventilation as a therapeutic intervention was first widely used during the poliomyelitis epidemic in Europe and the United States in the 1940s and 1950s. Since then there have been great advances in technology, so that negative-pressure ventilators that were used originally in the 1940s and 1950s have been replaced by increasingly sophisticated positive-pressure machines.

The purpose of mechanical ventilation is to provide ventilation support partially or fully by an external device to patients who cannot maintain an adequate gas exchange, as for example in acute respiratory failure. Ventilator support also reduces the oxygen cost of breathing. Mechanical ventilator support however has its own hazards; these include ventilator-induced lung injury, barotrauma, adverse hemodynamic changes and the potential for serious nosocomial infection.

Ventilator support to any critically ill individual requires expertise and round-the-clock supervision and care. Life in many such patients is totally dependent on the efficient working of a machine. A mechanical failure, accidental disconnection of the machine from the patient, or a sudden obstruction of the airway, are all potential disasters which can lead to sudden death or brain damage from protracted hypoxia. A patient on mechanical ventilator support must therefore never be left unattended even for a minute. Thus the optimal and safe use of mechanical ventilation is only possible in intensive care units (ICUs). Though the standard of critical care (which includes ventilator support) has improved and continues to improve significantly at least in the large metropolitan cities of India, care provided in large public and district hospitals in India and many other developing countries leaves much to be desired. In fact critical care units in the poor countries of the world are often mere apologies of what they ought to be, or are nonexistent. In the absence of a full-fledged ICU, the next best option is to use ventilator support in a patient who needs it, in a special or even a general ward, provided that the medical registrar and nurses are well trained in ventilator management. We managed to do this at one of the large public teaching hospitals in Mumbai, and salvaged a number of very ill patients who would otherwise have died. The need for all medical registrars (at least in the large hospitals of India and other developing countries) to be familiar with the use of mechanical ventilators is thus imperative. It is the duty of the medical and administrative staff of such hospitals to provide basic facilities, and train a team of doctors and nurses who can manage critically ill patients on ventilator support, even in the absence of well-equipped ICUs.

This chapter to start with briefly tabulates the physiological effects of mechanical ventilation. It then proceeds to discuss the indications and criteria for ventilator support, types of ventilators for intermittent positive-pressure ventilation (IPPV),

and the management of ventilatory support. This is followed by a description of the different modes of ventilator support, and the use of positive end-expiratory pressure (PEEP) as an adjunct. Then comes a section on the complications of mechanical ventilation, followed by a discussion on weaning from ventilator support. The chapter ends with a discussion on non-invasive ventilator support and of respiratory monitoring during mechanical ventilation.

INDICATIONS FOR MECHANICAL VENTILATION

In many ICUs in Mumbai and India, there is yet a certain hesitation and trepidation observed regarding the use of mechanical ventilation in patients who need ventilator support. In other words, mechanical ventilation is started much later than it should have been in the natural history of a disease requiring ventilatory support. The other equally common misconception and error is to be in a tearing hurry to remove ventilator support in a critically ill patient. Such a premature withdrawal of ventilator support is love's labour lost—the patient regresses from near recovery to a critical state, which again necessitates the use of the ventilator.

Established Acute Respiratory Failure

Early ventilator support is now initiated by all good units in patients with acute respiratory failure. The criteria and timing for initiating support depend on the aetiological agent producing acute respiratory failure, and above all, on the rate at which respiratory function is observed to deteriorate. Different diseases producing acute respiratory failure present their own special problems with regard to initiating mechanical ventilation, technicalities in maintaining ventilation, and difficulties in weaning the patient from ventilator support. It is therefore best from the practical point of view to consider the indications in acute respiratory failure, with reference to the different groups of diseases frequently encountered in the ICU.

VENTILATOR SUPPORT IN PRIMARY VENTILATORY FAILURE
The commonest indication for mechanical ventilation is acute primary failure of ventilation. Ventilatory failure occurs commonly in poisonings that depress the central nervous system (CNS), in acute inflammatory and other diseases involving the CNS, in some patients with head injury, increased intracranial tension, poliomyelitis, acute infective polyneuritis, and myasthenia gravis. Severe tetanus is an important cause of ventilatory failure in India. Neuromuscular paralysis following a krait or cobra bite is particularly common in South India. The lungs are normal to start with, but changes within the lungs

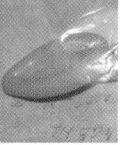

(chiefly increasing widespread atelectasis), almost always occur if treatment is delayed. In many patients with neuromuscular disease, deterioration can occur suddenly, almost precipitously, with disastrous consequences. It is therefore wise to start early ventilatory support in these patients.

VENTILATOR SUPPORT IN A HYPOVENTILATING COMATOSE PATIENT

Deep coma is an indication for securing the airways with an endotracheal tube or a tracheostomy. Hypoventilation in such patients may be due to depressed respiratory drive or secretions causing obstructed airways or patchy atelectasis. Hypoxia and hypercapnia resulting from hypoventilation may further impair the conscious state, which in turn may further depress ventilation. Unless the patient is clearly hyperventilating, a deeply comatose patient is safer on mechanical ventilation.

VENTILATOR SUPPORT IN ACUTE PULMONARY DISEASE

These patients are hypoxic due to hypoxaemic acute respiratory failure. Typical examples are in acute lung injury (ARDS), and fulminant pneumonia. Patients with acute pulmonary disease are difficult to ventilate. They have a strong respiratory drive, are often severely hypoxic, and 'fight' the ventilator. An inability to maintain a PaO_2 of > 55 mm Hg while on oxygen at a flow rate of 6–8 l/min, is an indication for initiating ventilator support. Other criteria for starting mechanical ventilation in these patients are dealt with later.

VENTILATOR SUPPORT IN FULMINANT PULMONARY OEDEMA

Acute pulmonary oedema, if fulminant, literally chokes the patient at the level of the alveoli. Mechanical ventilation is life-saving not only because it allows the maintenance of an adequate PaO_2, but perhaps because the high inflation pressures used to ventilate the lungs reduces the transudation of fluid from the alveolar capillaries into the alveoli. Ventilator support buys time during which diuretics like furosemide have a chance to act, and other corrective measures to treat the underlying cause of acute pulmonary oedema may be profitably undertaken.

VENTILATOR SUPPORT IN ACUTE THROMBOEMBOLIC LUNG DISEASE

Ventilator support is indicated if the PaO_2 is < 60 mm Hg on supplemental oxygen, particularly in the presence of shock.

VENTILATOR SUPPORT IN ACUTE ON CHRONIC RESPIRATORY FAILURE IN PATIENTS WITH CHRONIC AIRWAYS OBSTRUCTION

Many patients in this group are used to a low PaO_2 < 65 mm Hg, and a high $PaCO_2$ > 50–60 mm Hg. Ventilator support should not be used unless all other modalities of treatment have been of no avail, clinical deterioration is evident, and there is a further deterioration in the arterial blood gases and arterial pH. In such patients ventilatory support is fraught with difficulty, and requires experience and expertise.

VENTILATOR SUPPORT IN ACUTE SEVERE ASTHMA

Acute severe asthma is probably one of the most difficult problems for effective mechanical ventilation. Yet ventilator support is life-saving in those cases of acute severe asthma not responding to corticosteroids, nebulized bronchodilators and other medical therapy.

VENTILATOR SUPPORT IN PATIENTS WITH SEVERE MUSCLE FATIGUE

Severe muscle fatigue (involving the muscles of respiration), is an increasingly recognized and important cause of hypoventilation and respiratory failure. Muscle fatigue can occur in patients with primary neuromuscular disease involving the respiratory muscles. It occurs much more frequently in lung disease and in any condition (not necessarily involving the lungs), where ventilatory demands are excessive. The timing of initiating ventilator support in these patients is a matter of fine judgment. Altered blood gases or feeble ventilatory efforts are of course an immediate indication. Irregular breathing patterns, or the presence of a respiratory paradox in which the abdominal muscles move inwards rather than outwards during inspiration, point to excessive muscle fatigue. Respiratory alternans is characterized by alternate excursions involving the diaphragm and the intercostals, and is also a pointer to muscle fatigue. Another important pointer to impending disaster is the presence of apnoeic spells which are often forerunners of prolonged respiratory arrest. It is better to ventilate such patients even if the arterial blood gases are not significantly distorted, rather than wait for disaster to occur.

Factors which precipitate and contribute to respiratory muscle fatigue are hypoperfusion of the muscles, hypermetabolic states leading to an increased work load on the muscles of respiration, hypoxia, electrolyte and acid-base disturbances, poor nutrition as in alcoholics or those with chronic liver or renal diseases, and in old, feeble, debilitated patients.

Incipient Respiratory Failure

Mechanical ventilation is increasingly being used in patients in whom some degree of respiratory failure is anticipated. Perhaps the most important group comprises patients who have to meet increased ventilatory demands, and who therefore sooner or later show evidence of respiratory muscle fatigue. This is typically seen in acute severe asthma, but can occur in numerous medical and surgical problems. It is difficult for a seriously ill patient to sustain a ventilatory rate of > 35–40/min or a minute ventilation >10–12 l/min for any prolonged period of time without increasing muscle fatigue and the danger of impending sudden respiratory failure.

There is a special category of surgical patients who frequently require ventilator support for impending or insidious respiratory failure. These are obese individuals who have undergone upper abdominal surgery. This often leads to 'fixed' or 'splinted' domes of the diaphragm resulting in a loss of volume in both lower lobes. These patients are markedly tachypnoeic, particularly in the presence of fever and infection; their minute ventilation is often as high as 12–15 l/min, and their respiratory rates between 35–45/min. They maintain their arterial blood gases within the normal range for some length of time, but not uncommonly these patients go into sudden respiratory failure, deteriorate sharply, and pose problems in emergency intubation and ventilation. A quick anticipation of worsening problems calls for early intubation and ventilator support before such a disaster occurs.

Other susceptible patients in whom hypoventilation is a likely sequel include poor-risk surgical patients whose recovery from surgery or trauma is hindered by obesity, chronic lung disease, old age, debility, and electrolyte imbalance. In all these patients postoperative ventilatory support is merely an extension of surgical care in the operation theatre. They may require mechanical ventilation for a period varying from a few hours to a few days, and are weaned off ventilator support when they can maintain adequate gas exchange on spontaneous breathing.

Similarly, in acute or fulminant parenchymal lung disease where the tempo of impairment of respiratory reserve and respiratory function is very rapid, it is best to anticipate events in advance to allow for elective intubation and ventilatory support.

Low-Output States and Septic Shock

Ventilator support is now always indicated in low cardiac output states as in cardiogenic shock, or for that matter in shock from any aetiology. It is often used in septic shock, at times quite early in the natural history, when the march of events signifies a rapidly evolving dangerous clinical state. In shock from any cause, and in low-output states of any aetiology (for example, in advanced liver cell failure or multiorgan failure), tissue perfusion is inadequate in relation to tissue oxygen needs. Also, a low cardiac output is generally associated with a low PvO_2, which in turn is responsible for a low PaO_2. Shock of any aetiology which results in low pulmonary artery pressure and diminished perfusion of the lungs leads to an increase both in the VD/VT ratio, as well as to a V/Q imbalance. Ventilator support helps in two ways: (i) with an increase in FIO_2 (if needs be to 70–80%), the PaO_2 increases, and therefore both the arterial oxygenation and the arterial oxygen content rise; (ii) the muscles of respiration are rested once the ventilator takes over the function of ventilation. This prevents incipient respiratory failure from progressing to frank ventilatory failure, and even ventilatory arrest. In patients who breathe excessively, the oxygen cost of breathing is considerably increased. At rest, the normal work of breathing accounts for 2–3% of total oxygen consumption. This can increase in acute respiratory failure to as high as 35–40%. In low-output states, resting the overworked respiratory muscles through mechanical ventilation sharply reduces the oxygen cost of breathing and allows more oxygen to be diverted to vital organs starved of their oxygen supply. However, in critically ill patients it is equally important to control fever, shivering, constant movement and restlessness, as these can all contribute to increased oxygen consumption, and thereby reduce the already meagre available oxygen supply to the vital organs.

Mechanical Ventilation for the Specific Purpose of Hyperventilation

A comparatively rare indication for mechanical ventilation is to hyperventilate patients with head injury, when associated with increased intracranial pressure. Hyperventilating these patients reduces the $PaCO_2$ which leads to reduction in the cerebral blood flow, and hence in the intracranial pressure. Hyperventilation is generally combined with sedation and muscle paralysis to prevent coughing and clashing with the ventilator, as these could lead to a rise in intracranial pressure. Clinicians often prefer to manage unconscious neurological and neurosurgical patients with increased intracranial pressure, with controlled mechanical hyperventilation. The same approach is sometimes used to counter cerebral oedema following resuscitation after a cardiopulmonary arrest or in patients with cerebral oedema consequent to a massive cerebrovascular accident. However, the efficacy of hyperventilation in all the above-mentioned situations is temporary (generally not exceeding 48 hours) and debatable.

Table 55.1: Indications for mechanical ventilation
A. Established Acute Respiratory Failure
• Primary ventilatory failure where lungs are normal to start with e.g. poisonings that depress the CNS, CNS and neuromuscular disorders (poliomelitis, infective polyneuritis, myasthenia), snake bite, severe tetanus
• Hypoventilating comatose patients
• Acute pulmonary disease e.g. fulminant pneumonia, acute lung injury (ARDS)
• Fulminant pulmonary oedema
• Major or massive pulmonary embolism
• Major or massive atelectasis
• Patients with COPD in acute crisis, unresponsive to conventional therapy
• Patients with acute severe asthma unresponsive to conventional therapy
• Patients with severe respiratory muscle fatigue
B. Incipient Respiratory Failure
• Patients with excessive ventilatory demands
• Obese patients who have undergone upper abdominal surgery, or poor risk surgical patients
• Patients with acute/fulminant parenchymal lung disease with rapidly progressive impairment of pulmonary function and reserve
• Respiratory muscle fatigue in critical illnesses
C. Low-Output States—Shock of any Aetiology
D. Purposeful Hyperventilation
To decrease intracranial tension in patients with head injury associated with increased intracranial tension
To reduce cerebral oedema after CPR or massive CVA

OBJECTIVE CRITERIA FOR INITIATING VENTILATOR SUPPORT IN ADULTS

The criteria enumerated in Table 55.2 are mere guidelines, and not sacrosanct rules. It is crucial to take the clinical picture, the evolution of the disease in a given patient, and the trend and rate of change in the parameters outlined below, into consideration.

The parameters given in Table 55.2 apply to patients in ventilatory failure, and to respiratory failure occurring with acute lung disease; they are not applicable to patients with chronic

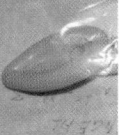

Table 55.2: Criteria for initiating ventilator support in adults
Respiratory rate > 35/min
VC < 10–15 ml/kg
MV > 10–12 l/min over a prolonged period
Maximum Inspiratory Force < –20 cm H_2O
PaO_2 < 60 mm Hg on nasal oxygen at 6–8 l/min and/or $PaCO_2$ > 55 mm Hg
Alveolar-arterial oxygen gradient > 300–350 mm Hg on FIO_2 of 1
V_D/V_T > 0.6
Visible excessive work of breathing in critically ill or debiliated patients
Clinical evidence of respiratory muscle fatigue • Poor chest excursions • Tachypnoea • Respiratory muscle paradox, 'respiratory alternans' • Apnoeic spells

Table 55.3: Comparison between Volume-controlled (Volume-targeted) and Pressure-controlled (Pressure-targeted) Ventilation		
	Volume-targeted	Pressure-targeted
Rate	Set or variable	Set or variable
Tidal volume (VT)	Set	Variable
Peak Airway Pressure	Variable	Set
Peak Alveolar Pressure	Variable	Set
Peak Flow	Set	Variable
I:E Ratio	Variable	Set

obstructive airways disease. These patients even under normal or basal conditions may have a PaO_2 of 60 mm Hg, and a $PaCO_2$ between 55–60 mm Hg. They are used to hypoxia and hypercapnia, and tolerate both rather well.

TYPES OF VENTILATORS FOR INTERMITTENT POSITIVE PRESSURE VENTILATION

Ventilators in intensive care units are either volume-cycled or pressure-cycled or time-cycled.

A volume-cycled, i.e. a volume-targeted ventilator, delivers a preset volume and continues to do so regardless of a change in the patient's airway resistance or lung compliance.

A pressure-cycled, i.e. a pressure-targeted ventilator, cycles to expiration after a specified preset pressure has been attained. Thus, gas flows into the lungs until a preset pressure limit is reached. The volume delivered will therefore change if the airway resistance and/or the lung compliance change.

In a time-cycled ventilator, the inspiratory phase ends when a predetermined time has elapsed. This time remains fixed, and is controlled by a timing mechanism within the ventilator, which is unaffected by conditions in the patient's lungs.

Volume-targeted ventilatory support is more flexible, easier to learn, and easier to manage than pressure-targeted or time-cycled ventilator support. All modern ventilators are capable of delivering adequate minute ventilation and of varying the oxygen concentration (FIO_2) from 25–100%.

Most modern ventilators incorporate within a single unit, mechanisms that allow either volume-targeted or pressure-targeted ventilatory support, the use of positive end-expiratory pressure (PEEP), and the choice of several modes of ventilator support, detailed later. Adjustment of minute ventilation, respiratory rates, flow rates, inspiratory-expiratory ratios are also possible. The ventilator is fitted with a series of alarms for better patient care, and can be fitted with modules that can monitor and display lung mechanics (compliance, airway resistance, waveforms, flow-volume loops) and the end-tidal PCO_2.

From the clinical viewpoint, neither volume-targeted, nor pressure-targeted ventilation offers a distinct advantage with regard to gas exchange, hemodynamic stability, and pulmonary mechanics.

The major advantage of volume-targeted ventilatory support is its ease of application, and the provision of a fixed tidal volume in spite of changing airway resistance or pulmonary compliance.

The main advantage of pressure-cycled or pressure-targeted ventilation is that gas is delivered at a fixed preset pressure; if there is increased impedance to ventilation (either due to increased airways resistance or to a lowered pulmonary compliance), the tidal volume delivered falls. Overstretching of the alveoli with resulting volutrauma, barotraumas and biotrauma is thus prevented. Pressure-control ventilation may also be able to answer the high inspiratory flow demands of some critically ill patients.

MANAGEMENT OF MECHANICAL VENTILATION

Initiating Ventilation—Basics of Initial Ventilator Setup

There are a number of ventilator modes available to help ventilate a patient. We generally initiate ventilator support with volume-controlled or volume-targeted ventilation using the assist-control mode. In assist-control ventilation, the patient triggers the inspiration by a spontaneous effort which is enhanced by the ventilator. In this mode, if for some reason the patient fails to trigger the machine, the machine takes over, initiates inspiration and takes over full ventilatory support. Most patients with different respiratory problems can be adequately ventilated by the volume-targeted, assist-control mode.

TIDAL VOLUME (V_T)

The tidal volume for an individual patient should be set between 5–10 ml/kg body weight. Selection of tidal volume in a given patient is influenced by the nature of the disease, the approximate minute ventilation requirement, pulmonary compliance, airway resistance, airway pressure, PaO_2 and $PaCO_2$.

Very low tidal volumes result in atelectasis, hypoventilation, hypoxaemia. On the other hand, very high tidal volumes can cause respiratory alkalosis, decrease cardiac output by reducing venous return and predispose to barotrauma, volutrauma and biotrauma. There is definite evidence that overstretch of alveolar walls through very large tidal volumes can induce lung 'injury'.

In patients with normal lungs to start with (as in neuromuscular disease causing respiratory failure, CNS disease, coma, poisoning, and immediate postoperative conditions), the tidal volume is set at 10 ml/kg.

In patients whose lungs are stiff because of abnormal respiratory mechanics (as in acute lung injury, pneumonia) tidal volumes are set at 5–7 ml/kg. A convenient algorithm is to start with 10 ml/kg, stabilize the patient and then progressively reduce the tidal volume to 5–7 ml/kg so that the plateau pressure does not exceed 30 cm H_2O.

RESPIRATORY RATE

The rate is generally set between 10–14 breaths per minute, if the patient is clinically stable. Higher rates may be required (20–25/minute) in patients with stiff lungs (e.g. acute respiratory distress syndrome (ARDS)), so as to match the machine to the spontaneous breathing pattern of the patient. Lower rates may be necessary in chronic obstructive pulmonary disease (COPD) patients where minute ventilation needs to be restricted. If the respiratory rate is too high, respiratory alkalosis, auto-PEEP and barotrauma can result. If too low, hypoventilation, hypoxaemia and patient discomfort are observed.

MINUTE VENTILATION

Minute ventilation is set according to the approximate ventilatory requirements of a patient and to start with is set at 5–10 l/minute. The minute ventilation decided upon is also influenced by the nature of the disease and the altered respiratory mechanics for which ventilatory support is offered.

INSPIRATION-EXPIRATION RATIO (I: E RATIO)

The I: E ratio to start with, is set at 1: 2 or 1: 3 to allow sufficient time for expiration.

OXYGEN CONCENTRATION

If the patient is hypoxic, the FIO_2 to start with should be 1.0. After 15 to 20 minutes, this is gradually reduced to a level which allows a $PaO_2 \geq 60$ mm Hg, and an O_2 saturation $\geq 90\%$.

INSPIRATORY FLOW RATE

The inspiratory flow rate is usually set at 40–60 l/minute in volume-targeted ventilation. This can be increased to 60–100 l/min in patients with high inspiratory demands. However, higher inspiratory flow rates would cause an increase in the peak inspiratory pressure. Lower flow rates can be used to decrease peak inspiratory pressure in patients who to start with have high peak inspiratory pressures (as in ARDS). Lowering inspiratory flow rates would increase inspiratory time, but decrease expiratory time—this could lead to air trapping, auto-PEEP, patient discomfort and barotrauma.

PEEP

PEEP may need to be used if the O_2 saturation is < 90% on an $FIO_2 > 0.5$. (See subsequent section on PEEP.)

It needs to be stressed that the tidal volume, respiratory rate, minute ventilation, I: E ratio and inspiratory flow rates are so adjusted as to enable good exchange of gases and yet maintain a plateau pressure ≤ 30 cm H_2O. This lung protection strategy minimizes the risk of barotrauma and volutrauma.

All alarms on the ventilator provided both for patient safety and as indicators of proper functioning of the ventilator should be activated—in particular, the high pressure, low pressure alarm and the apnoea alarm.

Problems at Initiation of Ventilator Support

1. *The major and the commonest problem is difficulty in synchronizing the patient's respiration with the ventilator.* In an unconscious or apnoeic patient this presents no difficulty. The problem is also easily surmountable in patients with respiratory failure due to poisoning, neuromuscular disease or other CNS problems. The following points are helpful in management:

   (i) Allay anxiety and fright in the patient by explaining the situation in a gentle and confident manner, and by the use of a tranquillizer. Diazepam, 5 to 10 mg intravenously is of great help.

   (ii) The commonest cause of difficulty in synchronizing is inadequate alveolar minute ventilation. The minute ventilation selected should result in a $PaCO_2$ between 35–40 mm Hg. Ordinarily a tidal volume of 10 ml/kg with a respiratory rate of 12–15/min is adequate. However, many patients with lung disease require higher minute ventilations than that stated above.

   (iii) If the patient continuously clashes with what appear to be reasonable ventilator settings, it is advisable to proceed as follows:

   (a) Use a high FIO_2 temporarily to ensure that there is no hypoxia—this can be easily checked by noting the oxygen saturation on the pulse oximeter.

   (b) If a very strong respiratory drive is responsible for asynchrony between the patient and the machine, the tidal volume is increased, and the respiratory rate increased to well beyond the patient's spontaneous rate. Once the patient is taken over by the machine, the settings are gradually lowered and modified to the desired values. Generally, if alveolar ventilation is adequate, and if other causes contributing to restlessness and increased respiratory drive are looked into and taken care of, the patient does not fight the machine and is relaxed. The only way to determine whether the alveolar ventilation is adequate is by monitoring the $PaCO_2$. A $PaCO_2 > 45$ mm Hg denotes alveolar hypoventilation; that < 35 mm Hg, alveolar hyperventilation. Hyperventilation in the initial stages reduces the respiratory drive and helps the machine to take over. Once this is achieved minute ventilation is adjusted so that the $PaCO_2$ is maintained around 35 mm Hg, and preferably not < 30 mm Hg.

   (c) In tachypnoeic patients with a strong respiratory drive, the patient's inspiratory flow rate is generally higher than the usual 40–60 l/min set on the machine. Increasing the inspiratory flow rate appropriately, or decreasing the I: E ratio, prevents 'clashing' and allows smoother ventilatory support in these patients.

   (d) Manual control of ventilation by using 100% oxygen for 5 minutes is a useful method for

abolishing the patient's respiratory effort, by ensuring oxygenation, and proper alveolar ventilation.

(e) Besides a strong respiratory drive chiefly related to altered mechanics of the lungs, there are other contributory factors which increase the degree of 'clash' between the machine and the patient. These may be present at the very outset, or may evolve during the critical care of a patient. They are briefly discussed later, and should be recognized and treated for more efficient ventilator support.

(iv) Asynchrony between the machine and the patient may persist, however, in spite of appropriate ventilator settings, the use of corrective measures, and despite all attempts to match the machine to the patient. This generally happens in patients with severe parenchymal lung disease producing very stiff lungs, tachypnoea and severe hypoxia. In many of these patients the spontaneous respiratory rate is > 40 per minute. It is unwise to even attempt to 'match' the machine to this spontaneous respiratory rate. What is more, these patients are critically ill, often with multiorgan failure and cardiovascular instability. It is important that the respiratory muscles are rested in such circumstances. Effective ventilation can be achieved only by depressing respiration, or by inducing neuromuscular paralysis. The respiration can be depressed by the use of 2–4 mg morphine, or 0.2–0.4 mg buprenorphine intravenously, repeated as and when necessary. An alternative is to use 10 mg intravenous diazepam or 2.4 mg midazolam intravenously or an intravenous combination of midazolam and fentanyl titrated to produce the desired effect. The main disadvantage of morphine is hypotension, which should be countered by vasopressors or by a volume load. In patients where morphine or a morphine derivative or diazepam or midazolam or fentanyl is unsuitable or ineffective, particularly in ventilating patients with severe lung injury, it is necessary to use intravenous pancuronium or an intravenous bolus dose of vecuronium 0.08–0.1 mg/kg. After an intravenous bolus dose, vecuronium is given as a 0.8–1.2-μg/kg/min continuous infusion, to induce neuromuscular paralysis and thereby abolish or sharply reduce spontaneous ventilatory support. Pancuronium is given as an intravenous bolus dose of 0.06–0.1 mg/kg and repeated as and when necessary to allow smooth takeover by the machine. It is unwise and often unnecessary to produce total paralysis with curare-like drugs.

2. *Other important problems* occurring within the first few minutes or hours of initiating ventilator support are (i) malposition of the airways; (ii) aspiration of stomach contents; (iii) hypotension. These are dealt with at length under complications of ventilator support.

OBJECTIVES OF VENTILATOR SUPPORT

1. Regulate gas exchange
2. Overcome mechanical problems

Table 55.4: Common problems encountered during initiation of ventilator support
A. Difficulty in synchronising patient's respiration with the ventilator
• Reassure patient and use tranquillizers (diazepam 5–10 mg IV)
• Use adequate alveolar minute ventilation to maintain PaCO$_2$ at 35–40 mm Hg
• Use high FIO$_2$ temporarily to ensure there is no hypoxia
• Increase TV and RR beyond patient's spontaneous rate. Once patient is taken over by machine, setting gradually lowered to desired values
• Use high FIO$_2$ temporarily to ensure there is no hypoxia
• Recognize and treat other factors contributing to 'clash' between machine and patient
• If in spite of above measures asynchrony between patient and machine persists (as in patients with severe parenchymal disease producing stiff lungs), sedate and depress respiration by 2–4 mg IV morphine, or IV diazepam or IV midazolam, IV fentanyl or IV propofol or induce neuromuscular paralysis by 4 mg IV bolus of pancuronium
B. Other Problems
• Malposition of endotracheal tube
• Aspiration of stomach contents
• Hypotension

3. Increase lung volumes—particularly in conditions in which the functional residual capacity (FRC) is reduced.

Regulate Gas Exchange

OXYGENATION

(i) Most patients requiring ventilator support have uneven ventilation and disturbed ventilation-perfusion ratios. Only a small minority on ventilator support can be adequately oxygenated with room air or 20% oxygen; most require an increased concentration of oxygen in the inspired air.

(ii) It is best to use an inspired oxygen concentration (FIO$_2$) sufficient to maintain an O$_2$ saturation $\geq$ 90% and a PaO$_2$ $\geq$ 60 mm Hg. In severe lung disease, high oxygen concentrations are necessary; oxygen concentrations > 70% for a prolonged period are a hazard as they contribute to lung injury. In very severe lung injury, an FIO$_2$ of 100% may be necessary to prevent death from hypoxia. If this is indeed so, 100% oxygen should be used, notwithstanding the fear of oxygen toxicity.

(iii) Use of PEEP. PEEP is indicated when the PaO$_2$ < 60 mm Hg despite inspired oxygen concentrations exceeding 50%.

CARBON DIOXIDE ELIMINATION AND REGULATION

The physiological dead space in patients with lung disease is often increased. The increase in dead space in relation to tidal volume may in fact be so large, that in some patients on ventilators 50–70% or even more of the tidal volume becomes dead space ventilation. It is therefore important to note the following points:

(i) It is impossible to predict the ventilation requirements of patients on ventilatory support as most patients have an increase in physiological dead space. Their ventilation requirements are invariably in considerable excess of that predicted by standard nomograms.

(ii) The only certain way to ensure adequate ventilation is to measure the $PaCO_2$ and to adjust volume exchange so that the $PaCO_2$ is close to normal.

(iii) It needs to be re-stressed that a disturbance in ventilatory exchange may be as much due to a fault in the pulmonary circulation as to a fall in alveolar ventilation.

(iv) Ventilator support can also be manipulated so as to purposely induce hyperventilation (with a low $PaCO_2$) in patients with raised intracranial pressure, or to purposely settle for hypoventilation (permissive hypercapnia) in certain clinical situations (ARDS and airways obstruction).

Overcome mechanical problems

Mechanical ventilation is of use to rest fatigued respiratory muscles, to overcome the abnormal mechanics of the thoracic cage in flail chest and to prevent or treat atelectasis.

Increase in Lung Volumes in Patients with a Low FRC

Use of PEEP improves ventilation—perfusion ratios and reduces the right to left shunt within the lungs.

SUMMARY OF VENTILATORY PATTERNS IN DIFFERENT GROUPS OF RESPIRATORY DISEASES REQUIRING VENTILATOR SUPPORT

(i) In patients with normal lungs: Tidal volumes of 10 ml/kg with respiratory rates between 10–14/min, a flow rate of 40–60 l/min, and a I: E ratio of 1: 2 to 1: 3 are recommended.

(ii) Patients with trauma to the chest wall causing a flail chest, and often haematoma or injury to the lung: These patients may need controlled ventilation for which sedation or neuromuscular paralysis becomes necessary. Tidal volumes of 10 ml/kg, with a respiratory rate between 12–14/min are recommended. The minute ventilation is adjusted to maintain a $PaCO_2$ between 30–40 mm Hg.

(iii) Acute hypoxaemic respiratory failure due to severe lung disease e.g. acute lung injury (ARDS), pneumonia: The principle is to avoid as far as possible high inflation pressures and to use small tidal volumes of 5–7 ml/kg. In mild to moderately severe cases, smaller tidal volumes of 6–8 ml/kg with a higher respiratory rate of 20–25/min are used to match the patient's breathing pattern. The inspiratory flow rates are adjusted to between 40–60 l/min. An increased FIO_2 and the use of PEEP are necessary. If adequate or efficient ventilation is not possible, particularly so in severely hypoxic, tachypnoeic, critically ill individuals, heavy sedation or even muscle paralysis with controlled ventilation becomes necessary, the principle again being not to exceed a plateau pressure of 30 cm H_2O as far as possible, even if this entails a rise in $PaCO_2$ (permissive hypercapnia). If pressure-controlled or pressure-targeted ventilator support is given to these patients, the peak inspiratory pressure should as far as possible not exceed 30 cm H_2O. PEEP is used in all patients. Inverse ratio ventilator support is occasionally tried when gas exchange remains unsatisfactory with the usual volume-targeted or pressure-targeted ventilatory support. The inverse ratio in our opinion should not be increased to > 1:1.

(iv) Acute on chronic respiratory failure in patients with chronic airways' obstruction: Small tidal volumes of 6 ml/kg with a respiratory rate and minute ventilation enough to allow a $PaCO_2$ between 45–55 mm Hg are adequate. These patients are used to a high $PaCO_2$ and it is unwise to aim at a $PaCO_2$ of 40 mm Hg, as their $PaCO_2$ even under ordinary conditions is significantly elevated. Sedation or at times induced paralysis is often necessary for ventilator support to be effectively maintained. Moderately low inspiratory flow rates (50 l/min), an I: E ratio of 1: 3, and avoidance of high inflation pressures by using a low tidal volume is recommended. Hypoxia is countered by an appropriate increase in the FIO_2.

(v) Acute severe asthma: These patients also require low tidal volumes (350–400 ml), and comparatively low minute ventilation (often < 5 l/min) to prevent hyperinflation of the lungs. A rise in $PaCO_2$ does not matter as long as hypoxia is relieved by an appropriate increase in the FIO_2. Ventilation in these patients can at times prove extremely difficult.

Table 55.5: Chart of ventilator settings and blood gases in the ICU														
Name of Patients: _____ Bed No.: _____														
Date	Time	Rate	MV	Tidal Volume	FIO₂	Peak Pressure	Pause Pressure	PEEP	pH	PaCO₂	PaO₂	Std Bicarb	Base exc/def	O₂ Sat

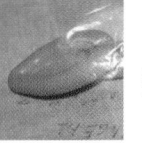

Lung protection strategies (outlined in the chapter on 'Acute Respiratory Distress Syndrome') should always be kept in mind in the management of mechanical ventilator support.

It is constant practice that allows the clinician to adjust ventilatory requirements to the need of each individual patient so as to allow adequate gas exchange and yet prevent as far as possible the hazards of mechanical ventilator support.

Three more points need to be stressed—

1. Hypovolaemia contributes to poor gas exchange, and accentuates or precipitates hypotension in patients on mechanical ventilation. It is therefore important to ensure normal circulatory volume, good pump function, a normal blood pressure and an adequate haemoglobin concentration.
2. Humidification of inspired gas, aseptic suction of secretions through the tracheobronchial tree at frequent intervals, and good chest physiotherapy are all vitally important. Good physiotherapy often spells the difference between life and death in critically ill patients on ventilator support.
3. Efficiently carried out mechanical ventilation can only ensure a satisfactory gas exchange. More often than not, a critically ill patient on ventilator support in the ICU has numerous other complications that pose potential hazards to life. Circulatory failure, renal dysfunction, gastrointestinal bleeding, acid-base disturbances, overwhelming sepsis, and in our country, a poor nutritional state, singly or in combination with other factors, can be dangerous enough to cause death. Therefore to concentrate solely on the correct and efficient working of a machine and on a single aspect of deranged physiology, constitutes bad medicine. An overall perspective should never be lost sight of in the management of a critically ill patient.

MODES OF INVASIVE VENTILATOR SUPPORT

The commonest modes in use are Volume-Controlled Ventilatory (VCV) mode, Pressure-Controlled Ventilatory (PCV) mode, Synchronized Intermittent Mandatory Ventilatory (SIMV) support, and Pressure Support Ventilation (PSV). These modes and the use of PEEP are considered to start with in this section, followed by a brief explanation of the more recent modes. It is very important for the clinician or the intensivist to be thoroughly familiar with the basic modes of ventilator support before attempting familiarity with the numerous other modes that modern ventilators are able to provide.

Volume-Targeted Support

CONTROLLED MODE (CMV)
In CMV, the ventilator completely controls the patient's ventilation, delivering a set tidal volume (or a preset peak pressure) at a set frequency. It is indicated in individuals who are apnoeic, or in those with respiratory muscle paralysis. It is also indicated in patients who are heavily sedated or those paralysed with neuromuscular agents so that ventilatory support is mandatory—a classic example of this situation is fulminant tetanus. Patients receiving CMV cannot increase their minute

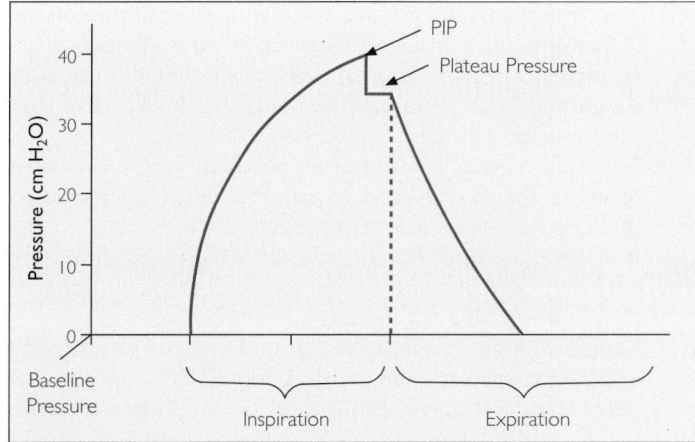

Fig 55.1: The airway pressures (peak and plateau) during a positive pressure breath. Pressure rises during inspiration to peak inspiratory pressure (PIP). With a breath hold, the plateau pressure can be measured. Pressures fall back to baseline during expiration. (Reproduced with permission from Pilbeam SP. 1992. *Mechanical Ventilation, Physiological and Clinical Applications.* Mosby Year Book, MO © Elsevier).

ventilation (VE) voluntarily; their ventilator needs should therefore be closely monitored, and changing needs should be met by suitable adjustments on the machine.

ASSIST/CONTROL (A/C) MODE
This is the most commonly used mode. The machine delivers a preset volume (or pressure) in response to a patient-initiated breath. To prevent the patient from being totally dependent on 'triggered' breaths, a backup minimum respiratory rate is set. The requisite VE can then be provided even if for some reason or the other the patient fails to trigger the machine. The main advantage of this mode is that the patient can increase his VE by increasing his respiratory rate. The disadvantages include the production of respiratory alkalosis and of dynamic hyperinflation (particularly in COPD patients), if the machine is triggered too frequently, and the possibility of asynchrony between the ventilator and the patient. Initial ventilator settings are a VE of 8–10 l/min, respiratory rate at 10–14/min, a sensitivity of –2 cm usually. If the patient triggers the machine too frequently, the sensitivity is set at –2 to –6 cm and the patient is sedated to reduce his respiratory drive. Most ventilators allow adjustment of the inspiratory flow rate or the inspiration expiration (I:E) ratio, the inspiratory rise time, end-inspiratory pause time and the flow pattern during inspiration.

Pressure-Controlled Ventilation (PCV)

In this mode the maximum peak pressure is preset, so that the ventilator increases the pressure to this preset level with each inspiratory breath. The tidal volume (V_T) obtained depends on the preset pressure (the higher the preset pressure, the higher the V_T), the stiffness of the lungs, (greater the stiffness, the lower the V_T for a preset pressure) and resistance to airflow (the greater the resistance, the lower the V_T). The adjustable parameters are preset pressures delivered by the ventilator and the inspiratory time. The flow pattern is decelerating, in that the

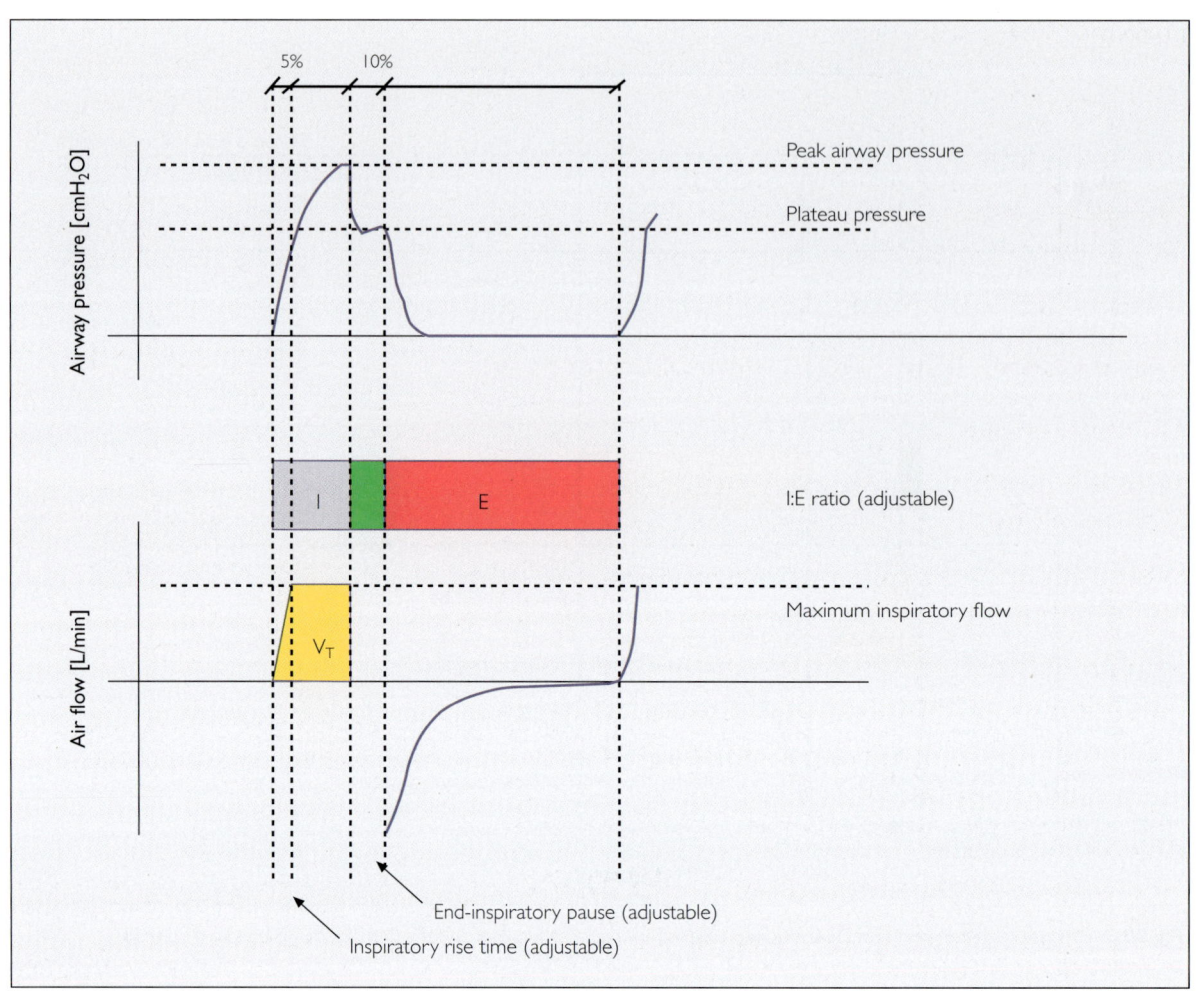

Fig 55.2: Volume targeted ventilation. Tidal volume is preset and the machine delivers the preset tidal volume regardless of change in compliance or airway resistance. Pressure rises during inspiration to peak inspiratory pressure (PIP). With a breath hold, the plateau pressure can be measured. Pressures fall back to baseline during expiration.

flow is high to start with but decreases as the preset pressure is about to be reached.

Synchronized Intermittent Mandatory Ventilation (SIMV)

In this mode, the ventilator delivers synchronized breaths at a set rate at either a preset tidal volume (V_T) or a preset pressure, in addition to allowing the patient to breathe spontaneously. The tidal volume and rate are determined by the patient. If for any reason, the patient does not breathe for a predetermined period, a machine breath is delivered. SIMV can be used with pressure support for spontaneous breaths. PEEP can be introduced in this mode, in which case the machine breaths will be combined with PEEP and the spontaneous ones with continuous positive airways pressure (CPAP).

The advantages claimed for the SIMV mode are as follows:

(i) Decreased asynchrony with the machine and less sedation requirements.

(ii) Less chances of hyperventilation as compared to the A/C mode.
(iii) Greater patient comfort
(iv) Continued use of respiratory muscles, which is believed to prevent respiratory muscle dysfunction.
(v) Reduced mean airway pressure even with the simultaneous use of PEEP, because many respiratory cycles are related to spontaneous breaths. This minimizes the cardiovascular effects of mechanical ventilation and is less likely to cause a fall in cardiac output or in arterial blood pressure.

In our opinion, the advantages ascribed to SIMV with or without PEEP are theoretical, and except in occasional instances, most patients are more comfortably and more satisfactorily ventilated with the A/C mode of ventilator support. In fact, the more ill the patient greater the necessity to rest the respiratory muscles rather than exercise them. The VO_2 by overworked respiratory muscles can be as high as 15–40% of the total oxygen consumption and this is certainly undesirable. The SIMV mode

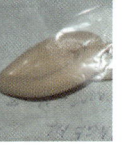

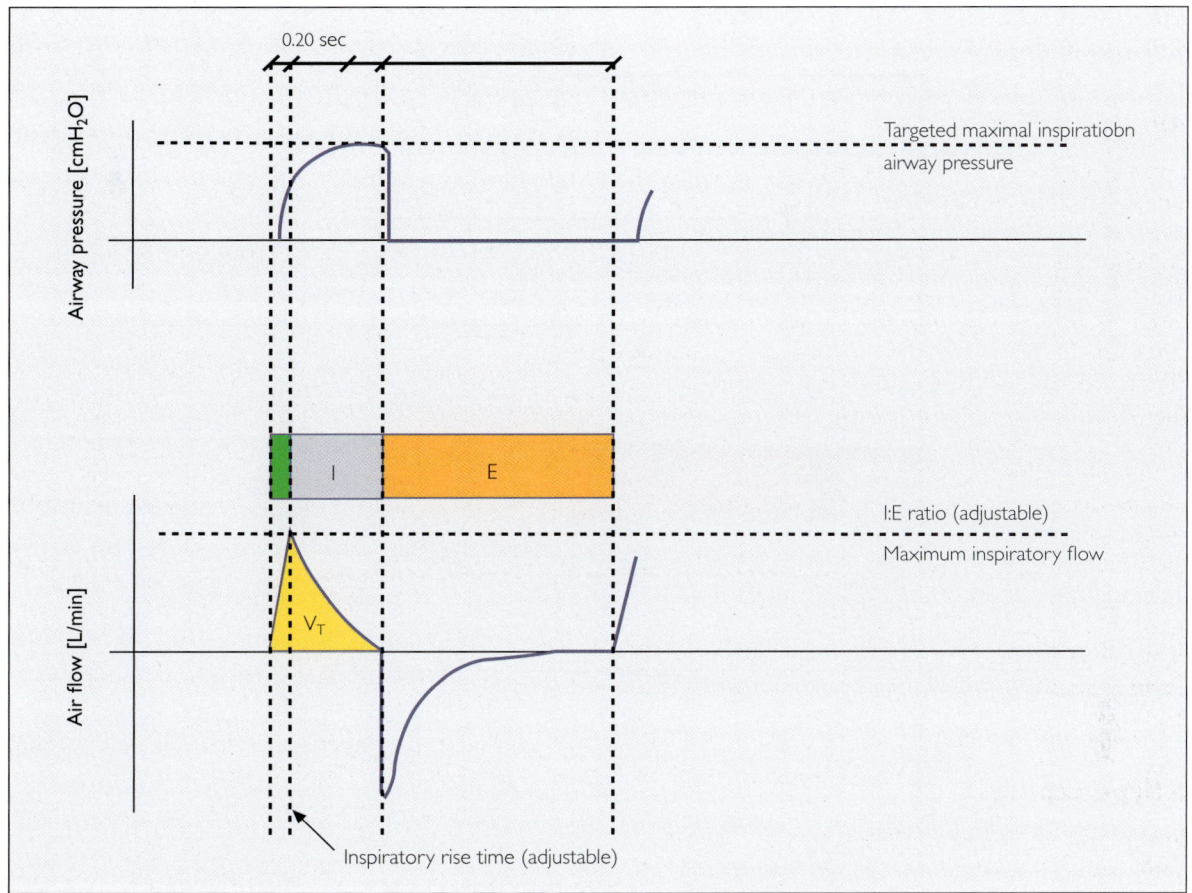

Fig 55.3: Pressure targeted ventilation. The maximum inspiratory pressure is preset and the tidal volume will depend upon lung compliance and airway resistance. I:E ratio and the inspiratory rise time is adjustable.

cannot also respond to changes in the patient's condition, and therefore needs close monitoring.

The chief uses of this mode in our opinion are stated below:

(i) In patients who develop hypotension while on the A/C mode or CMV mode with PEEP. The use of SIMV in such patients is associated with a lower mean airway pressure and this may restore cardiovascular stability.

(ii) In patients on the A/C mode who develop respiratory alkalosis. This can be countered by either sedation or by changing to the SIMV mode.

(iii) To prevent auto-PEEP in certain situations.

(iv) In patients with respiratory failure and a bronchopleural fistula. In this situation, one would desire the lowest mean airway pressure that does not adversely affect ventilation and gas exchange, yet allows the bronchopleural fistula to heal and get sealed. Low tidal volumes with increased respiratory rates to allow for adequate minute ventilation, the avoidance of PEEP, and the use of the SIMV mode may be ideally suited to these patients. This should be combined with the lowest effective chest drainage tube suction.

(v) For weaning purposes.

INITIAL SETTING

Settings to deliver a V_E of 6–10 l/min or a preset pressure (sufficient to allow a V_E of 6–10 l/min) with 10–12 mandatory breaths.

Pressure Support Ventilation (PSV)

In this mode a patient inspiratory effort triggers a response from the ventilator. The ventilator delivers a preset positive pressure to the airways, reducing the work of breathing and helping in patient comfort. Once the predefined percentage of the maximal inspiratory flow is reached, the ventilator stops inspiration and opens the expiratory valve. The respiratory rate and inspiratory flow rate are determined by the patient. This mode cannot be used in an apnoeic patient or in one who lacks an adequate spontaneous respiratory drive. It is chiefly used in selected COPD patients and as a weaning procedure.

INITIAL SETTING

Set a pressure of 10–12 cm of H_2O, ensuring a V_T of 7–10 ml/kg. The pressure support is gradually decreased to 5–7 cm H_2O provided an adequate V_T is maintained. Once this occurs, the patient can be weaned and allowed to breath spontaneously.

Continuous Positive Airways Pressure (CPAP)

CPAP is a mode of spontaneous breathing in which the airway pressure is maintained at levels greater than the ambient pressure throughout the entire respiratory cycle. A PEEP may be added as an adjunct to CPAP. All modern volume ventilators incorporate CPAP as a ventilatory mode. The ventilator does not provide any machine-generated breaths, but its humidification

and alarm systems are available for use. Special CPAP systems without a ventilator are also available.

Inverse Ratio Ventilation

Inverse ratio ventilation can be volume-targeted or pressure targeted. Whereas the normal I: E ratio is 1: 3 or 1: 2, in inverse ratio ventilation the I: E ratio is 1: 1 or even less. Ordinarily, one hesitates to go beyond 1:1.

This is used in patients with acute lung injury (ALI), ARDS, pneumonia, atelectasis, who show refractory hypoxaemia (O_2 saturation < 90% on an $FIO_2 \geq$ 60% on A/C mode in spite of suitable PEEP). In volume-controlled inverse ratio ventilation (VC-IRV), the inverse ratio of I: E is achieved by lowering inspiratory flow rate (and thereby lengthening inspiration) or by introducing a suitable end-inspiratory pause. The tidal volume is lowered sufficiently so as not to exceed a plateau pressure of 30 cm H_2O. In pressure-controlled IRV (PC-IRV), the I: E ratio is set to the desired level. The peak pressure should preferably not exceed 30 cm H_2O, or at most 35 cm H_2O.

PEEP is used with both VC-IRV and PC-IRV.

The advantages attributed to IRV are better relief of hypoxaemia and promotion of lung protection strategy that reduces the risk of both barotrauma and volutrauma.

Permissive Hypercapnia

The principle behind this approach is to protect the lung from both volutrauma and barotrauma when using either volume-targeted or pressure-targeted ventilatory support. Small tidal volumes (5–7 ml/kg) are used in certain groups of patients in volume-targeted ventilatory support, so that plateau pressures do not exceed 30 cm H_2O. When pressure-targeted ventilator support is used, peak pressures are generally set to not more than 30cm H_2O. This lung protection strategy can lead to hypoventilation and thereby hypercapnia. The hypercapnia is generally well tolerated by the patient and is permissible as an offshoot of the lung protection strategy stated above.

Use of PEEP

The use of PEEP is a valuable adjunct to every mode of volume-targeted ventilatory support, pressure-targeted ventilator support, pressure support ventilation and to the SIMV support. The effects of PEEP are listed in Table 55.6.

INDICATIONS FOR USE OF PEEP

PEEP is indicated in patients with severe hypoxic respiratory failure who have poorly compliant lungs and a large degree of ventilation-perfusion mismatch so that hypoxia persists despite using an FIO_2 of 50–60% or more to ventilate the lungs.

It is invariably indicated in patients with ALI, severe pneumonia, in patients with pulmonary oedema who require ventilatory support and in hypoxemic respiratory failure due to flail chest and marked obesity. All these patients have a reduced FRC leading to alveolar and small airways collapse thereby causing a ventilation-perfusion mismatch with a right to left shut within the lungs. In these patients PEEP increases the FRC, opens up collapsed alveoli, particularly in the dependent lung regions, prevents derecruitment of opened alveoli during expiration,

Table 55.6: Physiological effects and complications of PEEP
A. Physiological Effects
1. On Lungs
• Opening up of fluid-filled atelectatic alveoli, with increase in FRC and TLC
• Decrease in shunt causing increase in PaO_2
• Increase in V_A/Q units
• Increase in dead space and V_D/V_T ratio
• Increase in compliance upto a point; later fall in compliance
2. On Heart
Decrease in cardiac output; this can decrease shunt, and thereby increase PaO_2. Thus rise in PaO_2 may also result from a fall in cardiac output, and not necessarily from improvement in lung function
B. Complications
• Barotrauma—pneumothorax, pneumomediastinum, interstitial emphysema
• Fall in cardiac output—hypotension, poor oxygen transport with inadequate tissue perfusion
• Fall in PaO_2 due to overdistension of compliant alveoli, and increase in V/Q abnormalities
• Increase in intracranial pressure
• Water retention

Table 55.7: Conventional modes of ventilator support
1. Controlled Mode (CMV)
2. Assist/Control Mode (A/C)
3. Pressure Controlled Ventilation (PCV)
4. Synchronized Intermittent Mandatory Ventilation (SIMV)
5. Pressure Support Ventilation (PSV)
6. Continuous Positive Airways Pressure (CPAP)
7. Inverse Ratio Ventilation (VC IRV) and (PC IRV)

redistributes fluid within the alveoli and is believed to protect surfactant. The overall effect is to improve the ventilation-perfusion mismatch, reduce the absolute right to left shunt (also termed the true venous admixture) within the lungs, thereby increasing PaO_2, O_2 saturation, so that need for high FIO_2 is reduced. The danger of oxygen toxicity caused by prolonged use of high FIO_2 in these patients is thus obviated. The prevention of derecruitment or collapse of alveoli during expiration with PEEP allows breathing to occur in the favourable range of the pressure volume curve, reducing the work of breathing.

At one time PEEP was strictly contraindicated in patients with respiratory failure due to severe asthma or following an acute exacerbation of COPD requiring ventilator support. Many of these patients have dynamic hyperinflation of the lungs. The FRC is high and the alveolar pressure at the end

of expiration exceeds atmospheric pressure, resulting in auto-PEEP or intrinsic PEEP. Also, because of dynamic hyperinflation this auto-PEEP progressively increases. A high auto-PEEP increases the inspiratory work of breathing and ultimately leads to respiratory muscle fatigue that can progress to respiratory arrest. The principle of ventilatory support is to use small tidal volumes with an I: E ratio of 1: 3 and a rate preferably not more than 12 to 14/minute to help reduce dynamic hyperinflation. The application of extrinsic PEEP is also indicated in patients with severe airways obstruction who are on ventilatory support and develop a high auto-PEEP. The proper application of external PEEP will then counter the effect of auto-PEEP on the work of breathing, chiefly in relation to inspiratory effort. It is important however to set the level of extrinsic PEEP below that of the auto-PEEP observed in the patient.

In the past the main focus of attention in the use of PEEP was to improve oxygenation by reducing ventilation-perfusion mismatch and right to left shunt within the lung. *An equally important concept on the use of PEEP today is that it prevents the concertina-like opening and closing of alveoli during inspiration and expiration, keeps the alveoli open all through the respiratory cycle, thereby reducing the sheer forces acting on the alveoli and hence reducing ventilator-induced injury.*

SELECTION OF THE DEGREE OF PEEP USED

A variety of methods have been used to determine the optimal level of PEEP. In busy ICUs, the simplest, safest and most practical method is to use the lowest level of PEEP which maintains the PaO_2 equal to or > 60 mm Hg, on an FIO_2 equal to or < 0.6.

Other methods of selecting an optimum level of PEEP include the following:

1. Optimal Oxygenation
   It is wrong to aim at an ever increasing PaO_2 by increasing the levels of PEEP. A high PEEP can cause an increasing rise in the PaO_2 and yet can result in a sharp drop in the cardiac output. This fall in cardiac output further reduces oxygen transport to the tissues, in spite of the increase in the PaO_2; this can have disastrous consequences.

2. Maximal Oxygen Transport
   Adjusting the PEEP so as to obtain maximal oxygen transport (i.e. the product of arterial oxygen content and the cardiac output), takes the PaO_2, the haemoglobin and the cardiac output into consideration. Nevertheless, frequent measurements of cardiac output often pose problems in critically ill individuals.

3. Best Compliance
   With the use of PEEP, the reduced FRC increases, and the compliance increases up to a point. If static compliance is measured with a graded increase in PEEP, a level of PEEP which produces an optimal increase in the compliance can be arrived at. Further increase in PEEP beyond this point now leads to a fall in static compliance pointing to over-distension of the alveoli. An optimal compliance produced by a particular level of PEEP in any particular patient, is generally associated with an optimal rise in the PaO_2.

4. Lowest Q_S/Q_T
   As long as the level of PEEP does not significantly reduce the cardiac output, the optimal level of PEEP correlates with the lowest level of Q_S/Q_T. Many workers aim at reducing the shunt fraction to 15%, or aim at a PaO_2/FIO_2 ratio of 300 or more.

5. Lowest V_D/V_T and Lowest $PaCO_2$-$PETCO_2$
   The lowest V_D/V_T ratio and the lowest $PaCO_2$-$PETCO_2$ gradient are other parameters used by some workers to arrive at an optimal PEEP setting.

COMPLICATIONS OF PEEP

The three major complications are barotrauma, a fall in cardiac output, and at times a fall instead of the expected rise in PaO_2. PEEP used over a number of days, can result in an increase in intracranial tension, and to an increase in water retention, and a decrease in renal and portal blood flow.

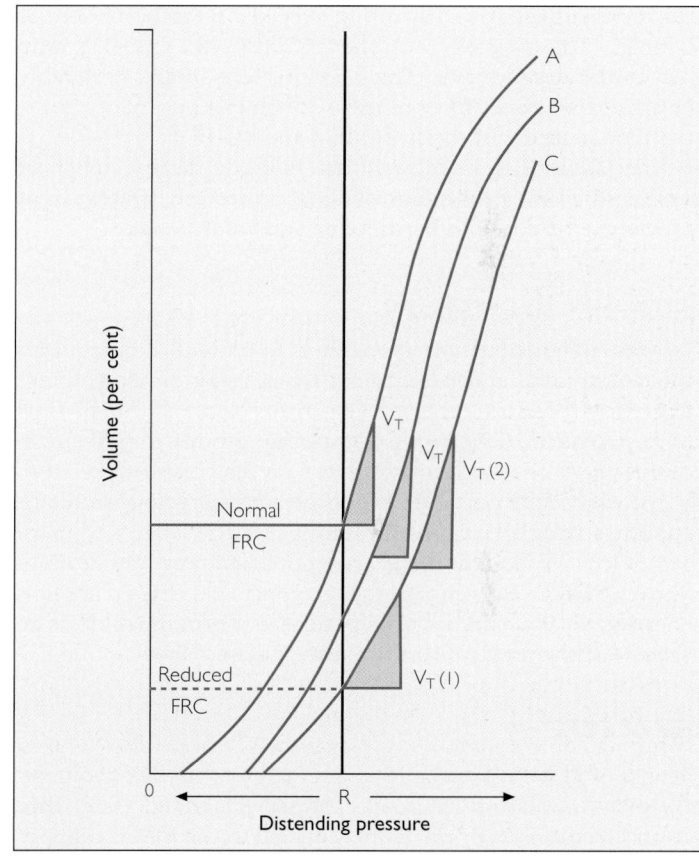

Fig 55.4: Effect of positive end-expiratory pressure on functional residual capacity (FRC) in patients with reduced compliance e.g. acute lung injury. Curve A represents a normal pressure-volume curve, wherein a relatively small distending pressure is required to achieve a given tidal volume (V_T). Curve C represents a pressure-volume curve in a patient with reduced compliance (as in acute lung injury) with decreased FRC. This is a more flattened curve and requires a greater distending pressure to achieve the same V_T (1). With the addition of PEEP, the FRC may be improved along the same abnormal compliance curve (2) or would shift to curve B, so that lesser distending pressures are required to achieve the same V_T, but the absolute value of the distending pressure is still greater than that required for curve A.

1. Barotrauma

The risk of barotrauma depends on the end-inspiratory airway pressure and regional overinflation of parts of the lung. End-inspiratory pressure is a function of the tidal volume, the FRC,

the inspiratory flow rate, the total compliance of the lungs, and the level of PEEP used. High tidal volumes, high inspiratory flow rates and high levels of PEEP, in association with a reduced FRC and compliance, potentiate the risk of barotrauma. Even in severely diseased lungs, there are some regional areas which are more compliant than others. With high levels of PEEP, these alveoli get enlarged and overdistended, and have a lower recoil pressure than the smaller, poorly compliant alveoli. High alveolar pressures in such distended alveoli predispose to rupture. On the other hand, the smaller, poorly compliant alveoli have a larger recoil pressure, and can therefore withstand high alveolar pressures and are less liable to rupture.

Alveolar rupture can lead to interstitial emphysema, pneumothorax, mediastinal emphysema, and surgical emphysema of the soft tissues which may involve the neck, face and trunk. Pneumothorax on high levels of PEEP is a disaster which often leads to death.

2. Fall in Cardiac Output

High levels of inflation pressure and PEEP are transmitted to the pleural space. The rise in the intrapleural and intrathoracic pressures leads to a fall in the venous return to the right heart, and a poor filling of the left heart due to a decrease in the transmural pressure across the left ventricular wall. Overinflation of the alveoli also increases the pulmonary vascular resistance with right heart strain, which further reduces the cardiac output. Also, right ventricular strain produces a shift of the interventricular septum to the left, thereby distorting and diminishing the size of the left ventricular cavity, and further impairing left ventricular filling and cardiac output. A sharp fall in the cardiac output leads to hypotension, poor oxygen transport, and inadequate tissue perfusion. A volume load together with dopamine support may be necessary in some patients to restore the cardiac output and oxygen transport to desired levels.

3. Fall in PaO_2

A paradoxical fall in the PaO_2 is sometimes observed with PEEP. This occurs when there are regional areas of normally compliant or overcompliant lung in patients with hypoxemic respiratory failure due to parenchymal lung disease. Overdistension of compliant alveoli leads to a decrease in the blood flow to these alveoli, and a shift of blood flow to the non-ventilated, non-compliant areas of the lung. This causes a further increase in the shunt and a fall in the PaO_2. Ventilatory settings and PEEP levels should be adjusted to allow less distension of the compliant alveoli, and better distribution of inspired gas to the poorly compliant portions of the lungs.

Open Lung Concept

The 'Open lung concept' is being increasingly used in some critical care units in ALI and ARDS and in postoperative atelectasis (see chapter on ARDS). The principle behind this concept is to 'open' the lung and keep it 'open' with the least changes in pressure so as to minimize alveolar shear forces. This serves to improve gas exchange and serves as a lung protection mechanism by avoiding the concertina-like opening of the alveoli during inspiration and their collapse and closure during expiration.

Sequential settings in a patient with ARDS on whom the open lung concept is used are given below.

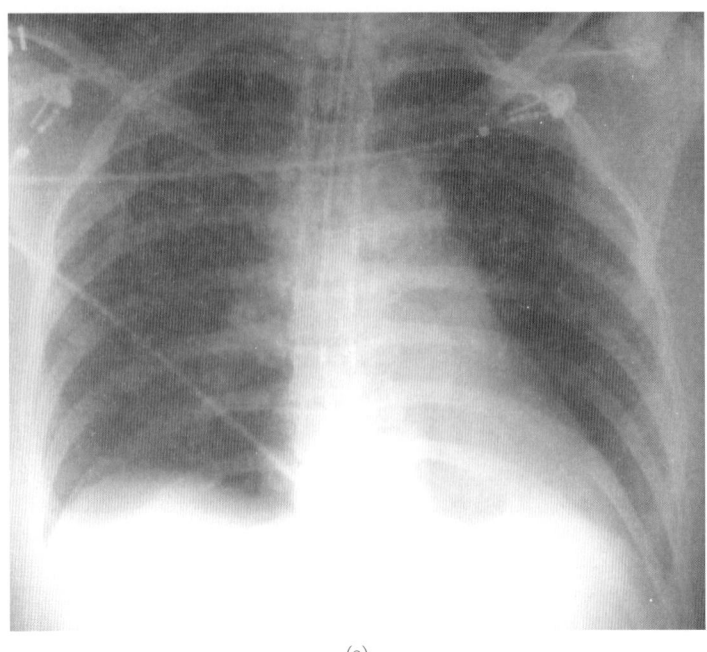

(a)

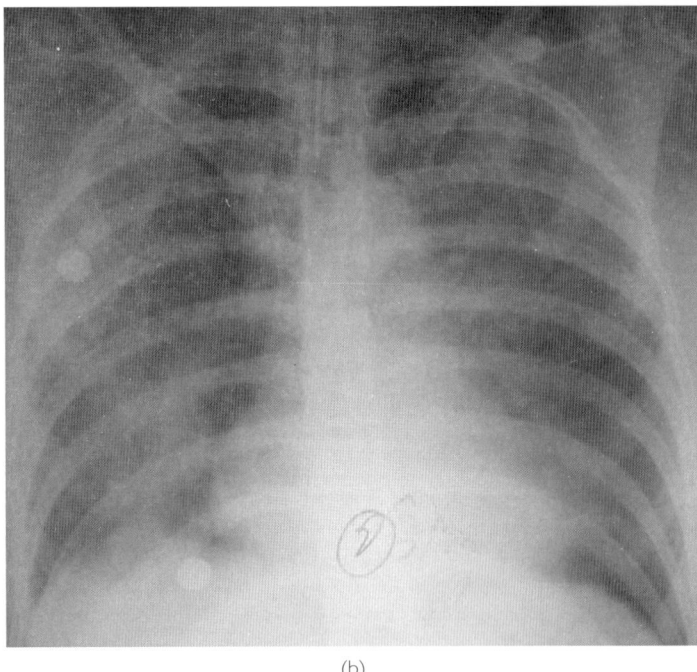

(b)

Fig 55.5: PEEP effect. Chest X-ray (a) demonstrates overinflated lungs with a tubular-shaped heart (b) Chest X-ray after removal of PEEP. The lungs are not inflated as much as with PEEP, the heart is not tubular. The apparent clearing of opacities on the X-ray (a) is a PEEP effect.

1. *Use pressure control* and set upper pressure limit to 50 cm H_2O. Set PEEP at 10–15 cm H_2O. Set pressure control level above PEEP to a value which gives a V_T of 10–15 ml/kg. Set respiratory rate at 15/min. Inspiratory time 50% or I:E 1:1.

2. *Determine opening pressure.* Raise peak inspiratory pressure step-wise by 2 cm H_2O at a time, allowing 10–15 breaths at each step-wise increase, till the lung is fully 'open'. This

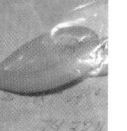

Table 55.8:
Practical guidelines for the use of PEEP

PEEP only helps to counter hypoxia in acute hypoxemic respiratory failure due to lung injury; it does not alter the natural history of acute lung pathologies requiring ventilator support

PEEP should not be used as a preventive measure, except after open heart surgery to prevent mediastinal bleeding, or to open up atelectatic segments chiefly present in the lower lobes

It is not necessarily indicated if conventional ventilator support with FIO_2 of 50–60 per cent maintains $PaO_2 > 60$–65 mm Hg

Start with PEEP levels of +5 cm H_2O, gauge effect, and then increase; do not exceed levels of +15 cm H_2O in Indian patients as barotrauma invariably results

Use the lowest PEEP that allows a PaO_2 of 60 mm Hg on $FIO_2 <$ 0.6 Ascertain that the rise in PaO_2 following the use of PEEP is not associated with a fall in CO as this will lead to poor oxygen transport and poor tissue oxygenation

If hypotension or decrease in CO is associated with use of PEEP, the PEEP level should be reduced, or even discontinued. The BP and CO are raised with volume load and/or inotropic support, and PEEP may then be better tolerated

PEEP may rarely cause a fall in PaO_2—it then needs to be reduced, or even discontinued

PEEP should be gradually tapered off, before discontinuing ventilator support

few breaths for each setting to enable a stabilized reading. The 'closing pressure' is that pressure at which the alveoli collapse or close. This is signified by an abrupt fall in the high PaO_2 and a sharp decline in tidal volume. Note 'closing pressure'.

4. *Reopen the lung fully* by repeating the steps outlined in II.
5. *Keep the lung open.* Slowly, step-wise, reduce the peak inspiratory pressure once more to a level which is 1–2 cm above the closing pressure. Now the lung has been opened and is being *kept open*. The tidal volume should remain stable, and the arterial blood gases good and constant.

PEEP is generally set at 10–15 cm H_2O. Some units prefer to set PEEP at higher levels of 15–25 cm H_2O. It is, however, not known if this high PEEP is necessary. Therefore the same procedure as described above to determine ideal peak inspiratory pressure is now performed to find the lowest level of PEEP. After once again opening the lung, the peak inspiratory pressure and the PEEP are adjusted to just above closing pressures, so that the lungs remain 'open'.

Avoid unnecessary ventilatory disconnects, or changes in ventilator settings. If ventilator disconnects occur or there is a change in lung condition to suggest further atelectasis, the whole procedure described above to reopen lung and keep it open is repeated. Table 55.9 describes the step-wise open lung procedure.

NEWER MODES OF VENTILATOR SUPPORT

The conventional modes that assist spontaneous ventilation have been described above. They deliver a fixed, uniform, predetermined degree of assist without taking into account the variability of the breathing pattern present in different individuals in different situations and at different times in the same patient. Therefore, ideal synchrony between the patient and the ventilator is often absent. Asynchrony between the patient and ventilator can result in an increase in the workload on

generally requires a rise in the peak inspiratory pressure to 40–60 cm H_2O. The features that signify a fully 'open' lung are a sudden and sustained jump of the PaO_2, so that the $PaO_2/FIO_2 > 400$, and also the sharp disproportionate increase in tidal volume in relation to the step-wise increase in peak pressure.

3. *Determine closing pressure* of the lung. Decrease peak inspiratory pressure step-wise by 2 cm H_2O, allowing a

Table 55.9:	
Open lung procedure	
Open lung and determine the 'opening pressure'	Use Pressure Control Mode; rate 15/min I:E 1:1, PEEP 10–15 cm H_2O Raise PIP stepwise to 40-60 cm H_2O to open the lung. Allow 10–15 breaths for each stepwise increase in PIP.
	Open lung—signified by a sharp sustained jump of PaO_2, PaO_2/FIO_2 and disproportionate increase in tidal volume. Note PIP for opening lung.
Determine 'closing pressure'	Lower PIP stepwise 2 cm at a time (allowing a few breaths at each reduction) till alveoli again start to close. This is signified by a sharp fall in PaO_2 and in tidal volume.
Reopen lung	Reopen lung as described above.
Now set PIP to just above closing pressure so that lung which has been opened is kept open	Stepwise reduce PIP to a level just above closing pressure to keep lung open. Check PaO_2, PaO_2/FIO_2 and tidal volume. Adjust respiratory rate for adequate ventilation.

respiratory muscles, an undesirable event in critically ill patients. New technologies have therefore been developed that allow the ventilator to provide assistance in proportion to the patient's demand, which may vary from breath to breath. These newer modes of ventilator support are briefly considered below.

Airway Pressure Release Ventilation (APRV)

This ventilatory mode comprises CPAP that is intermittently released to allow a brief expiratory interval. The advantage is a lower mean alveolar pressure as compared to that during positive pressure ventilation. It has been used in patients with ARDS, and postoperatively in some patients, and has been found to be effective in providing adequate oxygenation.

Proportional Assist Ventilator (PAV)

The ventilator in PAV has the ability to sense every inspiratory effort breath by breath and adjust ventilator support accordingly. It does this by delivering positive pressure throughout inspiration in proportion to inspiratory airflow and volume generated by the patient. In conventional ventilatory modes, peak inspiratory pressures and tidal volumes are relatively constant. In PAV there is a direct constant relationship between the inspiratory effort of the patient and the peak inspiratory pressure generated by the ventilator from breath to breath. The tidal volume and peak inspiratory pressure are thus dependent variables. The PAV mode necessitates that the patient is capable of performing a portion of the respiratory work. It demands that the ventilator should be able to determine the elastance and resistance of the respiratory system in spontaneously breathing patients.

Pressure Regulated Volume Control (PRVC) and Volume Support (VS)

In the PRVC mode a pressure-targeted ventilation is used to achieve a desired tidal volume. In the volume support mode a pressure support is given by the ventilator to achieve a predesigned tidal volume. This is done from breath to breath. The major concern with both these assist modes is that if because of inspiratory respiratory demands (for example fever or increased metabolism from any cause) there results increased effort in breathing, the level of assistance offered by the ventilator will paradoxically decrease. Also, the machine delivers a predesigned tidal volume; however, in spontaneously breathing patients the tidal volume is not constant and may vary breath to breath.

Neurally Adjusted Ventilatory Assist (NAVA)

This mode uses the electrical activity of the diaphragm (Edi) to control the ventilator. It is based on the concept that electrical activity of the diaphragm (triggered through the phrenic nerve) is representative of the overall neural respiratory effort both in timing and amplitude. In NAVA positive pressure generated by the ventilator is in direct proportion to the amplitude of the electrical activity of the diaphragm, sensed by the ventilator. The patient's respiratory control mechanisms including feedback from various receptors adjust the electrical activity of the diaphragm thereby regulating both tidal volume and the peak

inspiratory pressure. NAVA has been tried out in specialized ICUs, and has been shown to enhance ventilator-patient synchrony, provide adequate gas exchange, unload respiratory muscles without alteration in circulatory haemodynamics, both during invasive and non-invasive ventilatory support.

We have no experience with either the PAV or the NAVA ventilator modes and would rather wait for more clinical trials to define their optimum use.

Bilevel Positive Airway Pressure (BiPAP)

In BiPAP ventilation, two levels of continuous positive pressure are used, the patient being allowed to spontaneously breathe at both pressure levels. Assistance to spontaneous breathing can be given optimally at the low pressure level, high pressure level or at both levels. The change from low pressure level to high pressure level is coordinated by the patient's breathing effort. The BiPAP mode has its chief use in non-invasive ventilator support rather than in the invasive form.

High-Frequency Ventilation (HFV)

Several modes of HFV have been employed. The basic feature in common is the use of tidal volumes which are smaller than the dead space volume. Gas exchange does not occur through convection as in conventional ventilatory modes, but by molecular diffusion, non-convective mixing, and by other mechanisms. The two important modes of HFV are high-frequency oscillatory ventilation, and high-frequency jet ventilation. The advantages claimed for HFV include a decreased risk of barotrauma, and efficient gas exchange. This mode is believed to be best suited for healing of bronchopleural fistulae. Controlled trials however have shown no distinct benefit with this mode as compared to other conventional modes. The risk of complications is also significant.

Differential Lung Ventilation

Patients in respiratory failure due to severe asymmetrical lung disease may fail to be adequately ventilated by conventional ventilatory modes. In such patients adequate gas exchange can be provided by differential lung ventilation.

Clinical examples include patients with bronchopleural fistulae, unilateral trauma, scoliosis, or marked asymmetrical degree of parenchymal inflammatory disease in each lung (one lung being grossly affected, and the other only slightly so). When there is a large difference in compliance, resistance, or both parameters between the two lungs, a larger proportion of each tidal breath (using conventional ventilatory modes), is distributed to the comparatively unaffected lung. This results in a mismatching of ventilation and perfusion, an increase in the shunt, and poor gas exchange.

The initiation of differential lung ventilation requires the patient to be intubated with a double-lumen endotracheal tube (Carlen, Robert-Shaw, Univent, or Bronchocath). Different tidal volumes, flow rates, minute ventilation, and if necessary even PEEP, are set for each lung. Differential lung ventilation can be through two asynchronous ventilators each with its own circuit and its own settings, or through two synchronized ventilators which deliver tidal breaths to both lungs through

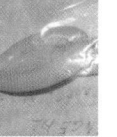

two independent circuits. The tidal volumes, FIO_2 and other ventilatory settings for each lung are independently adjustable.

Extracorporeal Membrane Oxygenation (ECMO)

The prohibitive cost and laborious technique of ECMO preclude its use in most critical care settings. In fact, a large multicenter trial using ECMO in patients with ALI, showed that there was no reduction in mortality in the ECMO-treated group; rather there was a significantly greater incidence of complications in this group of patients. Hence till such time as ECMO is shown to significantly improve survival, it cannot be recommended for routine use.

Table 55.10: Newer modes of ventilatory support
Open Lung Concept
Airway Pressure Release Ventilation (APRV)
Proportional Assist Ventilation (PAV)
Pressure Regulated Volume control (PRVC) and Volume Support (VS)
Neurally Adjusted Ventilatory Assist (NAVA)
High Frequency Ventilation (HFV)
Bilevel Positive Airway (Bi PAP)
Differential Lung Ventilation
Extracorporeal Membrane Oxygenation (ECMO)

COMPLICATIONS OF MECHANICAL VENTILATION

Alveolar Hyperventilation

A $PaCO_2$ of < 20 mm Hg can be dangerous. Respiratory alkalosis results in cramps, tetany, reduced cerebral blood flow, and hypotension. Electrolyte disturbances characterized by a sudden shift of potassium from the extracellular to the cellular compartment can trigger dangerous arrhythmias like ventricular tachycardia, or ventricular fibrillation. Prolonged alveolar hyperventilation makes weaning difficult as the respiratory centre gets used to a low arterial carbon dioxide tension, and cannot tolerate a rise of $PaCO_2$ to even normal levels.

Atelectasis

This may be of two kinds: (a) segmental, lobar, or even massive; (b) diffuse airspace collapse or atelectasis.

Lobar or massive atelectasis is easy to detect clinically as well as on X-ray. It produces distress with a rise in the static compliance (a rise in both peak and plateau pressures is observed). A slipping of the endotracheal tube into the right main bronchus is an important cause of collapse of part or whole of the left lung.

Diffuse airspace atelectasis is characterized by a collapse of very many scattered alveoli in both lungs, so that both the clinical examination, and the chest X-ray are essentially normal. It is at times observed when tidal volumes < 10 ml/

kg are used to ventilate the lungs. The use of tidal volumes of 10 ml/kg is the best prophylactic measure for this complication. Diffuse airspace atelectasis is suspected when there is a fall in the compliance, with an increase in the alveolar-arterial oxygen gradient, and a normal chest X-ray. When due to an increase in the water content of the lungs, the condition can be corrected by the prompt use of a diuretic like furosemide.

Uneven Compliances within Different Areas of the Lung

These produce uneven distribution of inspired gas. When some areas of the lung are normal or overcompliant, while others show a marked decrease in compliance, the problem in mechanical ventilation is immense. Inspired gas overventilates the compliant lung, and often fails to 'open' or ventilate the stiff or non-compliant parts of the lung. Overdistension of the compliant areas leads to increase in the physiological dead space, increasing Zone I conditions especially when large tidal volumes are used. The capillary perfusion in these areas is severely diminished, with blood being shunted to the less compliant, poorly ventilated areas. This produces an increased right-to-left shunt with a fall in the PaO_2. Lower tidal volumes with a judicious adjustment of PEEP are necessary, but the difficulties in providing adequate gas exchange are not always solved.

Auto-PEEP

An increase in PEEP occasionally occurs in patients on mechanical ventilation (auto-PEEP), even when PEEP is not used as an adjunct to ventilator support. Auto-PEEP (occult PEEP, intrinsic PEEP) is defined as an unintentional PEEP that occurs when a new inspiratory breath is delivered before expiration has ended, in patients on ventilator support. A progressively increasing auto-PEEP results in a 'dynamic hyperinflation' of the lung, which is merely another expression for increasing air-trapping within the lung. Auto-PEEP and dynamic hyperinflation are most commonly seen in patients with COPD, where narrowed obstructed airways lead to prolonged expiration and air trapping. Other factors that predispose to the occurrence of auto-PEEP are (a) V_E equal to or > 10 l/min; (b) patients > 60 years of age; (c) use of a small-sized endotracheal tube; (d) increase in V_T specially in patients with COPD; (e) increase in compliance; (f) increase in respiratory rate with increase in risk of air trapping, particularly when inspiratory time equals expiratory time; (g) reduced inspiratory flow rate with shorter expiratory time.

MEASUREMENT OF AUTO-PEEP

During normal mechanical ventilation, the auto-PEEP present in the patient's lungs at end-expiration is not registered on the ventilator manometer, as in most ventilators pressures during exhalation are measured internally on the inspiratory side of the machine. Also normally, the expiratory valve is open to the atmosphere during exhalation. Auto-PEEP can be measured by occluding the expiratory limb of the circuit just before the next positive pressure breath. When the exhalation valve is occluded, the manometer measures the pressure in the patient's airway as the pressure equilibrates with the circuit. This method of measuring auto-PEEP requires a quiet patient on controlled ventilation.

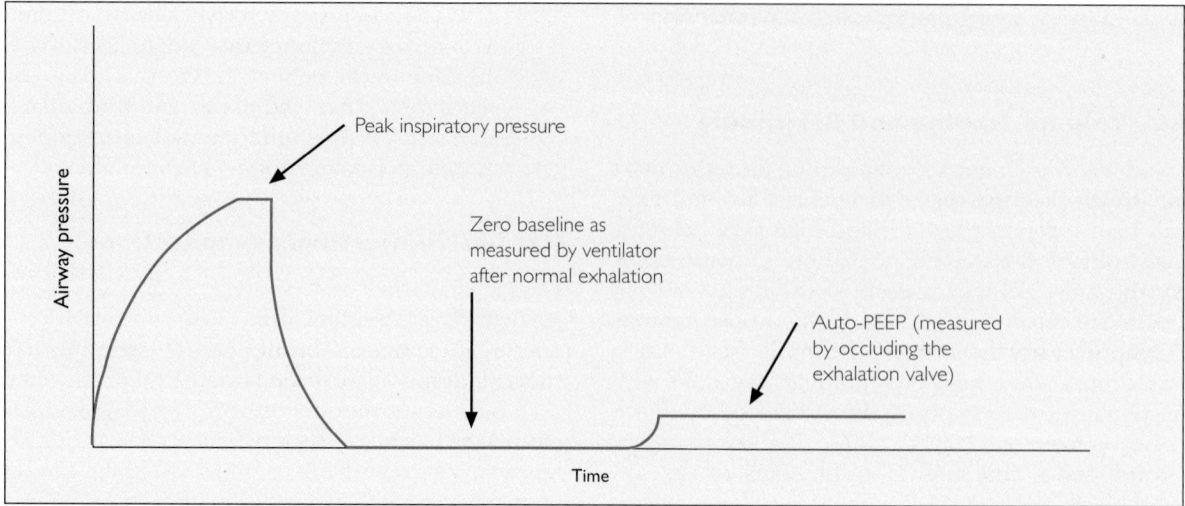

Fig 55.6: The airway pressure (peak and plateau) during a positive pressure breath. Pressure rises during inspiration to peak inspiratory pressure (PIP). With a breath hold, the plateau pressure can be measured. Pressures fall back to baseline during expiration. (Reproduced with permission from Pilbeam SP. 1992. *Mechanical Ventilation, Physiological and Clinical Applications.* Mosby Year Book, MO © Elsevier).

Some ventilators like the Siemens Servo 900C and the Ohmeda Advent have end-expiration pause buttons or controls. They are microprocessor ventilators that can time the closing of the exhalation valve. They close this valve just before the next positive breath is due, delay the next breath, and then measure the pressure in the circuit.

EFFECTS OF AUTO-PEEP
Effects of auto-PEEP are the same as those of PEEP used on purpose as an adjunct to ventilatory support. Deleterious effects include barotrauma, hypotension and a fall in PaO_2.

METHODS OF REDUCING AUTO-PEEP
Auto-PEEP can be reduced by the use of (a) higher inspiratory flow rates, thereby shortening the inspiratory time and allowing longer time for expiration; (b) increased expiratory time by using smaller VT and reduced respiratory rates; (c) low-resistance exhalation valves and large-bore endotracheal tubes to reduce air trapping; (d) low compressible volume ventilator patient circuit.

It must be mentioned that the occurrence of auto-PEEP is not confined to patients on ventilator support. It is frequently observed in spontaneously breathing patients who have severe airways obstruction that leads to air-trapping.

Infection

Nosocomial infection is an important complication and the following preventive measures are enumerated below:

(i) Cleanliness in the patient's room with scrupulous attention to avoiding cross-infection. Washing hands prior to examining the patient is important.

(ii) Care of the tracheostomy wound—spraying the wound with an antibiotic spray is useful.

(iii) Aseptic suction of secretions through the tracheostomy/ endotracheal tube—this should be done as often as is necessary.

(iv) Meticulous attention to prevention of atelectasis by physiotherapy and postural drainage. Prompt treatment of atelectasis and diffuse airspace collapse is mandatory.

(v) Frequent sterilization of humidifiers, tubings is essential.

(vi) Tracheostomy tubes should be changed every four days under aseptic conditions.

(vii) Proper nutrition, oxygenation, and perfusion should be well maintained, so as to increase resistance to infection.

In patients on ventilator support, growth of Gram-negative organisms (chiefly pseudomonas strains and klebsiella) is frequently observed on culture of tracheal secretions. A positive culture by itself does not indicate infection, and does not warrant treatment (see chapter on 'Nosocomial Pneumonia').

Hypotension

This is an important complication of mechanical ventilation. When it occurs soon after initiating ventilation, it is very likely to be related to the effects of the ventilator. In the presence of high inflation pressures, the use of PEEP, or in patients with overcompliant lungs as seen in emphysema, there may be a marked rise in intrapleural pressure. This reduces venous return and cardiac filling and induces a fall in blood pressure. Hypotension is often marked in hypovolaemic patients. The treatment in such patients is to reduce inflation pressures, reduce or go off PEEP totally (if this has been used), and give a volume load to expand the circulating volume. Hypotension can also result from barotrauma, for example a pneumothorax induced by ventilator support. This may occur at the time of initiation of ventilator support or at a later period.

When hypotension occurs later during mechanical ventilation (the patient having been haemodynamically stable for several days), the cause is generally unrelated to the ventilator. Severe hypoxia and hypocapnia should be looked for, as they can induce a fall in blood pressure. If the blood gases are normal, hypotension may be due to shock, blood loss, fluid or electrolyte imbalance, sepsis, metabolic acidosis or poor pump function. Only if all these factors have been excluded,

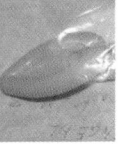

should the possibility of a ventilator-induced hypotension be considered.

Barotrauma, Volume Trauma and Biotrauma

Barotrauma and volume trauma (volutrauma) are the most important and dreaded complications of mechanical ventilation. Probably, both high inflation pressures and high tidal volumes, particularly when PEEP is also used, contribute to barotrauma. It is generally the more compliant parts of the lungs, and not the poorly compliant areas, that are susceptible to barotrauma. Barotrauma classically takes the form of pneumothorax—tension pneumothorax occurs when high tidal volumes are used with high inflation pressures. Unless promptly recognized, it causes cardiorespiratory collapse and death. Interstitial emphysema, mediastinal emphysema, and surgical emphysema of the soft tissues of the neck, spreading upwards to the face and downwards to the chest, may occur in the absence of pneumothorax.

A more subtle form of trauma to the alveolar walls can be caused by high tidal volumes (volume trauma or 'volutrauma'). High tidal volumes are as important in producing alveolar damage as high alveolar pressures. The over-stretched alveolar walls are damaged, so that alveoli (even those which were reasonably normal), are now thickened, distorted, and poorly compliant, thus adding to the overall stiffness and poor compliance of the lungs, and setting off a vicious cycle, which perpetuates respiratory failure to a point of no return. Over-stretch of alveoli with high tidal volumes is also believed to result in the production of cytokines that further injure the lung and perhaps also increase injury to other organs (biotrauma). The 'opening' and 'closing' of poorly compliant alveoli during inspiration and expiration results in shear forces that induce further lung injury (see chapter on ARDS).

Clashing with the Machine

This can occur at any time during mechanical ventilation, though it is most commonly observed during initiation of ventilator support. Clashing or fighting with the machine can be due to several causes, and each should be carefully evaluated prior to taking any decision on the management of the patient.

(i) Alveolar hypoventilation as stated earlier, is an important cause, if present, it should be corrected by increasing the minute ventilation.

(ii) Obstructed tracheostomy/endotracheal tube or obstructed airways due to bronchospasm or mucus plugging is an important cause of distress, leading to a 'clash' with the machine. A rise in peak pressure, with a fall in the dynamic compliance and a marked difference between the peak and pause pressures should point to the above cause.

(iii) Atelectasis, pneumonia, and pneumothorax are very important causes of a clash with the machine. Distress and high peak pressures with a fall in the compliance are observed.

(iv) Blood loss (as in bleeding within the gastrointestinal (GI) tract), shock from any cause, electrolyte imbalance, metabolic acidosis, high fever, pain, a distended bladder or colon, or a dilated stomach are other causes that aggravate difficulties in synchronization with the machine.

(v) A strong respiratory drive due to altered mechanics within diseased lungs may defy all efforts to match the machine to the patient. It is in this group that controlled ventilation after inducing neuromuscular paralysis or after depressing respiration with intravenous diazepam or morphine is mandatory.

(ix) Gastrointestinal Complications

Gastric dilatation and paralytic ileus are observed at times, particularly at the start of mechanical ventilation. The cause is obscure. Treatment is through gastric aspiration via a nasogastric tube, stopping all oral feeds, and using intravenous fluids till such time as gut motility returns. The maintenance of fluid and electrolyte balance in such patients is precarious. Hypokalaemia tends to aggravate the ileus, and needs to be carefully corrected by potassium replacement through intravenous infusions. Oral feeds are resumed once the gut motility returns.

GI bleeding occasionally occurs as a complication in patients on ventilator support. This is due to acute erosive gastroduodenitis in critically ill patients, particularly in those receiving corticosteroids. GI bleeding is particularly common with acute on chronic respiratory failure secondary to infection in patients with chronic bronchitis. These patients generally have a well-marked acidosis. Antacids and H_2-receptor antagonists, or sucralfate reduce gastric acidity, and thereby help stop bleeding. At times, laser therapy or endoscopic cauterization of bleeding points may be necessary. The blood loss should be replaced by transfusions.

Water Retention

Patients on prolonged ventilator support may retain water even in the clinical absence of left heart failure, or of a rise in venous pressure. Increase in the water content of the lungs may cause some degree of pulmonary oedema. This produces impaired gas exchange, and fluffy shadows in the lung on a chest X-ray. The problem is managed by restricting fluids to 1000 ml in 24 hours, and by the use of diuretics like furosemide.

WEANING FROM VENTILATOR SUPPORT

There are a number of patients who are electively intubated and mechanically ventilated for brief periods of time for reasons other than respiratory failure. These include those ventilated briefly after major surgery as an extension of intraoperative and postoperative surgical care, or those intubated for airway protection. An abrupt termination of ventilator support and often quick extubation is generally possible in such patients, if the following criteria are satisfied.

(i) The patient is awake, alert and can breathe well spontaneously. He should have a good 'blast' through the endotracheal tube, and if needs be, his tidal volume can be checked by connecting a spirometer to the endotracheal tube.

(ii) The clinical reason for ventilatory support no longer exists, or has resolved.

(iii) The airways are free of secretions through proper suction or spontaneous coughing, and the patient is capable of protecting the airways from aspiration.

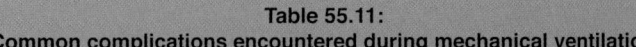

Table 55.11:
Common complications encountered during mechanical ventilation

Alveolar hyperventilation resulting in $PaCO_2 < 25$ mm Hg. This causes respiratory alkalosis (with decreased cerebral blood flow, tetany, hypotension), shift in K^+ from extracellular to cellular compartment causing arrhythmias, difficulties in weaning

Atelectasis—segmental, lobar or massive/diffuse airspace collapse

Uneven compliances in different areas of the lung resulting in uneven distribution of inspired gas and difficulty in mechanical ventilation

Occurrence of auto-PEEP

Nosocomial infection

Hypotension—Initially ventilator-related due to high inflation pressures; later, usually unrelated to ventilator support

Barotrauma/Volutrauma/Biotrauma—pneumothorax, pneumomediastinum, interstitial emphysema, damage to alveolar walls

'Clashing' with the machine

GI complications—paralytic ileus, gastric dilatation, GI bleeds

Water retention

(iv) The patient's chest X-ray is normal, and shows no atelectasis or pulmonary shadowing.

(v) In patients ventilated after open-heart surgery or following major surgical procedures, the arterial blood gases and arterial pH should be normal or near normal, both during ventilator support, and after discontinuing support.

(vi) The patient should remain under intensive care so that respiratory care can be continued in the form of humidification of inspired gas, nebulization therapy, physiotherapy, and if necessary, reintroduction of ventilator support.

The weaning parameters stated below are generally not required to be followed in these patients. When however postoperative pulmonary complications produce respiratory failure, or the presence of infection, bleeding or other complications leads to an increasingly critical state, the decision to wean is necessarily delayed. Clinical considerations together with the respiratory parameters discussed below, help to decide the appropriate time to commence weaning from ventilatory support in these patients.

Patients who require ventilator support for long periods of time, extending for a week or even months, are not easy to wean. Prolonged mechanical ventilation is often necessary in severe or fulminant tetanus, severe ALI, acute infective polyneuritis and poliomyelitis. The decision to wean such patients from ventilator support should first and foremost be a clinical one, based on clinical considerations. Parameters for weaning are useful, but they should support or supplement a clinical decision, and never be used as a substitute for it.

Clinical Considerations for Weaning

(i) As a general principle, mechanical ventilatory support can only be withdrawn when the reasons for initiating it are no longer present. This usually means that the underlying disease, whether it involves the lungs or not, has been cured or has markedly improved.

(ii) It is important that the patient on ventilator support maintains normal arterial blood gases at a FIO_2 of 0.4, before withdrawal of ventilator support is even contemplated. An important exception to this are patients with chronic airways obstruction who are being ventilated for acute on chronic respiratory failure. These patients are used to a PaO_2 of around 60 mm Hg and to a high $PaCO_2$, even under 'normal' conditions.

(iii) The lungs should be free of infection, atelectasis or oedema, as far as possible. Airways obstruction, either from mucus plugging or bronchospasm should be relieved as best as possible, as it significantly increases the work of breathing.

(iv) Disturbances in acid-base balance should be corrected before weaning is commenced. Metabolic acidosis can increase the work of breathing significantly, while alkalosis can result in mental obtundation, and depress respiration.

(v) A clinical judgment should be made whether the patient in the immediate future can withstand or cope with the demands imposed by the work of breathing. The general nutritional state and the neuromuscular status should be given careful consideration. Poor nutrition, electrolyte abnormalities, hypomagnesaemia and hypophosphataemia lead to difficulties in weaning. Severely catabolic states like tetanus result in marked weight loss and loss of muscle mass in spite of providing a large caloric and protein intake. High-carbohydrate diets lead to an increase in carbon dioxide production with increasing demands on ventilation, particularly in debilitated individuals, or in those with pre-existing lung disease. In such patients, less carbohydrates and more fats should be used for nutrition.

Patients with severe liver cell dysfunction, chronic renal failure, chronic alcoholics, and those who have weathered a prolonged critical illness, often pose great difficulties in weaning, chiefly because of their poor nutritional state, and their inability to cope with the work of breathing.

(vi) Haemodynamic stability, particularly in critically ill patients, is necessary before weaning can be commenced. As far as possible it is best to await the withdrawal of inotropic support before attempting to wean a seriously ill patient off ventilator support.

(vii) Ventilator support should be continued and weaning delayed in the presence of high fever, seizures, or when complications such as gastric dilatation, ileus, GI bleeding, or acute renal failure exist.

(viii) The patient should be awake, alert and cooperative, though there are exceptions to this consideration. The patient should also be prepared, indoctrinated and motivated to go off the ventilator.

Objective Respiratory Parameters for Weaning

The objective criteria used to supplement the clinical decision to wean a patient are a respiratory rate < 30/min, a V_E preferably < or equal to 8 l/min, and not > 10 l/min, a V_T of at least 5–7 ml/kg, a VC of at least 800–1000 ml, and a maximum inspiratory

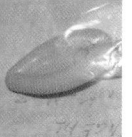

Table 55.12:
Clinical considerations for weaning patient from ventilator support

Mechanical ventilator support should be withdrawn only when the underlying disorder (pulmonary or extra-pulmonary) has completely resolved, or has improved markedly

Patient should maintain normal arterial blood gases on FIO_2 of 0.4 (except in patients with COPD whose basal P_aCO_2 values are raised, and P_aO_2 is around 60 mm Hg)

There should be no significant pulmonary infection, pulmonary oedema, atelectasis or airways obstruction

Acid-base and electrolyte balance should be corrected prior to weaning

The patient should generally be alert, co-operate and mentally prepared to be weaned; he must be haemodynamically stable and preferably off inotropic support

General nutritional state and neuromuscular status must be clinically assessed as to whether patient can cope with the work of breathing

In presence of high fever, seizures, gastric dilatation, paralytic ileus, GI bleeds, hepatic or acute renal failure, weaning should not be attempted.

On T-tube breathing, there should be no significant change in pulse rate, BP, no tachypnoea or respiratory distress, should maintain normal blood gases and a tidal volume of 5–7 ml/kg.

force > –20 cm H_2O. The arterial pH should be between 7.35–7.45, the PaO_2 between 75–100 mm Hg on an FIO_2 of 0.4, and the $PaCO_2$ should be normal, except in patients with chronic airways obstruction who are used to a higher $PaCO_2$. The finer niceties that may need to be looked into are a V_D/V_T ratio which should be < 0.6, and the alveolar-arterial gradient which should be < 250 on an FIO_2 of 1.

Weaning is not possible if the peak or the plateau pressures are high. The static compliance should preferably be equal to or > 30 ml/cm H_2O, and the airway resistance should not be significantly increased. PEEP should be withdrawn before starting to wean the patient off ventilator support.

Probably, the simplest bedside test to assess the feasibility of weaning is to note the respiratory rate after removing the

Table 55.13:
Objective respiratory parameters for weaning

1. Ventilatory Parameters

- RR < 30/minute

- V_E < 8 l/minute, and not > 10 l/minute

- V_T of minimum 5–7 ml/kg

- VC of minimum 800–1000 ml

- Maximum Inspiratory Force > – 20 cm H_2O

- V_D/V_T < 0.6

- Alveolar-arterial oxygen gradient on FIO_2 of 1 < 250 mm Hg

2. Arterial Blood Gases

- pH—7.35–7.45

- PaO_2—70–100 mm Hg on FIO_2 of 0.4

- $PaCO_2$—35–45 mm Hg

ventilator. Rapid (> 30 breaths/min) shallow (V_T < 300 ml) breathing is a clear indication for continuing ventilator support. An attempt has been made to compute a weaning index to predict whether attempts at weaning will be successful or not. This weaning index incorporates the efficiency of gas exchange, along with determination of load and neuromuscular competence. It is the product of a modified pressure-time index and a factor derived from the minute ventilation required to maintain an arterial $PaCO_2$ of 40 mm Hg. We feel that the use of such indices is confusing and unnecessary. Clinical considerations, simple bedside procedures and monitoring of arterial blood gases almost always suffice.

Method of Weaning or Withdrawal of Ventilatory Support

It matters little whether weaning is performed with SIMV at progressively lower rates, with the PS mode, or with a T-piece. We prefer the T-piece and have always managed to wean patients successfully even after months on ventilator support. Weaning requires to be very gradual in patients who have been on mechanical ventilation for prolonged periods of time, in those who have had a prolonged critical illness, and in those with muscle weakness or a poor nutritional state. It should start with just 15–30 minutes off the ventilator. The period is slowly but progressively increased under constant supervision, to reach a stage where the patient is off the ventilator for longer periods, than on it. In the next stage, the patient is weaned off all support during the day, but is kept on the ventilator at night. Finally, the patient is weaned off ventilator support at night as well.

Parameters to watch during the weaning process include the pulse rate, blood pressure, the respiratory rate and signs of respiratory muscle fatigue. Tachypnoea > 30/min during weaning, points to fatigue of the respiratory muscles, and weaning should be delayed or slowed down. Arterial blood gases should be satisfactory while the patient is off ventilator support. A fall in oxygen saturation to < 90% (as judged by pulse oximetry), or a rise in $PaCO_2$ to > 45 mm Hg whilst off ventilator support, are clear warnings that weaning should be slower.

Another method of weaning is to give a single daily trial of spontaneous breathing through a T-tube. This trial is carried out under close observation. If the patient can sustain spontaneous ventilation for 60 minutes without distress (a satisfactory respiratory rate, pulse, blood pressure, tidal volume), the patient can be extubated. If the patient shows features of distress, he or she is placed back on A/C mode of ventilator support for the next 24 hours. The patient is reassessed the next day for another trial of spontaneous breathing. In a recent study two-thirds of patients who were on ventilator support for about seven days, could be extubated by the above technique; without being 'weaned' in the strict sense of the word. It is doubtful if this technique would prove equally successful in patients who have been critically ill on ventilator support for several weeks or months.

Patients with chronic bronchitis who are under intensive care for an acute respiratory crisis, are often used to higher $PaCO_2$ levels ranging between 45–60 mm Hg. During weaning, these patients should be given controlled oxygen therapy at 1–2 l/min to provide an oxygen saturation of not more than 90%. Uncontrolled oxygen therapy can lead to progressive hypercapnia. Ventilator support may need to be restarted under these circumstances.

Some centres prefer to wean patients by using the IMV mode. The mandatory breaths in this mode are progressively decreased till almost all the breaths are spontaneous. This convinces and reassures the patient that ventilatory support can be dispensed with. Pressure support ventilation is also used at times as a mode to wean patients, particularly those with chronic airways obstruction. To start with, a pressure support of 20 cm or more is introduced. The pressure support is then reduced gradually, with a watch on the tidal volume and respiratory rate. If a patient can breathe comfortably with a good tidal volume when pressure support is down to 5 cm H_2O, spontaneous breathing through a T-tube is generally possible. Patients being weaned with this mode should be very carefully monitored—atelectasis, increased secretions or bronchospasm can result in low tidal volumes with disastrous consequences.

Two controlled prospective studies recently compared the efficacy of different weaning methods in 'difficult to wean' ventilator-dependent patients. In both studies IMV was noted to delay weaning. In one study, a single daily trial of spontaneous breathing through a T-tube was responsible for a two-fold increase in successful weaning and extubation compared to the use of pressure support. In the second trial pressure support was found to be superior to T-tube trials.

Experience with more than 1, 000 patients has convinced us that T-tube weaning is almost always successful, even in the most difficult cases. The IMV and PSV modes are indeed very rarely necessary; if handled ineptly these modes can aggravate rather than solve problems during the weaning process.

NON-INVASIVE POSITIVE PRESSURE VENTILATION

A number of critical care units attempt, in suitable patients, to offer ventilatory support through a nasal mask or through a fitting orofacial mask rather than through an endotracheal tube. The major advantage of non-invasive positive pressure ventilation (NIPPV) is the reduced incidence of nosocomial pneumonia and of other complications associated with endotracheal intubation.

The use of NIPPV has been standard therapy in patients with obstructive sleep apnoea and in many patients with central sleep apnoea. Other indications for NIPPV in acute respiratory failure are as follows:

(i)   Acute crisis in chronic airways obstruction. This is dealt with at length in the chapter on Management of COPD.
(ii) In some patients with mild to moderate cardiogenic or non-cardiogenic pulmonary oedema. The more severe forms need intubation and ventilatory support.
(iii) Community-acquired pneumonia with acute respiratory failure.
(iv) In AIDS with *Pneumocystis carinii* infection or with other forms of disseminated pulmonary infection.
(v)   Hypercapnic respiratory failure due to progressive chronic airways obstruction, or due to the obesity hypoventilation syndrome.
(vi) Postoperative respiratory failure (chiefly due to atelectasis).

It is obvious that if NIPPV fails to effect efficient gas exchange, or cannot be tolerated by the patient, prompt intubation with ventilator support becomes necessary.

NIPPV is contraindicated under the following conditions:

(i)   In patients with a respiratory arrest or need for immediate intubation.
(ii) Inability to protect the airway.
(iii) In the presence of copious respiratory secretions.
(iv) Haemodynamic instability or persistent hypotension (systolic < 90 mm Hg).
(v)   Occurrence of dangerous or persistent arrhythmia.
(vi) Inability to cooperate or tolerate either the nasal or facial mask.
(vii) In the presence of facial injuries.

NIPPV is also occasionally used after extubation in patients with marginal weaning criteria. NIPPV offers a transition from intubation to spontaneous breathing.

Different modes of ventilator support have been used with NIPPV. These include volume assist/control, pressure control, pressure support and the CPAP modes.

The major danger with NIPPV is the risk of aspiration of gastric contents. It is best not to exceed positive inspiratory peak pressures of 20–25 cm H_2O as gastric dilatation with fear of aspiration can become a major problem. The setting should allow a tidal volume of 7–10 ml/kg.

Bilevel pressure ventilators (BiPAP machine) should generally be used for long-term or chronic application of NIPPV as in patients with obstructive sleep apnoea or patients with chronic hypercapnic respiratory failure due to COPD. The expiratory positive airway pressure (EPAP) is set at 3–8 cm H_2O and the inspiratory airway pressure (IPAP) to +10 to +20 cm H_2O to provide effective ventilation. A backup assist rate should be set during sleep.

Table 55.14: Indications of NIPPV
1. Acute crisis in chronic airways obstruction
2. Mild to moderate cardiogenic or non-cardiogenic pulmonary oedema
3. Community acquired pneumonia with acute respiratory failure
4. AIDS with pneumocystis carinii infection or any other infection
5. Hypercapnic respiratory failure due to chronic airways obstruction or the obesity hypoventilation syndrome
6. Postoperative respiratory failure (chiefly due to atelectasis)

Table 55.15: Contraindications of NIPPV
1. Respiratory arrest or need for immediate intubation
2. Inability to protect the airway
3. Presence of copious respiratory secretions
4. Haemodynamic instability or persistent hypotension
5. Persistent arrhythmia
6. Inability to cooperate or tolerate either the nasal or facial mask
7. Presence of facial injuries

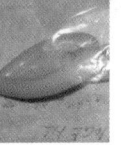

RESPIRATORY MONITORING DURING MECHANICAL VENTILATION

Monitoring of respiratory mechanics is only possible during volume-controlled ventilation, a ventilatory mode perhaps most often used in most ICUs at least at the start of invasive ventilatory support. The discussion below is limited to patients on volume-preset ventilation. Determining respiratory mechanics at the start and during mechanical ventilation is an important and necessary aspect of ventilatory management. It is important to note the peak pressures, the pause pressures, the tidal volumes, the PEEP, both extrinsic and intrinsic (if present), and to determine from these observations the dynamic compliance, static compliance and the resistance of the airway.

Airway Pressure and PEEP Measurement

Measurements are reasonably accurate when the patient is relaxed (preferably sedated) on volume-preset ventilatory support. The inspiratory airway pressure (P_{aw}) has three components–one, to overcome resistance of the airways during inspiration, the second, to overcome elastic recoil of the alveoli and expand them, the third, equal to end-expiratory alveolar pressure (PEEP) if this is present.

$$P_{aw} = P_R + P_{stat} + PEEP$$
where P_{stat} = static elastic pressure
P_R = resistive pressure component
$$P_{aw} = V_I \times R + V_T \times E + PEEP$$
where V_I = inspiratory flow
R = resistance of airways
E = elastance of the airways

The individual components of P_{aw} when separated provide significant diagnostic and therapeutic information. PEEP can be measured by the end-expiratory occlusion method. Most ventilators now provide an expiratory pause switch which allows a direct read-out of the PEEP. An error may creep into the measurement of intrinsic PEEP by this method if there is a leak around the endotracheal tubing or around the endotracheal tube cuff or when there is continuous nebulization with bronchodilators at the time of measurement, so that there is gas flow into the circuit, or if the patient is not completely taken over by the machine, and is not relaxed. Extrinsic PEEP is measured as set by the machine. Once PEEP has been measured the remainder of the airways pressure ($\Delta P = Ppeak—PEEP$) can be apportioned between the pressure needed to overcome airways resistance (P_{res}) and pressure needed to overcome elastic recoil (P_{es}). This is done by stopping flow at end-inspiration and allowing the P_{aw} to drop to a plateau level (P_{plat}).

The difference between the peak pressure and the plateau pressure is a measure of the airway resistance. The greater the difference between the peak pressure and the plateau pressure the greater the airways resistance.

If the inspiratory flow rate (V_I) is 60 l/min or 1 l/sec the airways resistance during inspiration (P_{res}) is between 4 to 10 cm H_2O. A rise in airways resistance denoted by an increase in the difference between peak airway pressure and plateau pressure is observed with bronchospasm, obstruction of the large airways or mucus plugging of the bronchi, bronchioles and small airways. An increase in airways resistance (increased difference between the peak and plateau pressures) also occurs if there is obstruction of the endotracheal tube or tracheostomy tube or the trachea. In patients with bronchospasm the airways resistance may fall after nebulization with a bronchodilator and this is evinced by a narrowing of the gap between the peak pressure and the plateau pressure.

There now remains the need to determine the resistance offered by the elastic recoil of the lungs. This is indirectly determined by computing the compliance of the lung.

Dynamic compliance = Tidal volume / Peak pressure – PEEP (if present)
Static compliance = Tidal volume / Plateau pressure – PEEP (if present)
The normal compliance is about 70 ml/cm H_2O.

A reduced static compliance means increased elastic recoil of the lungs—i.e. 'stiff lungs' as in pulmonary fibrosis, pulmonary oedema, areas of atelectasis, ALI and consolidation. Static compliance is also reduced when a patient on ventilator support develops a pneumothorax, collapsed lobe or lung or when there is increased stiffness of the chest wall or in the presence of abdominal distension.

A significant fall in compliance (the causes of which are listed above) will cause a sharp rise in both peak and pause pressures, pointing thereby to stiff lungs but no increase in the airways resistance (since there will be no increase in the difference between peak and pause pressure).

An increased compliance is observed in emphysema in which there is a loss of elastic recoil within the lungs. If the cause of ventilatory failure in a patient is undetermined at the time of intubation an assessment of the peak and plateau pressure, and of the compliance will help to determine the nature of the problem. A normal peak and plateau pressure in a patient intubated and ventilated for ventilatory failure should make the physician suspect an impaired central drive to breath or neuromuscular weakness as the underlying cause of ventilatory failure.

SUGGESTED READING

Calfee CS. Recent advances in mechanical ventilation. *Am J Med.* 1 Jun. 2005; 118(6): 584–91.

Haitsma JJ. Physiology of mechanical ventilation. *Crit Care Clin.* 1 Apr. 2007; 23(2): 117–34, vii.

Papadakos PJ. The open lung concept of mechanical ventilation: the role of recruitment and stabilization. *Crit Care Clin.* 1 Apr. 2007; 23(2): 241–50, ix–x.

Ramnath VR. Conventional mechanical ventilation in acute lung injury and acute respiratory distress syndrome. *Clin Chest Med.* 1 Dec. 2006; 27(4): 601–13; abstract viii.

Santanilla JI. Mechanical ventilation. *Emerg Med Clin North Am.* 1 Aug. 2008; 26(3): 849–62, x.

ACUTE RESPIRATORY DISTRESS SYNDROME

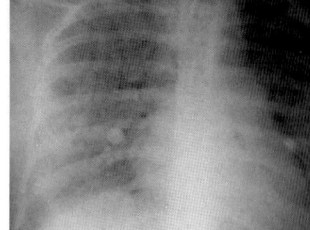

CHAPTER **56** **Acute Respiratory Distress Syndrome**

GENERAL CONSIDERATIONS

The Acute Respiratory Distress Syndrome (ARDS) is an important condition characterized by non-cardiogenic increased permeability, inflammatory pulmonary oedema, with diffuse alveolar damage; it leads to hypoxemic respiratory failure necessitating ventilator support and prolonged intensive care.

The first description of what probably was ARDS was given by Osler in his Textbook of Medicine in 1927. He wrote of 'uncontrolled septicaemia leading to pulmonary oedema' and went on to describe the clinical features and autopsy findings very nearly as we know them today. In 1967, Ashbaugh, Bigelow and Petty reported in the *Lancet* the occurrence of non-cardiogenic pulmonary oedema and acute respiratory failure in a number of diverse pathologies not directly involving the lungs. They termed this condition the adult respiratory distress syndrome. Semantically speaking, this was an unfortunate term. The syndrome can occur at all ages and is not related in its pathogenesis and pathology to the respiratory distress syndrome of the newborn. Also, the connotation of 'respiratory distress' is both vague and common to numerous other unrelated pathologies in cardiorespiratory medicine. The syndrome is now termed the Acute Respiratory Distress Syndrome (ARDS). Semantic confusion would have been avoided if from the very outset the condition had been termed Acute Lung Injury. Since 1967, the syndrome has been reported from many countries, including India. The precipitating factors have been recognized and the pathology of the lung has been elucidated. However, the pathogenesis after more than 40 years of research remains unclear and the mortality in spite of expert intensive care, even today is as high as 30–60%.

EPIDEMIOLOGY

The incidence of ARDS even in Western countries has not been clearly established. The National Heart, Lung and Blood Institute-sponsored ARDS Network of 20 hospitals estimated that the incidence could be as high as 64 cases per 100,000 population. The prevalence in developing countries including India is unknown. ARDS constituted a little over 4 % of ICU admissions in our unit over a five-year period. It is unquestionably a problem that is likely to be encountered with increasing frequency by all physicians who look after critically ill patients.

DEFINITION AND CONCEPT

ARDS is characterized by (i) an antecedent history of a precipitating condition; (ii) respiratory distress and refractory hypoxaemia not responding satisfactorily to supplemental oxygen and invariably necessitating the use of mechanical ventilatory support; (iii) radiographic evidence of newly evolving bilateral pulmonary infiltrates; and (iv) pulmonary artery occlusion pressure (PAOP) < 18 mm Hg in the presence of a normal colloid oncotic pressure.

The physiological changes underlying the above clinical definition include a reduced functional residual capacity (FRC), stiff lungs (reduced pulmonary compliance), increased ventilation-perfusion inequalities, an increase in the right to left shunt within the lungs, and an increase in the extravascular water content of the lungs with, as already mentioned, a normal PAOP. *The underlying pathological abnormality is damage to the alveolar capillary membrane with increased capillary permeability, leading to oedema, inflammation and subsequent fibrosis.*

The American–European Consensus Conference in 1994 clinically defined and distinguished between acute lung injury (ALI) and acute respiratory distress syndrome (ARDS), so as to avoid semantic confusion. The American–European Consensus Definition of ALI and ARDS is given in Table 56.1.

Table 56.1: The Americal–European Consensus Definition of Acute Lung Injury (ALI) and Acute Respiratory Distress Syndrome (ARDS)	
Acute Lung Injury (ALI)	Acute Respiratory Distress Syndrome (ARDS)
1. Acute onset respiratory failure	1. Acure onset respiratory failure
2. Bilateral chest infiltrates on frontal radiogaphs	2. Bilateral chest infiltrates on frontal radiographs
3. $PaO_2/FIO_2 < 300$	3. $PaO_2/FIO_2 < 200$
4. Absence of elevated left heart filling pressure (PAOP < 19 mm Hg)	4. Absence of elevated left heart filling pressure (PAOP < 18 mm Hg)

A more recent definition has been proposed through a Delphi method. This definition again primarily relies on hypoxemia ($PaO_2/FIO_2 < 200$, with a positive end-expiratory pressure [PEEP] > 10 cm H_2O), and the presence of bilateral chest infiltrates as detected on chest radiography. All definitions exclude the presence of unilateral lung injury and the presence of cardiogenic pulmonary oedema detected either through clinical judgement or through measurement of PAOP.

The most widely accepted definition is that proposed by the American-European Consensus Conference in 1994. Though there is a definite advantage in an internationally accepted definition, this definition has both lacunae and limitations.

These need to be considered for a balanced perspective of the syndrome.

1. The present definition does not include any aetiology or responsible risk factors. Perhaps this is because there are many (and a growing number of) background risk factors—some common and others uncommon. Also there may be more than one responsible factor in a patient.

2. Though ARDS signifies non-cardiogenic pulmonary oedema, patients with a background of left ventricular dysfunction and raised left atrial pressure may fortuitously suffer from a risk factor such as sepsis which could further evolve into ARDS. Both ARDS and cardiogenic pulmonary oedema may thus coexist. This is uncommon, but has been observed in our intensive care unit. Again, in the natural history of ARDS due to severe sepsis, cardiac function is often seriously compromised with a sharply reduced ejection fraction and raised filling pressures. When a patient is seen for the first time at this juncture, diagnosis is difficult.

3. 'Bilateral chest infiltrates' have been taken as a surrogate marker for the increased permeability inflammatory pulmonary oedema that characterizes ARDS. Meade and colleagues have shown that the specificity of a chest radiograph in indicating inflammatory oedema is questionable. Similar infiltrates on a chest radiography can occur with atelectasis, consolidation, interstitial and intra-acinar oedema.

4. The concept of ARDS as stated by the American–European Congress Conference is narrow in its perspective. An expanded concept should include not only the severity of the acute lung injury, but also the background factor causing or precipitating the syndrome, and most importantly the associated or evolving dysfunction of organ systems. *Most investigators consider ALI/ARDS as merely one facet of the multiple organ dysfunction syndrome.*

5. The diagnostic accuracy of the different definitions of ARDS has been recently assessed using as a reference or gold standard the finding of diffuse alveolar damage at autopsy. The commonly accepted criteria for the diagnosis of ARDS as stated by the American-European Congress Conference showed an acceptable sensitivity (0.83%) but a poor specificity (0.51%).

We therefore feel that the correct definition of ARDS is still an unsettled issue. Randomized trials using different ventilatory and other strategies to test for improved survival have been based on enrolling patients according to a given definition. It is obvious that an inappropriate definition of ARDS would lead to inappropriate enrollment of patients in trials, which in turn could lead to biased and misleading results.

AETIOLOGY

A variety of clinical disorders and risk factors can lead to ALI and ARDS. The incidence of various risk factors in relation to ARDS will depend on the geographical areas and the population that is studied. In India and in other tropical developing countries in addition to the risk factors observed in the West, there are special important risk factors chiefly confined to tropical poor countries.

The various clinical disorders that can lead to ALI or ARDS may do so by directly involving the lung (direct injury), or may involve the lung indirectly (indirect injury). Our experience on ARDS with regard to aetiology, and mortality in relation to each aetiological factor is summarized in the table below:

Table 56.2: The aetiology of ARDS as observed in our unit with observed mortality for each aetiological factor. Note the differece in mortality between ARDS (and MODS) in 'tropical problems' and 'non-tropical problems'			
Severe Acute Lung Injury Data	Total	Expired	Mortality
Total no. of patients	187	91	49%
Patients with tropical problems	52	14	27%
Patients with non-tropical problems	135	77	57%
Patients with non-tropical problems (n = 135)			
1. Direct Injury			
Acute pulmonary infection	33	23	70%
Aspiration pneumonia	18	11	61%
Direct trauma	7	2	29%
Noxious	5	0	0%
Pulmonary vasculitis	4	0	0%
Total	67	36	54%
2. Indirect Injury			
Severe sepsis	36	24	67%
Pancreatitis	9	5	56%
Burns	4	3	75%
Extrathoracic injury	4	0	0%
Poisoning	2	0	0%
Miscellaneous	13	8	62%
Total	68	41	60%
Patients with tropical problems			
Tetanus	9	4	44%
OP poisoning	10	1	10%
Cerebral malaria	10	3	30%
Gram negative sepsis from contaminated food	5	0	0%
Miliary/Disseminated Haematogenous tuberculosis	8	3	38%
Amoebiasis	5	2	40%
Salmonella infections	3	0	0%
Rabies	1	1	100%
Leptospirosis	1	0	0%
Total	52	14	27%

In 187 patients of ARDS studied over several years in our intensive care unit, 'direct injury' was the'aetiological factor in 67 patients; 'indirect injury' was the causative factor in 68 patients; and 51 patients developed ARDS due to fulminant infections and problems peculiar to the tropical and developing countries of the world. For convenience, these 51 patients were categorized under ARDS due to tropical problems. The first two groups of patients, for convenience, were categorized under non-tropical problems i.e. problems more or less common to the whole world. Though the exact incidence of various clinical disorders causing ALI/ARDS in different critical care units in India may vary for several reasons, the nature of risk factors is by and large common to critical care units in the large metropolitan centres of the country.

The most important cause of direct injury perhaps all over the world is acute pulmonary infection (chiefly bacterial or viral pneumonia). Aspiration pneumonia is also an important risk factor, both aspirated gastric acid and enzymes contributing to lung injury. After aspiration, lung injury may take some hours to evolve and manifest. Direct trauma to the chest with contusions within the lung is an important cause, particularly in trauma units. Polytrauma even when not directly involving the chest is an even more important cause and is probably due to inflammatory mediators released from trauma sites acting on the lungs.

Sepsis is unquestionably the most important cause of ALI/ARDS all over the world. In sepsis ALI and ARDS form merely one facet of the multi-organ dysfunction syndrome. The incidence of ALI and ARDS in severe sepsis or septic shock is over 25 %. Sepsis not only initiates acute lung injury but also perpetuates it. Even when ARDS is caused by a direct injury or insult to the lung, sepsis may subsequently supervene as a major complication and can worsen lung injury and cause multiple organ dysfunction. When sepsis is the indirect cause of acute lung injury, the source of sepsis is most frequently intra-abdominal. On the other hand, when sepsis is a supervening complication in a patient suffering from acute lung injury due to any other aetiology, the source of sepsis is most frequently within the lung itself.

Acute pancreatitis, burns, poisoning (in particular organo-phosphorus poisoning) are other important causes of ARDS.

There are a number of varying miscellaneous causes being reported with increasing frequency from different parts of the world. Among these, multiple blood transfusions head the list. ARDS following multiple blood transfusion has been reported in both trauma patients as also in non-trauma patients, such as patients transfused following massive GI bleeds. In trauma patients, systemic inflammatory mediators may perhaps play a greater or equal role as multiple blood transfusion in causing ALI/ARDS. Current evidence suggests that the risk of lung injury increases with the duration of stored blood.

Transfusion-related acute lung injury (TRALI) resembles ALI/ARDS, yet is not the same. This form of injury can be caused by transfusion of even small quantities of whole blood or any blood product. The cause is believed to be due to passively transfused antibodies that act as leukagglutins attaching to antigens on the recipient leucocytes, thereby causing lung injury. TRALI manifests with breathlessness during or after transfusion of whole blood or a blood product accompanied by shadows in the mid and lower zones of both lung fields.

Tachycardia and a fall in oxygen saturation are often observed. TRALI is often mistaken for acute left ventricular failure.

TROPICAL INFECTIONS AND PROBLEMS

It is pertinent and important to briefly outline tropical problems causing ALI and ARDS. These, in our experience, include fulminant *P. falciparum* infections, severe tetanus, severe typhoid infections, fulminant Gram-negative infections following ingestion of contaminated food, acute miliary tuberculosis, acute disseminated haematogenous tuberculosis, fulminant amoebic infections of the liver and large bowel, fulminant leptospirosis, haemorrhagic fevers and rabies. Severe organophosphorus poisoning is the most frequently encountered poisoning causing ARDS in western India. In the north, aluminium phosphide (added generally for the preservation of food grains) poisoning is an important cause of severe ARDS which invariably ends fatally. Each of these tropical problems can lead not only to ARDS, but to progressive multiple organ failure and death. The most important of these causes are fulminant P. falciparum infections, tetanus, acute miliary tuberculosis, acute haematogenous disseminated tuberculosis, leptospiral infections and fulminant B. typhosus infections.

The following clinical forms of ARDS have been noted in relation to severe P. falciparum malaria:

(i) Acute pulmonary oedema due to hyperpyrexia (temperature > 107°F).
(ii) Progressive bilateral shadowing within the lungs characterized physiologically by marked ventilation-perfusion inequalities, but by only a slight increase in the right to left shunt within the lungs—recovery is possible with good management.
(iii) Progressive bilateral fluffy shadows characterized physiologically by a marked increase in the right to left shunt—prognosis of patients in this category is grim.
(iv) ARDS caused by disseminated intravascular coagulopathy complicating falciparum infection.
(v) ARDS due to aspiration of gastric contents in obtunded patients.

The time from the original insult (direct or indirect), to the development of full-blown ALI has been studied in many large series. In Petty's original group it ranged from 1 to 96 hours. In a comprehensive, recent epidemiological study, 80% of patients had developed ALI within 48 hours of the initial insult, and 90% by 80 hours. This latent period offers a window of opportunity for therapeutic interventions, when effective blockers of the inflammatory process can be identified. Indeed, today there is a massive search for circulating markers of ALI which can be identified in the serum or bronchoalveolar lavage (BAL) fluid.

PATHOLOGY

The work of Gattioni and his colleagues on computed tomography (CT) scans in ARDS has brought forth important new concepts. The first of these concepts is that the lung in ARDS is not homogeneously affected. The most affected part

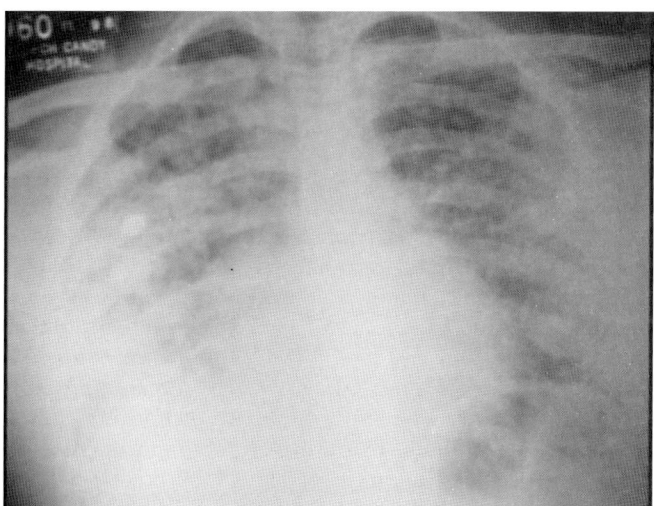

Fig 56.1: ARDS in typhoid; note extensive bilateral shadowing.

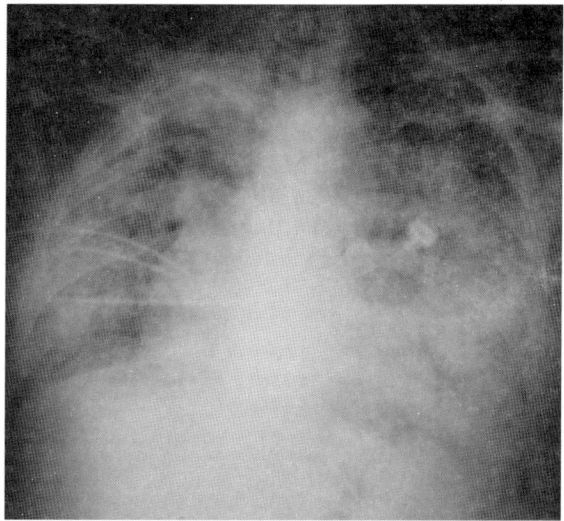

Fig 56.3: ARDS in malaria, showing extensive bilateral fluffy shadows.

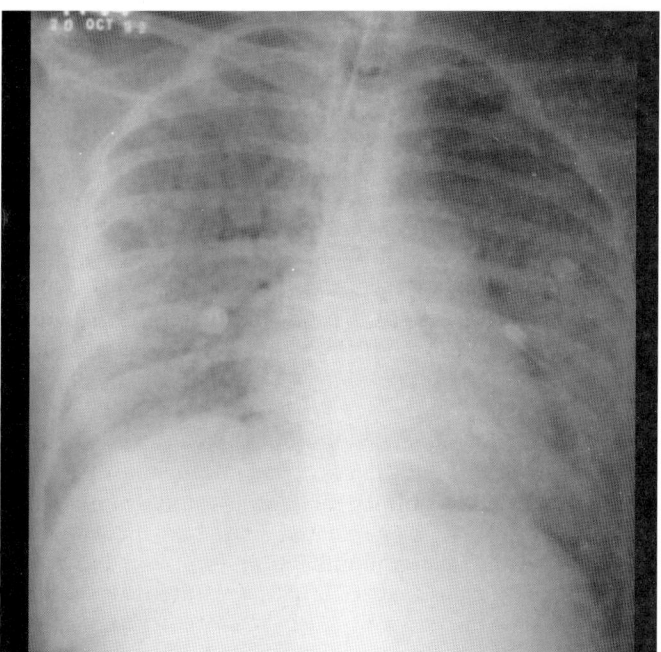

Fig 56.2: ARDS in tetanus.

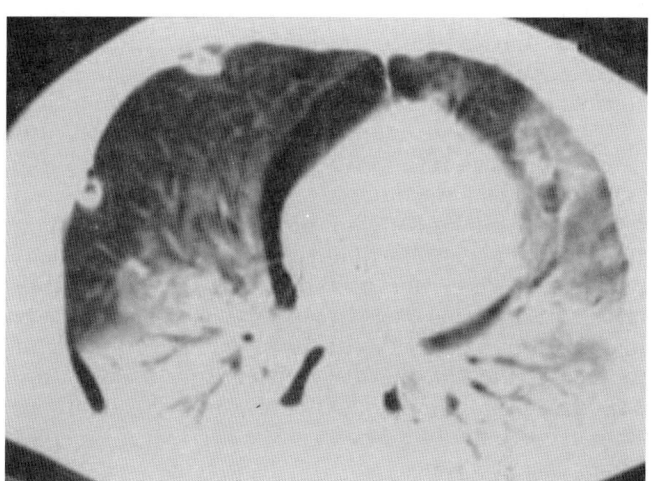

Fig 56.4: HRCT of the chest in ARDS. The most dependent part of the lung is dense and consolidated; above this is inflammatory oedema; right at the top is normally aerated lung.

of the lung is the most dependent portion. This dependent area is consolidated and represents 'core' disease, generally constituting about 24% of lung weight. The part or zone above this dependent portion is 'collapsed lung', the collapse being due to the weight of inflammatory oedema which is the hallmark of ARDS; still above the 'collapsed lung' is the zone of normally areated or even over-ventilated lung. (Figures 56.4, 56.5) The extent of the zone constituting collapsed lung varies. Of importance is the fact that this collapsed lung is capable of being opened up, that is to say it is recruitable by ventilatory measures (raising inspiratory pressure from +5 to 45 cm H_2O). The greater the recruitability, the greater the inflammatory oedema, the more severe the disease and worse the prognosis. The lesser the recruitability, the lesser the inflammatory oedema; the disease is then milder and the prognosis better.

The above views put forth by Gattioni not only allow a better conceptualization of ARDS, but also better prognostication, and perhaps most importantly may further guide ventilatory strategies in the management of this syndrome.

The basic pathological feature is damage to the alveolar capillary membrane leading to an increased permeability, inflammatory interstitial and alveolar oedema, alveolar atelectasis, consolidation and diffuse alveolar damage. Three overlapping phases are observed:

(i) Exudative phase in which there is an alveolar exudate with hyaline membrane formation along the alveolar ducts and within the alveoli.

(ii) Proliferative phase in which there is a proliferation of inflammatory cells, lymphocytes and Type 2 pneumocytes. Organization of the inflammatory exudate, combined with damage to the surfactant leads to obliteration of air spaces, atelectatic alveoli and a poorly compliant lung.

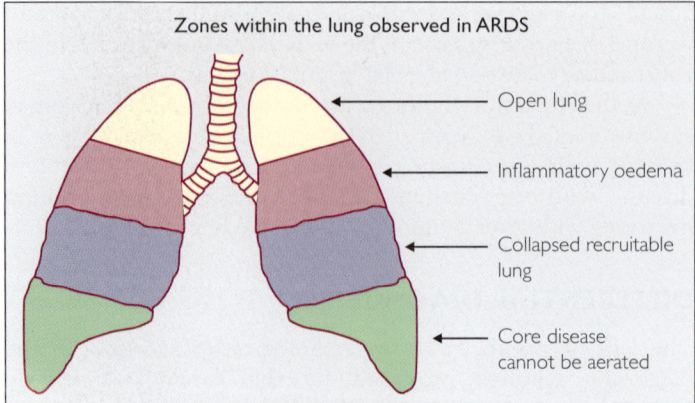

Fig 56.5: A schematic representation of 'zones' within the lungs in ARDS. The most dependant zone is consolidated lung which cannot be aerated; above this is collapsed but recruitable lung; still above is the zone of inflammatory oedema, the weight of which is responsible for the zone of collapsed recruitable lung; right at the top is normally ventilated or even hyperventilated lung.

(iii) Fibrotic phase which follows soon upon the proliferative phase, and is characterized by fibroblasts laying down fibrous tissue that strangles alveoli, and further reduces pulmonary compliance.

Severe lung injury distorts the pulmonary vasculature. Distortion with remodelling of the vasculature is due to fibrous tissue formation, thromboembolism, and increased muscularization with thickening and intimal fibrosis of the larger arteries. Thrombi may be present in the microcirculation and in the larger vessels. They may form in situ, or may have an embolic source. The end-result is an obstructed, distorted pulmonary circulation with increased pulmonary vascular resistance, causing pulmonary hypertension. (Figure 56.6).

PATHOGENESIS

The pathogenesis of ALI continues to remain unclear. Even so, current research allows a better comprehension of what transpires in this syndrome at a cellular and molecular level. Research into molecular genetics has revealed a complex network of interacting factors at the cellular level. It is clear that the cascade of mediators is far more complex than we thought, and many of yesterday's putative mediators are in reality modulators and regulators that finetune the inflammatory cascade, rather than cause it. Figure 56.6 illustrates the basic steps in the pathogenesis of ALI.

Role of Cytokines, Neutrophils and the Coagulation System

Cytokines, which are cell-derived peptide compounds, are the main mediators. Recombinant cDNA technology has permitted identification of the existence, structure and function of several cytokines. The cytokine on which most attention is currently focussed is the tumour necrosis factor (TNF). This cytokine has a molecular weight of 17 kD and is released from macrophages in response to Gram-negative bacterial endotoxin. TNF is one of the main mediators of the septic state. After injection of

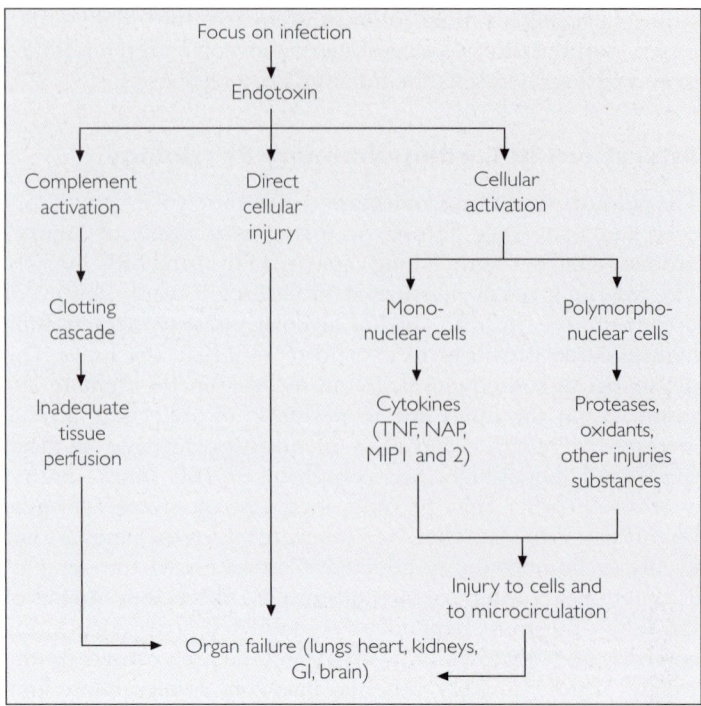

Fig 56.6: Pathogenesis of acute lung injury acute lung injury/ARDS due to sepsis.

endotoxin into animals or humans, TNF can be detected in the serum, the levels peaking at 2 hours. When TNF is infused into the sheep model, ALI is produced. Three other cytokines of importance mediating inflammatory response include neutrophil activating peptide (NAP), interleukin (IL)-6, IL-8 and macrophage inflammatory proteins (MIP 1 and 2). The neutrophil plays a vital role in the inflammatory response, and TNF is the chief mediator that promotes adherence of the neutrophils to the vascular endothelium and together with interleukin-8 causes and enhances neutrophil activation. The primed neutrophils degranulate, releasing proteases, reactive oxygen species, leukotrienes, all harmful to lung structure and function. The lipid mediators and platelet-activating factors also enhance inflammation. (Figure 56.6).

The activation of the coagulation and complement systems promotes coagulation and decreases fibrinolysis. Endothelial damage results in pulmonary oedema with a disturbance in pulmonary microcirculation. The end result is increasing respiratory failure with an increasing poverty of gas exchange, often leading to death. As mentioned earlier, changes in the lung often form just one facet of similar changes in other organs of the body.

There is a complex, poorly understood interaction at the molecular and cellular level as the syndrome continues to evolve. This interaction and inter-relation will continue to be the subject of future research.

Unfortunately, there is no definite biomarker which can reliably identify patients at risk, or assess the prognosis in ARDS. IL-6 and IL-8 can be found in alveolar fluid and in plasma but these are non-specific markers of lung inflammation. The ARDS network trial showed that high levels of IL-6 and IL-8 were associated with increased morbidity and mortality and that the

strategy of using low tidal volumes attenuated the inflammatory response of the disease, suggesting that alveolar stretch is linked to and perhaps worsens the inflammatory response.

Alterations in Cardiopulmonary Physiology

The pulmonary oedema, atelectasis, proliferation of inflammatory cells and increasing fibrosis occurring as a result of 'injury', produce a fall in the total lung capacity (TLC) and FRC by 50%. The low lung recoil pressure at FRC leads to early closure of the small airways, with further alveolar collapse, necessitating high inflation pressures to expand or re-inflate the lungs. The physiological consequences are an increase in the right to left shunt within the lungs due to perfusion of atelectatic alveoli, increased ventilation-perfusion inequalities, increase in dead space, and increasingly non-compliant or stiff lungs. 'Injury' as stressed earlier, may be mild, moderate or severe. Of equal importance is the fact that even in severe injury, the lungs are not evenly or homogenously affected. Computerized tomography, as mentioned earlier, has demonstrated a three-zone model of the lung—the most dependent consolidated area representing core disease, above which is an atelectatic area caused by the weight of inflammatory oedema. This zone is recruitable lung i.e. can be opened up by ventilatory measures; finally there is the least dependent zone of normal or even over-inflated alveoli.

Severe lung injury is sooner or later associated with increasing pulmonary hypertension. The latter is due to hypoxia and an obstructed, distorted pulmonary circulation. The resultant increase in right ventricular afterload can not only lead to right heart failure, but also cause a shift of the septum to the left. The septal shift can significantly reduce left ventricular filling and stroke volume.

Myocardial dysfunction is an important feature of ALI. It is contributed to by a circulating myocardial depressant factor (probably the same as TNF) in patients with sepsis. A significant fall in cardiac output is frequently observed in these patients, particularly when the mean pulmonary artery pressure exceeds 35 mm Hg. A fall in cardiac output, particularly when combined with a low oxygen tension in arterial blood, can cause a significant reduction in oxygen transport to the tissues. A decreased oxygen transport in association with a possible abnormality of oxygen uptake by the tissues, so frequently observed in ARDS, invariably spells disaster.

CLINICAL FEATURES

Against a background of one of the aetiologies mentioned earlier, the patient with ARDS presents with rapidly worsening dyspnoea and restlessness. On examination, such a patient has tachycardia, tachypnoea, and increasing hypoxaemia despite supplemental oxygen. Auscultation reveals scattered crackles and occasionally a wheeze. The condition may evolve rapidly over a few hours, or may take a few days to reach its maximum intensity. Respiratory distress is obvious, and the accessory muscles of respiration are active. Cyanosis may occur, but is not always evident in spite of severe hypoxaemia.

In the early stages, a slight but disproportionate tachypnoea may be the only warning sign of early ALI, and in an appropriate setting this must never be ignored, even in the absence of auscultatory crackles, and with a normal chest X-ray. An important warning diagnostic feature in the early phase is a slight fall in the PaO_2 and an increased alveolar-arterial oxygen gradient.

As the respiratory failure worsens, one or more other organ systems may show signs of dysfunction and failure. This is in keeping with the current concept that ALI is a multi-system disease, with the changes in the pulmonary endothelium mirroring widespread endothelial damage in other organs.

DIFFERENTIAL DIAGNOSIS

The lack of specificity in the radiological picture and in the diagnostic features proposed by the American-European Congress Conference has already been commented upon. The differential diagnosis includes:

1. Other causes of air space consolidation—multiple pulmonary infarcts, multiple areas of atelectasis (as after major upper abdominal or cardiothoracic surgery), pneumonia, atypical pneumonia, Legionnaire's disease, alveolar haemorrhage, alveolar proteinosis, eosinophilic pneumonia and bronchiolitis obliterans organizing pneumonia (BOOP).
2. Acute exacerbation of previously unrecognized low-grade interstitial lung disease, or acute interstitial pneumonia. The latter may be impossibly difficult to differentiate from ARDS without a lung biopsy.
3. Cardiogenic pulmonary oedema. Cardiac enlargement, the presence of more centralized oedema, Kerley's lines, help in radiological differentiation. Clinical history and examination of the cardiovascular system are of critical importance. In difficult problems, a Swan-Ganz catheter may be used to determine PAOP. It is to be noted that in intra-abdominal pathologies, the rise in intra-abdominal pressure may cause a rise in the PAOP and mislead the clinician.

COMPLICATIONS

Death is uncommon from severe refractory hypoxia, provided the patient receives good ventilator support. In our unit it occurs in not more than 10 per cent of patients.

Nosocomial Pneumonia

This is an extremely important complication. The incidence of this complication in severe acute lung injury (ARDS) varies in different units, and in our ICU is about 15%. The incidence increases with the length of time on ventilator support, and in our experience, is most marked when ALI is due to severe abdominal sepsis. It is less than 10% when ALI is caused by a direct insult—e.g. inhalation of noxious fumes, near-drowning, chest trauma, even when ventilator support is prolonged for weeks.

The lung injury per se, together with improper ventilatory management (such as use of high inflation pressures, high tidal volumes, high FIO_2), and the prolonged use of PEEP, also probably impair local immune and other defence mechanisms within the lung, and predispose to iatrogenic infection and sepsis. Background illnesses which impair immune function, and malnutrition, either present before the ALI, or occurring during the evolution of the syndrome, are other important

predisposing factors. Colonization of the upper respiratory tract and of the gastrointestinal tract by Gram≠-negative organisms remains an important source of infection.

The diagnosis of nosocomial pneumonia is difficult in the presence of shadows caused by atelectasis and oedema. We have missed a good-sized lung abscess causing an empyema in a patient with ARDS due to severe tetanus, the diagnosis being apparent only at autopsy. Suspicion of a nosocomial infection should prompt a CT of the chest which may reveal an abscess or an empyema undetected on an X-ray. The choice of antibiotics in the management of nosocomial pneumonia is empiric, and will depend on the nature of bacteria causing nosocomial pneumonia and their sensitivity to antibiotics in a critical care unit.

Multiple Organ Dysfunction

The better and more intensive the care offered to the patient, and hence the longer he is kept alive, the more often is the complication of multiple organ dysfunction observed. It occurs early and most frequently when sepsis is the cause of ALI. It can however complicate the course of ALI from any cause.

In our experience, renal dysfunction occurs in 30–40% of patients, cardiovascular dysfunction necessitating inotropic support in 50–70% of patients, and liver cell dysfunction occurs in about 50% of patients. Complications and dysfunction involving the gastrointestinal tract are observed in 20–30% of patients. There is an obvious inter-relation between various organ systems, so that impairment of one organ system induces, amplifies and modulates impairment in other organ systems.

Translocation of bacteria from the lumen of the gut to the lymphatics, peritoneal cavity and even the bloodstream, plays an important role in perpetuating the inflammatory cascade that underlies multiple organ dysfunction. This is observed when the protective barrier normally provided by the wall of the gut is breached. The problem is markedly worsened in the presence of associated liver cell dysfunction. In fact when ARDS occurs against the background of liver cell failure, death invariably results.

INVESTIGATIONS

Chest X-ray (Figures 56.1, 56.2, 56.3)

The chest radiograph shows interstitial oedema in the early stages, and full-blown pulmonary oedema in established cases. The pulmonary oedema causes bilaterally symmetrical shadowing, but the shadowing may initially be predominantly unilateral, depending on the position of the patient. The absence of cardiomegaly, of Kerley's lines and of vascular redistribution towards the upper lobes, help distinguish the pattern from cardiogenic pulmonary oedema. The absence of lobar consolidation helps differentiate it from infection. Having said this, cardiac failure, pneumonia and pulmonary emboli may all cause diagnostic confusion. ARDS does not necessarily involve both lungs symmetrically; one lung may be considerably more involved than the other. This adds to the problem of effective ventilation.

Arterial Blood Gases

Blood gas estimation is essential in the initial diagnosis and subsequent monitoring of ALI. In the initial stages, varying degrees of hypoxia are seen with hypocapnia. In late stages, hypercapnia may be seen. The pH disturbances range from respiratory alkalosis in the initial stages, to respiratory acidosis and metabolic acidosis in the later stages. The hypoxia is refractory to supplemental oxygen, indicating that in addition to ventilation-perfusion mismatch, increased right to left shunt and dead space ventilation also play major roles.

Haemodynamic Measurements

The insertion of a Swan-Ganz catheter is not essential for the diagnosis of ALI; however, it may on occasion be the only way to conclusively distinguish ALI from cardiogenic pulmonary oedema. Insertion of a Swan-Ganz catheter may also prove invaluable in the management of an individual patient. Much has been written concerning the wisdom of invasive monitoring in such patients, and there are some who feel that this technology may itself contribute to poor patient outcome. We now use the Swan-Ganz catheter infrequently. A Swan-Ganz catheter should only be inserted by doctors familiar with its use, to obtain specific answers to specific diagnostic or therapeutic dilemmas for example, assessing the adequacy of volume resuscitation, for titrating inotropic support, for assessing left ventricular dysfunction, degree of intrapulmonary shunting, or for assessing adequacy of oxygen delivery in problem patients.

Pulmonary oedema with pulmonary wedge pressure < 18 mm Hg in the presence of a normal colloid oncotic pressure is diagnostic of acute lung injury (ARDS). It should be noted that estimations of wedge pressure may be affected by the position of the catheter tip (which should be below the left atrium in Zone 3 lung), and the presence or absence of PEEP. All patients ill enough to require a Swan-Ganz catheter, are ill enough to require at least 10 cm H_2O of PEEP. In critically ill hypoxaemic patients, it may not be wise to switch off PEEP even while the necessary haemodynamic measurements are being made. Some authors have advocated subtracting 50% of the PEEP value from the measured wedge pressure, but a study by Teboul and associates suggested that PEEP did not affect the correlation between wedge pressure and left ventricular end-diastolic measurements, even in patients with severe ALI. To avoid iatrogenic complications, we prefer to remove a Swan-Ganz catheter within three days.

Pulmonary Compliance

Lung compliance is usually decreased to < 30 ml/cm H_2O. Compliance can easily be measured in patients on mechanical ventilator support.

Routine Tests

Tests for evidence of other organ dysfunction, for example renal, hepatic, haematological parameters, should be done.

Full Bacteriological Screen

This should include blood culture, cultures of tracheal aspirates, and in some patients with nosocomial pneumonia, culture of BAL fluid or culture of protected brush samples obtained bronchoscopically, to determine the nature of the infecting organism. Cultures of urine and other body secretions and discharges are often necessary.

Table 56.3: Investigations in ARDS
ALI/ARDS
1. Chest X-ray
2. Arterial pH and blood gases
3. Haemodynamic Measurements using a Swan-Ganz catheter in selected cases
4. Pulmonary compliance
5. Routine biochemistry to evaluate other organ dysfunction
6. Full bacteriological screen
• Blood culture
• Urine culture
• Culture of tracheal aspirates
• Culture of BAL
• Culture of any other secretions/discharges

MORTALITY AND PROGNOSIS

Some studies suggest a fall in mortality figures in ARDS compared to earlier years. But mortality depends on the population under study. Even in the ARDS network study of 861 patients, the mortality of 31% in the group using lung protection measures (6 ml/kg TV) is significantly underestimated because many severely ill patients were excluded—those with advanced liver disease, bone marrow transplant, severe chronic respiratory disease, burns > 30% BSA and those not expected to live > 6 months.

Mortality remains quite high in population-based studies. Several multicenter studies in France, Sweden, Australia, Argentina defined mortality and prognostic variables in observational population-based studies rather than clinical trial participants. Mortality varied –32% in ALI to 58–60% ARDS. The highest mortality, close to 60%, was seen in the French study.

In other studies, mortality was highest in sepsis (43%), intermediate in pneumonia (36%) or aspiration (37%), and lowest in multiple trauma (11%). Low tidal volumes were effective in reducing mortality across all cases of ALI/ARDS.

Four factors determine prognosis in ALI/ARDS:

(i) severity of the lung injury (judged by PaO_2/FIO_2 ratio);
(ii) nature and severity of the precipitating factor;
(iii) presence and degree of dysfunction of other organ systems;
(iv) background or associated disease.

In our experience, prognosis depends less on the severity of ALI and more on the other three factors listed above. Uncontrollable sepsis, particularly uncontrollable intra-abdominal sepsis, has a hopeless prognosis with 100% mortality. Severe sepsis even when controlled can set into motion a chain of events that may carry a mortality of > 60%. Prognosis is worse in the presence of septic shock. On the other hand, direct injury to the lungs as in drowning, inhalation of noxious fumes, mild to moderate aspiration of gastric contents, in our experience, has a mortality of < 20%, provided there is no nosocomial infection and no other major complication. Severe nosocomial pneumonia occurring in ARDS has a mortality of about 30%.

In the West, the reported mortality for single organ failure is 15–30%, for two-organ failure it is 45–55%, and for three or more organ failure lasting for more than four days, > 85%. In our experience we have found this true only for Gram-negative sepsis. These figures are unnecessarily pessimistic and are not true when multiple organ failure complicates fulminant Pl falciparum infection, fulminant tetanus and other severe tropical infections. Fulminant tetanus with excellent intensive care has a mortality of less than 10%, and in fulminant Pl falciparum infection the mortality even with severe prolonged multiple organ dysfunction is below 30%.

MANAGEMENT

Despite the many recent advances in intensive care, severe ALI continues to carry an overall mortality of 30–60%. As mentioned earlier, patients with ALI and ARDS do not usually die of respiratory failure (only 16% of all deaths in one large series were due to refractory hypoxaemia and hypercapnia). The majority of patients die of sepsis and multiple organ failure. Intensive care is mandatory for efficient management. The following management principles apply:

Treatment of the Underlying Condition

This should be identified promptly and treated aggressively. Unfortunately, the treatment of many diseases causing ARDS is largely supportive. Sepsis is an important exception and should be promptly recognized and treated. Studies have shown that the prompt use of an appropriate antibiotic or antibiotics significantly improves morbidity and mortality. Surgical drainage of an abscess and prompt surgery for abdominal sepsis are mandatory. Specific therapy for fulminant tropical problems causing ARDS should be immediate—in particular the use of quinine for severe *Plasmodium falciparum* infections.

Respiratory Support

This forms the cornerstone in the management of ALI and ARDS. Yet it needs to be stressed that mechanical ventilation is purely supportive, allowing the lungs time to recover from the acute insult. Mechanical ventilation in patients with severe acute lung injury (ARDS) presents complex problems and difficulties. To be effective, the intensivist must be aware of the changes in cardiorespiratory physiopathology, the interaction between the heart and the lungs, the importance not only of effective gas exchange but of efficient oxygen transport and the dangers and complications of ventilator support.

INITIATING VENTILATOR SUPPORT

There are two important indications for initiating ventilator support in an evolving ARDS. The first is progressive hypoxaemia not responding to oxygen inhalation; the second is a marked, unsustainable increase in the work of breathing, as when the respiratory rate is > 35 to 40/minute and the minute volume exceeds 12 l/minute. Lowered lung compliance adds even more to the work of breathing. Under the above circumstances, it is best to electively intubate and initiate ventilatory support even if the PaO_2 is greater than 60 mm Hg on supplemental oxygen. Elective intubation and ventilatory support is also preferred in the presence of haemodynamic instability and if for any reason the patient is unable to maintain and protect the airway.

NON-INVASIVE VENTILATOR SUPPORT

Severe acute lung injury (ARDS) always needs intubation and mechanical ventilation. A very small subset of patients with mild ALI may however be adequately oxygenated with the help of continuous positive airway pressure (CPAP) or by the use of a BiPAP ventilator, using a tight-fitting face mask. A recent multi-centre observational study has reported the merits of NIV in early ARDS from three ICUs in Italy and Spain. One-third of the patients were given NIV (the remaining two-thirds were already intubated and ventilated) The NIV patients had less ventilator-associated pneumonias and a lower mortality. This was not a randomized controlled trial and though the study showed that NIV was effective in early cases, no definite conclusions are possible.

If NIV is decided upon, CPAP levels are kept between 10–12 cm of H_2O. In order to maintain intra-thoracic pressure at the required level of CPAP throughout the respiratory cycle, high gas flows in excess of 70 l/min are required. With a BiPAP machine, reasonable initial ventilator settings are EPAP of 7 to 10 cm H_2O and IPAP of around 15 to 18 cm, the settings being adjusted both for patient comfort and for providing and maintaining an SaO_2 of greater than 90%. Non-invasive mechanical ventilation in patients with mild ALI recruits collapsed alveoli, increases the FRC and lung compliance, thereby unloading the respiratory muscles and reducing the work of breathing. A good response to non-invasive positive pressure ventilation is generally observed within 30 minutes of its initiation and is characterized by improved oxygen saturation, a fall in respiratory rate and less patient distress. An inability to maintain SaO_2 to ≥ 90% or the presence of haemodynamic instability, or a worsening clinical state are indications for intubation and mechanical ventilation.

DANGERS OF ENDOTRACHEAL INTUBATION IN ALI AND ARDS

The major danger during intubation is a severe increase in hypoxia, in an individual who is already hypoxic to start with. Haemodynamic instability and the danger of gastric aspiration form additional risks during intubation.

Endotracheal intubation should therefore be performed by an expert, preferably with the patient awake, using mild sedation with a benzodiapine or a narcotic. In an acute crisis, succinylcholine along with intravenous propofol may be used.

Changing of the endotracheal tube in a patient with ARDS following rupture of the cuff, or due to obstruction of the tube is also risky. A sudden loss of PEEP during this procedure may cause rapid desaturation with dangerous sequelae.

Principles of Mechanical Ventilation

The last several years have seen the evolution of two fundamental concepts in the ventilatory support of patients with ARDS. First is the prevention of over-distension of the alveoli by limiting tidal volume and the pause pressure. Second is to choose a level of positive end-expiratory pressure (PEEP) which is sufficiently high to prevent derecruitment of the alveoli at end expiration. *The fundamental concepts that guide ventilator support in ARDS are these two lung-protection goals.* Avoidance of oxygen toxicity to the lungs and prevention of haemodynamic instability of the cardiovascular system are two other important conditions guiding ventilator support in these patients.

LIMITING TIDAL VOLUME

The lung protection strategies have been firmly established following the result of the landmark ARDS Clinical Trials Network (ARDS net). In this large prospective randomized controlled trial, patients were randomly assigned to receive a tidal volume (V_T) of 6 ml/kg of predicted body weight or 12 ml/kg of predicted body weight. The plateau pressure (the airway pressure under no flow conditions maintaining the tidal volume) was not to exceed 30 cm H_2O. If it did so, the tidal volume was further reduced to 5 ml/kg of predicted body weight or even to a minimum of 4 ml/kg of predicted body weight. Patients receiving lower tidal volume had a lower mortality (31%) compared to those receiving higher tidal volume (mortality 40%). There was relative reduction in mortality of 22%.

The established principle is therefore to use low tidal volumes (6 ml/kg) and ensure that the pause pressure does not exceed 30 cm of H_2O when using a volume-regulated mode of ventilatory support. This strategy prevents over-distension of alveoli and undue increase in intra-alveolar pressure. In fact large tidal volumes (10–15 ml/kg) in patients with ARDS are dangerous. It is accepted that over-distension of alveoli in these patients can cause an amplification of the already existing lung injury (volutrauma), presumably by increasing oedema and pulmonary cytokine production. In addition to 'volutrauma', high intra-alveolar and inspiratory pressures can lead to an increased incidence of barotraumas. The concept of barotrauma is not new, but its spectrum includes not just pneumothorax, but also pneumomediastinum, interstitial emphysema, subcutaneous emphysema, and pulmonary haemorrhage. A frequent consequence of a limitation of the tidal volume in the above manner is a rise in the $PaCO_2$ to above 40 mm Hg. The $PaCO_2$ is allowed to rise—a condition called permissive hypercapnia.

This difference in mortality between the low tidal volume group and the high tidal volume group in the ARDS network trial was related to a greater reduction in IL-6 levels in patients with low tidal volumes. Rainieri and co-workers have also shown lower levels of TNF, IL-1, IL-6, and IL-8 in the broncho-alveolar lavage fluid of patients treated with the 'lung protective' ventilatory strategies, when compared to patients treated with the more conventional ventilatory techniques. These cytokines can produce further lung injury; they also gain entry into the bloodstream and produce 'injury' at distant sites, perhaps contributing to multiple organ dysfunction and multiple organ failure.

THE USE OF PEEP

PEEP is not a new ventilatory strategy but a mainstay of oxygenation in ALI and ARDS ever since the original description of the syndrome. It acts by recruiting collapsed alveoli, restoring FRC to normal, thus increasing compliance. It also causes redistribution of lung water within the alveolar space, improving V/Q mismatch and decreasing the shunt and venous admixture. By improving oxygenation, PEEP allows the oxygen concentration delivered to the patient to be reduced, thus decreasing the chances of oxygen toxicity, which in itself can worsen lung injury.

Of recent interest, is the likelihood that PEEP, if properly adjusted, also prevents further lung injury during mechanical ventilation of patients with ARDS. How does it do so? The concertina effect of opening of the alveoli during the inspiratory phase of mechanical ventilation, followed by well-nigh total closure of alveoli during the expiratory derecruitment, generates strong shear forces that worsen and perpetuate lung injury. Choosing the exact level of PEEP that can prevent the derecruitment of alveoli during mechanical ventilation is a difficult but an important 'lung protection' goal in patients with ALI and ARDS. In the ARDS network trial, the level of PEEP and FiO_2 were adjusted with a predetermined PaO_2/FiO_2 ratio in a step-wise fashion, so as to keep the PaO_2 and SaO_2 at a satisfactory desired range. Ideally, PEEP should be individualized for each patient. One can attempt to do so by plotting the pressure volume curve in a given patient, noting the upper and lower inflection points and adjusting the PEEP level at 1–2 cm above the lower inflection point. There is however often an observer difference in determining the exact lower inflection point (which is a slope rather than a point). Again the pressure volume curve relates to the whole of the lung but does not reflect regional differences (some alveoli are over-distended, others collapsed or consolidated). It is obvious that PEEP is more likely to be useful in patients with ARDS where a good proportion of the affected lungs are 'recruitable'. On the other hand if in a patient the 'recruitable lung' is very small, PEEP will be of little use. In fact it may be harmful as it may only serve to over-distend alveoli, thus contributing to lung injury. Gattioni determined the degree of recruitability of lungs through CT studies, a luxury denied to most ICUs in the developing world. Perhaps the simplest approach is to use the least PEEP that provides adequate oxygenation at an FiO_2 of < 0.6, starting with a PEEP of 10 cm and not exceeding 15 cm, as the risk of barotrauma, particularly in Indian patients is then significant. If oxygenation does not improve as judged by the PaO_2/FiO_2 ratio, and if there is no increase in compliance, PEEP should be reduced and not allowed to exceed 5 cm H_2O.

Three large randomized control trials (ARDS network trial, LOVS study, Express study) have compared the effects of higher PEEP to lower PEEP levels. All demonstrated increased oxygenation in the higher PEEP group, but there was neither a decrease in mortality nor in ventilator-free days. This suggests that the use of modest PEEP levels is to be generally preferred and is adequate to prevent ventilator-induced lung injury. High PEEP may perhaps open more atelectatic alveoli but over-distend normal alveoli, contributing further to lung injury.

VENTILATOR MODES

There are a large number of modes offered by currently available ventilators. These include pressure control ventilation, airway pressure release ventilation, high-frequency oscillatory ventilation and open-lung ventilation. Whichever mode one uses, the focus should be on preventing alveolar over-distention, countering alveolar derecruitment, minimizing cardiovascular instability and avoiding oxygen toxicity. The volume-controlled mode (with lung protection strategies) was used in the ARDS network trial and remains the one most commonly adopted. There is no evidence to suggest that any of the other ventilatory modes are superior to the volume-controlled mode in the management of ARDS. Many units use pressure-controlled mode; it is important when using this mode to ensure low tidal volumes (6 ml/kg body weight) and not to exceed a peak pressure of 30 cm H_2O. Inverse ratio respiration has been used generally with pressure-controlled ventilatory support. The inspiration-expiration ratio should be preferably 1:2 or 1:1 and not lower. The increased inspiratory time may allow better oxygenation in these patients.

High Frequency Oscillating Ventilation (HFOV) theoretically should offer lung protection as the tidal volumes delivered are very small (less than the dead space) and at a high frequency, gas exchange being promoted by diffusion. Its efficacy as a ventilatory mode in children is generally accepted. It remains to be established whether it reduces morbidity and mortality in ARDS when compared to the lung protection strategies adopted with the volume-controlled mode. A multicentre randomized controlled trial studying HFOV organized by the Canadian Critical Trial Group (CCTG) is in progress.

USE OF PRONE POSTURE

It was not until an original report by Piehl and Brown in 1976, that the benefits of a switch from the supine to the prone position were appreciated. The improvement in oxygenation may be dramatic, occurring soon after the patients are made prone. In their initial series, five patients of Piehl and Brown with ALI showed a mean rise in PaO_2 of 47 mm Hg. The question at issue is whether ventilating a patient with ARDS in the prone position improves either morbidity or mortality. There is no evidence to suggest this. A large multicentre RCT from Italy compared patients with ARDS ventilated and nursed in a supine position to those in the prone position for six hours in the day. Though oxygenation improved in the prone position, there was no benefit in the ultimate outcome.

The generally accepted explanation for improved oxygenation in the prone position is improved perfusion to less damaged portions of the lung. The disadvantages of this method are the great difficulty in nursing such patients in the prone posture, the danger of disconnection of life-supporting lines, of obstruction to the airway, the occurrence of facial-dependent oedema and even pressure sores. Even so, the prone position should be utilized when conventional modes of ventilator support do not result in adequate oxygenation. It has been suggested that improvement with prone posture ventilation may be more significant if it is used early in patients with a large shunt.

PERMISSIVE HYPERCAPNIA

When patients with ARDS are ventilated with the lung protection goal of low tidal volumes and pressure-limited ventilation, alveolar hypoventilation frequently occurs, causing a rise in $PaCO_2$ to 60 to 70 mm Hg or even more. Increasing $PaCO_2$ with respiratory acidosis can have potential adverse physiological

effects such as arrhythmias, cardiovascular and central nervous system depression. However, these effects are not generally encountered in clinical practice. In fact, high $PaCO_2$ levels seem to be very well tolerated in adequately sedated patients. Most clinicians and intensivists favour permissive hypercapnia to the injurious effects of over-distended alveoli and high inspiratory inflation pressures. The $PaCO_2$ in permissive hypercapnia should preferably be allowed to rise slowly at the rate of 10 mm Hg/h. Hypercapnia needs correction only if there is a significant fall in the pH. In the ARDS network trial, if the pH fell to < 7.30, the respiratory rate was increased till the pH was > 7.30 or the respiratory rate equalled 35/min. If the pH was < 7.3 in spite of the respiratory rate being increased to 35/min, an intravenous bicarbonate infusion was administered. We feel that this is a sensible approach in management. IV bicarbonate may temporarily correct the pH but could add substantially to the CO_2 that needs to be excreted by the patient via the lungs. Intravenous sodium bicarbonate could also lead to volume overload and potassium depletion in critically ill patients who already have an increase in intrapulmonary extravascular water content.

THE OPEN LUNG CONCEPT

The open lung concept though described first by Lachmann in 1977 has been adopted as a ventilatory strategy for ARDS over a little more than the last decade. Gattinoni and co-workers showed that patients with ARDS had multiple areas of atelectasis chiefly in the dependent lung regions, due to reduced volume of the aerated lung. The ventilatory strategy of an open lung opens up the atelectatic areas and keeps them open. Thereby the cyclic shear forces of alveolar opening and closing are minimized and optimal gas exchange is achieved (PaO_2 > 450 mm Hg on an FIO_2 of 1). The 'open lung' procedure is always attempted using pressure-controlled ventilation with a I:E ratio of 1:1 and with an FIO_2 of 1. To start with PEEP is applied at 15 to 20 cm H_2O in patients with ARDS, and the lung is opened with slow progressive increase (by 2 cm at a time) in the peak inspiratory pressure up to 40–60 cm H_2O. The 'opening pressure' is the peak inspiratory pressure at which the lung is 'opened'. The success of recruitment of closed alveoli is gauged either by noting the sudden sharp increase in PaO_2 > 450 mm Hg when the lung fully 'opens up' or by the proportional increase in tidal volume following increase in the peak inspiratory pressure. The peak inspiratory pressure and PEEP are now adjusted to the lowest pressure which keeps the lung open. This lowest pressure is realized when the tidal volumes are stable and the arterial blood gases continue to show a high constant PaO_2. The ideal pressure is generally 15 to 30 cm H_2O less than the required recruitment 'opening' peak pressure. After opening the lung and finding the lowest pressure to keep it open, the resultant pressure amplitude is minimized and gas exchange maximized. The ventilatory strategy described above enables a reduction in FIO_2 and protects the lung from further injury. It is possible that an open lung is less likely to produce cytokines injurious to itself as also to other organ systems.

The open lung strategy, if adopted, should preferably be put to use in the first 24 to 48 hours of mechanical ventilation in ARDS. Amato and co-workers showed a reduced mortality

in ARDS patients using the open lung ventilatory strategy as compared to ARDS patients on conventional modes. A recent Canadian Critical Care Trial Group Study of 1000 patients—The Lung Open Ventilation Study (LOVS) compared the ARDS network protocol to a regimen using pressure-controlled ventilation, recruitment manoeuvres combined with levels of PEEP of 5–7 cm higher for a given PaO_2 than that used in the ARDS network trial. There was no statistically significant increase in survival in the interventional arm, though no adverse effects were observed.

A number of critical care units use the open lung concept strategy as their first choice in ARDS. However, the open lung strategy requires experience, close attention to ventilator settings and extra care. It is possible that the chief benefit of open lung ventilation may be related more to the low tidal volumes and low peak pressure during ventilation rather than in 'opening' the lung.

Other Measures

Fluid Balance It is important not to over-hydrate the patient as this worsens pulmonary oedema. In established ALI/ARDS we have always preferred to keep filling pressures of the left ventricle on the lesser side of normal (PAOP < 12 mm Hg), central venous pressure (CVP) not more 6 mm Hg provided perfusion of vital organs is satisfactory. The ARDS Network Fluid and Catheter Treatment trial has recently shown that a conservative fluid management strategy increased the mean number of ventilator-free days (14.8 vs. 12.1). There was a 2.9% reduction in mortality rate in the conservative arm but this was not statistically significant. This study showed that the conservative fluid strategy did not increase the incidence of renal failure or shock. Also, the use of a pulmonary artery catheter or a central venous catheter in monitoring management was associated with the same mortality.

The above strategy applies to patients who are not in shock or whose shock has been effectively countered with appropriate fluid management. Unquestionably, a patient in shock will require the initial fluid resuscitation emergency measures outlined by Rivers and colleagues.

Other Fluid Management Strategies In the particular setting of hypoproteinemia and ALI/ARDS, the combination therapy of albumin and frusemide may be useful in improving pulmonary physiology. There is however no evidence that outcome is favourably influenced. Hypoproteinemia is a documented risk factor in the development of ALI/ARDS as also for poor outcome in critical illness in general. This in our opinion is reason enough to counter hypoalbuminemia with infusions of albumin in patients with ARDS.

Circulatory Support It is important to ensure adequate oxygen transport or delivery to the tissues. Oxygen transport or delivery (DO_2) is not only dependent on an adequate PaO_2, but is also dependent on cardiac output and the haemoglobin (Hb) concentration. The Hb concentration should be kept around 10 g/dl with a haematocrit of 35%. Inotropic support should be given even in patients with moderate lung injury. Dobutamine is preferred if the cardiac output is low as it generally does not induce tachycardia. If the systolic blood pressure is < 90

mm Hg, or if the systemic vascular resistance is low, dopamine is to be preferred. Nor-epinephrine is often necessary in hypotensive patients.

Supramaximal oxygen transport (cardiac index > 4.5 l/min/m^2 and oxygen delivery above 600 ml/min/m^2), was earlier thought to reduce oxygen debt in the tissues, prevent hypoxic injury and organ system failure. This is however by no means certain, and there are a number of conflicting studies that support or refute this suggestion. It is possible that increasing oxygen delivery to supramaximal levels reduces mortality in just a subgroup of patients, such as high-risk surgical patients. In our experience and in the experience of most critical care units, supramaximal oxygen delivery does not reduce mortality in ALI. Volume-loading patients with ALI to maintain PAOP at upper normal limits (15–18 mm Hg) in an attempt to raise the cardiac output, invariably does harm by potentiating the lung injury.

Support to Other Organ Systems

All organ systems often need support, in particular the kidney. Ultrafiltration or dialysis may be necessary to treat volume overload or renal failure.

NUTRITIONAL SUPPORT

Good nutrition is vital, particularly when ALI is due to excessively catabolic states as in fulminant tetanus, burns or severe sepsis. Severely catabolic states require a caloric intake of 2,500 or more calories/day, and this could lead to excessive fluid intake in a clinical situation which often necessitates fluid restriction. Under these circumstances, nutritional requirements are sacrificed on a short-term basis to allow fluid restriction. The alternative is to remove additional water by the use of loop diuretics if renal function is good or by the use of ultrafiltration if renal function is impaired. Enteral feeding is always to be preferred. In the presence of ileus, and abdominal sepsis, parenteral feeding becomes necessary.

Treatment of Complications

These can involve any organ system; they should be promptly diagnosed and treated. Iatrogenic sepsis and nosocomial pneumonias are of ominous significance.

Role of Corticosteroids in ARDS

Corticosteroids would appear to be ideal therapy for ARDS in view of their anti-inflammatory and anti-fibrotic properties. Soon after the description of ARDS, corticosteroids were used with rather gay abandon. Later, in Bone's study of 382 patients with sepsis and ARDS, those with impaired renal function had a higher mortality when given steroids compared to a control group given placebo. Corticosteroids fell out of favour. Interest was revived when Meduri and colleagues in 1994 reported in study of 20 patients that intravenous methylprednisolone instituted seven days after the onset of ARDS helped recovery and improved survival. Most recently, the NHLBI Acute Respiratory Distress Syndrome Network published a randomized controlled trial on the effect of methylprednisolone in ARDS patients of at least seven days

duration. Methylprednisolone was noted to decrease the ventilator-free, shock-free and ICU-free days during the first month. It was however associated with a significant increase in 60 and 180 days mortality among the patients enrolled after two weeks of ARDS. This increased mortality was probably because many patients enrolled after two weeks required re-intubation and return to ventilator support, raising the criticism that this group might perhaps have been extubated earlier than warranted. Methylprednisolone did reduce the 60-day mortality in patients with elevated BAL fluid levels of procollagen which is a biological marker of collagen synthesis in the lung.

We prefer to use methylprednislone 40 mg IV thrice daily after seven to ten days of onset of ARDS and prefer on current evidence not to use it two weeks after the onset of ARDS. The last word on the use of corticosteroids in ARDS is yet to be written.

New Potential Therapies for ARDS

1. *Use of Activated Protein* C   Though useful in a selected group of patients with sepsis, the use of Activated Protein C has not been proven in ARDS not related to sepsis. There is growing evidence of increased coagulation and decreased fibrinolysis in the pathogenesis of ARDS. Activated Protein C counters both decreased fibrinolysis and increased coagulation; it is also anti-inflammatory. This has prompted a trial of Activated Protein C in patients with ARDS. The results are awaited.

2. *Granulocyte-macrophage Colony-Stimulating Factor (GM-CSF)* is another therapy being evaluated as possible treatment for ARDS. GM-CSF is believed to encourage homeostasis of alveolar macrophages and to prevent apoptosis of alveolar epithelium. Further studies will decide the value of this therapy.

3. *Use of* β_2 *agonists*   A small single-centre randomized trial of IV salbutamol reduced the extravascular lung water, thereby increasing alveolar fluid clearance in ARDS. There was however a higher incidence of arrhythmias in the treatment group. The ARDS network is initiating a multi-centre randomized trial on the efficacy of inhaled β_2-agonist therapy in ARDS patients.

4. *Other Pharmaceutics Measures*   A great deal of research continues on pharmaceutical measures that could reduce or counter the inflammatory cascade that initiates and perpetuates injury to the lung and other organ systems. The use of anticytokines, anti-TNF antibodies, soluble TNF receptors, cyclogenase inhibitors is of unproven benefit. Surfactant replacement, nitric oxide inhalation, platelet activating factor antagonist, pentoxyfylline and antiproteases have all proved of no avail. None of these drugs can be recommended at this stage.

5. *Immunonutrition* has attracted attention in recent years. Addition of linoleic acid to the diet, as also arginine, glutamine, nucleotides and omega fatty acids is reported to reduce infection rates in critically ill patients treated with enteral immune-enhanced diets. There is no evidence that these diets influence ultimate outcome.

SUGGESTED READING

Avecillas JF. Clinical epidemiology of acute lung injury and acute respiratory distress syndrome: incidence, diagnosis, and outcomes. *Clin Chest Med.* 1 Dec. 2006; 27(4): 549–57; abstract vii.

de Hemptinne Q. ARDS—a clinicopatholological confrontation. *Chest.* 1 Apr. 2009; 135(4): 944–9.

Gattinoni L. The role of CT-scan studies for the diagnosis and therapy for acute respiratory distress syndrome. *Clin Chest Med.* 1 Dec. 2006; 27(4): 559–70; abstract vii.

Girard TD. Mechanical ventilation in ARDS: a state-of-the-art review. *Chest.* 1 Mar. 2007; 131(3): 921–9.

Jia X. Risk factors for ARDS in patients receiving mechanical ventilation for > 48 hours. *Chest.* 1 Apr. 2008; 133(4): 853–61.

Martin GS, Moss M, Wheeler AP, Mealer M, Morris JA, Bernard GR. A randomized, controlled trial of furosemide with or without albumin in hypoproteinemic patients with acute lung injury. *Crit Care Med.* 2005; 33: 1681–7.

The ARDS Network. Ventilation with lower tidal volumes as compared with traditional lung volumes for acute lung injury and acute respiratory distress syndrome. *NEJM.* 2000; 342: 1301–8.

The National Heart, Lung, and Blood Institute Acute Respiratory Distress Syndrome (ARDS) Clinical Trials Network. Efficacy and Safety of corticosteroids for persistent acute respiratory distress syndrome. *N Engl J Med.* 2006; 354: 1671–84.

The National Heart, Lung, and Blood Institurte. Acute Respiratory Distress Syndrome (ARDS) Clinical Trials Network. Comparison of two fluid-management strategies in acute lung injury. *N Engl J Med.* 2006; 354: 2564–75.

The National Heart, Lung, and Blood Institute Acute Respiratory Distress Syndrome (ARDS) Clinical Trials Network. Pulmonary-artery versus central venous catheter to guide treatment of acute lung injury. *N Engl J Med.* 2006; 354: 2213–24.

The National Heart, Lung, and Blood Institute Acute Respiratory Distress Syndrome (ARDS) Clinical Trials Network. Higher versus lower positive end-expiratory pressures in patients with the acute respiratory distress syndrome. *N Engl J Med.* 2004; 351: 326–36.

Vincent JL. New management strategies in ARDS. Immunomodulation. *Crit Care Clin.* 1 Jan. 2002; 18(1): 69–78.

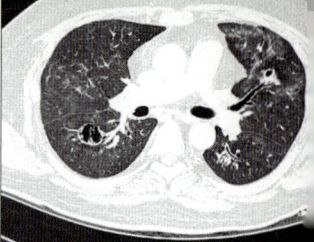

CHAPTER

57 Pulmonary Manifestations of Connective Tissue Disorders

GENERAL CONSIDERATIONS

Connective tissue disorders are a group of diseases characterized by an abnormality in the collagen or elastic framework of the body. There is a disturbance in immune function leading to the formation of autoimmune bodies in these diseases. Connective tissue disorders (also termed as collagen disorders) consist of rheumatoid arthritis (RA), systemic sclerosis (SSc), systemic lupus erythematosis (SLE), dermatomyositis (DM), polymyositis (PM), mixed connective tissue disease (MCD), Sjogren's syndrome (SS), ankylosing spondylitis and relapsing polychondritis.

Pulmonary involvement is commonly observed in connective tissue disorders. This involvement is more frequent than is clinically apparent and affects all components of the respiratory system. The airways, the alveoli, the interstitium, pulmonary vasculature and the pleura may all be involved singly or in various combinations depending on the nature of the connective tissue disorder.

Pulmonary disease has emerged as a major cause of death in collagen vascular disease. In SSc and DM/PM, pulmonary disease is now the most common cause of death.

The prevalence rate of pulmonary complications in connective tissue disorders varies in different studies. No estimate is available for India. Any estimate will depend on the geographical area and the population studied and more so perhaps on the investigational methods used to detect abnormalities within the respiratory system. Thus for example, dyspnoea on exertion is a common symptom in SSc but some patients because of musculoskeletal involvement in SSc may not be able to exercise sufficiently to report dyspnoea. Conversely, patients with RA or PM may be breathless secondary to increased work of locomotion, secondary to arthritis or myositis. Chest radiography is also an imprecise tool when it comes to diagnosing interstitial lung disease (ILD) in these patients. Studies which involve computed tomography (CT) of the chest, lung biopsies and autopsy studies will unquestionably show a much higher prevalence rate when compared to mere clinical studies coupled with a basic radiological examination of the chest.

Due to lack of evidence, it is impossible to compare the incidence of connective tissue disorders in India vis-à-vis the West. Pulmonary complications are however frequently encountered, their incidence in connective tissue disorders being probably similar to that in the West.

Interstitial pneumonia is perhaps the most important form of pulmonary involvement in most connective tissue disorders stated above. Systemic sclerosis has the highest prevalence rate of interstitial pneumonia which more often is of the non-specific type. Autopsy studies in the West show that close to 75% of patients with SSc show some degree of pulmonary fibrosis and 30% show some degree of vascular involvement. Yet overt disease is reported in just 5% of these patients. Rheumatoid disease and DM/PM also show a high prevalence rate of interstitial pulmonary fibrosis on autopsy studies, though overt disease again is about 5%. The interstitial pneumonia that complicates RA and DM/PM is more frequently a usual interstitial pneumonia (UIP) and organizing pneumonia.

Pleural disease is perhaps the most frequent and common pulmonary manifestation of connective tissue disorders, particularly of SLE and RA. A rough estimate of the relative frequency of different pulmonary manifestations in different connective tissue disorders is given in the accompanying table.

Table 57.1: Relative frequency of different pulmonary manifestations in various connective tissue disorders				
Pulmonary manifestations	**RA**	**SSc**	**DM/PM**	**SLE**
Interstitial pneumonia	++	+++	++	+
Pleural involvement	+++			+++
Pulmonary hypertension		+++	+	++
Alveolar haemorrahge	**			+
Constrictive bronchiolitis	+		**	**

Source: Modified from *Clinical Respiratory Medicine* (2008), third edition, Mosby Inc.
Note: +++ Common, ++ Fairly frequent, + Occasional, ** Rare.

Currently, genetic risk factors are being studied in relation to pulmonary complications of connective tissue disorders. A number of genes have been shown to be associated with pulmonary complications in SLE and RA. Thus the carriage of HLA-DRB1* 11 (04) and DPB1* 1301 alleles is believed to be associated with lung fibrosis and that of DRB1*04 and DRB1*08 with pulmonary hypertension, which is linked to the presence of antricentromere antibodies (ACAs). The ACAs are associated with the carriage of a functional tumour necrosis factor (TNF) variant which may perhaps exert a pathological role in SSc. In RA there is an association between obliterative bronchiolitis and the histocompatability antigens HLA-B40 and DR1. As yet, these and other genetic studies do not necessarily have clinical implications; further work in genetic and molecular biology may perhaps clarify this issue.

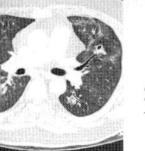

CLINICAL FEATURES
RHEUMATOID ARTHRITIS

Pulmonary disease generally occurs in patients with well-marked rheumatoid arthritis. Occasionally, it may precede clinical evidence of joint disease by several months. A strongly positive RA factor in the serum of these patients may however suggest the link with rheumatoid disease. Pulmonary manifestations in RA may form the sole overt systemic complication or involvement. On the other hand pulmonary manifestations may be associated with other extra-articular complications, notably rheumatoid nodules and occasionally with digital vasculitis.

Pleural Effusion

Pleural effusion is the most common respiratory manifestation of rheumatoid disease. At autopsy, histological evidence of pleural disease is present in 50% of patients. The majority are clinically silent. Clinically significant effusions occur in about 5% of RA patients, the majority resolving spontaneously. It is most often asymptomatic but may be associated with pleuritic pain and breathlessness. The effusion is generally small; it may however be moderate and in rare instances large in size. It may precede RA by several months in which case the diagnosis is often underdetermined. The main differential diagnosis is from tuberculosis and malignancy. A diagnostic pleural tap should always be done. A rheumatoid effusion is an exudate with a high protein content, low glucose (≤ 60 mg/dl), a pH often < 7.2 and a high lactate dehydrogenase (LDH); the cell count generally shows a lymphocytosis, though a significant number of polymorphs may also be present. The RA factor is positive in a high titre in the pleural fluid. In fact the immunoglobulin M (IgM) rheumatoid factor may be higher in the pleural fluid than in the serum suggesting local pleural production of this factor by mononuclear cells.

A pleural biopsy (preferably a thoracoscopic biopsy) is often necessary, particularly when the pleural effusion precedes the joint pains and joint swellings of rheumatoid disease. Video-assisted thoracoscopy may reveal granular pleural surfaces. Histological examination in typical cases shows granulomatous inflammation with mesothelial pleural cells being replaced by pallisading histocytes. Unfortunately, more often than not, pleural biopsy merely shows non-specific inflammatory changes with accompanying fibrosis. A pleural biopsy does however help to exclude other diseases, notably malignancy. A CT of the chest may reveal pulmonary nodules or subpleural nodules not visible on plain radiography; these findings may suggest the correct diagnosis.

Most pleural effusions, particularly when small, resolve spontaneously. Larger effusions may persist and may require paracentesis. Response to corticosteroids is unpredictable. Rarely, pleurodesis is necessary to prevent recurrence of the effusion particularly if it is large enough to cause symptoms.

Occasionally, a pleural effusion in rheumatoid disease becomes secondarily infected resulting in an empyema. Fever with chills, leucocytosis, and marked polymorphoneuclear leucocytosis of the pleural fluid is observed. The empyema is treated on conventional lines—systemic antibiotics, pleural aspiration, and if this is unsuccessful, tube drainage or rib resection and tube drainage.

Interstitial Pneumonia

This pulmonary manifestation is perhaps the most important because it is invariably progressive and can lead to respiratory disability and respiratory failure. The pattern of interstitial pneumonia observed in RA is often that of UIP. However, ILD in RA is quite heterogeneous with significant prevalence of non-specific interstitial pneumonia (NSIP) and lymphoid interstitial pneumonia. There are no clinical, radiological, and histopathological differences between cryptogenic fibrosing alveolitis (UIP) and the fibrosing alveolitis in a patient with rheumatoid arthritis. The pathogenesis of UIP in rheumatoid disease is unclear. It is almost certainly related to the immune complexes deposited within the pulmonary capillaries. Respiratory symptoms of increasing breathlessness on exertion and cough develop a little later when compared to cryptogenic fibrosing alveolitis, probably because of limited exertion imposed by arthritis.

Clinical features are characterized by breathlessness on exertion, end-inspiratory velcro crackles at the bases which with time generally extend upwards. Clubbing may be present. There may be no symptoms in some patients, yet the typical basal crackles in established rheumatoid disease are the single most important clinical diagnostic feature. In advanced interstitial pulmonary fibrosis, central cyanosis, and marked breathlessness with hypoxic respiratory failure result. The lung functions show a restrictive pattern with a reduced diffusion lung capacity for carbon monoxide (DLCO) with no reduction in expiratory flow

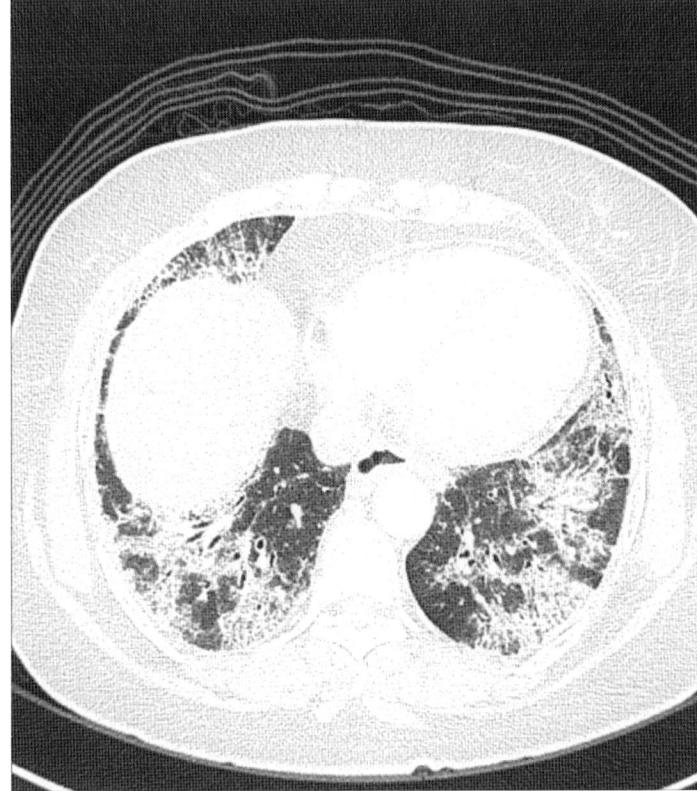

Fig 57.1: RA with NSIP. HRCT demonstrates ill-defined reticular opacities and ground-glass densities in both lung bases in a subpleural and peribronchovascular location. This pattern is of NSIP as significant fibrosis and honeycomb changes are absent. UIP would demonstrate fibrosis, honeycomb cysts and architectural distortion.

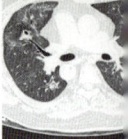

rates. Bronchoalveolar lavage (BAL) usually shows an increase in eosinophils and neurophils; the Gallium scan shows increased uptake pointing to an alveolitis. It is not necessary to perform a lung biopsy in these patients.

The X-ray chest shows interstitial lesions starting at the lung bases and slowly extending upwards. CT chest shows classical subpleural fibrosis with nodules, reticular lesions and honeycombing, again most marked over the bases. A minor degree of ground-glass shadowing is often present. At times these changes are associated with small bullae generally in the lower lobes, but also involving other areas of the lung pointing to small airways' obstruction produced by inflammatory disease. Such patients in addition to the usual restrictive pattern in lung function tests show a reduction in expiratory flow rates and an increase in the residual volume.

The course of interstitial pneumonia is unpredictable. It is not as relentlessly progressive as in cryptogenic fibrosing alveolitis (UIP). Some patients with interstitial pneumonia remain stable with little or slow progression of the disease. In others the disease continues to progress causing crippling interstitial pulmonary fibrosis with hypoxemic respiratory failure.

Cryptogenic Organizing Pneumonia

Some patients with RA develop organizing pneumonia. In a series of 40 patients with RA undergoing open-lung biopsy, cryptogenic organizing pneumonia (COP) was the second most common histological abnormality. Symptoms include fever, cough, weight loss and a sharp increase in an already high erythrocyte sedimentation rate (ESR). Breathlessness on exertion may be present. A chest X-ray shows one or more areas of pneumonic consolidation, often situated peripherally. A CT may reveal areas of consolidation not visible on an X-ray chest. The condition can be confirmed by a lung biopsy; the tissue obtained reveals the classical feature of intra-alveolar buds of granulation tissue. The terminal bronchioles may show inflammatory changes.

Pulmonary Nodules

Rheumatoid nodules may occur within the lungs or may be subpleural in position. They are most frequently found in a peripheral or subpleural distribution. They are similar to the subcutaneous rheumatoid nodules with which they may be associated. The prevalence of rheumatoid nodules in the lung depends on whether chest X-ray is used to identify them (1%) or HRCT. A recent HRCT series of 77 patients with RA found 22% of patients had rheumatoid nodules. Pulmonary nodules in RA are invariably silent and are discovered fortuitously on an X-ray chest. They may remain unchanged, increase in size or may even disappear. Rarely, they cavitate and then may cause haemoptysis. Their proximity to the pleural surface accounts for some of their rare complications including pneumothorax, pleural effusions, and bronchopleural fistula. The main difficulty is in differentiating them from other pulmonary pathologies. A cavitating nodule needs in particular to be distinguished from tuberculosis and from a squamous cell carcinoma. Sputum examination, bronchoscopy, BAL and a CT-guided biopsy may all help in the diagnosis. Even so, the diagnosis at times is uncertain and is made only after a lobectomy.

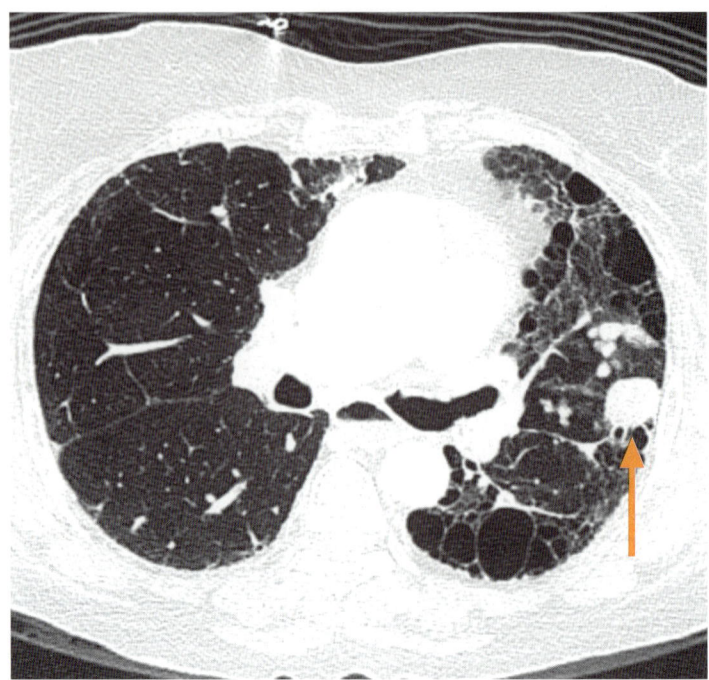

Fig 57.2: Rheumatoid arthritis. HRCT chest in a patient with rheumatoid arthritis demonstrating subpleural interstitial thickening with honeycomb changes due to UIP. Additionally noted are well–defined rheumatoid nodules within the lung parenchyma.

Kaplan's syndrome

This syndrome develops in patients with RA who develop coal workers' pneumoconiosis or other pneumoconiosis. It is characterized by the appearance of nodules within the lung on an X-ray chest. They occur in crops; at times the nodules fuse to give the appearance of progressive massive fibrosis. The nodules may cavitate and cause problems in diagnosis. The pathogenesis of this syndrome is unclear; it could be related to an overactive response of the hyperimmune rheumatoid lung to the coal dust or other dust particles within it. Histologically, the nodules in Kaplan's syndrome resemble the subcutaneous necrotic nodules of rheumatoid disease; in addition the lesions contain coal dust particles. Amazingly, similar nodules are found in the lungs of coal-miners who are sero-positive for rheumatoid disease but who have no arthritis. The diagnosis can pose problems, with the need to consider both inflammatory and neoplastic pathologies in the differential diagnosis. No treatment is necessary.

Airway Disease

Some patients with rheumatoid disease develop an arthritis of the crycoarytenoid joints. This leads to hoarseness, dyspnoea, cough and supraglottic stenosis. An indirect laryngoscopy together with a flow-volume loop determination will enable an accurate diagnosis. At times a tracheostomy becomes necessary to keep the airway patent. A rare but dangerous airway complication in rheumatoid disease is *obliterative bronchiolitis*. Pathologically, it is characterized by inflammation of the walls of the small airways with the formation of obliterative scar tissue. The patient gets progressively breathless and may die within some months from respiratory failure due to increasing unremitting obstruction of small airways. There may be no physical signs at all and the

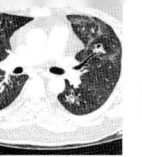

diagnosis of functional breathlessness may be made in the early stages of this disease if the patient is not carefully evaluated. In some patients there is an audible inspiratory squeak together with a few crackles during end-inspiration. The lung functions show small airways' obstruction with increased residual volumes and total lung capacity, but a preserved transfer factor of the lung for carbon monoxide (TLCO). Radiological examination of the chest shows over-inflated lungs. CT scan shows areas of decreased attenuation and vascularity and areas of increased attenuation and vascularity (mosaic pattern) which is brought out best in expiratory scans. Treatment is generally ineffective and prognosis poor. Young patients with severe progressive disease should be considered for lung transplant surgery.

There are some who attribute *obliterative bronchiolitis* in RA to the use of penicillamine. This may be so in rare instances but *obliterative bronchiolitis* has occurred in rheumatoid patients who have not been given penicillamine. Also, this complication has not been observed when penicillamine has been used for the treatment of biliary cirrhosis or Wilson's disease.

Follicular Bronchiolitis   Follicular bronchiolitis is a disorder of unknown aetiology with lymphoid follicles being reported in airway walls. It is a rare entity most commonly found in RA. It may mimic ILD but is more steroid-responsive than obliterative bronchiolitis or RA-related ILD.

Pulmonary infections appear to occur more frequently in rheumatoid disease. There is also an increased incidence of both *bronchitis and bronchiectasis*. Perhaps this may be related to immune suppression caused both by the disease and its treatment. Poor local host defences and difficulty in coughing and expectorating because of increasing debility and arthritic pain are other contributing factors. Finally, a very small minority of patients with rheumatoid disease develop relapsing polychondritis.

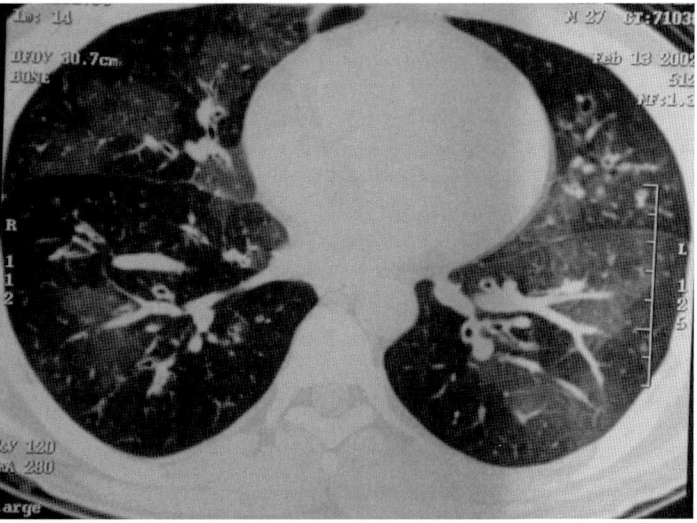

Fig 57.3: Obliterative bronchioloitis, marked areas of mosaic perfusion due to air trapping seen in a patient with rheumatoid disease.

Pulmonary Hypertension

Very rarely, pulmonary hypertension has been reported as an isolated pulmonary complication of rheumatoid disease. There is widespread intimal fibrosis in the medium-sized pulmonary vessels observed on histopathological studies. Pulmonary hypertension when present is more often related to severe interstitial pulmonary fibrosis than to direct vascular involvement.

Drug Toxicity

Added to the pulmonary manifestations produced by rheumatoid disease are the toxic effects of the drugs used in the treatment of this disease. Gold is known to produce pulmonary fibrosis, in addition to other toxic effects on other systems. Penicillamine has been reported to cause *obliterative bronchiolitis* and has been suspect for causing alveolar haemorrhage. Aspirin and non-steroidal anti-inflammatory drugs can exacerbate asthma in patients with bronchial hypersensitivity. Methotrexate lung occurs in about 5% of patients receiving this drug for their RA. This condition carries a mortality of up to 20%. A BAL lymphocytosis of up to 68% of the total cell count together with an increase in CD_4 lymphocytes is observed.

SYSTEMIC LUPUS ERYTHEMATOSUS

SLE often involves many organ systems. Pleuropulmonary manifestations are common, being more frequent when compared to any of the other connective tissue disorders. They occur both in the spontaneously occurring form as well as in the drug-induced form.

Pleural Disease

Pleural effusion is the commonest pulmonary manifestation of SLE. Clinically or radiologically overt pleural involvement is found in 20% of newly diagnosed SLE. In fact it is often the presenting feature. Pleurisy may be dry, but more often there is pleurisy with effusion, which may be small, moderate and rarely, large. Pleuritic pain, breathlessness and fever are the presenting clinical features. The effusion may be unilateral, is bilateral in close to 50% of cases, and at times is consecutive, involvement of one pleural space being followed after a lapse of days or weeks by involvement of the other. The differential diagnosis (particularly in patients where a pleural effusion is the presenting feature) is from tuberculosis. Even though tuberculosis is rife in India, in our experience bilateral pleural effusion in young females with no parenchymal lung lesion on imaging is more frequently due to SLE than due to tuberculosis. Pleural effusion may be accompanied by pericardial effusion so that there is an enlargement of the cardiac silhouette on an X-ray chest.

Pleural fluid examination shows sterile lymphocytic exudates. In the early stages neutrophilic exudates may occur and a preponderance of mononuclear cells has been reported in studies where pleural aspiration has been done after one week. A pH of >7.33 and a normal glucose content distinguish this exudate from that seen in rheumatoid disease. The anti-nuclear antibody (ANA) factor in the pleural fluid may be strongly positive, LE cells may be present and the complement level may be low.

Pleural effusion in SLE responds dramatically to corticosteroids, in contrast to pleural effusion in RA where the response is not predictable.

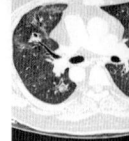

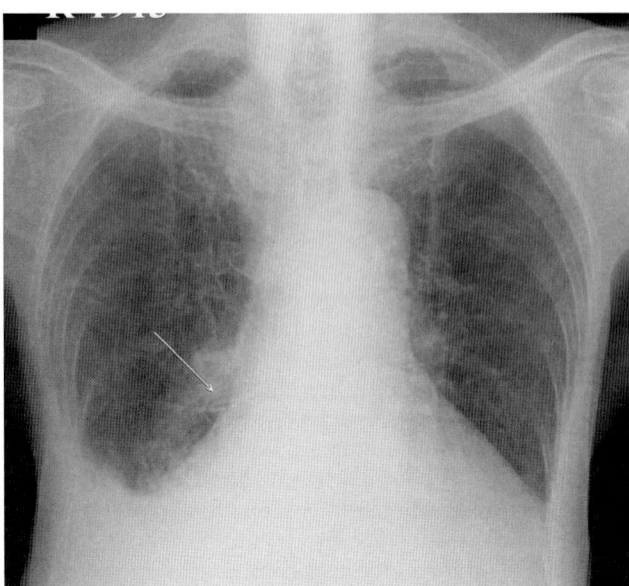

Fig 57.4: SLE. Chest X-Ray demonstrates bilateral pleural effusions with a pericardial effusion in a patient with SLE.

Pulmonary Involvement

Atelectasis is frequently observed in SLE. It takes the form of a plate atelectasis (about 2–4 cm in length), a little above the diaphragm and it may be associated with pleurisy. Restriction of breathing because of pain coupled with poor diaphragmatic movements probably explains the atelectasis, though an abnormality in surfactant has also been postulated. The differential diagnosis is chiefly from pulmonary embolism and infarction.

Shrinking Lung Syndrome

The shrinking lung syndrome observed in SLE is characterized by shrinkage of both lungs in size and volume with a progressive rise in the level of both domes of the diaphragm. This syndrome and the related rise in the diaphragm is due to progressive

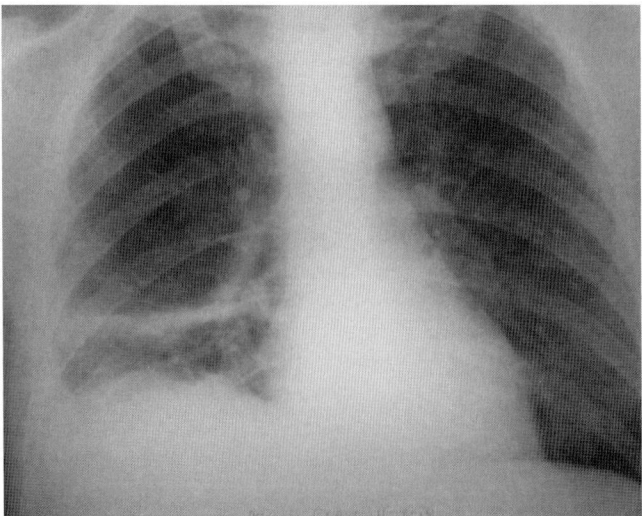

Fig 57.5: SLE. X-ray chest showing plate atelectasis above the right dome of the diaphragm in a patient with SLE. Note the small right-sided pleural effusion.

weakness and fibrosis of the muscles of diaphragmatic leaflets. When sufficiently advanced it causes breathlessness and marked orthopnoea. The latter symptom is an important diagnostic clue. On fluoroscopy the movements of the diaphragm are markedly restricted. Forced vital capacity (FVC) in the supine position is significantly (20%) lower than FVC in the upright position and this simple test may be an early pointer to diaphragmatic weakness. The syndrome may remain stable, or may be characterized by periodic exacerbations of breathlessness which partially respond to corticosteroids, though dyspnoea and orthopnoea persist.

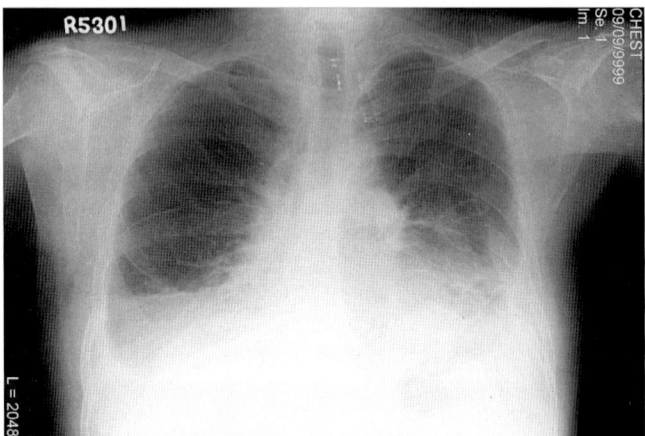

Fig 57.6: X-ray chest reveals bilateral basal atelectasis in a case of shrinking lung syndrome.

Interstitial Pneumonia (Fibrosing Alveolitis)

Interstitial pneumonia is less common in SLE compared to all other connective tissue disorders. When it occurs it is more likely to be of the NSIP variety than the UIP variety. It is

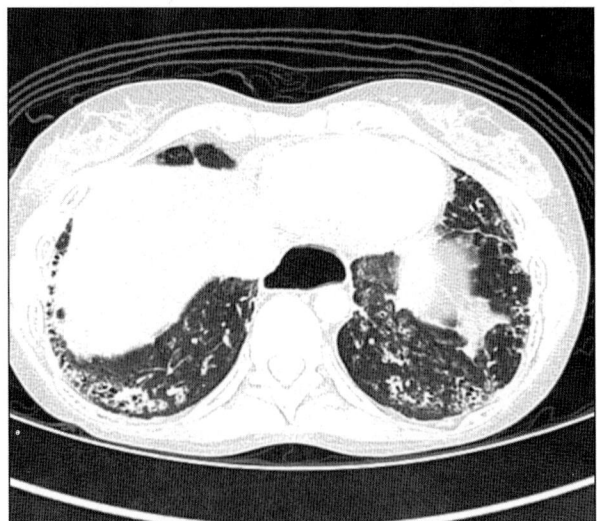

Fig 57.7: SLE with NSIP. HRCT demonstrates bilateral basal posterior interstitial thickening essentially in a peribronchovascular and subpleural location. The peribronchovascular location is well demonstrated as the bronchi are seen well-surrounded by the interstitial thickening. There are no honeycomb changes or fibrosis to suggest UIP pattern.

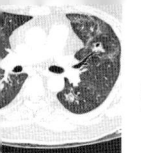

characterized as expected by breathlessness, clubbing of fingers, basal velcro crackles, restrictive lung function pattern and the presence of nodular and reticular basal shadows. The response to corticosteroids is generally better than in cryptogenic fibrosing alveolitis but is not predictable.

Acute Lupoid Pneumonia

Acute lupoid pneumonia is a rare complication of SLE. The features are those of a usual pneumonia, only it is non-infective in nature. It is characterized by fever, cough, breathlessness, tachypnoea and hypoxemia. Auscultatory crackles over the involved lung are present. An X-ray chest shows patchy shadows in one or both lungs or extensive alveolar consolidation involving one or both lungs. The differential diagnosis is from an infective pneumonia. A study of BAL fluid may be necessary to exclude infection. A well-marked leucocytosis is a point against the diagnosis of acute lupoid pneumonia. Corticosteroids have a dramatic effect on lupoid pneumonia. There is a prompt defervescence in the illness as also a resolution of the pulmonary shadows. Relapses may however occur and a maintenance dose of prednisolone may be necessary for a significant length of time.

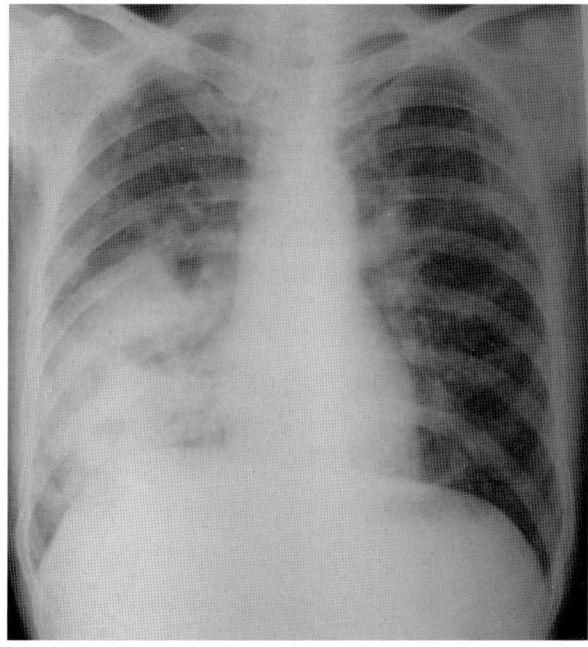

Fig 57.8: Lupoid pneumonia. Chest x-ray shows an ill-defined area of consolidation in a patient with SLE demonstrating a lupoid pneumonia. There was prompt resolution after the use of corticosteroids.

Pulmonary Vascular Involvement

Pulmonary vascular involvement in SLE may take two forms—alveolar haemorrhage and pulmonary hypertension. Alveolar haemorrhage is related to an underlying pulmonary capillaritis. We have seen this very rarely as a presenting feature of SLE. Acutely evolving breathlessness, tachypnoea, increasing hypoxia, and bilateral alveolar shadows that may be mistaken

for ARDS may be observed. Tachycardia and hypertension may be present and there is a fall in the haemoglobin. Haemoptysis may or may not be present, though a BAL study shows blood-stained fluid with macrophages filled with hemosiderin. The differential diagnosis is from other causes of intra-alveolar haemorrhage, notably from Wegener's granulomatosis, and in our country, from leptospirosis.

Pulmonary hypertension is caused by intimal fibrosis and sclerosis involving medium and small-sized vessels within the lungs. Though rare in our study, it has been reported in 4–14 % of patients in the West with an overall mortality of 20–50% at two years from the time of diagnosis. It occasionally dominates the disease and rarely may be its presenting feature. Breathlessness, evidence of right ventricular hypertrophy, and right-sided heart failure are observed. X-ray chest shows clear lung fields; the pulmonary function tests may be normal. It needs to be stressed that a diagnosis of idiopathic pulmonary hypertension in a young girl should not be accepted without doing relevant tests for SLE. Echocardiography may demonstrate right ventricular hypertrophy with pulmonary hypertension only when the disease is well advanced. In the few cases studied in our unit we noticed a definite response to corticosteroids. Perhaps this is observed only when steroids are used in the early part of the natural history of this complication. When severe irreversible pulmonary hypertension is the dominant feature of SLE, a lung transplant should be considered.

ANTIPHOSPHOLIPID ANTIBODY SYNDROME

The antiphospholipid antibody syndrome shows positivity for lupus anticoagulant and the antiphospholipid antibody test. It is characterized by a tendency to thrombosis, chiefly in the veins but also in the smaller arteries. Clinical features consists of a history of multiple abortions, Raynaud's phenomenon, thrombotic episodes in veins and arteries, thrombocytopenia and a prolonged partial thromboplastin time. Thrombotic episodes in pulmonary vessels can lead to pulmonary hypertension. This syndrome is often associated with SLE.

Besides lung involvement due to the direct effects of SLE on the lungs, respiratory manifestations and pleuropulmonary complications may result from a) pulmonary infections to which these patients are very prone; b) drugs used in the treatment of SLE; c) lung complications secondary to SLE involvement of other organ systems e.g. cardiac involvement, renal involvement, and thrombocytopenia.

SYSTEMIC SCLEROSIS

Involvement of the skin which may be localized or diffuse is generally the presenting feature of SSc. Nevertheless the disease often involves other organ systems, notably the heart, kidneys and the lungs. Pulmonary involvement is an important cause of morbidity and mortality. Pulmonary involvement is more likely in the presence of Scl 70 antibodies. In contrast the presence of anticentromere antibodies is generally associated with limited disease without pulmonary involvement. The two main pulmonary manifestations of SSc are interstitial pneumonia and pulmonary hypertension. Other manifestations include aspiration pneumonia when there is involvement of the lower end of the oesophagus in the sclerodermatous process

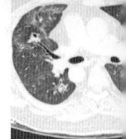

and alveolar hypoventilation caused by very thickened tight scleroderma-affected skin over the thorax which acts as cuirass sharply restricting respiratory movements.

Interstitial Pneumonia

Interstitial pneumonia is most frequently observed in SSc—much more frequently than in any other connective tissue disease. Patients dying of SSc invariably have clinical or autopsy evidence of pulmonary fibrosis. The symptoms and signs are similar to those detailed earlier. Pulmonary involvement should be suspected whenever the CO diffusion is impaired or lung functions show a mildly restrictive pattern. Lung function changes may be observed even in the presence of a normal X-ray chest. CT studies are far more sensitive in revealing interstitial pneumonia. It used to be believed that the fibrosing alveolitis in SSc was indistinguishable from cryptogenic fibrosing alveolitis i.e. UIP. Studies over the last decade suggest that the pattern of involvement is more akin to NSIP than to UIP. The latter pattern may also however occur. In a recent study of 80 patients of SSc who had undergone open-lung biopsies, 66 (78%) had NSIP whilst only six patients had UIP. Response to corticosteroids and immunosupprants is unpredictable. Some patients respond well and the lung lesion may remain stable for months and occasionally years and then show a sudden exacerbation. Exacerbations may occur spontaneously or may be triggered by respiratory infections or non-compliance with regard to therapy.

Pulmonary Hypertension

Pulmonary hypertension (like interstitial pneumonia) is more frequently associated with SSc than with any other connective tissue disease. In fact it may be the sole pulmonary manifestation of the disease and then dominates the clinical picture. It is caused by intimal fibrosis and muscular hypertrophy and hyperplasia of the precapillary vessels. The incidence of pulmonary hypertension both isolated and in association with ILD in diffuse scleroderma is close to 30%. It is found in 60% of

patients with the CREST (calcinosis, Raynaud phenomenon, oesophageal dysmotility, sclerodactyly, and telangiectasia) syndrome. These are Western figures; there are no reliable figures of the incidence of pulmonary hypertension in SSc in India. There is histological evidence of pulmonary vasculopathy in up to 65% of patients with limited SSc, although less than 10% develop clinically overt pulmonary hypertension during life.

Pulmonary hypertension in SSc can also occur from increasing interstitial pulmonary fibrosis. Pulmonary hypertension worsens prognosis. Survival rates in patients with SSc and pulmonary hypertension are similar to those observed in idiopathic pulmonary hypertension (a two-year survival rate of 50%).

Other Pulmonary Manifestations

1. Patients with SSc who also have oesophageal involvement are prone to aspiration pneumonia because of regurgitation of gastric contents from a fibrotic oesophagus and an incompetent oesophagogastric junction.
2. Traction bronchiectasis is a common feature in patients with interstitial fibrosis. Bronchiectasis together with the immunosuppressants used in the treatment of interstitial fibrosis predispose to pulmonary infection.
3. When the skin over the thorax is markedly involved in the sclerodermatous process, respiratory excursions are hindered. Alveolar hypoventilation results in hypercapnic respiratory failure.
4. Pleural involvement in SSc is very rare. It manifests as pleural thickening or a small pleural effusion.
5. Bronchogenic carcinoma may develop when there is well-marked interstitial pulmonary fibrosis.

DERMATOMYOSITIS, POLYMYOSITIS

This is an inflammatory connective tissue disorder involving the skin and the muscles. There is generally symmetrical skeletal

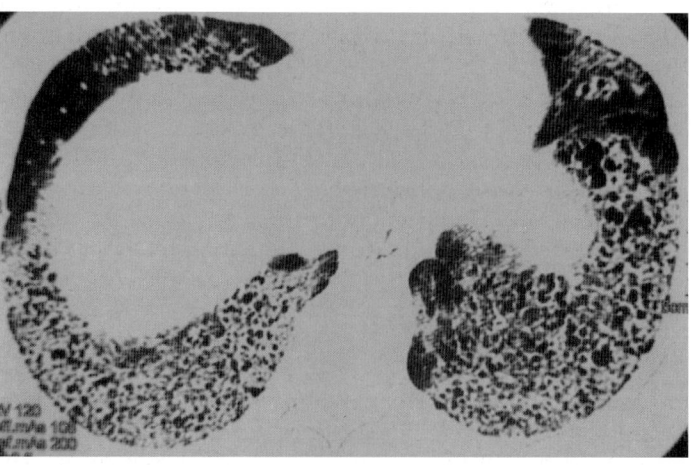
(a)

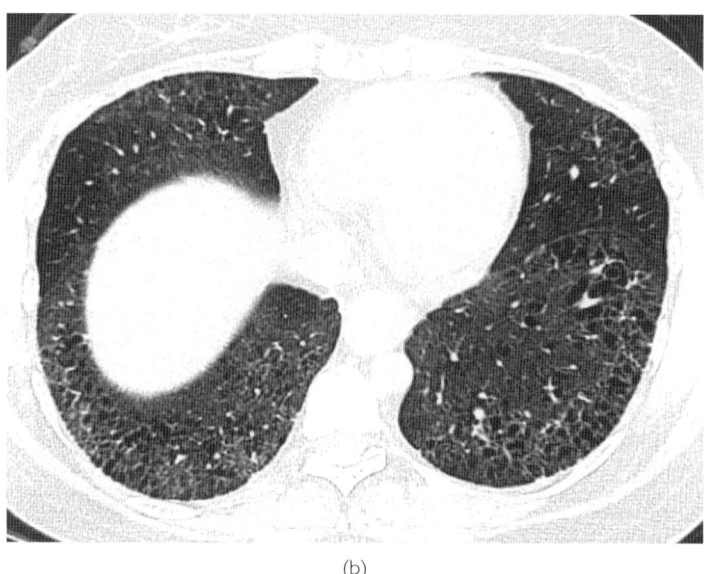
(b)

Fig 57.9: Systemic Sclerosis. Interstitial pneumonia in a patient with systemic sclerosis (a) There is extensive reticular thickening with honeycomb cysts and bronchiolectasis in both lung bases posteriorly (b) Resolution of interstitial pneumonia following treatment with corticosteroids, the previously visualized extensive reticular opacities have resolved now with only residual honeycomb cysts.

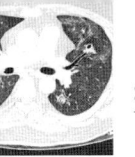

muscle weakness. Difficulty in swallowing is due to weakness of pharyngeal muscles and this may precede, accompany or follow weakness of the proximal muscles of the upper and lower limbs. In about 10% of patients, PM and DM present as a paraneoplastic syndrome consequent to an underlying malignancy within the body. Autoantibodies are frequently present in this connective tissue disorder. Anti-synthetase (anti-Jo) antibodies when present are often associated with interstitial pneumonias. Pulmonary complications are chiefly due to muscle weakness and to interstitial pneumonia leading to interstitial pulmonary fibrosis.

Complications due to Muscle Weakness

Weakness of pharyngeal muscles causes difficulty in swallowing with a risk of aspiration pneumonia. The patient may be unable to protect the airway; when this is well-marked a tracheostomy may be necessary to keep the airway patent and prevent aspiration. When muscle weakness involves the intercostal muscles and occasionally the diaphragm there is risk of hypoventilation causing both hypoxia and hypercapnia (hypercapnic respiratory failure). An increase in respiratory rate, a progressive fall in the tidal volume, in the vital capacity and in the maximal inspiratory force, are pointers to impending danger. Hypercapnic respiratory failure may develop in up to 5% of patients with DM/PM due to respiratory muscle weakness from muscle inflammation.

Interstitial Pneumonia

Interstitial pneumonia is commonly observed, particularly in the presence of antisynthetase antibodies. It is critical to note that interstitial pneumonia may be the first manifestation of DM or PM and may precede skin manifestations and/or muscle

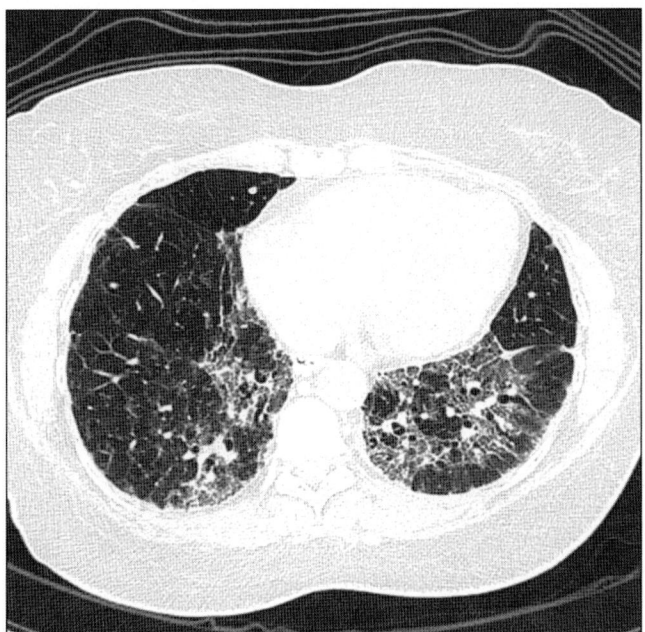

Fig 57.10: Dermatomyositis. HRCT chest demonstrates ill-defined areas of ground-glass densities in both lung bases with subpleural and peribronchovascular interstitial thickening; there is also traction bronchiectasis secondary to the peribronchial interstitial thickening. There are also areas of air trapping interspersed between the areas of interstitial thickening.

weakness by months or rarely by a few years. This happens in about 20% of patients with this connective tissue disorder. In these circumstances the interstitial pneumonia is often diagnosed as idiopathic or cryptogenic. The presence of autoantibodies and in particular of anti-synthetase antibodies should forewarn of the future evolution of skin or muscle manifestations. The pattern of ILD in PM/DM is heterogeneous with a recent study of 22 biopsied patients demonstrating NSIP in the majority (82%) with the remainder having diffuse alveolar damage or organizing pneumonia. Many other series have confirmed a significant prevalence of organizing pneumonia in PM/DM.

Rarely, the interstitial pneumonia presents acutely or subacutely with cough, rapidly progressive dyspnoea, rapidly evolving crackles all over the lungs and with increasing hypoxemic respiratory failure. The clinical features resemble an acute interstitial pneumonia and more often than not the course is inexorably downhill, unresponsive to all therapy.

Treatment of both muscular manifestations of the disease and of interstitial pneumonia is with corticosteroids and the use of immunosuppressants.

MIXED CONNECTIVE TISSUE DISEASE

As the name signifies this connective tissue disease partakes of more than one of the connective tissue disorders discussed above. It is also termed the "overlap syndrome". Thus features of SLE may be associated with those of SSc and/or DM or PM. It is therefore difficult to semantically label such patients as belonging to one single connective tissue disorder. Mixed connective tissue disease is generally characterized by antibodies in high titre to nuclear ribonucleoprotein antigen.

Pulmonary manifestations are common in the overlap syndrome. Pleural involvement takes the form of pleural effusion. Pulmonary involvement is chiefly characterized by interstitial pneumonia, generally NSIP. Organizing pneumonia with or without involvement of the respiratory bronchioles though rare may also occur. Intra-alveolar haemorrhage due to pulmonary capillaritis (as in SLE) has also been observed. Perhaps the most dreaded complication is of rapidly progressive pulmonary hypertension due to intimal fibrosis and medial hypertrophy affecting medium-sized pulmonary arterioles. The clinical features and course of pulmonary hypertension are indistinguishable from idiopathic pulmonary hypertension. Increasing interstitial fibrosis may contribute to or may itself be responsible for pulmonary hypertension in some patients. Mixed connective tissue disease which has features of SLE may be associated with antiphospholipid antibodies. Pulmonary thromboembolic complications can then occur, and if extensive can lead to crippling pulmonary hypertension.

SJOGREN'S SYNDROME

This autoimmune disorder may occur as a primary disorder or is secondary to any one of the other connective tissue disorders. It affects the exocrine glands at different sites within the body, causing diminished glandular secretions and a drying of the mucosa. It typically involves the lacrymal glands leading to dry eyes which fail to secrete tears, and the salivary glands leading to a diminished salivary secretion. This may be so marked as to cause difficulty in swallowing. Upper and lower airways

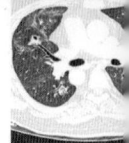

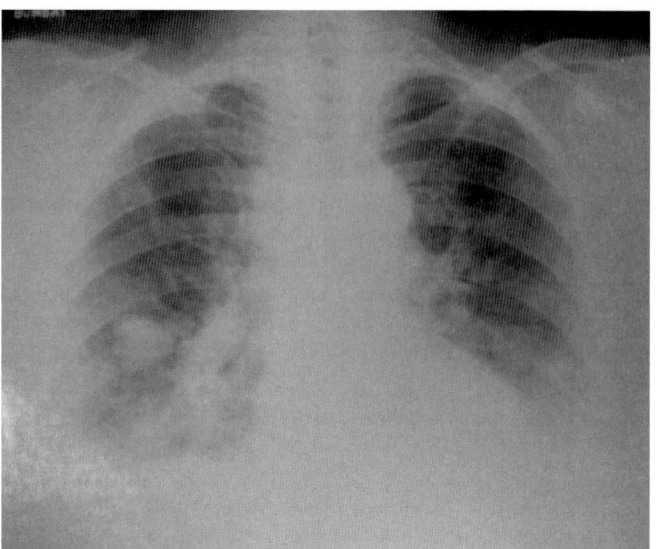

Fig 57.11: Sjogren's syndrome. B-cell lymphoma. Chest X-ray demonstrates a well-defined mass lesion in the right lower zone which on CT-guided biopsy revealed a lymphoma.

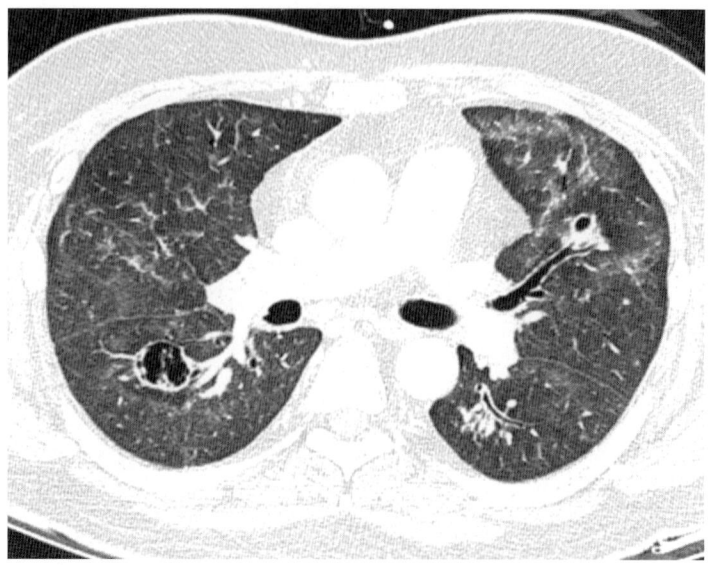

Fig 57.12: Ankylosing spondylitis with aspergilliomas. HRCT chest demonstrates multiple well-defined cavities in the apical segments of both lower lobes and the lingula. Linear densities and crescents are seen within the cavities representing hyphae due to aspergillus.

involvement may take the form of nasal mucosal infiltration with dryness (rhina sicca), lymphocytic infiltration of the tracheobronchial submucosal glands (xerotrachea) and lymphocytic subepithelial bronchial and bronchiolar infiltration. Tracheal disease is one of the most common respiratory manifestations in Sjogren's syndrome. It usually takes the form of xerotrachea, with loss of mucous secretions secondary to atrophy of tracheobronchial mucous glands. Patients present with a dry irritating cough and endobronchial inflammation at bronchoscopic biopsy. This dryness also predisposes these patients to recurrent bronchial infections which occur in about 20% of patients.

Pulmonary parenchymal manifestations have been reported in the primary and secondary forms of the disease. They include the different forms of interstitial pneumonia and lymphocytic interstitial pneumonia. Lymphoproliferative disorders may take the form of lymphomatoid granulomatosis or B-cell non-Hodgkin's lymphoma. In secondary Sjogren's syndrome, the pulmonary manifestations are influenced by the coexisting connective tissue disorders.

ANKYLOSING SPONDYLITIS

Ankylosing spondylitis is a seronegative spondyloarthritis involving the sacroiliac joints, the spine and the large joints, chiefly of the lower limbs. The majority of patients with this disease are HLAB27-positive though the incidence of this positivity in Indians is not as high as is reported in the West. The disease is also characterized by the occurrence of uveitis in 20%, aortic incompetence (in 10%), and a symptomatic inflammation of the thoracic aorta (10–15%).

Pulmonary complications take the form of bilateral upper lobe fibrosis with upward retraction of the hila. Bullous areas or cavities may be associated with the upper lobe fibrosis, so that a wrong diagnosis of pulmonary tuberculosis is often made. A fungal ball, chiefly an aspergilloma may be present in a bulla or a cavity. The aspergilloma may be silent or cause haemoptysis. Rarely, the haemoptysis is exsanguinating and can result in death.

In advanced ankylosing spondylitis chest excursions are markedly restricted due to fusion of the costovertebral joints and ankylosis of the thoracic spine; this leads to alveolar hyperventilation and hypercapnic respiratory failure. The limited chest movements, together with restricted cough also predispose to atelectasis and pulmonary infection.

There is no treatment for upper lobe fibrosis; corticosteroids are generally ineffective. Haemoptysis resulting from an aspergilloma is best treated conservatively. When severe, bronchial embolism is the treatment of choice, and if this fails one may be forced into surgery, which more often than not takes the form of a lobectomy. Surgery, however, carries a high mortality and morbidity.

Hypercapnic respiratory failure may require ventilatory support; non-invasive ventilatory support is generally possible and is to be preferred.

BEHÇET'S DISEASE

Behcet's disease is classified by some as a form of connective tissue disorder. It is an inflammatory disorder of unknown aetiology affecting blood vessels of all sizes and therefore can manifest with involvement of a number of organ systems. It is more prevalent in the Mediterranean zone and in the Far East, but is also observed in India occurring generally in the 20–30 years age group. It is often associated with HLA B5 antigen.

Its typical features are orogenital ulcers, ocular manifestations (chiefly anterior or posterior uvertis, retinitis), arthralgias and arthritis involving the large joints chiefly of the lower limbs and venous thromobophlebitis. Central nervous system involvement is fairly frequent, manifesting chiefly with headache, meningoencephalitis, cranial nerve involvement and seizures. Skin involvement takes the form of various forms of rashes, the disease often being first recognized in the skin department of hospitals.

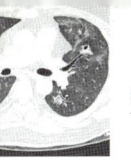

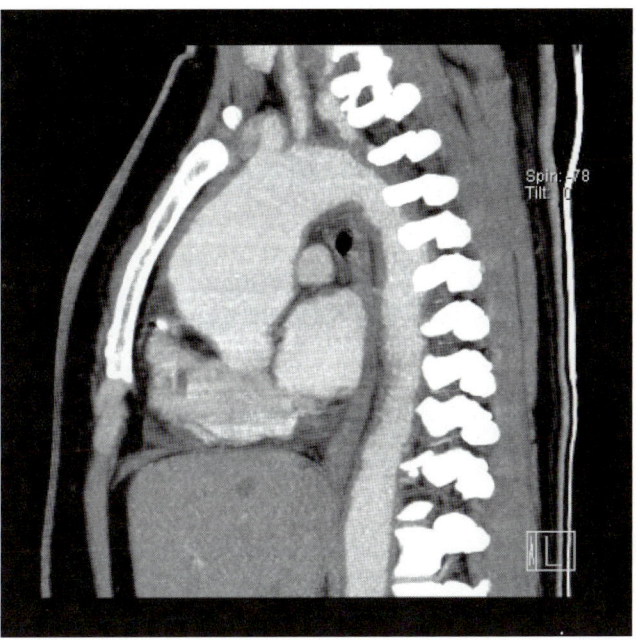

Fig 57.13: Ascending aortic aneurysm in a patient with Behçet's disease.

Pulmonary involvement is rare and is characterized by pulmonary artery aneurysm or thromboembolic disease affecting pulmonary vessels. Chest pain, dyspnoea, haemoptysis are the main symptoms. The pulmonary artery aneurysm is due to an inflammatory weakening of the vessel wall. Thromboembolic disease is due to inflammation of the pulmonary arterioles, leading to multiple pulmonary thrombi with pulmonary infarction. Thromboembolic disease requires the use of anti-coagulants; the latter can however lead to catastrophe in patients with a pulmonary artery aneurysm. Corticosteroids and immunosuppressants form the mainstay of therapy. Just as involvement of the pulmonary artery wall can lead to an aneurysmal dilatation of the pulmonary artery, involvement of the aortic wall can lead to an aneurysm of the aorta.

The Hughes Stovin Syndrome is considered by some to be a variant of Behçet's disease. It is characterized by the presence of a pulmonary artery aneurysm, systemic venous thrombosis often involving the vena cava and causing a rise in the intracranial pressure, but no other extrapulmonary features generally associated with Behçet's disease.

SUGGESTED READING

Celenk C. Pulmonary alterations in Behçet's disease. *Eur J Radiol.* 1 May 2009; 70(2): 317–19.

Fujisawa T. Differences in clinical featurs and prognosis of interstitial lung diseases between polymyositis and dermatomyositis. *J Rheumatol.* 1 Jan. 2005; 32(1): 58–64.

Kakati S. Pulmonary manifestations in systemic lupus erythematosus (SLE) with special reference to HRCT. *J Assoc Physicians India.* 1 Dec. 2007; 55: 839–41.

Kim EJ. Rheumatoid arthritis-associated interstitial lung disease: the relevance of histopathologic and radiographic pattern. *Chest.* 1 Nov. 2009; 136(5): 1397–405.

Parambil JG. Diffuse alveolar damage: uncommon manifestation of pulmonary inolvement in patients with connective tissue disease. *Chest.* 1 Aug. 2006; 130(2): 553–8.

Strange C. Interstitial Lung disease in the patient who has connective tissue disease. *Clin Chest Med.* 1 Sep. 2004; 25(3): 549–59, vii.

Won Huh J. Two distinct clinical types of interstitial lung disease associated with polymyositis-dermatomyositis. *Respir Med.* 1 Aug. 2007; 101(8): 1761–9.

Woodhead F. Pulmonary complications of connective tissue diseases. *Clin Chest Med.* 1 Mar. 2008; 29(1): 149–64, vii.

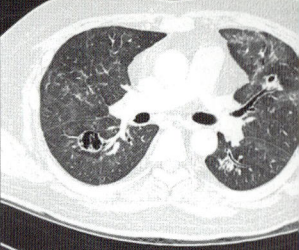

CHAPTER **58** # Pulmonary Manifestations of Hepatobiliary and Pancreatic Diseases

CHRONIC HEPATIC DISEASES

The pulmonary complications of chronic liver disorders may involve the pleura, the pulmonary vasculature or the pulmonary parenchyma.

Pleural effusions particularly in the right pleural space are common. They are secondary to ascites present in liver cirrhosis. Fenestrations within the domes of diaphragm (in particular the right dome) allow ascitic fluid entry into the pleural space. The pleural effusion is a transudate; it could be mild, moderate or massive. Hypoalbuminaemia present in liver cell dysfunction reduces plasma oncotic pressure and contributes to the formation of the transudate.

The Budd-Chiari syndrome characterized by hepatic vein thrombosis is a rare but often missed cause of a recurrent pleural effusion. The effusion is a transudate, large, often right-sided and recurs quickly on being tapped. The diagnosis is occasionally stumbled upon when liver functions show some degree of derangement. The TIPS (trans intrahepatic porto-systemic shunt) procedure, if successfully performed is the treatment of choice. The porto-systemic shunt decongests the systemic veins and thereby stops accumulation of fluid within the pleural space.

The most dangerous though infrequent complications in chronic liver disease are the hepatopulmonary syndrome and portopulmonary hypertension.

HEPATOPULMONARY SYNDROME

This syndrome is observed in patients with cirrhosis of the liver with portal hypertension. It can occur in all forms of cirrhosis including Wilson's disease. It has also been reported in non-cirrhotic portal hypertension, chronic active hepatitis, biliary cirrhosis and primary biliary atresia.

Clinical Features

There is a background of liver disease, both clinically and on liver function tests. Spider nevi are invariably present and are markers of spider nevi in the lungs and on the pleural surface, known to be present in these patients.

Breathlessness on exertion is the cardinal symptom. It is related to hypoxia which in some patients is so marked as to cause clinically evident central cyanosis. Clubbing is an early feature and in advanced cases is severe. Interestingly, these patients suffer from platypnoea, the patient being increasingly breathless in the standing position and less in the supine position. Another characteristic finding in the hepatopulmonary syndrome is orthodexia which is defined as a significant decrease in the PaO_2 ($PaO_2 < 3$ mm but often up to 30 mm Hg) when the patient moves from the supine to the standing posture. For reasons to be shortly explained, inhalation of oxygen does not bring complete relief and in severe cases hypoxia persists even when oxygen is delivered at high flow rates. Death occurs from hypoxic respiratory failure.

Not all cases are very severe and probably not all cases get progressively worse. Also, not all patients with this syndrome are so severely hypoxic as to be clinically cyanosed. *The combination of cirrhosis of the liver with a $PaO_2 < 55$ mm Hg should suggest a hepatopulmonary syndrome. The association of portal hypertension, cutaneous spider nevi and clubbing is also suggestive of the hepatopulmonary syndrome and should necessitate further tests.*

Pathophysiology

The hypoxia and the associated breathlessness in the hepatopulmonary syndrome are due to several factors of which the first two listed below are the most important.

1. V/Q abnormality This syndrome is characterized by a marked hyperdynamic circulation with marked dilation of the precapillary and capillary vessels perfusing the alveoli. The perfusion is both quick (hyperdynamic) and excessive in relation to ventilation so that there is fall in the V/Q ratio of alveoli so perfused. In fact, the haemodynamics in the hepatopulmonary syndrome is characterized by tachycardia, increased cardiac output, reduced pulmonary vascular resistance and a normal or low pulmonary artery pressure.

2. Some patients with this syndrome develop new vessels within the lungs which shunt the unoxygenated blood to the left without allowing it to perfuse the alveoli—this results in an intrapulmonary right to left shunt, proven by the inability of 100% oxygen to abolish the alveolar arterial oxygen gradient. On 100% oxygen many patients with the hepatopulmonary syndrome will have a PaO_2 of < 300 mm Hg.

3. The syndrome is also known to be associated at times with a thickening of the walls of the dilated pulmonary vessels, causing a diffusion defect that adds to hypoxia.

4. One other reason for hypoxia is a diffusion-perfusion defect. With the increased dilatation and width of precapillary vessels, oxygen molecules have a difficult time reaching the centre of the mixed venous stream. Mid-stream erythrocytes fail to oxygenate, leading to a varying degree of hypoxia.

5. Finally, hypoxemia may be increased by the decreased transit time of blood through the hyperdynamic pulmonary circulation, not allowing enough time for oxygen to reach the mid-stream *red blood cells* (RBCs) within the pulmonary capillaries.

Diagnosis

1. A positive contrast-enhanced transthoracic echocardiography points to the passage of microbubbles (normally absorbed via the lungs during a first pass) through dilated

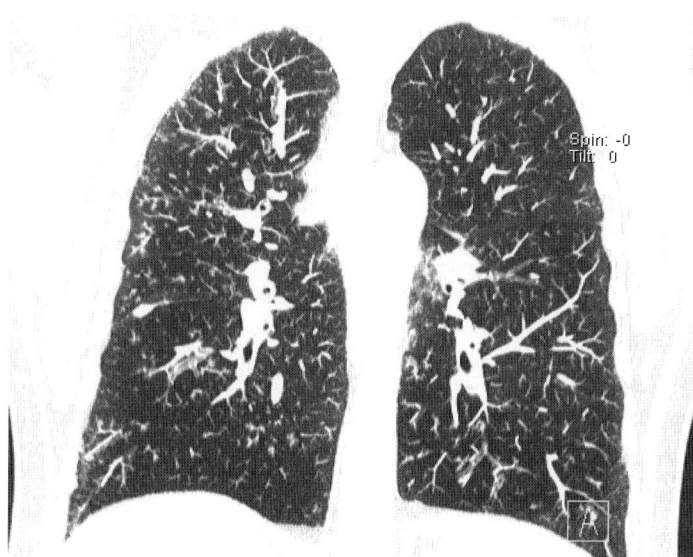

Fig 58.1: Patient with hepatopulmonary syndrome. Note vessels extending up to the subpleural space due to AV shunting.

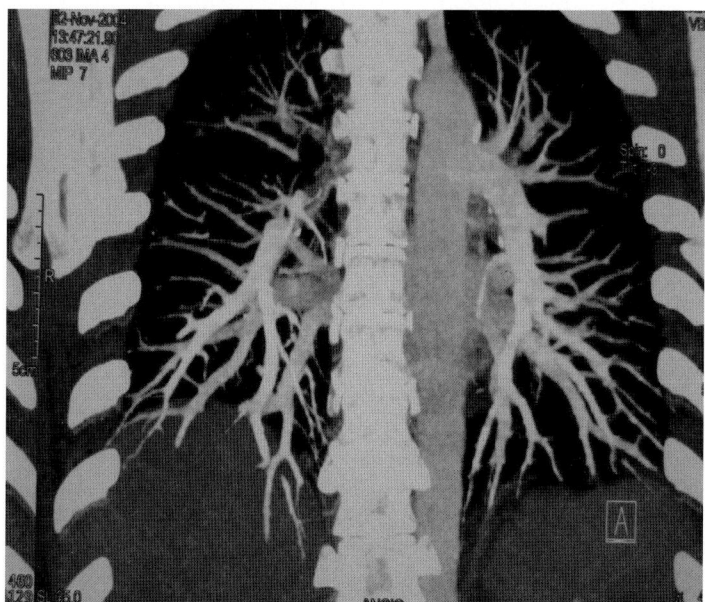

Fig 58.2: Patient with hepatopulmonary syndrome. Note vessels extending to the subpleural space due to AV shunting.

pulmonary vessels and a hyperdynamic pulmonary circulation so as to be detected in the left atrium. This is probably the most sensitive of all diagnostic tests.

2. A perfusion scan using technetium-labelled macroaggregate albumin reveals an increased uptake in the brain (> 6%) after lung perfusion. This again points to a quickened dilated pulmonary circulation.
3. Pulmonary angiography may delineate the vascular abnormalities in this syndrome. Two angiographic pictures have been reported; Type I diffuse vascular abnormalities and Type II focal vascular abnormalities.

Pulmonary angiography may however miss small arteriovenous malformations that are indirectly demonstrated by contrast-enhanced echocardiography and technetium[99] macro-aggregated albumin perfusion scans.

Management

The only definitive treatment is a liver transplant. One could embolize some of the right to left shunts provided these could be demonstrated by pulmonary angiography and provided they do not show a very diffuse distribution.

PORTOPULMONARY HYPERTENSION

Portopulmonary hypertension is characterized by an obstruction to the pulmonary vasculature caused by extensive intimal fibrosis and by medial hypertrophy of the pulmonary arterioles. Porto-systemic and portopulmonary collaterals could transport vasomotor factors like for example, endothelin-1 to the pulmonary circulation causing pulmonary vasoconstriction. Thrombosis occurring *in situ* within the pulmonary vessels adds to pulmonary hypertension. Clinically, the pulmonary second sound is loud, a right ventricular heave is present, a wave in the jugular pulse is prominent. Right ventricular failure is the end result.

Transthoracic Doppler echocardiography should identify pulmonary hypertension. Increased right ventricular systolic pressure > 50 mm Hg suggests the diagnosis. A right heart catheter study is generally performed for confirmation. A mean pulmonary artery pressure > 25 mm Hg, pulmonary vascular resistance > 240 dyn·s/cm[5] are definitive criteria for pulmonary hypertension.

Calcium channel blockers, bosentan, sildenafil and a continuous 24-hour infusion of epoprostenol have all been tried in the management but with poor results.

PULMONARY PARENCHYMAL INVOLVEMENT IN PRIMARY BILIARY CIRRHOSIS

Primary biliary cirrhosis has been known to be associated with pulmonary granulomas, lymphocytic interstitial pneumonia and rarely with organizing pneumonia. Alpha-1 anti-trypsin deficiency (ZZ or SZ type) can cause both liver cirrhosis and pulmonary emphysema. When either one or the other is found in a younger age group with no obvious risk factor, this genetic defect should be kept in mind.

Autoimmune hepatitis has been associated with interstitial pneumonia (UIP or NSIP).

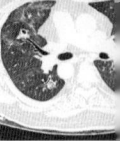

FULMINANT HEPATIC FAILURE

Fulminant hepatic failure, acute hepatic failure and acute on chronic hepatic failure are characterized chiefly by encephalopathy, coagulation defects and hyperbilirubinemia. Multiple organ failure follows, chiefly involving renal, pulmonary, cerebral and haematological systems. Fulminant hepatic failure is associated with a hyperdynamic circulation evidenced by tachycardia, a high pulse pressure, an increased cardiac output with a low systemic vascular resistance and a low pulmonary vascular resistance. There may be a fair degree of passive pulmonary hypertension. Hypoxia is frequently present and has many causes. It could be caused by pulmonary infection, by bleeding into the lungs, by aspiration in a comatose patient and by pulmonary oedema caused by overhydration. Perhaps the most dreaded pulmonary complication is the development of ARDS related to increased capillary permeability. Severe ARDS occurring against the background of fulminant hepatic failure has a dreadful prognosis and is generally fatal.

Table 58.1: Pulmonary complication in hepatobiliary diseases
I Complications in association with liver cirrhosis
Pleural effusion
Hepatopulmonary syndrome
Portopulmonary hypertension
Portosystemic shunt causing cyanosis and clubbing
Emphysema and cirrhosis related to alpha-1 antitrypsin deficiency
Frequent pulmonary infections
Interstitial pneumonia (associated with chronic active hepatitis)
II Complications in fulminant hepatic failure or acute on chronic hepatic failure
Pulmonary infections
Aspiration pneumonia
Pulmonary oedema
Intra-alveolar haemorrhage
ARDS
III Complications associated with primary biliary cirrhosis
Fibrosing alveolitis
Lymphocytic interstitial pneumonia
Pulmonary granulomas
Organising pneumonia
Bronchiectasis

ACUTE PANCREATITIS

Respiratory complications are frequent in acute pancreatitis and are responsible for 50–70% of deaths. The end-result of these complications is hypoxia of varying degree. In fact the severity of the hypoxia reflects the severity of the disease.

The respiratory features of acute pancreatitis have been classified by Basras and colleagues as follows:

Group I Hypoxemia with a normal chest X-ray

Hypoxemia is a common and important presenting feature even in the absence of radiological shadows. The PaO_2 may fall even below 60 mm Hg. The severity of the hypoxia is directly related to the prognosis—the more severe the hypoxia, the worse the prognosis. The hypoxia is obviously related to pancreatic inflammation as it is not generally present in other similar acute abdominal conditions. The hypoxia is partly due to ventilation perfusion abnormalities and partly to an increased shunt. Though the pathogenesis is not clear it may be related to release of cytokines such as TNFα, Interleukin-6 (IL-6), and platelet-activating factor. Fatty acids liberated from the inflamed pancreas may not only damage pulmonary capillaries but may shift the oxygen dissociation curve to the left, worsening hypoxia.

Group II Hypoxemia with pleural effusion and localized abnormalities on X-ray chest

Localized radiological abnormalities are common and occur in 30–40% of patients. The more severe the pancreatitis, the more likely are local radiological abnormalities within the chest. The commonest abnormality observed is a pleural effusion, generally left-sided but at times bilateral. This is invariably associated with a raised diaphragm involving chiefly the left dome, but at times to a lesser extent the right as well, so that the lung volumes seem small. The pleural fluid on tapping is a haemorrhagic exudate with a high neutrophil count and markedly raised amylase content. The amylase in the pleural fluid is far higher than in the serum. Other radiological abnormalities include basal, segmental or even lobar atelectasis.

Localized alveolar shadows and interstitial shadows probably reflect pulmonary oedema. The mechanism of pleural effusion as also of the pulmonary shadows is unclear. It is most likely related to the transport of the pancreatic inflammatory exudates through the diaphragm into the chest.

Group III Hypoxemia with diffuse bilateral pulmonary shadows due to ARDS

In our unit, 15–20% of patients with acute pancreatitis develop ARDS within three to seven days of the onset of the disease. The pathogenesis is complex and is discussed elsewhere. Perhaps liberation of pancreatic trypsin, lipase and fatty acids together with kinins may play a special role in causing the increased permeability inflammatory pulmonary oedema that characterizes the syndrome. Ventilatory support is mandatory and the mortality is significantly increased in spite of good critical care.

Late Pulmonary Complications

Pulmonary complications arising in the course of acute pancreatitis (after two weeks or more) are due to infection with the formation of a pseudocyst or a pancreatic abscess. Pancreatic pseudocysts present with abdominal complaints, fever, and a raised hemi-diaphragm with atelectatic bands or segmental atelectasis in the left lower lobe. They may track through the diaphragm to the mediastinum and may rupture into the pleural space. Treatment is conservative with the use of hyperalimentaion and pleural drainage. A pancreatic abscess

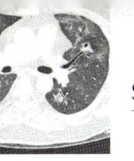

may also be associated with a pleural exudate which may graduate into an empyema. Surgical drainage of the abscess and the empyema becomes necessary.

PULMONARY COMPLICATIONS OF CHRONIC PANCREATITIS

The chief complication is pleural effusion, generally left-sided but occasionally bilateral. The effusions may be large, recurrent and often cause breathlessness and cough. The pleural aspirate is an exudate with high amylase content, the amylase level in the pleural fluid being much higher than in the serum. Pleural effusion in chronic pancreatitis is due to a pancreato-pleural fistula. It could also occur in the presence of pancreatic ascites, the ascitic fluid being drawn into the pleural space through fenestrations within the diaphragm.

Treatment consists of hyperalimentation, the use of octreotide and tube drainage of the pleural space. Surgical advice is necessary to identify and treat a pancreato-pleural fistula.

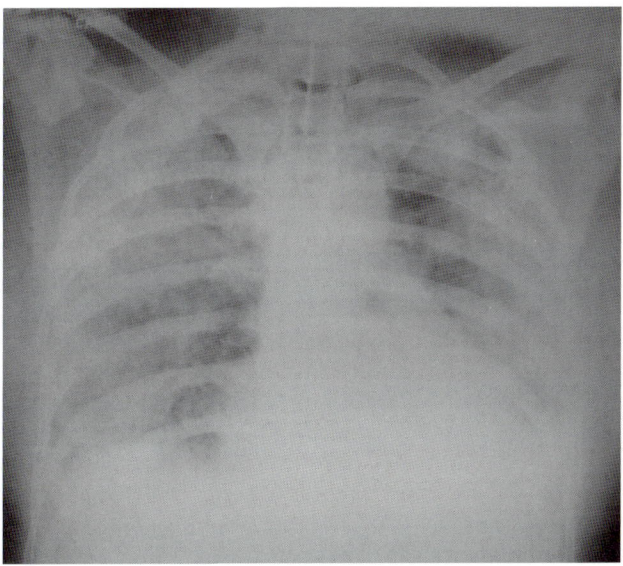

Fig 58.3: Patient with acute pancreatitis having acute lung injury.

SUGGESTED READING

Arguedas MR. Hepatopulmonary Syndrome. *Clin Lever Dis*. 1 Nov. 2005; 9(4): 733–46, vii.

Golbin JM. Portopulmonary hypertension. *Clin Chest Med*. 1 Mar. 2007; 28(1): 203–18, ix.

Layden TJ. Hepatic manifestation of pulmonary disease. *Clin Liver Dis*. 1 Nov. 2002; 6(4): 969–79, ix.

Pastor CM. Pancreatitis-associated acute lung injury: new insights. *Chest*. 1 Dec. 2003; 124(6): 2341–51.

Zhou MT. Acute lung injury and ARDS in acute pancreatitis: mechanisms and potential intervention. *World J Gastroenterol*. 7 May 2010; 16(17): 2094–9.

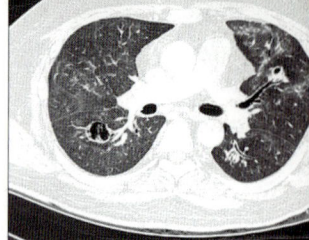

CHAPTER **59**   # Pulmonary Manifestations of Renal Disease

Pulmonary manifestations in renal disease may be related to renal disease per se or to the treatment of renal disease such as the use of peritoneal dialysis, haemodialysis or following a renal transplant. These pulmonary manifestations deserve serious consideration.

Pleural Effusion

This is probably the most frequent association with renal disease. The effusion is generally a transudate and several factors may contribute towards it. In the nephrotic syndrome, a pleural transudate, often bilateral is due to hypoalbuminaemia resulting in a lowered oncotic pressure. Both acute and chronic renal failure and end-stage renal disease may be associated with pleural transudates caused by congestive cardiac failure and/or hypervolaemia. Peritoneal dialysis is occasionally complicated by a large pleural effusion, the pleural fluid chemically resembling the peritoneal dialysate. In these cases structural defects in the diaphragm are responsible for allowing the peritoneal dialysate to enter the pleural spaces. If the effusion is large the peritoneal dialysis should be stopped. Pleural fluid may need to be tapped. The abdominal catheter should be left in place as it helps drainage of pleural fluid. Invariably peritoneal dialysis will need to be discontinued.

Pleural exudates may also be occasionally encountered. These are due to 'uraemic' pleural inflammation. The effusions are generally bilateral, haemorrhagic and are often associated with pleuritic pain and a pleural rub. 'Uraemic' effusions generally resolve spontaneously after some weeks. They may however result in pleural thickening with well-marked pleural fibrosis.

URAEMIC LUNG

An important respiratory association of uraemia is 'uraemic lung'—pulmonary oedema with or without pneumonitis. The pulmonary oedema is central; giving a typical 'bat-wing' appearance on a radiological examination of the chest. The periphery of the lung remains translucent. This appearance is not specific for a uraemic lung; it is also observed in chronic left ventricular failure which is a fairly frequent accompaniment of chronic renal disease and in early pulmonary oedema caused by hypervolaemia.

There are probably several factors responsible for the typical radiological picture of uraemic lung:

1. Possible fluid overload.
2. Increased pulmonary artery occlusion pressure, which may also be associated with an increased right atrial pressure.
3. Hypoproteinaemia, more often related to poor nutrition in end-stage renal disease rather than to loss of protein in the urine.
4. Impaired myocardial function.
5. Increased capillary permeability.

The last factor may indeed play a major pathogenic role if haemodynamic pressure studies show normal right and left atrial pressures. Pulmonary oedema fluid in some patients with uraemic lung has high protein content, and increased capillary permeability to technetium-labelled diethylene triamine pentaacetic acid (DTPA) has been demonstrated in these patients.

The alveoli to start with contain fibrinous oedema with swollen alveolar cells and oedematous interlobular septa. If the oedema persists, a fair degree of interstitial fibrosis results. The characteristic distribution of the 'bat wing' oedema is not well understood. It has been thought to result from diversion of blood flow to the more central parts of the lung due to peripheral vasoconstriction of the longer peripheral pulmonary vessels.

'Uraemic' lung is also observed in patients on haemodialysis, particularly in patients on chronic haemodialysis. Failure to comply with fluid restriction is an important cause in these patients. If this cause is excluded the uraemic lung is either related to persistent elevation of left atrial or left and right atrial pressure or due to increased capillary permeability.

Uraemic lung may be associated with uraemic pleurisy or with a haemorrhagic pleural exudate.

URINOMA

Ureteric rupture (from whatever cause) or a percutaneous nephrostomy may result in a retroperitoneal collection of urine which may track into the pleural space (urinothorax). Pleural fluid has an ammoniacal smell; the creatinine content is the same as in the urine and higher than in the blood.

PULMONARY INFECTIONS

Renal failure is associated with an increased risk of pulmonary infections. This is related to immune suppression from poor host defences in patients with chronic renal disease. Besides usual bacterial and viral infections, there is an increased prevalence of tuberculosis which has a 15 times higher incidence than in the general population.

PULMONARY COMPLICATIONS FOLLOWING RENAL TRANSPLANTATION

Pulmonary complications may occur in as many as 15–20% of kidney allograft recipients. They are classified as being non-

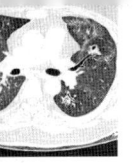

infectious or infectious in aetiology. The commonest non-infectious complication is pulmonary oedema due to allograft dysfunction, generally occurring within the first month after the transplant. An increased frequency of B-cell non-Hodgkin's lymphoma which may affect the lungs has been reported in transplant patients after prolonged immunosuppressive therapy. Finally, pulmonary thromboembolism is more frequent in the post-transplant period when compared to pre-transplant renal failure.

Infections are responsible for the large majority of pulmonary complications in the post-transplant period. Bacterial and cytomegalovirus infections are more frequent in the immediate post-transplant period. Opportunistic infections occur later—these include viral, nocardial, fungal infections and infection due to *Pneumocystis carinii*. The occurrence of pulmonary tuberculosis is several times greater than in the general population. It should be noted that renal dysfunction results in poor elimination of ethambutol and could thus add to its toxicity. Rifampicin when used in the treatment of tuberculosis may be the cause of renal dysfunction as it increases steroid catabolism and reduces the bioavailability of cyclosporin A.

Table 59.1:
Pulmonary associations of renal disease

Pulmonary Manifestations	Disease
Pleural Effusion (transudate)	Nephrotic syndrome Acute glomerulonephritis Acute renal failure Chronic renal failure (CRF) Peritoneal dialysis
Pulmonary Oedema	All of the above Haemodialysis
Pleural exudates	Uremic pleural inflammation
Uremic lung	CRF Long term haemodialysis
Respiratory infections, Tuberculosis	CRF Haemodialysis Peritoneal dialysis Renal transplant
Pulmonary alveolar haemorrhage	Pulmonary-renal syndrome
Malignancy	Renal Transplant
Pulmonary calcification	Haemodialysis Renal transplant CRF

PULMONARY HAEMORRHAGE COMPLICATING RENAL DISEASE

This is often termed the Pulmonary-Renal Syndrome and is characterized by alveolar haemorrhage and glomerulonephritis. Goodpasture's syndrome related to anti-glomerular basement membrane antibodies (anti-GBM disease) is one cause of the pulmonary-renal syndrome. The commonest causes however are systemic vasculitides associated with positive antineutrophilic cytoplasmic antibodies (ANCA-positive). These vasculitides include Wegener's granulomatosis, microscopic polyangiitis, and Churg-Strauss syndrome. Other rare systemic vasculitides (not associated with positive ANCA) have been reported to cause both pulmonary haemorrhage and glomerulonephritis (see accompanying table). Pulmonary-renal syndrome can also occur in vasculitis associated with connective tissue disorders such as SLE, mixed connective tissue disease, scleroderma and rarely in rheumatoid disease. Intra-alveolar bleeds have also been reported to occur in rapidly progressive glomerulonephritis and crescentric glomerulonephritis not associated with antibodies to glomerular basement membrane. Finally, drugs such as penicillamine/hydralazine have also been known to cause the pulmonary-renal syndrome.

A pulmonary-renal syndrome is suspected when there is a combination of haemoptysis due to alveolar haemorrhage and haematuria due to glomerulonephritis. The alveolar haemorrhage is confirmed radiologically by bilateral diffuse pulmonary shadows. Hypoxia, tachypnoea invariably result in patients with severe intra-alveolar haemorrhage. Haemoptysis is not always present, but bronchoscopy reveals haemorrhagic fluid which on microscopy shows macrophages laden with hemosiderin. The glomerulonephritis is confirmed on a urine examination and by a renal biopsy. In our part of the world fulminant leptospiral infection is an important cause of the pulmonary-renal syndrome.

Goodpasture's syndrome and the various ANCA-positive causes of the pulmonary-renal syndrome have been dealt with in a separate chapter.

Table 59.2:
Pulmonary-renal syndrome with alveolar haemorrhage

1. Goodpastures syndrome (positive for anti-GBM antibodies)

2. Rapidly progressive glomerulonephritis
   Cresentric glomerulonephritis
   (Both are negative for anti-GBM antibodies)

3. Connective Tissue Disorders
   Systemic lupus erythromatosis
   Mixed connective tissue disease
   Scleroderma
   Rheumatoid disease

4. Systemic vasculitides
   Wegener's granulomatosis
   Microscopic polyangiitis
   Churg-Strauss syndrome
   Cryoglobulinemia
   Henoch-Schönlein purpura
   Behçet's disease

5. Severe leptospiral infection

6. Drug induced
   Penicillamine

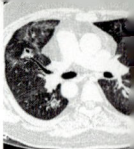

SUGGESTED READING

Bolton WK. Pulmonary renal syndrome and emergency therapy. *Contrib Nephrol*. 1 Jan. 2010; 165: 166–73.

Kotloff RM. Noninfectious pulmonary complications of liver, heart, and kidney transplantation. *Clin Chest Med*. 1 Dec. 2005; 26(4): 623–9, vii.

Papiris SA, Manali ED. Bench-to-bedside review: pulmonary-renal syndromes—an update for the intensivist. *Crit Care*. 2007; 11(3): 213.

Vandermarliere A. Mycobacterial infection after renal transplntation in a Western population. *Transpl Infect Dis*. 1 Mar. 2003; 5(1): 9–15.

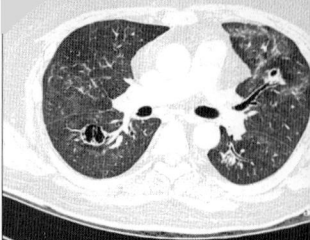
CHAPTER **60** **Pulmonary Manifestations of Inflammatory Bowel Disease**

Extraintestinal complications of ulcerative colitis and Crohn's disease have been known for several years. They include erythema nodosum, pyoderma granulosum, uveitis, sacroiliac arthritis, ankylosing spondylitis and hepatitis. To these can now be added a number of pulmonary complications that are being increasingly reported. Both ulcerative colitis and Crohn's disease are being met with increasing frequency in our country though their incidence is not high as in the West. Pulmonary complications are rare but it is important to be aware of their possible occurrence.

Pulmonary complications have been reported much more frequently with ulcerative colitis (85%) when compared to Crohn's disease. These complications in most cases (80%) follow the inflammatory bowel disease. Occasionally, they have been concomitant with the disease and in less than 10% of patients they may precede the bowel disease. Though pulmonary complications invariably produce overt manifestations, studies have shown the occurrence of sub-clinical abnormalities. These include a reduced forced expiratory volume in one second (FEV_1), small airways' obstruction and a reduced TLCO. A sub-clinical lymphocytic alveolitis similar to that in sarcoidosis has been observed in Crohn's disease. Perhaps more extensive studies on the lungs in inflammatory bowel disease may reveal the actual incidence of sub-clinical involvement and the natural history of this involvement.

Inflammatory Airway Disease

Inflammation of the airways is the commonest complication of inflammatory bowel disease. Inflammation may involve the glottis, epiglottis area, the large airways or the small airways. Rarely, the whole tracheobronchial tree is involved. Involvement of the upper airways produces cough, noisy breathing, stridor and may lead to asphyxia necessitating tracheostomy. Tracheo-bronchial involvement causes chronic cough which is dry or associated with mucopurulent sputum. Chronic inflammation of the airways can lead to bronchiectasis. Small airways may also be involved resulting in a diffuse inflammatory obstruction of the airways. Endoscopy reveals erythema and oedema of the mucosa. Biopsy shows granulation tissue with many neutrophils together with a lymphocytic and plasma cell infiltrate. When inflammation is marked it leads to tracheal or bronchial stenosis. The histology described above bears a resemblance to the histology of the bowel lesion in ulcerative colitis, suggesting that a common antigen target is shared by the gut and the lung.

Bronchiolitis and Organizing Pneumonia

These are rare associations which however cannot be ignored. Bronchiolitis causes increasing breathlessness, air-trapping, a fall in the FEV_1 and a poor response to corticosteroids. Organizing pneumonia presents with fever, cough, breathlessness, and a high ESR with radiological opacities. These shadows are multiple, peripherally placed and subpleural in location. The histology on biopsy is similar to organizing pneumonia observed in other conditions and the response to corticosteroids is excellent, though relapses do occur on withdrawal of steroids.

Interstitial Pneumonia (Fibrosing Alveolitis) and Vasculitis

Fibrosing alveolitis of the pattern of desquamative interstitial pneumonia is a rare but reported association of inflammatory bowel disease. The response to steroids is satisfactory. Withdrawal of sulphasalazine used in the treatment of inflammatory bowel disease is recommended as these drugs are known to cause interstitial pneumonia in some instances.

Vasculitic lesions have been reported in ulcerative colitis. These include necrobiotic nodules within the lung with a histology resembling pyoderma gangrenosum. Patients present with fever, chest pain, dyspnoea with multiple rounded

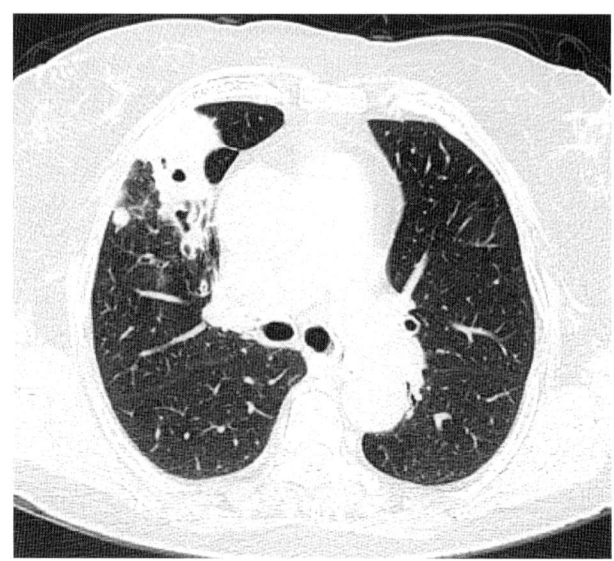

Fig 60.1: CT chest demonstrates an ill-defined consolidation with cavitation representing necrobiotic nodules in a patient with Crohn's disease.

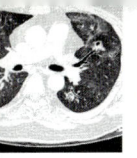

parenchymal opacities on imaging. The nodules may cavitate and then resolve, leaving a residual scar. Lung nodules may be associated with necrotic ulcerating nodules within the dermis.

Eosinophilic infiltration of the lungs observed in some patients is generally due to drugs used in the treatment of inflammatory bowel disease.

Pleuritis, Pericarditis

Western literature reports a serositis in as many as 30% of patients. The effusion is small, is an exudate and responds well to corticosteroids.

Thromboembolic Disease

The risk of thromboembolism is believed to be greater in patients with inflammatory bowel disease. It must be noted that sulphasalazine used in the treatment of inflammatory bowel disease can by itself produce various pulmonary complications. These include fibrosing alveolitis, organizing pneumonia, granulomatous lung disease and pulmonary eosinophilia. To separate the effects of the disease per se from complications caused by drugs used to treat the disease may at times be impossibly difficult.

Diagnosis and Management

An acute awareness that pulmonary symptoms in inflammatory bowel disease are often related to the latter is vital. Clinical examination and endoscopies with biopsies in patients with upper airways and tracheobronchial involvement will prove the inflammatory nature of the lesions. Imaging which should include CT chest reveals parenchymal lesions of ILD, organizing pneumonia and necrobiotic nodules. Transbronchial or CT-guided biopsies may further clinch the diagnosis.

Steroids form the mainstay of management. Airways inflammation is chiefly tackled by the use of inhaled steroids. Acute inflammation may necessitate a course of oral prednisolone therapy. Parenchymal lesions within the lung respond fairly well to oral corticosteroids.

Table 60.1: Pulmonary complications in inflammatory bowel disease

1. Inflammation of the airways
   a) Upper airways-glottis
   b) Tracheobronchitis
   c) Bronchial stenosis
   d) Bronchitis; purulent bronchitis
   e) Small airways

2. Bronchiolitis
3. Organizing pneumonia
4. Interstitial pneumonia (fibrosing alveolitis)
5. Necrobiotic nodules
6. Pulmonary eosinophilia (drug induced)
7. Thromboembolic disease

SUGGESTED READING

Black H. Thoracic manifestations of inflammatory bowel disease. *Chest.* 1 Feb. 2007; 131(2): 524–32.

Karadag F. Is it possible to detect ulcerative colitis-related respiratory syndrome early? *Respiratory.* 1 Dec. 2001; 6(4): 341–6.

Songür N. Pulmonary function tests and high-resolution CT in the detection of pulmonary involvement in inflammatory bowel diseases. *J Clin Gastroenterol.* 1 Oct. 2003; 37(4): 292–8.

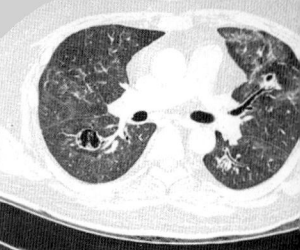

CHAPTER **61** Pulmonary Manifestations in Obstetric and Gynaecological Conditions

PHYSIOLOGICAL CHANGES IN THE RESPIRATORY SYSTEM IN PREGNANCY

Breathlessness is a frequent complaint in the first trimester. It is due to hyperventilation caused by an increased ventilatory drive due to the increased concentration of progesterone. An awareness of hyperventilation is translated into a feeling of breathlessness. A degree of hyperventilation persists throughout pregnancy so that $PaCO_2$ is low and the pH may be a little on the alkaline side. The PaO_2 is normal or may show a small rise.

In the last trimester of pregnancy breathlessness is related to the effects produced by the enlarging uterus which leads to increased intra-abdominal pressure and a significant rise in the diaphragm. There is no change in the vital capacity, there is a 25% reduction in the FRC chiefly related to a fall in the expiratory reserve volume. These changes may be observed by the sixth month of pregnancy. Expiratory flow rates are unaffected but chest wall and total pulmonary compliance are reduced in the third trimester. The TLCO increases slightly during the first and second trimester; it then returns to normal in spite of changes in haemoglobin concentration and in the circulatory volume.

Though the PaO_2 as mentioned above is generally normal or slightly raised, at full term, particularly when the uterus is very large, there could be mild hypoxia with an increased alveolar-arterial O_2 gradient. When the patient is supine, this is related to premature closure of the small airways related to the reduced FRC. Oxygen consumption is increased during pregnancy being 25–30% above the normal at full term. The combination of increased oxygen consumption and reduced FRC diminishes oxygen reserve so that any emergency or catastrophe that causes apnoea or alveolar hypoventilation can render both the mother and foetus dangerously hypoxic.

During labour there is further increase in tachypnoea and minute ventilation (due to increased muscular effort coupled with anxiety) so that there is increasing respiratory alkalosis. Alkalosis can reduce uterine blood flow because of vasoconstriction, thereby adversely affecting foetal oxygenation. This may be of importance if foetal blood flow is already jeopardized for other reasons.

In some patients, pain during and after delivery or after caesarean section may lead to rapid shallow breathing with resultant areas of atelectasis within the lungs, leading to some degree of hypoxia. This is particularly observed in obese older women. Physiotherapy and providing adequate pain relief during and after labour corrects this problem easily. Lung function changes during pregnancy start reverting to normal soon after delivery and reach baseline values within a few weeks.

DYSPNOEA DUE TO PATHOLOGICAL CONDITIONS ARISING DURING PREGNANCY, LABOUR OR THE POST-PARTUM PERIOD

Though breathlessness is a frequent complaint during normal pregnancy, dyspnoea is also an important symptom of an underlying pulmonary pathology. When acute and severe, it invariably points to the presence of a life-threatening emergency. The following pregnancy-related conditions should come to mind–pulmonary thromboembolism, pulmonary oedema due to preeclampsia or eclampsia, aspiration pneumonia, amniotic fluid embolism, pneumomediastinum, cardiomyopathy of pregnancy, ARDS related to eclampsia and drug-induced pulmonary oedema.

Progressively increasing dyspnoea could also be the early manifestation of sepsis unrelated to pregnancy or related to complicated labour, to impending liver cell failure in a pregnancy-related hepatic pathology, or to the co-incidence of an acute respiratory infection such as pneumonia occurring around this period.

A few pregnancy-specific problems causing pulmonary complications will now be considered.

PULMONARY THROMBOEMBOLIC DISEASE

Venous thromboembolic disease in our experience is the most frequent respiratory emergency related to pregnancy and the post-partum period. The incidence is four to five times greater in the post-partum period (particularly in early post-partum) than in pregnancy. Deep vein thrombosis involving the lower limbs results from a hypercoagulable state of the blood related to pregnancy, a hormone-related venous stasis in the lower limbs combined with pressure effect of the enlarged uterus on the inferior vena cava.

Clinical Diagnosis

Though the clinical features are the same as in non-pregnant women, it is amazing how often this diagnosis is missed in clinical practice. This is probably because the symptoms of breathlessness, vague unease, and chest discomfort are often

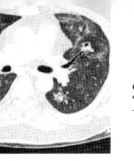

associated or confused with anxiety symptoms, which may also be present. Even the slightest suspicion of this potentially fatal condition necessitates investigation. A venous Doppler may occasionally give false positive results because of venous obstruction due to an enlarged uterus. A Doppler ultrasound may be more revealing. A d-dimer test is useful, as a negative test is a point against thromboembolic disease. If there is no immediate life-threatening emergency and if facilities are available, a lung perfusion scan with < 50 mrad exposure to the foetus may help. In an emergency and for definite specific evidence, a CT pulmonary angiography should be done with less foetal exposure. Notwithstanding the danger of teratogenicity to the foetus, (an increased incidence of childhood leukaemia has been reported with as low a radiation exposure as 2–5 rad) a definite diagnosis of pulmonary embolism is a must because of the hazard to the mother's life if correct treatment is not instituted, as also because of the potential hazard of unnecessary treatment of pulmonary embolism if pulmonary embolism is not present.

Treatment

Warfarin should not be used, as it can cause embryopathy and central nervous changes during the second or third trimester. Low-molecular heparin does not cross the placental barrier, is effective and does not need monitoring in relation to clotting parameters.

In patients who are haemodynamically very unstable or in shock, streptokinase or urokinase or tissue plasminogen activator should never be withheld. There should be no hesitation to use an inferior vena cava filter. Placement may be difficult because of possible dislodgment due to the dilated vena cava and increased pressure within the venous system during labour.

Women who have had thromboembolism before or those with known hypercoaguable states should receive heparin prophylaxis during pregnancy.

PULMONARY OEDEMA IN PREECLAMPSIA

Preeclampsia is characterized by hypertension, oedema, albuminuria, hypoalbuminaemia, together with some degree of liver cell and renal dysfunction. Pulmonary oedema is uncommon in preeclampsia because patients with preeclampsia are more often than not volume-depleted. More than one factor is generally responsible when pulmonary oedema does occur. More often than not, well-marked hypertension during or even before pregnancy, is present. Systolic cum diastolic myocardial dysfunction is an important cause of pulmonary oedema. When oedema occurs in the immediate post-partum period it is often precipitated by over-vigorous intravenous infusion of fluids during labour. A background of diastolic myocardial dysfunction caused by hypertension worsens matters. Hypoalbuminaemia when present is another contributory cause. Increased capillary permeability is another factor that has been incriminated, particularly in the presence of associated sepsis and multiple blood transfusions.

Clinical Features

Tachypnoea, respiratory distress, hypoxia, crackles over the bases and the radiological features of pulmonary oedema are present. Tachypnoea with a slight fall in oxygen saturation are early signs that are of ominous significance.

Treatment

Treatment consists of fluid restriction, use of oxygen, use of diuretics and in severe cases the initiation of ventilatory support. Inotropic support needs to be given in the presence of poor cardiac function. Vasopressor support is rarely necessary, diuretic therapy needs to be given cautiously, for if the patient becomes hypovolaemic it could worsen renal function, reduce cardiac output and jeopardize placental perfusion. We have generally managed patients with a central venous catheter monitoring central venous pressure, without using a pulmonary artery catheter. Ultimately, urgent delivery of the foetus as soon as is feasible is probably the best treatment of both preeclampsia and eclampsia.

AMNIOTIC FLUID EMBOLISM

Amniotic fluid embolism is a rare disastrous obstetric emergency which is very often fatal. In our experience we have witnessed it about once every eight to ten years. Western figures give the incidence between 1 in 8,000 to 1 in 80,000 live births with a mortality of 10–80%. This complication in the West is believed to account for 10% of all maternal deaths.

Amniotic fluid embolism occurs classically during labour and delivery. Rarely, it occurs in the early post-partum period. Amniotic fluid contains cell debris, cells, and humoral factors. When perhaps purely by chance this fluid gains entry into the venous circulation through enlarged uterine venous sinuses or through small or large uterine tears, disaster strikes. The cellular debris together with the amniotic fluid and its contents result in two major disturbances. The first is obstruction together with severe vasoconstriction of the pulmonary vasculature leading to sudden severe pulmonary hypertension. The other is an anaphylactic reaction caused by sensitivity to the amniotic fluid debris and to the humoral factors within the fluid.

Clinical Features

Clinical features are characterized by sudden severe dyspnoea, progressive profound hypoxemia coupled with cardiovascular collapse. Hypotension, tachycardia, an imperceptible pulse and increasing metabolic acidosis occur; seizures may supervene. In severe cases death occurs within minutes or a few hours from cardiac arrest, allowing very little time for resuscitative efforts. In fact when amniotic fluid embolism occurs at or immediately after caesarean section, cardiovascular collapse and arrest occur very often on the table.

Not all cases are as severe. The ones we have witnessed and who have recovered had sudden onset breathlessness, hypoxia, hypotension, tachycardia and developed within six to eight hours the clinical features of ARDS. Coagulation abnormalities in the form of a raised prothrombin time and partial thromboplastin time were observed.

Differential Diagnosis

Myocardial infarction, left ventricular failure, pulmonary thromboembolism, and tension pneumothorax can all simulate

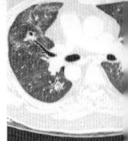

amniotic fluid embolism. ARDS from aspiration or sepsis needs to be considered in the differential diagnosis in the presence of pulmonary oedema.

Management

Urgent cardiorespiratory resuscitation is important for survival. Central venous pressures as also filling pressure of the left heart need to be measured and monitored for optimum fluid therapy. Inotropes and vasopressors are both necessary. Immediate intubation and ventilatory support with a high fraction of inspired oxygen (FIO_2) are mandatory. The occurrence of ARDS will need optimal ventilatory support for several days. Coagulation abnormalities if present should be appropriately corrected.

PERIPARTUM CARDIOMYOPATHY

Peripartum cardiomyopathy is an important cause of dyspnoea before, during or after delivery. Cardiac failure in the absence of pre-existing cardiac disease is either due to hypertension of pregnancy or cardiomyopathy.

It is important to exclude pre-existing causes of cardiac disease (e.g. valvular heart disease, ischaemic cardiomyopathy) before making a diagnosis of peripartum cardiomyopathy. Besides tachycardia and dyspnoea, orthopnoea, dry cough, epigastric discomfort and vomiting are important symptoms. The heart is enlarged on clinical examination. A diastolic third heart sound at the apex, a systolic murmur of functional mitral incompetence (due to a dilated mitral annulus) and an accentuated pulmonary second sound are often audible. Basal crackles are invariably present. The jugular venous pressure is elevated and the liver though difficult to feel may be palpable and tender. Oedema over the feet may or may not be present.

2-D echocardiography shows the presence of a dilated cardiomyopthy with an ejection fraction which may be as low as 15–20%. A radiographic examination of the chest shows an enlarged heart with pulmonary congestion or even pulmonary oedema.

During labour and immediately after, the exertion and the increased demand on the heart often triggers severe left ventricular failure with pulmonary oedema. Pulmonary thromboembolic complications are frequent.

Management

Diuretics, and reducing the after-load on the heart are both important. However angiotension-converting enzyme inhibitors should not be used during pregnancy as these drugs cause foetal renal dysfunction. Aldactone, the judicious use of carvedilol, and digoxin are recommended in appropriate doses. Patients with severe pump dysfuction should be tided over with inotropic support using both dopamine and dobutamine. Low molecular weight heparin should be used in all patients.

Over 50% of patients gradually improve with regard to cardiac function over six months after delivery. A significant proportion, however, remains unchanged or may even worsen. Even in those who improve, future pregnancy is fraught with danger as cardiomyopathy may recur as the pregnancy progresses. Cardiac transplantation may be offered to patients with severe persistent cardiomyopathy.

DRUG-INDUCED PULMONARY OEDEMA (TOCOLYTIC PULMONARY OEDEMA)

β agonists in particular terbutaline are often used to reduce uterine contractions in premature labour. In pregnancy, a rather unique complication of β agonist therapy is pulmonary oedema. The frequency of this complication varies in reported studies between 1–9%. It is postulated that terbutaline used over a prolonged period causes both myocardial dysfunction and increased capillary permeability. Intravenous infusion of large quantities of fluid and reduced oncotic pressure due to hypoalbuminaemia aggravate the oedema. Corticosteroids often administered to these patients also worsen the problem.

Clinical Features and Diagnosis

Sudden onset of dyspnoea in the setting described above points to pulmonary oedema. Tachypnoea, basal crackles, a fall in oxygen saturation and the radiological presence of shadows consistent with pulmonary oedema confirm the diagnosis.

Treatment

The β agonist is promptly stopped following which pulmonary oedema resolves. Diuretics need to be given; over-diuresis is dangerous as this may reduce placental flow with further danger to the foetus. With gross pulmonary oedema, mechanical ventilation support is given. This is however rarely necessary if the condition is promptly recognized.

TROPHOBLASTIC DISEASE IN PREGNANCY

A benign hydatiform mole can rarely lead to trophoblastic embolism, particularly during evacuation of the mole in the last trimester of pregnancy. Pulmonary hypertension and pulmonary oedema indistinguishable from ARDS result. Choriocarcinoma may be associated with a hydatiform mole and can lead to pulmonary or mediastinal metastasis and/or to malignant pleural effusion.

There are four other conditions in obstetrics and gynaecology practice which can lead to pulmonary complications. These are the ovarian hyperstimulation syndrome, Meig's syndrome and catamenial pneumothorax with or without thoracic endometriosis. Meig's syndrome has been described in the section on 'Diseases of the Pleura'.

OVARIAN HYPERSTIMULATION SYNDROME

The increasing practice of *in-vitro* pregnancy has led to awareness of the increasing frequency of this syndrome. It is caused by the artificial induction of ovulation, being observed in about 1% of these cases. The syndrome evolves following the use of follicle stimulating hormone and human menopausal gonadotropin together with pituitary suppression with leuprolide acetate. It is characterized by massive ovarian enlargement (often felt as abdominal masses), and by increased capillary permeability leading to volume depletion, massive oedema, ascites and pleural transudates. Pulmonary oedema similar to that observed in ARDS occurs. Oliguria, renal and liver dysfunction may be present. Breathlessness, crackles over both lungs, hypoxia and

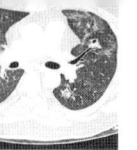

hypotension are frequent. In severe cases, death occurs from hypotension or multiple organ failure.

Management consists of paracentesis of ascites and pleural fluid, volume repletion with crystalloids and colloids, use of oxygen and ventilator support if there is marked pulmonary oedema. When ovarian enlargement is very large, drainage of the ovarian cyst helps. Diuretics are useful and hypotension may need to be corrected by inotropes and vasopressors. Once diuresis starts recovery generally ensues. The pathogenesis of this syndrome is unclear but is believed to be caused by high plasma rennin-like activity and increased capillary permeability mediated by vasoactive substances of ovarian origin releasing cytokines such as TNF, interleukin (IL)-6 and endothelial growth factor.

CATAMENIAL PNEUMOTHORAX

This is rare and is suspected if pneumothorax occurs within 48 hours of menstruation. Recurrence of pneumothorax occurring with the menstrual cycle is well-nigh diagnostic. Catamenial pneumothorax generally occurs in women over 30 years, is most often right-sided but may occur on the left side as well. The mechanism of catamenial pneumothorax has been described in the chapter on 'Pneumothorax' in the section on 'Diseases of the Pleura'. A contraceptive pill to suppress ovulation is the treatment of choice for catamenial pneumothorax, but if this is contraindicated or if pregnancy is desired, surgical advice is sought. At thoracotomy, diaphragmatic defects or pores may be identified and repaired; areas of pleural and diaphragmatic endometriosis if present can be surgically removed.

ARDS IN PREGNANCY

A number of pregnancy-specific or pregnancy-associated problems render a pregnant woman at risk. The most important of pregnancy-specific diseases causing ARDS in our part of the world is *eclampsia*. ARDS may also occur in preeclamptic states. The term eclampsia is applied to grand mal seizures in a patient with preeclampsia in whom the seizures could not be attributed to any other cause. Seizures are not necessarily related to the degree of hypertension but to microangioopathic changes in cerebral vessels. ARDS, disseminated intravascular coagulopathy and multi-organ failure result in severe disease and have a high mortality.

ARDS also results from amniotic fluid embolism, from the rare occurrence of trophoblastic embolism and from the administration of multiple transfusions to counter severe post-partum haemorrhage. In our part of the world, the commonest cause of ARDS with multiple organ failure in pregnancy is fulminant sepsis following septic abortion or following sepsis after full-term delivery. Aspiration of gastric contents particularly during labour is an important cause of aspiration pneumonia, followed by ARDS. Pregnancy predisposes to aspiration because of lowered tone of the oesophageal sphincter, increased abdominal pressure and the supine position during delivery.

Clinical Features and Diagnosis

The clinical history and diagnostic features are the same as in non-pregnant patients; these have been discussed in an earlier section.

Management

Management is no different when compared to non-pregnant patients. When administering drugs it is important to consider effects not only on the mother but also on the foetus. Alkalosis during ventilator support should be avoided as alkalosis reduces placental flow. Delivery of the foetus in our experience helps the mother and perhaps even the child. This is particularly so in patients with eclampsia.

SUGGESTED READING

Bandi VD. Acute lung injury and acute respiratory distress syndrome in pregnancy. *Crit Care Clin.* 1 Oct. 2004; 20(4): 577–607.

Moore J. Amniotic fluid embolism. *Crit Care Med.* 1 Oct. 2005 33(10 Suppl): S279–85.

Pereira A. Pulmonary complications of pregnancy. *Clin Chest Med.* 1 Jun. 2004; 25(2): 299–310.

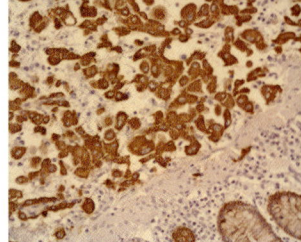

CHAPTER **62** **Pleural Effusions, Empyema**

GENERAL CONSIDERATIONS

The pleura is a thin double-layered membranous structure lining the inner thoracic surface as also the whole lung. It is lined by mesothelial cells which secrete a surfactant that enables the pleural surfaces to glide smoothly over each other during respiration. The parietal pleura is connected to the chest wall by a thin endothoracic fascia which fixes the pleura to the chest and provides it blood supply.

In healthy individuals the pleural space contains 10–30 ml of pleural fluid. This is a plasma ultrafiltrate across the pleural surface formed at the rate of 0.3 to 0.5 ml/kg/day with a protein content of 0.9 to 1.2 g/dl. There is an equivalent daily clearance of this fluid by lymphatics draining the visceral and parietal pleura, chiefly the latter.

The pleural space which is approximately 10–20 microns in width and lined by a single layer of mesothelial cells comprises a surface area of approximately 2000 cm^2 in a 70-kg man.

Functions of the pleura: The pleurae are absent in some mammalian species raising the question of what their exact function is in humans. They serve as a 'coupling organ' between the lungs and the chest wall. Their lubricant action allows for smooth movement of the lungs in the thoracic cage. Also, they may serve as a convenient 'drip pan' in patients who develop pulmonary oedema.

EPIDEMIOLOGY

It is estimated that close to 30% of diseases affecting the respiratory system involve the pleura. This involvement invariably takes the form of a pleural effusion. It has also been estimated that 30–40% of all pleural effusions are due to systemic diseases such as heart failure, liver and renal disease in which the pleura per se is uninvolved and normal. There are indeed numerous causes of pleural effusion (see accompanying table). The relative frequency of these causes will depend on the geographic areas and the population under study. In India, Pakistan, South East Asia, China and developing countries such as Africa the most important causes are congestive heart failure, pneumonia, tuberculosis and malignancy. Western countries would include viral infection in this list though viral infections are difficult to prove. Tuberculous pleural effusions do occur in the West but not with the same frequency.

In the US about 1 million pleural effusions occur a year. There is no such available data from India, so a look at the incidence of effusions in the West is informative. In order of decreasing frequency these would be as follows.

Type	Incidence
CCF	500,000
Parapneumonic	300,000
Neoplastic	200,000
PE	150,000
Viral	100,000
Cirrhosis/GI	100,000
CABG	50,000
TB	2500
Mesothelioma	2300

Table 62.1:
Causes of pleural effusion in the US, according to a study

Source: Richard W, Light MD. Pleural Effusion. *NEJM*. 2002; 346: 1971–77.

A glaring difference from India is that tuberculosis would be, by far, the commonest cause of a pleural effusion in this country.

PATHOPHYSIOLOGY

Pleural effusion can occur under two situations:

1. When there is an increase in the hydrostatic filtration pressure and/or a decrease in the plasma oncotic pressure. This leads to the formation of a transudate.
2. When the pleura is involved in a pathological process which increases capillary permeability leading to the formation of a pleural exudate.

Pleural pathology may be primary but is more often secondary to pulmonary disease. It could arise from a pathology within the mediastinum (e.g. oesophageal perforation) or from a subdiaphragmatic pathology (e.g. a liver abscess). Pleural effusion could also occur from abnormal communication or blockage of the thoracic duct and its main draining channels (chylothorax), or from communication transdiaphragmatically with peritoneal fluid, or from communication with the pancreas or the kidney (urinothorax).

CLINICAL FEATURES

The main clinical symptom is dyspnoea; at times cough is an important symptom. The degree of dyspnoea depends not just

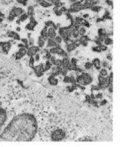

on the size of the effusion but the speed at which the pleural space is filled. Therefore a very slow accumulation of even a litre of fluid may not be subjectively noted by the patient unless the clinical presentation is determined by the underlying cause of the pleural effusion such as pneumonia or cardiac failure. Dyspnoea is generally perceived when half the hemothorax is filled with fluid. It occurs with smaller effusions when they are bilateral.

There needs to be at least 300 ml of fluid in the pleural space before it is detected on clinical examination. With a small to moderate pleural effusion, the important physical findings are a stony dull note over the fluid on percussion, diminished breath sounds and diminished vocal fremitus. Decreased chest movements over the lower chest on the affected side may afford a valuable clue.

With larger effusions, there may be bulging of the intercostal spaces with marked diminution of chest movements on the affected side, a shift of the apex beat and the trachea to the opposite side, stony dullness over the fluid with absent breath sounds and diminished vocal fremitus.

Large unilateral pleural effusions or moderate-sized pleural effusions if bilateral will cause tachypnoea and hypoxic respiratory failure. Massive unilateral pleural effusions produce a severe mediastinal shift to the opposite side. There is a reduced return of venous blood flow into the heart due to raised intrapleural pressure leading to a low cardiac output, hypotension, alveolar hypoventilation with increasing hypoxic plus hypercapnic respiratory failure.

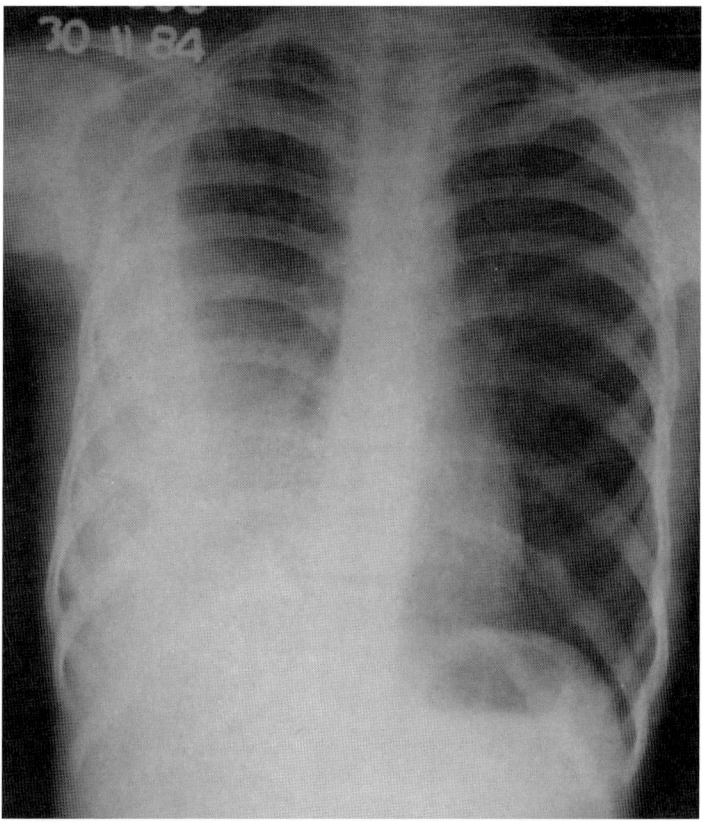

Fig 62.1: Pleural Effusion. Chest x-ray reveals a well-defined homogenous opacity in the right hemithorax.

DIAGNOSTIC APPROACH

1. Clinical Evaluation The first step in the evaluation of a patient with pleural effusion is a detailed history and a complete physical examination. This is because the cause of a pleural effusion may well lie outside the thorax; also, examination of the pleural fluid does not necessarily point to a specific cause. In fact even imaging findings or pleural biopsy may be non-contributory unless viewed in an overall perspective with the history and clinical findings.

2. Imaging A radiographic examination (postero-anterior view) of the chest shows a fairly dense shadow on the side of the effusion; the upper border may be slightly concave rising upwards towards the axilla. Large effusions push the heart and trachea to the opposite side. Very small effusions show a blunting of the costophrenic angle. The same effect can also be produced by pleural fibrosis and pleural adhesions in that area. Walled-off effusions over the anterior or lateral pleural surfaces are easily evident, but loculated effusions behind the heart or along the mediastinum as also subpulmonic effusions are difficult to diagnose.

Ultrasonography can detect even small pleural effusions; it has a sensitivity of nearly 100%. It is an invaluable mode to detect pleural effusion in critically ill patients in the intensive care units where basal shadows within the lung may be due to various factors—atelectasis, consolidation, fluid, or may result from a combination of one or more of the above factors. Ultrasound also distinguishes fluid from pleural thickening and is useful to demonstrate loculations and septa within the pleural fluid.

High-resolution computed tomography (HRCT) of the chest with pleural phase contrast enchancement provides better detection of pleuro-pulmonary pathologies. It may reveal, for example, an underlying pneumonia, a lung abscess, tuberculosis, mediastinal disease or a subdiaphragmatic pathology that may be responsible for a pleural effusion.

Pleural Fluid Examination

A diagnostic thoracocentesis with an examination of the pleural fluid is a must in the investigation of a pleural effusion where the diagnosis is even in the slightest doubt. A thoracocentesis is generally safe. Complications include a vasovagal syncope, bleeding due to injury to a vessel, and pneumothorax. Removal of large quantities of pleural fluid can cause re-expansion pulmonary oedema. The procedure should be promptly stopped if the patient complains of chest pain or develops cough.

APPEARANCE OF THE PLEURAL FLUID

Pleural fluid can be straw-coloured, turbid, blood-tinged or frankly haemorrhagic. Frank pus drawn from the pleural space points to an empyema. Milky fluid suggests a chylothorax or pseudochylothorax. Food particles in the fluid point to an oesophageal perforation. An ammonical smell suggests a urinothorax.

DISTINGUISHING A PLEURAL TRANSUDATE FROM AN EXUDATE

After noting the appearance of the pleural fluid, the next step is to determine whether it is a transudate or exudate. A transudate

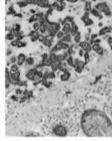

points to systemic disease, the three most important and common being congestive heart failure, cirrhosis of the liver and the nephrotic syndrome. Patients with severe hypoalbuminaemia from any cause, those on peritoneal dialysis, patients with myxoedema or with superior vena caval obstruction may also develop pleural transudates. The focus then is on the treatment of these systemic diseases.

If the pleural fluid is an exudate it could arise from diseases within the thorax or from sub-diaphragmatic causes or from other systemic causes. The diagnostic focus is to determine which of these several possible causes has produced a pleural pathology.

Pleural exudates are defined by Light's criteria, and have one or more of the following features:

(i)   The total protein in the pleural fluid divided by the total serum protein is > 0.5;
(ii) The lactate dehydrogenase (LDH) of the pleural fluid divided by the serum LDH is > 0.6;
(iii) The LDH of the pleural fluid is greater than two-thirds of the upper limit of the normal LDH in blood.

Pleural transudates have none of the above features. In addition pleural exudates have high cell counts.

Light's criteria have stood the test of time and remain the most robust biochemical criteria for distinguishing a transudate from an exudate. They retain a high sensitivity of 98%, specificity of 83% and overall accuracy of 95% in achieving this crucial distinction. The only occasional drawback of Light's criteria is that they sometimes falsely label a transudate an exudate, especially in patients with congestive cardiac failure (CCF) who are on diuretics. This important clinical pitfall of Light's criteria was elegantly demonstrated by Chako et al. (Chest 1989) where thoracocentesis was performed before and after six days of diuretics in patients with CCF. The diuresis resulted in significant increase in protein and LDH so that 30% of all transudates were now falsely classified as 'exudates'. This occurs because diuresis causes water to leave the pleural space faster than protein and LDH. The longer the patient is on diuresis, the more likely that this will occur. Combining Light's criteria with this knowledge of when 'transudate by aetiology' turns 'exudate by biochemistry' render these criteria well-nigh perfect. Light's criteria maximize sensitivity over specificity. It is better to occasionally misdiagnose a transudate as an exudate than vice versa.

A number of newer criteria have been looked at to see if these have greater sensitivity and specificity when it comes to differentiating a transudate from an exudate. These include the following 'Post-Light' criteria:

1. Pleural cholesterol > 60 mg/dl
2. Pleural fluid to serum albumin gradient of < 1.2 g/dl
3. Pleural bilirubin ÷ serum bilirubin > 0.6
4. Pleural to serum cholinesterase ratio > 0.6

None of these have been shown to have any great superiority over Light's criteria and are clearly more complex to perform.

DIFFERENTIAL LEUCOCYTE COUNT
A neutrophilic or predominantly neutrophilic exudate is seen in a parapneumonic effusion, in an empyema, or soon after pulmonary infarction. A lymphocytic exudate is often due to tuberculosis, malignancy and in other systemic disorders like connective tissue diseases. Tuberculous pleural effusions, particularly in the early part of their natural history, may show a predominance of polymorphs. An increase in the eosinophil count (> 10% of cells) is observed following a hemothorax, longstanding tuberculous effusions, drug-induced pleural disease, Churg-Strauss syndrome and eosinophilic pneumonia.

pH AND BLOOD GLUCOSE
A low pH and a lowered blood glucose (< 60 mg/dl) are found chiefly with empyema, malignancy, rheumatoid disease and other connective tissue diseases involving the lung or pleura. pH values below 7.2 in the presence of a normal pH in the blood are due to H^+ ion accumulation and increased anaerobic metabolism of bacteria, leucocytes or tumour cells. In malignant pleural effusions, a lowered pH is said to relate to more extensive pleural involvement, a greater chance of a positive cytology, a lowered success rate for pleurodesis and a poorer prognosis.

SPECIFIC TESTS
These depend on the disease causing pleural effusion and are detailed later under specific diseases. They include (among many others) relevant tests for an infective aetiology (bacterial, viral, fungal, tubercular), cytology for suspected malignancy, cytogenic studies to characterize chromosomal markers of suspected haematolymphoid and mesenchymal malignancies, and flow cytometry for the rare involvement of the pleura in lymphoma.

PLEURAL BIOPSY
If in spite of the above tests, the diagnosis of a pleural effusion is in doubt a pleural biopsy becomes necessary. The histological examination of the pleura together with other tests on the pleural tissue may help in a difficult diagnosis. A pleural biopsy can be done as a blind procedure using Abrams needle or a CT or ultrasound-guided biopsy, or done under direct vision through a thoracoscope or following a thoracotomy. With the advent of video-assisted thoracoscopy, thoracotomy as a diagnostic procedure is rarely necessary. Percutaneous blind biopsies using Abrams needle have a fair yield in the diagnosis of diseases causing a diffuse involvement of the pleura. CT-guided or ultrasound-guided biopsies are particularly useful to target focal lesions within the pleura (e.g. malignancy) revealed through imaging studies. The biopsy of choice however in most undiagnosed pleural disease is a video-assisted thoracoscopic biopsy. This is because a thoracoscopy is a simple procedure in expert hands, performed most often under local anaesthesia. It has few complications even when carried out on critically ill

Table 62.2: Light's criteria to distinguish exudates from transudates
A pleural fluid is an exudate if any of these criteria are met—
1. Protein in pleural fluid to protein in the serum ratio > 0.5
2. Pleural fluid LDH to serum LDH ratio > 0.6
3. Pleural fluid LDH more than two-thirds of the upper limit of normal LDH in serum.

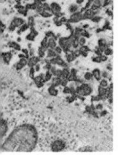

Table 62.3: Differential leucocyte counts in relation to the aetiology of pleural exudates	
Pleural Diseases	**Remarks**
Polymorphonuclear leucocytosis	
Complicated parapneumonic effusion; empyema	In chronic empyema there may be a significant lymphocytosis
Pleural fluid Lymphocytosis (≥ 80%)	
Tuberculosis	Lymphocytes predominate (85–95% of lymphocytes). In early exudative phase polymorphs may constitute 1/3 to 1/2 of the leukocyte count
Malignancies	In over 50% of cases, but generally < 80% lymphocytes
Rheumatoid disease	–
Lymphoma	95–100% lymphocytes
Chylothorax	Fluid has milky appearance
Sarcoidosis	A very rare cause of pleural effusion, > 90% lymphocytes
Pleural fluid Eosinophilia (>10%)	
Pneumothorax	Commonest cause when a pneumothorax is associated with an effusion—due to blood
Haemothorax	Occurs some days after the event
Previous thoracocentesis	Related to bleeding caused by needle trauma
Parasitic disease	Generally seen
Pulmonary embolism	Haemorrhagic fluid
Lymphoma	Rare occurrence in Hodgkin's disease
Drug-induced	–
Churg-Strauss Syndrome	Eosinophilia in blood and in pleural exudate
Tuberculosis	Rarely seen in old tuberculous effusions

Table 62.4: Diseases often associated with low pH (<7.3) and low glucose (≤ 60 mg/dl) in the pleural exudate
Empyema, complicated parapneumonic effusion
Malignant effusion
Tuberculosis
SLE involving the pleura
Rheumatoid disease involving the pleura
Chylothorax

patients. It gives a full visualization of the entire pleural surface allowing multiple biopsies from appropriate sites. Diagnosis of malignancy involving the pleura can be made with well-nigh 100% accuracy. It has one added advantage—drainage of pleural fluid and (if indicated) pleurodesis can be performed in the same procedure.

Tissue obtained through a biopsy should be submitted for histopathological examination, appropriately stained to detect infections, and should also be cultured, particularly when there is suspicion of tuberculosis.

SPECIFIC DISEASES ASSOCIATED WITH PLEURAL EFFUSION

Conditions Associated with Pleural Transudates

Congestive cardiac failure is the commonest and most frequent cause of pleural transudates all over the world. The effusion is generally bilateral; if unilateral it occurs more frequently in the right than in the left pleural space. Left ventricular failure causes a rise in the endcapillary pressure. There is increased filtration of a transudate into the interstitial tissue of the lung which then seeps through the visceral pleura into the pleural space. Though pleural transudates are more common in congestive heart failure, they are also observed frequently in isolated left heart failure.

The diagnosis rests on the clinical features of left heart failure or CCF, the frequent presence of an enlarged heart with clinical and radiological evidence of pulmonary congestion. Transudative pleural effusions also occur in veno-occlusive disease and in constrictive pericarditis.

Management consists in the treatment of congestive heart failure. Pleurodesis may be of help in some patients with persistent pleural effusion.

It is to be remembered that a patient with congestive heart failure could also have an exudative pleural effusion due to a separate pathology. If the pleural effusion does not clear with successful treatment of congestive heart failure or if the effusion is large (or particularly if large and unilateral) a pleural fluid examination with other relevant tests are necessary.

Occasionally, as discussed earlier, the pleural transudate in congestive heart failure may be mistaken as an exudate. This happens when the patient is on diuretic therapy; a preferential drainage of fluid over protein molecules may lead to an increased protein content in the pleural fluid. A plasma-to-effusion protein gradient of > 3 g/dl suggests that the fluid to start with was a transudate.

HEPATIC DISEASE

Pleural effusions due to hepatic disease are due to two causes.

a) Transdiaphragmatic migration of ascitic fluid;
b) a lowered oncotic pressure associated with hypoalbunemia. Most pleural transudates due to hepatic disease are right-sided because of the frequency of 'pores' in the right dome of the diaphragm which allow ascitic fluid to seep into the right pleural space. Ascites is generally present but is not an absolute prerequisite. Large diaphragmatic defects can lead to large pleural effusions, the significance of which is missed, particularly if there is little or no ascites.

Management is directed towards the treatment of hepatic disease—the use of diuretics, low-sodium diet and treatment of portal hypertension. Symptomatic relief may be often necessary through repeated paracentesis. Pleurodesis may also

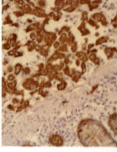

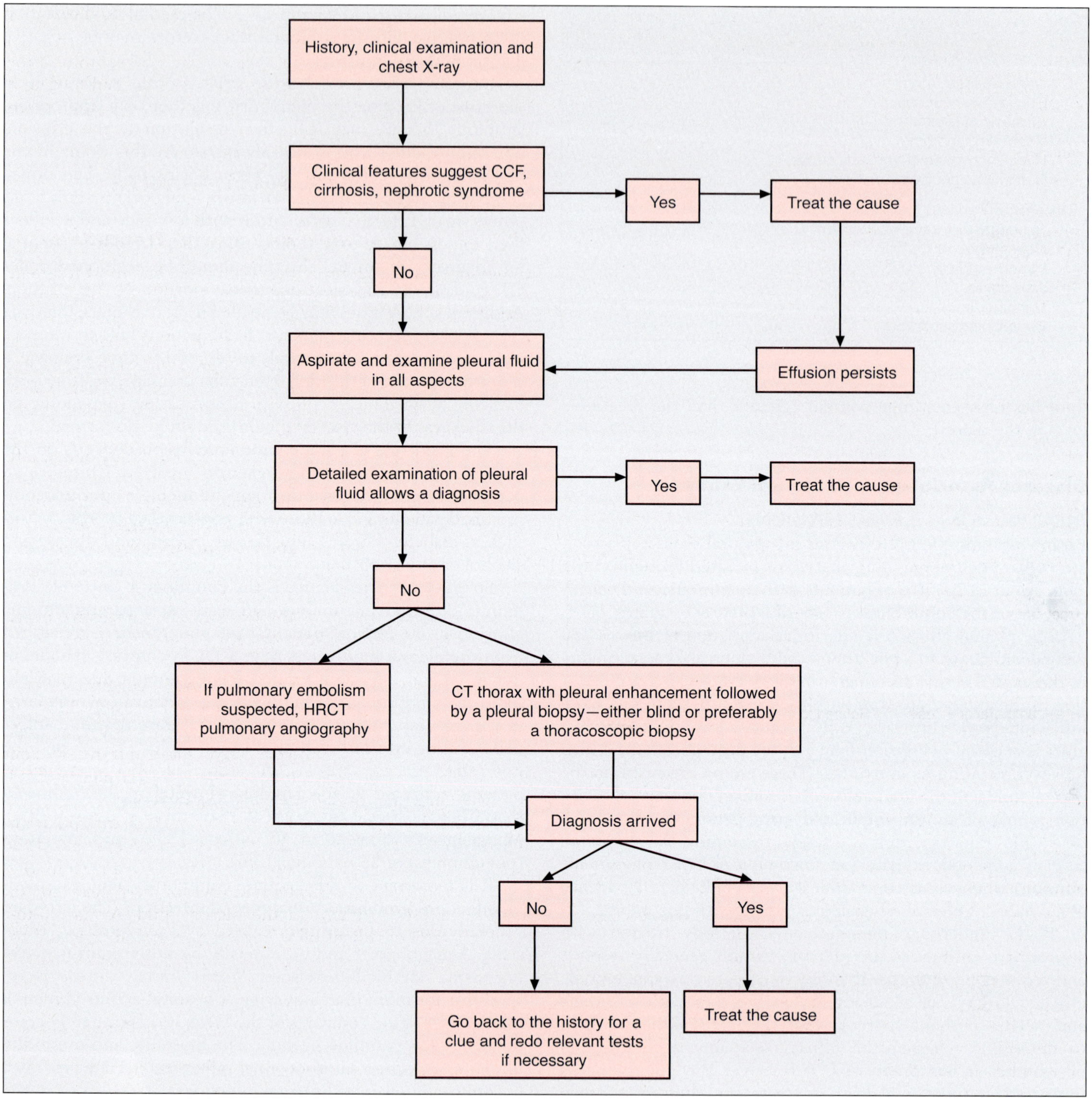

```
                ┌─────────────────────────────┐
                │ History, clinical examination│
                │       and chest X-ray        │
                └─────────────────────────────┘
                              │
                              ▼
        ┌─────────────────────────────┐        ┌───────┐      ┌──────────────┐
        │ Clinical features suggest CCF,│─────▶│  Yes  │────▶│ Treat the cause│
        │ cirrhosis, nephrotic syndrome │       └───────┘      └──────────────┘
        └─────────────────────────────┘                              │
                    │                                                 │
                 ┌─────┐                                              │
                 │ No  │                                              │
                 └─────┘                                              │
                    │                                                 ▼
                    ▼                                        ┌──────────────┐
        ┌─────────────────────────────┐                    │Effusion persists│
        │ Aspirate and examine pleural │◀───────────────────└──────────────┘
        │   fluid in all aspects       │
        └─────────────────────────────┘
                    │
                    ▼
        ┌─────────────────────────────┐        ┌───────┐      ┌──────────────┐
        │ Detailed examination of pleural│────▶│  Yes  │────▶│ Treat the cause│
        │   fluid allows a diagnosis   │       └───────┘      └──────────────┘
        └─────────────────────────────┘
                    │
                 ┌─────┐
                 │ No  │
                 └─────┘
                ╱        ╲
               ╱          ╲
   ┌──────────────────┐   ┌─────────────────────────────┐
   │ If pulmonary      │   │ CT thorax with pleural       │
   │ embolism suspected,│   │ enhancement followed by a   │
   │ HRCT pulmonary    │   │ pleural biopsy—either blind  │
   │ angiography       │   │ or preferably a thoracoscopic│
   └──────────────────┘   │ biopsy                       │
          │               └─────────────────────────────┘
          │                          │
          │                          ▼
          │               ┌──────────────────┐
          └──────────────▶│ Diagnosis arrived │
                          └──────────────────┘
                              ╱        ╲
                          ┌─────┐    ┌─────┐
                          │ No  │    │ Yes │
                          └─────┘    └─────┘
                             │          │
                             ▼          ▼
              ┌──────────────────────┐  ┌──────────────┐
              │ Go back to the history│  │Treat the cause│
              │ for a clue and redo   │  └──────────────┘
              │ relevant tests if     │
              │ necessary             │
              └──────────────────────┘
```

Fig 62.2: Diagnostic flowchart for a pleural effusion.

be tried. Transjugular hepatic porto-venous shunting (TIPS) when indicated for relief of portal hypertension has been noted to reduce the hydrothorax. A liver transplant when indicated is followed by disappearance of the hydrothorax.

RENAL DISEASES

Hydrothorax is typically observed in the nephrotic syndrome, due to hypoalbunaemia causing a lowered oncotic pressure. It can also occur in glomerulonephritis and in patients on peri-

toneal dialysis. Dialysis fluid generally seeps through communications (pores) in the right dome of the diaphragm into the right pleural space. Examination of the pleural fluid resembles dialysis fluid.

A urinothorax is a rare occurrence when there is renal obstruction with consequent retroperitoneal urine collection, which then seeps into the ipsilateral pleural space. The pleural fluid has an ammonical smell. A urinothroax should always be suspected when a pleural transudate has a low pH. The pleural

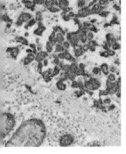

Table 62.5:
Causes of pleural transudate

Common Causes
  Congestive heart failure
  Cirrhosis of liver
  Nephrotic syndrome
  Hypoalbuminaemia from any cause
  Continuous peritoneal dialysis

Uncommon causes
  Superior vena caval obstruction
  Constrictive pericarditis
  Hypothyroidism
  Atelectasis
  Urinothorax
  Budd-Chiari syndrome

fluid has high creatinine content (greater than the creatinine level in the blood).

Diseases Associated with Pleural Exudates

PARAPNEUMONIC PLEURAL EFFUSIONS

Parapneumonic pleural effusions are pleural exudates associated with pneumonia, lung abscess or infected bronchiectasis. They occur in 20–50% of patients with pneumonia, and constitute one of the commonest causes of a pleural exudate.

The pleural effusion is due to inflammation of the visceral pleura contiguous to a pneumonic patch. Increased permeability of the pleural vessels secondary to inflammation leads to formation of the exudate. To start with the fluid appears serous, has a low white blood corpuscle (WBC) count, a low LDH, a normal glucose content, pH greater than 7.3; the protein content is high however, pointing to an exudate. There are no organisms in the pleural fluid and the fluid culture is negative. The above description is that of an 'uncomplicated' parapneumonic effusion. A diagnostic thoracocentesis is essential to confirm the sterile nature of a pleural exudate (an uncomplicated parapneumonic effusion) whenever there is clinical and/or radiological evidence of a significant pleural effusion in a patient with pneumonia.

If the underlying pneumonia is correctly treated with appropriate antibiotics the pleural effusion generally resolves and requires no drainage. If an uncomplicated parapneumonic effusion is large or recurs, a therapeutic tap with a syringe and needle perhaps hastens resolution. This will also help to determine whether the effusion remains uncomplicated or whether it has progressed. If however the pneumonia is untreated or there is a delay in treatment, there is a strong chance of the development of an infected pleural effusion, also called a complicated parapneumonic effusion. A point to note is that pleural infection with microorganisms can occur in spite of adequate therapy in patients with severe pneumonia, particularly in the presence of co-morbid factors. Recent genetic studies suggest that a variant of the protein tyrosine phosphatase (PTPN 22 Trp 620) is associated with increased susceptibility to invasive pneumococcal disease and empyema.

The exudate in a complicated parapneumonic effusion is often turbid; it will show a significant polymorphonuclear leucocytosis, generally over 100/mm^3, at times over 1000/mm^3. Besides a high protein content, the pleural fluid has a glucose < 60 mg/dl, a raised LDH, pH < 7.2. The pleural fluid culture is often positive. However, pleural fluid culture may be negative if antibiotics are in use.

Repeated paracentesis with strict aseptic precaution in the hope of keeping the pleura dry, together with appropriate antibiotic therapy may still effect resolution of the effusion, but unfortunately this is not always so. At this point in the natural history of the disease, fibrin begins to be laid down, compartmentalizing the effusion into several pockets, some large, others small. Effective paracentesis with a syringe and needle is then impossible. A tube thoracotomy then becomes essential for adequate treatment. The tube should be positioned under CT guidance in the most dependent portion of the effusion. Additional chest tubes may be needed if there is more than one large pocket requiring drainage. If the patient fails to improve or if the loculated effusion fails to respond to tube drainage, a thoracoscopically performed open-tube drainage, together with breaking of fibrinous loculi with decortication (depending on the thickness of the visceral pleura) should be performed.

The incidence of parapneumonic effusion depends on the case-mix of a study and the organisms involved. Complicated parapneumonic effusions are more frequent in immunocompromised patients and in those with associated co-morbid factors such as diabetes, chronic lung disease, rheumatoid disease and alcohol or other substance abuse.

Streptococcus pneumoniae is the commonest cause of community-acquired pneumonia and leads to a parapneumonic effusion in 30–50% of patients. Yet pneumococci are grown from the pleural fluid is less than 10%. In contrast, parapneumonic pleural infections related to pneumonia due to Klebsiella or Pseudomonas or Staphylococci often show organisms in the pleural fluid on culture. Other gram-negative infections causing infected pleural effusions include *E. coli* and the Enterobacteriaceae species. A study of 263 consecutive patients admitted to the Hinduja Hospital in 2005 showed that tuberculosis was the cause of 75 of these effusions (29%). Malignancies followed in 46 patients (17%) and infections (pneumonias) in 33 patients (13%).

It is important to differentiate community-acquired pleural infections from nosocomial pleural infections. The latter are generally due to pneumonia caused by Pseudomonas, Klebsiella, Acinetobacter and occasionally by other gram-negative organisms. Methicillin-resistant *Staphylococcus aureus* is responsible for more than a quarter of hospital-acquired pleural infections in some countries of the West; it is fortunately comparatively less common in India. The mortality and morbidity of pleural infection in nosocomial infections is far worse than in community-acquired pleural infections.

EMPYEMA

Empyema is a suppurative pleural effusion leading to pus within the pleural space. When the pus is localised within the pleura it forms an intrapleural abscess. Empyema can occur at any age but is most frequent in the middle-aged and elderly. Though the commonest cause of an empyema is an underlying bacterial pneumonia, other important causes need to be kept in mind. A lung abscess or infected bronchiectasis may occasionally cause an empyema. Tuberculosis involving the lung may lead not just to a tuberculous pleural effusion but also a tuberculous

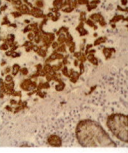

Table 62.6: Causes of pleural exudate

1. Infections
    Tuberculosis
    Other infections
        Bacterial
        Viral
        Nocardial
        Fungal
        Parasitic

2. Malignancies
    Pleural metastasis
    Lymphoma
    Pleural mesothelioma

3. Vascular
    Pulmonary embolism
    Vasculitides

4. GI diseases
    Pancreatitis
    Pancreatic pseudocyst
    Perforation of the oesophagus
    Intra-hepatic or subphrenic abscess

5. Inflammatory (non-infectious)
    Asbestosis
    Radiation
    Uremic
    Post-thoracotomy
    Post-transplant

6. Connective tissue diseases
7. Iatrogenic, traumatic (including haemothorax)

8. Miscellaneous
    Lymphangioleiomyomatosis
    Meig's syndrome
    Yellow nail syndrome
    Chylothorax

Table 62.7: Causes of empyema

1) Pulmonary Infection
    a) Bacterial pneumonia
    b) Tuberculous infection
    c) Pneumonia due to other microorganisms (including fungi)
    d) Lung abscess, infected bronchiectasis
    e) Infection distal to an obstructed bronchus—bronchogenic carcinoma, foreign body

2) Postoperative complication of cardiothoracic surgery
3) Penetrating or blunt trauma to the chest
4) Oesophageal perforation
5) Sub-diaphragmatic abscess
6) Hepatic abscess—pyogenic or amoebic
7) Primary pleural involvement—bacteremic or pyemic state

empyema. An empyema can also result from infection distal to a bronchus obstructed by a foreign body or by a bronchogenic carcinoma. It can occur as a postoperative complication of cardiothoracic surgery, following penetrating or blunt trauma or an oesophageal tear. A subdiaphragmatic abscess may involve the pleura either directly or via the lymphatics. A liver abscess, in particular an amoebic liver abscess can rupture into the pleura, or into the lung (from where infection spreads into the pleura) or into the lung and pleura. The empyema that then follows is not bacterial in origin but is due to *Entamoeba histolytica*. Primary direct pleural infection causing empyema must indeed be very rare. It may occur in bacteremic or pyaemic states. Even here, the possibility of a small subpleural abscess rupturing into the pleura rather than a direct pleural infection remains a possibility.

Predisposing Factors

Co-morbid states associated with empyema have been mentioned under 'Parapneumonic effusions'. In Western studies, alcoholism is the most important risk factor and is present in 20–40% of cases in some studies. In our part of the world, diabetes, immunocompromised states (in particular AIDS), neurological disorders favouring aspiration and underlying chronic lung disease are the important predisposing factors.

Bacteriology

Gram-positive cocci, in particular *Streptococcus pneumoniae*, other streptococcal species, *Haemophilus influenzae*, staphylococci and anaerobic infections from aspiration pneumonia are the important community-acquired causes of pneumonia that can lead to empyema. Empyema due to Legionella infection is rare in our experience; perhaps it is being missed. Empyemas due to nosocomial pneumonias are chiefly due to Pseudomonas, Klebsiella, Acinetobacter, Enterobacteria. Nosocomial staphylococcal infection is rare compared to its incidence in Western countries.

In a study of 60 consecutive cases in one of our units in Mumbai, over five years from 2001–06, the three commonest aetiologies of empyema based on pleural culture were; *S. pneumoniae, S. aureus* and *M. tuberculosis*.

Natural History and Pathogenesis

The natural history of empyema complicating pneumonia is a sequence of events or stages. The first stage is the formation of a sterile pleural exudate with few leucocytes. This stage graduates within a few days into an intermediate stage of infective pleurisy characterized by increased quantities of turbid pleural fluid, marked leucocytosis with many bacteria, a characteristic biochemical profile of the pleural fluid (described under complicated parapneumonic effusion), and by the formation of fibrous septa that loculate the pleural fluid into several compartments. The final stage is the presence of frank pus which is generally loculated. The whole collection within the pleura may be walled off from the rest of the pleural space forming thereby an intrapleural abscess with several loculations. Different locations in which an empyema may be encysted within the pleural space are illustrated in the accompanying figure.

If death has not occurred from pleuropulmonary infection the empyema becomes chronic. Fibrous tissue is laid down in peels, at times encircling the lung in a tight vice (fibrothorax)

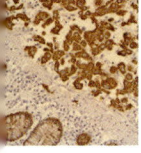

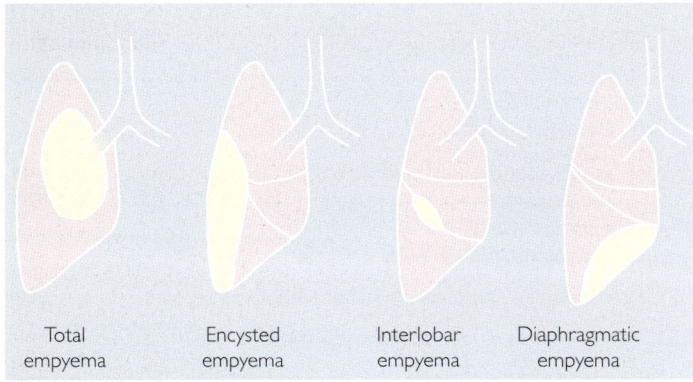

| Total empyema | Encysted empyema | Interlobar empyema | Diaphragmatic empyema |

Fig 62.3: Different locations of an empyema.

rendering it well-nigh functionless. A walled-off empyema, particularly situated anterolaterally within the thorax may point outwards causing an empyema necessitatis. A bulge is observed over the chest; there is an impulse over the bulge on coughing, and the bulge may be seen to pulsate. An 'empyema necessitatis' may open outside leading to a purulent discharge.

Clinical Features

An acutely evolving empyema is characterized by fever with chills, tachycardia, and tachypnoea if the pleural effusion is large or if an underlying pneumonia still persists. There is a well-marked leucocytosis. If undetected and not appropriately drained, all the features of increasing sepsis with progressive multiorgan dysfunction will appear. Hypotension and septic shock are of ominous significance. Pneumonia is an important cause of the acute respiratory distress syndrome (ARDS). An empyema in a patient with ARDS may be impossible to detect clinically or on a routine X-ray of the chest. A CT of the chest can however detect loculated fluid in ARDS; CT chest is indicated when a patient with ARDS fares poorly or when a patient with pneumonia fails to respond to therapy.

Not uncommonly, an empyema presents in a subacute or chronic form. In the subacute form the patient apparently recovers from a lower respiratory tract infection but continues to run a low-grade evening fever. Some degree of leucocytosis is present. At times the patient is afebrile for a few days or even weeks and then again runs low-grade or high fever. The relation of this fever to a recent lower respiratory tract infection may be missed. If the empyema is posteriorly placed, signs of fluid are apparent. If it is tucked away anteriorly and laterally physical signs are difficult to elicit. The empyema is however apparent on imaging—both on a PA and lateral X-ray and always on a CT chest.

A patient with chronic empyema generally presents with pyrexia of unknown origin (PUO). Leucocytosis and a raised C-reactive protein are generally present but not always so. In fact the WBC count may be normal in about 20% and some patients with chronic empyema may be afebrile (silent empyema). At times there are periods of low-grade fever followed by afebrile periods, the clinical pattern closely mimicking a Pel Ebstein type of pyrexia. There may be no physical signs in the chest; even an X-ray chest may be reported as normal if the empyema

is tucked away in the paravertebral space behind the heart. A CT of the chest is essential in all patients with a PUO if a loculated walled-off empyema tucked away in the chest is not to be missed.

In summary, an empyema should be suspected under the following conditions:

1. Pneumonia unresponsive to treatment or unexplained fever after the patient has received adequate treatment with resolution of the pneumonia.
2. Persistent leucocytosis and raised erythrocyte sedimentation rate (ESR) after pneumonia.
3. In a patient with PUO.
4. In an ill patient who has had cardiothoracic surgery, oesophageal surgery or any other procedure (such as a thoracocentesis) where an empyema is a possible complication.
5. In the presence of a foul malodorous at times feculent sputum suggestive of a bronchopleural fistula.
6. Imaging findings that strongly suggest an empyema.

A routine chest X-ray may show a convex border to the fluid in the pleural space, pointing to 'walled-off' fluid rather than the typical concave crescent of free fluid within the pleural cavity.

CT chest reveals thickened parietal and visceral pleura, multiloculated effusion with multiple fibrin strands within the walled-off pleural fluid. These features distinguish an empyema from an exudative pleural effusion. Multiloculation occurs in more than 80% of empyemas. It is a fairly sensitive criterion but not very specific, because it is observed with equal frequency in untreated and improperly treated tuberculous pleural effusions. There may be an air-fluid level within the empyema if there is a bronchopleural fistula, or if the empyema is caused by anaerobic organisms, or if air has been inadvertently introduced during paracentesis.

An empyema with an air-fluid level may closely resemble a lung abscess on imaging studies. The differentiation is critical from the point of view of management. The following imaging features on a contrast CT of the chest may help in the differential diagnosis.

An empyema often has the following features:

1. Thickened visceral and parietal pleurae separated ('dissected') by the fluid.
2. Compression of the adjacent lung.
3. Formation of a blunt angle with the chest wall.
4. No vessel markings within the opacity.

A peripherally situated lung abscess often has the following features:

1. A rounded opacity.
2. Absence of compression of adjacent lung.
3. Walls not smooth (as with an empyema) but often irregular and thickened (except in some patients with a staphylococcal lung abscess).
4. Presence of vasculature around the abscess—if present this is sure proof of a suppurative lung abscess, rather than an empyema.
5. A sharp angle with the chest wall.

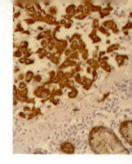

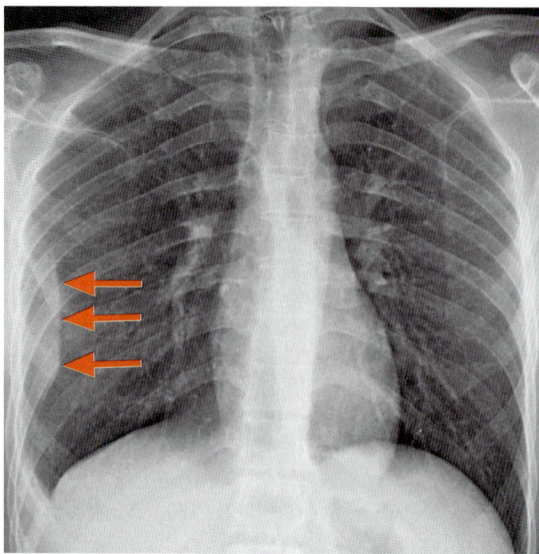

Fig 62.4: Empyema. X-Ray chest reveals a well-defined homogenous opacity along the right chest wall representing an empyema.

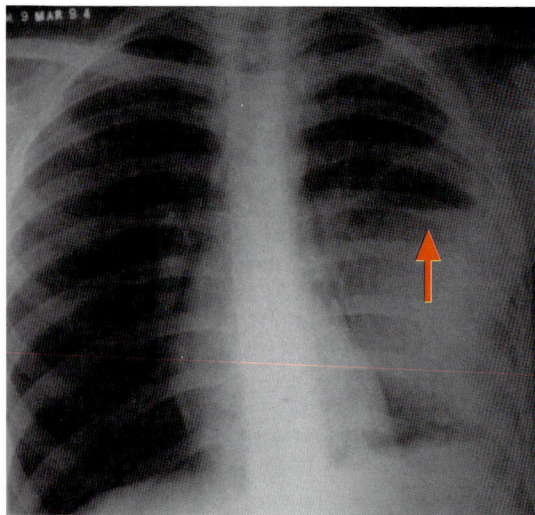

Fig 62.5: Empyema. X-ray chest demonstrates a homogenous opacity in the left hemi-thorax with an air-fluid level. The differential diagnosis for this would be between an empyema and lung abscess. The lesion is not spherical, the diameters are unequal, as well as the angles the lesion makes with the chest wall are obtuse (arrows) indicating an empyema.

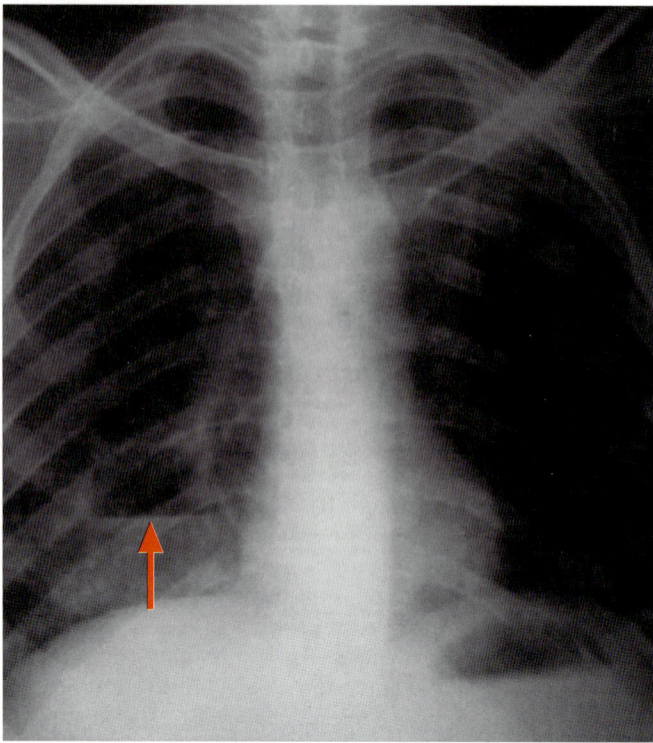

Fig 62.6: Lung abscess. Chest X-ray demonstrates a well-defined round opacity in the right paracardiac region with an air-fluid level. The diameters of this lesion are equal, as well as angles are acute indicating a lung abscess.

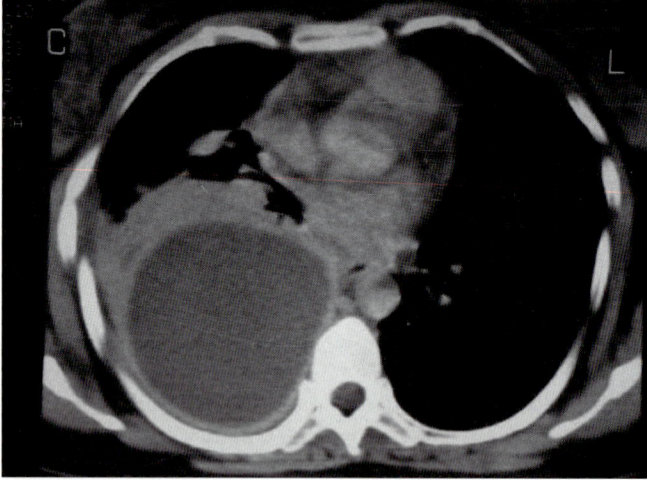

Fig 62.7: Empyema. CT chest demonstrates a well-defined and thick walled rounded opacity in the right pleural cavity with hypodense contents within it indicating an empyema.

Pleural Fluid Examination

A suspicion of empyema necessitates a prompt thoracocentesis. The presence of pus in the pleural aspirate confirms empyema. A foul odour points to a likely anaerobic infection. When an empyema is loculated it is extremely important to sample more than one location because the thoracocentesis may occasionally reveal clear fluid in one loculus and frank pus in a neighbouring loculus. This is because the fibrinous partition may prevent bacteria crossing from one Loculus A to the neighbouring Loculus B, so that the latter will have no or few pus cells, even though Loculus A will have multiplying bacteria, and numerous pus cells. The actively metabolizing bacteria in Loculus A will cause a sharp fall in the glucose content of the fluid and CO_2 produced by active metabolism will cause a sharp fall in the pH of the fluid. Though bacteria may not penetrate into Loculus B, glucose and CO_2 may do so. Thus fluid in Loculus B may be sterile yet have a lowered glucose content and a lowered pH.

Light's criteria give the characteristics of the pleural fluid in an uncomplicated parapneumonic effusion and in both a

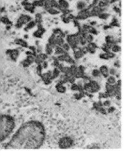

complicated parapneumonic effusion and a frank empyema, helping to distinguish one from the other. Complicated parapneumonic effusion and empyema are characterized by a low pH (7.1) a low glucose (<40 mg/dl), a raised LDH (>1000 IU/L) and an elevated WBC count. The presence of an elevated amylase in a pleural exudate points either to the possibility of a pancreatic aetiology to the fluid or an oesophageal perforation.

Light's criteria have important clinical significance in the management of bacterial pleural exudates. Uncomplicated parapneumonic pleural effusions almost always resolve spontaneously; complicated parapneumonic effusions and empyema require drainage.

Cultures are invariably positive in untreated patients with empyema but may be negative in those who have received antibiotics. While gram-positive cultures predominate in empyema due to community-acquired pneumonias, gram-negative cultures are far more frequent in empyemas consequent to nosocomial pneumonia. Gram-negative cultures are increasingly observed in elderly patients or in immunocompromised patients with empyema complicating community-acquired pneumonia. Anaerobic organisms are rarely encountered except in empyema following aspiration pneumonia or consequent to a lung abscess. Multiple infections have been reported in the Western literature but are uncommon in our experience.

When an empyema in an untreated patient is negative for bacterial infection the possibility of a tuberculosis infection should be kept in mind. Cultures for acid-fast bacilli should always be done.

Sputum cultures and cultures of BAL fluid may be of help in identifying organisms responsible for an empyema. Occasionally, in a tuberculous empyema, BAL cultures are positive for acid-fast bacilli even though the empyema fluid is sterile.

Bronchoscopy is useful in the following conditions:

1. To determine obstruction to a bronchus by a foreign body or a tumour. A bronchogenic carcinoma is an important underlying cause of an empyema. In our country an aspirated betel nut or 'supari'(of which the patient has no recollection) is also an important cause of a necrotizing pneumonia with an empyema.
2. To perform a microbiological study on the BAL fluid in a pneumonic consolidation complicated by an empyema.
3. To determine the presence, exact location of a bronchopleural fistula or an oesophageotracheobronchial fistula.
4. To aspirate bronchial secretions in those with excessive secretions or in those who are unable to cough up secretions.

Management

The principles of management are:

1. Use of appropriate antibiotic therapy.
2. Efficient drainage of the pleural cavity.
3. Use of fibrinolytic agents.
4. Surgery under certain select circumstances.

Antibiotic Therapy In severely ill septic patients, the sooner antibiotics are given the better. Empiric antibiotic therapy should preferably be started after the pleural fluid is sent for microbiological examination and culture but should never await the result of a laboratory report. Antibiotics used in critically ill patients should cover gram-positive infections, gram-negative infections and also anaerobes if there is reason to suspect anaerobic infection. A protocol followed in our unit is the use of a combination of amoxycillin and piperacillin-tazobactum in the appropriate dosage. If anaerobes are suspected, clindamycin or metronidazole is added. The regime is altered if necessary after culture sensitivity reports are available.

Instillation of antibiotics into the pleural space is not recommended for two reasons—the risk of introducing fresh infection, and because when the pleura is inflamed many studies have shown concentrations of antibiotics well above the minimal inhibitory concentration in the empyema fluid.

DRAINAGE

Tube drainage of purulent fluid is imperative for cure. Four questions need to be answered with regard to drainage of an empyema.

1. *When should one drain?*
2. *How should one drain?*
3. *Where should one drain?*
4. *How long should one drain?*

When should one drain? a) Drainage is always indicated when there is localized frank pus in the pleural cavity; b) in an acutely forming empyema when the patient is septic and when fluid is large in quantity, >1.5 L, or when fluid rapidly refills after more than one or two paracentesis; c) when there is a bronchopleural fistula (air-fluid level in the pleural space); d) following an assessment of pleural fluid examination by Light's criteria. Drainage should be done early. In the words of Stephen Sahn and Richard Light in 1989; 'The sun should never set on a parapneumonic effusion—because time is of the essence.'

How should one drain? Drainage should be through a fair-sized drainage tube of 20-Fr size. Though a good-sized drainage tube inserted through the appropriate intercostal space suffices in the formative maturing stage of an empyema (as in a complicated parapneumonic effusion), thick pus is best drained (particularly in a chronic empyema) by an appropriate rib resection followed by insertion of a large drainage tube.

Where should one drain? The drain is inserted at the most dependent portion of the empyema. Imaging studies (CT scan) can easily identify the most dependent portion. In poor countries or in areas where CT scan facilities are not available, PA and lateral X-ray of the chest helps. A few drops of an iodine dye injected into the pleural space will sink to the bottom of the empyema and thus helps localize the site of tube insertion.

How long should one drain? Drainage is continued till the empyema cavity closes and there is next to no fluid drainage. The lung as it expands approaches the chest wall so that the tube is well-nigh pushed out into the dressing. This may take weeks or a few months.

USE OF FIBRINOLYTIC AGENTS

The principle of evacuating infected pleural fluid was established 2000 years ago. The formation of multiple fibrinous septae in

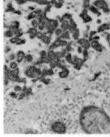

an empyema is thought to contribute to chest drain failure. Intrapleural thrombolytics have been investigated as potential agents to increase fluid drainage thereby potentially decreasing mortality and the need for surgery. Breaking down loculations to allow complete evacuation of pleural pus is traditionally considered the key to successful treatment. Fibrinolytics have gained popularity and are regarded as part of standard treatment. Successful intrapleural fibrinolysis can reduce the need for surgery and benefit patients in countries with limited surgical facilities and patients too sick for surgery.

The value of fibrinolytic agents has been shown in a few prospective trials. Even so, there are a number of units which avoid their use. Instillation of streptokinase or urokinase is indicated in the presence of thick pus or the presence of many loculations; 200,000 to 250,000 IU streptokinase or 30,000 to 100,000 IU of urokinase is instilled into the pleural space daily for five to six days. Occasionally, the instillation may be continued for longer—10–12 days. Some units use large-volume irrigation of the empyema cavity through a large drainage tube with the option of instillation of a fibrinolytic drug as well.

Fibrinolytic therapy with or without irrigation of the empyema cavity is not always successful. Failure of therapy is manifested by persistence of the empyema, persistence of loculations within the empyema cavity as judged by ultrasound or CT imaging and by persisting clinical features. Failure ratios vary from 15% (in those experienced in the use of fibrinolytics) to 30%.

Fibrinolytic therapy is contraindicated in patients with bronchopleural fistula (liquefied pleural secretions may then flood the lungs), in patients allergic to streptokinase, in septic patients with a deranged coagulation profile (for fear of excessive bleeding) and in patients with coagulation disorders.

EVIDENCE FOR AND AGAINST FIBRINOLYTIC THERAPY

Many case reports, several small series and four small randomized trials have confirmed the important impact fibrinolytics have in empyema. However, the results of the landmark Multicenter Intrapleural Streptokinase Study (MIST 1) published in 2005 *(Ref: First Multicenter Intrapleural Sepsis Trial (MIST1), by Maskell et al. Intrapleural streptokinase for pleural infection. N Engl J Med 2005; 352:865–74.),* failed to show significant benefit following the use of streptokinase in empyema. This study, by far the largest in the field, enrolled 454 patients with empyema, with 226 randomly assigned to streptokinase (SK) and the rest to placebo. The dose of intrapleural SK was 250,000 units twice a day for three days. The primary end points assessed were mortality and need for surgery while secondary end points were duration of hospital stay, lung function and radiographic clearing. Rather surprisingly, the MIST 1 trial concluded that SK offered no therapeutic benefits over placebo in terms of need for surgical intervention, mortality or length of hospital stay. Possible explanations for the negative results of the MIST 1 study are that an older population of patients was enrolled and sonography or CT was not used to define loculations. Perhaps more sophisticated thrombolytics like urokinase or human recombinant deoxyribonuclease might yield better results. The final verdict is thus not yet out on the role of intrapleural fibrinolytics.

SURGICAL TREATMENT

Indications for surgery are: Failure of medical treatment and failure of tube drainage to close the empyema cavity. Failure is generally due to incorrect drainage (too small a tube for proper drainage or tube inserted at the wrong site), multiple loculations within the empyema cavity, a persistent underlying cause for the empyema—for example a bronchogenic carcinoma, a foreign body such as a 'supari' aspirated within the bronchus, a persistent bronchopleural fistula or due to an oesophageotracheobronchial fistula. A chronic empyema cavity may persist and remain unclosed if there is thick fibrous tissue over the visceral pleura that prevents the lung from expanding.

Surgery may take several forms.

1. Rib resection with insertion of large-bore drainage tube at the appropriate site has already been mentioned.
2. A video-assisted thoracoscopic approach that breaks loculations within the empyema so that proper drainage now becomes possible through a large tube thereby promoting healing.
3. A thoracoscopic approach which not only breaks loculations but allows decortication of the lung surface followed by drainage through a large-bore tube. A rib resection to allow insertion of the large-sized drainage tube is invariably necessary.
4. An open thoracotomy for a full decortication of the lung, breaking down loculi within the empyema, a pleural toilet, followed by adequate drainage through a tube.

To conclude, 2400 years ago, in Hippocratic times the mortality from an empyema was 100%. To quote Hippocrates; 'If an empyema does not rupture, death will occur'. Today, in the modern antibiotic era, the mortality is closer to 15% but this is still a high rate for an infection. In the years to come, early diagnosis and appropriate treatment can bring down mortality further.

UNCOMMON PLEURAL INFECTIONS

Fungal infections are rare causes of pleural exudates. Invasive aspergillosis (due to *Aspergillus fumigatus*) may invade the pleural cavity causing pleural effusion. Pulmonary aspergillosis occurs under specific clinical settings—immunocompromised patients, HIV infections, longstanding bronchopleural fistulas, and chronic empyemas treated repeatedly with broad-spectrum antibiotics. The typical hyphae of *Aspergillus fumigatus* can be seen on smear and grown on culture. Amphotericin B is used systemically and can be used for local antifungal irrigation. Voriconazole is safer than and probably as effective as amphotericin B.

Histoplasmosis, coccidiomycosis infections of the lung causing pleural effusions occur against an epidemiological setting where these diseases are endemic, as for example in the American continent. Fungal pleural effusions resemble tuberculous pleural effusions in relation to fluid examination. Primary pleural infection or secondary infection related to a parenchymal lung pathology are both possible. Routine fungal cultures confirm diagnosis. Specific therapy includes azole therapy or amphotericin B.

Pleural effusions due to *Cryptoccoccus neoformans* are rare and occur only in immunocompromised patients, in particular AIDS. The disease may be localized to the lungs and pleura or be disseminated.

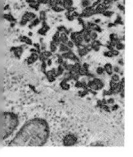

Rarely, *Actinomyces israeli* causes a pleural effusion. The diagnosis is suspected when there are multiple sinuses leading from the pleural cavity discharging on to the skin. The organism can be detected in the granules present in the discharge and can be cultured as well. Penicillin is the drug of choice.

Atypical mycobacterial infection of the lung is increasingly encountered in our country but pleural effusions are rare and if present are small collections. *Growth of atypical mycobacteria from pleural fluid should always arouse suspicion of contamination.*

Nocardial (*Nocardia asteroids*) pleural effusions result from a spread of nocardial parenchymal lung disease which may present as nodules or as small or large abscesses. These occur in immune-deficient states and in immunocompromised patients. One also encounters this infection in patients with longstanding chronic airways obstruction who have received corticosteroids and broad-spectrum antibiotics. Cotrimoxazole, doxycycline, rifampicin are effective drugs. Pleural effusions if they occur are always small in size.

Viral infections due to influenza virus, cytomegalovirus, coxsackie virus, adenovirus and other viruses can produce small acute pleural effusions. They remain unidentified because of difficulties in diagnosis. Perhaps quite a few small pleural effusions of undetermined aetiology are due to viruses, or due to *Chlamydiae pneumoniae*, and *Coxiella burnetii*. Diagnostic proof that this is indeed so in our part of the world is however lacking.

Parasitic pleural involvement is seen in defined epidemiological circumstances. Important parasitic pleural effusions are due to echinococcus (where this infection is endemic) and paragoniomiasis (common in South-east Asia). Amoebic involvement of the pleura is extremely common in India and several other countries. It is considered in the section on 'Tropical Infections Involving the Lung'.

TUBERCULOUS PLEURAL EFFUSION

Though in the West, tuberculosis accounts for less than 5% of all pleural effusions, in India and in poor developing countries where tuberculosis is rife, it remains perhaps the most common and important cause of a pleural exudate. In India, it is a disease of young adults, the mean age being between 15 and 30 years. In contrast, the mean age in the West lies between 47 to 56 years.

Tuberculous pleural effusions generally occur in the primary or in the post-primary phase of the disease. It is believed that rupture of a small subpleural tuberculous focus into the pleura leads to a marked exudative pleural reaction. Mycobacterial antigens within the pleural space elicit an intense immune response characterized initially by neutrophils and macrophages, followed by interferon-producing T helper cell (Th) Type I lymphocytes sensitized to tuberculous antigen. This results in a lymphocytic predominant exudative pleurisy. A recent study has shown that cells of an alternative T cell profile CD4+CD25+ FOXP3+ regulatory T cells are also increased in tuberculous pleural effusion. The role of these cells remains unclear.

Clinical Features

The onset may be insidious, subacute or occasionally acute. When acute, pleuritic pain is associated with fever ranging from 102°–104° F and with severe constitutional symptoms. Dry cough and dyspnoea are invariably present. When the onset is insidious the patient may have a low-grade fever, weight loss with very few respiratory symptoms. The effusion may be detected on a routine X-ray chest. Pleural effusion in tuberculosis may be small, moderate or massive. Bilateral pleural effusions though uncommon, can occur and often cause severe dyspnoea with respiratory failure. Large pleural effusions are invariably observed in the post-primary phase of tuberculosis. Imaging findings may reveal associated tuberculous mediastinal adenopathy but an obvious parenchymal lesion within the lung is often not observed.

Another form of tuberculous pleural effusion in the post-primary phase is caseous tuberculous involvement of the pleura. There are many who believe that caseous diffuse granulomatous involvement in the post-primary phase is the usual manifestation of pleural tuberculosis. This form of pleural involvement can produce severe pleural damage. A fibrous thickened pleura with calcification may envelop the lung resulting in a fibrothorax.

Tuberculous pleural effusion can also occur in reactivation tuberculosis with obvious parenchymal disease. Such tuberculous pleural effusions are generally small or at the most moderate in size—never large as at times observed in the post-primary phase of the disease. It is indeed a wonder why a patient with severe bilateral cavitative fibrocaseous tuberculosis involving the greater part of both lungs has generally little or no pleural involvement.

Miliary tuberculosis very often (though not necessarily) a post-primary event may have a pleural exudate, but again the effusion is generally small or moderate in size.

A tuberculous cavity within the lung may occasionally open into the pleura—the result is tuberculous pyopneumothorax. Tuberculous pleural effusion also occurs in HIV-related resurgence of tuberculosis. Pleurisy however occurs in the early stage of immune suppression with CD4 counts > 200 cell/dl, suggesting that a reasonably preserved immune competence is required for an exudative pleural response to occur.

Finally, tuberculous pleural exudates may evolve into pus leading to a tuberculous emphysema. *Tuberculosis should figure in the differential diagnosis of any empyema where the pus is reported to be sterile on routine aerobic and anaerobic cultures.*

Diagnosis

The pleural exudate shows an increase in leucocytes, at times as high as 500–750 cells/mm^3. There is a lymphocytic predominance though in the early stage polymorphs may form more than a third or half of the cellular count. The pH of the fluid may be low and the glucose content is often < 60 mg/dl. The pleural fluid is either straw-coloured or turbid and rarely, blood-tinged.

Acid-fast bacilli (AFB) are almost never found in the pleural exudate on smear. Positive cultures for AFB are rare, being found in not more than 5% of patients. A positive polymerase chain reaction (PCR) for tuberculosis in the pleural fluid is of help but should never be relied upon for a definite diagnosis.

The Mantoux test is generally strongly positive. In the early phase of the natural history of a tuberculous pleural effusion, particularly in a post-primary effusion the Mantoux test may be negative. But it is invariably positive after six to eight weeks of a pleural exudate.

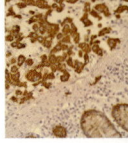

Non-specific Inflammatory Markers in the Diagnosis of Tuberculous Pleural Effusion

Adenosine Deaminase (ADA) released by activated lymphocytes and macrophages is a non-specific marker of inflammation. The ADA levels are found to be invariably raised in tuberculous pleural effusions. A convincingly raised ADA in the pleural fluid has a very high sensitivity (close to 100%) and good specificity (close to 90%) for a tuberculous pleural exudate. The higher the pleural fluid ADA level, the more likely the diagnosis of tuberculosis. In fact, low ADA levels in pleural fluid negate the diagnosis of tuberculosis. However, raised ADA levels have also been observed in parapneumonic empyemas, malignancies, lymphomas and rarely in rheumatoid and other connective tissue diseases. Even so, in countries where tuberculosis is endemic (high-prevalence settings), a positive ADA test provides a 99% post-test probability of tuberculosis. On the other hand, in countries with low or intermediate tuberculosis incidence, a positive ADA test does not have the same strong predictive value as in countries where tuberculosis is endemic. This illustrates the fact that the predictive value of a test is highly dependent on the prevalence of the disease.

ADA occurs in two different iso-enzymes, ADA 1 and ADA 2. Whilst the former is found in all cells, ADA 2 is present only in monocytes. The majority of ADA in tuberculous pleural effusion is ADA 2. Although the use of ratios of ADA 1 to ADA 2 have been advocated as a way of increasing the diagnostic value of the test in the diagnosis of tuberculous pleural effusions, the extra effort and cost does not justify the extra yield.

Other non-specific inflammatory markers whose levels are found to be raised in tuberculous pleural effusion include neopterin, leptin and lysozyme. They lack the sensitivity and specificity of ADA and are of no clinical importance.

The only cytokine in the pleural fluid which if raised is of diagnostic significance is interferon-γ (IFN-γ). A raised IFN-γ has a sensitivity of 89% and a specificity of 97% for a tuberculous pleural exudate. It is a difficult test to perform, extremely expensive and can never replace the easy-to-perform, cheap ADA test in countries where tuberculosis has a high prevalence rate.

Detection of Tuberculosis Nucleic Acid Sequences by Amplification Test

The detection of *Mycobacterium tuberculosis* nucleic acids from pleural fluid has a sensitivity of 62% but a very high specificity of 97%; the test therefore is not useful in excluding the disease.

In summary, a good history and clinical examination, imaging studies and examination of pleural fluid which should include ADA levels and AFB culture of the fluid suffice in the majority of cases to allow a diagnosis of tuberculous pleural effusion.

Pleural Biopsy

In the absence of a positive AFB culture of the pleural fluid, a confirmed diagnosis of tuberculosis can only be made by a pleural biopsy. A blind biopsy using Abram's needle is often negative and when malignancy is an important differential diagnosis a thoracoscopic biopsy is warranted.

Is a pleural biopsy mandatory for a diagnosis of a tuberculous pleural effusion when the fluid is negative for AFB culture? Not so. In a young individual with a pleural exudate compatible with tuberculosis, with raised ADA level, a positive Mantoux test, and no obvious lung pathology, the probability of tuberculosis is well-nigh certain. However, in an individual past 40 years, or in a heavy cigarette smoker, or when the ADA in the pleural fluid is marginally raised or when there is no response to specific anti-TB drugs, a definite diagnosis is necessary, because the characteristics of a malignant pleural effusion are very similar to tuberculous pleural effusion. Imaging studies, studies on the BAL fluid and on the cytology of the pleural fluid may help but not always so. A video-assisted thoracoscopy which enables the thoracoscopist to view the pleural cavity and take multiple biopsies will enable the physician to arrive at a correct diagnosis.

Spontaneous resolution is not uncommon in tuberculous pleural effusions. A follow-up of untreated patients over a five-year period reveals a high rate of recurrence of tuberculosis, chiefly in the lungs but occasionally at extra-pulmonary sites.

Large pleural effusions may require to be tapped more than once for symptom relief. The usual anti-TB drugs need to be given for a period of six to nine months. A course of corticosteroids starting with 30 mg prednisolone daily for a week and slowly tapered over a period of six weeks hastens resolution of a pleural effusion.

Untreated or incompletely treated pleural effusions may become loculated with thickened parietal and visceral pleura. Resolution and full expansion of the lung is possible in some of these patients only after thoracoscopic surgery which involves decortication and proper drainage of the fluid contents through a correctly placed drainage tube.

MALIGNANT PLEURAL EFFUSION

It is estimated that about one-third of all malignancies will develop a pleural effusion at some stage in their natural history. A malignant pleural effusion may be the initial presenting feature of underlying malignant disease. Except for pleural mesothelioma which is a primary malignancy of the pleura, all other pleural involvement is caused by secondaries from a primary situated elsewhere within the body. The commonest primary sites giving rise to pleural metastasis and malignant pleural effusion are the breast, lung, stomach and the rest of the gastrointestinal tract. These account for 60% of malignant pleural effusions. Nevertheless, primaries from almost any site are known to produce pleural metastasis. The pleura may be involved by direct spread (from the lung as an example), by haematogenous spread, or through lymphatics as in lymphoma. Non-Hodgkin's lymphoma involves the pleura far more frequently than Hodgkin's disease.

Pleural effusions (in patients with underlying malignancy) that show no detectable invasion of the pleura by malignant cells are often termed paramalignant effusions. These effusions may be due to tumour-related problems such as pneumonia, atelectasis, pulmonary embolism, lymphatic obstruction due to a malignant mediastinal adenopathy, radiation-induced pleural inflammation or may be transudative in nature due to hypoproteinemia, or associated cardiac, hepatic or renal disease. Distinction from a malignant pleural effusion is important as

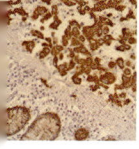

paramalignant pleural effusions do not negate surgical resection of a malignant tumour.

Pleural fluid in malignant involvement of the pleura is often haemorrhagic but not always so. It invariably reaccumulates after paracentesis. The pleural fluid cytology is positive in about 50–70% of patients. Absence of malignant cells in the pleural fluid should never exclude the diagnosis of malignancy.

Pleural biopsy either through a video-assisted thoracoscopy or a CT-guided biopsy if a lesion is clearly visible on imaging studies is absolutely necessary for a confirmed diagnosis.

A malignant pleural effusion in our country is often mistaken for a tuberculous pleural effusion. The mistake is often compounded if the PCR for tuberculosis is found positive in the pleural fluid and is relied upon to make a diagnosis of tuberculosis. A CT-guided or a thoracoscpopic biopsy is a must for the confirmation of either tubercle or malignancy, particularly in pleural effusions occurring in those over 40 years of age.

Except in patients where pleural involvement is due to a lymphoma (which can respond to chemotherapy), cure of the underlying malignancy is not possible once pleural involvement is confirmed. Management is then palliative and directed towards improving the quality of the patient's life.

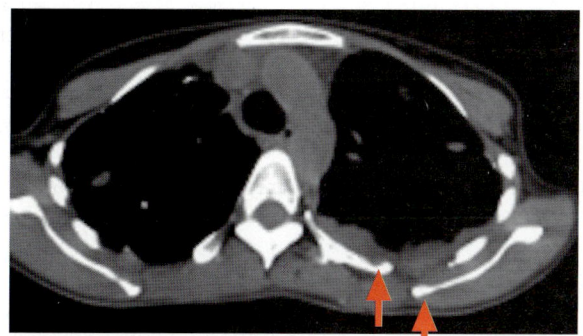

Fig 62.8: Pleural metastases. CT chest demonstrates multiple nodular lesions along the left pleural surface posteriorly in a patient with a renal cell carcinoma. These represent pleural metastasis.

PLEURAL EFFUSION IN GASTROINTESTINAL DISEASE

Acute pancreatitis is the commonest gastrointestinal disease causing a pleural exudate. The reported rate of a pleural effusion in acute pancreatitis is 3–17%. The effusion is left-sided in over two-thirds of patients because of the proximity of the pancreatic tail to the left dome of the diaphragm. The left dome is often elevated and immobile and examination of the pleural fluid reveals a raised amylase content often exceeding serum values. The effusion is generally small to moderate in size and clears as the pancreatitis subsides. Persistence of fluid over two weeks of therapy suggests a pancreatic pseudocyst, a pancreatopleural fistula or a pancreatic abscess. A pancreatopleural fistula is characterized by a direct sinus tract between the pancreas and the pleura, resulting at times in a massive pleural effusion. Pancreatic ascites due to communication of the pancreatic duct with the peritoneal cavity is also associated with pleural effusion which is often bilateral.

Pleural effusion occurring after major abdominal surgery should suggest a subphrenic or intrahepatic abscess. Pleural effusions are observed in 80% of subphrenic abscesses. The pleural effusion though an exudate is invariably sterile (sympathetic pleural effusion) and rarely leads to an empyema except when a subphrenic abscess breaches the diaphragm and opens into the pleura. Pleural effusions are common in amoebic abscesses of the liver. The subject is dealt with in the section on 'Tropical Infections Involving the Lung'.

Oesophageal perforation whatever be the cause produces a left-sided and occasionally, bilateral pleural exudates with a raised amylase content. Apart from the typical history, imaging findings and analysis of the pleural fluid with the raised amylase (of salivary origin on enzyme study) confirm the diagnosis. A pleural exudate following oesophageal perforation soon becomes an empyema.

PULMONARY EMBOLISM, PLEURAL EFFUSION FOLLOWING CORONARY BYPASS GRAFT SURGERY AND DRUG-INDUCED PLEURISY

Pulmonary Embolism

This is an important frequently missed cause of pleural effusion. The diagnosis rests on a keen awareness of this possibility particularly in specific clinical settings, as for example in critically ill patients under intensive care. The possibility of pulmonary embolism as a cause of a pleural effusion should always be considered where the aetiology of a pleural exudate remains undetermined. The effusion is often bloody but not always so. The presence of eosinophils in the pleural exudate should also arouse suspicion of an underlying pulmonary embolism.

Sickle cell crisis can lead to pleuritic chest pain with pleural effusions which may contain blood.

Post Coronary Bypass Graft Surgery (CABG)

Pleural effusion following CABG occasionally persists for weeks or months. The pathogenesis of such persistent effusions is unclear. They generally resolve after repeated paracentesis or drainage through an intercostal drain. Occasionally, pleurodesis becomes necessary.

Drug-induced Pleurisy

Drug-induced lupus or hypersensitivity reactions leading to a pleural exudate have been reported with isoniazid, nitrofurantoin, methylsergide, bromcriptine, procainamide, amiodarone, phenytoin and dantrolene. Drug-induced lupus is generally associated with antinuclear antibodies not only in the blood but also in the pleural exudate. Histone antibodies are considered to be specific for drug-induced lupus. Treatment consists in withdrawing the drug (even if there is a suspicion of drug hypersensitivity) and the use of a three to six-week course of corticosteroids. Thoracocentesis is necessary; eosinophils are often present in the pleural exudate. Failure to recognize drug-induced pleural effusion can lead to well-marked pleural fibrosis.

Hypersensitivity pleural exudates due to drugs can be associated with fever, well-marked constitutional symptoms

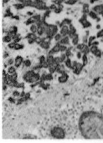

and with peripheral eosinophilia. This is particularly observed in hypersensitivity reactions to nitrofurantoin.

Ovarian Hyperstimulation Syndrome (OHSS)

Ovarian Hyperstimulation Syndrome (OHSS) is seen in 3–5% of women undergoing therapeutic ovarian stimulation through administration of ovarian hormones. The use of these hormones forms part of current reproductive techniques that help women to conceive. The syndrome is characterized by marked ovarian enlargement, the ovaries being often felt on palpating the abdomen. There is a marked increase in capillary permeability leading to depletion of intravascular volume. This results in hypotension, oliguria and the presence of oedema, ascites and at times massive hydrothorax. The pathogenesis of this syndrome is unclear. Treatment is supportive and is directed towards increasing intravascular volume through use of colloids and crystalloids.

HAEMOTHORAX

Haemothorax is characterized by a markedly blood-stained pleural effusion. The diagnosis of haemothorax however requires a pleural fluid haematocrit > 50% of that in the peripheral blood. This is important because many serosanguinous pleural effusions which appear as haemothorax may have haematocrits much lower than that stated above.

Aetiology Chest trauma (blunt or penetrating chest injury) is the single most important cause of haemothorax. Important medical causes include malignancy, severe forms of dengue, pulmonary infarction, rupture of an aortic aneurysm, in particular rupture of a dissecting aneurysm of the aorta. Haemothorax is also observed in bleeding disorders, coagulopathies and as a complication of anticoagulation therapy. Rarely, a spontaneous pneumothorax is followed by a small to moderate-sized haemothorax due to a rupture of a vessel within the tear. Finally, iatrogenic causes include cardiothoracic surgical procedures, pleural or lung biopsies, perforation of the subclavian vein or superior vena cava by a central venous catheter, and perforation of a pulmonary vessel by a Swan-Ganz catheter.

A small haemothorax has the usual signs of a pleural effusion. A large haemothorax besides causing cardiorespiratory embarrassment is associated with pallor, severe hypovolaemic shock, and a progressive fall in the haemoglobin.

Treatment

A large or moderate-sized haemothorax should be drained by insertion of a large-bore drainage tube. This allows the collapsed lung to expand, enables an estimation of continuing blood loss and prevents clotting of blood within the pleural cavity. Clots within the pleural space can get infected and lead to empyema. Organisation of clots leads to fibrosis with an unexpanded lung.

Surgical intervention is indicated under the following conditions:

1. Massive haemothorax, when the greater part of the haemothorax is opacified with blood;
2. when bleeding exceeds the rate of 200 ml/h continuously for three consecutive hours via the drain;
3. if a litre or more of blood is evacuated after insertion of the drainage tube; and
4. the presence of hypovolaemic shock even when the quantity of blood loss through the drain is not excessive. This point is of great importance. Blood gathered within the pleural space may occasionally not find egress through the drainage tube for several reasons, chiefly because of intrapleural clot formation and/or blockage of the drainage tube, so that the clinician gets a wrong impression of the quantum of blood loss.

It is advisable to administer broad-spectrum antibiotics to a patient with haemothorax to prevent infection or treat infection if it occurs. Infection often promotes fibrothorax—a lung trapped by a tight fibrous peel which sharply restricts its movement. Amazingly, even large blood clots within the pleural space, if uninfected, often resolve spontaneously, leaving behind very little pleural fibrosis.

CHYLOTHORAX

Chylothorax is a rare disorder characterized by chyle within the pleural exudate. The pleural fluid is milky and remains milky on centrifugation. Chyle in a milky pleural effusion is confirmed by the presence of triglycerides above 100 mg/dl on analysis and in doubtful cases by the demonstration of chylomicrons on lipid electrophoresis.

A chylous pleural effusion is due to injury to the thoracic duct with spillage of chyle through the mediastinal pleura into the pleural space. Besides surgical and non-surgical trauma, the two most important causes are malignancies which disrupt the thoracic duct and lymphomas. Tberculosis (a tuberculous adenopathy) is another cause, particularly in countries where tuberculosis is rife. Even so, it is a rare cause, and if imaging demonstrates adenopathy along the course of the thoracic duct, it is necessary to exclude a lymphoma through a biopsy before considering tuberculosis as the causative disease. Blockage of the thoracic duct by an adult filarial parasite (generally *Wucheria bancrofti*) should be considered in regions of the world where filariasis is endemic. Lymphoedema, fever with

Table 62.8: Causes of chylothorax
Trauma
Chest injury (blunt or penetrating)
Rarely following forceful vomiting, cough
Iatrogenic
Surgery, radiation
Malignancy
Lymphoma
Tuberculosis
Filariasis
Sarcoidosis
Lymphangioleiomyomatosis
Yellow Nail syndrome

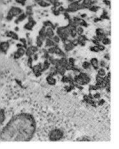

chills and demonstration of microfilaria in the peripheral blood are pointers to a filarial aetiology.

A rare but important cause of chylous pleural effusion is lymphangioleiomyomatosis; chylothorax occurs in about 20% of these patients. Not uncommonly in quite a few patients, the cause of a chylothorax, in spite of all investigations, remains obscure.

Clinical Features

A chylothorax invariably occurs on the right side because of the anatomical course of the thoracic duct. Escape of chyle into the pleural space leads to loss of nutrients, chiefly fats but also proteins. This can lead to severe inanition, weight loss and depressed immune function.

Diagnosis

Imaging, thoracoscopy and biopsy studies of manifest lesions may give the diagnosis of a lymphoma, malignancy or tuberculosis. The site of the leak is best determined by lymphangiography. A radioactive dye, injected into the web between two toes in both feet is carefully followed to determine the site of obstruction.

Treatment

Treatment for the underlying disease (such as a lymphoma, malignancy, tubercle or any other treatable cause) is mandatory. A low-fat diet with medium chained triglycerides is necessary as this reduces the production of chyle substantially. In patients who have become malnourished through the loss of chyle, parenteral nutrition is advised, thereby reducing the flow of chyle to a minimum; this may help to seal a leak in the thoracic duct, particularly in traumatic chylothorax.

Local measures are often necessary to prevent further weight loss and inanition. Chemical pleurodesis, pleuroperitoneal shunt, have their advocates, but the results are poor. Octreotide, a somatostatin analog has been tried (combined with a low-fat diet stated above) to reduce chyle production and help closure of the leak. It may be of help, particularly in post-traumatic chylothorax. Ligation of the thoracic duct a short distance above the diaphragm through a video-assisted thoracoscopy is usually effective. It obviates the often difficult or well-nigh impossible task of locating the leak. There are no long-term effects observed after ligation of the thoracic duct. Recently, percutaneous thoracic duct embolization under imaging guidance has been successfully attempted in special centres before advising surgical closure through video-assisted thoracoscopy. The percutaneous method may be of particular use in patients not fit for any surgical intervention. A prerequisite for percutaneous thoracic duct embolization is catheterization of the thoracic duct. Catheterization is contraindicated if the cysterni chyli or retroperitoneal lypmphatics are blocked.

PSEUDOCHYLOTHORAX

The term pseudochylothorax implies that the pleural fluid resembles chyle but in fact is not so. It results from accumulated cholesterol (> 200 mg/dl) or lecithin globulin complexes in a longstanding, often loculated pleural effusion. There are no chylomicrons within the fluid, distinguishing it from a true chylothorax. The most common cause is a longstanding tuberculous or post-traumatic effusion in which the pleura is fibrosed and at times calcified. Treatment is for the underlying disease.

MISCELLANEOUS CONDITIONS

Dressler's Syndrome

Dressler's syndrome is characterized by an aseptic inflammation chiefly of the pericardium but at times also involving the pleura. It can occur from 10 days to six weeks after a myocardial infarction or after cardiac surgery. The patient has precordial pain, fever, leucocytosis and a raised ESR, often as high as 100 mm/h. A pericardial rub may be present; pericardial effusion is often observed on a 2D-Echo study and on imaging studies. Small pleural effusions may occur. They are often left-sided, at times bilateral; the pleural aspirate is often bloody and may contain eosinophils. Cultures of both pericardial and pleural fluid are sterile.

Dressler's syndrome soon following upon a myocardial infarct is often misdiagnosed as a second infarct or as an increase in size of the previous infarct. When the syndrome occurs later (six weeks after an infarct or after cardiac surgery) its significance is often missed and a wrong diagnosis is entertained. The pathogenesis of Dressler's syndrome is uncertain; it is believed to be related to antibodies being developed against the patient's myocardial cells.

Non-steroidal anti-inflammatory drugs are generally effective. If they fail to resolve the problem, steroids always do so. Effusions may, however, return after steroids are withdrawn. Recurrences occasionally occur even after repeated courses of corticosteroids. Very rarely a pericardiectomy becomes necessary.

Vasculitis

Vasculitides involving the lung such as Wegener's granulomatosis or Churg-Strauss syndrome are rare causes of exudative pleural effusions. Parenchymal lesions within the lungs are invariably present. The exudate is inflammatory in nature often with a mixture of neutrophils and mononuclear cells; expectedly the protein level is raised. The pH of the fluid may be low. Eosinophils are characteristically high in the pleural aspirate in Churg-Strauss syndrome. Antineutrophilic cytoplasmicantibodies (ANCAs) if present are specific and of diagnostic significance. Pleural effusions in vasculitis are generally small and resolve with the use of corticosteroids.

AIDS

Pleural effusion in AIDS may be due to specific infections or due to neoplastic diseases like Kaposi's sarcoma and non-Hodgkin's lymphoma. At times the effusion is non-specific and of undetermined origin.

Organ Transplants

Organ transplantation is also at times followed by pleural effusion due to various specific infectious or non-infectious causes. The frequency of pleural effusion varies greatly. It is

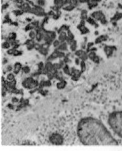

very high (>80 %) in chronic rejection of a lung transplant. A specific lesion in patients with chronic rejection is due to pleural involvement by a lymphoproliferative disorder.

Rheumatoid disease, SLE, other connective tissue diseases

Pleural effusions in these diseases are discussed in a separate chapter.

Uraemic pleurisy

This is a rare complication of uraemia in chronic renal failure. Unlike the transudative effusion encountered in renal failure, there occasionally occurs an inflammatory exudate which may be blood-stained and which may lead to significant pleural fibrosis. The exudate resolves with the correction of uraemia.

Meig's syndrome

Meig's syndrome consists of an ovarian tumour (generally a fibroma but also includes tumours with low-grade malignancies), associated with ascites and pleural effusion. The effusion is an exudate but is non-malignant. Fluid produced is derived directly from the tumour. Ascites occurs to start with; the ascitic fluid then seeps into one or both pleural spaces through pores within the diaphragm. The polyserositis disappears after removal of the ovarian tumour.

Yellow Nail Syndrome

Unilateral or bilateral lymphocytic pleural exudates in this syndrome are due to generalized hypoplasia of the lymphatics.

The syndrome in addition is characterized by yellow discolouration of the nails and peripheral lymphoedema. All these features may not occur simultaneously, but may occur one after the other, so that diagnosis may be difficult when the syndrome has not evolved in its entirety. Pleural effusions may be massive and may require pleurodesis.

Asbestosis

Exudative pleural effusion is a feature of asbestosis, and has been discussed in a separate chapter.

Sarcoidosis

Pleural effusions are very rare in sarcoidosis. They may be due to direct pleural involvement. Obstruction to lymphatic pathways can also lead to a pleural effusion which then is a transudate. Sarcoid glands can obstruct and disrupt the thoracic duct leading to a chylous pleural effusion.

Familial Mediterranean Fever

The diagnosis of this entity is suggested when transient small (at times recurrent) pleural effusions associated with fever occur in Sephardic Jews, Turks, Armenians and Arabs (Mediterranean communities). This entity is also associated with arthritis and recurrent attacks of abdominal pain occurring during bouts of fever.

SUGGESTED READING

Banales Jl, Pineda PR, *et al*. Adenosine deaminase in the diagnosis of tuberculous pleural effusions. A report of 218 patients and review of the literature. *Chest*. 1991; 99: 355–7.

British Thoracic Society Standards of Care Committee. BTS guidelines for the management of pleural disease. *Thorax*. 2003; 58 (Supp II): 1–59.

Colice GL, Curtis A, *et al*. Medical and surgical treatment of parapneumonic effusions. An evidenced based guideline. *Chest*. 2001; 118: 1158–71.

English JC. Pathology of the pleura. *Clin Chest Med*. 1 Jun. 2006; 27(2): 157–80.

First Multicenter Intrapleural Sepsis (MIST1) Group. UK Controlled Trial of Intrapleural Streptokinase for Pleural Infection. *NEJM*. 2005; 352: 865–74.

Kim HJ, Lee HJ, Kwon SY, *et al*. The prevalence of pulmonary parenchymal tuberculosis in patients with tuberculous pleuritis. *Chest*. 2006; 129: 1253–8.

Liam CK, Lim KH, Wong CM. Causes of pleural exudates in a region with a high incidence of tuberculosis. *Respirology*. 2000; 5: 33–8.

Light RW. The undiagnosed pleural effusion. *Clin Chest Med*. 1 Jun. 2006; 27(2): 309–19

Maskell NA, Davies CWH, Nunn AJ. UK. Controlled trial of intrapleural streptokinase for pleural infection. *N Engl J Med*. 2005; 352: 865–74.

Maritz FJ, Med M, *et al*. Comparative analysis of the biochemical parameters used to distinguish between pleural transudates and exudates. *Chest*. 1995; 107: 1604–9.

Porcel JM. Diagnostic approach to pleural effusion in adults. *Am Fam Physician*. 1 Apr. 2006; 73(7): 1211–20

Sahn SA. Pleural effusions of extravascular origin. *Clin Chest Med*. 1 Jun. 2006; 27(2): 285–308

Snider GL, Saleh SS. Empyema of the thorax in adults: review of 105 cases. *Chest*. 1968; 54: 12–17.

Wait MA, Sharma S, Hohn J, Dal Nogare A. A randomized trial of empyema therapy. *Chest*. 1997; 111: 1548–51.

63   Pneumothorax

Pneumothorax signifies air within the pleural space. Pneumothorax may be traumatic or spontaneous. Spontaneous pneumothorax can be either primary or secondary. Primary pneumothorax also called benign spontaneous pneumothorax occurs in apparently healthy individuals with no obvious evidence of lung disease. Secondary pneumothorax is secondary to an underlying lung pathology, the most common of which is chronic obstructive pulmonary disease.

PRIMARY SPONTANEOUS PNEUMOTHORAX (BENIGN SPONTANEOUS PNEUMOTHORAX)

Primary spontaneous pneumothorax usually occurs in young males between 20 and 40 years of age. It is fairly common in India though its exact incidence is not known and would probably be very difficult to establish. The reported incidence in the West is 7.4–8.6 per 100,000 in males and 1.2 per 100,000 in females. Cigarette smoking is an important risk factor of pneumothorax in healthy males, increasing the risk from 0.1% in non-smokers to 12% in smokers. The risk increases with the number of cigarettes smoked and is reported to be close to 100% higher in heavy cigarette smokers, smoking 20 or more cigarette per day.

Pathophysiology

Primary spontaneous pneumothorax is believed to be due to rupture of small subpleural blebs or bullae ('emphysematous-like changes') into the pleural space. A bleb is a small air-filled space between the visceral pleura and the lung parenchyma. A bulla is a small air-filled space within the parenchyma. When close to the visceral pleura, it could rupture through the pleura and produce a pneumothorax. These subpleural blebs and superficial small bullae have been observed in more than 75% of patients undergoing thoracoscopic treatment for primary spontaneous pneumothorax. They are of course not apparent clinically or on imaging so that the lungs outwardly are healthy. The blebs may well be due to an underlying bronchiolitis with rupture of a few alveolar walls due to non-specific infection which is more common in smokers. Air may then travel outwards along interstitial tissue planes to form a subpleural bleb. Damage to alveolar walls at the very periphery of the lung could result in small peripherally placed bullae. There is a clear tendency for primary spontaneous pneumothorax to occur in tall thin individuals (this includes patients with Marfan's syndrome), who have a high transpulmonary pressure at the lung apex. Ordinarily, primary pneumothorax is independent of intrathoracic pressure changes. Interestingly, emphysematous-like changes have been identified in close to 25% of control subjects; they do not necessarily lead to pneumothorax.

A recent concept in the pathogenesis of primary pneumothorax is the role played by increased lung porosity identified by fluorescein-enhanced autofluorescence techniques. Leakage from these porous areas can lead to air within the pleural space.

Genetic and hormonal factors may perhaps also be involved in the pathogenesis of a primary pneumothorax. A rare inherited autosomal dominant genetic condition (Birt-Hogg-Dube syndrome) is associated with pneumothorax, benign skin tumours and renal tumours.

Clinical Features

The presenting features of a primary pneumothorax are dyspnoea and pleuritic chest pain. A dry cough may be present in over a third of patients. Very exceptionally, a primary pneumothorax may be virtually silent.

Physical findings over the chest depend on the size of the pneumothorax. Typically, there is diminished movement over the affected side, with perhaps a slight bulging of the intercostal spaces. The trachea and the apex beat may be pushed to the opposite side. The percussion note on the affected side is hyperresonant; the breath sounds and vocal resonance are diminished. When the pneumothorax is small, the only reliable sign that may alert a discerning physician is the presence of diminished breath sounds on the affected side.

TENSION PNEUMOTHORAX

Tension pneumothorax may occur either in primary or secondary pneumothorax. It is characterized by air entering the pleural space during inspiration but because of a check valve mechanism at the site of rupture, little or no air can gain egress back into the lung and thence to the outside during expiration. The intrapleural pressure continues to increase and causes rapid cardiorespiratory collapse. The patient is tachypnoic, breathless, cold, clammy, extremely distressed, and gasping for air. The markedly increased intrapleural pressure together with the marked mediastinal shift hinders venous return. Hence there is increasing tachycardia and hypotension. The total collapse of the lung together with preservation of a fair degree of blood flow through it leads to a large right to left shunt within the collapsed lung so that there is increasing hypoxia, cyanosis and increasing respiratory failure. The markedly increased intrapleural pressure on the affected side is transmitted to an extent to the contralateral pleural space so that lung function of the contralateral side is also adversely affected. Ultimately,

if the tension pneumothorax is not promptly relieved there is well-nigh stoppage of venous return because of a tamponade-like effect on the heart. A cardiac arrest often associated with an electromechanical dissociation on the electrocardiogram (ECG) is the end result.

Diagnosis

An X-ray of the chest confirms the clinical diagnosis. An X-ray chest after full expiration is more sensitive in picking up a small pneumothorax. Mediastinal displacement to the opposite side is seen when the pneumothorax is of sufficient size. About 10% of patients may have an associated small pleural effusion. CT of the chest is generally unnecessary; it may however reveal a cyst or a bulla not visible on a routine X-ray. It may also help to distinguish between a large bulla and a pneumothorax.

The volume of a pneumothorax is quantified by the volume of the hemithorax the pneumothorax occupies and can be estimated by Light's index

$$\% \text{ of pneumothorax} = 100 - \frac{(\text{Hemithorax} - \text{interpleural distance})^3 \times 100}{\text{Hemithorax distance}^3}$$

Management

Small pneumothoraces with minimal symptoms and a stable cardiorespiratory system require only observation. The rate of spontaneous resorption of air from the pleural space is about 1.23% every 24 hours. This is of course obtained only if the tear in the visceral pleura has sealed. Oxygen administration at high flow rates is advocated in some centres as it theoretically helps air resorption by reducing the partial pressure of nitrogen in the blood. It is to be noted that partial pressure in the alveolar air and in the pneumothorax equates with arterial blood and is 760 mm Hg, whereas the total partial pressure of venous blood is 706 mm Hg. There is therefore a driving force of 54 mm Hg promoting resorption of air from the pleural space.

In a symptomatic pneumothorax or in a large pneumothorax, air needs to be withdrawn from the pleural space. The current trend is to do this by simple aspiration. This succeeds in over 60% of patients. Aspiration may be repeated once or twice.

If re-expansion of the lung is good, though not complete, the patient may just require further observation to ensure that the pneumothorax slowly resolves and does not increase. If aspiration is unsuccessful, or if the patient is markedly symptomatic, intercostal tube drainage is necessary. Small tube drains (10–14 Fr) are adequate, the drain being connected to an underwater seal. Gentle suction may be used to help re-expansion but should be avoided for the first 48 hours to reduce the risk of re-expansion oedema. Once the tube in the underwater seal ceases to bubble the tube is clamped for 24 hours and a radiographic examination of the chest is repeated to ensure that there is no slow air leak. The tube is then removed.

Surgical Treatment

Surgery is indicated when air leak persists in spite of tube drainage. This happens when the edges of the tear in the pleura and the lung beneath remain open so that air continues to have

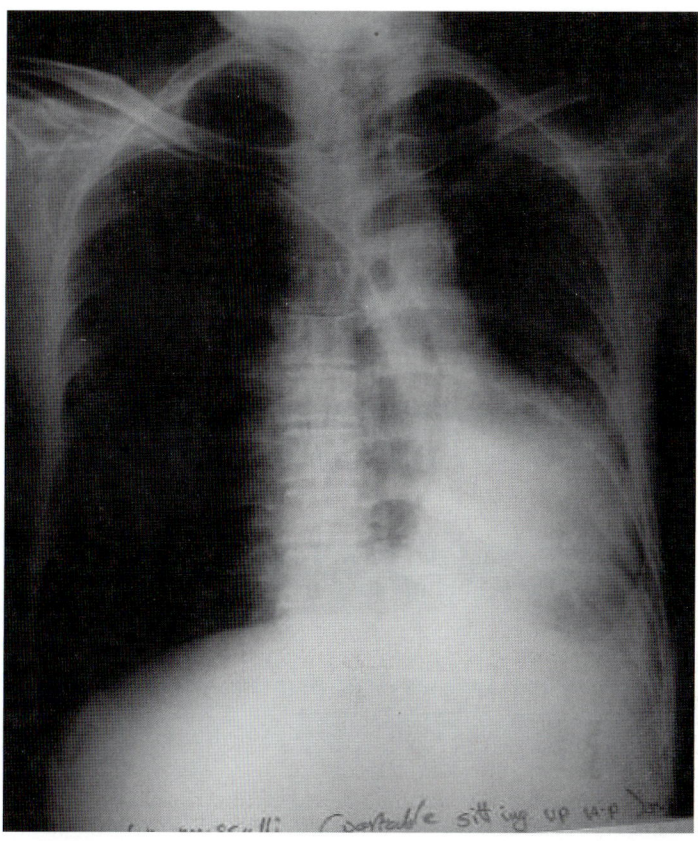

(a)

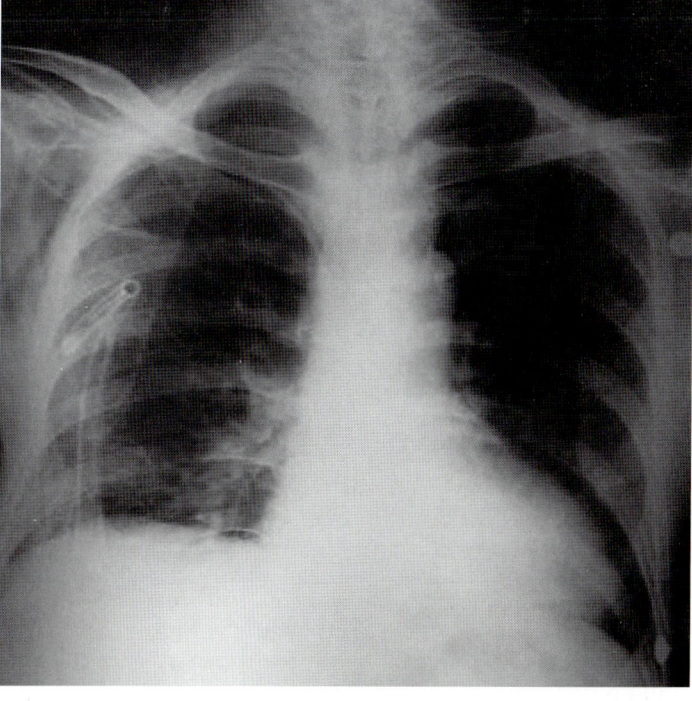

(b)

Fig 63.1: Tension pneumothorax. (a) Chest X-ray demonstrates a large pneumothorax on the right side which is under tension as the lung has herniated across the midline, the mediastinum is pushed to the left (b) X-ray chest after placement of intercostal tube on right side, the pneumothorax is no longer seen, the mediastinum is back in its normal location.

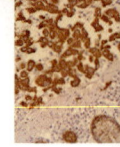

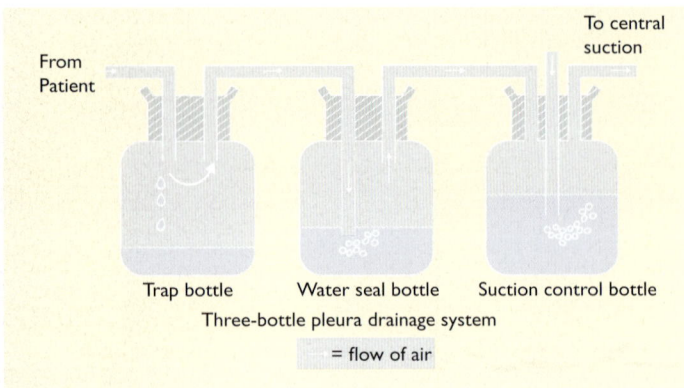

Fig 63.2: Three-bottle pleural drainage system.

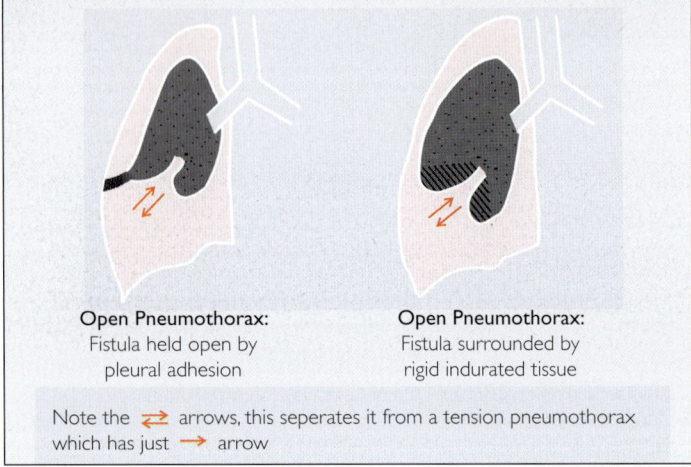

Fig 63.3: Open pneumothorax.

free egress into the pleural space. A persistent open tear may be due to a fibrotic thickened pleura in that area or a pleural adhesion holding the edges of the tear apart as show in Figure 63.3.

Surgery is also indicated with recurrent unilateral pneumothorax or following the occurrence of a first contralateral pneumothorax or the occurrence of bilateral synchronous pneumothorax. Surgery is also indicated in patients whose jobs (airline pilots, deep sea divers) demand that a recurrence is avoided as best as possible.

Video-assisted thoracoscopic surgery allows stapling of blebs and small bullae through the use of an endostapler, laser ablation or electrocoagulation. Following this, pleurodesis can be accomplished mechanically with pleural abrasion or partial pleurectomy or chemically through talc insufflation. Recurrence rates after the above procedures are very low (<5%). The new technology (not available in India) of fluorescence-enhanced autofluorescence thoracoscopy may help identify lesions not visible at routine thoracoscopy.

Prevention of Recurrence

The risk of a recurrence in a primary pneumothorax is about 30%; this risk is greatest in the first year. The recurrence rate is about 50% after one recurrence and over 80% after a third pneumothorax. The risk of a contralateral pneumothorax is about

10 to 15% after a primary event. Recurrence rate is higher in smokers and is believed to be also higher in tall thin individuals. Recurrences can be prevented either thorough pleurodesis using talc or tetracycline. This can be done at the bedside with an intercostal drain in place. Intervention through video-assisted thoracoscopy as outlined above reduces recurrence rates far more effectively than the use of chemical pleurodesis.

SECONDARY PNEUMOTHORAX

A pneumothorax is considered to be secondary when it occurs in patients with underlying lung disease. The incidence depends on the population under study. Secondary pneumothorax is observed in an older age group, the highest rate being in men over 70 years. Many lung diseases can cause a pneumothorax. The most common (perhaps in over 40 to 60% of cases) is chronic obstructive pulmonary disease (COPD), followed by bronchial asthma. Most patients with COPD have well-marked impairment of lung function before the event, with reduced forced vital capacity (FVC) and forced expiratory volume in the first second (FEV1)/FVC < 40%. Pneumothorax may result from rupture of a subpleural bulla or the opening of a large bulla into the pleural space. It could also result from rupture of pleural adhesions which tear and lay open the surface of an over-distended lung. A haemothorax may be associated because of bleeding from ruptured adhesions. Hyperdynamic inflation in patients with acute severe asthma may lead to alveolar rupture and pneumothorax.

Interstitial lung disease is another important underlying risk factor. Pneumothorax can also occur with tuberculosis, particularly in countries with a high prevalence rate. It is due to a rupture of a pleural adhesion allowing an air leak into the pleural space. It can be associated with either active tubercle or with old healed fibrotic tuberculosis.. *Pneumocystis carnii* infection in AIDS is another risk factor as are ARDS and aspiration pneumonia. Bilateral pneumothorax is not uncommon in ARDS and in *P. carinii* infection. Rare diseases like Langerhans' cell histicytosis and lymphangioleiomyomatosis may present with spontaneous pneumothorax or with recurrent pneumothorax.

An unusual type of secondary pneumothorax is catamenial pneumothorax characterized by recurrent pneumothorax

Table 63.1: Causes of pneumothorax	
Primary Spontaneous Pneumothorax	Traumatic Penetrating and non-penetrating chest injury
Secondary Spontaneous Pneumothorax Chronic obstructive airways disease Asthma Cysts and bullae within the lung Tuberculosis Interstitial lung disease Pneumatoceles in Staphylococcal pneumonia Whooping cough Oesophageal perforation *Pneumocystis carinii* infection Langerhan's cell histiocytosis Lymphangioleiomyomatosis	Iatrogenic Aspiration of pleural fluid Intercostal tube insertion Pleural/lung biopsy Transbronchial biopsy Central venous catheter insertion Pacemaker insertion Positive pressure ventilation External cardiac massage

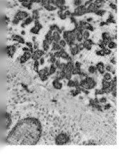

(generally on the right side) occurring in young women 48 to 72 hours after the onset of menstruation. It is due to the cyclic loss of cervical mucus plug during menstrual flow allowing air from outside to gain access through the uterus and fallopian tubes into the abdomen. This air may gain access to the pleura through pores generally present in the right dome of the diaphragm.

Pneumothorax can occur in advanced cystic fibrosis, a disease common in the West but less common in India. It is a marker of end-stage disease because most patients with an FEV1 < 30% are at risk. The list of diseases causing secondary pneumothorax observed in our unit is given in the accompanying table.

Clinical Features

The clinical features are often more severe than those observed in a primary pneumothorax. The significance of symptoms may be missed in patients with COPD as they may be attributed to an exacerbation of COPD rather than to a complicating pneumothorax. Any patient admitted to hospital with an exacerbation of asthma or COPD should have an X-ray chest done to ensure that a pneumothorax is not responsible for worsening symptoms. Even a shallow pneumothorax in these patients may prove dangerous; the over-inflated lung may fail to deflate even when the pressure in what appears as a small pneumothorax is significantly high. It therefore requires prompt drainage.

Diagnosis

Clinical diagnosis may be impossibly difficult in patients with COPD because of an over-inflated chest and also because unequal and reduced breath sounds are often heard in these patients even when there is no pneumothorax.

X-ray chest generally gives the diagnosis though it may be difficult to distinguish a large bulla from a pneumothorax. CT of the chest should help in differentiating one from the other.

Difficulties in diagnosis arise under the following conditions—

1. Localized or mediastinal pneumothorax.
2. Anteriorly located pneumothorax which requires CT imaging for recognition.
3. Pre-existing bullous or generalized emphysema. The contour sign may help to distinguish a pneumothorax from a bulla. A lung contour convex towards the chest wall suggests a pneumothorax; a concave edge suggests a bulla.
4. Small pneumothorax in a patient with consolidated lobe or lung.
5. Air-fluid level in a pneumothorax may be confused with an intrapulmonary cavity.
6. Pneumothorax in ARDS is often missed on a routine radiological examination and is evident only on a CT of chest.

Complications of Pneumothorax

These are more often observed in secondary pneumothorax (an overall complication rate of 60%) though they may occasionally be also seen in primary pneumothorax (an overall complication rate of 10%). Complications are listed in the accompanying table.

Tension pneumothorax is the most dangerous complication and has already been discussed. As an emergency measure, temporary drainage of the pneumothorax is done by inserting

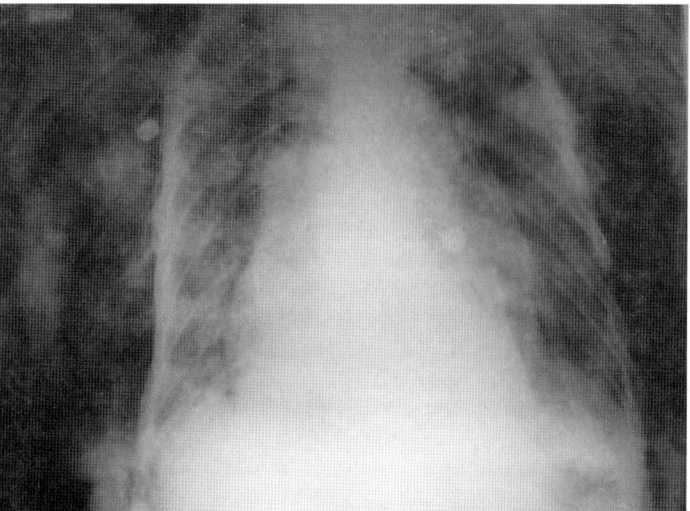

Fig 63.4: X-ray chest demonstrating a pneumothorax with extensive surgical and mediastinal emphysema.

Table 63.2: Complications of Pneumothorax (Primary and Secondary)	
Complications	**Remarks**
Tension pneumothorax	An emergency requiring prompt aspiration of air, followed immediately by insertion of an intercostal tube drain
Mediastinal emphysema Surgical emphysema of soft tissues of neck, chest, upper limbs	Almost always clears with time
Bilateral pneumothorax	An emergency—requires tapping
Bronchopleural fistula	May require special treatment—is difficult to close
Persistent alveolar leak	Generally closes with time if pneumothorax is adequately drained
Chronic pneumothorax	Determine the cause and treat it—generally due to a bronchopleural fistula or a persistent alveolar leak
Loculated pneumothorax	Leave alone if small, drain if large
Pyopneumothorax	Requires drainage of pus and air—use of appropriate antibiotics
Re-expansion oedema	Avoid immediate suction after a pneumothorax. Slow withdrawal of air

a large-bore needle into the pleural space through the second intercostal space. Then as quickly as possible the pneumothorax needs an intercostal tube drain connected to an underwater seal. Use of high-flow oxygen together with cardiorespiratory resuscitative measures are often necessary. Resuscitation is possible even in extreme cases with cardiac arrest and electromechanical dissociation, provided the pneumothorax is promptly and adequately drained.

Severe respiratory failure PaO_2 < 50 mm Hg, $PaCO_2$ > 50 mm Hg may be precipitated in patients with secondary pneumothorax.

Bilateral pneumothorax is a rare but dangerous complication and is observed particularly in AIDS, ARDS and in polytrauma.

Bronchopleural fistulas are difficult to heal, particularly in critically ill patients on ventilator support. They are caused by underlying pleural or lung disease, which keep the tear in the lung open, allowing the pleural space to communicate with a bronchiole or bronchus. Alveolar leaks are a nuisance and almost always heal on their own if the pneumothorax remains adequately drained.

MEDIASTINAL EMPHYSEMA
Air from the alveoli may track along the interstitial tissue planes, breach the mediastinal pleura and produce mediastinal emphysema followed by surgical emphysema of varying extent in the neck, upper limbs and chest wall. Mediastinal emphysema

and surgical emphysema of the soft tissues almost always resolve on their own. Extremely rarely it may be massive enough to produce a cardiorespiratory emergency. Decompressive measures are then indicated.

HAEMOTHORAX
Rupture of a pleural adhesion may result not only in a pneumothorax but also cause bleeding into the pleural space.

Management

Secondary pneumothorax must be drained, even if the pneumothorax is small. An intercostal tube drain should be promptly inserted. Aspiration should be considered only in asymptomatic small pneumothoraces. Air leaks often persist in a secondary pneumothorax so that the lung may take more

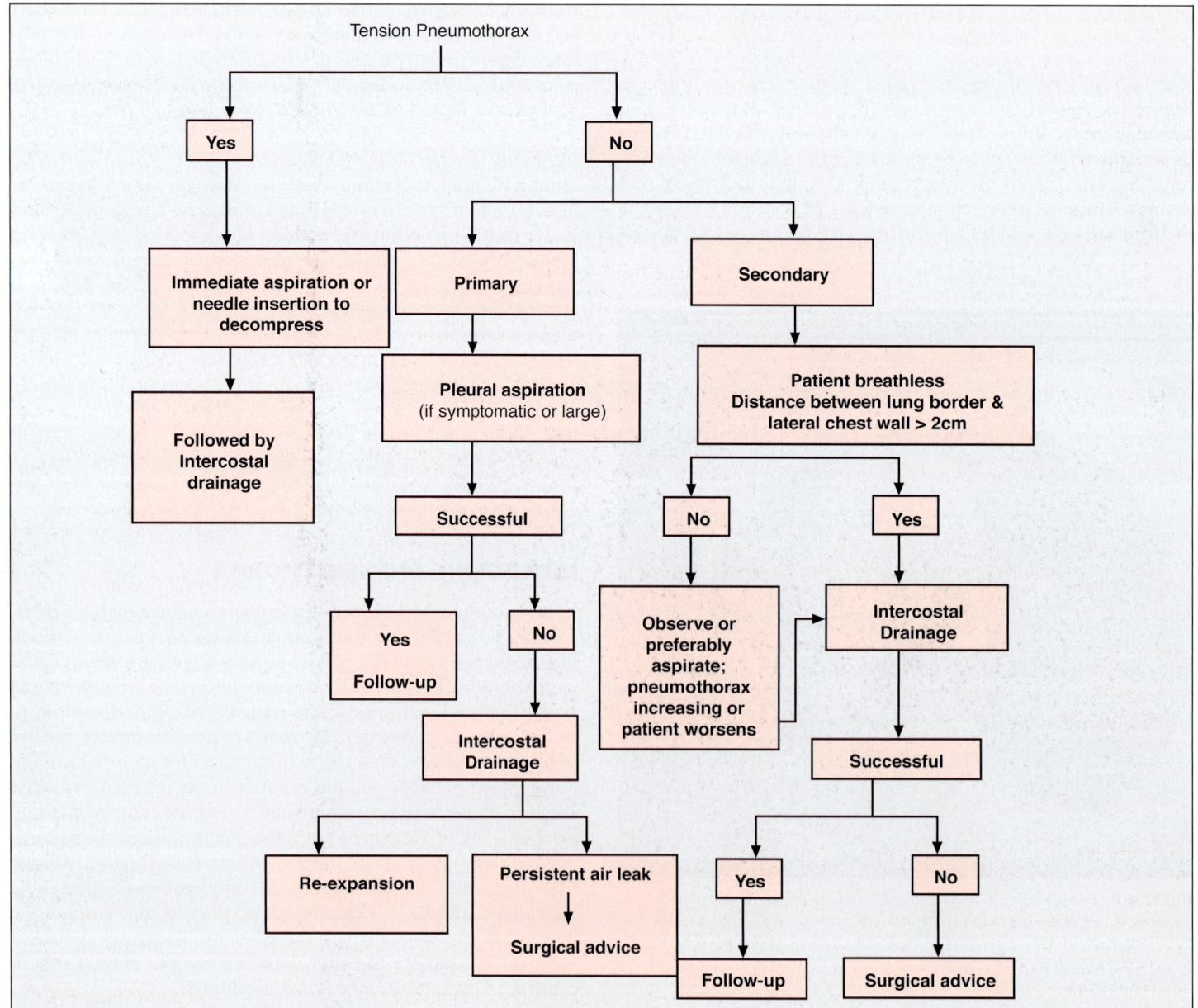

Fig 63.5: Management of spontaneous pneumothorax.

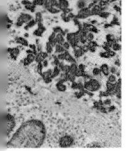

Table 63.3:
Management of pneumothorax with a bronchopleural fistula

1. Drain pneumothorax with a large-bore drain—avoid suction or use very soft suction—else air leak will increase.

2. Reduce 'steal flow' (which is the difference between inspired volume and expired volume) by keeping the diseased lung in dependent position.

3. Monitor 'steal flow'.

4. If on ventilator support
   a. Reduce tidal volume, go off positive end expiratory pressure (PEEP), reduce inspiratory time
   b. If possible allow spontaneous respiration, using BiPAP or CPAP.

5. If air leak is not reduced over time, attempt to seal site of leak with a fibrin seal through a bronchoscope.

6. If the above measures fail—
   a. Surgery if patient's condition allows
   b. Double lumen intubation for single lung or differential ventilation.

than seven days to expand even with adequate drainage. Surgical intervention is necessary if the leak persists. Video-assisted thoracoscopic surgery is generally well-tolerated except in patients with very poor respiratory reserve due to underlying lung disease. Chemical pleurodesis through the intercostal drainage tube is then an alternative approach. If chemical pleurodesis fails, a Hemlich flutter valve can be inserted with

good success rates. Management of a pneumothorax with a bronchopleural fistula is summarized in Table 63.3.

Prevention Strategies

The recurrence rate in secondary pneumothorax is close to 40%. It is about 60% after the first recurrence and about 80% after the third. Preventive strategies should therefore be seriously considered. Chemical pleurodesis through an intercoastal tube carries the least risk. Video-assisted thoracoscopy with pleural abrasion or surgical talc pleurodesis is the procedure of choice; it is more effective with a much lesser degree of recurrence. Open thoracotomy with pleurectomy has the lowest recurrence rate but is invariably unsuitable in patients with well-marked underlying pulmonary disease.

POST-DISCHARGE PRECAUTIONS

Patients should be instructed not to fly until radiography demonstrates complete resolution of a pneumothorax. Conventionally air travel should be avoided for six weeks. Diving should be prohibited permanently unless a surgical procedure such as pleural abrasion with pleurodesis or pleurectomy has been performed. The patient should be advised strongly against smoking.

TRAUMATIC PNEUMOTHORAX

Traumatic pneumothorax may be due to direct injury or indirect injury (as in a bomb blast) or may be iatrogenic. Direct injury may be penetrating resulting in what is termed an 'open pneumothorax' or a blunt injury. Traumatic pneumothorax does not require fracture of the rib or penetration of the pleura. It may result from compression of the chest leading to shear-force-related alveolar, bronchial rupture or even a rupture involving a main bronchus. Tachypnoea and respiratory distress in a trauma patient without evidence of a sharp penetrating injury should promptly raise suspicion of a pneumothorax, haemothorax or massive lung contusion. A pneumothorax in a trauma patient can in time develop into a tension pneumothorax and may be simultaneously associated or followed by haemothorax and pulmonary contusion. A close follow-up is warranted.

IATROGENIC PNEUMOTHORAX

Iatrogenic pneumothorax results from procedures such as central venous catheterization, thoracocentesis, transbronchial biopsies, pleural biopsies and CT-guided biopsies. It is an important cause of pneumothorax in critical care units. Iatrogenic pneumothorax is an important complication in patients on ventilator support. If not promptly recognized, tension pneumothorax results. Respiratory distress, clashing with the machine, deterioration of pulse, blood pressure and oxygenation together with a marked rise in both peak and pause pressures are important pointers to a possible underlying pneumothorax. Pneumothorax in patients on ventilator support is due to inhomogeneity of the lung pathology, some alveoli being more compliant and some having a very low compliance. More gas from the machine reaches the over-compliant alveoli which therefore have a greater chance of rupture. Volutrauma together with barotrauma plays a role in causing a ventilator-induced pneumothorax.

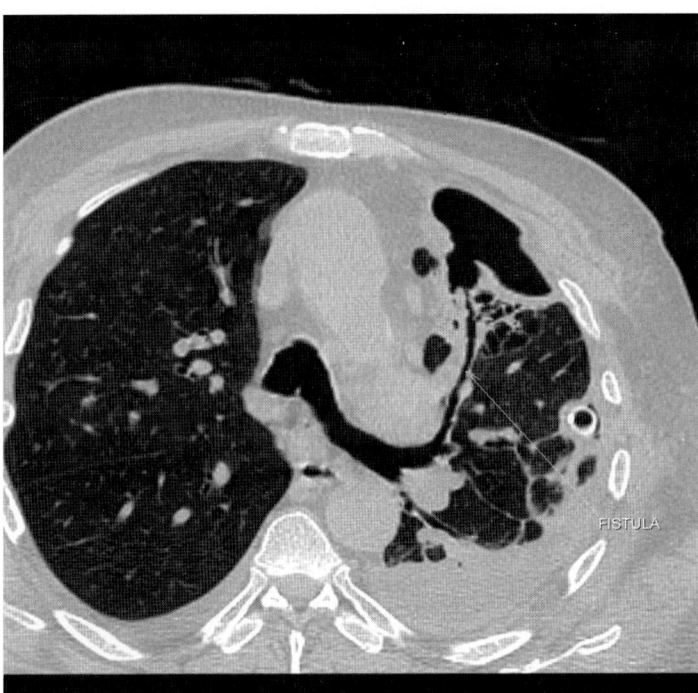

FISTULA

Fig 63.6: Bronchopleural fistula. Axial image reveals an abnormal communication between the left bronchus leading to the pleura as evidenced by the fistulous tract. Posteriorly an ICD tube is noted. Hence in a case of a persistent pneumothorax/hydropneumothorax in spite of an ICD tube in situ, the possibility of a bronchopleural fistula should always be thought of.

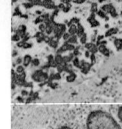

SUGGESTED READING

Baumann MH. Management of spontaneous pneumothorax. *Clin Chest Med*. 1 Jun. 2006; 27(2): 369–81.

Korom S. Catamenial pneumothorax revisited: clinical approach and systematic review of the literature. *J Thorac Cardiovasc Surg*. 1 Oct. 2004; 128(4): 502–8.

Marquette CH. Simplified stepwise management of primary spontaneous pneumothorax: a pilot study. *Eur Respir J*. 1 Mar. 2006; 27(3): 470–6.

Ricci ZJ, Haramati LB. Role of computed tomography in guiding the management of peripheral bronchopleural fistula. *J Thorac Imaging*. Jul. 2002;17(3): 214–8.

Tschopp JM, Rami-Porta R *et al*. Management of spontaneous pneumothorax: state of the art. *Eur Respir J*. Sep. 2006; 28(3): 637–50.

Varoli F, Roviaro G, Grignani F, *et al*. Endoscopic treatment of bronchopleural fistulas. *Ann Thorac Surg*. 1998; 65: 807–9.

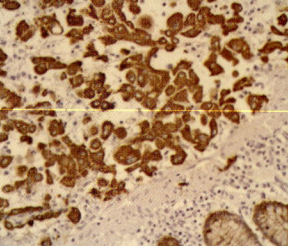
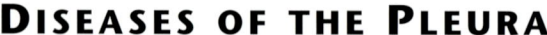

CHAPTER **64** # Malignant Pleural Mesothelioma

Malignant mesothelioma arises from the lining mesothelial cells of the pleura and peritoneal cavities, although rarely it can arise from the mesothelial cells of the pericardium and tunica vaginalis testis. Pleural mesothelioma is much more common than the peritoneal form. The ratio between the two varies in different studies from entirely pleural, to 2:1 in favour of pleural mesothelioma. The pleural tumour may be localized to a well-defined area, may be multi-focal or may involve the pleura as a continuous sheet. Pleural mesothelioma has been proven to be related to asbestos exposure. In 1960, Wagner and colleagues described 33 cases of pleural mesothelioma and all but one had been exposed to crocidolite. Several subsequent studies have confirmed the association between asbestos exposure and pleural mesothelioma.

AETIOLOGY

It is believed that even trivial exposure to asbestos carries the future risk of mesothelioma. The situations associated with non-industrial mild exposure include domestic contact with contaminated clothing or working in an office with a deteriorating crumbling asbestos ceiling or neighbourhood contact in an area which has asbestos factories. It must be noted that mesothelioma reported following non-occupational exposure occurred among a very large population at risk, so that risk associated with low-level exposure though present, is probably small. In people with heavy exposures as in asbestos factory workers, or with recurrent exposure the risk of mesothelioma is high. The West has taken stringent measures against occupational asbestos exposure and the coming decades will witness a further fall in the incidence of asbestos-related mesotheliomas. In India stringent anti-exposure measures are absent or not enforced, so the incidence of asbestos-related pleural mesothelioma will continue to rise.

Many studies support the view that the greater the concentration of asbestos to which a patient is exposed and the greater the duration of exposure, the greater is the future risk of pleural mesothelioma. Also, each brief period of exposure following the first causes an addition to the total, proportionate to the dose of asbestos received.

The average latent period between the first exposure to asbestos and death from pleural mesothelioma is 20–40 years. It is unlikely that the tumour grows during this latent period, as this would mean that the tumour has a very long doubling period. This would in turn imply a prolonged survival once clinical manifestations are observed. It is difficult to surmise the period between the start of growth of the mesothelioma and death. An indirect surmise is by a comparison with lung cancer.

It has been calculated that the period between the start of growth of a lung cancer and its clinical manifestation and death in both lung cancer and pleural mesothelioma is between 12–18 months. On this analogy, a pleural mesothelioma probably starts to grow 10 years before clinical manifestations appear.

Asbestos Fibre Type Involved

Evidence from various studies suggests that amphiboles are more potent than chrysolite, and among amphiboles, crocidolite is more potent than amosite in causing a mesothelioma.

Observations of differing incidence of mesothelioma in different industries involving exposure to asbestos suggest that the risk of mesothelioma is related to the fibre size and that fine fibres appear to be more dangerous. This has been substantiated by estimating the fibre content of lung tissue.

Non-industrial mesothelioma has been reported from Turkey, Cyprus, and Greece caused by naturally occurring asbestos minerals including tremolite and perhaps chrysolite. Endemic mesothelioma was first reported in 1978 from Karan, a remote village in central Turkey. Many deaths occurred in middle-aged adults but deaths were also reported in a 12-year-old boy and 15-year-old girl suggesting exposure to a carcinogenic agent from birth. The responsible agent was a fibrous zeolite called enonite. Other asbestos minerals including tremolite were found in the volcanic tuff which was quarried and used for building.

Pleural Mesothelioma in the Absence of Asbestos Exposure

Although exposure to asbestos is the main association and risk factor for a pleural mesothelioma, patients with pleural mesothelioma with no exposure to asbestos are not uncommon. An important causal factor (other than asbestos) is radiation exposure. In one reported series, five patients with Hodgkin's disease who received radiotherapy developed malignant pleural mesothelioma, the average interval from radiotherapy to the diagnosis of the disease being 15 years. The simian virus (SV40) has also been implicated in the aetiology of malignant pleural mesothelioma. This virus produces the disease in 100% of hamsters when injected intrapleurally. Also, using PCR analysis SV40 DNA sequences have been detected in 40–60% of malignant mesotheliomas in humans. The role of this virus however remains controversial.

It is of interest that the risk for mesothelioma is unrelated to smoking. The relative risk is not dependent on the age at which exposure begins but the absolute risk is greater with

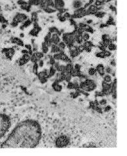

earlier exposure merely because it provides more time for a mesothelioma to occur.

PATHOGENESIS

Inhaled asbestos fibres go through the lung to reach the visceral pleura. They reach the parietal pleura either through lymphatics or perhaps through direct penetration of the visceral pleura. The exact mechanism of malignant transformation of the mesothelium of the pleura is not clear, but evidence suggests chromosomal damage including chromosomal depletion. Studies suggest a depletion of genetic material in the short arms of Chromosomes 1, 3, and 9 and the long arms of Chromosomes 6, 15, and 22. Some of these regions contain suppressor genes. It is believed that the large T antigen of SV40 is capable of inactivating suppressor genes and may well be responsible for inducing the chromosomal changes described above. Perhaps SV40 alone does not cause pleural mesothelioma; it may act as a co-carcinogen with asbestos. Epidemiological data from Turkey suggest that genetic predisposition may play a role in increasing the susceptibility to pleural mesothelioma though no specific gene or genetic alteration that identifies this susceptibility has been found as yet.

PATHOLOGY

The tumour can arise form either the parietal or visceral pleura. It occasionally presents as a localized mass, but more commonly is characterized by multiple nodules studding the pleural surface or by a continuous sheet of thickened neoplastic tissue which spreads by continuity to partially or completely encase the lung with retraction of the chest wall. Pleural effusion is often present. With advancing disease the pleural space may be obliterated and spread occurs through continuity and contiguity to involve the lung, chest wall, mediastinum, pericardium and diaphragm. The contralateral pleura may also be involved. Blood-borne distant metastases are also observed.

The histological appearance is varied. The main forms are epithelial, sarcomatous and mixed. The epithelial form resembles an adenocarcinoma and is characterized by tubule formation; the sarcomatous form consists of spindle-shaped cells with collagen deposition. The mixed form combines elements of each of the above in varying proportions. Pleural effusions are observed in about 70% of epithelial and mixed forms but in 16% of sarcomatous form. Distant metastasis is most often observed in the sarcomatous form but can occur in the other forms as well.

CLINICAL FEATURES

Malignant pleural mesothelioma is more common in men, (more than 70% of cases) perhaps due to their greater frequency of exposure to asbestos. Though most common between the fifth to the seventh decade, the disease may occur at any age.

The presenting features are dyspnoea and a dull chest pain of insidious onset. The dyspnoea is due to pleural effusion. The effusion invariably recurs when tapped. It is often blood-stained but may be serous and may continue to be so right up to the end. Chest pain is dull but is sometimes severe and pleuritic.

General systemic features include a low-grade fever, tiredness and weight loss.

Clinical examination often reveals the usual physical signs of a pleural effusion. Dullness over the base with diminished breath sounds may be present even in the absence of fluid because of a markedly thickened pleura. Chest wall retraction is observed when the tumour encases the lung like in a cuirass. Chest movements and breath sounds are diminished over the whole affected chest and there is a restrictive ventilatory defect. Tumour tissue may infiltrate needle tracts caused during pleural paracentesis or following a pleural biopsy.

Infiltration of the pericardium can cause constriction; involvement of the mediastinum, diaphragm, peritoneum and the chest wall may occur with advancing disease.

Death occurs chiefly from respiratory failure. Constrictive pericarditis, and cardiac arrhythmias due to pericardial invasion can also cause death. Extension of the pleural mesothelioma to involve the peritoneum can cause abdominal complications, chiefly intractable small bowel obstruction. Blood-borne distant metastasis may also occur.

INVESTIGATIONS

Imaging

The chest radiograph often reveals pleural effusion. A thickened pleura, often lobulated in appearance may be revealed after aspiration of the pleural fluid. As the disease advances and constricts the lung, the lung on the affected side is increasingly constricted with marked contraction of the affected hemithorax. A localized mass may be the only radiological abnormality in 5–10% of cases

Pleural and pulmonary changes due to asbestosis may also be present. These may be non-malignant though it may not be possible to distinguish non-malignant from malignant involvement.

CT of the chest demonstrates the above changes with greater clarity. Pleural thickening, nodularity of the pleura is observed in almost all cases. Thickening of the interlobar fissure is an important feature as is an associated pleural effusion. Extension of the tumour into the chest wall, lung, pericardium, mediastinum and peritoneum can be demonstrated clearly on CT imaging.

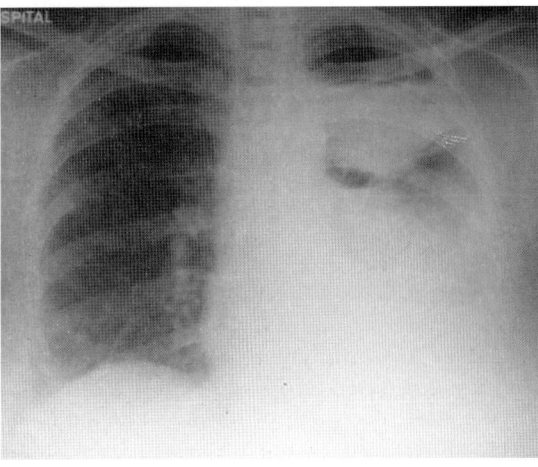

Fig 64.1: X-ray chest reveals a lobulated mass in the left hemithorax, biopsy of this mass showed a mesothelioma.

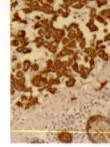

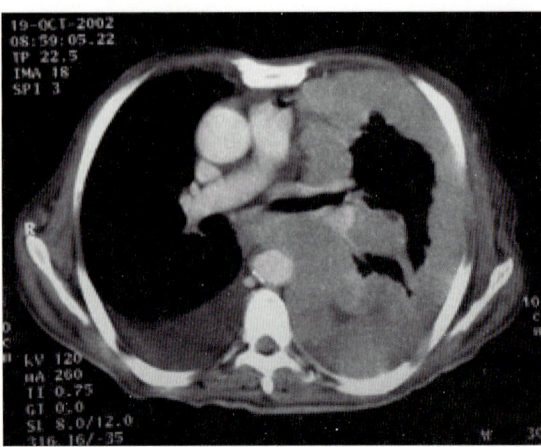

Fig 64.2: Mesothelioma. Chest CT reveals considerable thickening of the left pleura encasing the left lung with extension to the mediastinum encasing the mediastinal vasculature, as well as the left main bronchus. There is a right pleural effusion. Biopsy showed a mesothelioma.

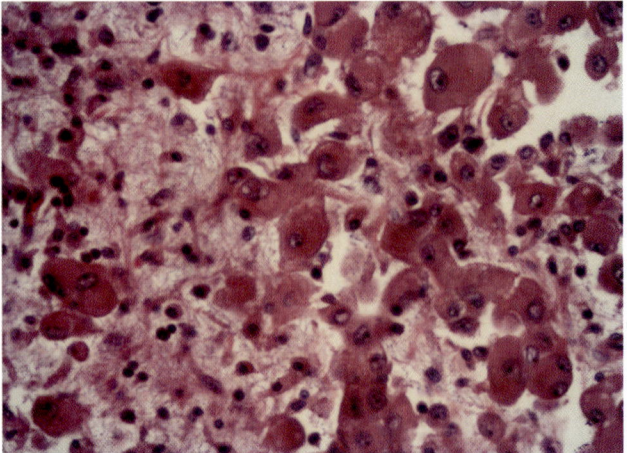

Fig 64.3: Malignant Mesothelioma. H&E 40x. Plump atypical mesothelial cells with enlarged nuclei are seen. Prominent nucleoli are also visible.

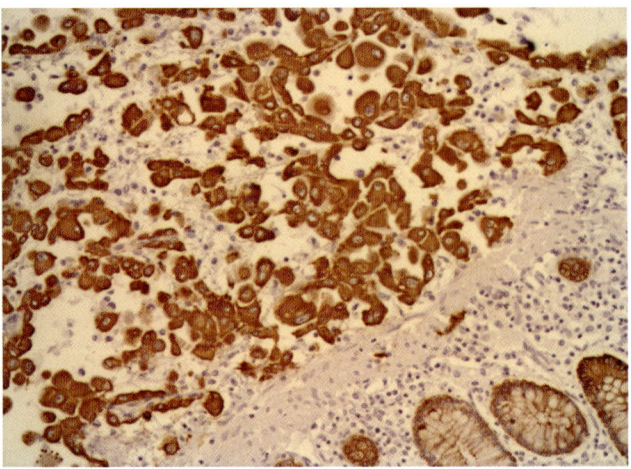

Fig 64.4: Immunohistochemistry. Strong positivity for mesothelial marker, Calretinin.

Magnetic resonance imaging of the chest using multi-dimensional planes is superior to CT scans for evaluating the relationship of the tumour to the great vessels, if surgery is contemplated.

Positron Emission Tomography (PET) scan

The PET scan is useful under the following circumstances:

1. To distinguish benign from malignant pleural lesions. A positive PET scan needs pathological confirmation but a negative scan lends reassurance and may permit close observation and follow-up without biopsy in a number of patients.
2. As a pre-treatment evaluation in patients with a pleural mesothelioma.
3. To identify distant metastasis in patients who are to undergo pleuropneumonectomy.
4. To assess response or lack of response to systemic treatment.

Pleural Aspiration

Examination of an aspirate (when pleural effusion is present) should be the next investigative step after an X-ray of the chest. The pleural fluid is an exudate; it is often blood-stained but not always so. Cytological examination may reveal malignant cells in 30–60% of cases depending on the expertise of the pathologist. It is difficult to distinguish reactive from malignant mesothelial cells. Even if malignant cells are present it may be difficult to determine whether they represent a pleural mesothelioma or pleural metastasis.

Pleural Biopsy

Histological confirmation of a pleural mesothelioma is almost always necessary. A blind pleural biopsy is generally unhelpful, adequate tissue being obtained in less than a third of patients. CT-guided biopsy gives a better diagnostic yield. Thoracoscopy with direct visualization of the pleura with biopsies from different sites is the procedure of choice. It has a diagnostic yield close to 90%. Even so, the diagnosis may not be definitive as problems are encountered both in sampling and in histopathological interpretation.

Tumour Markers

Two tumour markers reported recently in relation to pleural mesothelioma are mesothelin and osteoporin. Soluble mesothelin-related protein has been reported in 84% of patients with pleural mesothelioma and 2% of patients with other malignant tumours. Mesothelin levels may also be useful to evaluate response to treatment.

Osteoporin is a glycoprotein expressed in many cancers. Osteoporin levels have been reported to be significantly higher in patients with pleural mesothelioma compared to a group with exposure to asbestos but who did not have pleural mesothelioma. At an osteoporin value of 48 ng/ml the sensitivity and specificity at diagnosis was 78% and 86% respectively. The efficacy of the marker as a screening test is under investigation.

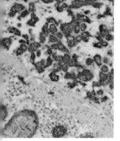

STAGING

The International Mesothelioma Interest Group proposed a staging system updating previous systems. This system has been adopted by the International Union Against Cancer and the American Joint Committee on Cancer. It has been validated by a study of a fairly large number of patients with pleural mesothelioma. Most patients were observed to be in advanced stage of the disease (Stage III and IV), very few were observed to be in the early stages (Stage I and II).

PROGNOSIS

The prognosis is poor. The median survival rate is between 8 to 12 months; fewer than 20% survive for more than two years. Patients with an epithelial histopathology fare better then the others. Poor prognostic factors arrived at by the Cancer and Leukaemia Group and the European Organization for the Research and Treatment of cancer include—non-epithelial histology, age > 75 years, chest pain, male gender, WBC > 8.3 × 10^4/L, platelets > 4,00,000 µL and LDH > 500 units/L.

TREATMENT

Treatment of pleural mesothelioma is unsatisfactory and produces little or no change in morbidity and mortality. The role of surgery is controversial. Pleurectomy with decortication or radical pleuropneumonectomy even in patients where surgery was feasible brought no significant increase in survival except in isolated instances. Surgery should only be reserved for patients with a localized tumour. Recent trials include a three-pronged attack–starting with chemotherapy, followed by extrapleural pleuropneumonectomy and then by radiation. Patients with Stage I and Stage II expectedly fared better than those with Stage IV disease. No single chemotherapeutic agent has proved very effective. Combination chemotherapy has been found to be superior to the use of a single agent though a number of chemotherapeutic agents are being tried. At present the standard combination therapy is primetrexed and cisplatin.

Palliative Therapy

In most patients the disease is too advanced for specific treatment. Pleural effusion produces increasing breathlessness. Repeated thoracocentesis brings temporary relief, but the fluid continues to refill and ultimately gets loculated. It is best to advise thoracoscopy with pleurodesis or chest tube drainage with chemical pleurodesis. A risk of thoracoscopy or tube drainage with pleurodesis is that after the pleural space is emptied, the lung if encased by tumour tissue would fail to expand (trapped lung). Pleurodesis would then be unsuccessful. It is only when the pleural space is obliterated after drainage that talc pleurodesis is possible. Currently, tunnelled pleural catheters with drainage by the patient, nurse or any caregiver into disposable bags affords relief. Pleurodesis often occurs (without the use of talc) with time, following which the catheter is removed. Control of pleural effusion by this method is satisfactory and affords symptomatic relief.

Pain relief is of great importance with advancing disease. Supportive treatment adds to patient comfort.

SUGGESTED READING

Pistolesi M. Malignant pleural mesothelioma: update, current management, and newer therapeutic strategies. *Chest.* 1 Oct. 2004; 126(4): 1318–29.

Ray M. Malignant pleural mesothelioma: an update on biomarkers and treatment. *Chest.* 1 Sep. 2009; 136(3): 888–96.

Scherpereel A, Astoul P, *et al.* Guidelines of the European Respiratory Society and the European Society of Thoracic Surgeons for the management of malignant pleural mesothelioma. *Eur Respir J.* Mar. 2010; 35(3): 479–95.

Vorobiof DA. Malignant pleural mesothelioma: medical treatment update. *Clin Lung Cancer.* 1 Mar. 2009; 10(2): 112–17.

CHAPTER **65** **Diseases of the Mediastinum**

GENERAL CONSIDERATIONS

The mediastinum is the vertical region within the middle of the thorax, between the two pleural cavities, thereby separating the lungs. It is bounded superiorly by the thoracic inlet, inferiorly by the diaphragm, posteriorly by the vertebral column and laterally by the mediastinal pleural reflections. The main structures within the mediastinum are the heart and great vessels, the trachea, the two main bronchi and the oesophagus. The phrenic and vagus nerves course through it; the sympathetic trunks lie one on each side of the vertebral column. These vital structures are all closely connected to one another by loose connective tissue. Hence air or infection can spread rapidly within the mediastinal space. Also fascial planes within the neck, mediastinum and retroperitoneum have both continuity and contiguity. Infection or air can therefore find easy egress from any one of these sites to the other. The mediastinum is rich in lymphatics and lymph glands, permitting both the dissemination of infection and neoplastic disease within it.

Traditionally, the mediastinum is divided into anterior, middle and posterior compartments based on the lateral chest X-ray.

This is not an actual anatomical division but is conceptualized to help in the differential diagnosis of mediastinal

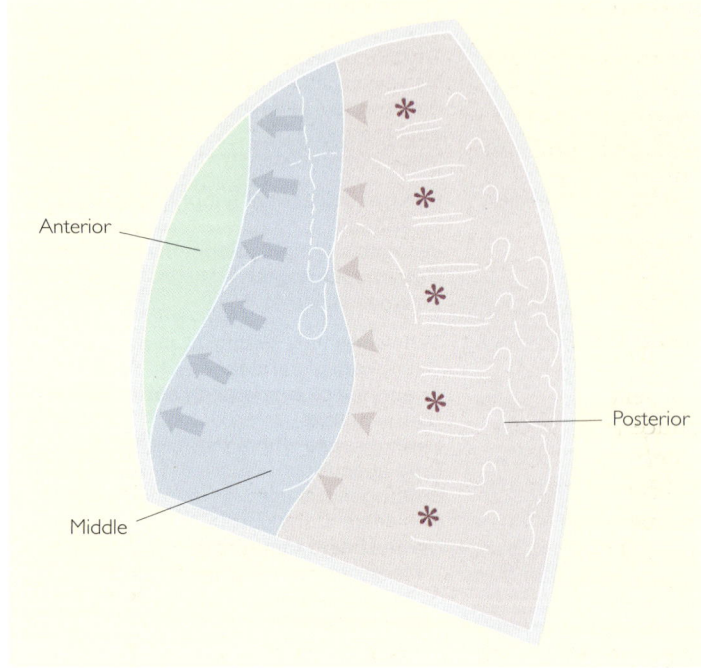

Fig 65.2: Illustration of mediastinal compartments according to this book.

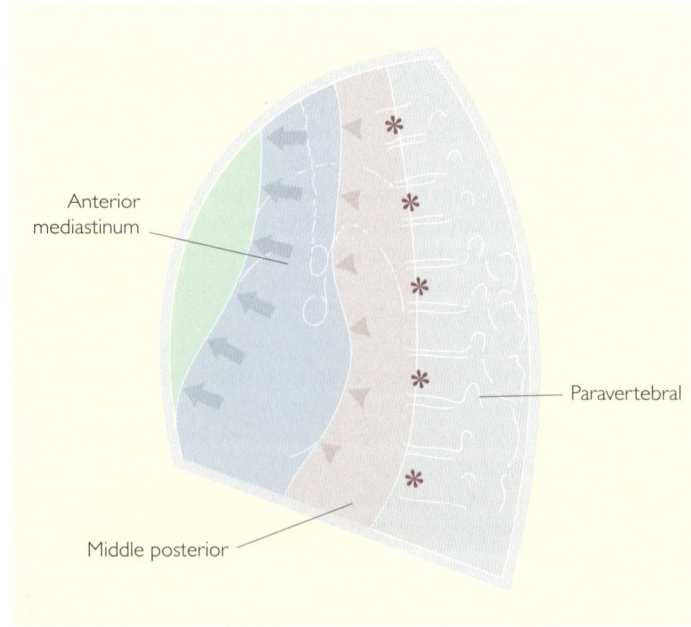

Fig 65.1: Illustration of mediastinal compartments as seen on lateral chest radiography.

tumours and masses since different mediastinal tumours, masses or cysts have generally a distinct predilection for one or the other of these compartments. In fact there is no consensus between clinicians on the boundaries of these compartments. The compartmental boundaries adopted for this book are as follows.

The anterior compartment is bounded anteriorly by the inner surface of the sternum and posteriorly by the anterior surface of the pericardium, the great vessels and the anterior surface of the trachea. Superiorly it extends to the thoracic inlet, inferiorly to the diaphragm. It contains the thymus gland, pericardial fat, lymph glands and connective tissue.

The middle or the visceral compartment is bounded anteriorly by the posterior limit of the anterior compartment and posteriorly by the posterior surface of the great vessels, posterior surface of the trachea and its division into the main bronchi and the posterior pericardial surface, extending upwards to the thoracic inlet and downwards up to the diaphragm. It contains the pericardium, heart, aorta and the great vessels, the superior vena cava (SVC) and the large veins draining into it, the pulmonary vessels, the trachea, major bronchi, the phrenic nerve and lymph glands.

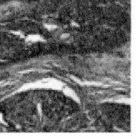

Table 65.1:
Mediastinal masses in relation to the anterior, middle and posterior mediastinal compartments

Anterior mediastinum	**Thymoma** **Thymic hyperplasia** **Thymic carcinoma** **Germ cell tumours** 　　**Teratoma** 　　**Seminoma** **Intrathoracic goitre** **Aneurysm of the ascending and root of aorta** Thymolipoma Thymic cyst Thymic carcinoid Non-seminomatous germ cell tumours Parathyroid adenoma Pericardial cyst Mesenchymal tumours
Middle Mediastinum	**Benign mediastinal lymphadenopathy** **Lymphoma** **Metastatic lymphadenopathy** **Bronchogenic cyst** Enterogenous cyst
Posterior mediastinum	**Schwannomas, Neurofibromas** **Oesophageal carcinoma** **Aneurysm of descending aorta** **Hiatus hernia** **Potts disease with a paravertebral** **Bold abscess** **Enterogenous cyst** **Achalasia of the cardia** **Nerve sheath tumours** 　　Malignant peripheral nerve tumours 　　Ganglioneuromas 　　Neuroblastomas 　　Paragangliomas 　　Neurofibromas **Extramedullary haematopoesis**

Note: 'Masses' in dark font are those more frequently encountered in our units.

The posterior compartment extends from the posterior aspect of the middle compartment to the anterior surface of the vertebral bodies including the paravertebral sulci. It contains the descending aorta, oesophagus, sympathetic trunk on each side of the vertebral column, the azygos, hemiazygos veins, the thoracic duct and intercostal nerves.

Some authors conceptualize the middle or visceral compartment as extending posteriorly right up to the anterior surface of the vertebral column. The oesophagus would then fall into the middle compartment. In this division the posterior compartment would include only the sympathetic trunk, thoracic duct, intercostals nerves, azygos and hemiazygos veins. Whichever of the two conceptualizations of mediastinal compartments one follows, the three compartments appear approximate to one another in the superior portion of the mediastinum.

A large study between January 1993 and June 2003 from Jaipur, India showed that among the 106 patients who underwent surgical treatment of a mediastinal mass, the male to female ratio was 1.9:1. Histopathologically, 39% patients had thymic pathology, 29% had lymphoma, 13% had germ cell tumours, 11% had neurofibroma, 4% had ganglioneuroma,

and 2% had bronchogenic cyst. (*Ref: Chandra P Shrivastava, Sanjeev Devgarha et al. Mediastinal Tumors: a Clinicopathological Analysis*: Asian Cardiovasc Thorac Ann 2006;14: 102–104).

CLINICAL FEATURES OF MEDIASTINAL MASSES

1. **Asymptomatic Presentation** Approximately one-third to half of patients with mediastinal masses are asymptomatic; the condition being discovered on a routine X-ray of the chest. Interestingly, only 15% of asymptomatic masses are malignant, whereas close to 60% of those producing symptoms are malignant.

2. **Compression of Neighbouring Structures** Though symptoms produced by compression of surrounding structures are more common with malignant tumours and masses, they may also be caused by large benign tumours. The site and extent of compression symptoms depend on the nature of the mediastinal mass and its situation within the mediastinum. The common symptoms of compression include cough, breathlessness and vague chest pain. Specific compression symptoms and signs depend on the anatomic structures compressed by a mediastinal mass. They are briefly detailed below.

   a) Pressure on the superior vena cava leads to the superior vena caval syndrome, characterized by increasingly distended jugular veins; pulsations in the veins are not evident, unlike the pulsatile engorged jugular veins seen in congestive heart failure. Subtle signs of venous engorgement include slight puffiness of the face, particularly around the eyes with chemosis of the conjunctiva in the early morning, a flushed feeling due to congestion of the face and neck on bending or stooping to pick up an object from the floor or when tying a shoelace.

   b) Compression of the trachea, major bronchus Compression of the trachea could lead to stridor; compression of the main bronchus could cause a unilateral monophonic wheeze; increasing pressure on the bronchus could cause atelectasis of a lobe or lung.

   c) Pressure on the oesophagus could cause dysphagia.

   d) Compression of the left recurrent laryngeal nerve could cause hoarseness of the voice due to abductor paralysis of the left vocal cord.

   e) Cardiac compression or pericardial invasion may lead to palpitations, pain and rhythm disturbances.

   f) Pressure on the sympathetic nerve trunk will cause Horner's syndrome, and is invariably due to a malignant tumour.

   g) Compression of the intercostal nerves as they emerge from their vertebral foraminae will lead to intercostal neuralgia, intraspinal extension of the mass could cause pressure on the spinal cord leading to varying neurological deficits.

   h) Pressure with erosion of the vertebra or ribs could cause bone pains and tenderness over the affected area.

A point of clinical importance is that however large a mediastinal tumour or cyst it does not obliterate an arterial pulse. Unequal pulses or an absent pulse in one or the other upper

Table 65.2:
Clinical features due to compression of neighbouring structures by mediastinal masses

Site of Compression	Features
Superior Vena Cava	Distended jugular veins, flushing and puffiness of face on bending (SVC syndrome)
Trachea	Stridor
Main bronchus	Unilateral monophonic wheeze, atelectasis of lobe/lung
Oesophagus	Dysphagia
Left recurrent laryngeal nerve	Hoarseness of voice
Cardiac compression, pericardial invasion	Cardiac pain, palpitations, arrhythmias
Sympathetic trunk	Horner's syndrome
Intercostal nerves	Intercostal neuralgia
Vertebra	Pain over affected area

limb in the presence of a mediastinal mass is invariably due to an aortic aneurysm. The position of a mediastinal mass within the mediastinum, its size and the direction of expansion will determine as to which organ or structure is subject to compression.

Other Systemic Features

1. Mediastinal masses when malignant may metastasize outside the mediastinum. A complete clinical examination is therefore important. One should particularly look out for pleural involvement (pleural effusion), lymphadenopathy (particularly in the neck and axilla) and hepatosplenomegaly. These features may provide a clue to a clinical diagnosis or allow an easy access for a biopsy procedure that establishes a diagnosis.
2. Specific clinical features may also occur depending on the nature of the mass. Thus myasthenia gravis may be the presenting feature in a thymoma, gynaecomastia in a germ cell tumour, and a Pel Ebstein fever in a patient with a mediastinal lymphoma.

Table 65.3:
Paraneoplastic syndromes associated with mediastinal masses

Diseases	Features
Thymoma	Myasthenia gravis, acquired hypogam maglobulinemia, red cell hypoplasia
Thymic carcinoid	Cushing's syndrome, SIADH
Germ cell tumours	Gynaecomastia, Klinefelter syndrome
Intrathoracic goitre	Hyper/hypothyroidism
Pheochromocytoma	Hypertension
Autonomic ganglion tumours	Horner's syndrome, diarrhoea, hypertension
Sarcoidosis	Hypercalcemia

3. Non-specific clinical features include low-grade fever, weight loss, and lassitude. Various paraneoplastic syndromes that may be encountered with different tumours and masses have been tabled below.

INVESTIGATION OF MEDIASTINAL MASSES

1. A good clinical history and a complete physical examination are vital. A careful search for compression syndromes, in particular the superior vena caval syndrome is helpful. A recurrent laryngeal nerve palsy or a Horner's syndrome due to a mediastinal mass invariably points to a malignancy. Paraneoplastic syndromes should be carefully sought for, particularly in masses known to cause them. An X-ray chest is considered part of the basic examination and gives a clue to the possible diagnosis.
2. High-resolution computed tomography (HRCT) has revolutionized accurate diagnosis of mediastinal masses. At times the appearances are so typical as with a pericardial cyst or an aortic aneurysm that further diagnostic proof may not be necessary. A CT scan also forms the most appropriate guide for a CT-guided fine needle biopsy or a core biopsy of a mediastinal mass.
3. Magnetic Resonance Imaging (MRI) as an imaging technique is particularly useful under the following circumstances:
   a) To determine invasion of vascular and neural structures or infiltration of tissue planes in malignant lesions. This information is of special significance if surgery is to be performed.
   b) T1 and T2 images may help to clearly delineate mediastinal masses from surrounding soft tissues.
   c) The difference between Tl and T2 values for bronchogenic carcinoma and inflammatory lesions is significant and may help in diagnosis.
   d) Lesions close to the thoracic inlet are better outlined with an MRI study as infiltration of the brachial plexus and the vertebral foramina are better visualized.

Radionucleotide Studies

Uptake of ^{131}I points to a substernal goitre while uptake of ^{131}I metaiodo benzyl guanidine can identify a pheochromocytoma either in the adrenals or in the mediastinum or other rare ectopic sites. Gallium scan (though not specific) may help in the identification of a lymphoma. It may help to distinguish a lymphoma in the anterior mediastinum from a thymoma, since a lymphoma picks up gallium avidly while a thymoma generally does not pick up gallium. Gallium is also picked up by any inflammatory mass or by a bronchogenic carcinoma. Carcinoids and germ cell tumours may or may not pick up gallium. Radioactive selenomethionine is picked up by a parathyroid adenoma and is therefore of particular help in the diagnosis of an ectopic mediastinal parathyroid adenoma.

Biochemical Markers

All patients with an anterior mediastinal mass should have a determination of the alphafoetoprotein (AFP), human chorionic gonadotropin (HCG) and the carcinoembryonic antigen

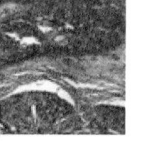
(CEA). Serum levels of HCG, AFP or both rise in the presence of non-seminomatous malignant germ cell tumour. Increased catecholamine secretion can be detected in pheochromocytomas through estimation of catecholamines, vanillyl mandelic acid, and metanephrine in the urine. Paragangliomas and neuroblastomas may occasionally secrete epinephrine and norepinephrine.

Biopsy Procedures Histological proof is very often (though not always) the sine qua non for a correct diagnosis. A CT-guided fine needle biopsy is most often used for diagnosis. It should, however, be avoided in a suspected well-encapsulated thymoma for fear of spillage of tumour cells that could prevent curative resection. Mediastinal adenopathy needs a CT-guided biopsy for diagnosis. Mediastinal biopsy or a thoracoscopic biopsy may at times be necessary. It is important to perform a biopsy in patients with mediastinal masses with raised AFP, HCG or CEA levels. This is because the treatment for patients with non-seminomatous germ cell tumours and for patients with small-cell carcinoma who show the above features is primarily chemotherapy followed by resection of residual disease. On the other hand, a biopsy procedure on a suspected pheochromocytoma is contraindicated.

Table 65.4: Investigation of mediastinal masses	
1) A good clinical history and examination	
2) Imaging Studies	X-ray chest—PA and lateral view, HRCT chest, MRI if necessary
3) Radionucleotide Studies (when necessary)	^{131}I uptake points to—substernal goitre, ^{131}I metaiodo benzyl guanidine uptake points to pheochromocytoma. Gallium scan—May help to distinguish thymoma from a lymphoma; gallium can also be picked up by an inflammatory mass or by a bronchogenic carcinoma Tc-99m Sestamibi—parathyroid adenoma
4) Biochemical markets	AFP, HCG and CEA in anterior mediastinal masses Catecholamine excretion in urine in suspected pheochromocytoma
5) Biopsy procedures	CT guided, fine needle or trucut biopsy Mediastinoscopic biopsy Thoracoscopic biopsy

ANTERIOR MEDIASTINAL MASSES

Thymoma

A thymoma consists of a neoplastic proliferation of thymic epithelial cells interspersed with mature (non-neoplastic) lymphocytes. It is the most common primary mediastinal neoplasm in adults and the most frequent neoplasm of the anterior mediastinum. It can occur at any age but generally affects adults over 40 years of age with no gender predilection. A thymoma is generally situated in front of the root of the aorta but may occasionally be found anywhere within the anterior mediastinum between the thoracic inlet and the diaphragm.

A thymoma may be totally confined within a surrounding capsule. It is then termed benign or non-invasive. On the other hand, a thymoma may break through the capsule and may further invade surrounding structures. It is then termed malignant or invasive. It is impossible on histopathological study to determine whether the cells comprising a thymoma are benign or malignant, hence it is more appropriate to use the terminology of non-invasive and invasive rather than benign and malignant when describing a thymoma. Most thymomas, (about 70%) are well-capsulated or non-invasive; the remaining break through the capsule to invade surrounding structures.

CLINICAL FEATURES

A thymoma may be asymptomatic, particularly when small, capsulated and non-invasive. Invasive thymomas as also large, non-invasive thymomas are often symptomatic, causing cough, vague chest pain and breathlessness. Pressure symptoms and signs are generally related to compression of the superior vena cava. Pressure on the recurrent laryngeal nerve causes hoarseness of the voice. These pressure symptoms generally occur with invasive thymomas. Invasive thymomas can produce symptoms and signs due to invasion of neighbouring structures. These include the mediastinum, the pericardium, the heart, the pleura and the pulmonary vessels. Pleural invasion may result in a pleural effusion or may spread to encase the lung on one side, entrapping the lung and mimicking a mesothelioma.

ASSOCIATION OF THYMOMAS WITH OTHER CLINICAL DISORDERS

1. Myasthenia Gravis. Myasthenia may be observed in one-third of patients, and is the most frequent disorder associated with a thymoma. It is estimated that 10% of patients with myasthenia may have a thymoma.
2. Haematological conditions. These include red-cell hypoplasia (5% of patients with thymomas), hypogammaglobulinaemia (in 10% with thymoma).
3. Collagen vascular diseases, such as polymyositis, scleroderma are reported to be rare associations.
4. Non-thymic malignancies including thyroid carcinoma, bronchogenic carcinoma, and lymphoma have also been reported.

IMAGING STUDIES

The location of the tumour in the anterior mediastinum generally in front of the aortic root, suggests the diagnosis. On cross-sectional HRCT imaging, the tumour is seen as a homogenous soft tissue mass. Large neoplasms may show heterogeneity due to necrosis, cystic changes or haemorrhage. Invasive thymomas, together with the nature and extent of invasion can generally be detected by CT scans. MRI scans are more effective in detecting vascular invasion. This is of importance before attempting surgical excision of invasive thymomas. Certain proof of invasiveness or non-invasiveness even in what appears to be a capsulated tumour can however only be judged at the time of surgical excision and by the demonstration of an unbroken capsule on histological study. Besides direct invasion, 'drop' metastasis leads to implantation of tumour seedlings into the ipsilateral pleura and pleural space. Imaging studies of pleural involvement are characterized by solid tumour tissue encasing the ipsilaterel lung or by an ipsilateral pleural effusion.

DIAGNOSIS

A definite diagnosis can be established by a CT-guided needle biopsy of the tumour mass, mediastinoscopic biopsy, and/or video-assisted thoracoscopy. In typical cases these diagnostic procedures are not always necessary.

PROGNOSIS

The staging classification of Masaoko and colleagues has been shown to correlate with resectability and survival. The revised 1999 World Health Organization (WHO) classification divides thymic epithelial neoplasms into Types A, B, C on the basis of epithelial cell morphology, the ratio of lymphocytes to epithelial cells and prognosis. Types A, B correlated with the usual major histological cell types of thymoma-epithelial cells, lymphocytes, lymphocytepithelial cells, and spindle cells. Type C refers to thymic carcinoma. Anatomical staging is based on the classification of Masaoko *et al.*

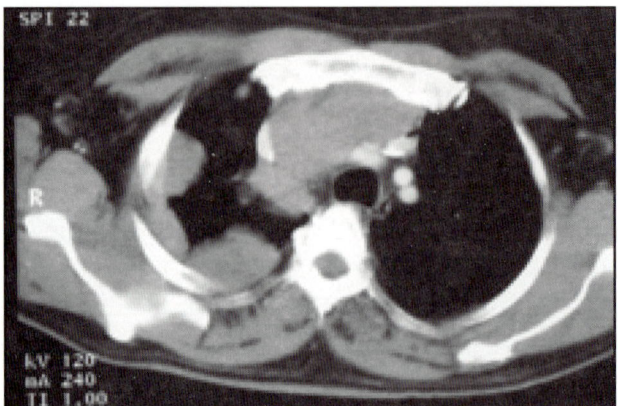

Fig 65.3: CT scan demonstrates an anterior mediastinal mass lesion in the midline displacing SVC to the right and great vessels to the left. Additionally, there are multiple pleural-based mass lesions. At surgery this mass lesion was an invasive thymoma.

Stage	Description	10-yr survival (%)
I	Encapsulated tumours without gross or microscopic invasion	85–100
II	Capsular or pleural invasion	60–84
III	Macroscopic invasion of lung, pericardium, vena cava or aorta	21–77
IV A	Disseminated disease within the chest	26–47
IV B	Distant metastasis	Unknown

Table 65.5: Staging of thymic malignancies

Source: Adapted from Masaoka A, *et al.* Follow-up study of thymoma with special reference in to their clinical stages. Cancer 48: 2485–92, 1981.

TREATMENT

Treatment is by excision of the thymic tumour mass. Excision of invasive tumour may involve resection of adjacent structures such as pericardium, part of the lung, major veins and the pleura. Radiotherapy is reserved for the unresectable invasive thymomas; chemotherapy involving protocols containing cisplatin may provide palliative relief.

The role of thymectomy in paraneoplastic syndromes related to thymomas is uncertain. In selected patients with myasthenia gravis (young patients with progressive symptoms) thymectomy is of use in the absence of a thymoma. There is complete remission in over one-third of patients and an improvement in more than half. Clinical improvement of myasthenia gravis is less likely in the presence of a thymoma. Thymectomy in patients with red-cell aplasia leads to 40–50% remission rates. Thymectomy is of no use in patients with hypogammaglobulinaemia.

Thymic Carcinoma

Thymic carcinomas are malignant epithelial tumours of the thymus (Type C of the revised WHO classification of thymic-epithelial tumours) which are locally invasive and metastasize to distant sites. Histopathologically, the cell types are either squamous cell or lymphoepithelial like carcinoma. Unlike

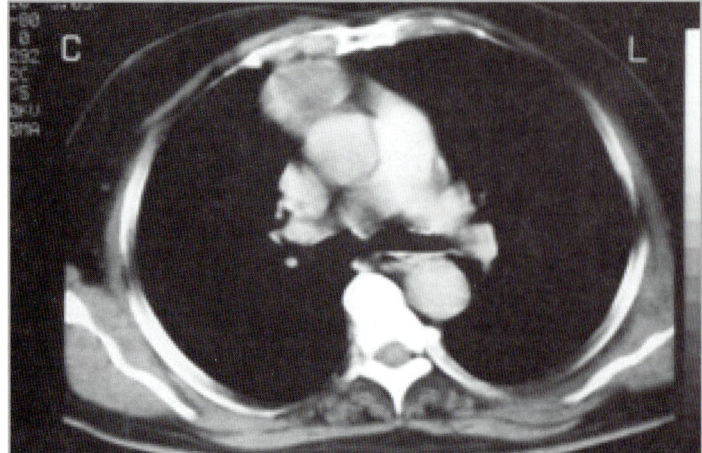

Fig 65.4: Non-invasive thymoma. Chest CT shows a well-defined mass lesion in the anterior mediastinum to the right of the midline. At surgery it was completely resectable with no invasion of surrounding structures nor any break in the capsule.

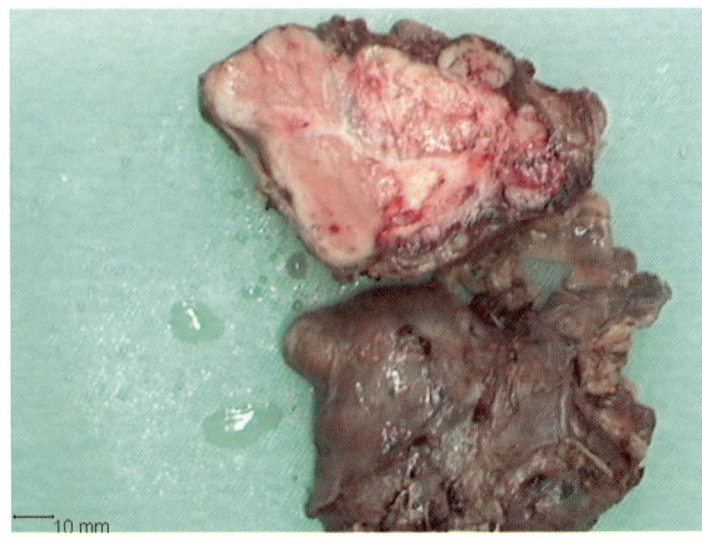

Fig 65.5: Gross section of a thymoma. External surface is smooth bosselated. Cut surface appears fleshy, lobulated with fibrous septae.

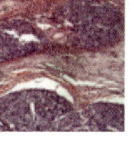

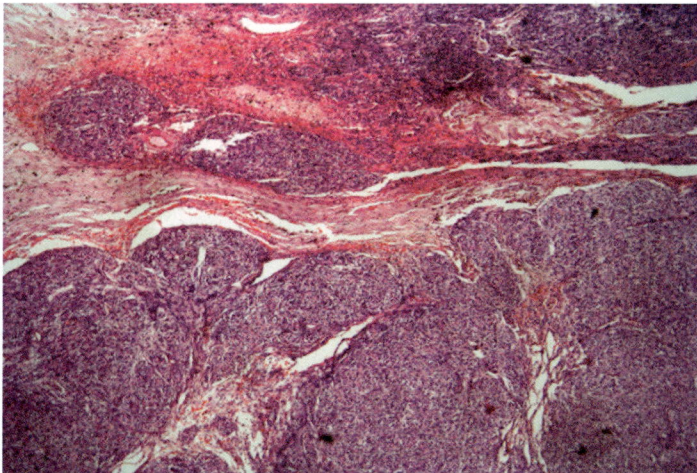

Fig 65.6: Microscopic picture of Type A thymoma. Multiple lobules separated by fibrous septae. This is the characteristic appearance of a thymoma.

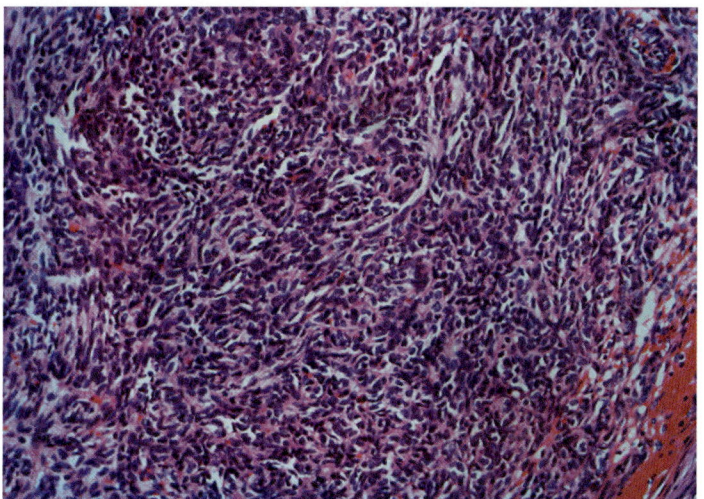

Fig 65.7: Microscopic picture of Type A thymoma. Spindle tumour cells in a vague fascicular arrangement, some cells being haphazardly distributed.

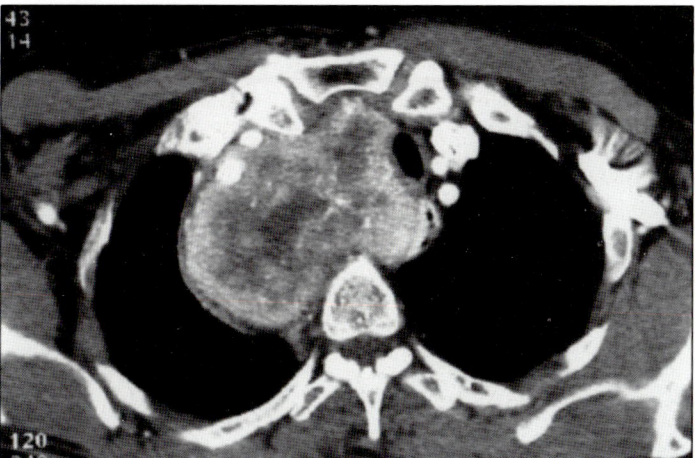

Fig 65.8: CT scan demonstrates a large heterogenous mass lesion in the anterior mediastinum displacing the trachea to the left and displacing and encasing the great vessels. The encasement is a strong sign of malignancy as benign lesions will displace and not encase. On biopsy this was a thyroid carcinoma.

thymomas, thymic carcinomas have the histological features of malignancy, and manifest as large anterior mediastinal masses with local infiltration, spread to lymph glands and to the lungs as also to distant sites.

Surgical resection (if possible) is the treatment of choice. Adjuvant radiotherapy plus cisplatin-based chemotherapy may help. The prognosis is poor even when total resection is possible, the five-year survival being less than 30%.

Thymic Carcinoids

Thymic carcinoids are aggressive neuroendocrine tumours, locally invasive with distant metastasis. They rarely produce the carcinoid syndrome but may be associated with the multiple endocrine neoplasia syndrome. Adenomas may be present in the parathyroids, adrenals and pituitary giving rise to hyperparathyroidism, Cushing's syndrome, or the inappropriate antidiuretic hormone secretion syndrome. Surgical treatment is advised in the absence of distant metastasis or extensive local invasion.

Thymolipoma

These are benign lipomatous tumours which may attain a large size but may have few or no compressive symptoms because of their softness. The HRCT of the chest shows a lobulated tumour of fat density. Surgical excision is necessary to establish a definite diagnosis and to prevent compressive symptoms.

Thymic Cysts

A thymic cyst is a benign rounded or ovoid cystic mass with sharply defined walls which may show calcification on an X-ray chest or on a CT examination. Thymic cysts usually occur in

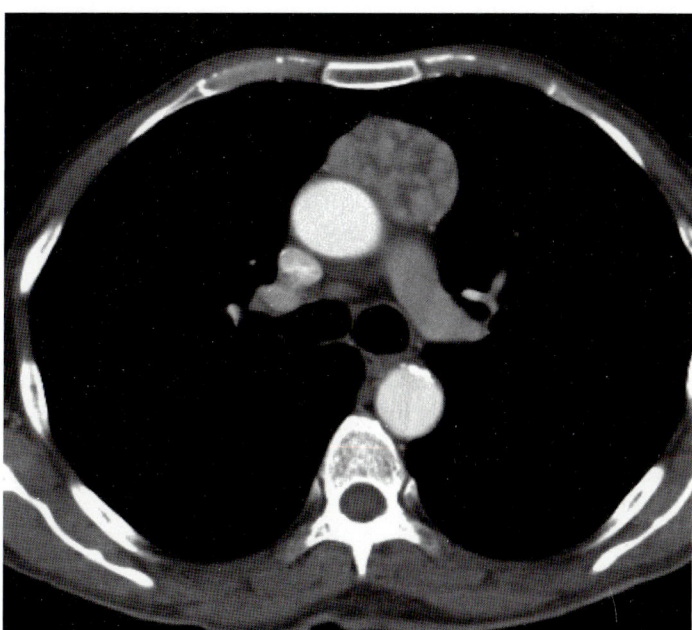

Fig 65.9: Thymic carcinoid. CT chest reveals a well-defined anterior mediastinal mass lesion with multiple well-defined nodular areas of enhancement within. Histopathology revealed this to be a thymic carcinoid.

children; they are asymptomatic and hardly ever produce compressive symptoms. They should be excised to establish a definite diagnosis so as not to miss out on a thymoma with cystic changes.

Thymic Hyperplasia

The thymus is relatively large in the newborn and the infant. It grows progressively up to puberty and then begins to involute so that it may be difficult to discern on imaging in the middle and older age group. If therefore the thymus gland appears larger than the range for a particular age group, and in particular if it is shown to progressively increase in size, it should be removed to exclude a thymoma. Thymic hyperplasia is the commonest histopathology found in thymic glands excised for myasthenia gravis. Thymic hyperplasia may also occur following chemotherapy for malignancies both in children and adults.

Mediastinal Germ Cell Tumour

Germ cell tumours generally originate in the testis or ovary; the commonest extra-gonadal site of this tumour is the anterior mediastinum. Mediastinal germ cell tumours are derived from primitive germ cells that fail to migrate during embryogenesis. They constitute about 15% of all mediastinal tumours in adults. It is always important to ensure that what appears to be a primary mediastinal germ cell tumour truly arises from the mediastinum and is not a metastatic lesion from an occult gonadal tumour. The latter may not always be clinically evident. Germ cell tumours are classified into teratomas, seminomas and non-seminomatous malignant germ cell tumours.

Mediastinal Teratoma

A mediastinal teratoma is invariably a benign tumour (mature teratomas or dermoid). It is the most frequent of germ cell tumours (over 50% of all cases) and consists of tissue from at least two of the three primitive germ cell layers. Ectodermal tissues generally predominate and include skin, hair, tooth, and sebaceous glands. Sebaceous secretions (when present within teratomas) are extremely irritant and result in a severe surrounding inflammatory reaction. Mesodermal tissue when present includes cartilage, bone, and smooth muscle. Tissues derived from the endoderm include respiratory and intestinal epithelium. Very rarely, teratomas are immature or malignant and are then classified as malignant teratomas or teratosarcomas.

Mature (benign) teratomas are histologically well-defined and benign. Though occurring at any age they typically occur in children and young adults. Patients are frequently asymptomatic, though large teratomas may produce pressure symptoms—notably cough, dyspnoea and vague chest pain. Rarely, a teratoma may open into a bronchus and the patient may cough up its contents, which may include clear or viscid fluid or even hair (trichophytosis).

Radiologically, teratomas present as well-defined spherical or lobulated anterior mediastinal masses which may show calcification of the wall or within the mass. Teeth and bone can occasionally be seen on imaging. A CT often shows multiloculation within the mass with fat attenuation.

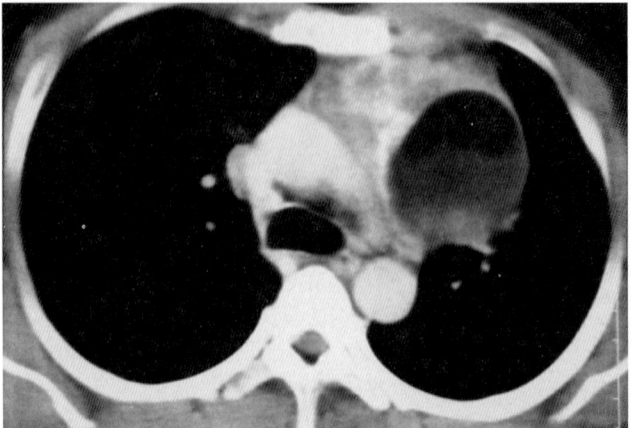

Fig 65.10: Teratoma. Chest contrast CT reveals an anterior mediastinal mass lesion to the left of the midline displacing vascular structures posteriorly. The mass contains solid as well as fat-density components. Histopathology showed teratoma.

Treatment of a teratoma is complete surgical excision, following which the prognosis is excellent.

Mediastinal Seminoma

Seminomas typically occur in adult males between the third and fifth decades and constitute 40–50% of malignant mediastinal germ cell tumours. It presents as a large lobulated homogenous anterior mediastinal mass, often causing dyspnoea, cough, and substernal pain. Gynaecomastia may be a presenting feature. Low-grade fever and weight loss may be the only symptoms, the mediastinal mass being detected as an investigative finding. Tumours may sometimes grow as large as 20–30 cm before pressure symptoms develop. About 10% of patients present with a superior vena caval syndrome. Seminomas are not associated with a rise in AFP levels, but a slight elevation of beta-HCG may be found. Invasion of mediastinal structures can occur particularly with large tumours; the tumour may spread to the lymph nodes and metastasize to the bones.

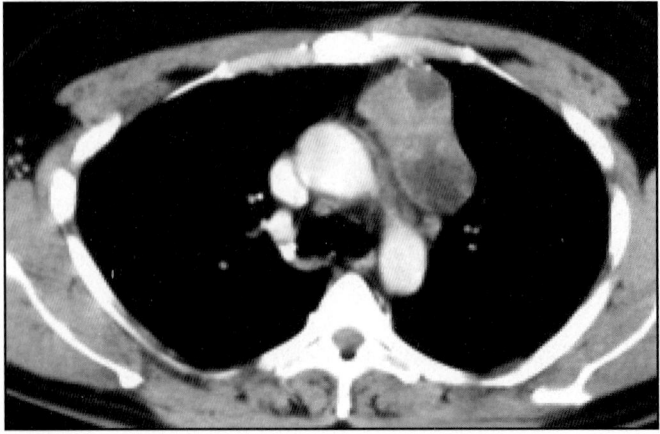

Fig 65.11: Malignant germ cell tumour. Chest CT with contrast demonstrates an anterior mediastinal mass to the left of the midline with internal areas of necrosis. Histopathology revealed a malignant germ cell tumour of the non-seminomatous variety. β-HCG was markedly elevated.

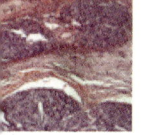

Cisplatin-based chemotherapy alone has led to a 90% disease-free survival rate. Additional radiation therapy offers only a slight further advantage in survival. Patients treated with radiation alone have a much higher rate of recurrence.

In patients with advanced disease, chemotherapy should be followed by excision of residual disease.

Mediastinal Non-seminomatous Germ Cell Tumour

These tumours are highly malignant and occur typically in young males invariably producing symptoms, either related to pressure on neighbouring structures or to local or distant spread. They are classified as choriocarcinoma, embryonal carcinoma, endodermal sinus (yolk-sac) tumour and mixed germ cell tumour. Tumour markers AFP and HCG are significantly elevated in choriocarcinoma, while AFP is significantly high in embryonic carcinoma. Non-seminomatous germ cell tumours may be associated with haematological disorders such as acute leukaemia and the myelodysplastic syndrome. Klinefelter's syndrome is another association in 20% of patients. Radiologically, these tumours manifest as large non-homogenous masses with areas of necrosis, haemorrhage, together with enhancing nodular soft tissue. Local invasion may lead to pericardial effusion and tamponade as also to pleural effusion. Lymph node and distant metastasis are frequently observed.

Treatment consists of courses of cisplatin-based chemotherapy followed if possible by resection of residual disease. The prognosis is worse when compared to a seminoma. The overall five-year survival being 48% compared to 86% in patients with seminomas.

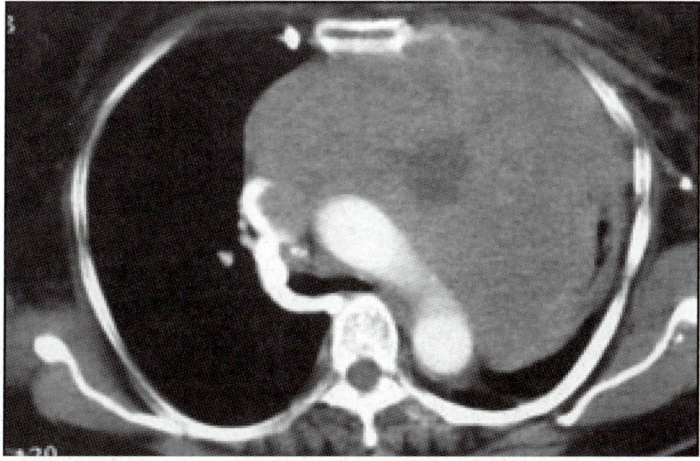

Fig 65.12: Malignant germ cell tumour of the seminomatous variety. A young man, 30 years old, presented with vague chest pain and shortness of breath. Chest X-ray showed a large mass involving the greater part of the left hemithorax. CT scan showed a large heterogeneous anterior mediastinal mass displacing vascular structures posteriorly as well as occupying a greater part of the left hemithorax. At surgery the entire mass was removed. Histopathology revealed a malignant germ cell tumour of the seminomatous variety.

Lymphomas

Lymphomas are best classified into Hodgkin's disease and non-Hodgkin's lymphoma. Lymphomas constitute 10–15% of all

mediastinal masses in adults; they occur in the anterior and/or middle mediastinal compartment but are rarely found in the posterior compartment. Approximately 20% of anterior mediastinal masses and 20% of middle mediastinal masses are lymphomas.

Mediastinal lymphomas are usually associated with generalized disease, lymph node involvement being present in one or more sites as well. Primary mediastinal lymphoma presenting as a solitary anterior mediastinal mass is uncommon comprising about 10% of all lymphomas.

The three most common forms of mediastinal lymphomas are the nodular sclerosing subtype of Hodgkin's disease, the large B-cell lymphoma and lymphoblastic lymphoma (subtypes of non-Hodgkin's lymphoma). Mediastinal lymphomas may be asymptomatic in about 25% of patients even when the glandular mass is fairly large. Symptomatic patients have systemic symptoms and/or present with pressure effects or with features of local invasion. Systemic features include fever, often of the Pel Ebstein type, weight loss, pruritus, anaemia and a significantly elevated erythrocyte sedimentation rate (often over 80mm/h). Local symptoms include chest discomfort, cough, and breathlessness. The superior vena caval compression syndrome may occur but is uncommon. Pressure on the trachea, bronchi can cause stridor, wheezing and dyspnoea.

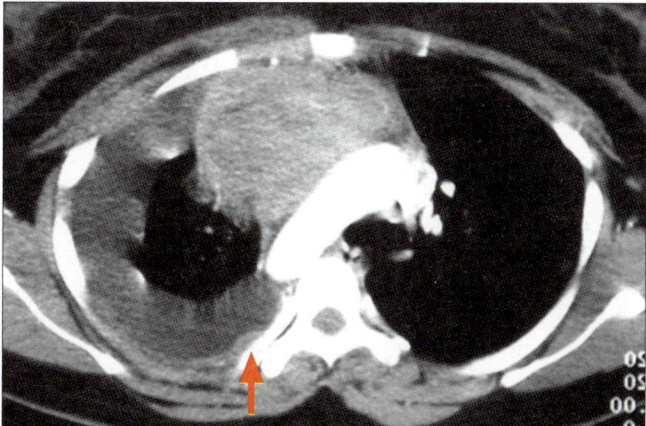

Fig 65.13: Non-Hodgkin's lymphoma. Chest CT reveals a heterogeneous anterior mediastinal mass lesion with an associated pleural effusion. Multiple pleural deposits are seen on the parietal surface of pleura (arrow). CT-guided biopsy showed Non-Hodgkin's lymphoma.

Hodgkin's Disease

The age distribution of patients with Hodgkin's disease is bimodal affecting individuals between 20–30 years of age or greater than 50 years of age. The nodular sclerosing subtype accounts for 90% of patients with Hodgkin's disease involving the mediastinum. Of these close to 50% have only mediastinal disease and the rest have involvement of other sites as well. The chest X-ray typically shows a superiorly placed mass in the anterior mediastinal compartment and/or in the middle compartment. Most often glands (pre-vascular and paratracheal) first appear in the anterior compartment and then spread by contiguity to the nodes of the middle compartment, to the hilar

nodes and then invade the lung. CT chest demonstrates this contiguous spread of disease. Skip involvement of lymph glands should prompt one to search for another diagnosis

Though systemic features are common in Hodgkin's disease, local invasion of the pleura, pericardium, and lungs generally occurs only when the mediastinal mass has reached a very large size.

The accompanying table gives the Ann Arbor classification of Hodgkin's disease. In Stages IA and IIA, radiotherapy generally suffices, though many centres now use limited chemotherapy. For advanced disease, Stage III, IV, chemotherapy is combined with radiotherapy. Cure rates of 90% are achieved in Stage I and Stage IIA. Even in patients with advanced disease, Stage III, and IV, cure rates as high as 60% have been observed.

Table 65.6: Ann Arbor classification of Hodgkin's Lymphoma	
Stage	**Features**
I	One lymph node region on either side of the diaphragm
II	Two or more lymph node regions on the same side of the diaphragm
III	Two or more lymph node regions on both sides of the diaphragm
IV	Disseminated organ involvement

Non-Hodgkin's Lymphoma

Non-Hodgkin's lymphoma involves cervical nodes, abdominal lymph nodes and lymphoid tissue of Waldreyer's rings far more often than the mediastinal nodes. Only 5% of non-Hodgkin's lymphoma present with a mediastinal mass. Thoracic lymphadenopathy can occur anywhere within the mediastinum and may involve unusual sites. Anterior mediastinal lymph node enlargement does occur but is less common than in Hodgkin's disease. These lymphomas are extremely aggressive so that pleural effusion, pericardial effusion and involvement of the lung parenchyma are commonly observed. Lymphoblastic lymphoma is commonly associated with an acute lymphoblastic leukaemia. Mediastinal spread (unlike in Hodgkin's disease) is typically non-contiguous and may occur in unusual sites, for example, in the posterior mediastinal, retrocrural sites. Non-Hodgkin's lymphomas consist of T-cell, B-cell, diffuse large cell lymphomas, and lymphoblastic lymphomas. According to the European American Classification of lymphoid neoplasms, non-Hodgkin's lymphomas are classified as indolent, aggressive or highly aggressive. Indolent lymphomas are more often associated with nodal disease; aggressive lymphomas are associated with extranodal involvement. Although untreated aggressive lymphomas have a poor prognosis, their potential for cure with chemotherapy is, remarkably enough, greater than indolent lymphomas. The treatment of indolent lymphomas depends on the stage of the disease and is often palliative.

DIAGNOSIS

Histological proof is imperative for a definite diagnosis. When the lymphoma is solely confined to the mediastinum histological proof is best provided by a video-assisted thoracoscopic biopsy, or a biopsy through mediastinoscopy or through an anterior mediastinomy. A CT-guided biopsy generally does not provide sufficient material to make both a correct histopathological diagnosis and typing of the lymphoma through immunohistochemical studies.

Lymphadenopathy within the mediastinum can be due to several other causes besides lymphoma. These must be considered in the differential diagnosis. Other causes of lymphadenopathy both benign and malignant are discussed in the section on masses in the middle mediastinum.

Intrathoracic Thyroid Masses

The commonest thyroid mass is an intrathoracic goitre resulting from an extension of a cervical goitre into the anterior superior mediastinum. Rarely, an ectopic-mediastinal thyroid goitre without any connection with a normally situated thyroid in the neck may also occur. Finally, cancer of the thyroid may extend into the anterior mediastinal compartment. A retrosternal goitre may be asymptomatic or if sufficiently large may compress the trachea causing dyspnoea, stridor, cough, or the superior vena caval syndrome. Dysphagia results from pressure on the oesophagus. The significance of a loud wheeze produced by pressure on the trachea has been occasionally missed and wrongly diagnosed as asthma. The wheeze is monophonic and though audible over both sides of the chest is best heard over the trachea and the manubrium.

X-ray of the chest in a patient with intrathoracic goitre demonstrates a cervicothoracic mass. CT demonstrates a well-defined lobular mass in the anterior-superior mediastinum, contiguous with the lower pole of the thyroid within the neck. The mass may be heterogeneous because of cystic changes or haemorrhage within it, is anterior to the trachea and generally to the right. Rarely, an intrathoracic goitre descends lateral to the trachea and may come to lie posterior to it. Pressure on the trachea if present is easily observed.

Marked enhancement of the mass generally follows after the administration of intravenous contrast. Isotope scans (^{131}I or technetium 99m) if positive are diagnostic. However, a

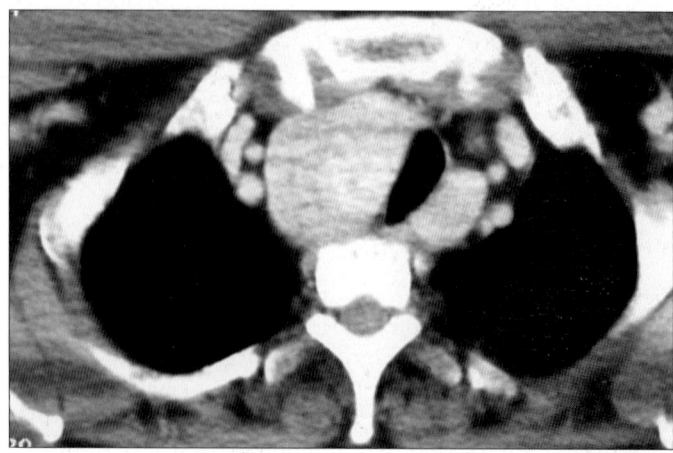

Fig 65.14: Retrosternal goitre. CT chest demonstrates a homogenously enhancing mass lesion in the prevertebral region displacing the trachea to the left and compressing it. This is a retrosternal goitre.

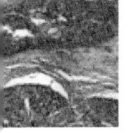

retrosternal goitre may be non-functioning; negative isotope scans do not therefore exclude a thyroid origin of a mass in the anterosuperior mediastinum.

If a thyroid mediastinal mass is symptomatic it should be excised. Even if asymptomatic and particularly if it is large, excision is advisable, as sudden haemorrhage into the gland can produce severe upper airways' obstruction.

Parathyroid Masses

A parathyroid mass may be an adenoma of one of the inferior parathyroid glands extending by continuity into the anterior mediastinum: It could also be due to an ectopic functioning parathyroid adenoma which is generally situated anteriorly in the mediastinum close to the thymus gland. It presents as a small encapsulated mass which is missed on an X-ray chest and often mistaken for a lymph node in a CT of the chest. Localization is achieved by radioisotope studies using ^{99m}Tc. Localization through radioisotopes should be correlated with CT or MRI. An ectopic parathyroid mass should be assiduously sought in patients with features of hyperparathyroidism who show neither an adenoma nor hyperplasia of the gland in the neck, or in patients in whom features of hyperparathyroidism persist even after removal of a parathyroid adenoma within the neck. A functioning parathyroid adenoma should be excised.

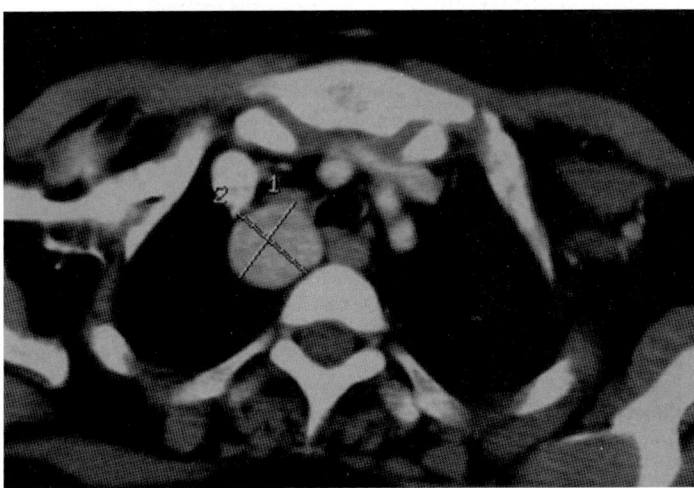

Fig 65.15: Parathyroid adenoma. Well-defined homogenously enhancing mass lesion in right paratracheal region. Excision biopsy showed parathyroid adenoma.

Pericardial Cysts

These are termed spring-water cysts because of the clear fluid contents. They are asymptomatic, most often found in middle-aged adults, and are discovered on a routine X-ray of the chest. A pericardial cyst is a developmental lesion typically found in the right cardiophrenic angle. CT demonstrates a non-enhancing cystic mass lesion of water attenuation, with a very thin barely perceptible cyst wall. It generally requires no treatment.

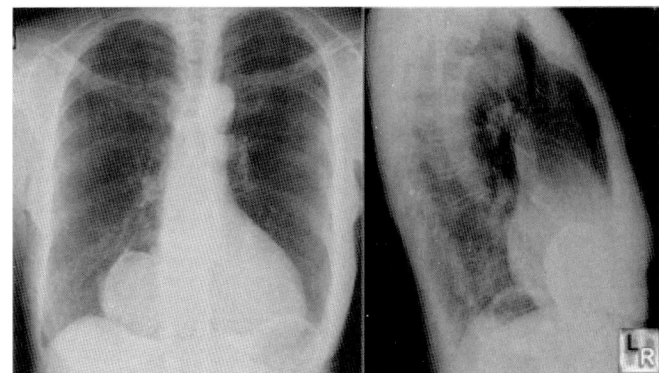

Fig 65.16: Pericardial cyst. (a) X-ray chest PA and (b) lateral demonstrate a well-defined homogenous opacity in the right paracardiac region with peripheral calcification representing a pericardial cyst.

Morgagni's Hernia

Hernia through the Foramen of Morgagni presents as a fairly large mass within the anteroinferior aspect of the anterior me-

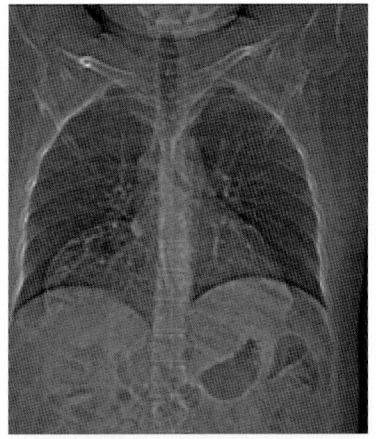

(a)

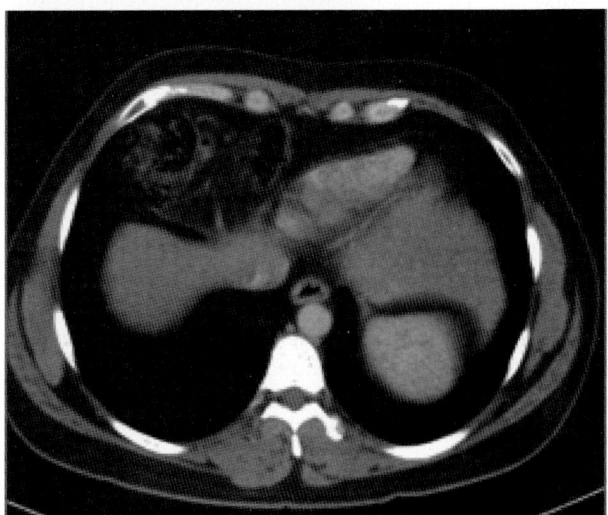

(b)

Fig 65.17: Morgagni's hernia. (a) CT scannogram demonstrates bowel loops in the right paracardiac region. These loops are anterior as there is no silhouetting with the diaphragm (b) This is confirmed on the CT and represents a Morgagni's hernia.

diastinum. It generally includes the large bowel and omentum, but other viscera may also be found. A barium study may disclose the contents of the hernia. A CT is diagnostic, revealing the fat attenuation produced by omentum and the pockets of air within the herniated gut. Surgery is necessary to reduce the contents of the hernia and to repair the defect through which herniation occurred.

Rare Mediastinal Tumours

An example of a rare anterior mediastinal tumour is a lipoma which can attain a huge size producing severe compression of the mediastinum, great vessels, heart and lungs.

MASSES IN THE MIDDLE MEDIASTINUM

Mediastinal Cysts

Congenital foregut cysts represent 12–20% of mediastinal masses. When related to the trachea or major bronchi they are termed bronchogenic cysts and when related to the oesophagus in its cervical or mediastinal course, they are termed gastroenteric and neuroenteric cysts.

Bronchogenic Cysts

These are formed during embryonic development following abnormal ventral budding of the foregut. A bronchogenic cyst is most commonly found in the subcarinal or paratracheal region and is lined with pseudostratified columnar epithelium. It contains bronchial mucus-secreting glands, cartilage and smooth muscle within its wall and is filled with serous fluid or mucus. Bronchogenic cysts can occur at any age but are most frequently seen in young adults. They often are asymptomatic but may produce symptoms, especially when large and in children. The commonest pressure symptoms are cough and breathlessness. Large cysts, particularly in children, can compress an airway causing air-trapping, atelectasis and infection in the atelectatic area.

Infection of the cyst contents converts the cyst into an abscess, causing fever with other systemic features of infection. When a bronchogenic cyst communicates with a bronchus, an air-fluid level is observed. Radiography reveals a well-defined spherical middle mediastinal mass, sometimes extending towards the posterior mediastinum. On CT these cysts are homogenous, without loculi and with varying attenuation, depending on the cyst contents. The cyst wall may show calcification; though generally non-enhancing, it may rarely enhance following the administration of contrast. An MRI may help to differentiate the lesion from other masses. A tissue diagnosis for a definite diagnosis can be made by tracheobronchial, CT-guided or a thoracoscopic needle aspiration. Aspirated fluid typically reveals mucus and bronchial epithelial cells.

Surgical excision is the treatment of choice. Small asymptomatic cysts with a confirmed diagnosis may be followed up clinically and by imaging studies, as surgery is not without some risk. In poor-risk symptomatic patients, the cyst can be drained through a CT-guided, transbronchial or thoracoscopic approach.

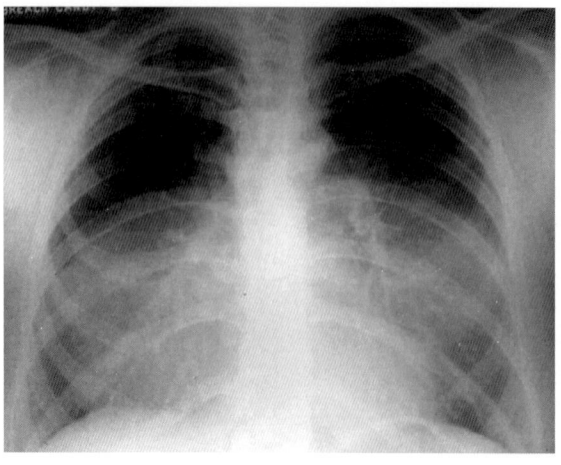
(a)

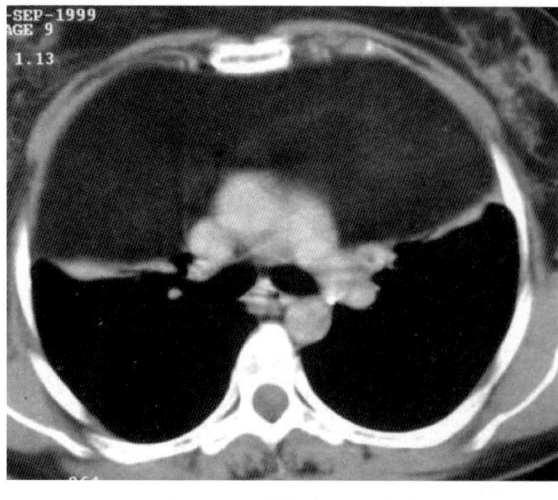
(b)

Fig 65.18: Mediastinal lipoma. Chest CT demonstrates the bilateral homogenous opacities seen on the chest X-ray (a) which are of fat density on the CT scan. (b) This was a mediastinal lipoma in a young 36-year-old lady who complained of marked breathlessness over some years. It was resected but postoperatively, she went into cardiorespiratory failure resistant to all support.

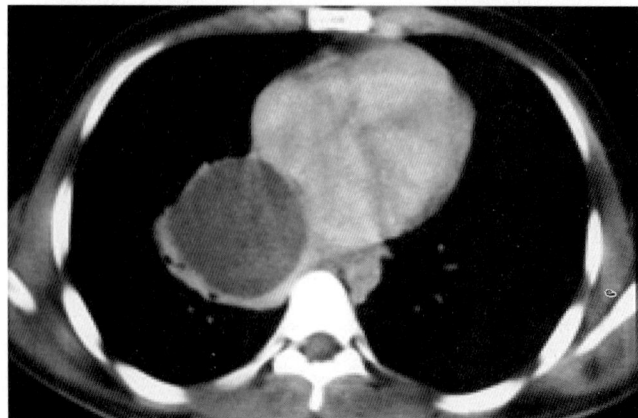

Fig 65.19: Bronchogenic cyst. Chest CT with contrast demonstrates a well-defined homogenous fluid-density lesion along the right paracardiac surface in the middle mediastinum causing compression of the adjacent lung. Surgery revealed a bronchogenic cyst.

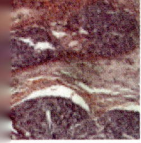

Enterogenous Cysts

Originate from the dorsal foregut and are located either in the middle or posterior mediastinum, more often in the latter. They are lined by squamous or enteric epithelium and may contain gastric or pancreatic tissue. Oesophageal duplication cysts are located in or are attached to the oesophageal wall and are associated with gastrointestinal malformations in 12% of cases.

Enterogenous cysts typically manifest in childhood as spherical well-defined cystic masses. Radiological features are indistinguishable from a bronchogenic cyst. Though often asymptomatic, haemorrhage or rupture may occur when gastric epithelium or pancreatic tissue is present.

Surgical excision is the treatment of choice. The prognosis after removal is excellent.

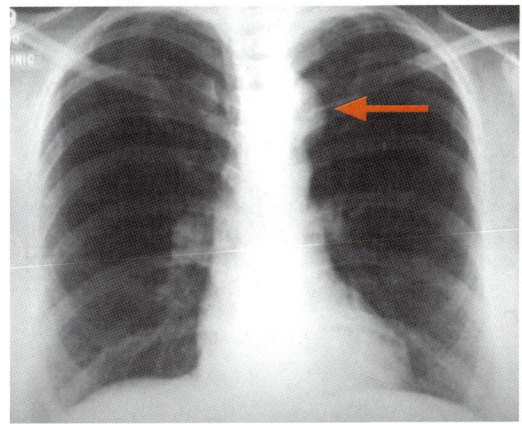

Fig 65.20a: Enterogenous cyst. Chest X-ray reveals a well-defined homogenous mass on the left side just above the aortic arch.

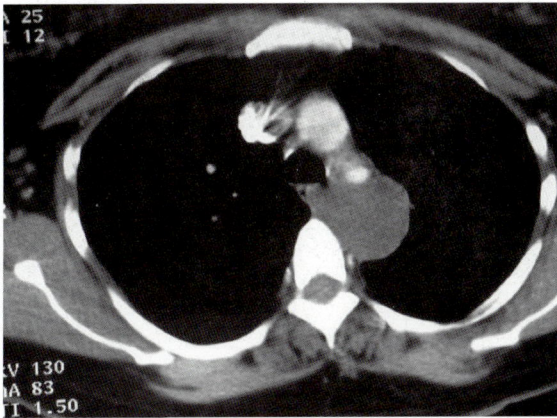

Fig 65.20b: CT reveals that the opacity seen on the chest X-ray is a well-defined homogenous cystic mass in close relation to the oesophagus representing an enterogenous cyst.

Aneurysm of Major Vessels

Aneurysm of the ascending aorta, the arch of the aorta and of any of the vessels arising from the arch may mimic a mediastinal mass within any compartment of the mediastinum. Thus an aneurysm of the ascending aorta, the aortic root or of the sinus of Valsalva may appear as an anterior mediastinal mass; an aneurysm of the arch may point anteriorly or extend into the posterior mediastinum while an aneurysm of the innominate or carotid vessels lies within the confines of the superior mediastinum and can extend in any direction.

Aneurysm of the ascending aorta is most often due to atherosclerosis but may occur with dissection of the aorta, syphilis or Marfan's syndrome. Aortic regurgitation may be an associated feature. A dissecting aneurysm involving the aorta proximal to the origin of the left subclavian needs surgery in spite of the hazard involved. An expanding aneurysm of the ascending or arch of the aorta may also require surgery.

Aneurysms of the pulmonary artery or its major branches also occupy the middle mediastinum.

A cardiac aneurysm following a myocardial infarction may arise from the anterolateral aspect or posterior aspect of the heart.

An aneurysm should be suspected when a mediastinal lesion or mass is adjacent to major vessels. CT with contrast enhancement of the involved vessel is diagnostic. Arteriography may still be necessary both for accurate diagnosis and planned treatment.

Benign Mediastinal Lymphadenopathy

Tuberculosis is unquestionably the commonest cause of infectious granulomatous mediastinal lymphadenopathy in our country and in most developing countries of the world. Areas of necrosis and liquefaction within the glands almost always point to tuberculosis. Histoplasmosis and Coccidiomycosis may cause granulomatous mediastinal lymphadenopathy in countries where these fungal infections are endemic. Bacterial and viral infections may rarely cause a benign lymphadenopathy. The viral infection to particularly bear in mind is an Epstein-Barr virus infection. Invariably, mediastinal adenopathy in this viral infection is associated with adenopathy elsewhere, in particular the cervical region.

The most important non-infectious granulomatous disease, perhaps all over the world including India is sarcoidosis. It typically produces bilateral hilar adenopathy with or without mediastinal adenopathy. Unilateral hilar adenopathy is uncommon and should prompt one to seek other causes. Also, bilateral hilar adenopathy can occur in tuberculosis and occasionally in lymphomas. Though an elevated serum angiotensin converting enzyme (SACE) level may help, it is not specific for sarcoidosis and is also observed in tuberculosis and lymphoma. Silicosis can also cause both hilar and mediastinal adenopathy. Egg shell calcification is not specific to silicosis; it can occur in sarcoidosis and in tuberculosis.

Other causes of benign masses in the middle mediastinum include drugs such as phenytoin, and Castleman's disease (angiofollicular lymphoid hyperplasia). Castleman's disease is an uncommon disease of unknown aetiology affecting young adult males; it generally produces no symptoms. Nodal enhancement after contrast can be marked because of hypervascularity. The hyaline vascular histologic type accounts for 90% of this disease. It is benign but may rarely produce compression symptoms. The plasma cell variety is associated with fever, weight loss, anaemia and hypergammaglobulinemia. Surgical exci-

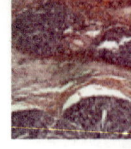

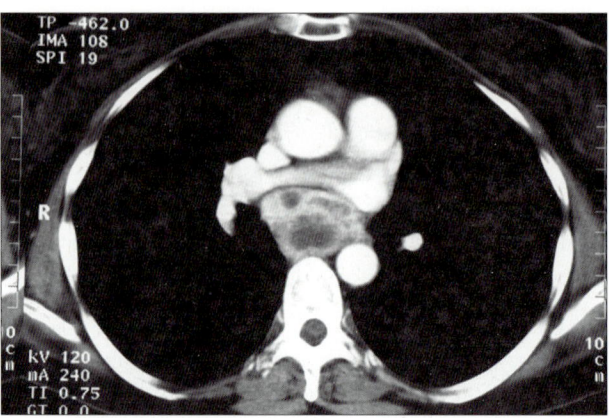

Fig 65.21: Tuberculous subcarinal lymphadenopathy. Note multiple areas of necrosis indicating a tubercular aetiology.

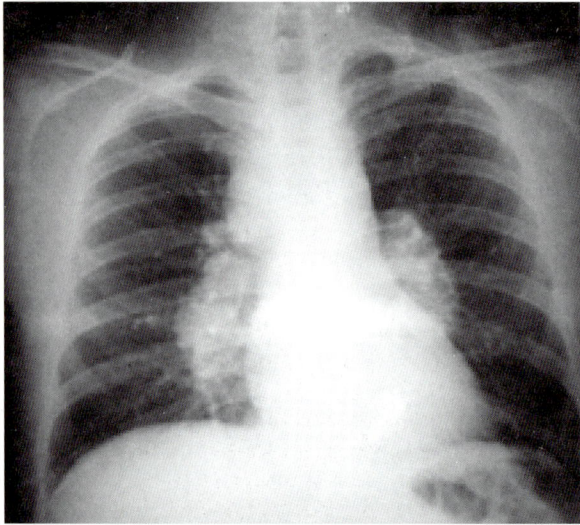

Fig 65.22: Sarcoidosis. Chest X-ray demonstrates large hilar and paratracheal adenopathy. Biopsy revealed sarcoidosis.

sion of nodes produces relief. The multicentric type is rare and is associated with severe systemic symptoms, generalized adenopathy, and hepatosplenomegaly. It graduates into a non-Hodgkin's lymphoma.

Metastatic Lymphadenopathy

Metastatic lymph node involvement is a common and important cause of mediastinal lymphadenopathy involving the middle mediastinal compartment. The common sites of a primary neoplasm are the lung, breast, gastrointestinal tract, kidney and prostate. Melanomas also metastasize to the mediastinum as do germ cell tumours arising within the testis or ovary. The secondaries in the mediastinum may involve just one group of glands or cause multifocal involvement.

Metastatic mediastinal lymphadenopathy should always enter the differential diagnosis of any mass within the mediastinum. A primary source if not evident should be assiduously sought. The diagnosis needs to be confirmed by a biopsy.

POSTERIOR MEDIASTINAL TUMOURS

Neurogenic Tumours

Neurogenic tumours arise from the tissue of the neural crest, including cells of the peripheral, autonomic and paraganglionic nervous system. They are classified according to cell type and constitute 12–20% of adult and 40% of all paediatric mediastinal tumours. Over 95% of these occur in the paravertebral region. Neurogenic tumours occurring in adults are most often benign; 50% of neurogenic tumours in the paediatric age group are malignant. Approximately 50% of patients affected are asymptomatic.

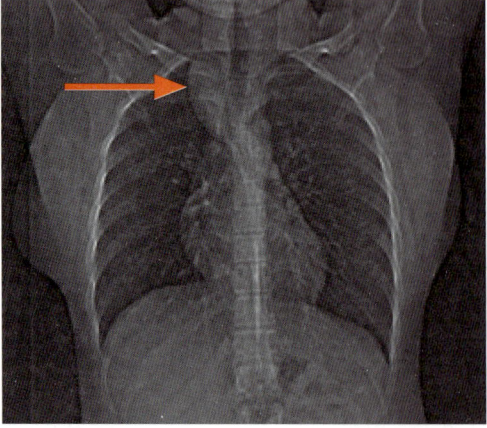

Fig 65.23a: Neurogenic tumour. X-ray demonstrates well-defined homogenous mass in right paratracheal region.

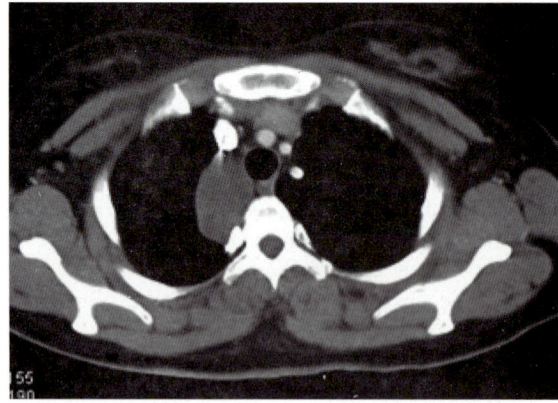

Fig 65.23b: Axial CT of the same patient demonstrates right paravertebral mass lesion representing a neurogenic tumour.

Nerve Sheath Tumours

Tumours arising from nerve sheaths are benign slowly-growing tumours comprising 40–60% of neurogenic mediastinal masses and are either schwannomas or neurofibromas. The latter may be associated with von Recklinghausen's neurofibromatosis. Both schwannomas and neurofibromas are generally asymptomatic and are discovered incidentally. Large tumours may however cause erosion and deformity of the ribs and vertebral bodies. Ten per cent of these tumours grow through the in-

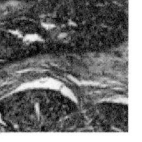
tervertebral foramina and create a dumb-bell-shaped appearance on imaging studies.

Radiologically, schwannomas and neurofibromas appear as spherical, sharply outlined, occasionally lobular masses extending one to three rib spaces. They could however attain a large size. Benign pressure erosion of one or more ribs, vertebral body or neural foramina may be observed. CT shows a sharply defined paravertebral mass which may be heterogeneous and show punctate calcification. An MRI should always be done to determine if there is an intraspinal extension of the growth. The treatment is surgical resection.

Malignant Peripheral Nerve Tumours

These are the malignant counterparts of schwannomas and neurofibromas. They are rare and occur equally in men and women between 30 to 50 years of age. Nearly half of mediastinal neurofibromas occur in patients with neurofibromatosis. The incidence of malignant change in neurogenic tumours in patients with neurofibromatosis is close to 5%.

Increasing pain due to pressure on the ribs and vertebrae are the usual symptoms. Intraspinal extension can result in pressure on the spinal cord. Radiologically on a CT, they may appear sharply defined fast-growing tumours often with manifest erosion of ribs and vertebral bodies.

Sympathetic Ganglion Neoplasms

Sympathetic ganglion neoplasms arise from the sympathetic ganglia in the paravertebral region. They affect both children and young adults; in children they are frequently malignant.

Ganglioneuromas

Ganglioneuromas are benign tumours affecting males and females equally. Pain from rib or vertebral erosion and intraspinal extension occurs in 50% of patients. Radiologically, they form well-defined, large paravertebral masses extending over three to five vertebrae. Pressure effects may be observed. MRI is necessary to determine the presence and extent of intraspinal extension which occurs far more frequently than with benign nerve sheath tumours. Surgical resection is the treatment of choice.

Ganglioneuroblastoma

Ganglioneuroblastomas are malignant neoplasms, generally occurring in children less than 10 years of age. Symptoms result from erosive pressure on neighbouring structures or from local and distant metastasis. Staging and treatment are as for a neuroblastoma. Prognosis however is more favourable when compared to neuroblastoma.

Neuroblastoma

Neuroblastoma is a tumour occurring in young children, with 95% of them occurring below five years of age. It is a highly aggressive, non-encapsulated, posterior mediastinal tumour that spreads locally and metastasizes quickly. The tumour on

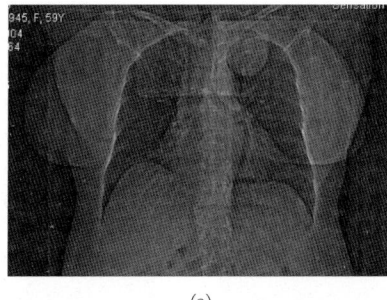

(a)

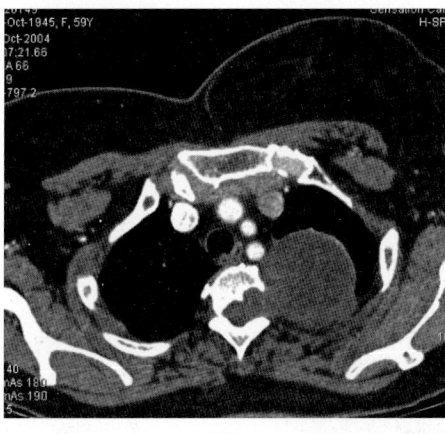

(b)

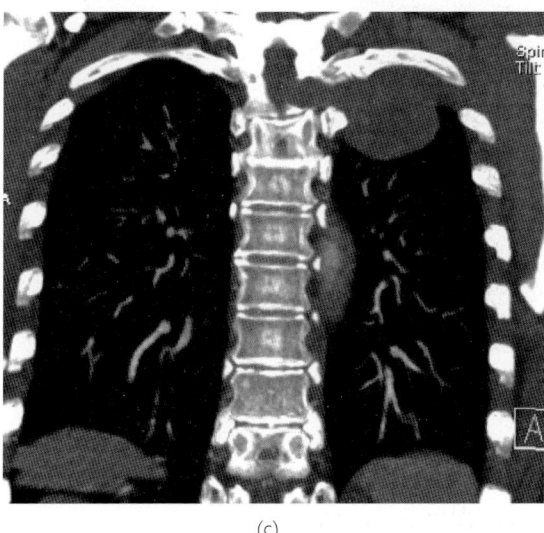

(c)

Fig 65.24: Neurofibroma. (a) Scannogram demonstrates a well-defined mediastinal mass in the left paravertebral region. (b) This is well seen on the axial images in the left paravertebral region extending into the spinal canal widening the neural foramen, scalloping the posterior surface of the vertebral body and compressing the dorsal cord, giving rise to long tract signs. (c) Similar features are seen on the coronal reconstructions. This was a neurofibroma extending through the neural foramen compressing the cord.

a macroscopic examination often shows necrosis, haemorrhage and cystic degeneration. Microscopically, it consists of mitotic small round cells arranged in sheets or rosettes.

Patients are invariably symptomatic either because of local spread and pressure effects or because of distant metastasis.

Pain due to erosion of vertebrae, cough and respiratory distress are commonly encountered. The tumour can invade and infiltrate through the foramina causing pressure and involvement of nerve roots and the spinal cord. Neurological deficits include paraplegia and Horner's syndrome. Neuroblastomas have a propensity to produce vasoactive substances like catecholamines and vasoactive intestinal peptides. The former result in tachycardia and hypertension; the latter cause flushing and severe watery diarrhoea. Radiologically, a neuroblastoma appears as a large paraspinal mass impinging on adjacent structures, crossing the midline, causing skeletal erosion and neurological damage. On a CT scan, 80% of these tumours show calcification; the tumours are heterogeneous because of haemorrhage and necrosis. An MRI should always be done to determine the presence and extent of intraspinal extension.

Neuroblastomas should be treated if possible by surgical resection. Chemotherapy and radiation may either follow resection to deal with residual disease, or may form primary therapy following which resection may be attempted.

The prognosis is poor and depends on the age at diagnosis, the size, the stage of the tumour and the histological differentiation.

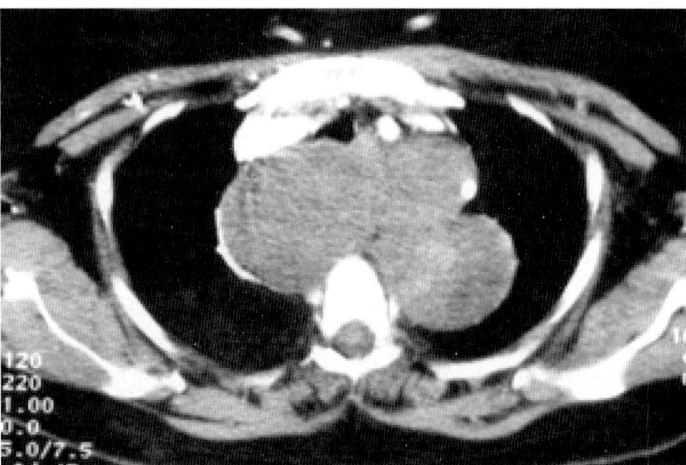

Fig 65.25: Neuroblastoma. Axial CT demonstrates a large lobulated mass in the posterior mediastinum displacing the trachea and vascular structures anteriorly, representing a neuroblastoma.

Paraganglionic Neoplasms

PHEOCHROMOCYTOMA
Paragangliomas are pheochromocytomas that most often arise from the adrenal glands. Two per cent of pheochromocytomas arise within the thorax, radiologically evident as enhancing well-localized posterior mediastinal masses. Pheochromocytomas occasionally occur as part of the multiple endocrine neoplasia (MEN2) syndrome. Symptoms are due to excessive catecholamine secretion or due to pressure on adjacent structures. Paroxysmal hypertension, hypertension with diabetes, hypermetabolic syndrome, and acute hypertension following anaesthesia for a surgical procedure are common presenting features due to excessive catecholamine secretion. Diagnosis is made by measuring urine catecholamines and their metabolites, in particular noting elevated levels of vanillylmandelic acid, metanephrine and norepinephrine in the urine. The diagnosis can be clinched if a tumour mass anywhere within the abdomen or thorax picks up the radioactive isotope, ^{131}I metaiodo benzyl guanidine (MIBG).

Treatment consists of the use of alpha and beta blockers for a couple of weeks before excision.

PARAGANGLIOMAS
Paragangliomas are rare tumours of paraganglion cells. They are benign, non-functioning, well-localized tumours situated in the posterior mediastinum in the paravertebral area or the middle mediastinum adjacent to the aorta or pulmonary artery. They show marked enhancement after contrast administration due to their vascularity. Treatment is by excision.

Other Posterior Mediastinal Masses

OESOPHAGEAL CANCER
An oesophageal cancer may extend outwards and produce a posterior mediastinal mass. Dysphagia is the prominent symptom. The relation of this mass to the oesophagus is easily determined by a CT study and also by oesophagoscopy. Surgery is the treatment of choice. In extensive disease chemotherapy is given to start with; residual disease can then be tackled whenever possible by surgery.

ANEURYSM OF THE DESCENDING AORTA
An aneurysm of the descending aorta is generally due to atherosclerosis or a dissection of the aorta which may extend below the origin of the subclavian artery to a varying extent. An aneurysm of the descending aorta often causes persistent pain over the thoracic spine due to erosion of one or more vertebrae. A systolic bruit may be heard over the spine generally to the left of the midline. The aneurysm may mimic a posterior mediastinal tumour mass but its relation with the aorta is easily determined by cross-sectional CT imaging. Whenever possible and particularly when symptomatic surgery is advised.

PARAVERTEBRAL TUBERCULAR ABSCESS
A paravertebral cold abscess should always be considered in the differential diagnosis of a posterior mediastinal mass. It could arise from tubercle involving the spine, or it could be due to tuberculosis involving the posterior end of the ribs or rarely from tuberculosis of the lymph glands in the posterior mediastinum. Spinal tuberculosis is evident on radiography and CT imaging of the spine. Erosion of endplates of adjacent vertebrae with involvement of the discs between vertebrae with a soft-tissue paraverterbral shadow are the diagnostic features. Pain in the back as also neurological symptoms and signs due to pressure on nerve roots or the spinal cord may be observed. Systemic symptoms of fever and weight loss are often seen and may precede local signs of pain in the back by weeks or even months. Bed rest for three to six weeks with the use of anti-tuberculosis drugs for a year invariably effects a cure. Large paravertebral cold abscesses need to be aspirated. Cord compression always necessitates surgical intervention.

HIATUS HERNIA
A large herniation of the stomach through the oesophageal hiatus into the chest manifests as a large retrocardiac posterior

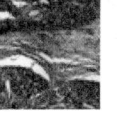

mediastinal mass. Diagnosis is confirmed by visualizing the stomach or other abdominal contents on a cross-sectional CT of the chest. Small or moderate-sized hernias can be managed conservatively. Symptomatic or large hernias need surgery.

EXTRAMEDULLARY HAEMATOPOIESIS

Extramedullary Haematopoiesis can present as a large posterior mediastinal mass. It produces no symptoms and is discovered on imaging. It develops only in those with abnormal bone marrow function and should be particularly considered in patients with thalassemia. A fine needle aspiration biopsy is pathologically characteristic; resection is not indicated.

MISCELLANEOUS DISORDERS OF THE MEDIASTINUM

Acute Mediastinitis

Acute mediastinitis carries significant morbidity and mortality. The mediastinum contains loose connective tissue enclosing and connecting organs and structures within. This allows an easy spread of infection within a mediastinal compartment as also spread from one compartment to the other. Acute infection may take the form of diffuse cellulitis or a mediastinal abscess.

Acute mediastinitis is due to the following causes—

1. **Postoperative** following trans-sternal operative procedures—chiefly cardiac procedures.
2. **Oesophageal perforation** A tear with perforation of the oesophagus can be due to forceful vomiting (Mallory Weiss syndrome), a tumour, a foreign body, or due to instrumental procedures such as endoscopy. Attempts at stenting an obstructed segment, or at dilatation of an oesophageal stricture or of an achalasia can result in an oesophageal tear. It can also occur after variceal sclerosis or following tube placements (Sengstaken Blakemore tube and very rarely a nasogastric tube).
3. **A descending infection** originating in the oral cavity, pharynx or cervical tissue. This infection can spread by continuity and contiguity along tissue planes, resulting in a necrotizing mediastinitis.
4. **An upward extension of a sub-diaphragmatic infection** into the mediastinum chiefly by way of tissue planes connecting the retroperitoneal space with the mediastinum.
5. **A direct extension of infection** from a necrotizing pneumonia into the mediastinum causing a mediastinitis is occasionally observed, particularly in immunocompromised patients.
6. **Penetrating injuries of the chest** close to the midline can also result in acute mediastinitis.
7. **Anthrax mediastinitis.**

OESOPHAGEAL PERFORATION

This is the commonest cause of acute mediastinitis in medical intensive care units through causes listed above. The Mallory Weiss syndrome and instrumental procedures are the commonest of these causes. Increasing substernal and upper abdominal pain is often associated with tachypnoea, tachycardia,

dysphagia and shock in severe cases. An important symptom often observed with a large perforation of the distal oesophagus is inability of the patient to lie down because of unbearable increase in severity of pain. Increasing tachyponea and desaturation is observed in these patients when they attempt to lie flat. The patient therefore sits leaning forward.

Two radiological criteria are helpful in diagnosis. The first is the presence of a pleural effusion—left-sided when the distal oesophagus is involved and right-sided when there is a perforation in the mid- or proximal oesophagus. At times a distal oesophageal perforation is associated with bilateral pleural effusion. The second radiological sign is the presence of pneumomediastinum. The air in the mediastinum may track up the tissue planes into the neck causing surgical emphysema with a crepitus on palpation. It is advisable never to perform an endoscopy to locate a tear as this can produce further trauma. A water-soluble contrast dye when swallowed generally outlines the tear but may fail to do so if the perforation is small. A barium swallow will however reveal a small perforation not identified by a water contrast agent.

Small perforations with normal haemodynamics and absence of sepsis may be treated conservatively with antibiotics, drainage of pleural fluid and with stoppage of all oral feeds. If symptoms worsen or there is increasing sepsis with mediastinitis, surgical repair is advised.

In patients who are severely symptomatic, show evidence of mediastinal sepsis with moderately large pleural effusions or who are haemodynamically unstable, surgery should be prompt. Early surgical management is critical for survival. Patients coming late into critical care after the onset of symptoms following a large tear in the oesophagus, have increased morbidity and mortality in spite of surgery.

Table 65.7: Etiology of acute mediastinitis
1. **Post-operative following trans-sternal operative procedures**

2. **Oesophageal performation:**
  (a) Mallory Weiss Syndrome
  (b) Iatrogenic
  (c) Tumour or foreign body

3. **Descending necrotizing mediastinitis**
4. **An upward extension of a sub-diaphragmatic infection**
5. **Direct extension of infection from a necrotizing pneumonia**
6. **Penetrating injuries of the chest**
7. **Anthrax mediastinitis**

DESCENDING NECROTIZING MEDIASTINITIS

A descending necrotizing mediastinitis is a complication of pharyngeal, tonsilar, retropharyngeal or cervical abscess. Infections can be due to beta-haemolytic streptococci, staphylococci, bacteroids or anaerobic streptococci. If these infections spread, are not drained, or remain uncontrolled in spite of treatment, they spread downwards along tissue planes into the mediasti-

num. Clinical features are characterized by increasing sepsis and substernal pain with tachypnoea.

The diagnosis is often clinical as there are no pathognomic radiological signs. The mediastinum may appear widened and there may be a widening of the retro-cervical space (if the infection has spread along the retrocervical tissue planes). The tracheal air column may be displaced anteriorly or laterally on a chest X-ray. A CT scan may demonstrate the spread of infection from the tissue planes of the neck into the mediastinum.

The principles of management are:

(i) A broad-spectrum antibiotic cover against gram-positive, gram-negative and anaerobic organisms.
(ii) Surgical drainage of the primary source—generally a cervical or retropharyngeal or odontogenic abscess. A review CT of the chest may help to decide whether more extensive drainage of the mediastinum is necessary. A localized mediastinal abscess must needs be drained. Surgical expertise from a thoracic and/or a cardiothoracic surgeon is vital for survival.
(iii) A tracheostomy becomes necessary only if there is a great deal of cervical inflammatory oedema that compromises the airway. A tracheostomy can however be treacherous even after the airway is secured as it further opens tissue planes in the neck that communicate with mediastinal tissue planes and thereby can perhaps worsen the mediastinitis.

The prognosis is grim in severe necrotizing mediastinitis which has a mortality of close to 50%. Death occurs from increasing sepsis with multiorgan failure, or from erosion of large vessels causing exsanguinating bleeds. Early diagnosis and prompt medical and surgical treatment are critical for survival.

DIRECT EXTENSION FROM THE RETROPERITONEAL SPACE

Mediastinitis can occur from a spread of infection along the retroperitoneal space in patients with suppurative, necrotizing pancreatitis. Pancreatic pseudocysts can extend into the mediastinum. Pleural effusion and occasionally pericardial effusion with high amylase content are noted. A pseudocyst should be drained into the stomach at the appropriate point in the natural history of pancreatitis.

MEDIASTINITIS FOLLOWING STERNOTOMY

Infection of the sternum is occasionally seen as a postoperative complication after surgery. Such infections heal poorly because of the poor vascularity in this area and are invariably associated with a varying degree of anterior compartment mediastinitis. When healing does not occur, surgeons prefer to do a wide sternal excision of dead or infected tissue, closing the dead space with transposed gastrocolic omentum. This is a vascular viable graft that promotes healing.

ANTHRAX MEDIASTINITIS

At one time anthrax was endemic in South India. It is rare today but may well return in the West and other parts of the world following the advent of bio-terrorism. Anthrax spores when inhaled gain entry into the lungs and from there

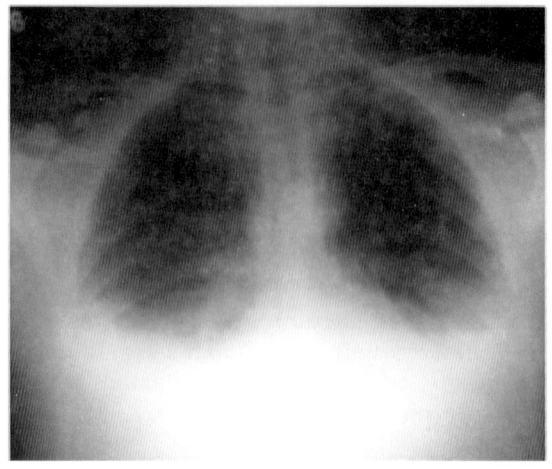

(a)

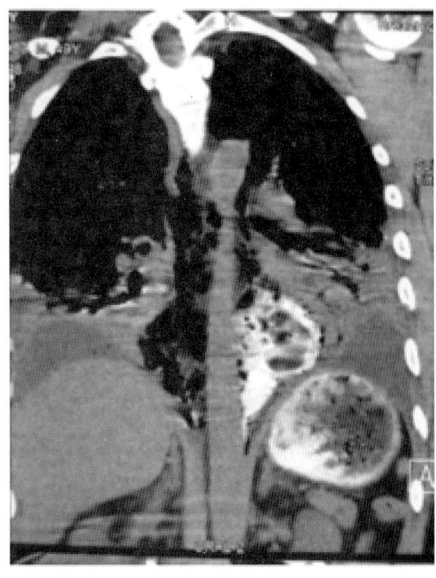

(b)

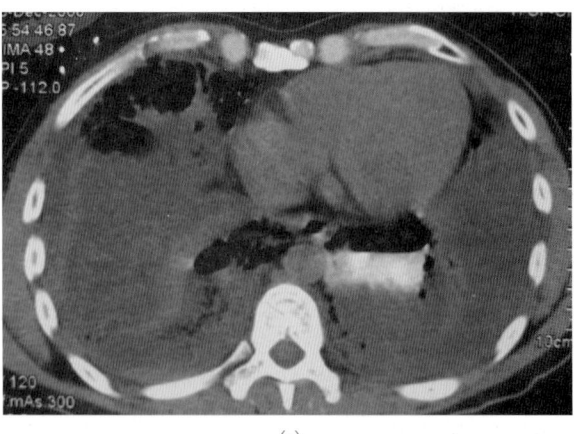

(c)

Fig 65.26: Young man with a bad oesophageal tear (Mallory Weiss syndrome) due to forceful vomiting. (a) Chest X-ray reveals bilateral pleural effusion. Pleural fluid aspiration revealed a markedly elevated amylase (b&c) Coronal and axial CT (b&c) shows a leak from the oesophagus, pleural effusion, mediastinal and surgical emphysema. Total oesophagectomy was necessary as two attempts at repair of the oesophagus were unsuccessful.

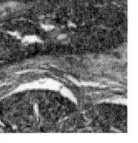

are transported to the regional lymph nodes. There ensues a necrotizing haemorrhagic mediastinitis with death within a few days. Ciprofloxacin, doxycyline plus other antibiotics effective against the anthrax bacillus should be promptly used.

FIBROSING MEDIASTINITIS

This is a rare disease characterized by the proliferation of dense fibrous tissue within the mediastinum. The extensive fibrosis compresses and strangles vital structures within the mediastinum. In most cases the aetiology is unknown. The two known infective causes are tuberculosis and histoplasmosis.

Out of the six cases encountered by our unit one was proven to be due to Histoplasma capsulatum (in an Indian patient living in the US but visiting India). The rest were of unknown aetiology. It is postulated that fibrosing mediastinitis results from a delayed hypersensitivity reaction to fungal, mycobacterial or other antigens. This remains a postulate. The disease has been however reported in association with autoimmune disorders and has been recorded following the use of the antimigraine drug methylsergide. Mediastinal fibrosis may be associated with retroperitoneal fibrosis. Either one could precede the other.

Pathologically, dense fibrosis is seen to compress the trachea, bronchi, the veins in the superior mediastinum, the hila, extending into the vessels (in particular the pulmonary vessels) and even infiltrating into the lungs.

CLINICAL COMPRESSION SYNDROMES

These depend on the site of the mediastinal fibrosis. Mediastinal fibrosis predominating in the superior mediastinum causes the **superior vena caval syndrome**. Though malignancy or large mediastinal tumours are the most important cause of this syndrome, fibrosing mediastinitis though infrequent, should be kept in mind as an important cause of this syndrome. Patients complain of puffiness of face and eyes with oedema of the neck and upper arms. Headache and visual disturbances are also observed. Symptoms worsen on bending or stooping to pick up an object. Clinical examination reveals a puffy plethoric face, puffy eyes; oedema may extend into the upper arms. Collaterals are observed over the upper chest and arms. The jugular veins are non-pulsatile and engorged—in severe cases right up to the angle of the jaw even in the sitting posture. Contrast CT or venography not only proves the diagnosis but also demonstrates the site and extent of blockage of contrast within the superior vena cava. It also helps to exclude pressure from a neoplasm as the cause of the superior vena caval syndrome.

In symptomatic patients, stenting of the stenosed superior vena cava may afford relief. Surgical bypass is offered to patients who have severe symptoms. It is done by connecting the unobstructed brachiocephalic vein to the right atrial appendage either through a saphenous vein graft or a prosthetic graft.

Hilar Compression   At times mediastinal fibrosis starts or remains confined to the hilar areas causing compression of one or more bronchi with resultant atelectasis or pressure on branches of the pulmonary vessels. When unilateral, the appearance is that of a large hilar mass indistinguishable from a neoplasm. In fact it is often misdiagnosed as a bronchogenic carcinoma. A

thoracoscopic or an open-lung biopsy is often necessary for a definite diagnosis.

Compression Within the Middle Mediastinal Compartment   (i) Increasing fibrosis could involve the tracheobronchial tree and lead to dyspnoea, wheezing, cough and compression atelectasis of a lobe. Bronchoplastic procedures or the placement of stents into the trachea and/or main bronchi may keep the large airways patent.

(ii) Mediastinal fibrosis around the pulmonary artery could lead to pulmonary hypertension, signs of right heart failure. If the fibrosis involves the pulmonary veins, the clinical picture resembles mitral stenosis or veno-occlusive disease, with cough, dyspnoea and attacks of pulmonary oedema. Constriction of the pulmonary veins at times produces a continuous murmur over the precordium, often also heard over the back. Constricted pulmonary veins could sharply reduce venous return to the left heart, the patient presents with fatigue, dyspnoea and angina on effort.

(iii) Mediastinal fibrosis starting or restricted to the posterior mediastinum constricts the oesophagus chiefly in the middle third. The fibrosis generally also involves the carina with compression of the main bronchi.

The diagnosis of mediastinal fibrosis is evident on an HRCT of the chest. It is even better visualized with an MRI. A histopathological diagnosis through a biopsy is advised as far as possible. The tissue should be stained for possible tubercular and fungal infections and should also be cultured.

We have found corticosteroids useful in two patients. There was significant regression of fibrosis on imaging and marked relief of symptoms. The use of azathioprine, methotrexate and cyclophosphamide has also been advocated; these drugs are however of unproven efficacy.

PNEUMOMEDIASTINUM

The commonest cause of pneumomediastinum is barotrauma causing alveolar rupture in patients on ventilator support. Spontaneous pneumomediastinum can also be due to rupture of alveoli because of increased intrathoracic volume and pressure in asthma or following trauma. Straining against a closed glottis as in vomiting, coughing or exercising can also lead to alveolar rupture. Obstruction to a large airway as with a foreign body or tumour can also increase alveolar volume and pressure leading to rupture. Pneumomediastinum has resulted from alveolar rupture during an epileptic fit. Following alveolar rupture, air dissects along the peribronchoalveolar tissue planes into the mediastinum and then frequently ascends upwards into the tissue planes of the neck. Air from alveolar rupture could also move towards the parietal pleura, break through it and cause pneumothorax.

Pneumomediastinum if not severe may be asymptomatic being discovered as translucent air streaks along the cardiac borders. If marked, it causes substernal pain which may be also felt in the neck or the back. Dyspnoea, dysphagia and dysphonia may present singly or in combination. Examination often reveals subcutaneous emphysema in the neck. Auscultation reveals a crunching clicking sound heard in systole and diastole (Hamman's sign). Non-specific ST-T changes may be present leading to a wrong diagnosis of myocardial infarction.

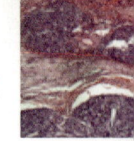

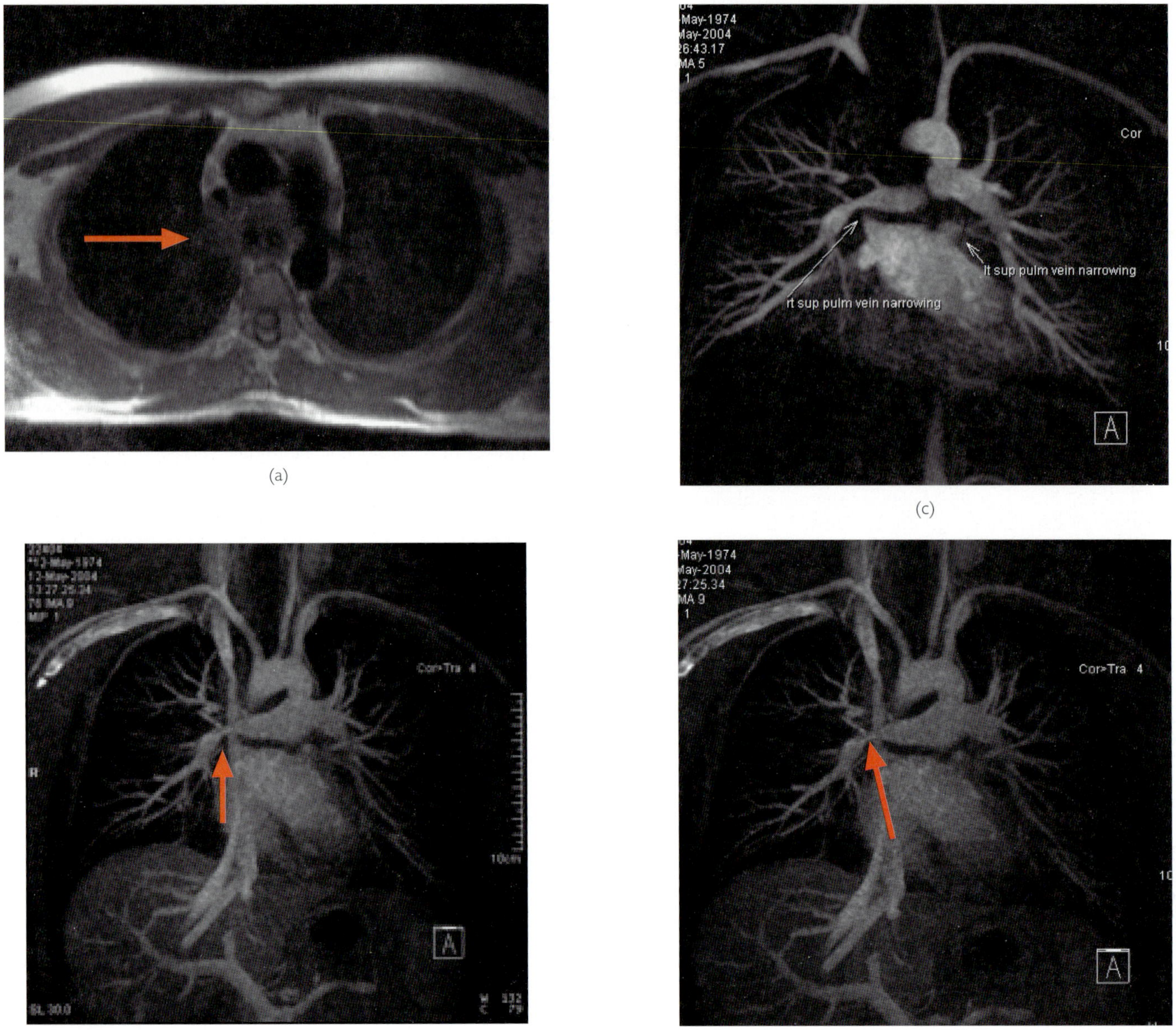

(a)

(c)

(b)

(d)

Fig 65.27: Mediastinal fibrosis. A 21-year-old man with dyspnoea on exertion and marked angina on exertion. Clinical examination revealed a soft continuous murmur over the bases of the lung, also heard over the back. (a) Axial MRI demonstrated soft tissue encircling carina and extending to posterior surface of SVC. (b, c, d) MR angiography revealed a long segment narrowing of the SVC, as well as focal narrowing of right and left superior pulmonary veins. His coronary angiography was normal, the angina was due to a marked diminishment of blood flow to the left heart due to marked constriction of pulmonary veins leading to markedly reduced cardiac output with decreased coronary flow. After treatment with steroids the soft tissue as well as vascular compression markedly reduced.

An X-ray chest reveals a translucent air streak most often along the left heart border and the left border of the mediastinum. CT defines the air with more clarity. There is often imaging evidence of air in the subcutaneous tissue of the neck and chest.

TREATMENT
When pneumomediastinitis results during mechanical ventilator support, it is important to reduce tidal volume thereby reducing both peak and pause pressure. An associated pneumothorax needs an intercostal drain.

Treatment of spontaneous pneumomediastinum with surgical emphysema is directed at pain relief and at treating the cause. Oxygen may be administered in dyspnoeic patients. Needle aspiration or skin incisions to relieve subcutaneous emphysema are almost never necessary. Air is fairly quickly absorbed over a period of a few days.

MEDIASTINAL HAEMORRHAGE
Haemorrhage into the mediastinum can occur spontaneously following rupture of an aneurysm, rupture or leak from a dissecting aneurysm of the aorta or from blunt or penetrating trauma or following invasive medical procedures.

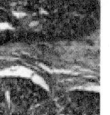

Severe blood loss can cause hypovolemic shock. Dyspnoea, chest pain and desaturation are observed. A CT-chest will reveal a dissecting aneurysm if this is the cause of the bleed, or a hyperdense area within the mediastinum or in the area of partial tear of the aortic wall (following blunt trauma as in a car crash). It could also reveal extravasated blood in the mediastinum, pericardium or pleura. Treatment is surgical and depends on the cause and site of the bleed.

SUGGESTED READING

Aquino SL, Taber KH, *et al*. Reconciliation of the anatomical, surgical, and radiographic classification of the mediastinum. *J. Comp Assist Tomogr*. 2001; 25: 489–92.

Casey EM. Clinical management of thymoma patients. *Hematol Oncol Clin North Am*. 1 Jun. 2008; 22(3): 457–73

Duwe BV. Tumors of the mediastinum. *Chest*. 1 Oct. 2005; 128(4): 2893–909

Holty JE. Anthrax: a systematic review of atypical presentations. *Ann Emerg Med*. 1 Aug. 2006; 48(2): 200–11

Jung K-J, Lee KS, Han J, *et al*. Malignant thymic epithelial tumors: CT-pathologic correlation. *AIR* 2001; 176: 433–9.

Macchiarini P. Uncommon primary mediastinal tumours *Lancet Oncol*. 1 Feb. 2004; 5(2): 107–18

Strollo DC, Rosado-de-Christenson ML. Primary mediastinal malignant germ cell neoplasms: Imaging features. *Chest Surg Clin North Am*. 2002; 12: 645–58.

Strollo DC, Rosado-de-Christenson ML, Jett JR. Primary mediastinal tumors. Part I. Tumors of the anterior mediastinum. *Chest*. 1997; 112: 511–58.

Strollo DC, Rosado-de-Christenson ML, Jett JR. Primary mediastinal tumors. Part II. Tumors of the middle and posterior mediastinum. *Chest*. 1997; 112: 1344–57.

Tormoehlen LM. Thymoma, myasthenia gravis, and other paraneoplastic syndromes. *Hematol Oncol Clin North Am*. 1 Jun. 2008; 22(3): 509–26

Wan JF. Superior vena cava syndrome. *Emerg Med Clin North Am*. 1 May 2009; 27(2): 243–55

OCCUPATIONAL AND ENVIRONMENTAL LUNG DISEASES

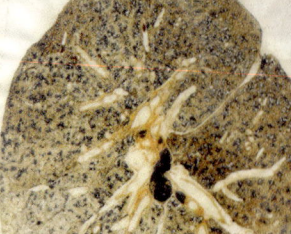

CHAPTER **66** Common Occupational Lung Diseases

INTRODUCTION

Occupational lung disease is any of a group of unusual problems in the lungs caused by breathing dusts, fumes, gases, or vapours in a place where a patient works.

Many types of work are associated with health hazards. Very few places in either industry or agriculture are completely free from gases, vapours, mists, fumes or dust and hence a great number of workers are exposed to air contaminants. As a major portal to the environment, the lung often bears the brunt of these toxic exposures.

Occupations especially at risk are: coal miners, farmers, asbestos workers, workers with epoxy resins or isocyanates. Other jobs associated with an increased risk of occupational lung disease include: construction, carpentry, baking, soldering, laboratory work, hairdressing, bird breeding, drug manufacture, processing textiles, forestry, horticulture and metalworking.

The physical properties of inhaled substances predict the site of deposition; irritants will produce symptoms at these sites. Large particles (10 to 20 μm) deposit in the nose and upper airways, smaller particles (5 to 10 μm) deposit in the trachea and bronchi, and particles less than 5 μm in size may reach the alveoli. Particles less than 0.5 μm are so small they behave like gases. Toxic gases deposit according to their solubility. A water-soluble gas will be adsorbed by the moist mucosa of the upper airway; less soluble gases will deposit more randomly throughout the respiratory tract.

Many host and environmental factors serve to modify the effects of inhaled chemicals, and the ultimate response is the result of their interaction. The main host factors are:

1. Age—older people with chronically reduced cardiovascular and respiratory function
2. Poor health status
3. Poor nutritional status
4. Immunological status
5. Sex and other genetic factors, for example, enzyme-related differences in biotransformation mechanisms
6. Psychological state, for example, stress, anxiety
7. Smoking—Cigarette smoking may affect normal defences, or may potentiate the effect of other chemicals.

OCCUPATIONAL LUNG DISEASES—BURDEN IN INDIA

The prevalence of occupational lung diseases in developed countries is not high and deaths due to such exposure are low when compared to developing countries.

The common occupational lung diseases in India include silicosis, asbestosis, byssinosis, bagassosis and coal workers' pneumoconiosis. Extrinsic allergic alveolitis and occupational asthma have been less well documented, and probably missed on account of lack of diagnostic facilities.

Silicosis in the unorganized sector has been reported to be as high as 25% among stone cutters, 22% in quarry workers, 16.7% in glass workers, 15.1% in ceramic workers, 27.2% in non-mechanized foundry workers, 28.7% in agate grinders, and 54.6% in slate pencil workers. In studies conducted in Ahmedabad, Mumbai and Delhi the prevalence of byssinosis among textile workers was estimated at 7–8%.

The National program for control and treatment of occupational diseases (National Institute of Health and Family Welfare, Government of India) estimates the following prevalence of occupational lung diseases in India.

Table 66.1: Prevalence of occupational lung diseases in India	
Occupational Lung Disease	**Prevalence**
Silicosis in mica miners	6.2–34%
Silicosis in manganese miners	4.1%
Silicosis in slate pencil workers	54.6%
Silicosis in lead and zinc miners	30.4%
Asbestosis	3% of miners and 21% in mill workers
Bysinossis	28–47%

Source: http://inihfw.nic.in/ndc-nihfw/html/Programmes/National Programme For Control Treatment.htm.

CLASSIFICATION OF OCCUPATIONAL LUNG DISEASES

Occupational lung diseases can be classified according to exposure to various agents.

Occupational lung diseases also depend on the toxicity potential of various compounds. Agents which are capable of causing lung toxicity after low to moderate exposure include the following as given in Table 66.3.

DIAGNOSIS OF AN OCCUPATIONAL LUNG DISORDER

The diagnosis of occupational lung disorders is usually based on a proven history of exposure to known agents, clinical

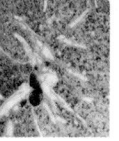

Table 66.2: Classification of occupational lung diseases		
General Agent	**Examples**	**Disorder**
Mineral dusts	Asbestos Silica Coal	Pneumoconiosis
Metal dusts	Iron Tin Barium Vanadium Cadmium Nickel Chromic salts Platinum salts Cobalt Cobalt Beryllium	'Inert dust' pneumoconiosis 'Inert dust' pneumoconiosis 'Inert dust' pneumoconiosis Irritant bronchitis Bronchitis, pneumoconiosis Asthma Asthma Asthma Asthma, Giant cell pneumonitis Granulomatous pneumonitis
Biological dusts	Spores Mycelia Bird droppings	Hypersensitivity pneumonitis
Toxic fumes	NO_2 SO_2 Chlorine Ammonia	Airways inflammation, ARDS ARDS, bronchiolitis abliteans Airways inflammation Airways inflammation
High molecular weight (Asthmatic agent)	Flour Dander	Asthma Asthma
Low molecular weight (Asthmatic agent)	Isocyanates Epoxy esins	Biphasic asthma Asthma
Infections	Viral Bacterial Fungal	Specific infection Specific infection Specific infection
Carcinogens	Asbestos Arsenic Chromium Coke oven Fumes Nickel Halo ethers Radon prodigy	Lung cancer and mesothelioma Lung caner—copper smelting Lung cancer—smelting process Lung cancer—steel making Lung cancer—smelting processing Lung cancer—engineered out the process Lung cancer—uanium mining

Repoduced with permission from Dr Gary R. Epler: Environmental and Occupational Lung Disease http://www.epler.com/occu_tab.html#1.

evaluation as well as specific tests including lung function tests, chest X-ray and computerized tomography (CT).

An investigation which can be done on-site with appropriate training is to conduct the lung function tests which can be carried out to determine the condition of the lungs. The resultant spirogram can be analysed to determine if the pulmonary functions have been compromised due to exposure to various substances at the workplace. The normal subdivisions of lung functions are depicted in Figure 66.1.

Lung function testing is an accepted way of diagnosing various conditions depending on the following parameters. The common deviations observed in occupational lung diseases include either a restrictive or an obstructive airway defect, or in many cases a combination of a restrictive cum obstructive defect depending on the type of exposure.

Condition	FEV_1	FVC	FEV_1/FVC	Interpretation
Silicosis, coal workers' pneumoconiosis, asbestosis, extrinsic allergic alveolitis (Farmer's lung, bagassosis, bird-handler's lung), beryllium disease	↓	↓	Normal/reduced	Restrictive or obstructive airways defect or a combination of both
Byssinosis, exposure to diisocyanates, COPD (Asthma, chronic bronchitis, emphysema)	↓	↓	↓	Obstructive airway defect

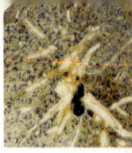

Table 66.3: Various agents causing lung toxicity		
Compound	**Source of exposure**	**Toxicity**
Arcolein	Plastics, textiles, pharmaceutical manufacturing, combustion products	Diffuse airways and parenchymal injury
Antimony trichloride; antimony pentachloride	Alloys, organic catalysts	Pneumonitis, non-cardiogenic pulmonary oedema
Cadmium	Alloys with zinc and lead, electroplating, batteries, insecticides	Tracheobronchitis, pulmonary oedema (often delayed onset over 24–48 hours), kidney damage: tubule proteinuria
Chloropicrin	Chemical manufacturing, fumigant components	Upper and lower airways inflammation
Chlorine	Bleaching, formation of chlorinated compounds, household cleaners	Upper and lower airway inflammation, pneumonitis and non-cardiogenic pulmonary oedema
Hydrogen sulphide	Natural gas wells, mines, manure	Ocular, upper and lower airway irritation, delayed pulmonary oedema, asphyxiation from systemic tissue hypoxia
Lithium hydride	Alloys, ceramics, electronics, chemical catalysts	Pneumonitis, non-cardiogenic pulmonary oedema
Methyl isocyanate	Pesticide synthesis	Upper and lower respiratory tract irritation, pulmonary oedema
Mercury	Electrolysis, ore and amalgam extraction, electronics manufacture	Ocular and respiratory tract inflammation, pneumonitis, CNS, kidney and systemic effects
Nickel carbonyl	Nickel refining, electroplating, chemical reagents	Lower respiratory irritation, pneumonitis, delayed systemic toxic effects
Nitrogen dioxide	Silos after new grain storage, fertilizer making, arc welding; combustion products	Ocular and upper airway inflammation, non-cardiogenic pulmonary oedema, delayed onset bronchiolitis
Nitrogen mustards, sulphur mustards	Military agents, vesicants	Ocular and respiratory tract inflammation, pneumonitis
Paraquat	Herbicides (ingested)	Selective damage to type-2 pneumocytes leading to RADS, pulmonary fibrosis; renal failure, GI irritation
Phosgene	Pesticide and other chemical manufacture, arc welding, paint removal	Upper airway inflammation and pneumonitis; delayed pulmonary oedema
Zinc chloride	Smoke grenades, artillery	Upper and lower airway irritation, fever, delayed onset pneumonitis

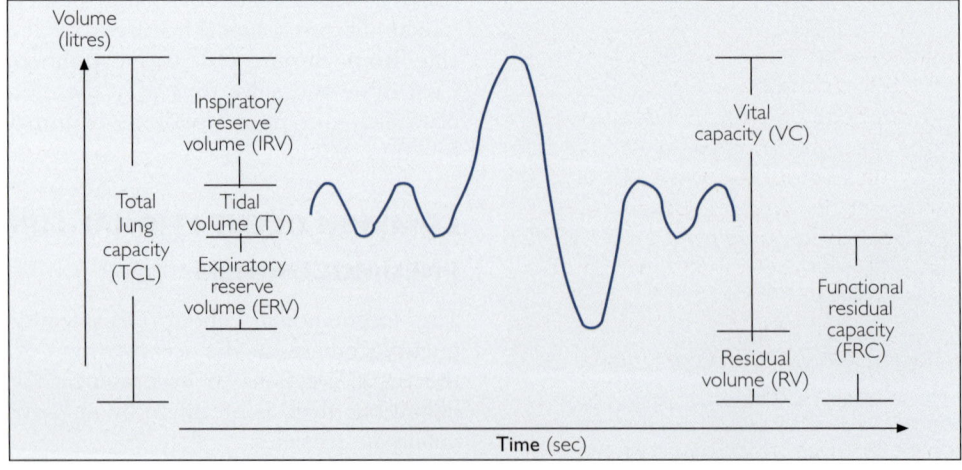

Fig 66.1: Spirogram labeled to show the subdivisions of the total lung capacity Inflammation.

Source: Ulf Ulfvarsoa and Monica Dahlqvist. *Lung function examination in Encyclopedia of occupational health and safety.* Fig. 10.10. Fourth edition. International Labour Office. 1998.

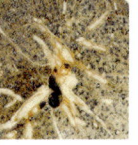

Although silicosis and coal workers' pneumoconiosis (CWP) are becoming less common, hypersensitivity pneumonitis is increasingly recognized as an occupational lung disease with new antigens being introduced annually.

Imaging, particularly high-resolution CT (HRCT), is central to the management of occupational lung disease and is useful in diagnosis, assessment of disease activity, and evaluating response to therapy.

Other important diagnostic tools include bronchoalveolar lavage (BAL). A predominance of lymphocytes could point to certain conditions like hypersensitivity pneumonia or beryllium disease. Characteristic multinucleated giant cells may be seen in those exposed to heavy metals. Transbronchial lung biopsies may also help in arriving at the diagnosis of the condition.

Figures 66.2, 66.3, 66.4 and 66.5 depict the histopathology of a few occupational lung diseases.

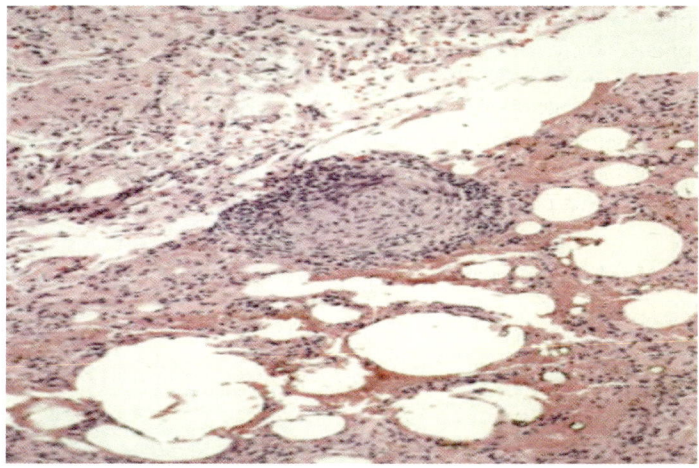

Fig 66.4: Chronic beryllium disease. The histopathology of the lung is indistinguishable from that observed in sarcoidosis. Non-caseating granulomas are observed (in the centre) together with some degree of fibrosis.

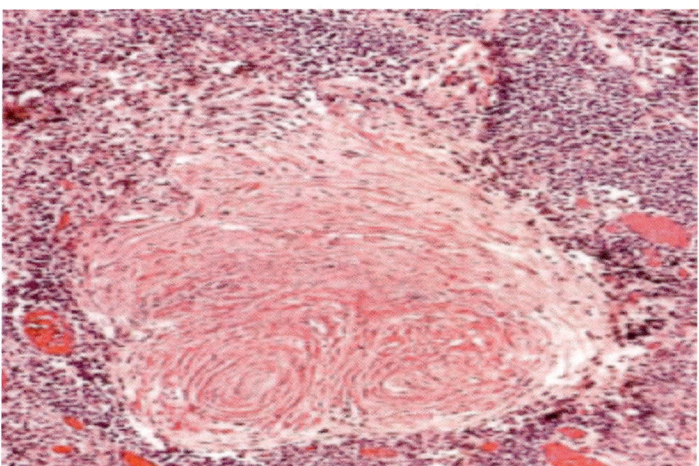

Fig 66.2: Silicosis. The lesion is characterized by a cell-free central area of concentrically arranged, whirled collagen fibres, surrounded by cellular connective tissue with reticular fibres.

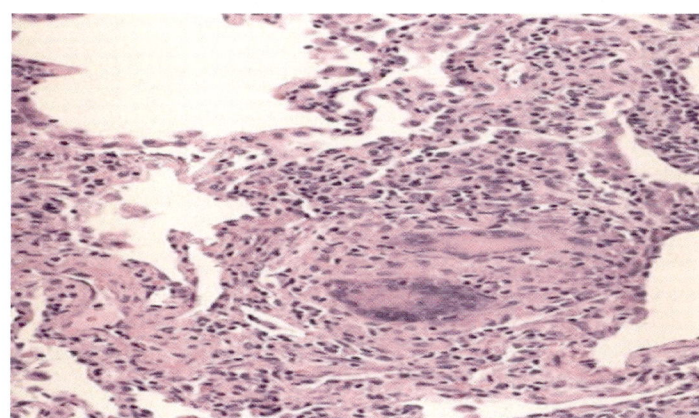

Fig 66.5: Hypersensitivity pneumonitis. The presence of non-caseating granulomas with giant cells, together with alveolitis, lymphocytic infiltration of bronchial walls and laying down of fibrous tissue is observed.

DIFFERENTIAL DIAGNOSIS

Exposure to silica and coal mine dusts may result in pulmonary scarring, with a ventilatory pattern that mimics idiopathic pulmonary fibrosis. Clinical features may at times be indistinguishable from chronic obstructive pulmonary disease (COPD). Coal mine and silica dust may therefore result in restrictive, obstructive, or mixed patterns of impairment on pulmonary function testing.

COMMON OCCUPATIONAL LUNG DISEASES

PNEUMOCONIOSIS

The International Labour Organization (ILO) has defined pneumoconiosis as 'the accumulation of dust in the lungs and the tissue reactions to its presence. For the purpose of this definition, 'dust' is meant to be an aerosol composed of solid inanimate particles.

Primary pneumoconiosis includes silicosis, coal workers' pneumoconiosis, and asbestosis. They are caused by inhalation

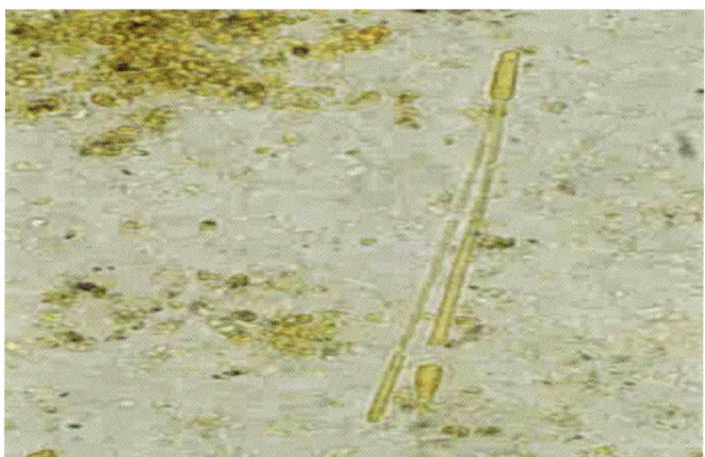

Fig 66.3: Asbestosis. Asbestos fibres (seen as parallel vertical yellowish streaks) inhaled deep into the lung parenchyma induce diffuse alveolar and interstitial fibrosis. Fibrosis is first evident in the respiratory bronchioles and this progresses to involve the alveolar walls. The subpleural portions of the lower lobes are first involved.

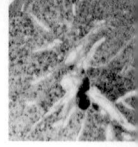

of silica dust, coal mine dust and asbestos fibres. Other forms of pneumoconiosis caused by inhalation of dusts containing aluminium, antimony, barium, graphite, iron, kaolin, mica, talc, among other dusts are encountered by the physician infrequently.

Byssinosis is another pulmonary disease caused by exposure to cotton dust and is sometimes included under pneumoconiosis, although its pattern of lung abnormality is different.

Aetiopathogenesis of Pneumoconiosis

Studies have shown four basic mechanisms in the aetiology of coal workers' pneumoconiosis and silicosis: a) direct cytotoxicity of coal dust or silica, resulting in lung cell damage, release of lipases and proteases, and eventual lung scarring; b) activation of oxidant production by pulmonary phagocytes, which overwhelms the antioxidant defences and leads to lipid peroxidation, protein nitrosation, cell injury, and lung scarring; c) activation of mediator release from alveolar macrophages and epithelial cells, which leads to recruitment of polymorphonuclear leukocytes and macrophages, resulting in the production of pro-inflammatory cytokines and reactive species and further lung injury and scarring; d) secretion of growth factors from alveolar macrophages and epithelial cells, stimulating fibroblast proliferation and eventual scarring. Results of *in vitro* and animal studies provide a basis for proposing these mechanisms for the initiation and progression of pneumoconiosis. Data obtained from exposed workers lend support to these mechanisms.

The exposure regimen seems to determine the time course of events. There is some indication that sufficiently low exposure regimens can in most cases limit the lung reaction to non-progressive lesions with no disability or impairment.

Typically, these three diseases (coal workers' pneumoconiosis, silicosis, and asbestosis) take many years to develop and manifest, although in some cases, in silicosis, particularly, rapidly progressive forms can occur after only short periods of intense exposure. When severe, the diseases often lead to lung impairment, disability, and premature death.

Clinical Manifestations and Diagnosis

Pneumoconiosis may be asymptomatic with only radiological abnormalities. Symptoms when they appear include cough (with or without expectoration), wheezing and shortness of breath, especially during exertion.

If pneumoconiosis causes severe lung fibrosis, breathing can become extremely difficult. Very advanced disease is associated with respiratory failure and right ventricular hypertrophy with congestive heart failure (cor pulmonale).

Pneumoconiosis is typically detected in individuals through the use of radiological imaging. Traditionally, this has been the chest X-ray, taken on film, but now increasingly being acquired through digital computer technology. The ILO provides guidelines for the systematic scientific classification of radiographs of pneumoconiosis.

A simplified format of the ILO classification of chest radiographs is given in Table 66.4.

Medical surveillance and screening have always been part of the strategies for the prevention of pneumoconiosis. In this context, the possibility of detecting some early lesions is advantageous.

Increased knowledge of pathogenesis paved the way for the development of several biomarkers and for the refinement and use of 'non-classical' pulmonary investigation techniques such as the measurement of the clearance rate of deposited 99 technetium diethylenetriamine-penta-acetate (99 Tc-DTPA) to assess pulmonary epithelial integrity, and quantitative gallium-67 lung scan to assess inflammatory activity.

Several biomarkers were considered in the field of pneumoconiosis: sputum macrophages, serum growth factors, serum Type III procollagen peptide, red blood cell antioxidants, fibronectin, leucocyte elastase, neutral metalloendopeptidase and elastin peptides in plasma, volatile hydrocarbons in exhaled air, and TNF (tumour necrosis factor) release by peripheral blood monocytes. Biomarkers are conceptually quite interesting, but many more studies are necessary to assess their precise significance. This validation effort will be quite demanding, since it will require investigators to conduct prospective epidemiological studies. Such an effort was carried out recently for TNF release by peripheral blood monocytes in CWP. TNF was found to be an interesting marker of CWP progression. Besides the scientific aspects of the significance of biomarkers in the pathogenesis of pneumoconiosis, other issues related to the use of biomarkers must be examined carefully, namely, opportunities for prevention, impact on occupational medicine and ethical and legal problems.

The impact of newer understanding of the cascade of events in the pathogenesis of pneumoconiosis has not modified the traditional approach to workers' surveillance, but has significantly helped physicians in their capacity to recognize the disease (pneumoconiosis) early, at a time when the disease has had only a limited impact on lung function. It is indeed workers in the early stage of disease who should be recognized and withdrawn from further significant exposure if prevention of disability is to be achieved by medical surveillance.

SILICOSIS

Silicosis is the commonest and one of the most serious occupational diseases. It is an irreversible fibrosis of the lungs caused by inhalation, retention and pulmonary reaction to free silica dust. It is estimated that about 3 million people working in various types of mines, ceramics, potteries, foundries, metal grinding, stone crushing, agate grinding, slate pencil industry etc. are occupationally exposed to free silica dust and are at potential risk of developing silicosis. Silica exposure also predisposes to development of pulmonary tuberculosis, which is an important public health problem in India.

In India, a prevalence of 55% was found in one group of workers, many of them very young, engaged in the quarrying of shale sedimentary rock and subsequent work in small, poorly ventilated sheds. Studies on silicotic pencil workers in central India demonstrated high mortality rates; the mean age at death was 35 years and the mean duration of the exposure was 12 years.

Occupational exposure to silica particles of respirable size (aerodynamic diameter of 0.5 to 5 μm) is associated with mining, quarrying, drilling, tunnelling and abrasive blasting with quartz-

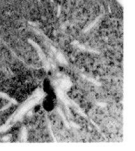

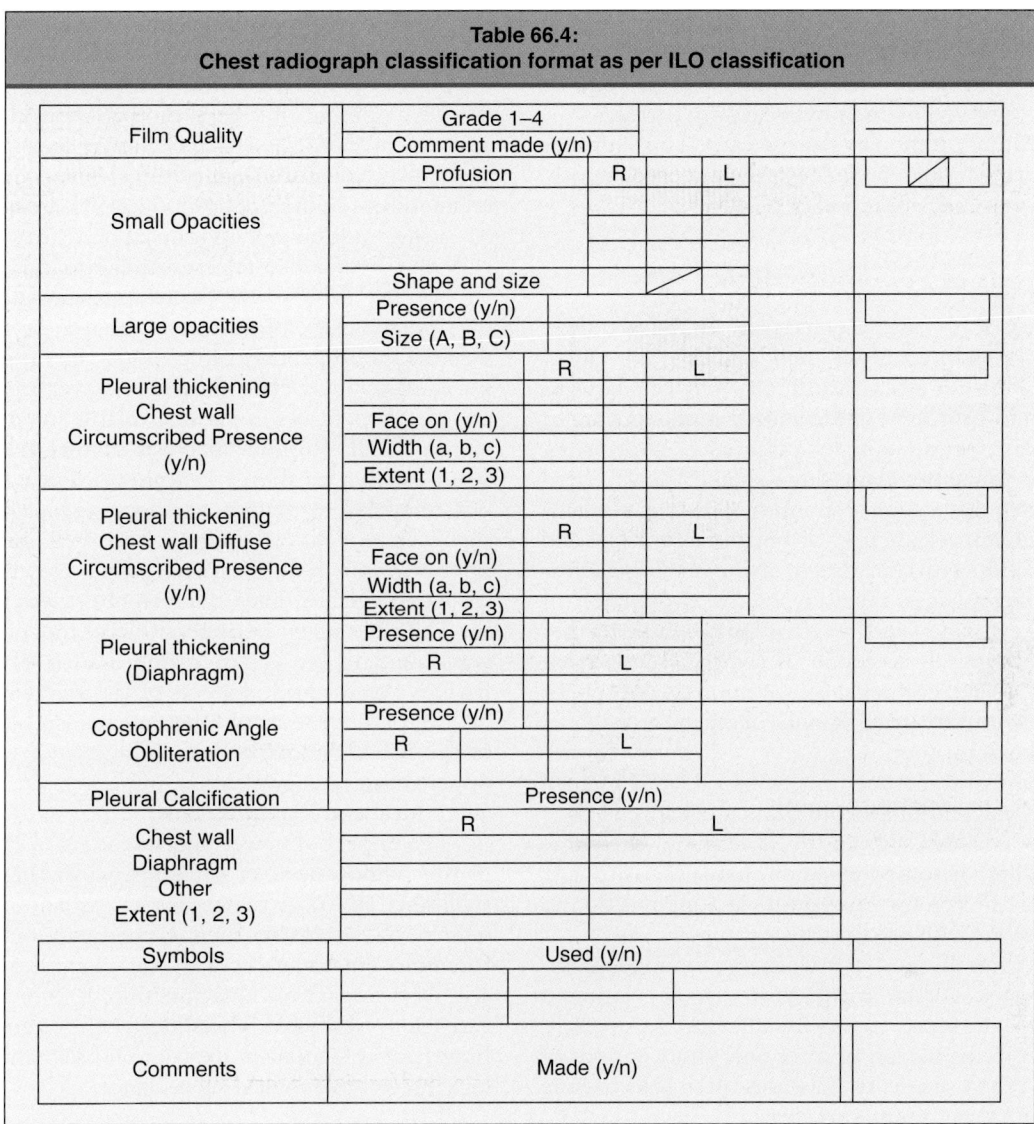

Table 66.4: Chest radiograph classification format as per ILO classification				
Film Quality	Grade 1–4			
	Comment made (y/n)			
Small Opacities	Profusion	R	L	
	Shape and size			
Large opacities	Presence (y/n)			
	Size (A, B, C)			
Pleural thickening Chest wall Circumscribed Presence (y/n)		R	L	
	Face on (y/n)			
	Width (a, b, c)			
	Extent (1, 2, 3)			
Pleural thickening Chest wall Diffuse Circumscribed Presence (y/n)		R	L	
	Face on (y/n)			
	Width (a, b, c)			
	Extent (1, 2, 3)			
Pleural thickening (Diaphragm)	Presence (y/n)			
	R		L	
Costophrenic Angle Obliteration	Presence (y/n)			
	R		L	
Pleural Calcification	Presence (y/n)			
Chest wall Diaphragm Other Extent (1, 2, 3)	R		L	
Symbols	Used (y/n)			
Comments	Made (y/n)			

containing materials (sandblasting). Silica exposure also poses a hazard to stonecutters, and pottery, foundry, ground silica and refractory workers. The true prevalence of the disease is unclear.

Pathology

The pathologic hallmark of the chronic form is the silicotic nodule. The lesion is characterized by a cell-free central area of concentrically arranged, whorled hyalinized collagen fibres, surrounded by cellular connective tissue with reticulin fibres.

The susceptibility of silicotic workers to infections, such as tuberculosis and Nocardia asteroides, is likely related to the toxic effect of silica on pulmonary macrophages. Active tuberculosis in silicotic workers may exceed 20% when community prevalence of tuberculosis is high. Again, people with acute silicosis appear to be at a considerable higher risk.

Clinical Manifestations and Diagnosis

Acute silicosis can occur within a few months to two years after massive exposures to dust in unregulated environments. This is characterized by severe dyspnoea, hypoxemia, weight loss, cough, fever and pleuritic pain.

Chronic silicosis occurs after 15–20 years of exposure to moderate to low levels of silica dust. Chronic silicosis itself is further subdivided into simple and complicated silicosis. This is the most common type of silicosis. Patients with this type of silicosis may not have obvious symptoms, so a chest X-ray is necessary to determine if there is lung damage. It presents as a radiographic abnormality with small (<10 mm), rounded opacities predominantly involving the upper lobes. Latency period of 15 years or more is quite common.

Accelerated silicosis is the condition where silicosis develops 5–10 years after high exposure to silica dust. Symptoms include severe shortness of breath, weakness, and weight loss.

Silicosis can lead to progressive massive fibrosis (PMF) which generally presents with exertional dyspnoea. This form of disease is characterized by nodular opacities greater than 1 cm on a chest radiograph and is associated with reduced carbon monoxide diffusing capacity, reduced arterial oxygen tension at rest or with exercise, and marked restriction on spirometry or lung volume measurement. Chronic silicosis can progress to

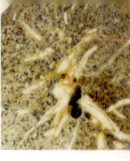

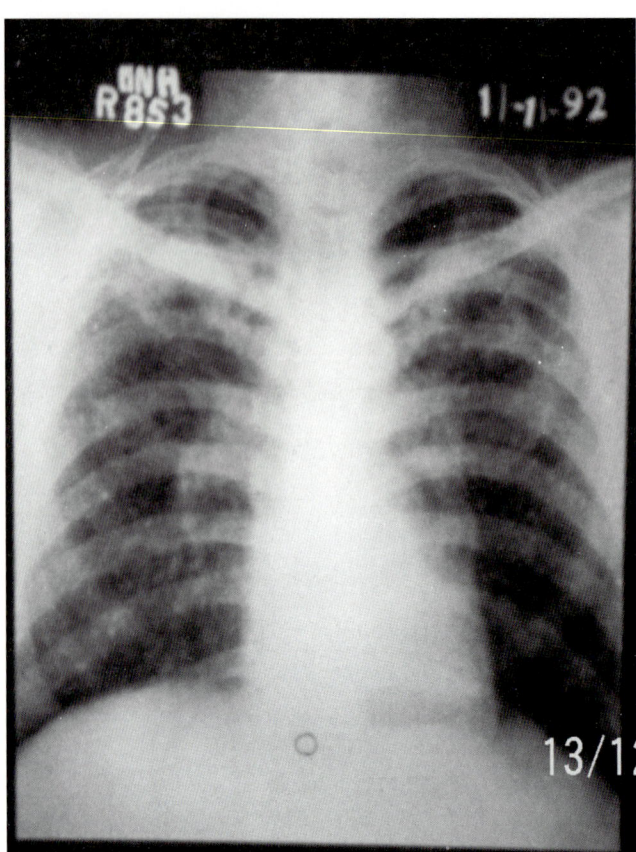

Fig 66.6: Chest X-ray of a subject who worked in an underground tungsten metal mine for 18 years as a labourer, rock drilling operator and material feeding helper involving exposure to silica dust. A known smoker for 25 years—the radiograph shows r/r type of small regular pneumoconiotic opacities in all zones with profusion 3/2 (Category 3). There is also evidence of healed tuberculosis in the upper zones. A few pneumoconiotic opacities show calcification and there is enlargement of the hilar lymph nodes.

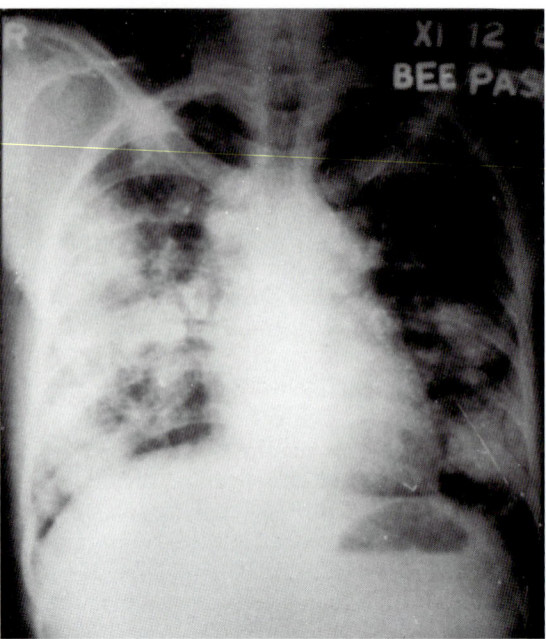

Fig 66.7: Chest X-ray of a 25-year-old woman with complaints of breathlessness and cough. X-ray revealed egg-shell calcification of the hilar lymph nodes in addition to bilateral fibrocaseous tuberculosis. She had a history of exposure to silica as a child when she used to play around a glass factory where the quartz-rich stone was manually crushed. Her X-ray reveals classical features of silicosis and tuberculosis.

PMF (sometimes referred to as complicated silicosis) even after exposure to silica-containing dust has ceased.

Patients with chronic disease may be asymptomatic with an abnormal chest radiograph or have dyspnoea. In some cases, the onset of dyspnoea signifies a complication, such as PMF, tuberculosis, or obstructive airway disease. Cough may be a feature of the disease or may signify chronic bronchitis, tuberculosis, or a complicating lung cancer. In chronic silicosis, lung function may be normal, or there may be an obstructive, restrictive, or a mixed obstructive/restrictive pattern. Impairment of function is more rapid in accelerated disease. In acute disease, impairment of gas exchange is a prominent feature.

In chest radiographs the usual early signs are those of rounded opacities and in line with the ILO classification of radiographs they are usually the 'q' and 'r' type of opacities. Hilar node involvement is frequent; the nodes may show egg-shell calcification. This form of calcification can also occur in other granulomatous diseases involving the lymph nodes. PMF is characterized by the formation of large opacities which are classified by the ILO as categories 'A', 'B' or 'C'. Pleural abnormalities are not a frequent feature on chest radiography. Occupational history along with chest radiographs is usually sufficient to make a diagnosis of silicosis. The possibility of coexisting tuberculosis should always be considered.

A frequent cause of death in people with silicosis is pulmonary tuberculosis (silico-tuberculosis). In acute silicosis, radiological progression is accompanied by increasing ventilatory impairment and gas exchange abnormalities, which lead to respiratory failure and eventually to death from severe intractable hypoxaemia. and/or right heart failure.

Treatment

No specific measures are available for treating silicosis. General measures are similar to those commonly used in the management of airway obstruction, infection, pneumothorax, hypoxaemia, and respiratory failure complicating other pulmonary disease. Coexisting tuberculosis should be evaluated and treated with multidrug therapy.

Prevention

Prevention should focus on improved ventilation and local exhaust, process enclosure, use of wet techniques, personal protection including the proper selection of respirators, and where possible, industrial substitution of agents less hazardous than silica. The education of workers and employers regarding the hazards of silica dust exposure and measures to control exposure are also important.

COAL WORKERS' LUNG DISEASE

Exposure to coal mine dust may cause pneumoconiosis, chronic bronchitis and chronic obstructive pulmonary disease.

In the developed countries, regulations have brought about a reduction in dust levels resulting in a substantial drop in disease prevalence since the 1970s.

COAL WORKERS' PNEUMOCONIOSIS (BLACK LUNG DISEASE)

Coal workers' pneumoconiosis (CWP) is a distinct pathologic entity resulting from the deposition of coal dust in the lungs. The tissue reactions to deposits of dust include the *coal macule* and the *coal nodule* (simple CWP), and PMF (complicated CWP).

Aetiopathogenesis

Alveolar macrophages engulf the dust, release cytokines that stimulate inflammation, and collect in the lung interstitium around bronchioles and alveoli (coal macules). Coal nodules develop as collagen accumulates, and focal emphysema develops as bronchiolar walls weaken and dilate. Fibrosis can occur but is usually limited to areas adjacent to coal macules. Distortion of lung architecture, airflow obstruction, and functional impairment are usually mild but can be highly destructive in some patients.

Two forms of CWP are described: Simple, with individual coal macules and Complicated, with coalescence of macules and PMF.

Patients with simple CWP develop PMF at a rate of about 1–2%. In PMF, nodules coalesce to form black, rubbery parenchymal masses usually in the upper posterior fields. The masses may encroach on and destroy the vascular supply and airways or may cavitate. PMF can develop and progress even after exposure to coal dust has ceased. Despite the similarity between coal-induced PMF and conglomerate silicosis, the development of PMF in coal workers is unrelated to the silica content of the coal.

Usually, CWP which is associated with mining coal takes about 10 years to develop and often much longer when exposures are less. However, over a period of time the disease could progress to massive pulmonary fibrosis.

Clinical Aspects

CWP does not usually cause symptoms. Most chronic pulmonary symptoms in coal miners are caused by other conditions, such as industrial bronchitis from coal dust or coincident chronic airways obstruction from smoking. Cough can be chronic and problematic in patients even after they leave the workplace, even in those who do not smoke.

PMF causes progressive dyspnoea. Occasionally, patients cough up black sputum (melanoptysis), which occurs as a result of rupture of PMF lesions into the airways. PMF often progresses to pulmonary hypertension with right ventricular and respiratory failure.

Diagnosis

Diagnosis depends on a history of exposure and chest X-ray or chest CT appearance. In patients with CWP, X-ray or CT reveals diffuse, small, rounded opacities or nodules. The finding of at least one opacity > 10 mm suggests PMF. The specificity of the chest X-ray for PMF is low, because up to one-third of the

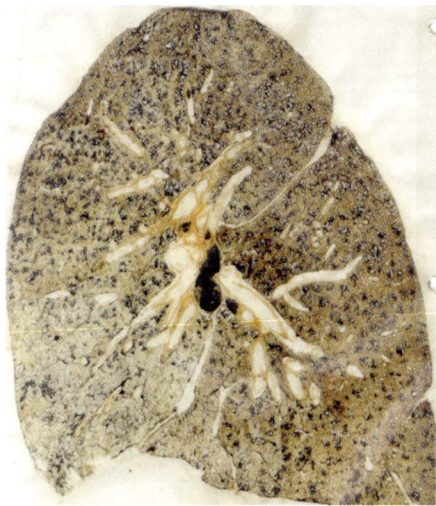

Fig 66.8: Simple coal workers' pneumoconiosis. Gross specimen shows that the lung is studded with nodules representing simple coal workers' pneumoconiosis. Focal areas of emphysema in relation to these nodules are clearly visible.

Source: Image reprinted with permission from eMedicine.com, 2009. Available at: http://emedicine.medscape.com/article/297887-overview. Copyright with eMedicine.com

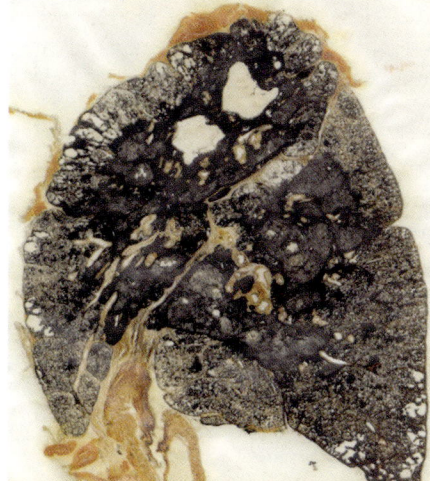

Fig 66.9: Progressive massive fibrosis. Gross specimen shows that in addition to nodules studding the lung surface, there are two conglomerate masses which characterize progressive massive fibrosis. Note thickened pleura over the apex and upper lobe and the increased density of nodules subpleurally and along the fissure.

Source: Image reprinted with permission from eMedicine.com, 2009. Available at: http://emedicine.medscape.com/article/297887-overview. Copyright with eMedicine.com

lesions identified as being PMF turn out to be cancers, scars, or other disorders. Chest CT is more sensitive than chest X-ray for detecting coalescing nodules, early PMF, and cavitation.

Pulmonary function tests are nondiagnostic but are useful for characterizing lung function in patients in whom obstructive, restrictive, or mixed defects may develop. Because abnormalities of gas exchange occur in some patients with extensive simple CWP and in those with complicated CWP, baseline and periodic measures of diffusing capacity for carbon monoxide (DLCO) and arterial blood gases at rest and during exercise are recommended.

Because patients with CWP often have had exposure to both silica dust as well as coal dust, surveillance for tuberculosis is usually done. Patients with CWP should have annual tuberculin skin testing. In those with positive test results, sputum culture and cytology, CT, and bronchoscopy with microbiological examination of BAL may be needed to confirm tuberculosis.

Treatment

Treatment should be geared towards symptom management and prevention of infectious complications of the affected miners. Miners should stop smoking. Treatment is usually for acute

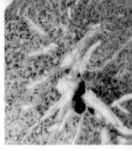

bronchitis, congestive cardiac failure and for complications arising out of respiratory failure.

Prevention

The key to prevention is the minimization of dust exposure. Various dust control methods include provision of ventilation, use of water sprays and modern mining methods. Respirator use should be the final resort and not the primary way of managing exposures. Ongoing health surveillance is also effective in monitoring the respiratory health of miners.

PROGRESSIVE MASSIVE FIBROSIS

Diagnosis

Progressive massive fibrosis (PMF) is characterized by the presence of one or more large fibrotic lesions (whose definition depends on the mode of detection) present in one or both lungs. PMF often becomes more severe over time, even in the absence of additional dust exposure. It can also develop after dust exposure has ceased, and may often cause disability and premature death.

Aetiopathogenesis

Despite extensive research, the actual cause of PMF development remains unclear. Over the years, various hypotheses have been proposed, but none is fully satisfactory. One prominent theory was that tuberculosis played a role. Indeed, tuberculosis is often present in miners with PMF, particularly in developing countries. However, PMF has been found to develop in miners in whom there was no sign of tuberculosis, and tuberculin reactivity has not been found to be elevated in miners with pneumoconiosis. Despite investigation, consistent evidence of the role of the immune system in the development of PMF is lacking.

PMF lesions may be unilateral or bilateral, and are most often found in the upper or middle lobes of the lung. The lesions are formed of collagen, reticulin, coal mine dust and dust-laden macrophages, while the centre may contain a black liquid which cavitates on occasion. US pathology standards require the lesions to be 2 cm in size or larger to be identified as PMF entities in surgical or autopsy specimens.

Clinical Aspects

Each individual miner with large chest opacities must be appropriately evaluated. Miners with progressive symptoms, risk factors for other disorders (e.g., tuberculosis), or atypical clinical features should undergo a thorough appropriate examination before being diagnosed as PMF.

Dyspnoea and other respiratory symptoms often accompany PMF, but may not necessarily be due to the disease itself. Congestive heart failure (due to pulmonary hypertension and cor pulmonale) is an infrequent complication. PMF leads to premature death.

Radiology

Large opacities (>1 cm) on the radiograph, coupled with a history of extensive coal mine dust exposure, are taken to imply the presence of PMF. However, other diseases such as lung cancer, tuberculosis and granulomas should also be considered. Large opacities are usually seen on a background of small opacities, but development of PMF from Category 0 profusion has been noted over a five-year period.

Treatment

Medical care should be organized around ameliorating the condition and associated lung illnesses, while protecting against infectious complications. Although maintaining functional stability may be more difficult in patients with PMF, in other respects, management is similar to simple CWP. The incidence and rate of CWP progression is related to the amount of respirable coal dust to which miners were exposed during their working lifetime. Early pneumoconiosis can be asymptomatic, but advanced disease often leads to disability and premature death.

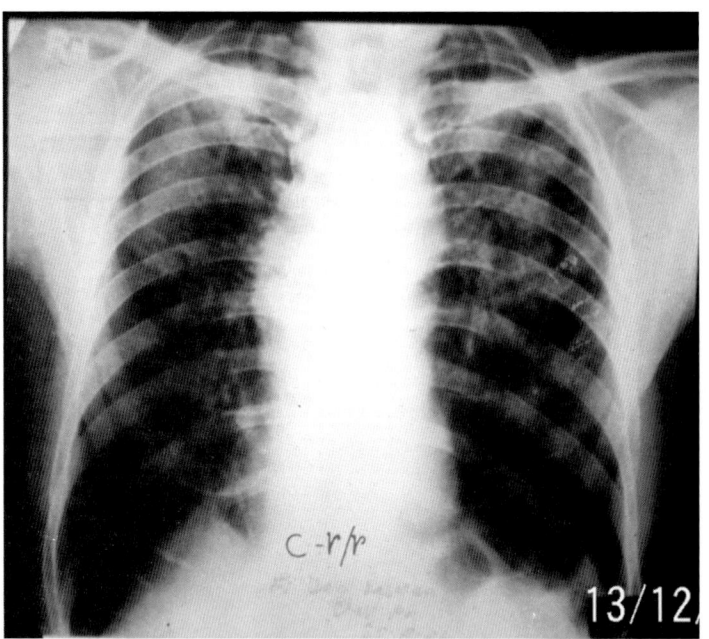

Fig 66.10: The radiograph shows r/r type of small regular pneumoconiotic opacities in all zones with profusion of 3/2 (Category 3). There is coalescence of pneumoconiotic opacities in both right upper zones; one opacity (80 × 30 mm) in the right upper zone, and another large opacity with dimensions of 50 × 40 mm mainly in the left upper zone indicate progressive massive fibrosis (PMF).

Prevention

Avoidance of dust exposure is the only way to prevent PMF. Since the risk of its development increases sharply with increasing category of simple CWP, a strategy for secondary prevention of PMF is for miners to undergo periodic chest X-rays and to terminate or reduce their exposure if simple CWP is detected. Although this approach appears valid and has been adopted in certain jurisdictions, its effectiveness has not been evaluated systematically.

Legal Exposure Limits in India (Coal Dust): 2mg/m^3, respirable dust fraction containing less than 5% quartz.

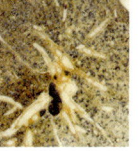
ASBESTOSIS

Definition and History

Asbestosis is a disease of interstitial pneumonitis and fibrosis caused by inhalation of asbestos fibres.

Asbestos is the name given to a group of six naturally occurring fibrous silicate minerals that have been widely used in commercial products. Asbestos is composed of silicate chains bonded with magnesium, iron, calcium, aluminium, and sodium or trace elements to form long, thin, separable fibres. These fibres are often arranged in parallel or matted masses. Asbestos occurs naturally but much of its presence in the environment stems from mining and commercial uses.

There are two classes of asbestos viz. serpentine and amphibole.

Asbestos was widely used commercially until the 1970s. Mining and milling of the raw material and production of asbestos has declined since the early 1970s, but asbestos is still used in some construction materials. Asbestos fibres are released into the air and dust when asbestos-containing materials are loose, crumbling, or disturbed. Until the 1970s, asbestos was widely used in the construction, shipbuilding, and automotive industries, among others. For example, asbestos was formerly used in the following items: boilers and heating vessels, cement pipes, clutch, brake, and transmission components, conduits for electrical wire, corrosive chemical containers, electric motor components, heat-protective pads, laboratory furniture, paper products, pipe covering, roofing products, sealants and coatings, insulation products, and textiles (including curtains).

Serpentine: long, flexible fibres	Amphiboles: brittle, rod or needle-shaped
Member: chrysotile	Members: crocidolite, amosite, anthophyllite, tremolite, actinolite, winchite, richterite
Accounts for 93% of world's commercial, purposeful use of asbestos	Accounts for 7% of commercial, purposeful use of asbestos

Today, asbestos is still used in brake pads, automobile clutches, roofing materials, vinyl tile and imported cement pipe and corrugated sheets. Other occupations at risk include those in the construction industry, automechanics, demolition workers, refinery and shipyard workers.

Although asbestos is no longer used in many products, it will remain a public health concern well into the 21st century.

Exposure to Asbestos

Exposure to asbestos can occur when asbestos-containing material (man-made or natural) is loose, crumbling or disturbed, releasing asbestos fibres into the air and dust.

The primary route of asbestos entry into the body is inhalation of air or dust that contains asbestos fibres. Asbestos can also enter the body via ingestion. With dermal exposure, asbestos fibres may lodge in the skin.

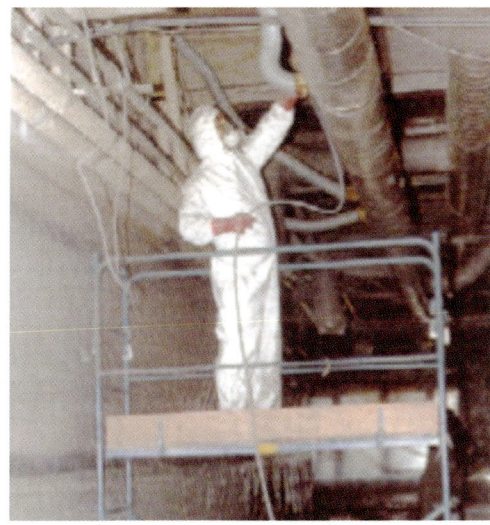

Fig 66.11: Building demolition presents an asbestos hazard when the insulation is disturbed [Picture courtesy—Dr G.K. Kulkarni].

Inhalation: Inhalation is the most important route of exposure to asbestos, and the route that most commonly leads to illness.

Ingestion: Swallowing material removed from the lungs via tracheociliary clearance by a person who had inhaled asbestos fibres into the lungs.

Drinking water contaminated with asbestos, for example from erosion of natural land sources, discarded mine and mill tailings, asbestos cement pipe, or disintegration of other asbestos-containing materials transported by rain.

Dermal: Today, dermal contact is rare. In the past, handling asbestos could result in heavy dermal contact and exposure. Asbestos fibres could become lodged in the skin, producing a callus or corn, but not any more serious health effects.

Asbestos-Related Lung Diseases

The inhalation of asbestos fibres may lead to a number of respiratory diseases, including asbestosis, lung cancer, pleural plaques, benign pleural effusion, and malignant mesothelioma. Although exposure is now regulated, patients continue to present with these diseases because of the long latent period between exposure and clinical disease Non-malignant asbestos-related disease refers to the following conditions: asbestosis, pleural thickening or asbestos-related pleural fibrosis (plaques or diffuse fibrosis), 'benign' (non-malignant) pleural effusion, and airflow obstruction.

The prognosis depends on the specific disease entity. Asbestosis generally progresses slowly, whereas malignant mesothelioma has an extremely poor prognosis. The treatment of patients with asbestos exposure and lung cancer is identical to that of any patient with lung cancer.

Aetiopathogenesis

Some of the inhaled asbestos fibres are deposited on the surface of the larger airways where some of them are cleared by mucociliary transport and swallowing. Other fibres are deposited further in the lung, especially in the bifurcations of the tracheobronchial tree and eventually in the alveolar sacs.

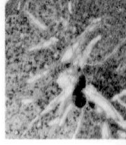

The dimensions of the asbestos fibre determine how easily and how far it penetrates the lungs and how quickly it is cleared. Wide fibres (diameter greater than 2 to 5 microns) tend to be deposited in the upper respiratory tract and cleared. Long thin asbestos fibres reach the lower airways and alveoli and tend to be retained in the lungs. However, it is important to remember that asbestos fibres of all lengths can induce pathological changes and cannot be excluded as contributors to asbestos-related disease.

The mechanisms by which asbestos causes disease are not fully understood. Currently, there are three hypotheses to account for asbestos's pathogenicity—direct interaction with cellular macromolecules, generation of reactive oxygen species, and other cell-mediated mechanisms (especially inflammation).

Clinical Features and Diagnosis

Depending on the level of exposure, inhalation of asbestos fibres can cause different diseases such as parenchymal asbestosis, asbestos-related pleural abnormalities, lung carcinoma, pleural mesothelioma.

Any combination of these syndromes (or all four of them) can be present in a single patient labelled as parenchymal asbestosis.

Parenchymal asbestosis is a diffuse interstitial fibrosis resulting from inhalation of asbestos fibres. Asbestos fibres inhaled deep into the lung parenchyma become lodged in the tissue, resulting in diffuse alveolar and interstitial fibrosis. The fibrosis first occurs in the respiratory bronchioles, particularly the sub-pleural portions of the lower lobes. The fibrosis can progress to include the alveolar walls. Fibrosis tends to progress even after exposure ceases. This fibrosis leads to a restrictive lung pathology, characterized by reduced lung volumes, diminished compliance, reduced CO diffusing capacity and impaired gas exchange. Airways' obstruction due to small airways disease may be present. Progressive disease may be present. Progressive dyspnoea on exertion, insidious in onset, is the prominent symptom.

Parenchymal asbestosis is characterized by the following radiographic changes: fine, irregular opacities in both lung fields (especially in the bases) and septal lines that progress to honeycombing and sometimes, in more severe disease, to obscuration of the heart border and hemi-diaphragm, the so-called shaggy heart sign. Radiographic changes depend on the duration, frequency, and intensity of exposure. Patients with parenchymal asbestosis may have elevated levels of antinuclear antibody and rheumatoid factor and a progressive decrease in total lymphocyte count with advancing fibrosis.

Parenchymal asbestosis has no unique pathognomonic signs or symptoms, but diagnosis is made by the constellation of clinical, functional, and radiographic findings as outlined by the American Thoracic Society criteria (American Thoracic Society 2004). These criteria include sufficient history of exposure to asbestos, appearance of disease with a consistent time interval from first exposure, clinical picture such as insidious onset of dyspnoea on exertion, bibasilar end-inspiratory crackles not cleared by coughing, lung function tests showing restrictive (occasionally obstructive) pattern with reduced diffusing capacity, characteristic X-ray appearance, exclusion of

Table 66.5: Natural history associated with parenchymal asbestosis	
Parameter	**Typical Findings**
Sufficient exposures	Usually associated with high-level occupational exposures
Latency periods	Radiographic changes: <20 years. Clinical manifestation: 20–40 years. Asbestosis appears earliest in those with the highest exposure levels.
Risk of asbestosis	Asbestosis develops in 49–52% of adults with occupational levels of asbestos exposure
Co-morbid conditions	Increased risk for lung cancer and mesothelioma, though both can occur without parenchymal asbestosis
Mortality and Morbidity	Severe asbestosis may lead to respiratory failure over 12–24 years. Many patients with asbestosis die of other causes such as asbestos-associated lung cancer (38%), mesothelioma (9%) and other causes (32%)

other causes of interstitial fibrosis or obstructive disease, such as usual interstitial pneumonia, connective tissue disease, and drug-related fibrosis.

Table 66.5 describes the natural history associated with parenchymal asbestosis. Table 66.6 lists the asbestos related pleural abnormalities.

ASBESTOS AND LUNG CARCINOMA

Exposure to asbestos is associated with all major histological types of lung carcinoma (adenocarcinoma, squamous cell carcinoma, and small-cell carcinoma). It is estimated that 4–12% of lung cancers are related to occupational levels of exposure to asbestos. It is estimated that 20–25% of heavily exposed asbestos workers will develop bronchogenic carcinomas. Whether asbestos exposure will lead to lung cancer depends on several factors—-level, duration, and frequency of asbestos exposure (cumulative exposure), time elapsed since exposure occurred, age when exposure occurred, history of tobacco use and individual susceptibility factors not yet determined.

Most asbestos-related lung cancers reflect the dual influence of asbestos exposure and smoking. Smoking and asbestos exposure have a multiplicative effect on the risk of lung cancer. Asbestos as the sole contributing factor for cancer in an individual patient can be difficult to prove especially when the patient has other risk factors for lung cancer. The presence of parenchymal asbestosis is an indicator of high-level asbestos exposure, but lung cancer can occur without asbestosis.

ASBESTOS AND PLEURAL MESOTHELIOMA

Pleural mesothelioma (see section 'Diseases of the Pleura')'is a signal tumour for asbestos exposure; other causes are uncommon. The risk of mesothelioma does depend on the amount of asbestos exposure. All types of asbestos can cause mesothelioma, but some researchers believe that the amphibole form is more likely to induce mesothelioma than the serpentine form.

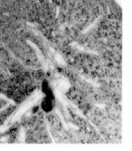

Table 66.6: Asbestos-related pleural abnormalities			
Type of pleural change	**Appearance**	**Occurrence or frequency**	**Symptoms**
Pleural plaques	Well-circumscribed	Very common (58% in insulation workers)	Asymptomatic
Benign asbestos pleural effusions	Small unilateral pleural effusions-blood stained with mesothelial and various other cells	Earliest manifestation	Asymptomatic
Diffuse pleural thickening	Noncircumscribed fibrous thickening of the visceral pleura with adherence to the parietal pleura	10% of patients with asbestosis	Progressive dyspnoea and chest pain
Rounded atelectasis (Folded lung)	Rounded pleural mass with bands of lung tissue radiating outwards	Least common	Asymptomatic

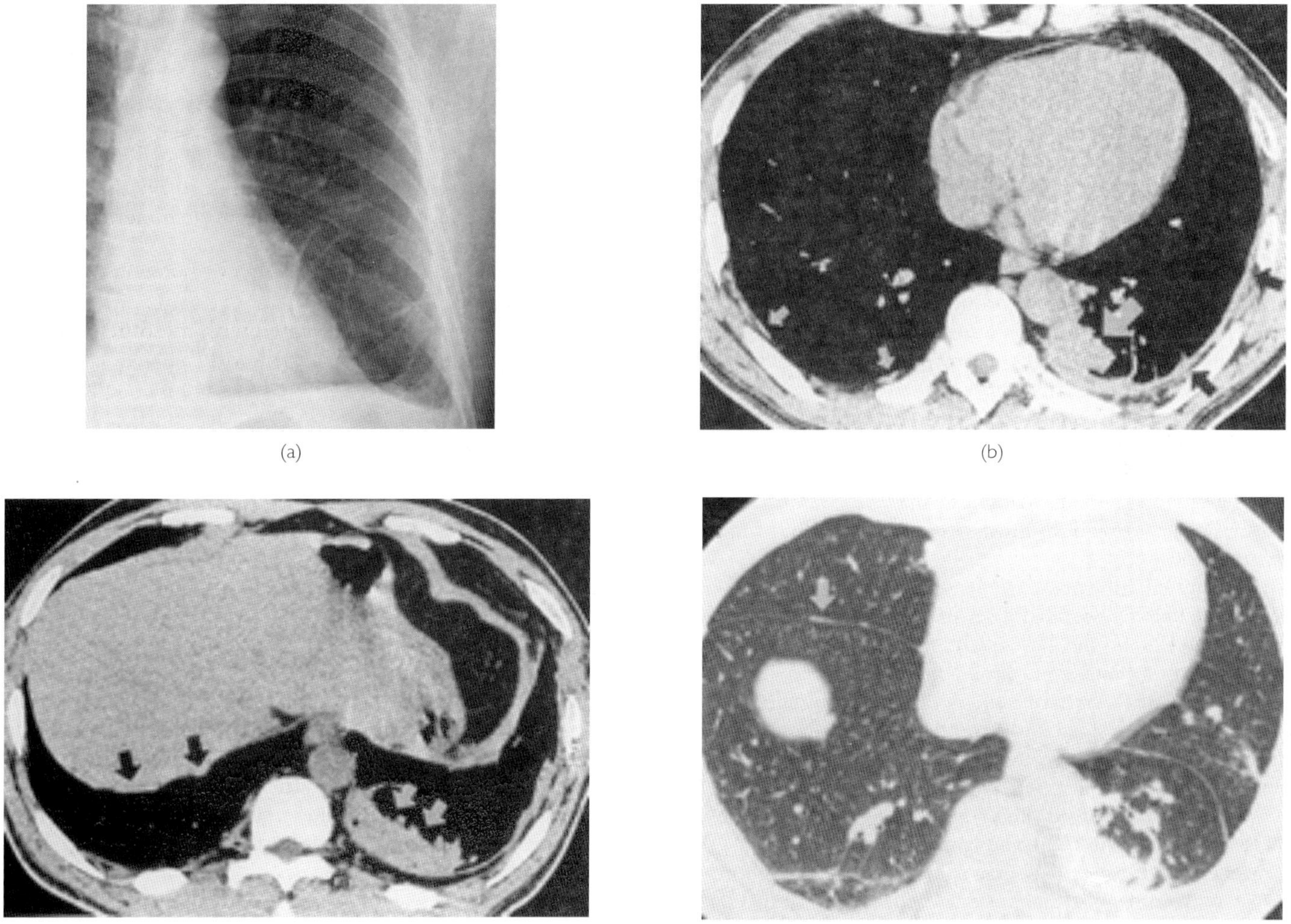

(a)

(b)

(c)

(d)

Fig 66.12: Pleural plaques, diffuse pleural thickening, rounded atelectasis, and asbestosis in a 50-year-old man with asbestos exposure from working in a brake lining production plant. (a) Chest radiograph shows diffuse thickening of the left pleura and curvilinear band opacities in the left lower lung zone (b) High-resolution CT scan (mediastinal windowing) shows pleural plaques on the right side (small white arrows) and rounded atelectasis (large white arrow) with adjacent diffuse pleural thickening (black arrows) on the left side (c) High-resolution CT scan obtained at a lower level than (b) demonstrates pleural plaques along the diaphragmatic contour (black arrows) and an irregular attenuation pattern, which is typical in rounded atelectasis (white arrows) (d) High-resolution CT scan (lung windowing) obtained at the level of the liver dome shows a visceral pleural plaque in the right major fissure (arrow) and curvilinear bands of hyperattenuation in the posterior subpleural area. Note also the rounded atelectasis with posterior displacement of the left major fissure. The diagnosis of asbestosis was proved by open-lung biopsy.

Source: (Reproduced with permission. Fig. 66.12: Kim KI, Kim CW, Lee MK et al. Imaging of Occupational Lung Disease, *Radiographics* 2001; 21:1371–1391. The Radiological Society of North America (RSNA®)

Table 66.7:
Typical findings associated with lung carcinoma

Typical exposures	Large cumulative exposure (short term, high-level exposures or long-term, moderate-level exposures)
Latency periods	20–30 years
Clinical presentation	Only 5–15% of patients are asymptomatic when diagnosed. Most present with cough, hemoptysis, wheeze, dyspnoea
Comorbid conditions	Asbestosis, other asbestos-related diseases
Mortality	Same as lung carcinoma from other causes—14% five year survival rate

Table 66.8:
Typical findings associated with pleural mesothelioma

Typical exposures	Short-term, high-level exposures or chronic low-level exposures, especially to amphibole asbestos; incidence increase in dose-related manner
Latency periods	10–57 years (30–40 years typical)
Clinical presentation	Frequently presents with chest pain accompanied by pleural mass or pleural effusion on chest X-ray
Mortality	High. The typical 1-year survival rate is <30%. Average survival time is 8–14 months after diagnosis

In the year 2000, about 3,000 people in the United States died of mesothelioma. According to the National Cancer Institute's SEER data, there was an increase in the incidence of mesothelioma in the United States from the early 1970s to the mid-1990s, as disease developed in people exposed during peak asbestos exposure years (1940–1970). Mesothelioma incidence has probably started to decline in the United States, although it may still be increasing in Europe and Australia because of more abundant and prolonged use of asbestos in these countries than in the United States.

Chest radiography in patients with malignant mesothelioma may show an effusion, pleural thickening, and as the tumour progresses, a more lobulated outline. CT can help identify the disease in its early stages. Asbestos-related cancers can occur anywhere in the lungs. Recognition of the clinical, radiological, and pathologic features of these diseases will be important for some years to come.

Clinical Evaluation of Patients with Asbestosis— Key Points

- Exposures to asbestos, smoking history and other respiratory conditions.
- The most typical abnormal finding on examination of patients with a history of asbestos exposure is bibasilar end-inspiratory râles on pulmonary auscultation. Patients with parenchymal asbestosis present to the clinician with the chief complaint of fatigue, insidious onset of dyspnoea on exertion.
- Asbestos-related pleural abnormalities typically do not cause symptoms, although some patients experience progressive dyspnoea and chest pain.
- Lung cancer can be asymptomatic, but in the later stages patients experience fatigue, weight loss, chest pain, dyspnoea, or haemoptysis.
- Mesothelioma is typically asymptomatic until later stages, at which point patients have dyspnoea and chest pain.

Pulmonary Function and Imaging Findings— Key Points

- Parenchymal asbestosis is associated with a reduction in forced vital capacity (FVC) and restrictive patterns on spirometry. Signs of parenchymal asbestosis on chest X-ray include irregular opacities, interstitial fibrosis, and the 'shaggy heart sign.'
- On chest X-ray, pleural plaques appear as well-circumscribed areas of pleural thickening, sometimes with calcification, pleural effusions have a cloudy or blood-stained appearance, diffuse pleural thickening appears as a lobulated prominence and interlobar fissure thickening.
- On chest X-ray, findings associated with rounded atelectasis appear as a rounded pleural mass with radiating bands of lung tissue.
- Asbestos-associated lung cancer has the same appearance as lung cancer from other causes.
- Chest X-ray findings associated with mesothelioma include pleural effusions or a pleural mass.
- CT and HRCT scans can be useful in diagnosing early changes associated with asbestosis, in helping to clarify questionable pleural or parenchymal findings and in diagnosing mesothelioma.

Management of Asbestosis

Management is entirely symptomatic as there is no specific treatment available. Intercurrent respiratory infections should be appropriately treated. Patients should be given pneumococcal vaccine and influenza vaccine at intervals recommended by the Centre for Disease Control (CDC). Patients should be strongly counselled against smoking. Pulmonary rehabilitation may provide symptomatic relief. The degree of patient disability needs to be carefully assessed and clinical, radiological and lung function test follow-up should be maintained with specific reference to development of lung cancer and pleural mesothelioma.

OCCUPATIONAL ASTHMA

Asthma is a respiratory disease characterized by airways obstruction and airflow limitation that is significantly or completely reversible, either spontaneously or with treatment. Occupational asthma (OA) is asthma that is caused by environmental exposures in the workplace.

Several hundred agents have been reported to cause OA. Pre-existing asthma or airway hyper-responsiveness, with symptoms worsened by work exposure to irritants or physi-

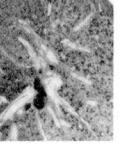
cal stimuli, is usually classified separately as work-aggravated asthma (WAA). There is general agreement that OA has become the most prevalent occupational lung disease in developed countries, although estimates of actual prevalence and incidence are quite variable. It is clear, however, that in many countries asthma of occupational aetiology causes a largely unrecognized burden of disease and disability with high economic and non-economic costs. Although occupational diseases such as asbestosis and silicosis may be eradicated with time because of better preventive measures, it is unlikely that occupational asthma will ever disappear, because of the constant introduction of new chemicals into workplaces. Much of this public health and economic burden is potentially preventable by identifying and controlling or eliminating the workplace exposures causing the asthma.

Magnitude of the Problem

Prevalence of asthma in adults generally ranges from 3–5%, depending on the definition of asthma and geographic variations, and may be considerably higher in some low-income urban populations. The proportion of adult asthma cases in the general population that is related to the work environment is reported to range from 2–23%, with recent estimates tending towards the higher end of this range.

Pathophysiology

OA is the result of an interaction between environmental factors at the workplace and individual susceptibility. Genetic factors probably play a role. Most genetic studies suggest the importance of HLA class II polymorphisms in controlling the risk for sensitization in OA. Glutathione S-transferase protects cells from oxidative stress. It is believed to play an important role in OA caused by exposure to isocyanates. Over 200 agents (specific substances, occupations or industrial processes) have been reported to cause OA based on epidemiological studies and/or clinical evidence. In OA airways inflammation and bronchoconstriction can be caused by the following mechanisms:

1. Immunological immunoglobulin E (IgE) mediated
2. Immunological non-IgE-mediated
3. Non-immunological
4. Direct pharmacological action—an example of agents which do so are organophosphorous insecticides.

Immunological IgE-Mediated OA

Many high molecular weight occupational agents, such as animal derived allergens, flour, act as complete antigens and induce specific IgE antibody formation. Low molecular weight agents, for example tricyclic anhydride and other acid anhydrides may also induce specific IgE antibodies resulting in a Type I hypersensitivity reaction. Some occupational agents give rise to IgG-specific antibodies. They act as haptens, bind with proteins to form complete antigens. These antigens are recognized by antigen-presenting cells and induce a CD4 response resulting in production of specific IgE antibodies by B-cells stimulated by interleukin (IL)-4. The antigen-IgE antibody

reaction leads to airways inflammation, mucosal oedema, airways constriction and increased bronchial hyper-reactivity similar to what is observed in non-occupational asthma. There is no pathogenetic difference in the mechanism operating in OA as compared to non-occupational asthma.

Immunological Non-IgE-Mediated OA

Many low molecular weight agents, notably isocyanates are known to cause OA without the presence of IgE antibodies. Specific IgG antibodies have been found to be associated with OA but their significance has not been exactly determined.

It has been suggested that T-lymphocytes may play an important role in the pathogenesis of OA. Bronchial mucosal biopsies show proliferation of activated T-cells. Cloning of cells from bronchial mucosal biopsy specimens show that most of the lymphocytes are of the CD8 phenotype. This is supportive of the possibility that CD8 lymphocytes play an important role in the pathogenesis of some forms of OA without the production of IgE antibodies.

The early asthmatic reaction in OA is characterized by constriction and mucosal oedema related to the release of histamine, histamine-related substances and leukotrienes. The late asthmatic reaction is characterized by the influx of inflammatory cells. The eosinophil of course is the key cell in both OA and non-occupational bronchial asthma. Current work also shows the importance of the neutrophils in the inflammatory response that characterizes asthma. In fact eosinophilis and neutrophil variants have been observed in cases of OA due to low molecular weight agents, especially isocyanates. Some low molecular weight agents, in particular isocyanates exert a variety of inflammatory effects to induce asthma. For example, isocyanates may block the β-adrenergic receptors and also stimulate sensory nerves to secrete substance P which inhibits endopeptides that are necessary for inactivation of neuropeptides. Neuropeptides are known to recruit inflammatory cells, cause mucosal oedema and bronchial constriction.

Non-Immunological

The features that characterize the non-immunologic form of OA is the absence of latency. Respiratory irritants often worsen symptoms in workers with pre-existing asthma, and at high levels of exposure can cause new-onset asthma—termed

Table 66.9: Agents causing immunologically mediated occupational asthma	
High molecular weight	**Low molecular weight**
Cereals	Isocyanates
Enzymes	Wood dusts
Gums	Anhydrides
Animal-derived allergents	Amines
Sea-foods	Sea-foods dyes
	Formaldehyde
	Metals
	Persulfate

reactive airways dysfunction syndrome (RADS) or irritant-induced asthma.

The exact mechanism of RADS is not known. The condition is characterized by extensive loss of mucosal epithelium of the airways leading to airways inflammation and hyper-responsiveness. Inflammation and hyper-responsiveness may well be due to exposure of nerve endings and non-specific activation of mast cells with release of inflammatory mediators and cytokines. Airways remodelling is induced as a result of growth factors for epithelial cells, smooth muscle and fibroblasts. In the chronic form of RADS there is marked thickening of the bronchial walls.

Clinical Presentation

The symptom spectrum of OA is similar to non-occupational asthma: wheeze, cough, chest tightness and shortness of breath. Patients sometimes present with cough-variant or nocturnal asthma. OA can be severe and disabling, and deaths have been reported. Onset of OA occurs due to a specific job environment, so identifying exposures that occurred at the time of onset of asthmatic symptoms is the key to an accurate diagnosis. In work aggravated asthma (WAA), workplace exposures cause a significant increase in frequency and/or severity of symptoms of pre-existing asthma.

Several features of the clinical history may suggest an occupational aetiology. Symptoms frequently worsen at work or at night after work, improve on days off, and recur on return to work. Symptoms may worsen progressively towards the end of the work week. The patient may note specific activities or agents in the workplace that reproducibly trigger symptoms. Work-related eye irritation or rhinitis may be associated with asthmatic symptoms. These typical symptom patterns may be present only in the initial stages of OA. Partial or complete resolution on weekends or vacations is common early in the course of OA, but with repeated exposures, the time required for recovery may increase to one or two weeks, or recovery may cease to occur. The majority of patients with OA whose exposures are terminated continue to have symptomatic asthma even years after cessation of exposure, with permanent impairment and disability. Continuing exposure is associated with further worsening of asthma. Brief duration and mild severity of symptoms at the time of cessation of exposure are good prognostic factors and decrease the likelihood of permanent asthma.

Several characteristic temporal patterns of symptoms have been reported for OA. Early asthmatic reactions typically occur shortly (less than one hour) after beginning work or the specific work exposure causing the asthma. Late asthmatic reactions begin 4 to 6 hours after exposure begins, and can last 24 to 48 hours. Combinations of these patterns occur as dual asthmatic reactions with spontaneous resolution of symptoms separating an early and late reaction, or as continuous asthmatic reactions with no resolution of symptoms between phases. With exceptions, early reactions tend to be IgE-mediated, and late reactions tend to be IgE-independent.

Increased non-specific bronchial responsiveness (NBR), generally measured by methacholine or histamine challenge, is considered a cardinal feature of OA. The time course and degree of NBR may be useful in diagnosis and monitoring. NBR may decrease within several weeks after cessation of exposure, although abnormal NBR commonly persists for months or years after exposures are terminated. In individuals with irritant-induced OA, NBR is not expected to vary with exposure and/or symptoms.

Diagnosis and Evaluation of Occupational Asthma

Occupational asthma is the most prevalent form of work-related lung disease in industrialized nations. Increasing numbers of new chemicals are being produced and new manufacturing processes are being introduced. The variety of environments in which individuals may become exposed to respiratory sensitizers and irritants makes diagnosing and treating this illness even more challenging. Clinicians must first document the presence of asthma, and then establish a relationship between asthma and the workplace.

The adult patient's occupational history is the key diagnostic tool. In addition, lung function assessments that include spirometry and bronchial responsiveness are now often coupled with immunological assessment and an evaluation of inflammation in the investigation of OA. Evaluations may include serial peak expiratory flow rate (PEFR) measurements and non-specific hypersensitivity challenges with histamine or methacholine. Serial PEFR monitoring while at work and away from work may be important in documenting whether asthma is work-related in selected people, work environment permitting. Information about workplace exposures to irritants and sensitizers may be useful. Specific challenge testing at tertiary referral centres providing specialized laboratories can also be helpful but is rarely necessary.

Since asthma is an inflammatory disease, a measure of the degree of inflammation would be helpful in quantifying severity and titrating of anti-inflammatory therapy. There is evidence that monitoring eosinophils and neutrophils in induced sputum can help in the management of asthma.

Treatment and Prevention

The medical management of OA is similar to that for non-occupational asthma. The key to managing OA is to ensure that the exposure which triggers asthma is optimally controlled. In many cases it may mean removal of a worker from the exposure source, especially in sensitizer-induced OA where the degree of symptoms could be disproportionate to the concentration of the sensitizer at the workplace. In some cases the employee may be able to continue in work with specific treatment and

Table 66.10:
Agents responsible for reactive airways dysfunction syndrome
Acetic acid
Spray point
Ammonia
Bleaching agent
Chlorine
Isocyanates
Sulphur dioxide

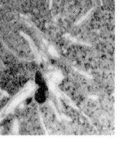

with lowering of the levels of the irritants at the workplace. It would be useful to institute a periodic follow-up of pulmonary functions along with a respiratory questionnaire to ensure appropriate follow-up.

Workplace environmental controls to avoid casual exposures and a system to record and deal with chemical spills can lead to prevention of sensitization of an employee. Substance-specific immunological tests can provide evidence of sensitization, although it is now accepted that sensitization is not the same as disease. In addition, the usual occupational health-related measures like substitution of the chemical, enclosure of processes, ensuring appropriate personal protective measures and employee education would all help in preventing OA at the workplace.

BYSSINOSIS

Byssinosis is an obstructive disease of the airways caused by prolonged exposure to cotton dust. It can also occur after similar exposure to jute, flax, hemp and sometimes sisal dust. In fact the jute industry ranks second in importance after the cotton industry, especially in West Bengal, Andhra Pradesh, Kerala.

China, USA, Russia, India, Pakistan, Egypt and Brazil are among the largest cotton-producing countries in the world. The growing of cotton and the manufacture of cotton textiles is a major industry in India. Weaving cloth is also a cottage industry and there are several lakh cotton handlooms in the country employing several million people. The large number of people exposed to cotton dust in the work environment in India is therefore staggering.

Prevalence and Epidemiological Studies in India

Kamat and colleagues devised a five-year prospective study of 1241 textile workers from three mills in Mumbai to determine the incidence, pattern and course of byssinosis in India. The prevalence rate in the carding section was 14%, 10% in the spinning section and 11% in the winding section. In these dusty sections, the prevalence of both byssinosis and bronchitis increased with longer duration of service.

Parikh and co-workers conducting a survey of 289 workers in four cotton gins in Gujarat noted that 39% of workers complained of work-related symptoms of chest tightness, cough and breathlessness. The pulmonary function tests showed significant decline in the short-staple cotton gin workers, but not in the long-staple cotton gin workers. The difference in lung functions was attributed to a higher content of bract in the short-staple cotton.

Pathogenesis

All phases of textile manufacture pose a risk for cotton dust exposure, and byssinosis particularly occurs in workers in the gins and those in the carding department. Exposure to cotton dust causing disease constitutes exposure not only to cotton fibre but to a variety of other substances many of which are biologically active. The dust present in the air may thus include ground up plant matter, bacteria, fungi and non-cotton contaminants that may accumulate during the growing, harvesting and processing of cotton. Physical irritation of the airways by the cotton fibre, bacterial contamination with increased levels of endotoxin in the work environment and cotton dust and the direct release of histamine by cotton extracts may all play a role in the airways' obstruction that characterizes byssinosis.

Clinical Features

The clinical features are the same the world over. The classic symptom is chest tightness and work-related breathing difficulty typically occurring on Monday mornings during the first shift after a holiday weekend. The symptoms start four to six hours after the start of work, increase in severity over the rest of the shift and subside in the evening after leaving the work environment. In some workers symptoms develop within a few hours of starting work, increase by the end of the first half of the shift and then improve towards the end of the shift. Exposure over a number of years leads to chest tightness on all days of the work week with increasing breathlessness and cough not only in the work environment but also outside the work environment. Finally, the patient develops permanent incapacity characterized by increasing breathlessness on exertion, wheezing and cough.

The severity of byssinosis has been graded by Schilling and is given below.

Table 66.11: Schilling's classification	
Grade	**Tightness**
0	Chest tightness on the first day of some working weeks
1	Chest tightness on the first day of every working week
2	Chest tightness on the first and other days of the working week
3	Grade 2 symptoms along with evidence of permanent incapacity in the form of diminished effort tolerance and/or reduced ventilatory capacity

Lung function studies have shown lower values of forced expiratory volume in one second (FEV_1) associated with increasing grades of byssinosis, as well as more acute reduction in FEV_1 particularly in Monday shifts in patients with byssinosis.

Kamat and co-workers in their study on byssinosis noted that 54% workers had chest tightness, 56% had work-related and exertional dyspnoea, 20% had wheezing and 36% had cough. During a five-year follow-up they noted that the atypical presentation of byssinosis with cough was more common in the carding department. The yearly decrease in FEV_1 in patients with work-related symptoms was 114 ml and was significantly higher than in those with non-specific chest symptoms. The decrease in FVC and FEV_1 was greater with increased dust loads.

It is of interest that though chest tightness and decline in lung function are often associated in byssinosis workers, this is not always so. At times individuals with chest tightness do not have a measurable decline in lung functions and occasionally patients with decline in lung functions may not have chest symptoms.

Radiographic examination of the chest in severe byssinosis may show over-inflated lungs as in chronic airways obstruction, but the appearances are not specific. Hyper-responsiveness to metacholine is also often noted.

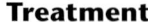

Treatment

Measures to avoid and reduce exposure of workers to cotton dust are of prime importance. Byssinosis is characterized by airways obstruction and airflow limitation. Inhaled β_2 agonists combined with inhaled corticosteroids as in asthma provide relief.

OCCUPATIONAL LUNG CANCER

The International Agency for Research on Cancer (IARC) has categorized certain substances as being human respiratory carcinogens. These include the following:

Individual Agents

- Asbestos
- Arsenic and arsenic compounds
- Beryllium and beryllium compounds
- Bis (chloromethyl) ether
- Cadmium and cadmium compounds
- Chlormethyl methyl ether
- Chromium (VI) compounds
- Nickel compounds
- Mustard gas
- Talc with asbestiform fibres

Complex Mixtures

- Coal tars, coal tar pitches, soot and tobacco smoke.

Other Occupations of Possible Risk

- Aluminium production
- Coal gasification and production
- Iron and Steel founding
- Painters
- Radon and its decay products

The signs and symptoms of lung cancer depend on the location of the tumour. The prognosis varies with the stage of the disease. In addition to the list enumerated above several agents which have been considered to be possible human carcinogens (IARC Group 2B) include inorganic lead compounds (IARC 1987), cobalt (IARC 1991b), man-made vitreous fibres (rockwool, slagwool and glasswool) (IARC 1988b) and welding fumes (IARC1990c). (See section on 'Lung Tumours'.)

EXTRINSIC ALLERGIC ALVEOLITIS

This subject has been dealt with in the section on 'Interstitial Lung Diseases and Other Diffuse Lung Diseases'.

SUGGESTED READING

Am J Respir Crit Care Med. 15 Sep. 2004; 170(6): 691–715, American Thoracic Society.

Dodson RF, Atkinson MA, Levin JL. Asbestos fiber length as related to potential pathogenicity: a critical review. *Am J Ind Med.* Sep. 2003; 44(3): 291–7.

Gary R, Epler MD. Environmental and Occupational Lung Diseases. http://www.epler.com/occu_tab.html#1 Retrieved 22/2/2010.

http://www.highbeam.com/doc/1P1-28737133.html Retrieved 22/2/2010.

Indian Journal of Occupational and Environmental Medicine (IJOWM), 2005; 9(1): 10–14.

Kamat SR, Lobo E, *et al.* Distinguishing byssinosis from COPD. Results of a prospective 5-year study of cotton mill workers in India. *Am Rev Respir Dis.* 1981; 124(1): 31–40.

LS David, Ryon and Rom William N. 1998. *Diseases caused by Respiratory Irritants and Toxic Chemicals.* Table 10.12, Table 10.5 and Table 10.15 in the *Encyclopedia of Occupational Health and Safety*, 4th edition, International Labour Office.

Pande N and Khilnani GC. *Indian Journal of Community Medicine*, 1993; 18(4): 137.

Respiratory research foundation of India.

http://www.rrfindia.org/occupational_lung_diseases.htm Retrieved 22/2/2010.